LFTs (liver function tests)	
Bilirubin	3–17 micromoles/L
Alanine aminotransferase (ALT)	3–35IU/L
Aspartate transaminase (AST)	3–35IU/L
Alkaline phosphatase	30–150IU/L *(non-pregnant adults)*

Lipids and other biochemical values	
Cholesterol	<6mmol/L *(desired)*
Triglycerides	0.5–1.9mmol/L *(desired)*
Amylase	0–180 somorgyi unit/dL
C-reactive protein (CRP)	<10mg/L
Glucose, fasting	3.5–5.5mmol/L
Prostate-specific antigen (PSA)	0–4ng/mL
T4 (total thyroxine)	70–140mmol/L
TSH	0.5–5 mu/L

Reproduced from Longmore *et al.*, *Oxford Handbook of Clinical Medicine* 7e (2007), with permission from Oxford University Press.

Oxford Handbook of

Infectious Diseases and Microbiology

Second edition

Dr M. Estée Török
Clinical Scientist Fellow & Senior Research Associate
University of Cambridge, UK

Dr Ed Moran
Consultant in Infectious Disease
Heartlands Hospital, Birmingham, UK

Dr Fiona J. Cooke
Consultant Medical Microbiologist
Addenbrooke's Hospital
Cambridge, UK

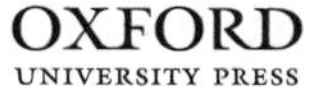

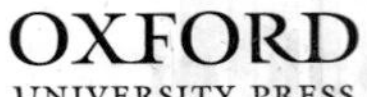

Great Clarendon Street, Oxford, OX2 6DP,
United Kingdom

Oxford University Press is a department of the University of Oxford. It furthers the University's objective of excellence in research, scholarship, and education by publishing worldwide. Oxford is a registered trade mark of Oxford University Press in the UK and in certain other countries

First Edition published in 2009
Second Edition published in 2017

Impression: 1

Published in the United States of America by Oxford University Press
198 Madison Avenue, New York, NY 10016, United States of America

British Library Cataloguing in Publication Data

Data available

Library of Congress Control Number: 2016936810

ISBN 978–0–19–967132–8

Printed and bound in China by
C&C Offset Printing Co., Ltd.

Foreword to the second edition

It is a great honour to be writing the foreword for the latest edition of the *Oxford Handbook Infectious Diseases and Microbiology*.

It is put together by a talented and committed group of authors who have direct experience and insight on the practicalities of delivering specialist clinical care in infectious diseases and microbiology, as well as in running expert laboratory support and advancing research in the field.

The latest edition of the Handbook provides an ideal and useful combination of being organized into chapters that are both organism-based and syndrome-based. The new edition importantly provides more information and detail on infection prevention which is increasingly important in the context of addressing antimicrobial resistance as well as protecting our patients and staff. Well laid out, user-friendly flow charts have been provided in this edition providing valuable rapid resources, for example in organism identification. A newly updated section on antibiotic resistance and antibiotic agents also provides critical information for the now combined ID/Microbiology trainees in the UK, but also valuable for any infection specialty trainees internationally.

It is marvellous to see that the Handbook is promoting cross-disciplinary working and provides a shared resource for all of those working in infectious diseases and clinical microbiology, whether they are students, trainees or senior doctors or ID pharmacists, nurses and biomedical scientists, infection nurses.

Alison Holmes,
Professor of Infectious Diseases,
Imperial College, UK

Preface to the second edition

Medicine is all about adapting to change as research is published and new therapies launched. In the years since the publication of the first edition of this book the treatment of viral hepatitis has transformed beyond recognition, to the extent that drugs have been introduced *and* withdrawn as obsolete, and novel classes of anti-virals and antibiotics are now mainstream. Those of us working in infection have additional challenges: the rise of entirely new diseases (MERS, Ebola, Chikungunya and Zika have each taken their turn in the spotlight), the failure of treatments that have served us faithfully for many years (multi-resistant organisms now attract the attention of Presidents and Prime Ministers), and the automation and molecular revolution in our diagnostic laboratories. UK infection training has responded with the distinction between classic 'Infectious Disease' and 'Microbiology' becoming ever harder to spot, recognized with the launch of Core Infection Training.

Whilst as ever no single book—or at least no single portable book—can tell you everything you need to know, we hope that this second edition of the *Oxford Handbook of Infectious Diseases and Microbiology* will continue to prompt, guide, and educate those caring for people with infections.

Estée Török,
Ed Moran, Fiona Cooke

Acknowledgements

With thanks to Lee Reed for significant revision contributions, and to Jane Stockley, Armine Sefton, Gemma Winzor, and George Trafford for providing valuable thoughts on the first draft. Mike Riste, Chris Green, and Rebecca Sutherland provided invaluable extra pairs of eyes in proof reading the final version.

Contents

Symbols and abbreviations *xiii*

Part 1 Antimicrobials

1	Basics of antimicrobials	3
2	Antibiotics	31
3	Antifungals	79
4	Antivirals	89
5	Antiparasitic therapy	111

Part 2 Infection control

6	Infection control	129

Part 3 Systematic microbiology

7	Bacteria	207
8	Viruses	365
9	Fungi	469
10	Protozoa	511
11	Helminths	541
12	Ectoparasites	571

Part 4 Clinical syndromes

13	Fever	579
14	Respiratory, head, and neck infections	589
15	Cardiovascular infections	629
16	Gastrointestinal infections	643
17	Urinary tract infections	677
18	Sexually transmitted infections	693
19	Neurological infections	717

20 Ophthalmological infections 745
21 Skin and soft tissue infections 757
22 Bone and joint infections 773
23 Pregnancy and childhood 785
24 Immunodeficiency and HIV 809
25 Health protection 843

Index 851

Symbols and abbreviations

A–a	alveolar–arterial
ABC HSR	abacavir hypersensitivity reaction
ABG	arterial blood gas
ABPA	allergic bronchopulmonary aspergillosis
ABPI	ankle–brachial pressure index
ACA	acrodermatitis chronica atrophicans
ACDP	Advisory Committee on Dangerous Pathogens
ACE	angiotensin-converting enzyme
ACT	artemisinin combination therapy; adenylate cyclase toxin
ADH	antidiuretic hormone
ADL	acute adenolymphangitis
AFB	acid-fast bacilli
AFLP	amplified fragment length polymorphism
AIDS	acquired immune deficiency syndrome
AKI	acute kidney injury
ALP	alkaline phosphatase
ALT	alanine aminotransferase
AME	aminoglycoside-modifying enzyme
AMP	adenosine monophosphate
AMRHAI	Antimicrobial Resistance and Healthcare Associated Infections Reference Unit
a.m.	*ante meridiem* (before noon)
ANA	antinuclear antibody
ANCA	antineutrophil cytoplasmic antibody
aP	acellular pertussis (vaccine)
APACHE	acute physiology and chronic health evaluation (score)
ARB	angiotensin receptor blocker
ARDS	acute respiratory distress syndrome
ARF	acute renal failure
ART	antiretroviral therapy
ASD	atrial septal defect
ASOT	anti-streptolysin O titre
AST	aspartate transaminase
ATL	adult T-cell leukaemia/lymphoma

ATN	antiretroviral toxic neuropathy
ATP	adenosine triphosphate
AUC	area under the curve
AV	atrioventricular
BA	blood agar; bacillary angiomatosis
BAL	bronchoalveolar lavage
BC	blood culture
BCG	bacillus Calmette–Guérin
BCYE	buffered charcoal yeast extract
bd	twice daily
BHIVA	British HIV Association
BIA	British Infection Association
BKV	BK virus
BLNAR	β-lactamase-negative ampicillin-resistant
BMT	bone marrow transplant/ation
BNF	*British National Formulary*
bp	base pair
BP	bacterial peliosis
BSAC	British Society for Antimicrobial Chemotherapy
BSE	bovine spongiform encephalopathy
BSI	bloodstream infection
BTS	British Thoracic Society
BV	bacterial vaginosis
Ca	calcium
cAMP	cyclic adenosine monophosphate
CA-MRSA	community-acquired meticillin-resistant *Staphylococcus aureus*
CAP	community-acquired pneumonia
CAPD	continuous ambulatory peritoneal dialysis
CATT	card agglutination tests for *Trypanosoma gambiense* trypanosomes
CBD	common bile duct
CCDC	Consultant in Communicable Disease Control
CCEY	cefoxitin cycloserine egg yolk
CCF	congestive cardiac failure
CCFA	cefoxitin cycloserine fructose agar
CCHF	Congo–Crimean haemorrhagic fever
ccr	cassette chromosome recombinase

CCU	clean-catch urine
CDAD	*Clostridium difficile*-associated disease/diarrhoea
CDC	Centers for Disease Control and Prevention
CDI	*Clostridium difficile* infection
cDNA	complementary deoxyribonucleic acid
CDRN	*Clostridium difficile* Ribotyping Network
CDSC	Communicable Disease Surveillance Centre
CE	California encephalitis
CEE	central European encephalitis
CF	cystic fibrosis
CFA	colonization factor antigen; circulating filarial antigen
CFTs	complement fixation tests
CFTR	cystic fibrosis transmembrane conductance regulator
cfu	colony-forming unit
CIN	Cefsulodin, Irgasan, Novobiocin; cervical intraepithelial neoplasia
CIS	Commonwealth of Independent States
CJD	Creutzfeldt–Jakob disease
CK	creatine kinase
CKD	chronic kidney disease
Cl^-	chloride ion
CL	containment level
CLED	cystine, lactose, electrolyte-deficient (agar)
CLSI	Clinical & Laboratory Standards Institute
cm	centimetre
CMI	cell-mediated immunity
CMV	cytomegalovirus
CNA	colistin nalidixic acid agar
CNS	central nervous system
CO_2	carbon dioxide
CoNS	coagulase-negative staphylococci
COPD	chronic obstructive pulmonary disease
COSHH	Control of Substances Hazardous to Health
CPA	Clinical Pathology Accreditation
CPE	carbapenemase-producing *Enterobacteriaceae*
CPK	creatine phosphokinase
CQC	Care Quality Commission

CT-BSI	catheter-related bloodstream infection
CrCl	creatinine clearance
CRE	carbapenem-resistant *Enterobacteriaceae*
CRF	circulating recombinant form
CRP	C-reactive protein
CSF	cerebrospinal fluid
CSSD	Centre for Surgical Sterilization and Disinfection
CSU	catheter specimen for urine
CT	computerized tomography
CVC	central venous catheter
CVID	common variable immunodeficiency
CVS	cardiovascular system
CXR	chest X-ray
DAA	direct-acting antiviral
DAIR	debridement and implant retention
DAT	direct agglutination test
DDT	dichlorodiphenyltrichloroethane
DEC	diethylcarbamazine
DEET	diethyltoluamide
DF	dengue fever
DFA	direct fluorescent antibody test
DH	Department of Health
DHF	dengue haemorrhagic fever
DHFR	dihydrofolate reductase
DHHS	Department of Health and Human Services
DHP-1	dehydropeptidase-1
DHPS	dihydropteroate synthase
DIC	disseminated intravascular coagulation
DIPC	Director of Infection Prevention and Control
DKA	diabetic ketoacidosis
dL	decilitre
DLA	acute dermatolymphangioadenitis
DMSA	dimercaptosuccinic acid (scan)
DNA	deoxyribonucleic acid
DNase	deoxyribonuclease
DNT	dermonecrotic toxin
DoH	Department of Health

dsDNA	double-stranded deoxyribonucleic acid
DSN	distal sensory neuropathy
DSP	dry sterilization process
DST	drug susceptibility testing
DTP	diphtheria, tetanus, polio (vaccine)
DVT	deep venous thrombosis
EASL	European Association for the Study of the Liver
EBNA	Epstein–Barr virus nuclear antigen
EBV	Epstein–Barr virus
ECDC	European Centre for Disease Prevention and Control
ECG	electrocardiogram
EDTA	ethylenediaminetetraacetic acid
EEE	eastern equine encephalitis
EEG	electroencephalography
EF	(o)edema factor
eGFR	estimated glomerular filtration rate
EI	erythema infectiosum
EIA	enzyme-linked immunoassay
EIEC	enteroinvasive *Escherichia coli*
EITB	enzyme-linked immunoelectrotransfer blot
ELISA	enzyme-linked immunosorbent assay
EM	electron microscopy; erythema chronicum migrans
EMG	electromyography
EMJH	Ellinghausen-McCullough-Johnson-Harris
ENT	ear, nose, and throat
EO	ethylene oxide
epo	erythropoietin
EPP	exposure-prone procedure
EQA	external quality assessment
ERCP	endoscopic retrograde cholangiopancreatography
ESBL	extended-spectrum β-lactamase
ESCAPPM	*Enterobacter* spp., *Serratia* spp., *Citrobacter freundii*, *Acinetobacter* spp., *Proteus vulgaris*, *Providencia* spp., *Morganella morganii*
ESR	erythrocyte sedimentation rate
ESRD	end-stage renal disease
ET	exfoliative toxin
ETEC	enterotoxigenic *Escherichia coli*

EUCAST	European Committee on Antimicrobial Susceptibility Testing
EVD	external ventricular drain
FAN	Fastidious Antibiotic Neutralization (bottle)
FAT	fluorescent antibody test
FBC	full blood count
FDA	Food and Drug Administration
FDG-PET	fluorodeoxyglucose positron emission tomography
FEV_1	forced expiratory volume in 1 second
FFI	fatal familial insomnia
FHA	filamentous haemagglutinin
FNA	fine-needle aspiration
FTA-ABS	fluorescent treponemal antibody absorption (test)
FUO	fever of unknown origin
g	gram
G6PD	glucose-6-phosphate dehydrogenase
GAM	granulomatous amoebic encephalitis
GAS	group A *Streptococcus*
GBS	group B *Streptococcus*; Guillain–Barré syndrome
GBV-C	GB virus type C
GCS	Glasgow coma scale
G-CSF	granulocyte-colony-stimulating factor
GDH	glutamate dehydrogenase
GDP	guanosine diphosphate
geq	genome equivalent
GFR	glomerular filtration rate
GGT	gamma-glutamyl transferase
GI	gastrointestinal
GISA	glycopeptide-intermediate *Staphylococcus aureus*
GMC	General Medical Council
GMP	good manufacturing practice
GNR	Gram-negative rod
GORD	gastro-oesophageal reflux disease
GP	general practitioner
GRE	glycopeptide-resistant *Enterococcus*
GSS	Gerstmann–Sträussler–Scheinker (disease)
GU	genitourinary

GUM	genitourinary medicine
GVHD	graft-versus-host disease
h	hour
HA	haemagglutinin
HAART	highly active antiretroviral therapy
HACCP	hazard analysis and critical control point
HAD	HIV-associated dementia
HAI	hospital-acquired infection
HA-MRSA	health care-acquired meticillin-resistant *Staphylococcus aureus*
HAP	hospital-acquired pneumonia
HAT	human African trypanosomiasis
HAV	hepatitis A virus
Hb	haemoglobin
HBcAg	hepatitis B core antigen
HBeAg	hepatitis B e antigen
HBIG	hepatitis B immune globulin
HBsAg	hepatitis B surface antigen
HBV	hepatitis B virus
HCAI	health care-associated infection
HCC	hepatocellular carcinoma
HCO_3^-	bicarbonate ion
HCoV	human coronavirus
HCV	hepatitis C virus
HCW	health-care worker
HDV	hepatitis D virus
H&E	haematoxylin and eosin (staining)
HE	Hektoen enteric
HELLP	haemolysis, elevated liver enzymes, low platelets (syndrome)
HEPA	high-efficiency particulate air
HEV	hepatitis E virus
HFM	hand, foot, and mouth (disease)
Hfr	high-frequency recombination
HHV	human herpesvirus
Hib	*Haemophilus influenzae* type b (vaccine)
HICPAC	Healthcare Infection Control Practices Advisory Committee

HIDA	hepatobiliary iminodiacetic acid
HII	High Impact Intervention: from 'Saving Lives' programme
HIV	human immunodeficiency virus
HIVAN	HIV-associated nephropathy
HLA	human leucocyte antigen
HNIG	human normal immunoglobulin
H_2O_2	hydrogen peroxide
HPA	Health Protection Agency
HPLC	high-pressure liquid chromatography
HPU	health protection unit
HPV	human papillomavirus
H_2S	hydrogen sulfide
HSE	Health and Safety Executive
HSP	Henoch–Schönlein purpura
HSV	herpes simplex virus
HTLV	human T-cell lymphotropic virus
HTM	health technical memorandum
HUS	haemolytic uraemic syndrome
IAS-USA	International Antiviral Society-USA
IBD	inflammatory bowel disease
ICC	infection control committee
ICD	infection control doctor
ICN	infection control nurse
ICP	intracranial pressure
ICT	infection control team
ICU	intensive care unit
ID	infectious diseases; implanted device
IDSA	Infectious Diseases Society of America
IDU	injecting drug user
IE	infective endocarditis
IFA	immunofluorescence assay/indirect fluorescent antibody
IFAT	immunofluorescence antibody test
IFN	interferon
Ig	immunoglobulin (IgA, IgE, IgG, IgM)
IGRA	interferon gamma release assay
IL	interleukin
IM	intramuscular

IMS	industrial methylated spirit
INH	inhaled
INR	international normalized ratio
IPV	inactivated polio vaccine
IQA	internal quality assurance
IQC	internal quality control
IRIS	immune reconstitution inflammatory syndrome
IS	insertion sequence
ISAGA	IgM immunosorbent agglutination assay
ITP	idiopathic thrombocytopenic purpura
IU	international unit
IUCD	intrauterine contraceptive device
IUGR	intrauterine growth restriction
IV	intravenously
IVC	intravascular catheter
IVIG	intravenous immunoglobulin
JCV	JC virus
JE	Japanese encephalitis
K	potassium
kb	kilobase
kg	kilogram
KOH	potassium hydroxide
kPa	kilopascal
KPC	*Klebsiella pneumoniae* carbapenemase
KS	Kaposi's sarcoma
L	litre
LAM	lipoarabinomannan
LAME	*Listeria*, 'atypical' organisms (*Mycoplasma, Chlamydia*), MRSA and enterococci
LCMV	lymphocytic choriomeningitis virus
LDH	lactate dehydrogenase
LES	Liverpool epidemic strain
LF	lethal factor
LFT	liver function test
LGV	lymphogranuloma venereum
LOS	lipo-oligosaccharide
LP	lumbar puncture

LPS	lipopolysaccharide
LRTI	lower respiratory tract infection
LTR	long tandem repeat
LTS	long-term storage
LVF	left ventricular failure
m	metre
MAC	*Mycobacterium avium* complex
MAI	*Mycobacterium avium intracellulare*
MALDI-TOF	matrix-assisted laser desorption/ionization time-of-flight mass spectroscopy
MALT	mucosa-associated lymphoid tissue
MAT	micro-agglutination test
MBC	minimum bactericidal concentration
MBL	metallo-β-lactamases
MC&S	microscopy, culture, and sensitivity
MCD	multicentric Castleman's disease; mild neurocognitive disorder
MDI	microbiological documented infection
MDR	multidrug-resistant
MDRD	modification of diet in renal disease
MDT	multidrug therapy
MEC	minimum effective concentration
mg	milligram
Mg	magnesium
MGE	mobile genetic element
MGIT	Mycobacteria Growth Indicator Tube
MHC	major histocompatibility complex
MIC	minimum inhibitory concentration
MIF	micro-immunofluorescent antibody
min	minute
mL	millilitre
MLEE	multilocus enzyme electrophoresis
MLS_B	macrolide-lincosamide-streptogramin B (resistance)
MLST	multiple locus sequence typing
MLVA	multiple loci variable number repeat tandem analysis
mm	millimetre
mmHg	millimetre of mercury

mmol	millimole
MMR	measles, mumps, rubella (vaccination)
MODS	multiple organ dysfunction syndrome
MOTT	mycobacteria other than tuberculosis
MR	magnetic resonance
MRCP	magnetic resonance cholangiopancreatography
MRI	magnetic resonance imaging
mRNA	messenger RNA
MRSA	meticillin-resistant *Staphylococcus aureus*
MSA	mannitol salt agar
MSCRAMM	microbial surface components recognizing adhesive matrix molecule
MSM	men who have sex with men
MSSA	meticillin-sensitive *Staphylococcus aureus*
MSU	midstream urine
MTB	*Mycobacterium tuberculosis*
NA	neuraminidase
NAAT	nucleic acid amplification test
NaCl	sodium chloride
NAD	nicotinamide adenine dinucleotide
NADPH	nicotinamide adenine dinucleotide phosphate oxidase
NASBA	nucleic acid sequence-based amplification
NASH	non-alcoholic steatohepatitis
ND	notifiable disease
NDM	New Delhi metallo-β-lactamase-1
neb	nebulized
NG	nasogastric
NGS	next-generation sequencing
NH_4^+	ammonium ions
NHL	non-Hodgkin's lymphoma
NHSBT	NHS Blood and Transplant (Tissue Services)
NICE	National Institute for Health and Care Excellence
NICU	neonatal intensive care unit
NINSS	Nosocomial Infection National Surveillance Scheme (UK)
NK	natural killer
nm	nanometre
NNRTI	non-nucleoside reverse transcriptase inhibitor

NPA	nasopharyngeal aspirate
NRTI	nucleoside/nucleotide analogue reverse transcriptase inhibitor
NSAID	non-steroidal anti-inflammatory drug
NTM	non-tuberculous mycobacteria
NTS	non-typhoidal *Salmonella* species
NYC	New York City (agar)
NVS	nutritionally variant streptococci
OCP	oral contraceptive pill
od	once a day
OHS	oral hydration salts
OLM	ocular larva migrans
OMP	outer membrane protein
ONPG	*o*-nitrophenyl-B-*D*-galactopyranoside
OPAT	outpatient antimicrobial therapy
OPSI	overwhelming post-splenectomy infection
OPV	oral polio vaccine
ORF	open reading frame
PA	protective antigen
PABA	para-aminobenzoic acid
PAE	post-antibiotic effect
PaO_2	partial pressure of arterial oxygen
PAS	para-aminosalicylic acid
PAS	periodic acid–Schiff (staining)
PBMC	peripheral blood mononuclear cell
PBP	penicillin-binding protein
PCNSL	primary central nervous system lymphoma
PCP	*Pneumocystis* pneumonia
PCR	polymerase chain reaction
PCV	pneumococcal conjugate vaccine
PD	peritoneal dialysis
PDA	patent ductus arteriosus
PDH	progressive disseminated histoplasmosis
PE	pulmonary embolism
PEA	phenyl ethanol agar
PEG-IFN	pegylated interferon
PEL	primary effusion lymphoma

PEP	post-exposure prophylaxis
PEPSE	post-exposure prophylaxis following sexual exposure
PfEMP1	*Plasmodium falciparum*-infected erythrocyte membrane protein 1
PFGE	pulsed-field gel electrophoresis
PGL	persistent generalized lymphadenopathy
PHE	Public Health England
PI	protease inhibitor
PIA	polysaccharide intracellular adhesion
PICC	peripherally inserted central catheter
PICU	paediatric intensive care unit
PID	pelvic inflammatory disease
PII	period of increased incidence
PJI	prosthetic joint infection
p.m.	*post meridiem* (after noon)
PML	progressive multifocal leukoencephalopathy
PO	orally
PPD	purified protein derivative
PPE	personal protective equipment
PPI	proton pump inhibitor
ppm	part per million
PR	per rectum
PRCA	pure red cell aplasia
PrEP	pre-exposure prophylaxis
PROM	premature rupture of the membranes
PrP	prion protein
PSA	prostate-specific antigen
PSS	post-splenectomy sepsis
PT	prothrombin time; pertussis toxin
PTC	percutaneous transhepatic cholangiography
PTLD	post-transplant lymphoproliferative disorder
PUO	pyrexia of unknown origin
PV	per vagina
PVC	peripheral venous catheter
PVE	prosthetic valve endocarditis
PVL	Panton–Valentine leucocidin
QAC	quaternary ammonium compound

qds	four times a day
qPCR	quantitative polymerase chain reaction
RAPD	random amplification of polymorphic DNA
RBC	red blood cell
RCT	randomized controlled trial
REA	restriction endonuclease analysis
rep-PCR	repetitive element polymerase chain reaction
RFLP	restriction fragment length polymorphism
RIDDOR	Reporting of Injuries, Diseases and Dangerous Occurrences Regulations
RMAT	rapid micro-agglutination test
RMSF	Rocky Mountain spotted fever
RNA	ribonucleic acid
RPR	rapid plasma reagin
rRNA	ribosomal ribonucleic acid
RSSE	Russian spring–summer encephalitis
RSV	respiratory syncytial virus
RT	reverse transcriptase
RT-PCR	reverse transcription polymerase chain reaction
RVF	Rift Valley fever
s	second
SaBTO	(Advisory Committee on the) Safety of Blood, Tissues and Organs
SaO_2	arterial oxygen saturation
SARS	severe acute respiratory syndrome
SBP	spontaneous bacterial peritonitis
s/c	subcutaneous
SCC	staphylococcal cassette chromosome
SCID	severe combined immunodeficiency disease
sCJD	sporadic Creutzfeldt–Jakob disease
SDD	selective decontamination of the digestive tract
SE	staphylococcal enterotoxin
SENIC	Study on Efficacy of Nosocomial Infection Control
SHOT	Serious Hazards of Transfusion
SIADH	syndrome of inappropriate antidiuretic hormone secretion
SIGN	Scottish Intercollegiate Guidelines Network
SIRS	systemic inflammatory response syndrome

SIV	simian immunodeficiency virus
SLE	systemic lupus erythematosus
SLST	single locus sequence typing
S-MAC	sorbitol MacConkey
SMI	Standards for Microbiology Investigations
SNP	single nucleotide polymorphism
slpAST	surface layer protein A gene sequence typing
SOP	standard operating procedure
spp.	species
SPA	suprapubic aspirate
SPS	sodium polyanetholesulphonate
SRSV	small round structured virus
SSA	streptococcal superantigen
SSI	surgical site infection
SSPE	subacute sclerosing panencephalitis
ssRNA	single-stranded ribonucleic acid
SSRI	selective serotonin reuptake inhibitor
SSSS	staphylococcal scalded skin syndrome
STD	sexually transmitted disease
STI	sexually transmitted infection
Stx	shiga toxin
SVR	sustained virological response
SVT	supraventricular tachycardia
TAC	transient aplastic crisis
TB	tuberculosis
TCBS	thiosulfate citrate bile salts sucrose
TCT	tracheal cytotoxin
Td	combined tetanus/low-dose diphtheria vaccine
tds	three times a day
TFT	thyroid function test
TINU	tubulointerstitial nephritis and uveitis
TK	thymidine kinase
TMA	transcription-mediated amplification
TNF	tumour necrosis factor
TOC	test of cure
TOE	transoesophageal echocardiography
TOP	topically

TP	tube precipitin
TPHA	*Treponema pallidum* haemagglutination assay
TPN	total parenteral nutrition
TPPA	*Treponema pallidum* particle assay
TQM	total quality management
TREM-1	triggering receptor expressed on myeloid cells-1
tRNA	transfer ribonucleic acid
TSE	transmissible spongiform encephalopathy
TSS	toxic shock syndrome
TSST	toxic shock syndrome toxin
TST	tuberculin skin test
TTE	transthoracic echocardiography
U&E	urea and electrolyte
UCD	unicentric Castleman's disease
UCV	ultraclean ventilation
UICP	universal infection control precautions
UK	United Kingdom
UKAP	UK Advisory Panel for health-care workers infected with blood-borne viruses
ULN	upper limit of normal
URTI	upper respiratory tract infection
US/USA	United States
USS	ultrasound scan
UTI	urinary tract infection
UV	ultraviolet
VA	ventriculo-atrial
VAP	ventilator-associated pneumonia
VATS	video-assisted thoracoscopic surgery
VCA	viral capsid antigen
vCJD	variant Creutzfeldt–Jakob disease
VDRL	Venereal Disease Research Laboratory (test)
VEE	Venezuelan equine encephalitis
VGK	Vogt–Koyanagi–Harada
VHF	viral haemorrhagic fever
VIP	visual infusion phlebitis (score)
VISA	vancomycin-intermediate *Staphylococcus aureus*
VLM	visceral larva migrans

VNTR	variable-number tandem repeat
VP	ventriculoperitoneal
VRE	vancomycin-resistant enterococci
VRSA	vancomycin-resistant *Staphylococcus aureus*
VSD	ventricular septal defect
VUR	vesico-ureteric reflux
v/v	volume by volume
VZIG	varicella-zoster immune globulin
VZV	varicella-zoster virus
WCC	white cell count
WGS	whole-genome sequencing
WHO	World Health Organization
XDR	extensively drug resistant
XLD	xylose lysine deoxycholate
ZN	Ziehl–Neelsen (stain)

Part 1

Antimicrobials

1 Basics of antimicrobials 3
2 Antibiotics 31
3 Antifungals 79
4 Antivirals 89
5 Antiparasitic therapy 111

Chapter 1

Basics of antimicrobials

A history of antibiotics *4*
Global antibiotic use *6*
Mechanisms of action *8*
Mechanisms of resistance *9*
Molecular genetics of resistance *11*
Clonal expansion *12*
Heteroresistance *13*
Susceptibility testing *13*
Pharmacokinetics *15*
Pharmacodynamics *16*
Routes of administration *18*
Antimicrobials in renal impairment *21*
Antimicrobials in liver disease *23*
Antimicrobials in pregnancy *24*
Antimicrobial prophylaxis *25*
Antimicrobial stewardship *27*
Outpatient parenteral antimicrobial therapy *28*

A history of antibiotics

To start, some definitions: an 'antimicrobial' is an umbrella term for drugs with activity against microorganisms (antibacterials, antivirals, antifungals, antiparasitic agents); an 'antibiotic' is, strictly speaking, a chemical compound made by a microorganism that inhibits or kills other microorganisms at low concentrations. This does not include synthetic agents, although, in practice, it is often used for any antibacterial; an 'antiparasitic' is used to treat parasitic diseases and includes antiprotozoals and antihelminthics.

A history

Substances with some form of anti-infective action have been used since ancient times. The Chinese used 'mouldy' soybean curd to treat boils and carbuncles. The South American Indians chewed cinchona tree bark (contains quinine) for malaria.

In Europe, one of the earliest recorded examples was the use of mercury to treat syphilis in the 1400s.

In 1877, Louis Pasteur showed that injections of extracts of soil bacteria cured anthrax in animals.

In 1908–1910, Paul Erlich, Nobel Prize winner and father of chemotherapy, synthesized arsenic compounds effective against syphilis.

In 1924, the compound actinomycetin, so named because it is produced by actinomycetes, was discovered.

In 1932, Domagk discovered the dye prontosil that cured streptococcal infections in animals. The active group turned out to be the sulfonamide attached to the dye, and, by 1945, over 5000 sulfonamide derivatives had been developed. Adverse effects and drug resistance have limited clinical use of these compounds.

In 1939, Dubos isolated two agents that were active against Gram-positive organisms (gramicidin and tyrocidin) from *Bacillus brevis*.

In 1944–1945, Waksman isolated streptomycin from the soil microbe *Streptomyces griseus*. It was active against *Mycobacterium tuberculosis* and some Gram-negative organisms, and Waksman was awarded the Nobel Prize.

History of penicillin

(See Table 1.1.) Alexander Fleming returned to St Mary's Hospital after a weekend away in 1928 to discover that the mould *Penicillium notatum* had contaminated his culture plates. He observed that the colonies of *Staphylococcus aureus* nearest to the mould had lysed, while those further away had not, and hypothesized that the *Penicillium* had released a product that caused bacterial cell lysis. He called this product penicillin. Although Fleming discovered penicillin, he was unable to purify sufficient quantities for clinical trials. In 1939, Howard Florey, Ernst Chain, and Norman Heatley, working in Oxford, obtained the *Penicillium* fungus from Fleming. They overcame the technical difficulties and conducted clinical trials to demonstrate the efficacy of penicillin. Mass production soon began in the United Kingdom (UK) and United States (USA). Initially, penicillin was used almost exclusively for soldiers injured during the Second World War. It became widely available by 1946. As soon as he discovered penicillin, Fleming warned of the development of penicillin resistance, and indeed resistance was seen almost immediately. Chemical modifications of the drug have since created derivatives (e.g. ampicillin) that are less susceptible to enzymatic degradation.

Table 1.1 A non-exhaustive antibiotic timeline

Year	Antibiotic	Class of antibiotic
1928	Penicillin discovered	β-lactam
1932	Prontosil discovered	Sulfonamide
1942	Penicillin introduced	β-lactam
1943	Streptomycin discovered	Aminoglycoside
1945	Cephalosporins discovered	β-lactam
1947	Chloramphenicol discovered	Protein synthesis inhibitor
1947	Chlortetracycline discovered	Tetracycline
1949	Neomycin discovered	Aminoglycoside
1952	Erythromycin discovered	Macrolide
1956	Vancomycin discovered	Glycopeptide
1960	Flucloxacillin introduced	β-lactam
1961	Ampicillin introduced	β-lactam
1963	Gentamicin discovered	Aminoglycoside
1964	Cephalosporins introduced	β-lactam
1964	Vancomycin introduced	Glycopeptide
1966	Doxycycline introduced	Tetracycline
1971	Rifampicin introduced	Rifamycin
1974	Co-trimoxazole introduced	Sulfonamide and trimethoprim
1976	Amikacin introduced	Aminoglycoside
1979	Ampicillin/clavulanate introduced	β-lactam/β-lactamase inhibitor
1987	Imipenem/cilastin introduced	Carbapenem
1987	Ciprofloxacin introduced	Quinolone
1993	Azithromycin and clarithromycin introduced	Macrolide
1999	Quinupristin/dalfopristin introduced	Streptogramin
2000	Linezolid introduced	Oxazolidinone
2003	Daptomycin introduced	Lipopeptide
2004	Telithromycin introduced	Ketolide
2005	Tigecycline introduced	Glycylcycline
2012	Fidaxomicin introduced	Macrocyclic

Global antibiotic use

National data on the quantity and trends of antibiotic usage are usually not available. However, it is generally thought that about 50% of all antimicrobials are used in human medicine, and about 50% for animals and crops. The total amount of antimicrobials used varies between countries; developed countries use proportionately more than developing countries. Different countries have different antibiotics available—just because an antibiotic is widely prescribed in one country, it does not mean it will be licensed in another, e.g. teicoplanin is not available in the USA.

Human use of antibiotics

Most infections are treated in the community by general practitioners (GPs) or through outpatient clinics; this accounts for the greatest number of antibiotic prescriptions. Some agents with antimicrobial activity are available over the counter (e.g. clotrimazole for vaginal thrush and topical aciclovir for cold sores). The quantity of antibiotics used varies between hospitals, depending on the specialist units there (e.g. hospitals with large intensive care units (ICUs) or a renal unit are likely to use more antibiotics). Hospitals with similar patient populations have different approaches to prescribing antibiotics, which may be influenced by local antimicrobial susceptibility data. In the first instance, you should follow your local hospital policy and consult microbiology/infectious diseases (ID) specialists for advice.

Problems with human use of antibiotics

Overuse of antibiotics has led to rising rates of resistance to antimicrobials, with the result that a few organisms have become virtually untreatable (e.g. vancomycin-resistant *S. aureus*, extensively drug-resistant (XDR) *M. tuberculosis* (MTB), carbapenemase-producing *Enterobacteriaceae*).

Resistance results in increased morbidity and mortality, with considerable economic and social consequences. In the USA, the Centers for Disease Control and Prevention (CDC) estimates that one-third of all outpatient antibiotic prescriptions is not required. Hence, many organizations have been working to try to reduce inappropriate prescribing, e.g. public education (e.g. most upper respiratory tract infections (URTIs) are caused by viruses), changing the practice of health-care prescribers (e.g. short course, narrow-spectrum agents where appropriate).

Other problems associated with the overuse of antibiotics include superinfection (e.g. with *Candida albicans, Clostridium difficile*), the unnecessary risk of adverse effects, drug interactions, and expense.

In the developing world, a number of additional problems exist:

- antibiotics are often available without prescription from a cornershop;
- if the patient does take an appropriate antibiotic, they may take the wrong dose for the incorrect duration;
- the purchased drug may be inappropriate, so the infection remains untreated, and patients may therefore develop a more severe or complicated infection before consulting a doctor;
- some drugs are 'fake', substandard, or past their expiry date;
- patients may take a combination of traditional therapy along with antibiotics that may lead to interactions and toxicity.

Non-human use of antibiotics

Antimicrobials have been used increasingly for the prevention and treatment of infections in animals (e.g. on farms, in fish factories, and for domestic pets) and in the environment (e.g. crop production). Since the discovery of their growth-promoting abilities, they have also been added to animal feed (particularly for pigs and poultry). In addition, some antibiotics increase feed efficiency (the amount of feed absorbed by an animal), increasing the chance that the animal reaches its target weight on time. Other examples of non-human use include:

- tetracycline sprayed on apple plantations to treat fireblight;
- oxytetracycline added to water in commercial fish farms to treat infections;
- antibiotics used to eliminate bacterial growth inside oil pipelines.

When farm animals consume antibiotics in their feed, they may excrete them into the environment. This may select for antibiotic-resistant organisms that may then infect other animal species. Antibiotics in the environment undoubtedly contribute to increasing antibiotic resistance, particularly amongst food-borne pathogens such as *Salmonella* species (spp.) and *Campylobacter* spp. Many organizations have developed strategies to try to control the non-human use of antibiotics (particularly in agriculture and animal husbandry) and thus reduce the development of resistance.

Responses to the problem of resistance

There is an increasing political awareness of the risk antibiotic resistance poses to human health. Travel and health tourism make it a global issue, from which no one country can isolate itself. England's chief medical officer described it as a 'catastrophic threat', and British and US premiers have backed national plans for research and control. The World Health Organization (WHO) recently conducted a worldwide 'country situation analysis' and is coordinating national responses. Table 1.2 gives sources of information on antimicrobial resistance.

Table 1.2 Sources of information on antimicrobial resistance

Information	Web address
Alliance for the Prudent Use of Antibiotics	www.tufts.edu/med/apua
World Health Organization Drug Resistance	www.who.int/drugresistance/en/
Antibiotic Action	www.Antibiotic-action.com
UK government bodies	www.gov.uk/defra www.gov.uk/phe www.hps.scot.nhs.uk/haiic/amr/
European data (Eurosurveillance)	www.eurosurveillance.org/
National Antimicrobial Resistance Monitoring System (USA)	www.cdc.gov/narms/
British Society for Antimicrobial Chemotherapy	www.bsac.org.uk

Mechanisms of action

Antimicrobial agents are classified by their specific modes of action against bacterial cells. The modes of action of antimicrobial agents against Gram-positive and Gram-negative bacteria are very similar and can be divided into five categories:

- inhibition of cell wall synthesis;
- inhibition of protein synthesis;
- inhibition of nucleic acid synthesis;
- inhibition of folate synthesis;
- disruption of the cytoplasmic membrane.

Inhibition of cell wall synthesis

Agents that interfere with cell wall synthesis block peptidoglycan synthesis or cross-linking. They are active against growing bacteria and are bactericidal.

Gram-negative bacteria—β-lactam antimicrobials enter the cell through porin channels in the outer membrane and bind to penicillin-binding proteins (PBPs) on the surface of the cytoplasmic membrane. This blocks their function, causing weakened or defective cell walls, and leads to cell lysis and death.

Gram-positive bacteria lack an outer membrane, so β-lactam antimicrobials diffuse directly through the cell wall and bind to PBPs, which results in weakened cell walls and cell lysis. Glycopeptides inhibit cell wall synthesis by binding to the D-ALA-D-ALA terminal end of peptidoglycan precursors, thus inhibiting the action of transglycosidase and transpeptidases.

Inhibition of protein synthesis

Tetracyclines bind to the 30S ribosomal subunit, and block attachment of transfer RNA (tRNA) and addition of amino acids to the protein chain. Tetracyclines are bacteriostatic.

Aminoglycosides also bind to the 30S ribosomal subunit and prevent its attachment to messenger RNA (mRNA). They can also cause misreading of the mRNA, resulting in insertion of the wrong amino acid or interference in the ability of amino acids to connect with each other. The combined effect of these two mechanisms is bactericidal.

Macrolides and lincosamides attach to the 50S ribosomal subunit, causing termination of the growing protein chain. They are bacteriostatic.

Chloramphenicol also binds to the 50S ribosomal subunit and interferes with binding of amino acids to the growing chain. It is also bacteriostatic.

Linezolid (an oxazolidinone) binds to the 23S ribosomal RNA (rRNA) of the 50S subunit and prevents formation of a functional 70S initiation complex which is necessary for protein synthesis. It is bacteriostatic.

Inhibition of nucleic acid synthesis

Fluoroquinolones interfere with DNA synthesis by blocking the enzyme DNA gyrase. This enzyme binds to DNA and introduces double-stranded breaks that allow the DNA complex to unwind. Fluoroquinolones bind to the DNA gyrase–DNA complex and allow broken DNA strands to be released into the cell, resulting in cell death.

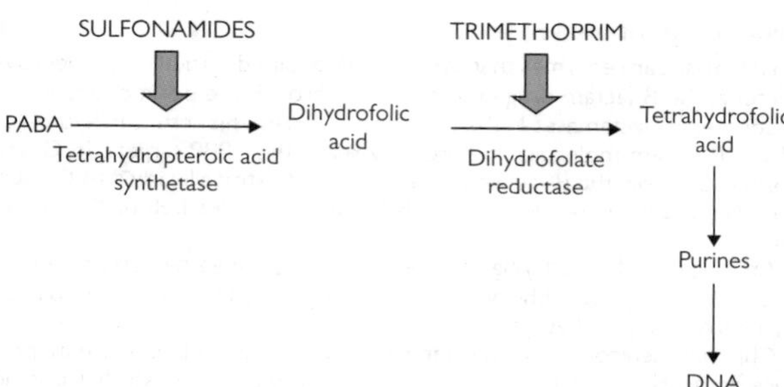

Fig. 1.1 Inhibition of folate synthesis.

Rifampicin binds to DNA-dependent RNA polymerase, which blocks synthesis of RNA and results in cell death.

Inhibition of folate synthesis

(See Fig. 1.1.)

For many organisms, para-aminobenzoic acid (PABA) is an essential metabolite which is involved in the synthesis of folic acid, an important precursor to the synthesis of nucleic acids.

Sulfonamides are structural analogues of PABA and compete with PABA for the enzyme dihydropteroate synthetase.

Trimethoprim acts on the folic acid synthesis pathway at a point after the sulfonamides, inhibiting the enzyme dihydrofolate reductase.

Both trimethoprim and sulfonamides are bacteriostatic. When they are used together (e.g. co-trimoxazole), they produce a sequential blockade of the folic acid synthesis pathway and have a synergistic effect.

Disruption of the cytoplasmic membrane

Polymyxin molecules diffuse through the outer membrane and cell wall of susceptible cells to the cytoplasmic membrane. They bind to the cytoplasmic membrane, and disrupt and destabilize it. This causes the cytoplasm to leak out of the cell, resulting in cell death.

Mechanisms of resistance

There are a number of ways by which microorganisms become resistant to antimicrobial agents. These include:

- production of enzymes;
- alteration in outer membrane permeability;
- alteration of target sites;
- efflux pumps;
- alteration of metabolic pathways.

Production of enzymes

β-lactamases are enzymes that hydrolyse β-lactam drugs. In Gram-negative bacteria, the β-lactam drug enters the cell through the porin channels and encounters β-lactamases in the periplasmic space. This results in hydrolysis of the β-lactam molecules, before they reach their PBP targets. In Gram-positive bacteria, the β-lactamases are secreted extracellularly into the surrounding medium and destroy the β-lactam molecules before they enter the cell.

Aminoglycoside-modifying enzymes—Gram-negative bacteria may produce adenylating, phosphorylating, or acetylating enzymes that modify an aminoglycoside, so that it is no longer active.

Chloramphenicol acetyl transferase—Gram-negative bacteria may produce an acetyl transferase that modifies chloramphenicol, so that it is no longer active.

Alteration in outer membrane permeability

Gram-negative bacteria may become resistant to β-lactam antibiotics by developing permeability barriers.

Mutations resulting in the loss of porin channels in the outer membrane no longer allow the entrance and passage of antibiotic molecules into the cell.

Alterations in proton motive force may result in reduced inner membrane permeability.

Alteration of target sites

PBPs in Gram-positive and Gram-negative bacteria may be altered through mutations, so that β-lactams can no longer bind to them.

Methylation of rRNA confers resistance to macrolides, lincosamides, and streptogramins

Mutations in the chromosomal genes for DNA gyrase and topoisomerase IV confer quinolone resistance.

Efflux pumps

A wide variety of efflux pumps produce antimicrobial resistance in both Gram-positive and Gram-negative bacteria. Transmembrane proteins form channels that actively export an antimicrobial agent out of the cell as fast as it enters. This is the main mechanism of resistance to tetracyclines.

Alteration of metabolic pathways

Some microorganisms develop an altered metabolic pathway that bypasses the reaction inhibited by the antimicrobial. Mutations that inactivate thymidylate synthetase block the conversion of deoxyuridylate to thymidylate. These mutants use exogenous thymine or thymidine for DNA synthesis and therefore are resistant to folate synthesis antagonists.

Molecular genetics of resistance

Genetic variability is essential for microbial evolution and may occur by a variety of mechanisms:

- point mutations;
- rearrangements of large segments of DNA from one location of a bacterial chromosome or plasmid to another;
- acquisition of foreign DNA from other bacteria, via a mobile genetic element (MGE).

Acquisition of resistance, in the presence of the antibiotic, confers a survival advantage on the host, thus leading to the emergence of resistant clones. The overuse, incorrect use, or injudicious use of antibiotics contributes to this problem, and explains why new resistance patterns tend to emerge in areas of the hospital with the greatest antibiotic consumption (e.g. ICUs). This antibiotic resistance may be passed vertically to future generations through clonal expansion, resulting in a bacterial population that is resistant to an antibiotic.

Point mutations

These are often referred to as single nucleotide polymorphisms (SNPs). The bacterial genome is dynamic, in that bacteria are constantly undergoing mutations. Some of these mutations will (by chance) result in a survival advantage to the organism, e.g. due to increased virulence or antibiotic resistance. In certain environments, these will be preferentially selected for; thus, the mutation that arose by chance will be retained and passed to future generations. Examples of point mutations include the generation of β-lactamase and fluoroquinolone resistance.

Mobile genetic elements

These are pieces of DNA that can move around between genomes. They may thus be involved in the horizontal transfer of resistance genes between bacteria, as opposed to the vertical transfer of resistance by clonal expansion (see list below). Bacterial genomes consist of core genes and accessory genes; it is the latter that are defined by acquisition and loss. There are several different MGEs described in the following list.

- Plasmids—these are extrachromosomal pieces of circular DNA, which vary in size from 10kb to over 400kb. In addition to carrying resistance genes, they may determine other functions, e.g. virulence factors and metabolic capabilities. They are autonomous self-replicating genetic elements that possess an origin for replication and genes that facilitate their maintenance in the host bacteria. Conjugative plasmids require additional genes to initiate self-transfer.
- Insertion sequences (IS)—these are short DNA sequences that are usually only 700–2500bp (base pairs) long. They encode an enzyme needed for transposition (i.e. to excise a segment of DNA from one position in the chromosome and insert it elsewhere) and a regulatory protein, which either stimulates or inhibits the transposition activity. They are thus different from transposons, which also carry accessory

genes such as antibiotic resistance genes. The coding region in an insertion sequence is usually flanked by inverted repeats.

- Transposons—these are often called 'jumping genes' and may contain IS. They cannot replicate independently but can move between one replicating piece of DNA to another, e.g. from a chromosome to a plasmid. Conjugative transposons mediate their own transfer between bacteria, whereas non-conjugative transposons need prior integration into a plasmid to be transferred.
- Integrons—these may be defined as a genetic element that possesses a site (*attI*) at which additional DNA in the form of gene cassettes can be integrated by site-specific mutation. They also encode a gene, integrase, which mediates these site-specific recombination events. Gene cassettes normally consist of an antibiotic resistance gene and a 59-base element that functions as a site-specific recombination site. The largest integrons (e.g. in *Vibrio cholerae*) can contain hundreds of gene cassettes.
- Bacteriophages—a bacteriophage is a virus that infects bacteria and may become integrated into the bacterial chromosome (and is then called a prophage). They typically consist of an outer protein enclosing genetic material (which may be single- or double-stranded DNA or RNA). Bacteriophages may be considered MGEs but are rarely involved in the transfer of resistance genes. They have been used as an alternative to antibiotics (phage therapy) in Eastern Europe and the former USSR for ~60 years.

Clonal expansion

Clonal expansion refers to the multiplication of a single 'ancestor' cell. This may result in the propagation of antibiotic resistance into daughter cells. The antibiotic resistance genes will be passed from one generation of bacteria to the next, which is also called vertical transfer of resistance. If an organism becomes resistant to an antibiotic, either by mutation or acquisition of an MGE, it will have a survival advantage in an environment where that antibiotic is present. Thus, the daughter cells that are generated will be positively selected for, over daughter cells from another antibiotic-sensitive strain of the bacteria, and future generations will be resistant to that agent. A bacterial clone refers to all organisms that are likely to have arisen from a common ancestor. This may not be immediately obvious. Examples of recent clonal expansion relating to the spread of antibiotic resistance genes are meticillin-resistant *S. aureus* (MRSA) and penicillin-resistant pneumococci.

Important definitions

Isolate: this refers to a pure culture. It says nothing about typing.

Clone: this refers to bacterial cultures which have been isolated independently, from different sources, in different places, and maybe at different times, but are so similar phenotypically and genotypically that the most likely explanation is that they arose from a common ancestor.

Strain: this refers to a phenotypically and/or genotypically distinctive group of isolates. It is dependent on the typing scheme used, and some experts suggest avoiding the use of this term.

Type: this refers to organisms with the same pattern or set of markers displayed by a strain, when the bacteria are subject to a particular typing system.

Heteroresistance

This is defined as the growth of one bacterial subpopulation at a higher antibiotic concentration than predicted by the minimum inhibitory concentration (MIC) for most cells. Heteroresistance may be difficult to diagnose and result in poor response to treatment. Examples include:

- *S. aureus* and vancomycin;
- *Cryptococcus neoformans* and azoles;
- MTB and rifampicin;
- *Enterococcus faecium* and vancomycin;
- *Acinetobacter baumanii* and carbapenems and colistimethate sodium;
- *Helicobacter pylori* and metronidazole and amoxicillin;
- *Streptococcus pneumoniae* and penicillin.

Susceptibility testing

Bacteriostatic

Antibiotics that inhibit growth and replication of bacteria, but are non-lethal (e.g. drugs that inhibit folic acid synthesis; ➲ see Trimethoprim, pp. 60–1; ➲ Co-trimoxazole, pp. 61–2; ➲ Quinolones, pp. 62–4).

Bactericidal

Antibiotics that cause bacterial cell death by inhibition of: (a) cell wall synthesis, (b) nucleic acid synthesis, or (c) protein synthesis. Some antibiotics may be bacteriostatic at low concentrations, but bactericidal at higher concentrations.

Minimum inhibitory concentration

This is the concentration of antimicrobial required to completely inhibit the growth of an organism after a defined time period (usually overnight). It is determined by agar dilution (incubation on multiple plates with differing antibiotic concentrations) or broth microdilution (liquid broth with varying concentrations of antibiotic—a technique used by many automated systems). Performing MIC testing on a number of strains of a single species allows estimation of the concentration that will inhibit 90% (MIC_{90}) or 50% (MIC_{50}) of that isolate *in vitro* and can detect shifts in antibiotic susceptibility in bacterial populations.

Minimum bactericidal concentration

This is the concentration of antimicrobial required to kill a bacterium. It can be determined from broth dilution tests by subculturing the overnight culture to agar containing no antibiotic. Minimum bactericidal concentration (MBC) is considered the lowest concentration capable of reducing the original inoculum by a factor of 1000 (e.g. from 10^5 cfu/mL to 10^2 or less).

Susceptibility testing techniques

Dilution methods—agar and broth dilution (➔ see Minimum inhibitory concentration, p. 13). The former is considered the gold standard due to good reproducibility. Both are labour-intensive, if performed manually. They should be performed, following the standardized guidelines of a reference body such as the British Society for Antimicrobial Chemotherapy (BSAC), the European Committee on Antimicrobial Susceptibility Testing (EUCAST), or the Clinical & Laboratory Standards Institute (CLSI).

Disc diffusion—efficient and cost-effective, and the most widely used manual method. There are a number of standard methods for performing disc diffusion (Kirby–Bauer, Stokes), and, as a number of factors can influence performance (e.g. agar depth, time, temperature), it is important they are followed. In essence, an agar preparation is evenly seeded with the organism of interest. Commercially prepared discs, each impregnated with a standard concentration of a relevant antibiotic, are placed on the agar surface. The antibiotic diffuses into the agar. After overnight incubation, the bacterial growth around each disc is observed. The zone around the disc with no growth ('zone of inhibition') contains sufficient agent to prevent growth. This zone is measured and compared to the published 'zone breakpoint diameter' for that particular organism/antibiotic combination. It is a qualitative test, and the MIC cannot be derived, but the organism is classed as susceptible, intermediate, or resistant.

E-test—a commercial product taking the form of a plastic strip impregnated with a steadily decreasing concentration of a single antibiotic. It is placed on an agar plate already seeded with the organism of interest. The MIC can then be read from the strip at the point at which bacterial growth is inhibited.

Automated systems—a number of commercial systems now exist that provide standard microdilution plates preloaded with antibiotics (and biochemical assays relevant to organism identification). They are costly to purchase and maintain, but they reduce technical errors and lengthy preparation time.

Mechanism-specific tests—certain phenotypic tests may enable inference of the presence of a resistance mechanism. For example, chromogenic systems for detection of MRSA or cephalosporinase.

Genotypic methods—specific genes encoding resistance mechanisms can be detected by techniques such as polymerase chain reaction (PCR) and DNA hybridization. However, the presence of a gene may not equate to treatment failure (its product may be expressed only at a low level), and its absence clearly does not exclude the presence of another means of resisting a particular agent.

Sensitive or resistant?

A 'breakpoint' is the antibiotic concentration used in the interpretation of susceptibility testing to define isolates as susceptible, intermediate, or resistant. This is not the same as the MIC and may take into account *in vitro* potency, pharmacokinetics/dynamics, clinical experience, and infection site. Increasingly, national authorities think in terms of 'clinical' breakpoints to guide prescribers for specific patients and 'microbiological' breakpoints which seek to identify strains that do not belong to the normal antibiotic-naïve population for the purposes of surveillance.

In January 2016, the BSAC ceased support and development of the BSAC disc diffusion method as part of a national move to the EUCAST disc diffusion method. The EUCAST method is based on the Kirby–Bauer method and uses Mueller–Hinton agar. Full details on the EUCAST method and breakpoint setting are available at www.eucast.org/clinical_breakpoints/.

Pharmacokinetics

This is what the body does to the drug; it comprises absorption, distribution, metabolism, and excretion (mnemonic ADME).

Absorption

To be effective, a drug must reach the site of the infection. In some cases, this is possible by topical application (e.g. nystatin pastilles for oral candidiasis), but, in most cases, drugs are transported around the body by the circulation.

Some drugs are poorly absorbed when given by mouth (e.g. aminoglycosides and glycopeptides) and are therefore given parenterally. Occasionally, oral drugs may be used to treat luminal infections, e.g. vancomycin for *C. difficile*.

If a drug is absorbed when given by mouth, the proportion that is absorbed into the systemic circulation is called the bioavailability. Drugs given intravenously (IV) have 100% bioavailability. The time profile of absorption versus elimination is usually more important than the total amount of drug absorbed (see Pharmacodynamics, pp. 16–8).

Absorption may be affected by interactions with other drugs or food that may bind the drug (e.g. tetracyclines should not be given with milk). Altered physiology (e.g. diarrhoea) may reduce absorption. None of the commonly prescribed antibiotics are subject to significant first-pass metabolism in the liver.

Distribution

The volume of distribution relates the drug concentration in the blood to the amount of drug given. A drug with a small volume of distribution is largely confined to the plasma. A drug with a large volume of distribution is widely distributed, e.g. fat-soluble drugs.

Box 1.1 Antimicrobials metabolized by CYP3A4

- Inducers—rifampicin.
- Inhibitors—ketoconazole, itraconazole, erythromycin, clarithromycin.
- Substrates—ritonavir, saquinavir, indinavir, nelfinavir.

Metabolism

Some antibiotics are metabolized in the liver by isoforms of cytochrome P450, of which the CYP3A4 isoform is the most abundant (see Box 1.1). Rifampicin induces the activity of CYP3A4, leading to increased metabolism (and reduced efficacy) of drugs that share this pathway, e.g. human immunodeficiency virus (HIV) protease inhibitors (PIs). In contrast, the azole antifungals and the macrolides inhibit the activity of CYP3A4, which will reduce the metabolism (and may increase toxicity) of drugs also metabolized by this isoform. Always check for interactions before starting or stopping antibiotics, and seek expert advice if unsure.

Excretion

This can be divided into renal (e.g. aminoglycosides, glycopeptides) and non-renal (biliary tree, e.g. ceftriaxone; gastrointestinal (GI) tract, e.g. azithromycin). Clearance determines the half-life of the drug (the time for the blood concentration to decrease by half). Steady state generally occurs when a patient has taken the drug for a period of time equal to 5–7 half-lives. Calculating the creatinine clearance (CrCl) (➔ see Antimicrobials in renal impairment, pp. 21–3) as a measure of renal function can be essential for safe dosing of some renally excreted drugs, such as once-daily aminoglycosides (➔ see Aminoglycosides, pp. 46–8).

Pharmacodynamics

The study of the biochemical and physiological effects of a drug on the body or microorganism, and the mechanism of drug action, including the link between concentration and effect.

Effects on the body

These may be desired (the therapeutic action of the agent) or undesirable (side effects, e.g. diarrhoea, neuropathy, ototoxicity, etc.). The balance between them is influenced by the therapeutic window—the difference between the dose that is effective (desired) and the dose that gives more adverse undesired effects than desired. Drugs with narrow windows may require therapeutic drug monitoring (e.g. gentamicin).

Synergism

This occurs when the activity of two drugs together is greater than the sum of their actions if each were given separately. An example is the use of ampicillin and gentamicin for enterococcal infections (➔ see Enterococci, pp. 245–7) where ampicillin acts on the cell wall to enable gentamicin to gain entry to the cell and act on the ribosome.

Antagonism

One drug diminishes the activity of another drug, so giving both antibiotics together may result in a worse clinical outcome than just giving one antibiotic. For example, co-administration of a bacteriostatic agent (e.g. tetracycline) with a β-lactam may inhibit cell growth and prevent the bactericidal activity of the β-lactam.

Concentration-dependent killing

The antibiotic kills the organism when its concentration is well above the MIC of the organism. The greater the peak, the greater the killing, e.g. once-daily dosing of gentamicin (➲ see Aminoglycosides, pp. 46–8).

Time-dependent killing

The antibiotic *only* kills the bacteria when its concentration is above the MIC of the organism, but increasing the concentration does not lead to increased killing. If the concentration rises above four times the MIC, any additional effect is negligible. Most recommended dosing schedules account for this (➲ see Penicillins, pp. 32–3; ➲ Cephalosporins, pp. 33–5; ➲ Macrolides, pp. 48–50). On a practical level, it is important when adjusting the dose of glycopeptides (➲ see Glycopeptides, pp. 42–4).

Post-antibiotic effect

The post-antibiotic effect (PAE) is defined as the time during which bacterial growth is inhibited after antibiotic concentrations have fallen below the MIC. The mechanism is unclear, but it may be due to a delay in the bacteria re-entering a log-growth period. Several factors influence the presence or duration of the PAE, including the type of organism, type of antimicrobial, concentration of antimicrobial, duration of antimicrobial exposure, and antimicrobial combinations. *In vitro*, β-lactam antimicrobials demonstrate a PAE against Gram-positive cocci, but not against Gram-negative bacilli. Antimicrobials that inhibit RNA or protein synthesis produce a PAE against Gram-positive cocci and Gram-negative bacilli. The clinical relevance of the PAE is probably most important when designing dosage regimens. The presence of a long PAE allows aminoglycosides to be dosed infrequently; the lack of an *in vivo* PAE suggests that β-lactam antimicrobials require frequent or continuous dosing.

Eagle effect

This is a paradoxical effect, first described by Eagle in 1948, whereby higher concentrations of penicillin resulted in decreased killing of staphylococci and streptococci. Eagle also showed that this paradoxical effect seen *in vitro* correlated with an adverse outcome *in vivo*. This effect has since been described with a number of other antimicrobials and organisms, e.g. ampicillin and *Enterococcus faecalis*, carbenacillin and *Proteus mirabilis*, mecillinam and *Providencia stuartii*, cefotaxime and *S. aureus* and *Pseudomonas aeruginosa*, and aminoglycosides and Gram-negative bacteria.

Preventing the development of resistance

Studies are focusing on defining the breakpoints that predict the emergence of resistance. An ideal antibiotic should have a low rate of resistance mutation, high-fitness cost of resistance, and low rate of fitness-restoring complementary mutation. Novel parameters that are being investigated include:

- mutant prevention concentration—the ability to restrict the selection of resistant mutants;
- mutant selection window—the concentration range between the minimal concentration required to block the growth of wild-type bacteria, up to the concentration needed to inhibit the growth of the least susceptible single-step mutant. There are different concentration ranges for each organism/drug combination.

Routes of administration

Oral administration

Most antibiotics used in human medicine are given orally (PO) in the community. If a drug is absorbed when given by mouth, the proportion that is absorbed into the systemic circulation is called the bioavailability (➲ see Pharmacokinetics, pp. 15–6). This depends on the formulation of the drug and how it is taken, e.g. some tetracyclines should not be taken with milk or antacids, as these decrease their absorption. Some drugs are not absorbed when given PO. This can be advantageous when treating luminal infections, e.g. oral vancomycin for *C. difficile* and neomycin in hepatic failure.

Intravenous administration

The IV route enables higher doses to be given and results in higher, more reliable drug concentrations (see Box 1.2).

Indications

Antimicrobials are given IV in the following situations:

- life-threatening infections, e.g. meningitis, septicaemia, endocarditis, require IV therapy. Antibiotics may be given as infusions or bolus doses, depending on the drug;
- inability to take/absorb oral medications, e.g. nil by mouth, severe vomiting or diarrhoea, oesophageal or intestinal obstruction, post-operative ileus;
- poor oral bioavailability—some drugs are not absorbed if given PO, e.g. aminoglycosides, glycopeptides, colistimethate sodium.

Box 1.2 Practical points

- Many people believe that IV antibiotics are somehow 'stronger' than oral antibiotics. This is not necessarily the case (e.g. ciprofloxacin is as effective when given PO as when given IV and much cheaper).
- The oral and IV doses of the same antibiotic may be different (e.g. metronidazole).

Disadvantages

IV therapy may be associated with a number of problems:

- side effects, which may be local (e.g. phlebitis) or systemic (e.g. rapid infusion may result in anaphylactoid reactions such as the 'red man syndrome' with vancomycin);
- line infections, which may be local (e.g. exit site, tunnel or pocket infections) or systemic (e.g. bacteraemia, endocarditis);
- inconvenience to the patient;
- need to stay in hospital. This may be overcome by the use of outpatient antimicrobial therapy (OPAT) which is now available in some regions of the UK;
- IV antibiotics are usually considerably more expensive than the oral formulation.

IV to oral switch

As a result of the problems associated with IV therapy, many hospitals employ 'IV to oral switch' protocols for certain conditions which encourage clinicians to change to oral antibiotics as soon as is safe. Criteria include:

- suitable oral agent available;
- the patient can tolerate, swallow, and absorb oral antibiotics;
- no symptoms or signs of ongoing sepsis;
- some conditions are specifically excluded (e.g. meningitis and endocarditis). If in doubt, consult an infection specialist.

Intramuscular administration

This is an infrequent method of administration, largely because absorption is unpredictable and the injection may be painful. Local side effects include irritation and development of a sterile abscess. The advantages are that there is no question of compliance and the agent can be administered easily in the community. Intramuscular (IM) administration is commonly used for vaccinations, in genitourinary (GU) clinics, and for tuberculosis (TB) treatment in the developing world.

Never give IM injections to patients with bleeding/clotting disorders, e.g. thrombocytopenia, haemophilia.

Examples of drugs given intramuscularly

Benzylpenicillin should be given immediately if a GP suspects bacterial meningitis (especially meningococcal disease) in the community, before transferring the patient urgently to hospital. If it cannot be administered IV, then deep IM injection is recommended.

Procaine penicillin (procaine benzylpenicillin) is given as daily IM injections in early syphilis or late latent syphilis. It is only available on a named patient basis.

Cefotaxime IM may be given as secondary prophylaxis for contacts of meningococcal disease, if the individual is unable to take rifampicin or ciprofloxacin (although it is not licensed for this indication).

Ceftriaxone IM is used for gonococcal infection (particularly pharyngeal or conjunctival infection).

Spectinomycin IM is occasionally given to patients who cannot take cephalosporins or quinolones (e.g. pregnant women with β-lactam allergy).

Streptomycin IM is commonly given for the treatment of TB in the developing world.

Gentamicin IM is sometimes given before changing a urinary catheter in a patient in the community.

Topical administration

Many antimicrobials are available as topical (TOP) preparations. They are most commonly used in general practice and dermatology. However, they are not without risk and should be used with caution. Before prescribing a topical drug, consider the following.

- Does the condition require treatment? Not all skin conditions that are oozing, crusted, or pustular are infected. Would improving hygiene resolve the situation? Even if an organism is cultured from a swab, it may represent colonization and not require treatment.
- Would systemic antibiotics be more appropriate? Some skin infections (e.g. erysipelas, cellulitis) require systemic antibiotics, as the infection is too deep for topical antibiotics to penetrate adequately.
- Development of resistance—topical antibacterials should be limited to those not used systemically, in order to prevent the development of resistance.
- Duration of treatment—topical agents should only be used for short periods in defined infections.

Examples of drugs given topically

Fusidic acid may be used to treat impetigo, although oral therapy is often required. It should not be used for >7–10 days.

Mupirocin may also be used to treat impetigo (if MRSA-positive) or given as part of MRSA decolonization regimens. It should not be used for >7–10 days.

Neomycin is also used to treat skin infection but may cause ototoxicity, if large areas of skin are treated, and sensitization.

Chloramphenicol may be given as eye drops or ear drops for conjunctivitis or otitis externa, respectively.

Aciclovir cream may be used for the treatment of oral and genital herpes simplex infections.

Nystatin pastilles can be used for oral candidiasis.

Clotrimazole cream is used for vulvovaginal candidiasis or athlete's foot.

Permethrin and malathion are used for scabies.

Malathion, pyrethroids, or dimeticone may be used for head lice.

Aerosolized administration

Aerosolized antibiotics are usually given for treatment or prophylaxis of respiratory infections. They are administered directly to the site of action and may have fewer systemic adverse effects. However, they are usually more difficult to give, and there may still be some systemic absorption. One of the main groups to benefit from aerosolized antibiotics are cystic fibrosis (CF) patients, who may acquire multiresistant organisms (➔ see Cystic fibrosis, pp. 623–5).

Examples of antimicrobials given by inhalation

Tobramycin (➡ see Aminoglycosides, pp. 46–8) is an aminoglycoside often given by nebulizer for chronic pulmonary infection with *P. aeruginosa* in CF patients. It is usually given cyclically (twice daily for 28 days, followed by a 28-day tobramycin-free period). Not all patients respond to treatment, and some become less responsive as drug resistance develops.

Colistimethate sodium (➡ see Polymyxins, pp. 68–9) is a polymyxin antibiotic active against many Gram-negative organisms, including *P. aeruginosa* and *Acinetobacter* spp. It is not absorbed PO and is toxic when given systemically, so inhalation of a nebulized (neb) solution is the preferred route for treating respiratory infections. It is mainly used as an adjunct to standard antibiotics in CF patients. It has also been used for the prevention and treatment of ventilator-associated pneumonia (VAP) due to *Acinetobacter* spp., although this practice is controversial.

Pentamidine isethionate (➡ see Antiprotozoal drugs, pp. 119–24) is used as a second-line agent for the treatment of *Pneumocystis jiroveci* pneumonia (➡ see *Pneumocystis jiroveci*, pp. 482–4). In mild disease, inhaled pentamidine may be used in patients who are unable to tolerate co-trimoxazole, but systemic absorption may occur. In severe disease, IV pentamidine is used in patients who are unable to tolerate, or have not responded to, co-trimoxazole. Side effects include hypotension following administration, and severe, sometimes fatal, reactions due to hypotension, hypoglycaemia, pancreatitis, and arrhythmias. Intermittent inhaled or IV pentamidine may be used as prophylaxis in patients unable to tolerate co-trimoxazole (although inhaled pentamidine does not protect against extrapulmonary disease).

Ribavirin (➡ see Antivirals for respiratory syncytial virus, p. 96) is licensed for the treatment of severe respiratory syncytial virus (RSV) bronchiolitis in infants and children, especially if they have other serious diseases. There is no evidence of mortality benefit. Side effects include worsening respiration, bacterial pneumonia, and pneumothorax. CAUTION: ribavirin is teratogenic, and exposure should be avoided in pregnant and breastfeeding women.

Antimicrobials in renal impairment

General principles

- Avoid nephrotoxic drugs in patients with renal impairment.
- Keep antibiotic prescriptions to a minimum for patients with severe renal disease.
- Some IV antibiotic preparations contain sodium (e.g. Tazocin®), which may cause difficulties in patients with renal impairment.
- The use of drugs in patients with renal impairment can cause several problems:
  - reduced excretion of a drug or its metabolites may cause toxicity;
  - increased sensitivity to some drugs;

- many side effects are poorly tolerated in patients with renal impairment;
- some drugs are not effective when renal function is impaired.

- Some of these problems may be avoided by reducing the dose (or using alternative drugs).

Assessment of renal function

Renal function can be assessed in a number of ways.

- Serum creatinine is the most commonly used parameter. It is affected by muscle mass which may be reduced in elderly patients (resulting in underestimation of renal impairment) or increased in certain races (e.g. blacks). Serum creatinine does not rise until 60% of total kidney function is lost.
- CrCl can be measured using a 24-h urine collection. Estimated CrCl is calculated using the Cockcroft and Gault formula (see Box 1.3), which is based on age, weight, sex, and serum creatinine. Thus, estimated CrCl may be inaccurate in patients who are obese or have acute renal failure.
- Glomerular filtration rate (GFR) is the volume of fluid filtered from the renal glomerular capillaries into the Bowman's capsule per unit time, and can be measured by injecting inulin into the plasma. Estimated GFR (eGFR) can be calculated using the modification of diet in renal disease (MDRD) formula (see Box 1.4), which is based on serum creatinine, age, sex, and race. Renal impairment was previously classified into three grades (mild, moderate, and severe); this has now been superseded by the use of CrCl or GFR.

Dose modification in renal impairment

- The level of renal function below which the dose of a drug must be reduced depends on the proportion of the drug eliminated by renal excretion and its toxicity.
- For drugs with only minor or no dose-related side effects, very precise modification of the dose regimen is unnecessary, and a simple scheme for dose reduction is sufficient.
- For more toxic drugs with a small safety margin, dose regimens based on GFR should be used.

Box 1.3 Cockcroft and Gault formula for estimated creatinine clearance

$$[CrCl\ (mL/min) = (140 - age) \times lean\ body\ weight\ (kg) \times N] / serum\ creatinine\ (micromole/L)$$

NB. N = 1.23 for males and 1.03 for females.

Box 1.4 MDRD formula for estimated glomerular filtration rate

$$\text{eGFR (mL/min/1.73m}^2\text{)} = 186 \times (\text{serum creatinine} / 88.4)^{-1.154} \times (\text{age})^{-0.203} \times (0.742 \text{ if female}) \text{ or } \times (1.21 \text{ if black})$$

- When both efficacy and toxicity are closely related to plasma drug concentration, recommended regimens should be regarded only as a guide to initial treatment; subsequent doses must be adjusted according to clinical response and plasma drug concentration (e.g. vancomycin, gentamicin).
- The total daily maintenance dose of a drug can be reduced either by reducing the size of the individual doses or by increasing the interval between doses. For some drugs, although the size of the maintenance dose is reduced, it is important to give a loading dose if an immediate effect is required. The loading dose should usually be the same size as the initial dose for a patient with normal renal function.
- Seek specialist advice from your hospital pharmacist for patients on haemodialysis, haemofiltration, or chronic ambulatory peritoneal dialysis.

Drugs to be used with caution

- For up-to-date guidance, always consult your hospital pharmacist, the *British National Formulary* (*BNF*), or the electronic *Medicines Compendium* (🔗 www.medicines.org.uk/emc/).
- A wide range of antimicrobials should be used with caution in patients with renal impairment, including:
  - antibacterials, e.g. aminoglycosides, aztreonam, cephalosporins, carbapenems, chloramphenicol, colistimethate sodium, ethambutol, isoniazid, linezolid, macrolides, ketolides, penicillins, quinolones, sulfonamides, tetracyclines, trimethoprim, vancomycin;
  - antifungals, e.g. amphotericin, flucytosine, fluconazole, itraconazole, voriconazole;
  - antimalarials, e.g. atovaquone, chloroquine, atovaquone/proguanil, proguanil, pyrimethamine, quinine, artemether with lumefantrine, sulfadiazine;
  - antivirals, e.g. aciclovir, adefovir, amantadine, antiretrovirals, famciclovir, foscarnet, ganciclovir, oseltamivir, pentamidine, ribavirin, valaciclovir, valganciclovir.

Antimicrobials in liver disease

Metabolism by the liver is the main route of elimination for many drugs, but hepatic reserve is large, and liver disease has to be severe before important changes in drug metabolism occur. Routine liver function tests (LFTs) are a poor guide to metabolic capacity, and it is not possible to predict the extent to which the metabolism of a particular drug may be impaired in an individual patient. Drug prescribing should be kept to a minimum in all patients with severe liver disease.

Effect of liver disease on response to drugs

Liver disease may alter the response to drugs in several ways:

- impaired drug metabolism may lead to increased toxicity;
- hypoproteinaemia results in reduced protein binding and increased toxicity of highly protein-bound drugs, e.g. phenytoin;

- reduced synthesis of clotting factors increases the sensitivity to oral anticoagulants;
- hepatic encephalopathy may be precipitated by certain drugs, e.g. sedative drugs, opioid analgesics, diuretics, and drugs that cause constipation;
- fluid overload (ascites, oedema) may be exacerbated by drugs that give rise to fluid retention, e.g. non-steroidals and corticosteroids;
- hepatotoxicity is either dose-related or unpredictable (idiosyncratic), and is more common in patients with liver disease.

Drugs to be used with caution

- For up-to-date guidance, always consult your hospital pharmacist or the *BNF*.
- The following antimicrobials should be used with caution in liver disease:
  - antibacterials, e.g. ceftriaxone, chloramphenicol, co-amoxiclav, co-trimoxazole, daptomycin, flucloxacillin, fusidic acid, isoniazid, macrolides, ketolides, linezolid, meropenem, metronidazole, moxifloxacin, neomycin, ofloxacin, rifamycins, sodium fusidate, quinupristin/dalfopristin, tetracyclines, tigecycline, tinidazole, ticarcillin/clavulanic acid;
  - antifungals, e.g. azoles, caspofungin, griseofulvin, terbinafine;
  - antimalarials, e.g. mefloquine, pyrimethamine, artemether with lumefantrine;
  - antivirals, e.g. antiretrovirals, interferons (IFNs), ribavirin, valaciclovir.

Antimicrobials in pregnancy

Caution should be exercised in prescribing any medication in pregnancy. When it is necessary to use antibiotics, the prescriber should bear in mind the gestational age and balance the risk of teratogenesis or other complication with the risk of failing to treat the mother effectively. Many antibiotic agents have very limited data available on their use in pregnancy. The following advice is general, and prescribers should check a current formulary (e.g. *BNF*) for the latest data on the agent they plan to use.

Specific agents

- Penicillins—considered safe in pregnancy. Trace amounts can be found in breast milk, but most are considered safe to use. Limited data regarding the use of piperacillin with tazobactam (Tazocin®) has led the manufacturer to recommend its use only if benefit outweighs risk.
- Cephalosporins—generally considered safe for use in pregnancy. Some may cross into breast milk at low levels. The manufacturers of cefixime and ceftaroline recommend avoiding use when breastfeeding.
- Carbapenems—manufacturers recommend use only if benefit outweighs the potential risk. All may be found in milk, and, while it is unlikely they would be absorbed, the manufacturer recommends avoiding.
- Tetracyclines—affect skeletal development in the first trimester in animal studies and deposit in growing bones and teeth. Should not be given to pregnant or breastfeeding women. Maternal hepatotoxicity has been reported.

- Aminoglycosides—avoid unless essential (in which case meticulous therapeutic monitoring is required) due to the risk of auditory and vestibular nerve damage. The risk is greatest in the second/third trimesters.
- Macrolides—erythromycin is not known to be harmful in pregnancy, and only small amounts are found in breast milk. The others, including clarithromycin, have more limited data and should only be used if there are no alternatives and benefit outweighs risk.
- Clindamycin—not known to be harmful in pregnancy, and only very small amounts cross into breast milk. Bloody diarrhoea has been reported in one infant.
- Glycopeptides—limited data. Use if benefit outweighs risk, and monitor levels carefully. Present in milk, but significant absorption by infant is unlikely.
- Co-trimoxazole and trimethoprim—avoid folate antagonists with a teratogenic risk in the first trimester. Co-trimoxazole has the additional risks of neonatal haemolysis and methaemoglobinaemia in the third trimester, and a small risk of kernicterus in jaundiced babies and haemolysis in the glucose-6-phosphate dehydrogenase (G6PD)-deficient baby if breastfed.
- Metronidazole—probably safe, but manufacturer recommends avoiding high-dose regimes.
- Quinolones—avoid in pregnancy. Associated with arthropathy in animal studies. Present in small amounts in breast milk. Probably harmless, but manufacturer recommends to avoid.
- Nitrofurantoin—safe to use in pregnancy, but avoid at term due to association with neonatal haemolysis.

Antimicrobial prophylaxis

Definitions

Prophylaxis is the administration of antibiotics to prevent the infection of a previously uninfected tissue. Primary prophylaxis aims to prevent initial infection or disease (e.g. to cover a surgical procedure), while secondary prophylaxis aims to prevent recurrent disease (e.g. giving penicillin to a patient who has had rheumatic fever). Surgical prophylaxis is usually primary and aims to target the operative period when the site may become contaminated.

Principles of antimicrobial prophylaxis

All hospitals should have a policy for prescribing antimicrobial prophylaxis for common procedures, which may be area-/unit-/surgeon-specific. The following factors should be considered.

- Before prescribing, always consider:
  - does the patient have any known drug allergies?
  - has the patient received any recent antibiotics?
  - is the patient known to be colonized with resistant organisms?

- Which drug? A bactericidal agent should be used which:
  - is active against the probable infecting organism(s);
  - penetrates the likely site of infection;
  - has a favourable safety profile.
- What dose? The aim is to maintain the drug concentration above the target MIC throughout the operative period. The number of doses usually depends on the length of procedure and likely blood loss.
- Which route? This depends on the nature of the procedure, whether or not the patient is nil by mouth, and the pharmacokinetics of the drug.
- Time of administration? Antimicrobial prophylaxis should be administered 0–2h prior to the procedure, in order to ensure adequate tissue levels.
- Duration? Prophylactic antibiotics should not usually be given for >24h. If there is evidence of infection, the patient should be carefully assessed, and appropriate cultures sent. The organisms responsible for post-operative infections are unlikely to be sensitive to the prophylactic antibiotics. Seek advice on antimicrobial therapy from an infection specialist in light of the clinical picture and likely infecting organisms.

Risks of antimicrobial prophylaxis

While the benefit of prophylactic antibiotics is clear, there are also potential risks. These include:

- adverse effects associated with specific drug (e.g. penicillin anaphylaxis);
- selection of antibiotic-resistant organisms;
- alteration of normal flora.

Before prescribing antimicrobial prophylaxis for a procedure, consider whether it is actually needed. Consult your local antibiotic policy, or seek advice from an infection specialist if unsure.

Detailed indications for prophylaxis

For up-to-date information, consult the *BNF*. Antimicrobial prophylaxis is currently recommended in the following situations:

- prevention of recurrence of rheumatic fever;
- prevention of a secondary case of group A streptococcal (GAS) infection;
- prevention of a secondary case of meningococcal infection;
- prevention of a secondary case of *Haemophilus influenzae* type b disease;
- prevention of a secondary case of diphtheria in a non-immune contact;
- prevention of a secondary case of pertussis in a non-immune or partially immune contact;
- prevention of pneumococcal infection in asplenia or sickle-cell disease;
- prevention of gas gangrene in high lower-limb amputations or following major trauma;
- prevention of TB in susceptible close contacts or those who become tuberculin skin test (TST)-positive;
- prevention of infection in certain GI procedures;
- prevention of infection in certain obstetric/gynaecological, orthopaedic, urological, and vascular surgery;

- prevention of endocarditis is now only recommended for 'at-risk' patients undergoing a GI or GU procedure where infection is suspected. At-risk groups include those with valve replacement, acquired valvular heart disease with stenosis or regurgitation, structural heart disease (excluding isolated atrial septal defects (ASDs), fully repaired ventricular septal defects (VSDs), fully repaired patent ductus arteriosus (PDA), and endothelialized closure devices), hypertrophic cardiomyopathy, or a previous episodes of endocarditis.

Other examples of antimicrobial prophylaxis

- Selective decontamination of the digestive tract (SDD)—administration of antibiotics that are poorly absorbed when given PO to eliminate normal GI flora. Some ICUs use it to prevent VAP. This practice is controversial.
- Local infiltration into wound/incision line—current data suggest this can lead to higher rates of infection, unless combined with systemic administration. There is no additional reduction in wound infections if antibiotics are given by both routes simultaneously, compared with systemic antibiotics alone.
- Antibiotic-impregnated materials—gentamicin cement is used routinely in joint replacement; this is also controversial. Antibiotic-soaked Dacron® vascular grafts are used in vascular surgery.

Antimicrobial stewardship

Antimicrobial stewardship is the practice of monitoring and improving the appropriate use of antibiotics by promoting best practice in the choice of regimen, duration, and route. Inappropriate use includes unnecessarily broad agents, unwarranted prophylaxis, and failing to administer by the route appropriate for the indication. Such use may lead to avoidable complications such as *C. difficile* diarrhoea, promotes the development of antibiotic resistance, and increases costs. The increase in prevalence of extended-spectrum β-lactamase (ESBL) organisms and the development of metallo-β-lactamase-1 (New Delhi metallo-β-lactamase-1, NDM-1) and other carbapenemase-mediated resistance raise the spectre of a return to a 'pre-antibiotic era', in which increasing resistance is not matched by the release of new drugs. Such concerns have prompted health systems across the world to promote stewardship interventions (e.g. the 'Start smart, then focus' toolkit in the UK). Evidence suggests that, just as the use of broad-spectrum agents promotes resistance, so changing prescribing practices to narrower agents is associated with a decline in resistant organisms such as MRSA.

Stewardship programmes

Successful implementation of such programmes requires leadership from senior hospital management and dedicated time from enthusiastic infection specialists and pharmacists. The UK Department of Health (DoH) recommends every hospital have an antibiotic prescribing and management group, publish treatment and prophylaxis guidelines, and ensure good practice in prescribing. A typical stewardship programme includes:

- guidance on when to start antibiotics and locally developed treatment guidelines that balance the use of focused-spectrum agents with clinical safety;
- education of the importance of taking appropriate cultures prior to initiating therapy, so that a switch can be made from broad empirical therapy with confidence;
- regular review of the diagnosis (are antibiotics really required?), antibiotic given (switch to narrower agent once culture results available?), route (can a switch to oral be made?), and stop date (shortest possible course);
- rigorous enforcement of single-dose surgical prophylaxis guidelines;
- bedside review of those patients on broad agents by infection specialists to assess clinical indication and need;
- audit of antibiotic use to identify areas requiring specific interventions.

The UK 5-year antimicrobial resistance strategy 2013–2018

This initiative spans government agencies, including environmental and animal health. The aims are to slow the development and spread of antimicrobial resistance through improving understanding of resistance, promoting stewardship to conserve the effectiveness of existing treatments, and stimulate the development of new agents, novel therapies, and diagnostics.

Guidelines

Infectious Diseases Society of America (IDSA) stewardship guidelines: www.idsociety.org/stewardship_policy/.

UK 'Start smart, then focus': www.gov.uk/government/publications/antimicrobial-stewardship-start-smart-then-focus.

Outpatient parenteral antimicrobial therapy

OPAT refers to the administration of IV antibiotics to those patients who require them but are otherwise well enough to remain in the community. Patients may attend an outpatient unit each day, or community teams may visit them at home to administer treatment.

The drive to reduce health costs has seen a rapid increase in OPAT, as health systems look for ways to avoid hospital admissions, reduce length of stay, and reduce health care-associated infections (HCAIs). Patients inevitably receive less supervision than they would as inpatients, and it is important that they are carefully selected and OPAT programmes have rigorous clinical oversight.

OPAT programme structure

Several national guidelines exist—all highlight the following key features.

- The team should have a medical lead, an infection specialist, an antimicrobial pharmacist, and a specialist nurse with expertise in IV drug administration and vascular access device management.
- Every patient should have a management plan agreed between the OPAT service and the referring specialty, with clearly defined lines of responsibility. Any primary care physician and community service would be kept fully informed, and systems should exist for urgent assessment or readmission, should it be required, while being managed by the service.
- Patient selection criteria should be well defined, and each patient assessed before acceptance. Criteria include physical nature of residence, accessibility/safety of visiting nurses, suitability and safety of any IV access device, and storage and safety of any prescribed medications in the home.
- The first dose should be administered by a professional competent and equipped to manage anaphylaxis. Records must be kept of drug administration.
- While on therapy, patients should be reviewed daily by a nurse or similar, with a view to oral switch. Patients should be reviewed weekly in a multidisciplinary team meeting. Those receiving extended therapy should be seen by a specialist nurse or doctor at agreed intervals and have appropriate blood tests performed.
- Data should be collected prospectively for the purposes of audit. This should be reviewed to detect issues relating to, for example, line infection, readmission, and drug reactions.

Guidelines

Chapman AL, Seaton RA, Cooper MA, *et al.* BSAC/BIA OPAT Project Good Practice Recommendations Working Group. (2012). Good practice recommendations for outpatient parenteral antimicrobial therapy (OPAT) in adults in the UK: a consensus statement. *J Antimicrob Chemother*. **67**:1053–62.

Tice AD, Rehm SJ, Dalovisio JR, *et al.*; IDSA. (2004). Practice guidelines for outpatient parenteral antimicrobial therapy. *Clin Infect Dis*. **38**:1651–71.

Chapter 2

Antibiotics

Penicillins *32*
Cephalosporins *33*
β-lactamases *35*
β-lactamase inhibitors *37*
Carbapenems *39*
Monobactams *41*
Other cell wall agents *41*
Glycopeptides *42*
Glycopeptide monitoring *44*
Lipoglycopeptides *45*
Fidaxomicin *45*
Aminoglycosides *46*
Macrolides *48*
Ketolides *50*
Lincosamides *51*
Streptogramins *52*
Lipopeptides *53*
Oxazolidinones *54*
Chloramphenicol *55*
Tetracyclines *56*
Sulfonamides *58*
Trimethoprim *60*
Co-trimoxazole *61*
Quinolones *62*
Nitroimidazoles *64*
Nitrofurans *66*
Novobiocin *67*
Rifamycins *67*
Polymyxins *68*
Fusidic acid *69*
Mupirocin *70*
Antituberculous agents *71*
Antileprotics *75*

Penicillins

Penicillin was discovered by Alexander Fleming in 1928 but did not become widely available until the 1940s. The penicillins are closely related compounds comprising a β-lactam ring, a five-membered thiozolidine ring, and a side chain (see Fig. 2.1). The ring structures are essential for antibacterial activity, and the side chain determines the spectrum and pharmacological properties. Most penicillins in current use are semi-synthetic derivatives of 6-aminopenicillic acid. They inhibit bacterial cell wall synthesis and are thus bactericidal.

Classification

- Group 1—benzylpenicillin and its long-acting parenteral forms.
- Group 2—orally absorbed penicillins, e.g. phenoxymethylpenicillin.
- Group 3—antistaphylococcal penicillin, e.g. meticillin, flucloxacillin.
- Group 4—extended-spectrum penicillins, e.g. amoxicillin.
- Group 5—antipseudomonal penicillins, e.g. ticarcillin, piperacillin.
- Group 6—β-lactamase-resistant penicillins.

Mode of action

The penicillins inhibit cell wall synthesis by binding to PBPs and inhibiting transpeptidation of peptidoglycans.

Resistance

Bacteria may become resistant to penicillins by a number of mechanisms:

- destruction of the antibiotic by β-lactamases (➔ see β-lactamases, pp. 35–7)—this is the commonest mechanism;
- failure to penetrate the outer membrane of Gram-negative bacteria;
- efflux across the outer membrane of Gram-negative bacteria;
- low-affinity binding of antibiotic to target PBPs.

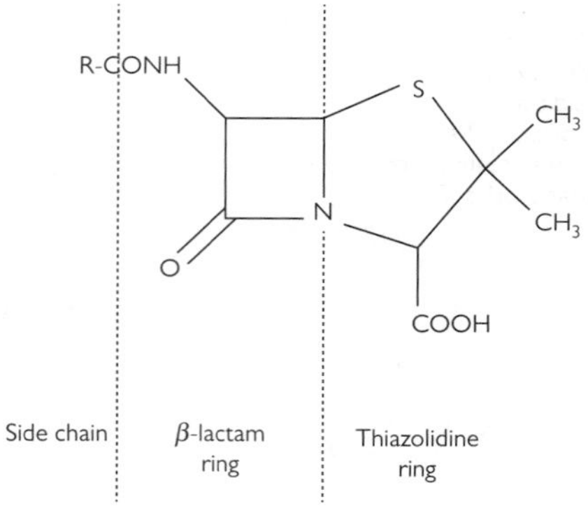

R-CONH
S
CH_3
CH_3
N
O
COOH
Side chain
β-lactam ring
Thiazolidine ring

Fig. 2.1 Structure of penicillin.

Some bacteria may display >1 resistance mechanism, e.g. in MRSA, the *mecA* gene encodes an additional PBP (i.e. altered target site), and most also produce a β-lactamase.

Clinical use

- Benzylpenicillin is used in infections due to group A and group B streptococci; meningitis due to *S. pneumoniae* (if penicillin-susceptible) and *Neisseria meningitidis*, streptococcal and enterococcal endocarditis, neurosyphilis.
- Aminopenicillins are used in respiratory tract infections, endocarditis, meningitis, and urinary tract infections (UTIs) caused by susceptible organisms, and treatment of *H. pylori*.
- Extended-spectrum and antipseudomonal penicillins are used in infections due to resistant Gram-negative bacteria, usually in combination with an aminoglycoside.
- Phenoxymethylpenicillin is also used prophylactically to prevent recurrent rheumatic fever, secondary cases in outbreaks of GAS disease, and pneumococcal and *H. influenzae* infections in asplenic patients.

Pharmacology

- Penicillins differ markedly in their oral absorption (phenoxymethylpenicillin 60%, amoxicillin 75%, antipseudomonal penicillins 0%).
- They vary in their degree of protein binding, and metabolism is minimal.
- They are rapidly excreted by renal tubular cells; excretion may be blocked by probenecid. Dose modification may be required in renal failure.

Toxicity and side effects

- Allergic reactions (skin rashes, serum sickness, delayed hypersensitivity)—occur in <10% of those exposed. Anaphylactic reactions are rare (0.004–0.4%).
- GI—diarrhoea, enterocolitis (2–5%, usually ampicillin).
- Haematological—haemolytic anaemia, neutropenia; thrombocytopenia (1–4%).
- Laboratory—elevated transaminases (usually flucloxacillin), electrolyte abnormalities (hypernatraemia, hypo- or hyperkalaemia).
- Renal—interstitial nephritis, haemorrhagic cystitis.
- Central nervous system (CNS)—encephalopathy or seizures are rare, but may occur in renal failure or if high, prolonged doses of penicillin are used.

Cephalosporins

Giuseppe Brotzu first demonstrated the antimicrobial activity of culture filtrates of the mould *Cephalosporium acremonium* in 1945. However, the cephalosporin class of antibiotics did not become widely used for another 20 years. Cephalosporins consist of a β-lactam ring and a six-membered dihydrothiazine ring modified at certain positions to produce different compounds. Most available cephalosporins are semi-synthetic derivatives of cephalosporin C.

Classification

The classification into 'generations' is the most commonly used with each successive generation acquiring better Gram-negative activity, usually at the expense of some Gram-positive, until more broad-spectrum activity appears in generations 4 and 5. Not every country agrees on which agent belongs in which generation.

- First generation—primarily active against Gram-positive bacteria, e.g. cefazolin, cefalotin, cefradine, cefalexin.
- Second generation—enhanced activity against Gram-negative bacteria, with varying degrees of activity against Gram-positive bacteria, e.g. cefuroxime, cefamandole, cefaclor. The cephamycin group (e.g. cefotetan and cefoxitin) have additional anaerobic activity against e.g. *Bacteroides fragilis*.
- Third generation—markedly increased activity against Gram-negative bacteria, e.g. cefotaxime, ceftriaxone, ceftazidime (NB. poor activity against Gram-positives), cefdinir, cefixime, cefpodoxime.
- Fourth generation—broad spectrum of activity against Gram-positive cocci, and Gram-negative bacteria, including *Pseudomonas* spp., e.g. cefepime, cefpirome.
- Fifth generation—active against MRSA, e.g. ceftaroline (no pseudomonal or vancomycin-resistant enterococci (VRE) activity) and ceftobiprole (active against *Pseudomonas* and enterococci).

Mode of action

They inhibit cell wall synthesis by binding to PBPs and inhibiting transpeptidation of peptidoglycans. They are bactericidal and exhibit significant post-antibiotic effect against Gram-positive (but not Gram-negative) bacteria.

Resistance

- Due to: destruction of the antibiotic by β-lactamases (➔ see β-lactamases, pp. 35–7), reduced penetration through the outer membrane of Gram-negative bacteria, and enhanced efflux or alteration in PBP target, resulting in reduced-affinity binding.
- *Listeria*, 'atypical' organisms (*Mycoplasma*, *Chlamydia*), MRSA and enterococci ('LAME') were considered intrinsically resistant to cephalosporins—however, some fifth-generation agents have activity against the latter two.

Clinical use

- First generation—staphylococcal and streptococcal skin and soft tissue infections, UTIs.
- Second generation—severe community-acquired pneumonia (CAP), otitis media, sinusitis, streptococcal pharyngitis, early Lyme disease.
- Cephamycins—intra-abdominal, pelvic, and gynaecological infections, infected decubitus ulcers, diabetic foot infections, mixed aerobic–anaerobic soft tissue infections.
- Third generation—penicillin-resistant pneumococci, meningitis, URTIs and lower respiratory tract infections (LRTIs), sinusitis, otitis media, nosocomial infections caused by Gram-negative bacilli, *Neisseria gonorrhoeae*, chancroid, Lyme disease, typhoid, severe *Shigella* spp. and

Box 2.1 CAUTION!

The second- and third-generation cephalosporins are susceptible to inactivation by inducible β-lactamases (➲ see β-lactamases, pp. 35–7). They should never be used to treat organisms that may have these enzymes, e.g. *Enterobacter* spp., *Serratia* spp., *Citrobacter freundii, Acinetobacter* spp., *Proteus vulgaris, Providencia* spp., *Morganella morganii* (ESCAPPM).

non-typhoidal *Salmonella* infection, outpatient antibiotic therapy for endocarditis and osteomyelitis.
- Fourth generation—role not yet clear, but effective in severe Gram-negative infections. Active against *P. aeruginosa, Enterobacter* spp., *Citrobacter* spp., and *Serratia* spp.

Pharmacology

May be given PO, IV, or IM. Fourth-generation drugs are all parenteral. Oral preparations have 80–95% bioavailability. Protein binding is variable (10–98%). Drugs are largely confined to the extracellular compartment. Poor cerebrospinal fluid (CSF) penetration, unless meningeal inflammation. Cross the placenta. Most drugs are not metabolized, except cefotaxime and cealothin which are metabolized in the liver. Most drugs are excreted by the kidneys. Ceftriaxone and cefoperazone are excreted by the biliary system (see Box 2.1).

Toxicity and side effects

- Hypersensitivity—rash (1–3%), urticaria and serum sickness (<1%), anaphylaxis (0.01%).
- GI—diarrhoea (1–19%), nausea and vomiting (1–6%), transient hepatitis (1–7%), biliary sludging (ceftriaxone).
- Haematological—eosinophilia (1–10%), neutropenia, thrombocytopenia, clotting abnormalities, platelet dysfunction, haemolytic anaemia.
- Renal—interstitial nephritis.
- CNS—seizures.
- False-positive laboratory tests—Coombs' test, glycosuria, serum creatinine.
- Other—drug fever, disulfiram-like reaction, phlebitis.

β-lactamases

β-lactamases are enzymes that bind covalently to the β-lactam ring, hydrolyse it, and make the antibiotic ineffective. Emergence of resistance to β-lactam antibiotics began even before penicillin was widely available, with the first β-lactamase (penicillinase) being described in *Escherichia coli* in 1940. This was followed by the emergence of resistance in *S. aureus*, due to plasmid-encoded penicillinase. Many genera of Gram-negative bacilli possess naturally occurring chromosomally mediated β-lactamases (AmpC); these enzymes are thought to have evolved from PBPs, to which they are very similar. The first plasmid-mediated β-lactamase in Gram-negative bacteria TEM-1 was described in 1960. Within a few years, it had spread worldwide and was found in many different species. Over the past 20 years, many antibiotics have been developed to be resistant to these β-lactamases. However, with each new class of drugs, new β-lactamases have emerged.

Classification

There are two classification systems for β-lactamases.

- Molecular (Ambler)—four classes (A to D) based on the nucleotide/amino acid sequences of the enzymes:
  - classes A, C, and D are serine β-lactamases;
  - class B are zinc-dependent enzymes (metallo-β-lactamases, MBLs) that hydrolyse the β-lactam ring by a different mechanism.
- Functional (Bush–Jacoby–Medeiros)—three groups, each with subgroups:
  - group 1 β-lactamases are cephalosporinases that are not inhibited by clavulanic acid. They correspond to Ambler group C;
  - group 2 β-lactamases are penicillinases and/or cephalosporinases that are inhibited by clavulanic acid. This group corresponds to Ambler groups A and D, and includes the TEM and SHV enzymes;
  - group 3 β-lactamases are zinc-dependent (MBLs) and are not inhibited by clavulanic acid. They correspond to Ambler group B;
  - group 4 is no longer used—it included enzymes that would have been included in one of the other groups, if more information had been available.

AmpC β-lactamases

These are chromosomally mediated β-lactamases that are active against third-generation cephalosporins and are not inhibited by clavulanic acid. They fall into molecular group C/functional group 1. They are found in the ESCAPPM group of organisms, e.g. *Enterobacter* spp., *Serratia* spp., *Citrobacter freundii, Acinetobacter* spp., *Proteus vulgaris, Providencia* spp., and *Morganella morganii*. The use of third-generation cephalosporins to treat these infections results in the selection of stably derepressed mutants that hyperproduce AmpC, and has been associated with clinical failure. These infections are therefore usually treated with carbapenems.

Extended-spectrum β-lactamases

These are β-lactamases which are capable of conferring bacterial resistance to the penicillins, first-, second-, and third-generation cephalosporins, and aztreonam (but not the cephamycins or carbapenems) by hydrolysis of these antibiotics, and which are inhibited by β-lactamase inhibitors such as clavulanic acid. They fall into functional groups 2be and 2d. ESBLs are most commonly found in *E. coli* and *Klebsiella pneumoniae*, but have been described in many other Gram-negative bacilli. Most ESBLs are derivatives of the TEM and SHV enzymes (see below).

- TEM β-lactamases—TEM-1 is the commonest β-lactamase in Gram-negative bacteria and is able to hydrolyse penicillins and early-generation cephalosporins. TEM-2 has a similar spectrum. TEM-3 was the first ESBL, reported in 1989. Since then, over 160 TEM enzymes have been described. Most of these are inhibited by clavulanic acid, but some inhibitor-resistant variants exist, particularly in Europe. TEM enzymes are commonest in *E. coli* and *K. pneumoniae*, but are increasingly found in other species of Gram-negative bacilli.

- SHV β-lactamases—the SHV-1 β-lactamase is most commonly found in *K. pneumoniae* and accounts for ≤20% of ampicillin resistance in this species. Unlike TEM, there are relatively few SHV-1 derivatives.
- CTX-M β-lactamases—this family of plasmid-mediated β-lactamases preferentially hydrolyses cefotaxime. They have been found in *Salmonella enterica* serovar Typhimurium and *E. coli*, as well as other enterobacteria. These enzymes are quite different to the TEM and SHV enzymes, and show greater similarity to chromosomal AmpC enzyme of *Kluyvera ascorbata*, suggesting CTX-M may have originated from this species. CTX-M β-lactamases have previously been associated with outbreaks in Europe, South America, and Japan, although they are now reported worldwide.
- OXA β-lactamases—these are characterized by their high hydrolytic activity against oxacillin and cloxacillin, and are poorly inhibited by clavulanic acid. They belong to molecular group D/functional group 2d. OXA-type ESBLs are mainly found in *P. aeruginosa* but have been detected in other Gram-negative bacteria. More recently, non-ESBL OXA derivatives have been described.
- Other ESBLs—a number of ESBLs that are unrelated to the established families of ESBLs have been described, e.g. PER-1, PER-2, VEB-1, GES, BES, TLA, SFO, and IBC.

ESBL detection methods

In general, ESBL detection methods use a β-lactamase inhibitor (clavulanate) in combination with an oximino-cephalosporin, e.g. ceftazidime or cefotaxime. Clavulanate inhibits the ESBL, thereby reducing the level of resistance to the cephalosporin. A number of methods exist, e.g. Jarlier double disc method, Etest® for ESBLs.

β-lactamase inhibitors

β-lactamase inhibitors are clavulanic acid and penicillanic acid sulfone derivatives. They have weak antibacterial activity but are potent inhibitors of many β-lactamases, e.g. penicillinases produced by *S. aureus, H. influenzae, Moraxella catarrhalis*, and *Bacteroides* spp., and of TEM and SHV β-lactamases produced by *Enterobacteriaceae*. They can restore the antibacterial activity of certain antibiotics, e.g. amoxicillin, ampicillin, piperacillin, mezlocillin, and cefoperazone. Three β-lactamase inhibitors are in clinical use: clavulanic acid, sulbactam, and tazobactam. All are only available in combination with a β-lactam antibiotic; the antibiotic spectrum is determined by the companion antibiotic. Although there are minor differences in potency, activity, and pharmacology between the three compounds, they can be considered therapeutically equivalent (except for some *Klebsiella* spp. where clavulanate inhibits isolates resistant to sulbactam and tazobactam).

Co-amoxiclav

- Clavulanate is a potent inhibitor of many plasmid-mediated β-lactamases and a weak inducer of some chromosomal β-lactamases.
- It is available as a combination with amoxicillin and used for the treatment of a wide range of infections where β-lactamase-producing organisms may be present. Examples include otitis media, sinusitis, pneumonia, skin and soft tissue infections, diabetic foot infections, and bite infections.
- It is available as oral or parenteral formulations. In the oral formulation, the ratio of amoxicillin to clavulanic acid is 2:1, e.g. 250mg/125mg, whereas, in the IV formulation, it is 5:1, e.g. 1000mg/200mg.
- Side effects are similar to ampicillin. Cholestatic jaundice may occur during/after therapy and is six times commoner than with amoxicillin alone.

Ticarcillin/clavulanic acid

- This combination is useful against infections caused by *Pseudomonas* spp. and *Proteus* spp.
- It has been used for the treatment of pneumonia, intra-abdominal infections, gynaecological infections, skin and soft tissue infections, and osteomyelitis.
- It is only available in parenteral form and is given IV.
- Side effects are similar to those of other β-lactams. Cholestatic jaundice may also occur because of the clavulanic acid component.

Ampicillin–sulbactam

- Sulbactam is 6-desaminopenicillin sulfone. It has a broader spectrum of activity but is less potent than clavulanic acid.
- In the USA, it is available as a combination with ampicillin and is given IV.
- It is used for the treatment of skin and soft tissue infections, intra-abdominal infections, and gynaecological infections caused by β-lactamase-producing bacteria. It has also recently been used to treat carbapenem-resistant *A. baumanii* infections.
- Side effects are similar to those of ampicillin.

Piperacillin–tazobactam

- Tazobactam is penicillanic acid sulfone β-lactamase inhibitor, with a similar structure to that of sulbactam. Its spectrum of activity is similar to that of sulbactam, but its potency is comparable to clavulanic acid.
- It is available as a combination with piperacillin (an antipseudomonal penicillin) and is given parenterally.
- It has a broad spectrum of activity and is used in the treatment of pneumonia (especially *P. aeruginosa*), skin and soft tissue infections, intra-abdominal infections, UTIs, polymicrobial infections, bacteraemia, and febrile neutropenia (in combination with an aminoglycoside).
- Side effects are similar to those of piperacillin.

Carbapenems

The carbapenems are β-lactam antibiotics derived from thienamycin, a compound produced by *Streptomyces cattleya*. Three carbapenems are licensed for use in the UK: imipenem, meropenem, and ertapenem. Other drugs in the same class include panipenem, doripenem, and faropenem.

Mode of action

These agents show high affinity to most high-molecular-weight PBPs of Gram-positive and Gram-negative bacteria. Carbapenems, particularly imipenem, traverse the outer membrane of Gram-negative bacteria through different outer membrane proteins (OprD) than those that are used by penicillins and cephalosporins (OmpC and OmpF). They also have excellent stability to β-lactamases. Consequently, carbapenems have the broadest antibacterial spectrum of all the β-lactam antibiotics. Imipenem is slightly more active against Gram-positive bacteria, whereas meropenem and ertapenem are slightly more active against Gram-negative species. Meropenem is the most active against *P. aeruginosa*. Ertapenem has poor activity against *P. aeruginosa* and *Acinetobacter* spp.

Resistance

Resistance is due to one of four mechanisms: the production of a low-affinity PBP target, reduced outer membrane permeability due to the absence of OprD in Gram-negative bacteria, efflux of the drug in Gram-negative bacteria, or the production of β-lactamases (➲ see β-lactamases, pp. 35–7) that hydrolyse carbapenems (carbapenemases). Carbapenem resistance in *Enterobacteriaceae* may be due to a combination of porin loss PLUS an ESBL or AmpC enzyme (such strains rarely spread) OR an acquired carbapenemase (such a strain being more likely to spread, and often occurring in strains already resistant to many antibiotics). For a summary of carbapenemases, see Table 2.1.

Clinical use

- Carbapenems may be used to treat a wide variety of severe infections, e.g. bacteraemia, pneumonia, intra-abdominal infections, obstetric and gynaecological infections, complicated UTIs, and soft tissue and bone infections.
- Imipenem and meropenem are most appropriate for treatment of infections caused by the cephalosporin-resistant AmpC-producing organisms, e.g. *Enterobacter* spp., *Serratia* spp., *C. freundii*, *Acinetobacter* spp., *P. vulgaris*, *Providencia* spp., *M. morganii* (the ESCAPPM group).
- Imipenem and meropenem are also used for the treatment of serious infections, e.g. patients with polymicrobial infections, febrile neutropenia, and nosocomial infections such as those caused by *P. aeruginosa* and *Acinetobacter* spp.
- Meropenem is also licensed for the treatment of bacterial meningitis—imipenem should not be used because of its propensity to cause seizures.
- Ertapenem has similar uses to those of imipenem and meropenem, but cannot be used in infections caused by *P. aeruginosa* and *Acinetobacter* spp. Its long plasma half-life means that it can be administered once daily, making it useful for OPAT.

Table 2.1 A summary of the main carbapenemases

Enzyme	Class	Characteristics
IMP-type	Metallo (class B)	Plasmid-mediated, at least 17 varieties, originated in Japan in 1990s in enterics. Now worldwide. Also found in *Pseudomonas* and *Acinetobacter*
VIM	Verona Integron-encoded metallo (class B)	Originally from Italy (1999), at least ten types, now wide geographic distribution. Mainly found in *P. aeruginosa* and *Pseudomonas putida*, only rarely in *Enterobacteriaceae*
OXA	Oxacillinase (class D)	Occurs mainly in *Acinetobacter*. Also OXA-48 *K. pneumoniae* in the Middle East, North Africa, and imported into the UK. Both plasmid and clonal spread
KPC	*K. pneumoniae* carbapenemase (class A)	Ten variants, KPC-2 to KPC-11 which differ by one or two amino acid substitutions. Also clonal spread, including global *K. pneumoniae* ST258 lineage
CMY	Class C	First class C carbapenemase, isolated from *Enterobacter aerogenes* in 2006 on plasmid pYMG-1
SME, IMI, NMC, CcrA	Class A	Little clinical significance at present
NDM-1	New Delhi metallo-β-lactamase	Described originally in New Delhi in 2009. Mainly plasmid spread in *E. coli* and *K. pneumoniae*

Pharmacology

- Imipenem, meropenem, and ertapenem have poor oral absorption and are given parenterally.
- Imipenem and meropenem are pharmacologically similar, with a plasma half-life of 1h, whereas ertapenem has a plasma half-life of 4h, which permits once-daily dosing.
- All carbapenems are widely distributed and penetrate inflamed meninges.
- All are renally excreted and require dose modification in renal failure.
- Imipenem is a substrate for renal dehydropeptidase-1 (DHP-1) enzyme and is therefore co-administered with cilastatin, a DHP-1 inhibitor.

Toxicity and side effects

- Carbapenems are generally well tolerated.
- β-lactam allergic reactions are the commonest side effects, e.g. rash, urticaria, immediate hypersensitivity, and cross-reactivity with penicillin.
- Imipenem causes nausea (if infused too quickly) and can cause seizures.

Carbapenemases

Carbapenem antibiotics (➔ see Carbapenems, pp. 39–40) are the cornerstone agents for treating ESBL infection. The emergence of carbapenem-hydrolysing β-lactamases has prompted great concern. Enzymes have been identified belonging to classes A and B (the MBLs) and can be chromosomally or plasmid-mediated, the latter facilitating transmission between strains and species. *K. pneumoniae* carbapenemase (KPC) is the most clinically important of class A carbapenemases—they are plasmid-mediated and confer resistance to all β-lactams. NDM-1, a novel MBL, was first described in 2009 in a European patient hospitalized in India with a *K. pneumoniae* infection. It has been identified in other *Enterobacteriaceae*, including *E. coli* and *Enterobacter*. In general, bacteria carrying NDM-1 are sensitive to colistimethate sodium or tigecycline.

Monobactams

The monobactams are monocyclic β-lactam antibiotics produced by some bacteria (e.g. *Chromobacterium violaceum*). They are only active against Gram-negative bacteria.

Aztreonam

- Aztreonam is the only commercially available compound.
- It is active against most *Enterobacteriaceae, H. influenzae*, and *Neisseria* spp. *Stenotrophomonas maltophilia, Burkholderia cepacia*, and many *Acinetobacter* spp. are resistant. Some strains of *P. aeruginosa, Enterobacter cloacae*, and *C. freundii* are resistant.
- Aztreonam passes through the outer membrane and binds to PBP3 of Gram-negative bacteria. It is resistant to hydrolysis by most β-lactamases, apart from AmpC β-lactamases.
- Aztreonam is not absorbed PO and is given IV or IM. It is widely distributed and penetrates inflamed meninges. It is mainly renally excreted and requires dose modification in renal failure.
- It is used for the treatment of a variety of infections, e.g. UTIs, pneumonia, septicaemia, skin and soft tissue infections, intra-abdominal infections, gynaecological infections, and wound and burn infections.
- Aztreonam should never be used alone as empiric therapy, as it has no activity against Gram-positive organisms.
- Side effects are similar to those of the other β-lactams, except for hypersensitivity which does not occur.

Other cell wall agents

Bacitracin

Bacitracin binds to isoprenyl phosphate and prevents dephosphorylation of the lipid carrier that transports the cell wall building block across the membrane. Without dephosphorylation, the native compound cannot be regenerated for another round of transfer. Similar reactions in eukaryotic cells may be why this agent is so toxic, and it is therefore used topically. It is also used to identify GAS (bacitracin-resistant) in the diagnostic laboratory.

Fosfomycin

Fosfomycin inhibits pyruvyl transferase, and therefore formation of *N*-acetylglucosamine from *N*-acetylmuramic acid. It is a naturally occurring antibiotic with a fairly broad spectrum, particularly against Gram-negative rods (GNRs). It is mainly used to treat UTIs.

Cycloserine

This drug is often part of the second-line regimen for drug-resistant TB. It is a structural analogue of *D*-alanine, and acts on alanine racemase and synthetase to inhibit the synthesis of terminal *D*-alanyl-*D*-alanine. It thus prevents formation of the pentapeptide chain of muramic acid (➲ see Antituberculous agents, second line, pp. 73–4).

Isoniazid and ethambutol

These are first-line drugs used in the treatment of TB. They interfere with mycolic acid synthesis in mycobacterial cell walls (➲ see Antituberculous agents, first line, pp. 71–3).

Glycopeptides

The glycopeptide antibiotics vancomycin and teicoplanin are bactericidal against most Gram-positive bacteria. Vancomycin was first isolated from *Nocardia orientalis* and introduced into clinical practice in 1958. Teicoplanin was obtained from *Actinoplanes teichomyceticus* in 1978 and is available in Europe and Asia, but not in the USA.

Mode of action

Glycopeptides inhibit cell synthesis by binding to the *D*-alanyl-*D*-alanine tail of the muramyl pentapeptide. This complex cannot be processed by the enzyme glycosyltransferase, inhibiting the incorporation of murein monomers (*N*-acetylmuramic acid and *N*-acetylglucosamine) into the growing peptidoglycan chain.

Antimicrobial activity

Glycopeptides have broad activity against Gram-positive organisms, e.g. staphylococci, *E. faecalis, S. pneumoniae*, groups A, B, C, and G streptococci, *Streptococcus bovis, Streptococcus mutans*, viridans group streptococci, *Listeria monocytogenes, Bacillus* spp., *Corynebacterium* spp., *Peptostreptococcus* spp., *Actinomyces* spp., *Propionibacterium* spp., and most *Clostridium* spp. Glycopeptides show no activity against Gram-negative species (except non-gonococcal *Neisseria* spp.). The MICs of teicoplanin against coagulase-negative staphylococci (CoNS) are more variable than that of vancomycin.

Resistance

Vancomycin resistance may be intrinsic or acquired.

- Intrinsic vancomycin resistance occurs in *Leuconostoc, Pediococcus, Lactobacillus*, and *Erysipelothrix rhusiopathiae*. Intrinsic teicoplanin resistance is seen in *Staphylococcus haemolyticus*.

Table 2.2 Vancomycin resistance in enterococci and staphylococci

	VanA	VanB	VanC	VanD	VanE	VanG
Vanc MIC	64–>500	4–>500	2–32	64–128	16	12–16
Teic MIC	16–>500	0.5–2	0.5–2	4–64	0.5	0.5
Expression	Inducible	Inducible	Constitutive, inducible	Constitutive	Inducible	
Location	P, C	P, C	C	C	C	C
Species	*E. faecalis, E. faecium, S. aureus*	*E. faecalis, E. faecium*	*E. gallinarum, E. casselflavius, E. flavescens*	*E. faecium*	*E. faecalis*	*E. faecalis*

C, chromosome; MIC, minimum inhibitory concentration (microgram/mL); P, plasmid; Teic, teicoplanin; Vanc, vancomycin.

- Enterococci—six types of glycopeptide resistance have been described (VanA, VanB, VanC, VanD, VanE, and VanG), named on the basis of their ligase genes (*vanA, vanB*, etc.; see Table 2.2). These result in the formation of a peptidoglycan precursor with decreased affinity for glycopeptides. Resistance may be intrinsic (e.g. in *Enterococcus gallinarum, Enterococcus casseliflavus*) or acquired (e.g. in *E. faecium* and *E. faecalis*).
- *S. aureus*—the first clinical isolate of *S. aureus* with diminished susceptibility to vancomycin was reported in Japan in 1997. This is referred to as a vancomycin-intermediate *S. aureus* (VISA) or glycopeptide-intermediate *S. aureus* (GISA). VISA isolates have a thickened cell wall which may prevent glycopeptides from reaching their target sites. In 2002, two isolates of truly vancomycin-resistant *S. aureus* (VRSA) were reported, both of which carried the *vanA* gene, suggesting horizontal transfer of this gene from enterococci.
- *S. pneumoniae*—vancomycin tolerance has recently been reported.

Clinical use

Glycopeptides are used to treat the following conditions:

- severe infections caused by MRSA;
- meningitis due to penicillin-resistant *S. pneumoniae*;
- *C. difficile*-associated diarrhoea (oral vancomycin);
- febrile neutropenia;
- continuous ambulatory peritoneal dialysis (CAPD) peritonitis;
- endophthalmitis;
- empiric treatment of intravascular catheter-related infections and cerebrospinal fluid (CSF) shunt infections.

Pharmacology

- Vancomycin is usually given intravenously but may also be given orally, intraperitoneally, intrathecally or intraocularly. It is widely distributed but has poor CSF penetration in the absence of meningeal inflammation. Vancomcyin is excreted unchanged in the kidneys, and dose reduction

is required in renal impairment. Vancomycin shows time-dependent killing: if the trough level is too high, it is better to reduce the dose rather than increase the dosing interval.
- Teicoplanin is usually administered IV and IM, but may also be given intraperitoneally. It has a long plasma half-life (83–168h), enabling daily dosing. Teicoplanin has better bone penetration than vancomcyin. It is excreted by the kidneys.

Toxicity and side effects

Toxicity is commoner with vancomycin than teicoplanin.
- Ototoxicity is rare, unless there is renal impairment.
- Nephrotoxicity occurs with high doses and is often associated with concomitant aminoglycoside usage.
- Infusion-related reactions can occur, e.g. 'red man syndrome' with rapid infusion of vancomcyin.
- Others, e.g. neutropenia, thrombocytopenia, rashes, drug fever.

Glycopeptide monitoring

Basic principles of glycopeptide monitoring are described on ➲ pp. 42–4. Please consult your hospital guidelines, antibiotic pharmacist, or infection specialist for specific advice.
- Recommended initial dose of vancomycin or teicoplanin depends on the type of infection, patient weight, and renal function. Loading doses (based on actual body weight) are commonly given, if CrCl >20mL/min.
- Vancomycin trough (pre-dose) levels are usually monitored to reduce the risk of nephrotoxicity and guide future dosing. Always review any other nephrotoxic drugs your patient is taking (e.g. gentamicin) (see Table 2.3).
- Teicoplanin trough (pre-dose) levels are usually monitored in severe infections to ensure therapeutic levels. Monitoring is not needed for toxicity (see Table 2.4).

Table 2.3 Interpretation of vancomycin pre-dose (trough) levels

<10mg/L	Subtherapeutic	Check sample timing. If a true sample, increase dose (usually by 500mg increments, either as once daily (od) or in divided doses)
10–20mg/L	Optimum dose*	Continue on current dose; re-assay 1–2 times a week if no change in renal function
20–25mg/L	Above recommended target level	Reassessment/extend dosing interval, e.g. from twice daily (bd) to od. Re-assay after third dose
>25mg/L	Above recommended target level	Omit further dosing until level <20mg/L. Reassessment/extend dosing interval

* For severe infections (e.g. MRSA pneumonia, osteomyelitis, endocarditis, and bacteraemias), many experts aim for a target concentration of 15–20mg/L.

Table 2.4 Interpretation of teicoplanin pre-dose (trough) levels

<20mg/L	Subtherapeutic level, especially if severe infections	Increase dose (usually by ~50%). Re-assay after five doses
20–60mg/L	Optimum dose	Continue on current dose, and re-assay in 1 month, if no change in renal function
>60mg/L	Above recommended target level	Reassess dose according to renal function. Consider reducing daily dose or extending the dosage interval (e.g. to every 48h)

- Information: always state the time of last dose, time of sample, and current dosing regimen, to aid interpretation of result.
- Timing of levels: vancomycin is usually monitored before the third dose (unless CrCl <10mL/min, then before second dose). Teicoplanin is usually monitored after 7 days of treatment.

Lipoglycopeptides

Dalbavancin, oritavancin, and telavancin are semi-synthetic lipoglycopeptides, not yet licensed in the UK. They have been developed to treat infections with multiresistant Gram-positive pathogens. The heptapeptide core (common to all glycopeptides) results in inhibition of cell wall synthesis (transglycosylation and transpeptidation), and the lipophilic side chain prolongs the half-life, helping to anchor the drug to the cell membrane. Telavancin and oritavancin also disrupt bacterial membrane integrity and increase membrane permeability, while oritavancin also inhibits RNA synthesis. All three agents are active *in vitro* against *S. aureus* (including MRSA), *Staphylococcus epidermidis, Streptococcus* spp., and VanB-VRE. Oritavancin is also active against VISA, VRSA, and VanA-VRE, while dalbavancin and telavancin are also active against VISA, but not against VanA-VRE or VRSA. These may be potential alternatives for complicated skin and skin structure infections, if cheaper options, such as vancomycin, have been ineffective or in cases of reduced vancomycin susceptibility or resistance. Dalbavancin is given once weekly which may facilitate outpatient treatment.

Fidaxomicin

Fidaxomicin is the fermentation product of the actinomycete *Dactylosporangium aurantiacum* subspecies *hamdenesis*. It is the first in a new class of macrocyclic antibiotics, and is bactericidal, poorly absorbed systemically, and more selective for *C. difficile*, with minimal disruption to normal gut flora. Evidence from two double-blind randomized controlled trials (RCTs) indicates it is non-inferior to vancomycin in curing patients with mild to severe *C. difficile* infection (CDI). It reduces the recurrence rate of CDI, and its side effect profile is similar to oral vancomycin. There are no clinical trials comparing fidaxomicin to metronidazole. The National Institute for Health and Care Excellence (NICE) guidance in 2012 recommended considering fidaxomicin for patients with severe or recurrent CDI.[1] Consult an infection expert, and weigh up the potential benefits alongside the medical need, risks of treatment, and relatively high cost of fidaxomicin (➔ see *Clostridium difficile* diarrhoea, pp. 654–6).

Reference

1 National Institute for Health and Care Excellence (2012). *Clostridium difficile infection: fidaxomicin.* Available at: http://www.nice.org.uk/advice/esnm1/chapter/Relevance-to-NICE-guidance-programmes.

Aminoglycosides

Streptomycin, produced by *Streptomyces griseus*, was the first aminoglycoside used in the initial treatment trials of TB in the 1940s. Today aminoglycosides remain an important part of the antibiotic arsenal. All aminoglycosides have an essential six-membered ring with amino group constituents (aminocyclitol). The term aminoglycoside results from glycosidic bonds between aminocyclitol and two or more sugars. They are active against many Gram-negative, and some Gram-positive, organisms. In the UK, the currently available aminoglycosides are: streptomycin, neomycin, kanamycin, paromomycin, gentamicin, tobramycin, amikacin, netilmicin, and spectinomycin. Other drugs (e.g. sisomicin, dibekacin, and isepamicin) are available in Japan and continental Europe.

Mode of action

Aminoglycosides bind to the A site of the 30S ribosomal subunit, resulting in a conformational change that interferes with mRNA translation and translocation, and hence inhibit protein synthesis. Avidity of binding varies between aminoglycosides. The transport of aminoglycosides into the cell by energy-dependent mechanisms (EDP-I and EDP-II) results in accumulation of high concentrations of the drug in the cell. The onset of cell death is coincident with the transition from EDP-I to EDP-II.

Resistance

Resistance to aminoglycosides may be intrinsic or acquired.

- Intrinsic resistance may be non-enzymatic or enzymatic:
  - anaerobes are unable to generate a sufficient electrical potential difference across the membrane and are intrinsically resistant;
  - mutations in the 16S ribosomal subunit can result in resistance to streptomycin in MTB;
  - methylating enzymes that modify 16S rRNA may cause intrinsic resistance; this has not yet been seen in clinical isolates.
- Acquired resistance may occur by a variety of mechanisms:
  - reduced drug uptake;
  - efflux pumps, e.g. activation of the Mex XY pump in *P. aeruginosa*;

- enzymatic modification of the drug may occur as a result of aminoglycoside-modifying enzymes (AMEs) that phosphorylate, acetylate, or adenylate exposed amino or hydroxyl groups. The enzymatically modified drugs bind poorly to ribosomes, resulting in high levels of resistance.

Clinical use

- Empiric therapy—aminoglycosides may be given as empiric therapy for serious infections suspected to be due to Gram-negative bacteria. Depending on the clinical indication, they are usually combined with a β-lactam, vancomycin, or an anaerobic agent.
- Specific therapy—once culture results are available, aminoglycosides may be useful for the specific treatment, e.g. infections due to *Pseudomonas* spp. or resistant Gram-negative species, endocarditis.
- Prophylaxis—aminoglycosides are sometimes used prophylactically, e.g. to prevent enterococcal endocarditis in 'at-risk' patients undergoing GU or GI procedures.
- Gentamicin is the most commonly used aminoglycoside in the UK. Its main use is in the empirical treatment of serious infections (e.g. septicaemia, febrile neutropenia, biliary sepsis, acute pyelonephritis, endocarditis). It is often incorporated into cement in orthopaedic procedures. Gentamicin drops are used in superficial eye infections and bacterial otitis externa.
- Amikacin is used in gentamicin-resistant infections, mycobacterial infections, or nocardiosis.
- Tobramycin is slightly better for *P. aeruginosa* than gentamicin, and may be used in CF patients.
- Neomycin is given PO for bowel sterilization pre-surgery or for selective decontamination of the digestive tract (➔ see Antimicrobial prophylaxis, pp. 25–7).
- Netilmicin is used in Gram-negative infections that are resistant to gentamicin.
- Streptomycin is used to treat TB, particularly in the developing world. It is sometimes used synergistically in enterococcal endocarditis (if there is gentamicin resistance).
- Spectinomycin is used to treat gonococcal infections.
- Paromomycin is used to treat cryptosporidiosis.

Pharmacology

- The aminoglycosides share a number of important characteristics (➔ see Pharmacodynamics, pp. 16–8):
  - concentration-dependent bactericidal activity;
  - significant PAE;
  - synergism particularly with cell wall-active agents.
- Aminoglycosides have poor oral absorption and are usually administered IV or IM. They may also be administered PO (e.g. neomycin, paromomycin), TOP, intrapleurally, intraperitonally, or intrathecally.

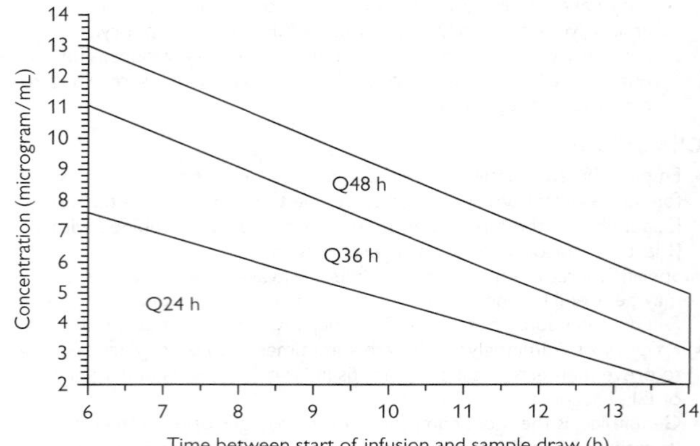

Fig. 2.2 Hartford nomogram for once-daily aminoglycosides.
Reproduced with permission from Nicolau *et al.* (1995). *Antimicrob Agents Chemother* **39**:650–5.

- Aminoglycosides are highly soluble with low protein binding, resulting in distribution in the vascular and interstitial compartments. CSF penetration is poor, apart from in neonates. Aminoglycosides are excreted unchanged in the urine (99%).
- Aminoglycosides may be given od or in multiple daily doses. od dosing is simpler and as efficacious as multiple dosing, and may lower the risk of drug-induced toxicity. The usual suggested dose of gentamicin is 5–7mg/kg/day. The dose is reduced in renal failure to 3mg/kg/day. Exceptions: children, pregnancy, burns, endocarditis. If patients need to continue therapy beyond 48h, trough drug levels should be monitored, and the dosing interval adjusted according to the Hartford nomogram (see Fig. 2.2).

Toxicity and side effects

- Nephrotoxicity is the commonest adverse effect (5–25%).
- Ototoxicity (cochlear and vestibular) may be irreversible.
- Neuromuscular blockade is rare.

Macrolides

The macrolides (erythromycin, clarithromycin, azithromycin) and the lincosamides (lincomycin and clindamycin), although chemically unrelated, have some similar properties such as antimicrobial activity, mechanisms of action, and resistance and pharmacology. The ketolides are a new class of antibiotics, derived from erythromycin, with activity against macrolide-resistant strains.

Erythromycin

- Erythromycin was derived from *Saccharopolyspora erythraea* in 1952. Erythromycin A is the active component. It consists of a 14-membered macrocyclic lactone ring attached to two sugars.
- Mode of action—inhibits RNA-dependent protein synthesis at the step of chain elongation by interacting with the peptidyl transferase site. It also inhibits the formation of the 50S ribosomal subunit.
- Resistance—there are four resistance mechanisms:
  - decreased outer membrane permeability, e.g. *Enterobacteriaceae, Pseudomonas* spp., *Acinetobacter* spp. are intrinsically resistant;
  - efflux pumps, e.g. *msr(A)* gene of *S. aureus* and *mef(A)* gene of *S. pneumoniae* and GAS;
  - alterations of 23S rRNA by methylation of adenine. This confers resistance to macrolides, lincosamides, and streptogramins type B, and is referred to as the MLS_B phenotype. It is encoded by *erm* (erythromycin ribosomal methylase) genes;
  - enzymatic inactivation by phosphotransferases, mediated by *mph* genes. Hydrolysis of the macrocyclic lactone is encoded by esterase genes *ere(A)* and *ere(B)* on plasmids.
- Clinical use—CAP, atypical pneumonia (e.g. *Mycoplasma pneumoniae, Chlamydia pneumoniae, Legionella pneumophila*), *Bordetella pertussis, Campylobacter* gastroenteritis.
- Pharmacology—given PO (stimulates GI motility) or IV. Widely distributed in tissues. Excreted in the bile and urine; some is inactivated in the liver.
- Toxicity and side effects—GI symptoms (nausea, vomiting, abdominal cramps, diarrhoea) are common; skin rash, fever, eosinophilia, cholestatic jaundice, transient hearing loss, QT prolongation, torsades de pointes, candidiasis, pseudomembranous colitis, infantile pyloric stenosis.

Clarithromycin

- Structure—14-membered ring with a methoxy group at position 6.
- Mode of action—same as erythromycin. More active than erythromycin against *S. pneumoniae*, GAS, MRSA, *M. catarrhalis*, and *L. pneumophila*. Also active against *Mycobacterium leprae, Mycobacterium* avium complex (MAC), and *Toxoplasma gondii*.
- Resistance—similar to erythromycin.
- Clinical use—similar to erythromycin. Treatment of MAC and other non-tuberculous mycobacterial (NTM) infections, *H. pylori* eradication, Lyme disease.
- Pharmacology—given PO or IV. Metabolized in the liver to active metabolites.

Azithromycin

- Structure—15-membered lactone ring (azalide).
- Mode of action—same as erythromycin. Greater activity against Gram-negative species than with erythromycin and clarithromcyin. Also active against MAC and *T. gondii*.
- Resistance—similar to erythromycin.

- Clinical use—similar to erythromycin. Also use for treatment of trachoma, *Babesia microti, Borrelia burgdorferi*, cryptosporidiosis.
- Pharmacology—given PO, but should be taken 1h before or 2h after food. Widely distributed in tissues, with a half-life of 2–4 days. Mostly not metabolized and excreted in the bile.
- Toxicity and side effects—similar to erythromycin.

Spiramycin

- Used in treatment of cryptosporidia and prevention of congenital toxoplasmosis.

Ketolides

Ketolides are a new class of antibiotics derived from erythromycin A that have increased potency against bacteria that have become resistant to macrolides, e.g. *S. pneumoniae* and *Streptococcus pyogenes*. Telithromycin is currently the only available drug.

Telithromycin

- Structure—a 14-membered ring with ketone, instead of l-cladinose, at position 3; this prevents induction of macrolide–lincosamide–streptogramin B (MLS_B) resistance (➔ see Lincosamides, pp. 51–2; see Box 2.2).
- Mode of action—similar to that of erythromycin.
- Resistance—this is uncommon, as ketolides are poor inducers of efflux pumps and MLS_B methylase genes. *S. aureus* strains with constitutive *erm* genes are resistant, whereas *S. pneumoniae* strains with constitutive *erm* genes remain sensitive.
- Toxicity and side effects—similar to clarithromycin and azithromycin. Reports of exacerbation of myasthenia gravis.
- Pharmacology—good oral absorption and bioavailability. Metabolized in the liver by CYP3A4.
- Clinical use—CAP, acute exacerbation of chronic obstructive pulmonary disease (COPD), tonsillitis, pharyngitis, and sinusitis.

Box 2.2 MLS_B resistance (also known as inducible resistance)

Macrolides, lincosamides, and streptogramin type B (MLS_B) antibiotics bind to closely related sites on the 50S ribosome of bacteria. One consequence is that some bacteria (e.g. staphylococci, streptococci, and enterococci) with inducible resistance to erythromycin also become resistant to the other MLS_B agents, in the presence of erythromycin. The methylase enzyme involved is not induced by lincosamides or streptogramins, which therefore remain active in the absence of macrolides. Over 20 *erm* genes encode the MLS_B resistance, and it is becoming commoner in GAS and pneumococci.

Lincosamides

This group of antibiotics includes lincomycin (not available in the UK) and clindamycin. Lincomycin was isolated from *Streptomyces lincolnensis* in 1962. Clindamycin, which was produced by the chemical modification of lincomycin, has better oral bioavailability and increased bacterial potency, compared with lincomycin. Although chemically unrelated to erythromycin, many of the biological properties of lincosamides are similar to the macrolides.

Mode of action

Lincosamides inhibit protein synthesis by interacting with the peptidyl transferase site of the 50S ribosomal subunit. They also inhibit the formation of the 50S ribosomal subunit. Clindamycin is highly active against anaerobes (e.g. *B. fragilis*), pneumococci, GAS, meticillin-sensitive *S. aureus* (MSSA), *T. gondii*, and *Plasmodium falciparum*.

Resistance

There are several resistance mechanisms.

- Alteration of 50S ribosomal proteins of the receptor site confers resistance to macrolides and lincosamides.
- Alteration in the 23S subunit by methylation of adenine results in the MLS_B phenotype (see Box 2.2) and confers resistance to macrolides, lincosamides, and type B streptogramins. This MLS_B phenotype is encoded by *erm* (erythromycin ribosomal methylase) genes.
- Inactivation by 3-lincomycin, 4-clindamycin 0-nucleotidyl transferase. This is plasmid-mediated and encoded by *linA* and *linA′* genes.
- Decreased membrane permeability in Gram-negative species, e.g. *Enterobacteriaceae*, *Pseudomonas* spp., *Acinetobacter* spp.

Clinical use

- Alternative to β-lactams in penicillin-allergic patients with skin and soft tissue infections.
- Staphylococcal bone and joint infections.
- Severe GAS infections, e.g. necrotizing fasciitis, toxic shock syndrome (TSS).
- Anaerobic infections, e.g. intra-abdominal sepsis, anaerobic bronchopulmonary infections.
- *P. jiroveci* pneumonia (in combination with primaquine).
- *P. falciparum* malaria (in combination with quinine).

Pharmacology

- Clindamycin is given PO or IV, or by deep IM injection.
- Well absorbed orally and widely distributed with good tissue penetration, especially bone. CSF penetration is negligible.
- Most of the drug is metabolized to products with variable antibacterial activity.
- Excreted in the bile and urine—dose modification required in severe renal and liver disease.

Toxicity and side effects

- *C. difficile* colitis—discontinue clindamycin.
- Allergic reactions—rashes, fever, erythema multiforme, anaphylaxis.
- Laboratory abnormalities—transient hepatitis, neutropenia, thrombocytopenia.

Streptogramins

Streptogramins are a group of antibiotics derived from various *Streptomyces* spp. They consist of two macrocyclic lactone peptolide components referred to as streptogramin A and streptogramin B. A number of compounds exist:

- quinupristin–dalfopristin is the only drug available in the UK and used for the treatment of resistant Gram-positive infections;
- pristinamycin (used for treatment of skin and soft tissue infections);
- virginiamycin (mainly used as an animal growth promoter);
- mikamycin.

Mode of action

Streptogramins exert their action on the second or elongation stage of protein synthesis. The two components act synergistically as follows:

- streptogramin A molecules (e.g. dalfopristin) bind to the 50S ribosomal subunit and prevent aminoacyl-tRNA from attaching to the catalytic site of the peptidyl transferase, thus inhibiting transfer of the growing peptide chain;
- streptogramin B molecules (e.g. quinupristin) prevent the peptide bond from forming, which leads to the premature release of incomplete polypeptides.

Quinupristin–dalfopristin is active against most Gram-positive organisms (except *E. faecalis*, which is intrinsically resistant).

Resistance

There are three mechanism of resistance:

- modification of the ribosomal target site (quinupristin). This results in resistance to macrolides, lincosamides, and streptogramin B (MLS_B phenotype) and is encoded by various *erm* genes (➔ see Lincosamides, pp. 51–2; see Box 2.2);
- enzymatic inactivation by acetyltransferases, encoded by *vat(A)*, *vat(B)*, *vat(C)* in staphylococci, and *vat(D)* in *E. faecium* (quinupristin and dalfopristin);
- active transport out of cells by efflux pumps, encoded by *vga(A)* and *vga(B)* genes in staphylococci (quinupristin and dalfopristin).

Clinical use

- Vancomycin-resistant *E. faecium* (not active against *E. faecalis*).
- Skin and soft tissue infection caused by MSSA or GAS.
- Serious Gram-positive infections where there is no alternative antibiotic available.

Pharmacology

- Quinupristin–dalfopristin is given IV, preferably into a central vein.
- Exhibits significant PAE: 2.8h for pneumococci, 4.7h for staphylococci, and 2.6–8.5h for enterococci.
- Wide volume of distribution, but poor CSF penetration.
- Metabolized in the liver and excreted in the faeces.

Toxicity and side effects

- Injection site reactions occur in >30%, so the drug should be given via a central vein.
- Arthralgia and myalgia are common.
- Nausea, vomiting, diarrhoea, skin rash, pruritus.
- Laboratory abnormalities—hepatitis, hyperbilirubinaemia.
- Inhibition of hepatic CYP3A4, resulting in increased levels of drugs metabolized by this enzyme.

Lipopeptides

Daptomycin, a fermentation product of *Streptomyces roseosporus*, was discovered in the 1980s. It is a 13-membered cyclic amino acid lipopeptide antibiotic with a lipophilic tail. It was approved in the UK in 2003 for the treatment of complicated skin and soft tissue infections.

Mode of action

The exact mechanism of action is unknown, although it appears to bind to the cell membrane of Gram-positive bacteria in a calcium-dependent manner, disrupting the cell membrane potential. Daptomycin is active against Gram-positive organisms, e.g. staphylococci and streptococci, including those that are glycopeptide-resistant.

Resistance

Resistance to daptomycin is rare, but strains with reduced susceptibility have been obtained after serial passage *in vitro*.

Clinical use

Daptomycin is used for complicated skin and soft tissue infections caused by Gram-positive bacteria.

Pharmacology

Daptomycin is given by IV infusion. The area under the curve (AUC)/MIC profile and prolonged PAE enable od dosing. Daptomycin is highly protein-bound and is eliminated largely unchanged by the kidneys.

Toxicity and side effects

- Common side effects—nausea, vomiting, diarrhoea, headache, rash, injection site reactions.
- Muscle toxicity—myalgia, muscle weakness, and myositis are uncommon; rhabdomyolysis is rare. Serum creatine kinase (CK) should

be checked before starting treatment, and weekly during treatment. Stop treatment if symptoms develop.

- Interference with prothrombin time (PT)/international normalized ratio (INR) assay—clotting sample should be taken just prior to administration of daptomycin.

Oxazolidinones

Oxazolidinones are a purely synthetic class of antimicrobials with activity against staphylococcal and streptococcal species. Linezolid was introduced in 2001. It is active against Gram-positive bacteria and is used for infections that are resistant to other antibiotics (e.g. MRSA and VRE). Always involve an infection specialist when initiating therapy.

Mode of action

Oxazolidinones are protein synthesis inhibitors that are bacteriostatic against Gram-positive organisms. They bind to the 50S ribosomal subunit at its interface with the 30S ribosomal subunit, preventing formation of the 70S initiation complex.

Resistance

Despite its recent introduction, resistance to linezolid among strains of MRSA and VRE has already been reported. The mechanism appears to be mutation in the 23S RNA domain V region. It is usually associated with long durations of therapy or prior exposure to linezolid.

Clinical use

- Linezolid is approved for use in Gram-positive pneumonia and complicated skin/soft tissue infections, and serious infections due to resistant Gram-positive bacteria (e.g. MRSA, VRE, and penicillin-resistant pneumococci).
- Tedizolid is a related agent currently approved for acute Gram-positive skin and skin structure infections only.

Pharmacology

Linezolid may be given PO (100% bioavailability) or IV. Linezolid is widely distributed, with good tissue and CSF penetration. It is metabolized by oxidation in the liver and excreted in the urine (85%) or faeces. No dose adjustment is required for renal or hepatic disease. It is given bd; tedizolid is given daily.

Toxicity and side effects

Linezolid is generally well tolerated.

- GI symptoms, e.g. nausea, vomiting, diarrhea, are common.
- Myelosuppression—thrombocytopenia, neutropenia, and pancytopenia have been reported. Commoner with prolonged therapy (>10 days) and usually reversible. Full blood count (FBC) should be monitored weekly in patients taking linezolid.

- Monoamine oxidase inhibition—linezolid is a monoamine oxidase inhibitor. Patients should be told to avoid tyramine-rich foods. Linezolid has been associated with serotonin syndrome in patients taking concomitant selective serotonin reuptake inhibitors (SSRIs).
- Optic neuropathy has been reported in patients taking >28 days' treatment. Patients should be told to report visual symptoms and referred to an ophthalmologist, if necessary.
- Lactic acidosis has been associated with prolonged treatment.

Chloramphenicol

Chloramphenicol, initially called chloromycetin®, was first isolated from *Streptomyces venezuelae* in 1947. It has a broad spectrum of activity against a wide range of bacteria, spirochaetes, rickettsiae, chlamydiae, and mycoplasmas. Soon after its introduction in 1949, reports of aplastic anaemia emerged, limiting its use. Furthermore, widespread use in the developing world has resulted in resistance, particularly in *Salmonella* typhi. Despite this, chloramphenicol remains useful for the treatment of serious infections that are resistant to other antibiotics.

Mode of action

Chloramphenicol inhibits protein synthesis by binding to the 50S subunit of the 70S ribosome at a site that prevents the attachment of tRNA—this prevents association of the amino acid with peptidyl transferase and peptide band formation. This is a bacteriostatic effect in most organisms but is bactericidal in some meningeal pathogens, e.g. *H. influenzae*, *S. pneumoniae*, and *N. meningitidis*.

Resistance

There are several resistance mechanisms:

- reduced permeability or uptake;
- ribosomal mutation;
- production of acetyl transferase, an enzyme that acetylates the antibiotic into an inactive form. This mechanism also confers resistance to tetracyclines (➔ see Tetracyclines, pp. 56–8) and is responsible for widespread epidemics of chloramphenicol resistance to *S.* Typhi and *Shigella dysenteriae* seen in the developing world.

Clinical use

In the developed world, chloramphenicol is rarely used (because of toxicity), but it remains a commonly used antibiotic in the developing world.

- Enteric fever due to *S.* Typhi and *S.* Paratyphi—high rates of drug resistance have been reported in India, Vietnam, and Central and South America.
- Severe infections such as meningitis, septicaemia, epiglottitis due to *H. influenzae*.
- Sometimes used in infective exacerbations of COPD.
- An alternative agent for infections in pregnancy, young children, or patients with immediate penicillin hypersensitivity.
- Eye drops/ointment are widely used for superficial eye infections.
- Ear drops are used for bacterial otitis externa.

Pharmacology

Chloramphenicol may be administered PO, IV, IM, or TOP. It has high lipid solubility and low protein binding, resulting in a wide volume of distribution in body fluids and tissues. CSF and ocular penetration is good. Chloramphenicol is metabolized in the liver by glucuronidation and excreted in the bile. Only 5–10% is excreted in the urine.

Toxicity and side effects

- Bone marrow suppression is common, dose-related, and reversible. It is a direct pharmacological effect of the antibiotic, resulting from inhibition of mitochondrial protein synthesis. Manifestations include anaemia, reticulocytosis, leucopenia, and thrombocytopenia. Monitor FBC twice weekly during treatment.
- Aplastic anaemia is a rare, idiosyncratic, and often fatal complication, which may occur during or after completion of therapy. It occurs in 1 in 25 000–40 000 patients. The pathogenesis of this condition is incompletely understood. Monitor FBC twice weekly during treatment, and discontinue the drug if the white cell count (WCC) falls below 2.5 $\times 10^9$/L.
- There are also reports of haemolytic anaemia in patients with G6PD deficiency and childhood leukaemia after chloramphenicol therapy.
- Grey baby syndrome—high doses in neonates may result in grey baby syndrome (abdominal distension, vomiting, cyanosis, circulatory collapse) due to inability to metabolize and excrete the drug. If the drug is required in neonates, the dose should be reduced and drug levels monitored.
- Other side effects—rash, fever, Jarisch–Herxheimer reactions, GI symptoms, glossitis, stomatitis, optic neuritis, bleeding disorders, acute intermittent porphyria, interference with development of immunity after immunization.

Tetracyclines

Tetracyclines are a group of broad-spectrum bacteriostatic antibiotics active against Gram-positive, Gram-negative, and intracellular organisms, e.g. *Chlamydia*, mycoplasmas, rickettsiae, and protozoan parasites. The first tetracycline chlortetracycline was isolated from *Streptomyces aureofaciens*, a soil organism. Since then, a number of other tetracyclines have been developed. Tetracyclines differ in their pharmacological properties, rather than their spectrum of cover, although minocycline has a slightly broader spectrum.

Classification

- First generation—tetracycline, chlortetracycline, oxytetracycline, demeclocycline, lymecycline, and metacycline.
- Second generation—doxycycline and minocycline.
- Third generation (glycylcyclines)—tigecycline.

Mode of action

- Tetracyclines inhibit bacterial protein synthesis by reversibly binding to the 30S ribosomal subunit. This blocks binding of aminoacyl-tRNA to the ribosomal 'A' site, preventing the addition of new amino acids. As their binding is reversible, these agents are mainly bacteriostatic.
- Tetracyclines also inhibit mitochondrial protein synthesis by binding to 70S ribosomal subunits in mitochondria in eukaryotic parasites. The mechanism of their antiprotozoal activity is unknown.

Resistance

The widespread use of tetracyclines has been accompanied by increasing drug resistance. This is mediated by acquisition of genes on MGEs (➔ see Molecular genetics of resistance, pp. 11–2). Many tetracycline resistance genes have been identified; most belong to the *tet* family, and some belong to the *otr* family. These genes confer resistance by the following mechanisms:

- efflux pumps—these membrane-associated proteins pump tetracyclines out of the cell. They confer resistance to first-generation tetracyclines;
- ribosomal protection proteins are cytoplasmic proteins that release tetracyclines from their binding site by guanosine diphosphate (GDP)-dependent mechanisms. They protect the ribosome from first- and second-generation tetracyclines;
- enzymatic inactivation—this mechanism is seen in *B. fragilis* where the *tet(X)* gene codes for a protein that modifies tetracyclines in the presence of nicotinamide adenine dinucleotide phosphate oxidase (NADPH) and oxygen.

Clinical use

- Chlamydial infections—trachoma, psittacosis, salpingitis, urethritis, lymphogranuloma venereum (LGV).
- Rickettsial infections.
- Q fever.
- Brucellosis (doxycycline with either streptomycin or rifampicin).
- Lyme disease (*B. burgdorferi*).
- *Mycoplasma* spp. infections.
- Infective exacerbations of COPD (due to their activity against *H. influenzae*).
- Also used in acne, destructive (refractory) periodontal diseases, sinusitis, chronic prostatitis, pelvic inflammatory disease (PID), melioidosis.

Pharmacology

- Tetracyclines are usually given PO. Absorption of tetracycline and oxytetracycline is reduced by milk, antacids, and some salts. Doxycycline and minocycline are highly bioavailable.
- They are sometimes divided into three groups on the basis of their half-lives: short-acting (tetracycline, oxytetracycline), intermediate-acting (demeclocycline), and long-acting (doxycycline, minocycline).
- Tetracyclines are widely distributed and show good tissue penetration.
- Tetracycline is eliminated in the urine. Minocycline is metabolized in the liver. Doxycycline is mainly eliminated in the faeces.

Toxicity and side effects

- Nausea, vomiting, diarrhoea, dysphagia, and oesophageal irritation are common.
- Photosensitivity reactions are common and appear to be toxic, rather than allergic.
- Prolonged minocycline administration can cause skin, nail, and scleral pigmentation.
- Deposition occurs in growing bones and teeth, so tetracyclines should not be given to children <12 years or pregnant/breastfeeding women.
- Hepatotoxicity due to fatty change may be fatal.
- Tetracyclines exacerbate renal impairment. All tetracyclines (except minocycline and doxycycline) should be avoided in renal failure. Demeclocycline causes nephrogenic diabetes insipidus and is used as a treatment for inappropriate antidiuretic hormone (ADH) secretion.
- Vertigo is unique to minocycline.
- Benign intracranial hypertension has been described with all tetracyclines.
- Superinfection—mucocutaneous candidiasis is common. *C. difficile* colitis may occur.
- Allergic reactions (rashes, urticaria, anaphylaxis) are uncommon.

Tigecycline

- A glycylcycline antibiotic, structurally related to tetracyclines.
- Active against Gram-positive and Gram-negative bacteria, including tetracycline-resistant organisms, and some anaerobes. It is also active against MRSA and VRE, but not against *P. aeruginosa* and *Proteus* spp.
- Reserved for the treatment of complicated skin and soft tissue infections, and complicated abdominal infections caused by multidrug-resistant (MDR) organisms. The UK MHRA and US FDA advise use only if it is known or suspected that other antibiotics are unsuitable—pooled analysis of phase 3 and 4 trials suggested higher death rates in patients receiving tigecycline compared to those receiving comparator drugs.
- Side effects are similar to those of tetracyclines.

Sulfonamides

Prontosil was discovered in 1932, the result of 5 years of testing dyes for antimicrobial activity. It exerted its antibacterial effect through the release of sulfanilamide, an analogue of PABA. PABA is essential for bacterial folate synthesis (see Fig. 2.3). Although many sulfonamide drugs were developed, relatively few are in clinical use today, mainly because of their toxicity and increasing drug resistance. Those currently available in the UK include sulfamethoxazole, sulfadiazine, sulfadoxine, sulfasalazine, mafenide acetate, and sulfacetamide sodium.

Classification

The sulfonamides can be classified as follows:

- short-/medium-acting sulfonamides, e.g. sulfamethoxazole, sulfadiazine;
- long-acting sulfonamides, e.g. sulfadoxine;

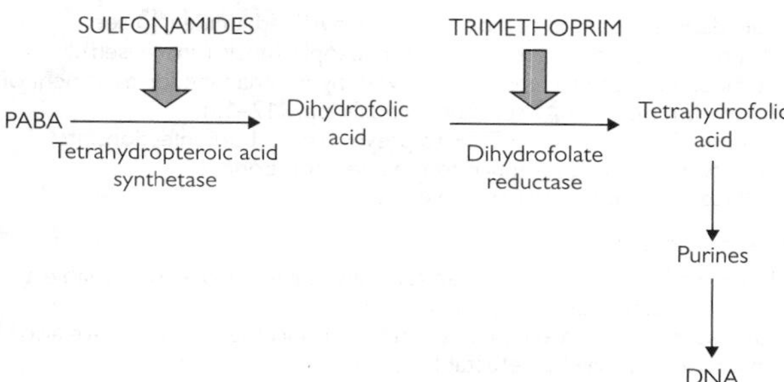

Fig. 2.3 Action of sulfonamides and trimethoprim on the bacterial folate synthesis pathway.

- sulfonamides limited to the GI tract, e.g. sulfasalazine;
- topical sulfonamides, e.g. silver sulfadiazine, mafenide acetate, sulfacetamide sodium.

Mode of action

Sulfonamides inhibit bacterial growth by competitive inhibition of the incorporation of PABA into tetrahydropteroic acid by the enzyme tetrahydropteroic acid synthetase. They are bacteriostatic and slow to act—several generations of bacterial growth are required to deplete the folate pool. They are active against a broad spectrum of Gram-positive and Gram-negative bacteria, *Actinomyces, Chlamydia, Plasmodium*, and *Toxoplasma* spp. Activity against enterococci (which are auxotrophic for folic acid), *Pseudomonas* spp. (possess drug efflux pumps), and anaerobes is poor.

Resistance

Resistance to sulfonamides is widespread and increasingly common; cross-resistance between different sulfonamides occurs. Resistance may be due to:

- chromosomal mutations that result in overproduction of PABA (e.g. *S. aureus, N. gonorrhoeae*) or alterations in dihydropteroate synthetase resulting in reduced affinity for sulfonamides (e.g. *E. coli*);
- plasmids that carry genes coding for the production of drug-resistant enzymes or decreased bacterial permeability.

Plasmid-mediated sulfonamide resistance is common in *Enterobacteriaceae* and has increased greatly in recent years, often in conjunction with trimethoprim resistance.

Clinical use

They have only a limited role as single-agent antimicrobials but are still found in combination products with trimethoprim, pyrimethamine, etc. Sulfasalazine is used for its anti-inflammatory properties (e.g. ulcerative colitis, rheumatoid arthritis)—which are probably a result of its breakdown product 5-aminosalicylic acid.

- Sulfadiazine is used in combination with pyrimethamine (➲ see Antiprotozoal drugs, pp. 119–24) for toxoplasmosis (unlicensed).
- Sulfadoxine is used in combination with pyrimethamine for treatment of falciparum malaria (➲ see Antimalarials, pp. 112–13).
- Silver sulfadiazine is used TOP to prevent/treat burn infections. Its activity is likely to owe much to the silver component.
- Sulfacetamide is used TOP in eye drops.

Pharmacology

- Usually administered PO. Sulfadiazine and sulfisoxazole are available as IV or subcutaneous (s/c) preparations.
- Oral sulfonamides are rapidly absorbed. Topical sulfonamides are also absorbed and may be detectable in blood.
- Widely distributed, with high concentrations in body fluids, including CSF.
- Metabolized in the liver and excreted in the urine. Dose modification is required in renal impairment.

Toxicity and side effects

Around 3% of people experience some form of side effect, much higher in patients with HIV. Hypersensitivity reactions are usually a class effect.

- General—nausea, vomiting, diarrhoea, rash, fever, headache, depression, jaundice, hepatic necrosis, drug-induced lupus, serum sickness-like syndrome.
- Haematological—acute haemolytic anaemia, aplastic anaemia, agranulocytosis, leucopenia, thrombocytopenia.
- Hypersensitivity reactions—drug eruption, vasculitis, erythema nodosum, erythema multiforme, Stevens–Johnson syndrome, anaphylaxis.
- Neonatal kernicterus if given in the last month of pregnancy.

Trimethoprim

Trimethoprim is a diaminopyrimidine. The other members of this class are pyrimethamine (an antiprotozoal), cycloguanil (a product of proguanil; ➲ see Antimalarials, pp. 112–13), and flucytosine (an antifungal). Trimethoprim has a fairly broad spectrum of activity against many Gram-positive bacteria and most Gram-negative rods, except *P. aeruginosa* and *Bacteroides* spp.

Mode of action

Trimethoprim inhibits the bacterial enzyme dihydrofolate reductase (DHFR), preventing the conversion of dihydrofolate to the active form of the vitamin tetrahydrofolate (➲ see Sulfonamides, pp. 58–60; see Fig. 2.3). It works on the pathway at a later point than the sulfonamides, and their combination is synergistic. It is bactericidal or bacteriostatic, depending on the organism and drug concentration.

Resistance

Resistance is common in *Enterobacteriaceae*. May be caused by:

- chromosomal mutations in the gene for DHFR (or its promoter), resulting in overproduction or modification of the target enzyme;

- plasmid-encoded resistance, e.g. *dfr* genes in *Enterobacteriaceae*, producing an additional trimethoprim-resistant DHFR enzyme;
- change in cell permeability/efflux pumps;
- alterations in metabolic pathway.

More than one mechanism can occur in the same cell, resulting in higher resistance levels.

Clinical use

- UTIs—treatment and prophylaxis.
- Treatment of prostatitis and epididymo-orchitis.
- Option for oral MRSA treatment (in combination with rifampicin or fusidic acid).

Pharmacology

- Trimethoprim is given PO and is rapidly absorbed from the gut.
- Widely distributed in tissues and body fluids, including CSF. High concentrations are achieved in the kidney, lung, sputum, and prostatic fluid.
- Sixty to 80% is excreted in the urine within 24h, the remainder excreted as urinary metabolites or in the bile.
- Synergy with sulfamethoxazole, polymyxins, and aminoglycosides.

Toxicity and side effects

- Avoid in pregnancy, especially first trimester (antifolate).
- Contraindicated in blood dyscrasias.
- Side effects are similar to those of co-trimoxazole, but less severe and less frequent with trimethoprim alone.
- Other side effects include GI disturbance, pruritus, rashes, and hyperkalaemia.
- Known to decrease the tubular secretion of creatinine which can lead to rises in serum creatinine that do not reflect a true fall in the GFR.

Co-trimoxazole

Co-trimoxazole is a synergistic combination of trimethoprim and sulfamethoxazole, in the ratio of 1:5.

Mode of action

Sequential inhibition of two enzymes (tetrahydropteroic acid synthetase and dihydrofolate reductase) in the bacterial folate synthesis pathway (➲ see Sulfonamides, pp. 58–60).

Resistance

Resistance may be due to a variety of mechanisms (for details, ➲ see Sulfonamides, pp. 58–60; ➲ Trimethoprim, pp. 60–1). Increasing drug resistance rates have been seen in *S. aureus*, many *Enterobacteriaceae*, and *Pneumocystis jiroveci*.

Clinical use

Apart from the following exceptions, consider using standard trimethoprim when possible—it is often as effective an antibacterial as co-trimoxazole, with fewer side effects:

- *Pneumocystis jiroveci* pneumonia (treatment and prophylaxis);
- toxoplasmosis (prophylaxis and second-line therapy);
- nocardiosis (second-line therapy);
- MDR organisms, e.g. *Acinetobacter* spp.; *B. cepacia; Stenotrophomonas maltophilia; Mycobacterium marinum; Mycobacterium kansasii*. Seek advice from an infection specialist;
- acute exacerbations of COPD (if sensitive and no other options);
- UTIs (if sensitive and no other options);
- acute otitis media in children (if sensitive and no other options).

Pharmacology

Co-trimoxazole may be given PO or IV. Oral bioavailability is around 85%. Components have different volumes of distribution, so seek advice if treating complicated cases (e.g. at an unusual site).

Toxicity and side effects

Avoid in blood disorders, infants <6 weeks, hepatic impairment, renal impairment, pregnancy, and breastfeeding. Side effects are mainly due to the sulfonamide component, may be more severe in the elderly, and are more frequent in those with HIV. See also individual agents (➲ see Sulfonamides, pp. 58–60; ➲ Trimethoprim, pp. 60–1).

- Common: nausea, vomiting, diarrhoea, anorexia, and hypersensitivity.
- Rashes: rare but can be severe, including erythema multiforme, Stevens–Johnson syndrome, and toxic epidermal necrolysis.
- Other: haematological toxicity, renal dysfunction, interstitial nephritis, hyperkalaemia, drug-induced hepatitis, pancreatitis, hepatic failure.
- Patients with low urine output and low urinary pH may be at increased risk of urinary tract crystal formation due to the sulfa component.

Quinolones

Nalidixic acid, the first quinolone antibiotic, was produced as a side product of attempts to manufacture chloroquine. The majority of quinolones now in use are fluoroquinolones (fluorine atom attached to the central molecular ring) with an expanded spectrum of activity and greater potency.

Mode of action

The only antibiotics in clinical use that directly inhibit bacterial DNA synthesis. This is via inhibition of DNA gyrase (primary target in Gram-negatives) and topoisomerase IV (primary target in Gram-positives). DNA gyrase consists of α- and β-subunits (encoded by the *gyrA* and *gyrB* genes, respectively), and is responsible for DNA supercoiling. Topoisomerase IV also consists of two subunits, encoded by the *parC* and *parE* genes, and is involved in DNA relaxation and chromosomal segregation. Quinolones bind to the complex of enzyme with DNA, blocking progress of the DNA replication enzyme, damaging bacterial DNA—they are thus bactericidal.

Resistance

The likelihood of developing resistance is related to the duration of therapy (as little as 5 days in *in vitro* conditions) and may be a result of:

- spontaneous chromosomal mutations occurring in genes that either alter target enzymes (with increasing resistance occurring by selection of resistant strains produced by sequential mutations in *gyrA*, *gyrB*, *parC*, or *parE*) or alter cell membrane permeability by mutations that reduce entry through porin channels or increase efflux. In *P. aeruginosa*, resistance has been shown to be due to overexpression of genes that encode the MexAB–OprM efflux pump;
- plasmid-encoded proteins, e.g. Qnr proteins that protect DNA gyrase from quinolone action. They have been reported in *K. pneumoniae*, *E. coli*, *Enterobacter*, and other enteric bacteria. While alone conferring only low-level resistance, they are often found in strains with additional chromosomal mutations leading to high-level MDR. Other plasmid-mediated mechanisms include efflux pumps (QepA) and antibiotic-modifying enzymes;
- acquired fluoroquinolone resistance may be seen with MRSA and *P. aeruginosa*. They are no longer recommended for the treatment of gonorrhoea in the UK or USA, and treatment failures are well recognized with *S.* Typhi strains of decreased susceptibility.

Clinical use

- The greatest activity of quinolones is against aerobic Gram-negative bacilli (*Enterobacteriaceae*, *Haemophilus* spp., and certain Gram-negative cocci, e.g. *Neisseria* spp.).
- Fluoroquinolones are active against non-enteric Gram-negatives (e.g. *P. aeruginosa*), staphylococci, and the common causes of atypical pneumonia (*L. pneumophilia*, *M. pneumoniae*, *C. pneumoniae*).
    - Ciprofloxacin is the most potent against Gram-negatives but has limited activity against streptococci (see Box 2.3).
    - Levofloxacin (the active *L*-racemer of ofloxacin) is more potent against Gram-positives but sacrifices some *Pseudomonas* activity.
    - Moxifloxacin has enhanced activity against anaerobes and streptococci, but further loss of activity against *P. aeruginosa* (not reliable for clinical treatment), *Proteus* spp., and *Serratia marcescens*, compared to ciprofloxacin.
    - Mycobacteria—great potential in the treatment of resistant TB (moxifloxacin has early bactericidal activity similar to that of ethambutol in patients with pulmonary TB); active against a number of NTM species (➔ see Non-tuberculous mycobacteria, pp. 361–2).

Box 2.3 Indications for consideration of higher-dose ciprofloxacin

Serious infections in which antibiotic penetration may be suboptimal, e.g. septic arthritis, osteomyelitis, pseudomonal pneumonia, neurological and intraocular infections.

- Note that activity against enterococci is marginal, and, while most MSSA strains are sensitive, many MRSA strains have high-level resistance to the class as a whole.
- Not recommended for routine use in those <18 years (animal studies demonstrate arthropathy), but often used in those with CF and complicated UTIs under specialist guidance.

Pharmacology

- Well absorbed, with bioavailability ranging from 50% to 100%. Oral bioavailability is reduced by co-administration of antacids.
- Moxifloxacin, nalidixic acid, and norfloxacin are only given PO; ciprofloxacin and levofloxacin may also be given IV. Protein binding is low, and volumes of distribution are high. Concentrations in the prostate, lung, bile, and stool may exceed plasma concentrations.
- Ofloxacin, levofloxacin, and gatifloxacin are renally eliminated. Nalidixic acid and moxifloxacin undergo hepatic metabolism. Most others are excreted by renal and non-renal pathways. Dose adjustments may be required in renal or liver disease.

Toxicity and side effects

- GI—common (3–17%), e.g. nausea, vomiting, abdominal discomfort, diarrhoea (risk factor for *C. difficile* disease).
- CNS (0.9–11%), e.g. headache, dizziness, insomnia, altered mood. Rarely hallucinations, delirium, seizures (lower threshold in those prone to them, thus should not be given to epileptics), and profound muscle weakness in those with myasthenia gravis (avoid use).
- Allergic reactions—rash, photosensitivity, drug fever, urticaria, angio-oedema, vasculitis, serum sickness, interstitial nephritis.
- Arthropathy and tendon rupture (usually Achilles) in adults. Not recommended in adults with a history of tendon disorders.
- Arrhythmias—moxifloxacin is contraindicated in those with risk factors for prolonged QT, and other agents should be used with caution.
- Laboratory abnormalities (vary with agents) include leucopenia, eosinophilia, hepatitis (severe with moxifloxacin), and dysglycaemia.

Nitroimidazoles

Metronidazole

The imidazoles are remarkable in that members of the class are effective across the whole microbiological spectrum: bacteria, fungi, protozoa, and helminths. Metronidazole, a 5-nitroimidazole, was introduced for the treatment of *Trichomonas vaginalis* infections in 1959 and subsequently found to be bactericidal for most anaerobic and facultatively anaerobic bacteria (when a patient's acute ulcerative gingivitis 'spontaneously' improved, while receiving therapy) and protozoa. Related compounds (e.g. tinidazole) share its properties but have longer half-lives.

Mode of action

Metronidazole has a low molecular weight and enters the bacterial cell by passive diffusion. It is a pro-drug and activated intracellularly by reduction of its nitro group by a nitroreductase under conditions achievable only in anaerobes. The highly reactive resulting compounds interact with nucleic acids and proteins, causing breakage, destabilization, and cell death.

Resistance

Resistance to metronidazole is rare, and a combination of mechanisms is required. Both chromosomally mediated and plasmid-mediated resistance have been described. Reports of resistance in *Bacteroides* spp. have been attributed to the transferable genes *nimA* and *nimD*. Metronidazole resistance in *H. pylori* is associated with mutational inactivation of the *rdxA*, *frxA*, and *fdxB* genes. Metronidazole resistance in *T. vaginalis* and *Giardia* is probably multifactorial, with reduced activation of metronidazole and/or reduced transcription of the ferredoxin gene.

Clinical use

- Parasitic infections, e.g. bacterial vaginosis, intestinal amoebiasis, giardiasis, amoebic liver abscess.
- Anaerobic infections, including *C. difficile* colitis, *H. pylori* eradication therapy, small bowel bacterial overgrowth, pouchitis (inflammatory bowel disease, IBD), infected leg ulcers and pressure sores, PID, dental infections, and acute ulcerative gingivitis (see Box 2.4).
- Surgical prophylaxis.

Pharmacology

- Metronidazole may be given PO, IV, per vagina (PV), per rectum (PR), or TOP. *It should never be taken with alcohol because of the risk of a disulfiram-like reaction* (➔ see Toxicity and side effects below).
- When given PO, it is absorbed rapidly and almost completely.
- Protein binding is low, and the drug is widely distributed in fluids and tissues. Metronidazole shows excellent penetration into abscesses.
- It is metabolized in the liver by the CYP450 enzyme system.
- Metronidazole and its metabolites are primarily eliminated by the kidneys.

Toxicity and side effects

- Metronidazole is generally well tolerated.
- Abnormal metallic taste is commonly reported.

Box 2.4 Antibiotics with anaerobic cover

If your patient is on one of the following drugs, seek advice about whether it is necessary to continue metronidazole:

- co-amoxiclav;
- imipenem or meropenem;
- clindamycin;
- piperacillin–tazobactam.

- GI—nausea, anorexia, epigastric discomfort, vomiting, diarrhoea, constipation.
- Peripheral neuropathy occurs with prolonged treatment.
- Disulfiram-like reaction with alcohol, e.g. nausea, vomiting, flushing, tachycardia, hypotension, acute confusion/psychosis, sudden death.
- GU—transient darkening of the urine, dysuria, cystitis, incontinence.
- Allergic reactions—rash, urticaria, flushing, bronchospasm, serum sickness.
- CNS symptoms include headache, dizziness, syncope, vertigo, sleep disturbance, confusion, excitation, and depression. Cerebellar toxicity has been seen with high doses and/or prolonged therapy.
- Other—fever, mucocutaneous candidiasis, neutropenia, thrombophlebitis with IV infusion.

Nitrofurans

The nitrofuran group of antibiotics comprises nitrofurantoin, furazolidone, and nitrofurazone (the latter two are not available in the UK).

Mode of action

The mechanism of action is poorly understood but requires enzymatic reduction within the bacterial cell (like metronidazole). The reduced derivatives bind to ribosomal proteins and block translation. They also appear to directly damage bacterial DNA (like quinolones) and inhibit DNA repair. Nitrofurans are bactericidal against urinary pathogens such as *E. coli*, *Citrobacter*, group B streptococci (GBS), *Staphylococcus saprophyticus*, *E. faecalis*, and *E. faecium*. However, note that only a minority of *Enterobacter* spp. are sensitive, and most members of *Proteus*, *Providencia*, *Morganella*, *Serratia*, *Acinetobacter*, and *Pseudomonas* spp. are resistant.

Resistance

Resistance is rare. In *E. coli*, resistance may be chromosomal or plasmid-mediated, and is associated with inhibition of nitrofuran reductase activity.

Clinical use

It is rapidly excreted into the urine after oral absorption and achieves no useful blood or tissue level. It is therefore restricted to the treatment of lower UTIs in those with adequate renal function.

- Acute uncomplicated cystitis (not pyelonephritis)—3 days;
- Treatment of recurrent UTIs—7 days;
- Prophylaxis of recurrent UTIs.

Pharmacology

- Nitrofurantoin has good oral absorption, which is enhanced by food.
- Serum concentrations are low, but urine concentrations are high.
- Activity is enhanced by acid conditions.

Toxicity and side effects

- GI—nausea, vomiting.
- Pulmonary—acute hypersensitivity (fever, cough, dyspnoea, pulmonary infiltrates, myalgia, eosinophilia), chronic (pulmonary fibrosis, bronchiolitis obliterans organizing pneumonia).

Novobiocin

This was once commonly used as a reserve drug for staphylococcal infections but is now out of favour because of problems with resistance and toxicity. It acts on the β-subunit of DNA gyrase (like quinolones). It is used in the diagnostic microbiology laboratory to identify *S. saprophyticus* (coagulase-negative, novobiocin-resistant), a urinary pathogen.

Rifamycins

These are semi-synthetic derivatives of rifamycin B, one of a number of antibiotic compounds produced by *Streptomyces mediterranei*. They bind to the β-subunit of DNA-dependent RNA polymerase, resulting in inhibition and bactericidal activity against a variety of bacteria. Resistance arises readily by mutation in the *rpoB* gene (encoding the subunit), and they are therefore used in combination with other agents to suppress the emergence of resistance. They stimulate hepatic metabolism by the CYP450 enzyme system and are primarily excreted in the bile.

Rifampicin (rifampin)

This is the most important rifamycin and is widely used for the treatment of TB, leprosy, and other bacterial infections.

- Activity—bactericidal against *S. aureus* (including MRSA), GAS, *S. pneumoniae, N. gonorrhoeae, N. meningitidis, H. influenzae*, MTB, *M. kansasii, M. marinum, M. leprae, Legionella* spp., *L. monocytogenes, Brucella* spp.
- Clinical use—TB, leprosy, serious or device-related infections with antibiotic-resistant staphylococci, pneumococci, *Legionella*, elimination of nasopharyngeal carriage of *N. meningitidis* and *H. influenzae*.
- Pharmacology—>90% oral absorption, widely distributed, low CSF penetration unless meningeal inflammation, metabolized in the liver (cytochrome P450), predominantly excreted in the bile and undergoes enterohepatic circulation, some excreted in the urine. Dose reduction in renal failure.
- Interactions—enhances its own metabolism and that of other drugs, e.g. warfarin, oral contraceptives, corticosteroids, PIs.
- Toxicity and side effects—orange discoloration of body fluids (contact lenses may discolour), skin rashes, GI upset, hepatitis, thrombocytopenia, purpura (stop drug), 'rifampicin flu' 2–3h after taking (worse with intermittent therapy than daily regimes), 'red man syndrome' (overdose).

Rifabutin

Longer half-life and some activity against rifampicin-resistant organisms. Good *in vitro* activity against MAC.

- Clinical use—prophylaxis against MAC in acquired immune deficiency syndrome (AIDS) patients, treatment of NTM disease, treatment of TB in those who cannot have rifampicin (unacceptable interactions, e.g. with certain antiretrovirals; intolerance).
- Pharmacology—12–20% oral absorption, widely distributed with concentrations in organs being higher than in plasma.
- Interactions—clarithromycin and ritonavir inhibit CYP450, increasing rifabutin levels.
- Toxicity and side effects—skin rashes, GI upset, hepatitis, neutropenia, uveitis, and arthralgia (with higher doses).

Rifapentine

Not widely used in the UK. Similar to rifampicin, its prolonged half-life allows once-weekly dosing for the continuation phase of TB treatment in non-cavitatory, drug-susceptible, smear-negative (at 2 months) TB. It can be used weekly with isoniazid for the supervised treatment of latent TB and may help improve compliance. Should not be given in HIV-infected patients, as it has high treatment failure rates.

- Pharmacology—70% oral absorption; well distributed, with tissue concentration exceeding plasma concentrations, except in CSF and bone.
- Interactions—potent inducer of CYP450, resulting in reduced concentrations of co-administered drugs, e.g. PIs.
- Toxicity and side effects—neutropenia, hepatitis, animal evidence of teratogenicity and fetal toxicity (avoid in pregnancy).

Other rifamycins

- Rifamide—used in staphylococcal and biliary infections (limited availability).
- Rifamycin SV—can be given parenterally or TOP (not available in the UK).
- Rifaximin—used in traveller's diarrhoea, hepatic encephalopathy (not available in the UK). May have a role in *C. difficile*-associated disease (CDAD).

Polymyxins

The polymyxins (polymyxin B, and polymyxin E or colistimethate sodium) are produced by *Bacillus polymyxa*. They were used parenterally until the development of aminoglycosides and fell into disuse in the 1980s. With the emergence of MDR Gram-negative organisms, e.g. *Pseudomonas* spp. and *Acinetobacter* spp., injectable polymyxins began playing a greater role. Colistimethate sodium is available as colistin sulfate (TOP and non-absorbable PO products) and colistimethate sodium (IV). Polymyxin B is available TOP and as a parenteral preparation that can be given IV or IM.

Mode of action

Polymyxins are cyclic cationic polypeptide detergents. They penetrate cell membranes and interact with phospholipids, disrupting the membranes and causing cytoplasmic leakage. They are rapidly bactericidal. The effect is not very selective, explaining their toxicity. Their spectrum of action includes many GNRs (exceptions include *Proteus* spp., *S. marcescens, M. catarrhalis*, and *B. cepacia*). Gram-positive bacteria and Gram-negative cocci are inherently resistant. They are primarily used in the treatment of multiresistant *P. aeruginosa* and *A. baumanii*, in which acquired resistance is uncommon.

Clinical use

- Polymyxins are used for the treatment of severe infections caused by MDR Gram-negative organisms, e.g. VAP, joint infection.
- Colistin sulfate has been used for intestinal decontamination.
- Aerosolized colistimethate has been used to treat multiresistant VAP and CF patients with pulmonary colonization or infection with MDR *Pseudomonas* spp.—usually in combination with additional IV agents. There is, however, minimal evidence of outcome benefit of the neb route over IV when used in patients with MDR VAP.
- Greater use has seen a rise in resistance—polymyxin-resistant variants of the *K. pneumoniae* KPC clone have been reported from Greece, the UK, and other countries. The BSAC Respiratory Surveillance (2011/2012) reported 15% colistin resistance (mostly MIC >64mg/L) in *Enterobacter* spp.

Pharmacology

Not absorbed PO. Good serum levels after IV administration, but poor penetration of CSF, biliary tract, pleural fluid, and joint fluid. Renally excreted—reduce the dose in renal impairment.

Toxicity and side effects

Dose-related nephrotoxicity and neurotoxicity (paraesthesiae, peripheral neuropathy, and neuromuscular blockade). Bronchospasm with inhalation.

Fusidic acid

Fusidic acid is a member of the fusidane class of antibiotics, derived from the fungus *Fusidium coccineum* and chemically related to cephalosporin P. The sodium salt of fusidic acid (fucidin) was introduced into clinical practice in 1962.

Mode of action

Bacteriostatic, inhibiting protein synthesis by blocking elongation factor G. Fusidic acid also has *in vitro* and *in vivo* immunosuppressive effects. It is active against *S. aureus*, most CoNS, β-haemolytic streptococci, *Corynebacterium* spp. and most *Clostridium* spp. It is active against *M. leprae*, but not useful against MTB.

Resistance

Occurs by chromosomal mutations in the *fusA* gene which codes for elongation factor, and by plasmid-mediated resistance resulting in reduced permeability to the drug. This is of particular concern with long-term monotherapy, so fusidic acid is often combined with another agent.

Clinical use

Fusidic acid is mainly used for the treatment of staphylococcal infections, and many MRSA strains remain sensitive. In most clinical settings, it should be used in combination with another agent to reduce the risk of resistance developing. Useful in skin and soft tissue infections, bacteraemia, endocarditis, septic arthritis, osteomyelitis, and LRTIs in CF patients. It has been used to treat erythrasma due to *Corynebacterium minutissimum* and lepromatous leprosy.

Pharmacology

Fusidic acid may be given PO, TOP, or IV. Oral absorption is rapid and almost complete. It is highly protein-bound and widely distributed in most tissues. Metabolized in the liver by CYP450 and eliminated in the bile.

Toxicity and side effects

Generally well tolerated, but the oral form may cause nausea, vomiting, and reversible jaundice (6%). The IV form is associated with thrombophlebitis and jaundice (17%). Ophthalmic preparations may cause itching or stinging. A drug-induced immune-mediated thrombocytopenia has been described.

Systemic fusidic acid should not be given with statins because of the risk of serious and potentially fatal rhabdomyolysis.

Mupirocin

Mupirocin is a pseudomonic acid, produced by *Pseudomonas fluorescens*, that is not related to any other antibiotic in clinical use. Available preparations are for external use only.

Mode of action

Bacteriostatic—inhibits bacterial RNA and protein synthesis by binding to bacterial isoleucyl tRNA synthetase, preventing the incorporation of isoleucine into protein chains in the bacterial cell wall. It is active against staphylococci and certain other Gram-positive organisms.

Resistance

Low-level resistance is due to spontaneous mutation resulting in altered access to binding sites in isoleucyl tRNA synthetase. High-level resistance is mediated on transferable plasmids by the *mupA* gene, which codes for a modified enzyme. Mupirocin resistance in MRSA has been associated with widespread use—prolonged use (>7 days) is discouraged.

Clinical use

Primarily used for skin infections, e.g. impetigo and folliculitis, and for nasal decolonization of *S. aureus* or MRSA carriage. Mupirocin has also been used for treatment of secondarily infected eczema, burns, lacerations, and ulcers.

Pharmacology

Given TOP as a cream or nasal ointment.

Toxicity and side effects

Local reactions, such as pruritus, burning sensation, rash, and urticarial, may occur, particularly if used on broken skin.

Antituberculous agents

The traditional first-line drugs (rifampicin, isoniazid, pyrazinamide, and ethambutol) remain the most effective and least toxic. Agents vary in their activity under different conditions. In classic pulmonary TB, most organisms are in cavities open to the bronchi (oxygenated, more alkaline, actively multiplying), with a smaller less active population in necrotic tissue or inside macrophages (less oxygen and more acidic). An agent's bactericidal activity against rapidly multiplying bacteria determines the effectiveness of the early response to treatment, whereas sterilizing activity against less active persisters influences the risk of relapse after treatment finishes. Rifampicin acts against intra- and extracellular organisms, in addition to those dormant in nodules. Isoniazid and streptomycin are bactericidal against replicating tubercle bacilli in cavities. Pyrazinamide is active against intracellular organisms in acidic environments (e.g. necrosis—hence its importance in the induction phase of 'short-course' therapy). For treatment guidelines, ➲ see Pulmonary tuberculosis, pp. 627–8.

First line

Isoniazid (H)

- Isonicotinic acid hydrazide, synthetic agent. Penetrates rapidly into tissues and lesions.
- Mode of action—inhibits mycolic acid synthesis. Rapidly bactericidal against actively replicating MTB (MIC 0.01–2mg/L). Most other mycobacteria are resistant.
- Resistance—isoniazid resistance is one of the two most frequent forms of resistance (5.5% of isolates mono-resistant in 2014 in England). Associated with mutations in *inhA* (mycolic acid synthesis), *katG* (catalase peroxidase), and *oryR-ahpC* genes.
- Clinical usage—treatment of all forms of TB infection, chemoprophylaxis in contacts and highly susceptible patients. LFTs should be measured before starting treatment, as a comparison for any subsequent adverse reactions.
- Pharmacology—>95% oral absorption, widely distributed, good CSF penetration (50–80% of serum levels), metabolized in liver (*N*-acetyltransferase), excreted in urine. Given as a single daily dose, as high peak concentrations are more important than a continuously

inhibitory level. Patients may be fast or slow acetylators, depending on genetic polymorphism—this is of clinical significance only if intermittent weekly regimes are considered. Dose reduction in renal failure.
- Toxicity and side effects—neurotoxicity (interferes competitively with pyridoxine metabolism; reduced by co-administration of the vitamin), hepatitis (potentially serious and risk increases with age; for management, ➔ see Acute hepatitis, pp. 671–3), arthralgia, hypersensitivity, antinuclear antibody-positive lupus-like syndrome; inhibits the hepatic metabolism of several drugs, increasing plasma levels (e.g. warfarin, diazepam, phenytoin, carbamazepine).

Rifampicin (R)

(➔ see Rifamycins, pp. 67–8.)
- Highly potent and effective TB drug; 1.4% of English isolates mono-resistant in 2014, much higher (>20%) in Thailand and countries of the former Soviet Union.
- Bactericidal against actively replicating MTB and other mycobacteria (*M. kansasii, M. marinum, M. leprae*).

Pyrazinamide (Z)
- Pyrazinoic acid amide, synthetic nicotinamide analogue. Particularly effective against intracellular tubercle organisms in acidic environments (e.g. necrotic inflammatory foci) and an essential component of the first 2 months of 'short-course' (6-month) treatment regimes.
- Mode of action—unknown. Activity requires conversion to pyrazinoic acid by mycobacterial pyrazinamidase.
- Resistance—uncommon and is due to mutations in the *pncA* (pyrazinamidase) gene. *Mycobacterium bovis* is inherently resistant; consider this organism if preliminary sensitivities of a presumed TB culture indicated pyrazinamide mono-resistance.
- Pharmacology—>90% oral absorption, widely distributed, good CSF penetration. Metabolized in the liver; excreted by kidneys. Dose reduction in renal failure. Increase the dose in dialysis patients.
- Toxicity and side effects—rare but include GI upset, hepatotoxicity, gout (inhibits excretion of uric acid), arthralgia, photosensitivity.

Ethambutol (E)
- Hydroxymethylpropylethylene diamine, synthetic compound.
- Mechanism of action—inhibits arabinosyl transferase enzymes (synthesis of arabinogalactan and lipoarabinomannan). Bacteriostatic and active against mycobacteria (MTB, *M. kansasii, M. xenopi, M. malmoense*) and *Nocardia*.
- Resistance is uncommon—develops slowly during therapy, caused by point mutations in the genes encoding arabinosyl transferase enzyme (*embA*, *embB*, and *embC*).
- Pharmacology—75–80% oral absorption, widely distributed, 25–40% CSF penetration. Metabolized in the liver, renal excretion. Dose modification in renal failure.
- Adverse effects—optic neuritis (dose-dependent, resulting in changes in acuity and colour vision; reversible in early stages if treatment discontinued promptly; measure acuity before, and monitor during, treatment), peripheral neuropathy, arthralgia, hyperuricaemia, rashes.

Streptomycin (S)

(➔ see Aminoglycosides, pp. 46–8.)

- An aminoglycoside. Use limited by toxicity and resistance. pH-dependent activity, thus antimicrobial effect reduced in lung secretions (low pH). Bactericidal against MTB in the proliferative phase.
- Resistance—emerged rapidly in the past when given as a single agent. Due to mutations in ribosomal binding protein or the ribosomal binding site (e.g. *rpsL* gene encodes ribosomal protein S12). Primary resistance is seen in populations with a high incidence of isoniazid resistance.
- Pharmacology—not absorbed from the GI tract, administered IM. Widely distributed, but poor penetration of CSF (better if meninges inflamed), bone, aqueous humour, and abscesses; 99% renal excretion. Monitor serum levels in those over 40 years old.
- Adverse effects—ototoxicity is the most important problem, with vestibular damage in <30%. Perform baseline testing. Other—injection site reactions, hypersensitivity, neuromuscular blockade, peripheral neuritis, optic neuritis.

Second line

Considered to have less favourable pharmacokinetic profiles, a relative lack of clinical data, or an increased incidence/severity of adverse events, compared to first-line agents. Some are considerably more expensive. They are used in cases of intolerance or resistance to first-line drugs. Treatment in these situations may be complicated, and advice should be sought from a specialist experienced in treating such patients. Certain agents are used in the treatment of atypical mycobacterial infections (➔ see Non-tuberculous mycobacteria, pp. 361–2).

Para-aminosalicylic acid (PAS)

- Mode of action—interferes with folate synthesis and iron uptake (by inhibition of the salicylate-dependent biosynthesis of iron-chelating 'mycobactins'). Bacteriostatic against MTB.
- Clinical usage—used for MDR-TB in developed countries. Cost limits use elsewhere. Evidence for its effectiveness compares unfavourably with that for cycloserine or the thioamides.
- Pharmacology—incomplete oral absorption, hepatic metabolism, renal excretion (metabolites accumulate in severe renal impairment and contraindicated, unless no alternative).
- Adverse effects—GI upset, interferes with iodine metabolism (check thyroid function tests (TFTs) at baseline and 3-month intervals), hepatitis (check LFTs at baseline), coagulopathy.

Capreomycin

- Cyclic polypeptide antibiotic, produced by *Streptomyces capreolus*; its mode of action is unknown.
- Resistance—mechanism unknown. No cross-resistance with streptomycin, but some kanamycin/amikacin-resistant isolates are cross-resistant to capreomycin.
- Clinical usage—first-line injectable agent in MDR-TB, particularly if streptomycin-resistant.

- Pharmacology—administered IM or IV daily (lower dose for those over 60 years). It may be possible to reduce frequency once the sputum is culture-negative. Renally excreted (reduce the dose and frequency in renal impairment); no useful CSF penetration. Toxicities may be potentiated by aminoglycoside use.
- Adverse effects—injection site reactions, ototoxicity, nephrotoxicity (potassium (K) and magnesium (Mg) wasting, proteinuria), neuromuscular blockade. Perform baseline audiometry and vestibular testing. Monthly renal function, and K/Mg and audiology testing while on therapy.

Cycloserine

- Naturally occurring amino acid that inhibits cell wall synthesis. Derived from *Streptomyces orchidaceus*. Mechanism of resistance unknown.
- Activity—broad: *S aureus*, streptococci, enterococci, *Enterobacteriaceae*, *Nocardia* spp., *Chlamydia* spp., and mycobacteria.
- Clinical use—usually given bd; start with a low dose, and increase as tolerated. No data to support intermittent therapy.
- Pharmacology—well absorbed PO; widely distributed, including CSF; 50% metabolized, 50% excreted unchanged in the urine (dose modification required in renal impairment).
- Adverse events—CNS (psychosis, depression, convulsions); pyridoxine may help. Assess the neuropsychiatric status monthly.

Thioamides (ethionamide, prothionamide)

- Thioisonicotinic acid derivatives that inhibit mycolic acid synthesis. Bacteriostatic for TB, weakly bactericidal to *M. leprae*. Resistance mechanism unknown. Some isolates are resistant to both isoniazid and the thioamides which may be associated with mutations in the *inhA* gene promoter region (involved in mycolic acid synthesis).
- Pharmacology—well absorbed; widely distributed, including CSF; metabolized in the liver, 99% excreted as metabolites in the urine (dose reduction in renal failure). Contraindicated in pregnancy.
- Adverse effects—GI upset (nausea may be severe enough to require bedtime administration with anti-emetic), hypersensitivity, hepatitis, CNS (pyridoxine may help).

Thiacetazone

- Acetylaminobenzaldehyde thiosemicarbazone.
- Mode of action—poorly understood, inhibits mycolic acid synthesis.
- Resistance—mechanism unknown. Primary and acquired resistance are common in developing countries where it has been used widely.
- Clinical usage—rarely used because of low efficacy and frequency of adverse effects. Should never be given to an HIV-infected patient.
- Pharmacology—well absorbed, 20% eliminated in the urine.
- Adverse events—rash, exfoliative dermatitis, Stevens–Johnson syndrome (especially in HIV patients), GI upset, vertigo, conjunctivitis.

Others

- Fluoroquinolones (➔ see Quinolones, pp. 62–4)—later-generation drugs (e.g. moxifloxacin) are significantly associated with cure in MDR-TB. Their use is recommended in the treatment of such patients.

- Aminoglycosides (➲ see Aminoglycosides, pp. 46–8)—kanamycin and amikacin. Ototoxic and nephrotoxic—perform baseline audiometry and vestibular testing.
- Viomycin—a cyclic polypeptide antibiotic, related to capreomycin with which it displays cross-resistance. Limited usage.
- Bedaquiline—a novel agent which acts by inhibiting mycobacterial ATP synthase. Approved in 2012 for the treatment of MDR-XDR-TB and on the WHO essential drugs list. For specialist use only—risk of increased mortality and prolonged QT interval.
- Delamanid—approved in 2014 for the treatment of MDR-XDR-TB. Blocks synthesis of mycolic acids. On the WHO essential drug list. Limited data on effectiveness.
- Drugs with limited evidence base used in the treatment of MDR-TB and XDR-TB include linezolid (increasing evidence supporting its effectiveness may see it used more routinely in resistant TB), co-amoxiclav, clarithromycin, imipenem, clofazimine, carbapenems, thioacetazone.
- Always seek specialist advice when managing resistant TB. The British Thoracic Society (BTS) operate an online clinical advice service on the following link: forums.brit-thoracic.org.uk.

Antileprotics

Introduced by the WHO in 1982, multidrug therapy (MDT) with a combination of dapsone, clofazimine, and rifampicin is the current treatment for infections with *M. leprae* (see Table 2.5). It has been very successful, with a high cure rate, few side effects, and low relapse rate. However, disability caused by leprotic neuropathy and eye damage may not be reversible.

Dapsone

Since first used to treat leprosy by Cochrane in 1947, dapsone has remained the cornerstone of treatment. The emergence of drug resistance in the 1960s led to the MDT recommendations.

Table 2.5 MDT regimens for the treatment of *M. leprae* infections

Regimen	Drug	Duration
Paucibacillary leprosy (TT, BT)	Dapsone 100mg daily	6 months
	Rifampicin 600mg monthly	
Multibacillary leprosy (LL, BL, BT)	Dapsone 100mg daily	2 years
	Clofazimine 50mg daily and 300mg monthly	
	Rifampicin 600mg monthly	

BL, borderline lepromatous leprosy; BT, borderline tuberculoid leprosy; LL, lepromatous leprosy; TT, tuberculoid leprosy.

NB. The regimens shown in Table 2.5 are those of the WHO. The guidance of the American National Hansen's Disease Programme differs with longer durations (12 months for paucibacillary, 24 months for multibacillary) and daily rifampicin dosing.

- Mode of action—a diaminodiphenyl sulfone which is active against many bacteria and some protozoa. It inhibits the synthesis of dihydrofolic acid. Bacteriostatic and weakly bactericidal. Resistance acquired by sequential mutations.
- Pharmacology—>90% oral absorption; widely distributed, but selectively retained in the skin, kidneys, and liver; metabolized by oxidation and acetylation; mostly renally excreted.
- Toxicity and side effects—GI upset, anorexia, headaches, dizziness, insomnia, 'dapsone syndrome' (fever, skin rash ± lymphadenopathy, jaundice, hepatomegaly), haemolysis (especially if G6PD deficiency), methaemoglobinaemia, sulfhaemoglobinaemia.
- Clinical use—leprosy, malaria (treatment and prophylaxis), toxoplasmosis (prophylaxis), pneumocystis pneumonia (PCP) (treatment and prophylaxis), dermatitis herpetiformis. Patients should be screened for G6PD deficiency before treating.

Clofazimine

- Mode of action—unknown. An iminophenazine dye with anti-inflammatory properties, active against mycobacteria (MTB, *M. scrofulaceum, M. leprae, M. avium intracellulare* (MAI), *M. fortuitum, M. chelonae*), *Actinomyces* spp., and *Nocardia* spp. While weakly bactericidal alone, it displays pronounced synergy with dapsone. Resistance is rare.
- Pharmacology—well absorbed PO, taken up by adipose tissue and monocytes/macrophages, long half-life (10–70 days), excreted in the urine and faeces.
- Adverse effects—GI upset, skin discoloration (dose-related, reversible, and particularly pronounced in leprotic skin lesions, as the drug is lipophilic and accumulates in the organism's mycolic cell wall), small bowel oedema/subacute obstruction (prolonged use).
- Clinical use—leprosy.

Rifampicin

- Most effective antileprotic; highly bactericidal, even with monthly dosing. Renders the patient non-infectious within days of starting therapy (➔ see Rifamycins, pp. 67–8).

Alternative agents

Evidence for the use of alternative combinations is limited. Other antibiotics with bactericidal activity against *M. leprae* are shown below; all are less bactericidal than rifampicin.

- Minocycline (the only tetracycline with significant activity; ➔ see Tetracyclines, pp. 56–8);
- Ofloxacin (levofloxacin and moxifloxacin are also effective, but there are less clinical data; ➔ see Quinolones, pp. 62–4);
- Clarithromycin (the only effective macrolide; ➔ see Macrolides, pp. 48–50).

Short-course therapy

Recent research has focused on determining alternative regimens of shorter duration. A single-dose regimen of rifampicin, ofloxacin, and minocycline has been trialled for single-lesion paucibacillary leprosy and is slightly less effective.

Immunological reactions

Systemic inflammatory complications can occur before, during, or years after treatment. Symptoms include: fatigue, malaise, fever, neuritis, arthritis, and iritis. Neuritis must be treated aggressively, in an effort to avoid nerve damage and disability.

- Reversal reactions (type 1 reactions) can be treated with aspirin (if mild) or prednisolone (if moderate to severe). Up to 60mg prednisolone for 20 weeks or more may be required. Around 70% of patients improve; second-line: ciclosporin.
- Erythema nodosum leprosum (type 2 reactions) can be treated with aspirin (if mild), prednisolone, or thalidomide (if severe; may require years of treatment). Clofazimine may have a role in chronic cases.

Antifungals

Antifungals: introduction *80*
Polyenes *80*
Imidazoles *82*
Triazoles *83*
Echinocandins *85*
Other antifungals *86*

Antifungals: introduction

A number of antifungal agents are available:

- alkylamines inhibit ergosterol biosynthesis by inhibiting squalene epoxidase, e.g. terbinafine;
- antimetabolites that interfere with DNA synthesis, e.g. flucytosine;
- azoles inhibit ergosterol synthesis by blocking 14-α-demethylase, e.g. imidazoles and triazoles;
- glucan synthesis inhibitors, e.g. echinocandins;
- polyenes bind to the fungal cell membrane and cause it to leak electrolytes, e.g. nystatin, amphotericin;
- miscellaneous agents, e.g. griseofulvin.

Polyenes

Two are in clinical use—nystatin and amphotericin. Neither is absorbed PO, and only amphotericin can be administered IV. Amphotericin acts against a wide range of pathogenic fungi. It is a cornerstone in the treatment of invasive fungal infections (e.g. disseminated candidiasis, cryptococcosis, aspergillosis), including the dimorphic fungi. Organisms intrinsically resistant to amphotericin are: dermatophytes, *Aspergillus terreus, Fusarium* spp., *Pseudallescheria boydii, Scedosporium prolificans, Trichosporon beigelii*, and some mucormycoses.

Mode of action

Polyenes bind to ergosterol in the fungal cell membrane, resulting in increased membrane permeability. Essential cell contents leak and the cell dies.

Resistance

- *Candida lusitaniae* may develop resistance to amphotericin B during treatment.
- Otherwise acquired resistance is rare, apart from in AIDS patients with relapsing cryptococcal disease, and cancer patients with prolonged neutropenia and yeast infections.

Clinical use

Amphotericin

- Conventional IV amphotericin deoxycholate may be used to treat systemic fungal infections. It is the drug of choice for aspergillosis and also commonly used for disseminated candidiasis and cryptococcosis, either alone or with flucytosine (➔ see Other antifungals, pp. 86–7).
- Toxicity is a major problem with systemic therapy. Lipid formulations of amphotericin are better tolerated and recommended if toxicity or renal impairment preclude the use of conventional amphotericin. Other licensed indications include:
  - Abelcet® for systemic fungal infections not responding to conventional amphotericin or other antifungals (it can be given at a higher dose than the other lipid formulations);

  - AmBisome® for infections in febrile neutropenia unresponsive to broad-spectrum antibacterials, and visceral leishmaniasis.
- Amphotericin is used for mucosal candidiasis, and a solution can be used for continuous bladder irrigation in mycotic infections.

Nystatin

- Nystatin is limited to topical treatment of mucosal infections, and *Candida* infections of the oropharynx, oesophagus, intestinal tract, and vagina.
- Drops are used for mucosal *Candida*.
- Nystatin cream or pessaries are used to treat vaginal candidiasis. It stains clothes yellow and damages latex condoms and diaphragms.

Pharmacology

Amphotericin is usually given IV with a carrier (e.g. deoxycholate). It is highly protein-bound and penetrates the CSF and other body fluids poorly. Liver or renal impairment and dialysis have little effect on serum levels. The lipid formulations have widely diverse pharmacokinetics.

Toxicity and side effects

- Despite the theoretical selective toxicity to fungal cell membranes, compared to human cell membranes, conventional amphotericin is associated with infusion-related reactions (chills, fever, headache, nausea, vomiting) and nephrotoxicity. A test dose is required (because of the risk of anaphylaxis), and close supervision is necessary (monitor FBC, LFTs, renal function, and electrolytes). Prophylactic antipyretics or hydrocortisone may be tried in patients with previous acute adverse reactions, in whom ongoing treatment is essential. Toxicity has driven the development of new lipid formulations (see Table 3.1) that may be preferred in well-resourced health systems.
- Additional side effects of IV amphotericin include GI (anorexia, nausea and vomiting, diarrhoea, epigastric pain), muscle and joint pain, anaemia and other blood disorders, cardiovascular toxicity (including arrhythmias, especially if infused too quickly), neurological disorders, abnormal LFTs, and rash and pain at the infusion site.

Table 3.1 Lipid formulations of amphotericin

Name	Formulation
Liposomal amphotericin(AmBisome®)	Drug encapsulated in phospholipid-containing liposomes
Amphotericin colloidal dispersion (ABCD; Amphocil®)	Drug complexed with cholesterol sulfate to form small lipid discs
Amphotericin lipid complex (ABLC; Abelcet®)	Drug is complexed with phospholipids to form ribbon-like structures

Imidazoles

Commonly used imidazoles include clotrimazole, miconazole, and ketoconazole. Other rarely used agents: econazole, fenticonazole, sulconazole, and tioconazole. They should be considered for topical use only; ketoconazole can be given PO but has been implicated in fatal hepatotoxicity, and the triazoles are now preferred for the treatment of systemic fungal infections.

Mode of action

The imidazoles inhibit the synthesis of ergosterol, the main sterol in fungal cell membranes, by inhibiting the cytochrome P450-dependent enzyme 14-α-demethylase. The damaged cell membrane becomes permeable, leading to cell lysis. However, the imidazoles should be considered fungistatic, although some may be fungicidal at high concentrations.

Resistance

Acquired ketoconazole resistance is rare, but there are case reports of ketoconazole resistance in patients treated for chronic mucocutaneous candidiasis, and AIDS patients with mucosal candidiasis.

Clinical use

- Ketoconazole—oral use for systemic mycoses, serious chronic resistant mucocutaneous candidiasis (including vaginal), serious resistant GI mycoses, and resistant dermatophyte infections of fingernail skin (not toe), non-life-threatening infections with dimorphic fungi. Largely replaced by triazoles. It should not be used for trivial dermatophyte infections due to potentially fatal hepatotoxicity.
- Miconazole—oral gel for the treatment or prophylaxis of oral and intestinal fungal infections. Hold in the mouth near localized lesions, after food.
- Clotrimazole or miconazole cream/pessaries are used to treat vaginal candidiasis. They can damage latex condoms and diaphragms. Topical preparations are used for many fungal skin infections, e.g. dermatophyte infections, pityriasis versicolor, and candidiasis.
- Clotrimazole solution is used for fungal otitis externa infections.

Pharmacology

- Ketoconazole is better absorbed by mouth than the other imidazoles, but levels are highly variable. It is only available PO, and co-administration of antacids should be avoided. Poor CSF penetration.
- Miconazole is available as an oral gel for mouth infections, but systemic absorption may result in significant drug interactions. Clotrimazole is used topically.

Toxicity and side effects

Ketoconazole has been associated with fatal hepatotoxicity—consult an expert before use, and monitor liver function. Ketoconazole and miconazole are contraindicated in hepatic impairment, pregnancy, and breastfeeding. Side effects of these two drugs include GI (nausea, vomiting, abdominal pain), rashes, and headache. With topical preparations, avoid contact with eyes and mucous membranes, and discontinue if severe local irritation or hypersensitivity reactions occur.

Triazoles

The triazoles are important agents in the treatment of systemic mycoses. They differ widely in their spectrum of activity. Varying kinetics, with potential for significant drug interactions—check product details. Avoid in pregnancy.

Mode of action

As for imidazoles. Essentially fungistatic, but voriconazole is fungicidal against *Aspergillus*. Well absorbed PO, but only fluconazole and voriconazole penetrate into the CSF in useful concentrations.

Fluconazole

- Active against yeasts, but no meaningful activity against *Aspergillus* spp. or most other moulds.
  - Useful against most *Candida* spp. (not *Candida krusei*), *Cryptococcus* spp., *Coccidioides immitis*.
  - Limited activity against *Histoplasma capsulatum, Blastomyces dermatitidis*, and *Sporothrix schenkii*.
- Resistance—*C. krusei* is intrinsically resistant to fluconazole. *Candida glabrata* has high fluconazole MICs; 10–15% are resistant. Acquired resistance to fluconazole has been reported in *C. albicans* in HIV patients.
- Pharmacology—available as PO and IV preparations. Well absorbed PO (90% bioavailable); CSF levels of 60–80% of serum CSF. Renal excretion; reduce the dose in impairment.
- Clinical use—treatment of oropharyngeal, vulvovaginal, and invasive candidiasis. Also used for prophylaxis in transplant patients.
- Side effects and toxicity—generally well tolerated. May cause abnormal LFTs.

Itraconazole

- Active against yeasts (including fluconazole-resistant *C. krusei* and *C. glabrata*), moulds, and dimorphic fungi.
  - Useful against: *Candida* spp., *Cryptococcus* spp., *Aspergillus* spp., *P. boydii, S. schenkii, H. capsulatum, B. dermatitidis, C. immitis, Paracoccidioides brasiliensis, Penicillium marneffei*, and dermatophytes.
  - Limited activity against *Fusarium* spp. and *Zygomycetes*.
- Resistance—detectable in most of the aforementioned species, as well as others.
- Pharmacology—available as oral capsule, oral suspension, or IV formulation. Absorption differs between formulations and is highly variable—suspension is best, but GI upset is common. Gastric acidity and food affect absorption. Highly lipophilic; achieves high concentrations in fatty tissues and purulent exudates.
- Clinical use—used in the treatment of yeast and mould infections, especially fluconazole-resistant *Candida* spp. and *Aspergillus* spp. Variable bioavailability limits its use in the severely ill.

- Side effects and toxicity—side effects are rare and similar to those of fluconazole. Hypertension, hypokalaemia, oedema, headache, and altered mental state have been reported. Seek advice before giving itraconazole to patients at risk of heart failure (e.g. elderly, those with cardiac disease or on negative inotropes, e.g. calcium channel blockers, or those on long courses/high doses of itraconazole).

Voriconazole

- Structurally similar to fluconazole. Inhibits P45014DM to a greater extent than fluconazole and enhanced activity against *Aspergillus* spp.
  - Widely active: *Candida* spp. (fungistatic), *Cryptococcus* spp. (fungistatic), *Aspergillus* spp. (fungicidal), *B. dermatitidis, C. immitis, H. capsulatum, Fusarium* spp., and *P. marneffei*. Active against fluconazole-resistant *C. krusei, C. glabrata*, and *Candida guilliermondii*.
  - Not useful for *Zygomycetes*, e.g. *Mucor* spp. and *Rhizomucor* spp., due to high MICs.
- Pharmacology—available PO or IV; 90% PO bioavailability. IV formulation contains a vehicle known to accumulate in renal failure, thus limited to those with CrCl of >50mL/min. Non-linear pharmacokinetics, and therapeutic drug monitoring may be useful.
- Clinical use—licensed for treatment of invasive aspergillosis and invasive candidiasis. Salvage therapy of *Scedosporium apiospermum* and *Fusarium* spp.
- Side effects and toxicity—dose-related, transient visual disturbance, skin rash, abnormal LFTs, visual hallucinations.

Posaconazole

- The only azole with consistent activity against *Zygomycetes*.
  - Excellent activity against *Candida* spp. (including those with reduced fluconazole susceptibility), *Aspergillus* spp., *S. schenkii, H. capsulatum, B. dermatitidis, C. immitis, P. brasiliensis, P. marneffei*, and many causative agents of chromoblastomycosis, mycetoma, and phaeohyphomycosis.
- Pharmacology—oral suspension available. IV formulation under development.
- Clinical use—used in prevention of invasive antifungal infections in high-risk patients with neutropenia or graft-versus-host disease (GVHD). Also used as salvage therapy in patients with invasive fungal infections that failed primary therapy (usually amphotericin). Preliminary data suggest that posaconazole may be effective for zygomycosis unresponsive to amphotericin.
- Toxicity and side effects—more favourable side effect profile than that of the other triazoles; nausea, headache, rash, dry skin, taste disturbance, abdominal pain, dizziness, and flushing may occur.

Ravuconazole

- Currently in phase II trials as oral formulation.
- Active against *Candida* spp., *C. neoformans, Aspergillus fumigatus*, and dermatophytes. Likely to be active against fluconazole-resistant *Candida* spp.

Echinocandins

Target the fungal cell wall. They are rapidly fungicidal for yeasts, but more bacteriostatic for filamentous fungi. They are primarily effective against *Candida* and *Aspergillus* spp.—their relatively weak action against other fungi may reflect differences in fungal wall construction. A large lipopeptide molecule; all agents are for IV administration.

Mode of action

Blocks the synthesis of glucan (a fungal cell wall component) by inhibiting the β-1,3-D-glucan synthase enzyme complex. β-glucans contribute to cell wall integrity. They account for <60% of the cell wall mass in yeasts, and depletion results in cell lysis. Filamentous fungi (e.g. *Aspergillus*) concentrate their β-glucan synthesis in the tips and hyphal branching points; thus, echinocandins merely result in impeded growth. Selective fungal-specific targeting results in fewer side effects, fewer drug interactions, and lack of cross-resistance with other antifungals. Agents differ in pharmacokinetics but have similar spectrums of activity.

Spectrum of activity

- *Candida*—potent activity against *Candida* spp. Thought to be particularly effective against biofilm-embedded organisms (a setting in which the MIC for amphotericin and fluconazole rises dramatically). Active against fluconazole-resistant *C. glabrata* and *C. krusei*.
    - *C. albicans, C. glabrata*, and *C.tropicalis* are highly susceptible.
    - Elevated MICs have been seen for *C. parapsilosis, C. guilliermondii*.
    - Resistance is rare overall. Sporadic acquired resistance occurs.
- *Aspergillus*—growth is inhibited; most species susceptible. Rather than 'MICs', the 'MEC' (minimum effective concentration) endpoint is determined by the lowest concentration, resulting in grossly abnormal hyphal forms.
- Other—not considered useful against dimorphic fungi, *Cryptococcus* or non-*Aspergillus* moulds. No role in treatment or prevention of *Pneumocystis* (glucan synthase is expressed only during the cystic, not trophic, part of the life cycle).

Clinical use

All are approved for invasive candidiasis (adults) and oesophageal candidiasis. Further specific approvals are as follows.

Caspofungin

- Pharmacology—protein binding is >90%. Widely distributed, with high levels in the lungs, liver, spleen, and kidneys, and lower levels in the CSF. Loading dose is followed by lower daily dosing. Metabolized by the liver. Reduce the dose in moderate hepatic impairment. Metabolites eliminated in the urine and faeces. No dose adjustment is required in renal impairment. Dose increase may be needed with rifampicin and potent inducers of cytochrome P450.
- Clinical use—as with pharmacology plus: invasive *Aspergillus* infections where other therapies fail or are not tolerated; empirical therapy in neutropenic patients.

- Toxicity and side effects—nausea, vomiting, abdominal pain, diarrhoea, flushing, fever, headache, and injection site reactions. Transient LFT abnormalities occur in 11–24% of patients.

Anidulafungin

- Pharmacology—loading dose necessary for rapid therapeutic concentrations. No dose adjustment needed for renal or liver impairment.
- Toxicity and side effects—abnormal LFTs.

Micafungin

- Clinical use—as with anidulafungin plus: prevention of *Candida* infections post-bone marrow transplantation (BMT).
- Toxicity and side effects—fever, electrolyte disturbances, abnormal LFTs.

Other antifungals

Flucytosine

A fluorine analogue of cytosine (pyrimidine) that inhibits DNA synthesis.

- Mode of action—inhibits thymidylate synthetase. Also converted to 5-fluorouracil which is incorporated into fungal RNA. Active against yeasts—no useful action on filamentous fungi.
- Resistance—emerges rapidly with monotherapy, thus usually given with amphotericin (may facilitate entry of flucytosine into the cell). May be due to loss of cytosine permease (that permits entry of the drug) or loss of enzymes that convert it into its active metabolites.
- Clinical use—cryptococcosis, candidiasis, chromoblastomycosis, in combination therapy with amphotericin or fluconazole.
- Pharmacology—given IV or PO. Rapidly and almost completely absorbed. Low protein binding. CSF concentrations are 74% of plasma concentrations; 90% is excreted unchanged in the urine—dose reduction required in renal impairment.
- Toxicity and side effects—rash, diarrhoea, and abnormal LFTs. Leucopenia, thrombocytopenia, and enterocolitis may occur in patients with renal impairment—monitor FBC, renal function, LFTs, and serum flucytosine concentrations weekly during treatment. Flucytosine is teratogenic in rats and contraindicated in pregnancy.

Griseofulvin

Griseofulvin was previously used for fungal nail infections, but poor response rates and significant relapse rates have limited its use. Used in children for tinea capitis. Given PO.

- Mode of action—disruption of fungal cellular microtubules.
- Clinical use—tinea capitis in children. Dermatophyte infections of skin, scalp, nails, and hair where topical therapy has failed or is inappropriate.
- Toxicity and side effects—impaired performance of skilled tasks, enhancement of effects of alcohol, headache, nausea, vomiting, and rashes. May diminish the anticoagulant effect of warfarin. Avoid in pregnancy, breastfeeding, systemic lupus erythematosus (SLE) (risk of exacerbation), and liver disease.

Terbinafine

- Mode of action—acts on the enzyme squalene epoxidase, blocking the transformation of squalene to lanosterol and thus inhibiting ergosterol synthesis. The intracellular accumulation of squalene also results in disruption of fungal cell membranes. Accumulates in keratin.
- Resistance—not yet reported.
- Clinical use—dermatophyte and ringworm infections (including tinea pedis, cruris, and corporis) where oral therapy is appropriate. Fingernail infections need a 6-week course, toenails usually 12 weeks. Also available TOP to treat fungal skin infections.
- Pharmacology—given PO or TOP. Metabolized by cytochrome P450 enzymes.
- Toxicity and side effects—abdominal discomfort, anorexia, nausea, diarrhoea, headache, rash, and urticaria. Rare events include liver toxicity and serious skin reactions (e.g. Stevens–Johnson syndrome).

Chapter 4

Antivirals

Antivirals for herpes simplex virus and varicella-zoster virus 90
Antivirals for cytomegalovirus 92
Antivirals for influenza 94
Antivirals for respiratory syncytial virus 96
Antivirals for hepatitis B 97
Antivirals for hepatitis C 99
Principles of HIV treatment 101
Nucleoside/nucleotide analogue reverse transcriptase inhibitors 104
Non-nucleoside reverse transcriptase inhibitors 106
HIV protease inhibitors 108
Other HIV therapies 109

Antivirals for herpes simplex virus and varicella-zoster virus

For therapy, see Table 4.1.

Aciclovir and analogues

Aciclovir was the first agent with demonstrated effectiveness against herpes simplex virus (HSV) infection. Valaciclovir is the *l*-valyl ester pro-drug of aciclovir and is preferred due to its better oral bioavailability. It is rapidly and nearly completely converted to aciclovir in first-pass enzymatic hydrolysis in the liver. Penciclovir and its pro-drug famciclovir are similar to aciclovir.

Mode of action

- A nucleoside analogue and substrate for HSV-specific thymidine kinase (TK); it is phosphorylated only in HSV-infected cells to form aciclovir triphosphate, a competitive inhibitor of viral DNA polymerase.
- Incorporated into viral DNA chain. Causes chain termination. Chain–enzyme complex formation may irreversibly inactivate the polymerase.
- Most active against HSV 1 and 2, then varicella-zoster virus (VZV) and Epstein–Barr virus (EBV). Cytomegalovirus (CMV) (does not encode TK) is resistant at standard therapeutic levels—it has been used for CMV prophylaxis.

Table 4.1 Antiviral therapy for HSV and VZV

Drug	Preparations	Use
Aciclovir	Oral	Treatment and prophylaxis for HSV, treatment of VZV
	IV	Treatment of HSV in the immunocompromised; treatment of severe genital herpes, VZV, and HSV encephalitis
	Topical	Skin and eye infections (e.g. dendritic corneal ulcer)
Valaciclovir	Oral	Treatment of herpes zoster and HSV infections of skin and mucous membranes. Prevention of CMV disease following solid organ transplantation
Penciclovir (acyclic guanosine analogue)	Topical	Similar to aciclovir in potency and spectrum of activity. Cross-resistance common. Labial HSV treatment
Famciclovir (penciclovir pro-drug)	Oral	Treatment of herpes zoster, acute and recurrent genital HSV
Cidofovir (➲ see Cidofovir, pp. 93–4)	IV	Aciclovir-resistant HSV strains, as activation is not dependent on virus-specified enzymes

Resistance

- Rarely seen in the immunocompetent host. Mechanisms include:
  - reduced/absent TK or altered activity of TK for aciclovir—these strains may exhibit reduced virulence;
  - decreased affinity of viral DNA polymerase for aciclovir triphosphate—emerge particularly in those receiving repeated or prolonged treatment (e.g. HIV patients).
- HSV may show cross-resistance to related agents (valaciclovir, famciclovir, penciclovir), and, where resistance is due to TK deficiency, this may extend to ganciclovir (requires phosphorylation for activity). Foscarnet tends to be used for the treatment of aciclover-resistant infections. Resistant HSV is seen in <1% of immunocompetent patients, 6–8% of immunocompromised patients, and up to 17% of patients with AIDS and transplantation patients receiving over 2 weeks of aciclovir therapy.
- Aciclovir-resistant VZV is less common—increased risk in chronic suppressive therapy with subtherapeutic doses.

Pharmacology

- Oral bioavailability: aciclovir 15–20%, valaciclovir up to 54%.
- Oral valaciclovir achieves total aciclovir exposure similar to that of IV aciclovir, but with lower peak plasma concentrations.
- Sixty to 90% renally excreted, the remainder metabolized. Removed by haemodialysis. Reduce the dose in renal impairment.
- Topical absorption low.
- Crosses the placenta, high levels in breast milk. Not known to be harmful in pregnancy, but manufacturers advise caution.

Interactions

- Zidovudine—lethargy.
- Ciclosporin and other nephrotoxic agents—renal impairment.
- Probenecid—decreased clearance and prolonged half-life.
- May decrease the clearance of other drugs eliminated by active renal secretion (e.g. methotrexate).

Side effects and toxicity

- Topical may cause skin irritation.
- Nausea, rash, headache.
- Neurotoxicity in 1–4% of those receiving IV aciclovir, increased in renal impairment.
- Reversible renal impairment in up to 5% receiving IV aciclovir.
- High-dose valaciclovir may cause GI disturbance, confusion, and hallucinations.

Other agents

- Foscarnet (➔ see Foscarnet, p. 93)—used to treat mucocutaneous HSV infections unresponsive to aciclovir.
- Inosine pranobex—effectiveness in HSV unproven.

Antivirals for cytomegalovirus

Ganciclovir, foscarnet, and cidofovir act by inhibiting viral DNA polymerase and are used to treat CMV end-organ disease.

Ganciclovir

Inhibits herpesviruses (including HSV and VZV). Particularly potent inhibition of CMV replication; ~33% of patients receiving IV therapy interrupt or prematurely stop therapy due to marrow or CNS toxicity. Due to its side effects, it is restricted to life-threatening or sight-threatening CMV infections in immunocompromised patients, or to prevention of CMV disease during immunosuppressive therapy after organ transplantation. It is the preferred agent for the treatment of symptomatic simian herpes B.

- Mode of action—nucleoside analogue of guanosine. Phosphorylated by a CMV viral protein kinase (not TK as in HSV). Inhibits viral DNA chain elongation but does not necessarily cause chain termination (unlike aciclovir), leading to accumulation of short non-infectious viral DNA fragments. Unlike aciclovir (phosphorylated only by viral TK in HSV-infected cells), cellular enzymes also phosphorylate ganciclovir, resulting in much greater toxicity than the former drug.
- Resistance—due to mutations in the protein kinase or DNA polymerase. High-level resistance seen in prolonged therapy for those with AIDS or transplantation-related disease (28% of patients acquired resistance after 9 months of treatment for CMV retinitis in one study).
- Pharmacology—ganciclovir oral bioavailability 5–10%, thus given IV only. Aqueous, vitreous, and subretinal levels similar to serum. Most eliminated unaltered renally (dose-adjust in impairment). Removed by haemodialysis. Available as intravitreal implant which requires replacing every 6 months—less used since advent of oral valganciclovir.
- Interactions—increases didanosine levels and may increase ciclosporin levels. Zidovudine and other cytotoxic agents—myelosuppression significantly increased; they should not normally be given together. Probenecid decreases clearance and prolongs half-life. Renal dysfunction with concurrent ciclosporin or amphotericin.
- Adverse effects—myelosuppression, e.g. neutropenia and thrombocytopenia occur in 15–20% of AIDS patients receiving IV therapy (less in transplantation patients). Usually seen in second week of therapy and reversible within 1 week of cessation in most cases. Recombinant granulocyte-colony-stimulating factor (G-CSF) may be useful. Note that CMV itself can cause marrow suppression which may improve with therapy; 5–15% have CNS effects—from headache to confusion and convulsions. Others—renal impairment, LFT abnormalities, rash, fever, phlebitis at IV site.
- Contraindications—pregnancy (ensure effective contraception up to 90 days after therapy), breastfeeding, low haemoglobin (Hb), low WCC or platelets.
- Monitoring—FBC and renal function during treatment.

Valganciclovir

An ester of ganciclovir that may be given PO; valganciclovir is licensed for induction and maintenance of CMV retinitis in AIDS and prevention of transplant-associated CMV disease. The bioavailability of ganciclovir from oral valganciclovir is 60%. Other properties as those of ganciclovir.

Foscarnet

Principal use is the treatment of ganciclovir-resistant CMV retinitis and aciclovir-resistant mucocutaneous HSV or VZV. Ninety per cent of retinitis patients experience clinical stabilization. In those with persistent or relapsed retinitis, combined foscarnet/ganciclovir delays progression longer than high doses of the individual agents.

- Mode of action—inorganic pyrophosphate analogue inhibitory for herpesviruses and HIV. No intracellular metabolism. Directly inhibits viral DNA polymerase or reverse transcriptase (RT) (100-fold greater effect, compared with cellular DNA polymerase). Active against most ganciclovir-resistant CMV strains (and aciclovir-resistant HSV/VZV).
- Resistance—due to point mutations in DNA polymerase of HSV/CMV or RT of HIV. Occurs in <5% of patients.
- Pharmacology—oral bioavailability 8%. Vitreous concentrations 1.4 times higher than plasma. Renal elimination—most unaltered (dose-adjust in impairment). Removed by haemodialysis. Prolonged terminal half-life due to bone deposition.
- Interactions—hypocalcaemia with concomitant IV pentamidine. Renal dysfunction with concurrent ciclosporin, amphotericin, and other nephrotoxic agents.
- Side effects and toxicity—nephrotoxicity, proteinuria, sometimes acute tubular necrosis (one-third develop significant renal impairment—reversible within 3–4 weeks of cessation of therapy). Saline loading may reduce incidence. Metabolic—hypo- and hypercalcaemia, hypo- and hyperphosphataemia, hypomagnesaemia, hypokalaemia. CNS—secondary to hypocalcaemia, and direct effects: seizures, hallucinations. Nausea, rash, abnormal LFTs, heart block.
- Contraindications—pregnancy and breastfeeding.
- Monitoring—electrolytes, calcium (Ca), Mg, phosphate, and renal function.

Cidofovir

Used in CMV retinitis in AIDS patients where ganciclovir or foscarnet therapy not tolerated or failed. Topical gel used in mucocutaneous lesions. Available intravitreally for CMV retinitis, but very toxic. Conflicting evidence for its use in the treatment of progressive multifocal leukoencephalopathy (PML).

- Mode of action—acyclic phosphonate nucleotide analogue of deoxycytidine monophosphate. Active against herpesviruses and other DNA viruses (e.g. hepatitis B). Activation does not require virus-specific enzymes, therefore inhibitory for certain aciclovir- and ganciclovir-resistant HSV and CMV strains. Cellular enzymes metabolize it to the active form—competitively inhibits viral DNA polymerase.

- Resistance—some ganciclovir and foscarnet cross-resistance associated with DNA polymerase mutations. Development of resistance secondary to cidofovir therapy uncommon.
- Pharmacology—oral bioavailability <5%. Renal elimination—active metabolite has a prolonged half-life, allowing fortnightly dosing.
- Side effects and toxicity—dose nephrotoxicity; concomitant probenecid and saline prehydration reduce incidence. Neutropenia 20%; Fanconi-like syndrome; intravitreal dosing can cause iritis/vitritis.
- Contraindications—renal impairment (CrCl <55mL/min, proteinuria 2+). Other nephrotoxic agents. Pregnancy and breastfeeding. Men should not father a child during, or within, 3 months of finishing treatment.

Antivirals for influenza

The neuraminidase inhibitors oseltamivir and zanamivir are licensed for the treatment and prophylaxis of influenza A and B. The adamantanes amantadine and rimantadine are only active against influenza A and, due to an increase in resistant strains, are no longer recommended. Vaccination is the most effective way of preventing influenza. In the UK, NICE (www.nice.org.uk) issues evidence-based guidance on the use of these agents (see Influenza—treatment/prevention, pp. 378–9).

Neuraminidase inhibitors

Sialic acid analogues that inhibit viral neuraminidase and are effective against both influenza A and B. They have been shown to shorten symptom duration by 1–3 days, the greatest benefit seen when given to febrile patients within 24h of symptom onset. Little to no benefit if given after 2 days of symptoms.

Oseltamivir

- Given PO, with good bioavailability. Shortens symptom duration and reduces the duration of viral shedding. May also reduce illness severity and frequency of complications. Some studies suggest a mortality benefit in severe influenza.
- Licensed for treatment within 48h of first symptoms, and prophylaxis within 48h of exposure—they may provide benefit beyond these times in severe cases or the immunocompromised.
- Resistance results from mutations in either the active site of neuraminidase (usually drug-specific) or in haemagglutinin at the site responsible for binding sialic acid residues (resulting in broader cross-resistance). It may arise during drug therapy, but resistant strains have spread widely, even in the absence of therapy.
  - Between 2007 and early 2009, oseltamivir resistance became widespread among seasonal H1N1 isolates (H274Y mutation)—90–100% of isolates in most regions. They remained susceptible to zanamivir and adamantanes.

 - This predominantly resistant strain was replaced in 2009 by the predominantly oseltamivir-susceptible (but adamantane-resistant) H1N1 influenza A pandemic strain.
 - Low levels of resistance have since been reported in the pandemic strain, often associated with immunocompromised patients, perhaps a result of prolonged viral shedding despite therapy.
 - In 2010/11, a variant of pandemic H1N1 with moderate resistance to both oseltamivir and zanamivir was detected. This was found to have a mutation in residue 247 of the neuraminidase gene (S247N). Strains possessing both this and the H274Y mutation have high-level resistance to both oseltamivir and zanamivir.
 - Resistance has been observed in influenza B only rarely.
- Toxicity and side effects—nausea, vomiting, abdominal pain, headache, fatigue, and insomnia. Rarely rashes, hypersensitivity, Stevens–Johnson syndrome.
- Contraindications—use only if benefit outweighs risks in pregnancy and breastfeeding. Avoid in severe renal impairment.

Zanamivir
- Inhaled. An IV preparation is in development. Poor oral bioavailability. Levels far above those required for viral inhibition achieved at the respiratory mucosa after inhalation.
- Licensed for treatment within 48h (36h in children) of first symptoms, or prophylaxis within 36h of exposure. Those with severe disease or immunocompromise may benefit after this time.
- Resistance is rare, and most oseltamivir resistance does not result in cross-resistance. It is the preferred agent for oseltamivir-resistant virus.
- Toxicity and side effects—GI disturbance. Rarely angio-oedema, rash, bronchospasm (use with care in those with asthma and COPD—bronchodilators should be available).
- Contraindications—asthma or other chronic respiratory disease, breastfeeding, caution in pregnancy.

Peramivir
In development. An IV neuraminidase inhibitor used on a compassionate use basis during the 2009 pandemic. No published large clinical trials at the time of writing. Preliminary data suggest it is as effective as oseltamivir.

Adamantanes
Amantadine and rimantadine are active only against influenza A. Initiating therapy within 2 days of symptoms caused by a susceptible virus reduces the duration of illness by 1–2 days. Their use is limited by side effects, limited antiviral spectrum, and the rapid development of resistance.
- Mode of action—block viral M2 protein at low concentrations, preventing viral uncoating in endosomes. Higher concentrations increase lysosomal pH and inhibit virus-induced membrane fusion.
- Resistance—often acquired in the course of treatment of seasonal flu, and the 2009 pandemic H1N1 strain was resistant.
- Pharmacology—well absorbed PO. Amantadine excreted unchanged by the kidney (decrease doses in the elderly and renally impaired).

Rimantadine extensively metabolized by the liver before renal excretion (reduce doses in those with severe liver or renal dysfunction).
- Interactions—increased CNS side effects with concomitant antihistamines or anticholinergics.
- Toxicity and side effects—diarrhoea, nausea, difficulty concentrating, neurotoxicity at high doses or in those with renal impairment, anticholinergic symptoms with high doses (dry mouth, pupillary dilation, toxic psychosis, and cardiac arrhythmias). It is a weak dopamine agonist with modest antiparkinsonian effects.
- Contraindications—epilepsy, pregnancy and breastfeeding, gastric ulceration, severe renal impairment. Use with caution in congestive cardiac failure (CCF). Not licensed for use in children <10 years.

Antivirals for respiratory syncytial virus

Ribavirin

Broad-spectrum antiviral, used in the treatment of RSV, hepatitis C, influenza, and Lassa fever. Studies assessing its role in the treatment of RSV infection in children have been small, and, although they show no reduction in hospital stay, there is a beneficial effect on pulmonary function at 1 year. Currently used in the treatment of RSV bronchiolitis and pneumonia in hospitalized children—especially those with complicated or severe disease.
- Mode of action—guanosine analogue: interferes with nucleic acid synthesis and may also block production of viral mRNA.
- Resistance—not demonstrated in RSV.
- Pharmacology—excreted renally (around 40%) and in faeces (15%), and metabolized by the liver. Some is retained in tissues (especially red blood cells (RBCs)). Given by nebulizer in bronchiolitis, PO or IV in other conditions.
- Toxicity and side effects—dose-related anaemia (extravascular haemolysis) and marrow suppression at high doses. Itch, nausea, depression, and cough. With aerosolized preparations—conjunctivitis, rash, bronchospasm.
- Contraindications—pregnancy (teratogenic risk—contraception for 6 months after therapy in both men and women, and condoms must be used if the partner of the male patient is pregnant, as ribavirin is present in semen) and breastfeeding. Avoid oral therapy in: severe cardiac disease, haemoglobinopathies, severe hepatic dysfunction, autoimmune disease.
- Monitoring—FBC and biochemistry on initiation of therapy, and at weeks 2 and 4. Electrocardiogram (ECG) if history of cardiac disease.

Other therapies for respiratory syncytial virus

These are discussed in more detail later (➔ see Bronchiolitis, pp. 609–11). Some authorities advocate the use of ribavirin in combination with RSV immunoglobulin, particularly in the immunosuppressed. This has not been well studied, however.

Antivirals for hepatitis B

A number of drugs are licensed for the treatment of chronic hepatitis B. The aim of therapy is to reduce the risk of progressive chronic liver disease, cirrhosis, and hepatocellular carcinoma, by suppressing hepatitis B virus (HBV) replication and hence histological activity, leading to biochemical remission and a reduced risk of cirrhosis. For details and treatment guidelines, ➲ see Hepatitis B virus, pp. 413–7. In the UK, NICE has approved the following for treatment of hepatitis B.

Interferon-α

- IFN-αs are part of the innate immune antiviral response and have a role in adaptive immunity. They induce genes that activate an antiviral state: blocking the synthesis of some viral proteins, decreasing viral RNA stability, and stimulating the adaptive immune response.
- Attaching polyethylene glycol to IFN (pegylated) slows both its absorption after s/c injection and renal clearance—enhancing its half-life, achieving higher steady-state concentrations, and allowing weekly dosing.
- Most likely to benefit those who are hepatitis B e antigen (HBeAg)-positive, with high alanine aminotransferase (ALT), and HBV DNA-positive but with low viral load. The course is 48 weeks. Seroconversion may occur months after therapy has stopped. Around 35% of HBeAg-positive patients become eAg-negative. Of these, 30–50% also become hepatitis B surface antigen (HBsAg)-negative (mostly genotype A), associated with a loss of HBV DNA in most cases. Response seems more durable than with lamivudine; <85% remain eAg-negative after 3 years.
- HBeAg-negative patients who are DNA-positive with high ALT require longer courses (12–24 months) and are more likely to relapse on cessation; 25% of patients have a durable virological response (HBV DNA <10 000 copies/mL).
- Pharmacology—IM or s/c 3 times weekly if standard, weekly if pegylated.
- Side effects—fever, chills, fatigue, myalgia, myelotoxicity (monitor FBC), impaired concentration, altered mood, exacerbation or development of autoimmune thyroid diseases, alopecia, arthralgia, hypersensitivity (rare), pulmonary infiltrates (rare).
- It should NOT be used in patients with decompensated cirrhosis—consider oral agents. Also avoid if a history of suicidal tendency, active psychiatric illness, autoimmune disease, severe leucopenia, or thrombocytopenia.

Lamivudine

- Nucleoside analogue used in the treatment of HIV and HBV infection.
- Mechanism—inhibits viral RT enzyme.
- Resistance emerges with monotherapy, the principal mutation occurring in the YMDD motif of the catalytic domain of HBV polymerase. Suspect it in previously well-suppressed patients with an increase in HBV DNA. Resistance rates of 24% at 1 year, and <65% at 5 years. Virological breakthrough leads to biochemical relapse within 2 years.
- Pharmacology—usual dose 100mg od (unless part of highly active antiretroviral therapy (HAART)), well absorbed, renal excretion (reduce the dose in renal impairment).

Telbivudine

- A thymidine nucleoside analogue. Inhibits viral DNA polymerase.
- Data suggest that it is slightly more effective than lamivudine at suppressing HBV DNA in HBeAg-positive patients, BUT this does not translate into a useful clinical benefit, as measured by HBeAg seroconversion or histological improvement.
- It may be more effective at viral suppression than adefovir.
- Displays cross-resistance with lamivudine and, to a lesser extent, entecavir.
- It cannot be used with pegylated IFN (PEG-IFN) due to a high risk of myopathy/neuropathy.
- NICE does not recommend telbivudine.

Adefovir

- Nucleotide analogue of adenosine monophosphate (AMP) that inhibits RT and DNA polymerase.
- Monotherapy achieves viral load reduction, but not as great as that caused by entecavir, tenofovir, or lamivudine.
- It should not be used in countries where tenofovir is available. Adefovir is less potent and shows cross-resistance.
- Lamivudine-resistant strains are sensitive to adefovir.
- Side effects—renal toxicity (rare at doses used), headache, abdominal pain.

Tenofovir

- A synthetic nucleotide analogue related to, and significantly more effective than, adefovir at achieving HBV DNA reduction (75% get HBV DNA levels of <400 copies/mL) and normalizing ALT. Rates of HBeAg seroconversion (20%) and histological improvements are similar, however.
- Effective at suppressing lamivudine-resistant HBV.
- Resistance—most cases of breakthrough currently attributed to compliance, rather than acquisition of resistance mutations.
- Pharmacology—25% oral absorption, not metabolized, renal excretion. Dose requires adjusting in renal insufficiency—caution.
- Side effects—GI symptoms, renal impairment, lactic acidosis, and hepatic steatosis (rare).

Entecavir

- An oral nucleoside analogue—inhibits HBV DNA polymerase.
- Superior to lamivudine and adefovir in achieving viral suppression.
- It is active against lamivudine-resistant strains, but less so than against wild-type virus. A higher dose (1mg daily) is used.
- Monotherapy achieves HBeAg seroconversion in 20% of HBeAg-positive treatment-naïve patients.
- Drops in HIV RNA have been noted in patients receiving entecavir monotherapy—thus it should not be used in HIV/HBV co-infected patients, unless they are on HAART.
- Virological resistance rate of 1% at 5 years of follow-up in treatment-naïve patients, but <50% after 5 years in lamivudine-resistant patients.
- Dosing should be decreased in those with renal impairment.
- Side effects—GI symptoms, lactic acidosis, hepatomegaly with steatosis, and CNS symptoms.

General prescribing points

- Entecavir or tenofovir are preferred in those requiring long-term therapy (e.g. HBeAg-negative patients, those with cirrhosis), as resistance is less likely to arise than with lamivudine.
- IFN cannot be used in patients with decompensated liver disease. Its main use is in the treatment of younger patients who do not wish to be on long-term therapy.
- Lamivudine achieves viral suppression more rapidly than adefovir, but not as potently as the other agents. There are increasing rates of drug resistance, but it is still frequently used in HIV/HBV co-infection.
- Adefovir is active against lamivudine-resistant virus, but up to 25% of patients show minimal viral suppression. Tenofovir has superseded it in most countries.
- Entecavir is potent, with low rates of drug resistance among the treatment-naïve. It is favoured in those with decompensated cirrhosis or renal insufficiency.
- Tenofovir is more potent than adefovir, and effective against wild-type and lamivudine-resistant virus. Its efficacy in those with adefovir-resistant HBV is limited.

Investigational treatments

- Selective targeting—conjugating antiviral agents to ligands that are selectively taken up by the liver.
- Viral entry inhibitors—a bile salt transporter (NTCP) is the host receptor for HBV. Trials of agents that block this receptor are ongoing.
- Interfering with transcription/translation of HBV DNA and RNA with antisense molecules or short interfering RNAs
- T-cell stimulation with thymic-derived peptides (thymosin)—studies suggest it increased the chance of clearing HBV DNA.
- HBV immunomodulatory vaccines—incorporating the pre-S antigens into hepatitis B vaccines might increase immunogenicity. A small trial suggested such a vaccine was associated with a higher rate of antiviral response, but its size and confounders made interpretation difficult. DNA and T-cell vaccines are in trials.
- Improving fibrosis—IFN-γ inhibits collagen synthesis and improved fibrosis scores in a small trial. Long-term significance is not clear.

Antivirals for hepatitis C

The aim of the treatment is the elimination of hepatitis C virus (HCV) RNA, predicted by achieving a 'sustained virological response' (SVR), defined as the absence of HCV RNA by PCR testing 6 months after stopping treatment. Treatment of genotype 1 infection has been revolutionized by the development of NS3/4A PIs and the direct-acting antivirals (DAAs). Dual therapy (IFN/ribavirin) saw only 40–50% of patients with genotype 1 HCV achieve an SVR. New combination therapies produce SVRs in 90% or more in some patient groups. Regimes vary with the genotype and nature of the initial response. For more details of treatment regimes and SVR rates, ➲ see Hepatitis C virus, pp. 418–21.

Interferon alfa

- IFN monotherapy has a role only in those who cannot tolerate ribavirin (e.g. severe haemoglobinopathies, renal failure). SVR rates are around 25% with genotype 1, and 54% with genotypes 2 and 3.

Ribavirin

- A guanosine analogue with broad-spectrum anti-RNA virus activity. Decreases hepatitis C infectivity by depletion of intracellular triphosphate pools and inhibition of viral-dependent RNA polymerase, potentiating IFN, and may induce mutations in viral RNA.
- Used in combination with peginterferon alfa (dual therapy) and, in some settings, a protease PI or DAA. No role as monotherapy outside special settings such as liver transplantation (modest improvement in histology does not improve morbidity/mortality).
- Cautions—it should not be used in those with severe renal insufficiency. It can cause haemolysis that may be severe in those with thalassaemia—transfusions may be required, and it may be appropriate to start chelation therapy before treatment in such patients.
- Pharmacology—rapidly absorbed PO, rapidly metabolized in the liver; excreted in the urine (50%) and faeces (15%), or retained in tissues.
- Side effects—haemolytic anaemia (monitor FBC; 10–15% require dose reduction, erythropoietin (epo) can help), pruritus, rash, hypersensitivity (rare), teratogenicity (accumulates in gonadal tissue—women AND men must adhere to strict contraception, while on therapy and for 6 months after), insomnia.

Protease inhibitors

The HCV RNA genome encodes a single polyprotein of 3000 amino acids. NS3/4A contains a serine protease that cleaves the viral protein.

- Telaprevir and boceprevir competitively inhibit the NS3 protease complex of HCV genotype 1.
    - Resistance—used alone, resistance emerges (within 2 weeks in some trials), due to the large number of quasi-species in an infected individual (poor fidelity of the RNA-dependent RNA polymerase).
    - Interactions—numerous. Cleared by CYP3A4/5 and should not be given in conjunction with medications that are inducers (carbamazepine, phenytoin, rifampicin, certain antiretrovirals) or are highly dependent upon it for clearance (methadone, certain triazoles, non-nucleoside reverse transcriptase inhibitors (NNRTIs), etc.). They also interfere with tacrolimus and ciclosporin dosing.
    - Side effects—*telaprevir* can cause rash, pruritus, anaemia, nausea, haemorrhoids, diarrhoea, anal discomfort, and fatigue. Severe rashes should prompt cessation of therapy with all three drugs. Stevens–Johnson syndrome/toxic epidermal necrolysis have occurred. Mild rashes may respond to topical steroids. *Boceprevir* may cause fatigue, anaemia, nausea, headache, diarrhoea, and QT prolongation. Neutropenia occurs more commonly in boceprevir than telaprevir regimes.
- Simeprevir is a second-generation PI used in combination for the treatment of genotype 1 or 4. Better tolerated, with fewer drug–drug interactions, than first-generation agents.

Other agents

- NS5A inhibitors—daclatasvir, ledipasvir. NS5A is a multifunction protein, important in viral replication and assembly. Inhibitors are active across genotypes, but with low barriers to resistance. Some agents available in fixed-dose combination tablets with other DAAs.
- NS5B inhibitors—NS5B is a viral RNA polymerase. Highly conserved across genotypes; thus agents have efficacy across all six genotypes. Two classes: nucleotide/side polymerase inhibitors and non-nucleoside analogues. The former group includes sofosbuvir and has a high barrier to resistance (NS5B active site intolerant to mutations). The latter class are less potent and more genotype-specific (mostly 1), e.g. dasabuvir available in a combination tablet.

Investigational treatments

- Ribavirin derivatives, e.g. taribavirin, modified with the intention of causing less anaemia and allowing higher doses. In trials.
- Novel viral targets, e.g. NS2/3 autoprotease, NS3 RNA helicase, NS5B RNA-dependent RNA polymerase (the development of the most promising NS5B polymerase inhibitors had to be halted due to severe neutropenia).
- Host factor targets—cyclophilin inhibitors (cyclophilin is a host cellular protein that modulates NS5A function; a non-immunosuppressive form of ciclosporin—alisporivir—is active against HCV and HIV in cell culture, but caused pancreatitis in clinical trials); microRNA (miR-122 is a liver microRNA which interacts with the HCV RNA genome, upregulating viral RNA in infected cells. An oligonucleotide designed to antagonize miR-122 has been shown to inhibit HCV RNA in chimpanzees).
- Vaccines—challenges include the substantial sequence diversity (six known genotypes), large number of viral quasi-species, and lack of an animal model. Several therapeutic vaccines in development (boosting the immune response with the aim of clearing a chronic infection).

Principles of HIV treatment

The development of potent combination antiretroviral drug therapies (ARTs) has resulted in dramatic falls in HIV-related morbidity and mortality. A number of problems remain: ongoing viral replication, emergence of drug resistance, high treatment failure rates, and concerns about the long-term metabolic complications of ART. Drug selection is more complex, with >20 agents now available. The benefits of ART in reducing morbidity and mortality in patients with CD4 counts of <200 cells/mm^3 are well established. Mounting evidence indicates that even earlier therapy leads to improved immunological recovery, and the treatment threshold is lowering steadily with the increasing number of better tolerated, more potent agents, and simpler regimes. Untreated HIV is itself a risk factor for coronary artery disease, kidney disease, neurological deficits, and malignancy, perhaps due to HIV-induced chronic inflammation. In 2012, the US Department of Health and Human Services (DHHS) and International Antiviral Society-USA

(IAS-USA) guidelines were revised to recommend ART to be offered to all HIV-infected, including asymptomatic, patients, regardless of the CD4 count. There is good evidence for this approach in those with CD4 counts of <500 cells/cm^3, and, while there are no RCTs comparing the treatment of those treated above 500 cells/cm^3 with those treated under, some observational data suggest a survival benefit.

Antiretroviral drugs

There are five main classes of antiretroviral drugs:

- nucleoside/nucleotide analogue reverse transcriptase inhibitors (NRTIs) (➔ see Nucleoside/nucleotide analogue reverse transcriptase inhibitors, pp. 104–6);
- NNRTIs (➔ see Non-nucleoside reverse transcriptase inhibitors, pp. 106–8);
- PIs (➔ see HIV protease inhibitors, pp. 108–9);
- entry inhibitors (➔ see Other HIV therapies, pp. 109–10);
- integrase strand transfer inhibitors (➔ Other HIV therapies, pp. 109–10).

Considerations when starting antiretroviral therapy

(See Table 4.2.)

Table 4.2 Recommendations for starting ART in adults

Disease stage	UK guidelines[a]	US guidelines[b]
Primary HIV infection	In AIDS-defining illness or CD4 <350 cells/mm^3 or neurological involvement	Consider treatment
Established infection, CD4 <350 cells/mm^3	Treat—strong RCT evidence	
Established infection, CD4 350–500 cells/mm^3	If HBV or HCV co-infection	Treat—observational evidence
Established infection, CD4 >500 cells/mm^3	Only in the situations below	Treat—expert opinion
Symptomatic disease or AIDS, including HIV nephropathy	Treat	Treat
Regardless of CD4, offer treatment to:	AIDS-defining condition, pregnant women, HBV co-infection (UK: only if HBV treatment is indicated if CD4 >500 cells/mm^3), those at risk of transmitting to an uninfected partner and they choose it, non-HIV-associated malignancy requiring immunosuppressive or radiotherapy	

CD4, CD4 T-cell count.

[a]BHIVA guidelines (2012). Available at: www.bhiva.org.

[b]US DHHS guidelines (2012). Available at: www.aidsinfo.nih.gov.

The aim of ART is to prolong and improve quality of life by maintaining viral load suppression and increasing the CD4 count for as long as possible. Suppression has the additional benefit of reducing the risk of onward transmission to an uninfected sexual partner. Factors determining when, and with what, to treat include:

- risk of disease progression (CD4 count, viral load);
- willingness of the patient to start therapy and ability to adhere;
- clinical effectiveness of the combination regimen;
- co-morbidity, e.g. TB, liver and cardiovascular disease, mental health;
- pill burden, dosing schedule, food considerations;
- adverse effects and drug–drug interactions (check the Liverpool interaction database at www.hiv-druginteractions.org; available as an app);
- gender, pregnancy potential, and CD4 count (if considering nevirapine);
- drug resistance potential/results of genotypic testing;
- future therapeutic options.

Primary HIV infection

The rationale for starting treatment during, or shortly after, infection is to attempt to maintain specific and robust CD4 T-cell responses, which are generally lost in chronic HIV infection. This should be balanced against the risks of toxicity, development of drug resistance, and difficulties of long-term adherence. It is not known whether treatment at this stage results in long-term benefit, and this remains an area of active research.

Established HIV infection

Any patient who is symptomatic or has a CD4 count of <500 cells/mm^3 should be offered therapy. The data supporting this recommendation are strongest for patients with a CD4 count of <200 cells/mm^3 or an AIDS-defining condition. It should be started, regardless of the CD4 cell count, in pregnant women, those with HIV-associated nephropathy, or HBV infection requiring treatment.

Initial regimen in treatment-naïve patients

Any antiretroviral regimen should be individualized to achieve the best potency, adherence, and tolerability, and to minimize drug interactions and toxicity. Although baseline drug resistance testing is recommended prior to starting ART, this is unavailable in developing countries. Regimens are described as having a 'backbone' and a 'base'. The backbone is usually two NRTIs, and the base an NNRTI or PI. A 2006 meta-analysis demonstrated that efavirenz-including regimes were superior to contemporary alternatives. More recent data have led the British HIV Association (BHIVA) (2013) to recommend efavirenz, raltegravir, ritonavir-boosted darunavir or atazanavir, or elvitegravir/cobicistat as suitable third agents in treatment-naïve patients. Mono- and dual therapy, or triple therapy with three NRTIs are not recommended. Recommended initial combinations are:

- NNRTI-based—NNRTI plus two NRTIs;
- PI-based—one to two PIs plus two NRTIs.

Nucleoside/nucleotide analogue reverse transcriptase inhibitors

HIV RT is an RNA-dependent DNA polymerase that is essential for virus replication. It enables transcription of viral RNA into a DNA copy, which is then integrated into the host genome. NRTIs are all nucleosides, with the exception of tenofovir which is a nucleotide. Within the cell, host enzymes phosphorylate the parent drug to an active triphosphate. This inhibits viral replication through competitive binding to the viral RT, resulting in termination of DNA chain elongation. They also inhibit mitochondrial DNA polymerase to a greater or lesser extent, resulting in toxicity. NRTIs (see Table 4.3) are commonly used in pairs as the backbone of HIV therapy in combination with an antiretroviral with a different mechanism of action (e.g. PI or NNRTI). Studies suggest the most effective pairing is tenofovir–emtricitabine. Certain pairing can be antagonistic, as they compete for phosphorylation, and should be avoided (zidovudine and stavudine; emtricitabine and lamivudine—both are cytosine analogues; didanosine and tenofovir—combined use associated with early virological failure and the selection of resistance mutations). For treatment guidelines, see ☞ www.bhiva.org and ☞ www.AIDSinfo.nih.gov.

Specific drugs

There are seven agents currently available. They vary in their efficacy and toxicity profiles.

- Didanosine (ddI) and stavudine (d4T) are no longer first choice, due to problems of mitochondrial toxicity (neuropathy, lactic acidosis) and relatively inferior potency, compared to other agents. They should not be used together, as they are synergistically toxic. d4T continues to be widely used in the developing world, but the 2010 WHO guidelines emphasize the need to eliminate its use, where possible, due to toxicity.
- Lamivudine (3TC) and emtricitabine (FTC) are both cytosine analogues and are essentially therapeutically interchangeable (and cannot be combined). They and tenofovir (TDF) have activity against hepatitis B and are useful in treating dual-infected patients.
- Abacavir (ABC), zidovudine (AZT, ZDV).

Resistance

- Caused by one or more mutations in the RT gene.
- Some specific mutations confer cross-resistance to other NRTIs.
- The rates of resistance in treatment-naïve patients in the UK is increasing, and the BHIVA recommends routine pre-therapy resistance testing. Knowledge of the predominant mutations present allows inference of resistance to various antiretrovirals.[1]

Pharmacology

- Variable oral absorption (25–93%), which may be reduced by food (ddI especially). Variable CSF penetration (12–50%).
- Pregnancy—cross the placenta, secreted in breast milk. 3TC and AZT have the most data on use in pregnancy and tend to be preferred. Other NRTIs, excepting tenofovir, are considered alternatives.

Table 4.3 Characteristics of NRTIs

Drug	Pharmacology	Adverse effects
Abacavir	83% oral bioavailability; metabolized in liver, thus useful in those with severe renal impairment. May be less effective in those with high viral loads	May be associated with an increased risk of myocardial infarction—use with caution in those at risk of cardiovascular disease. Potentially fatal hypersensitivity associated with HLA B5701. Usually appears within 6 weeks. Immediately discontinue, and NEVER rechallenge
Didanosine	Take 1h before, or 2h after, meals; 30–40% oral bioavailability; renal excretion 50%—adjust dose in renal impairment	Pancreatitis (<7%), peripheral neuropathy (25%). Co-administration with tenofovir increases didanosine levels
Emtricitabine	93% oral bioavailability, not affected by food; renal excretion—adjust dose in renal impairment	Minimal toxicity
Lamivudine	86% oral bioavailability, not affected by food; renal excretion—adjust dose in renal impairment. Can be given od or bd	Minimal toxicity
Stavudine	86% oral bioavailability; renal excretion 50%—adjust dose in renal impairment	Peripheral neuropathy, pancreatitis, lipodystrophy, rapidly progressive ascending neuromuscular weakness (rare)
Tenofovir	Bioavailability: 25% if fasting, 39% with high-fat meal; renal excretion—adjust dose in renal impairment, but best avoided in these cases, if possible, particularly in those receiving other nephrotoxic medications. Monitor renal function every 6–12 months in all patients	Renal insufficiency, Fanconi syndrome (glycosuria, hypophosphataemia, acute tubular necrosis). Co-administration with didanosine increases didanosine levels. Do not use with unboosted atazanavir (reduces atazanavir levels)
Zidovudine	60% oral bioavailability; metabolized to glucuronide, renal excretion of metabolite	Bone marrow suppression

- Excretion—most NRTIs are renally excreted, and doses must be reduced or dosing intervals extended in renal impairment. The exceptions are abacavir and zidovudine which are metabolized in the liver. They may not require dose change in renal impairment but may need reduction in hepatic impairment. Combination preparations are not recommended in renal impairment, as the components may need separate dose adjustments.
- Relatively few drug–drug interactions, as they do not interact with P450 enzymes.

Adverse effects

- Mitochondrial toxicity—neuropathy, pancreatitis, lipodystrophy, hepatic steatosis, lactic acidosis (rare but may be fatal). Risk depends on the relative affinity for the mitochondrial DNA polymerase—ddI and d4T are the worst.
- Other—myelosuppression (AZT), hypersensitivity (ABC).

Reference

1 Stanford University HIV Drug Resistance Database. Available at: hivdb.stanford.edu.

Non-nucleoside reverse transcriptase inhibitors

RT inhibitors that act at a site separate from that of NRTIs. Highly effective at reducing HIV-1 viraemia and increasing CD4 counts when included in combination therapy. Not active against HIV-2 (see Table 4.4).

Specific drugs

- First generation: efavirenz, nevirapine, and delaviridine. Nevirapine-containing regimens are as potent as efavirenz but have a higher incidence of serious adverse toxicities (hepatitis, Stevens–Johnson syndrome). It should be considered as an alternative to efavirenz, e.g. in those hoping to become pregnant.
- Second generation (diarylpyrimidines): etravirine, rilpivirine.

Resistance

- Associated with mutations in the RT gene. A mutation associated with resistance to one first-generation agent will show cross-resistance to the other two. Second-generation agents may remain effective, depending on the specific mutation.
- Potential for the emergence of resistance when an NNRTI-containing regime is discontinued, due to their long half-life ('the tail'). When a combination is stopped, the NRTI components are quickly cleared from the serum, while the NNRTI remains for 7–10 days. It is suggested that stopping the NNRTI 7 days before the NRTIs may prevent this.

Table 4.4 Characteristics of NNRTIs

Drug	Pharmacology	Adverse effects
Efavirenz	Take on an empty stomach at night (reduces levels and side effects); mixed CYP3A4 inducer and inhibitor; variable serum levels due to genetic variations in CYP metabolism; excretion: 14–34% in urine, 16–61% in faeces. No dose adjustment required in renal failure	CNS/neuropsychiatric symptoms (>50%, e.g. sleep disturbance, rarely agitation, hallucinations), increased transaminases. Most settle over 2–4 weeks. Also rash, false-positive cannabinoid test, teratogenic in monkeys, liver failure
Nevirapine	>90% oral bioavailability; CYP3A4 inducer, thus multiple drug interactions—rifampicin can reduce levels; excretion: 80% in urine, 10% in faeces. Used in pregnancy if CD4 <250 cells/mm^3	Rash, hepatitis, Stevens–Johnson syndrome, toxic epidermal necrolysis, DRESS syndrome (drug rash with eosinophilia and systemic symptoms)
Rilpivirine	Well absorbed with food. Inhibits CYP3A. Many interactions. Little data on renal or hepatic dosing. Do not use in patients on proton pump inhibitors	QT prolongation. Otherwise well tolerated, with less rash/CNS effects than efavirenz
Etravirine	Take with food; oral bioavailability not known; 99% protein-bound; metabolized by CYP3A4; eliminated in faeces and urine. Effective in those with documented NNRTI resistance mutations	Rash, GI symptoms, fatigue, peripheral neuropathy, headache, hypertension

Pharmacology and side effects

- Well absorbed PO and metabolized by cytochrome P450 system, thus multiple drug interactions. All have long half-lives.
- Excretion of metabolites in the urine and unchanged drug in the faeces.

Prescribing points

- Delaviridine—least potent NRTI, requires dosing three times daily (tds). Rarely used.
- Efavirenz—>50% of patients experience sleep disturbance and mild neuropsychiatric effects. Reduced by evening dosing on an empty stomach (reduces peak levels) and often settles over 2–4 weeks. Suitable for patients with high viral loads and high CD4s. Potentially teratogenic (animal data).
- Nevirapine—relatively high rates of hypersensitivity. Discontinue in any patient who presents with rash, fever, or weight loss. This usually occurs in the first 6 weeks. Risk factors include CD4 >250 cells/mm^3. Hepatotoxicity is commonest in the first 3 months, and the risk is increased in women with CD4 >250, and men with CD4 >400 cells/mm^3. However, treatment-experienced patients with high CD4 and viral suppression have no increased risk of hepatotoxicity when switching to nevirapine. It can be used in pregnancy.

- Nevirapine—induces its own metabolism (like efavirenz); thus, to reduce the incidence of side effects, it is started at a lower dose (200mg od) for 2 weeks before increasing to the standard dose (200mg bd). If treatment stops for >1 week, it should be started at the lower dose once again.
- Rilpivirine—for use only in patients with baseline viraemia of <100 000 copies/mL; studies comparing it to efavirenz demonstrated greater virologic failure in those with viral loads above this. Those developing virologic failure on rilpivirine are more likely to be cross-resistant to other NNRTIs than those who develop virologic failure on efavirenz. They are also more likely to develop resistance to their NRTIs. Available as od combination with tenofovir and emtricitabine.
- Etravirine—a flexible molecule that can fit into the RT active site in a number of ways, even in the presence of certain NNRTI resistance mutations. Thus, it may be effective where other members are not. Useful in highly treatment-experienced patients, but it should be combined with more than just two NRTIs (e.g. with a PI).

HIV protease inhibitors

Structurally related molecules that represent synthetic analogues of one of the HIV *gag-pol* cleavage sites. They are used in combination with NRTIs for treatment and post-exposure prophylaxis (PEP) of HIV infection. They differ widely in absorption, half-life, and metabolism, and thus also vary in administration (e.g. with/without food) and dosing frequency. Incorrect administration can reduce bioavailability significantly, predisposing to the development of resistance. There is also significant potential for drug interactions; even garlic supplements can drop levels by 50%, and proton pump inhibitors (PPIs) may increase (saquinavir) or dramatically decrease (atazanavir) levels.

Pharmacology

- Oral absorption varies with the agent. Metabolized by cytochrome P450. Eliminated primarily in the faeces. Poor CNS penetration.
- Ritonavir—rarely used simply therapeutically, is co-administered with other PIs to boost their levels through potent inhibition of hepatic CYP450 3A4 (which all PIs do to a greater or lesser extent). This results in better trough levels and less pills. Saquinavir, atazanavir, fosamprenavir, tipranavir, and darunavir are all approved for use in boosted regimes (ritonavir administered separately), and lopinavir is available in co-formulation with ritonavir (LPV/r, Kaletra®).

Mechanisms of action and resistance

Inhibits HIV protease-mediated cleavage of viral polypeptides into structural proteins and viral enzymes. Resistance emerges as a result of mutations in the HIV protease gene—many confer cross-resistance to other PIs. The newer PIs, especially if boosted with ritonavir, have a high genetic barrier to resistance (an accumulation of multiple mutations is required), and treatment failure is rarely due to PI resistance.

Prescribing points

- Lopinavir/ritonavir (Kaletra®)—the preferred PI for pregnant treatment-naïve patients.
- Saquinavir—may be used as an alternative to lopinavir/ritonavir in pregnancy. However, high pill burden (some formulations), GI side effects, and may cause PR/QT prolongation, thus not preferred.
- Fosamprenavir—pro-drug of amprenavir. Levels reduced by ranitidine.
- Atazanavir—a newer agent with favourable effects on lipids, compared to other PIs. Trials suggest it is as effective as efavirenz in treatment-naïve patients. Uniquely, it requires an acidic gastric pH for absorption.
- Tipranavir—active against strains of HIV resistant to other PIs. For use only in treatment-experienced patients with PI resistance.
- Darunavir—active against many PI-resistant HIV strains. od dosing possible for treatment-naïve patients. Higher dosing for those with resistance mutations.
- Indinavir and nelfinavir are older PIs with inconvenient dosing schedules and poor side effect profiles (e.g. renal stones in 25% with the former)—they are less widely used today.

Toxicity and side effects

- GI symptoms (nausea, vomiting, diarrhoea), hepatotoxicity.
- Neurological symptoms (headache, paraesthesiae).
- Skin rash, lipodystrophy (long-term).
- Metabolic (insulin resistance, diabetes, hyperlipidaemia).
- QT prolongation, bleeding in haemophilia patients.
- Darunavir, fosamprenavir, and tipranavir have a sulfa component and should be used cautiously in those with allergies to sulfonamides.

Interactions

There are numerous, potentially dangerous drug interactions. Check an online interaction database.[2] Common drugs that should *not* be administered with PIs include amiodarone, lidocaine (IV), terfenadine, ergot derivatives, midazolam, rifampicin, simvastatin, sildenafil, St John's wort.

Reference

2 University of Liverpool. HIV drug interactions. Available at: ℛ www.hiv-druginteractions.org.

Other HIV therapies

- The fusion entry inhibitor enfuvirtide (T20).
- Chemokine receptor antagonists—maraviroc, vicriviroc (in phase II trials).
- Integrase inhibitors—raltegravir, dolutegravir, elvitegravir.
- Experimental therapies such as therapeutic vaccines designed to boost host response to HIV and immunotherapy (interleukin (IL)-2 was thought promising but was of no clinical benefit, despite increases in CD4).

Enfuvirtide (T20)

- The first of a new class of drugs called the entry inhibitors; it binds to the HIV surface protein gp41, preventing binding of gp41 to CD4 cells.
- Reserved for use in treatment-experienced patients.
- Given bd by s/c injection.
- Side effects include injection site reactions, increased risk of bacterial pneumonia, and hypersensitivity reactions (<1%).

Maraviroc (MVC)

- HIV enters cells via CD4 and one of its co-receptors, either CCR5 or CXCR4. HIV viral strains from patients with early infection use CCR5, whereas about half of the strains in patients with advanced immunosuppression use CXCR4 or both.
- MVC is a chemokine receptor antagonist that prevents the binding of CCR5-tropic HIV virus to the CCR5 receptor on CD4 T cells.
- Used in highly treatment-experienced patients and requires a tropism assay prior to initiating treatment to determine if the virus is CCR5 (susceptible) or CXCR4 (not susceptible). This is determined by amplifying the HIV *env* gene from RNA in the patient's plasma to generate recombinant virions that are used to infect cell lines expressing CD4 and either CXCR4 or CCR5. Genotypic assays are in development.
- Given PO (no food effect), metabolized in the liver by CYP3A.
- Side effects—abdominal pain, cough, dizziness, musculoskeletal symptoms, pyrexia, rash, URTIs, hepatotoxicity, postural hypotension. Generally well tolerated.

Raltegravir (RAL) and dolutegravir (DTG)

- Inhibits HIV-1 integrase and hence prevents the insertion of viral genetic material into the human chromosome (strand transfer inhibitor). Used in treatment-experienced patients.

Chapter 5

Antiparasitic therapy

Antimalarials *112*
Quinolines *113*
Antifolates *116*
Other agents and combination therapies *116*
Artemisinin and its derivatives *117*
Antiprotozoal drugs *119*
Antihelminthic drugs *124*

Antimalarials

Antimalarial drugs are used for both the treatment and prevention of malaria (see Box 5.1). Most drugs act upon the erythrocytic stage of the parasite life cycle. Artemisinins additionally act on gametocytes—potentially reducing onward transmission—and have been shown to reduce mortality, compared to quinine. As ever, the emergence of resistance is a major threat to malaria control and treatment. Combination treatment can reduce the chance of resistance emerging, and the WHO has called for the banning of all oral artemisinin monotherapy.

Resistance

Arises through the selection of rare naturally occurring mutants with reduced drug susceptibility. Unlike bacteria, plasmodia do not have transferable resistance mechanisms, but they are eukaryotes, and can acquire or lose polygenic resistance mechanisms during meiosis. Individual mechanisms are discussed on ➔ *Plasmodium* species (malaria), pp. 512–4.

Combination therapy

Treating malaria with a suitably chosen drug combination increases efficacy, may shorten treatment duration (increasing compliance), and decreases the risk of resistant parasites arising by mutation. If each drug has a different mechanism of action, then the per-parasite probability of developing resistance is the product of their individual per-parasite probabilities. They are, however, more expensive (but short-term cost is easily outweighed by longer-term benefits), and, if there is already high resistance to one of the components (perhaps through previous monotherapy), then resistance can arise to the other.

Box 5.1 Guidelines for prevention and treatment of malaria

Treatment

- UK guidelines:
  - Lalloo D, Shingadia D, Pasvol G, *et al*. UK malaria treatment guidelines. *J Infect* 2016;72(6):635–64
  - Public Health England. Guideline for malaria prevention in travellers from the UK 2015
  - Both available at www.britishinfection.org/guidelines-resources/published-guidelines/
  - See also sections on treatment and prophylaxis of malaria in the *BNF* (www.bnf.org)
- US guidelines:
  - Treatment of malaria (guidelines for clinicians) 2013. Available at http://www.cdc.gov/malaria/resources/pdf/clinicalguidance.pdf
  - *The Yellow Book*. CDC health information for international travel 2016, Chapter 3, Malaria. Available at wwwnc.cdc.gov/travel/yellowbook/2016/infectious-diseases-related-to-travel/malaria
- World Health Organization:
  - 2015 *Guidelines for the treatment of malaria*, third edition. Available at www.who.int/malaria/publications/atoz/9789241549127/en/

Key prescribing points

- Uncomplicated non-falciparum malaria can be treated with chloroquine. Resistance should be considered in cases of *Plasmodium vivax* acquired from Indonesia or Papua New Guinea, or if parasitaemia fails to fall after 4 days of therapy.
- Where *P. falciparum* co-circulates with non-falciparum species, it is wise to treat with a falciparum-active agent.
- Following treatment of *P. vivax* or *Plasmodium ovale*, anti-relapse therapy should be given with primaquine (contraindicated in pregnancy)—the only quinoline with reliable activity on hypnozoites. It should ideally start after G6PD testing and near the start of chloroquine therapy. *P. vivax* is treated at a higher dose than *P. ovale*.
- While chloroquine-sensitive falciparum malaria does occur, it should only be used for treatment when there is certainty about the region of exposure and local parasite sensitivities.
- The WHO recommends artemisinin combination therapies (ACTs) as first-line treatment for uncomplicated falciparum malaria. They have the fastest parasite clearance times.
- Severe falciparum malaria should be treated with IV artesunate, if available (studies demonstrate mortality benefit, compared to quinine). It has a short half-life, and monotherapy of <5–7 days has been associated with parasite recrudescence. Thus, in practice, once patients are well enough to take oral medication, they should be switched to complete a full course of ACT (usually 3 days). Alternative—IV quinine (watch for hypoglycaemia), combined with a second agent (e.g. doxycycline, clindamycin), for 7 days or a complete course of ACT, once well enough to swallow.

Quinolines

Quinolines (not to be confused with quino*lones*) have been the mainstay of antimalarial therapy since the seventeenth century when Peruvian Indians used the bark of the cinchona tree. Chloroquine has succumbed to global resistance in *P. falciparum*. Quinine remains widely used. Primaquine is notable for its additional activity on intrahepatic forms and gametocytes.

Quinine

- A quinoline methanol derived from the bark of the cinchona tree. Inhibits erythrocytic stages of human malaria parasites, but not all liver stages. It is active against gametocytes of *P. vivax, P. ovale*, and *P. malariae*. It is the most widely available parenteral agent.
- Mode of action—accumulates in the parasite food vacuole, forming a complex with haem. This results in the inhibition of haem polymerase and accumulation of cytotoxic free haem.
- Resistance—widespread in South East Asia where some strains are also resistant to chloroquine, mefloquine, and sulfadoxine–pyrimethamine. Cross-resistance with mefloquine in Central Africa.
- Pharmacology—well absorbed PO; IM administration more predictable than IV administration. Hepatic metabolism. Urinary clearance <20%. Give a loading dose if the patient has not received a related agent.

- Adverse effects—cinchonism (tinnitus, vomiting, diarrhoea, headache), hypoglycaemia (stimulates insulin production—monitor blood glucose), hypotension, cardiac arrhythmias, haemolytic anaemia (blackwater fever). Cinchonism is observed in most patients, resolves upon completion, and should not prompt a change in dose.
- Use—treatment of falciparum malaria and can be given IV in severe disease. Quinidine (a stereoisomer of quinine) is more commonly used in the USA but has greater cardiotoxicity (QT prolongation, ventricular tachycardia).

Chloroquine

- A synthetic 4-aminoquinoline, active against erythrocytic stages of all four human malaria species and gametocytes of *P. vivax, P. ovale*, and *P. malariae*. However, *P. falciparum* resistance is now widespread, due to increased drug efflux (mutation in the *pfmdr1* gene) and/or decreased drug uptake (mutation in the *pfCRT* gene). It remains effective for the treatment of *P. ovale, P. malariae*, and *P. vivax* in most regions.
- Pharmacology—80–90% oral absorption. Widely distributed. Extensive tissue binding, with high affinity for melanin-containing tissues. Extensive metabolism to active metabolite; 50% renal excretion.
- Adverse effects—dizziness, headache, rashes, nausea, diarrhoea, pruritus. Long-term treatment may cause CNS effects and retinopathy. Rarely, photosensitivity, tinnitus, and deafness may occur.
- Use—prophylaxis and treatment of chloroquine-sensitive malaria.

Mefloquine

- A synthetic 4-quinoline methanol. Active against erythrocytic stages of *Plasmodium* spp. Effective against strains of *P. falciparum* that are resistant to chloroquine, sulfonamides, and pyrimethamine. Also active against bacteria (e.g. MRSA) and some fungi.
- Resistance—increasing; 15% high-grade resistance and 50% low-grade resistance in South East Asia. Cross-resistance with quinine and halofantrine. Inverse relationship with chloroquine resistance.
- Pharmacology—well absorbed PO, concentrated in erythrocytes, metabolites not active, predominantly excreted in the bile.
- Adverse effects—nausea, dizziness, fatigue, confusion, sleep disturbance, pneumonitis (steroids may be required). Psychosis, encephalopathy, and convulsions in 1/1200–1700 patients (thus, when used as prophylaxis, tends to be started 2–3 weeks before it is required, to assess tolerability); 1/10 000 risk of serious toxicity in prophylaxis.
- Use—prophylaxis in areas of chloroquine resistance. Treatment of uncomplicated MDR malaria.

Amodiaquine

- A 4-aminoquinoline, active against *P. falciparum* and *P. vivax*.
- Pharmacologically similar to chloroquine, with which it is cross-resistant. Elimination half-life of 1–3 weeks.
- Adverse effects appear to be related to immunogenic properties of its metabolites, rather than direct toxicity. Severe/life-threatening adverse events have been associated with prophylaxis—agranulocytosis,

hepatotoxicity, aplastic anaemia—but it is well tolerated when given as a 3-day treatment course. Adverse events increased in those with HIV.
- Use—treatment of falciparum malaria, often in combination with artesunate. No longer available in the USA.

Piperaquine
- A 4-aminoquinoline; structurally related to chloroquine, but active against chloroquine-resistant *P. falciparum*.
- Pharmacology—well absorbed PO; elimination half-life 17 days.
- Combination with dihydroartemisinin has shown excellent tolerability and high cure rates of MDR falciparum malaria.

Primaquine
- A synthetic 8-aminoquinoline, formulated as diphosphate. Active against hepatic stages of *Plasmodia* spp., including the hypnozoite stage of *P. vivax*. Poor activity against erythrocytic stages, but active against gametocytes. Also active against *Pneumocystis* spp., *Babesia* spp., *Leishmania* spp., and *Trypanosoma cruzi*.
- Resistance—failure rates of up to 35% reported in South East Asia in patients treated for *P. vivax*.
- Pharmacology—well absorbed PO, extensive tissue distribution, metabolized to carboxyprimaquine, methoxy and hydroxy metabolites; <4% excreted unchanged in the urine.
- Adverse effects are generally mild—abdominal cramps, anaemia, leucocytosis, methaemoglobinaemia. Haemolysis occurs in G6PD deficiency (check G6PD levels first).
- Use—treatment of *P. vivax* and *P. ovale*. Second line for treatment of *P. jiroveci* (in combination with clindamycin).

Tafenoquine
- An 8-aminoquinoline with activity against *P. falciparum* and hepatic stages of *P. vivax* and *P. ovale*.
- Pharmacology—similar to primaquine, but more potent, less toxic, and longer half-life (14 days), enabling weekly or monthly administration.
- Adverse effects—methaemoglobinaemia, haemolysis in G6PD deficiency.
- Use—prophylaxis and treatment of malaria.

Lumefantrine
- Similar structure to 4-methanol quinolines. Inhibits erythrocytic stages of *Plasmodium* spp., including most chloroquine-resistant parasites. Mostly used in combination with artemether derivatives. Halofantrine is a related compound with greater cardiac toxicity.
- Resistance reported in Central and West Africa and Thailand. Cross-resistance with mefloquine.
- Pharmacology—widely variable absorption, bioavailability increased by a fatty meal. Not concentrated in erythrocytes; 20–30% metabolized by the CYP450 enzyme system. Little excreted in the urine.
- Adverse effects—abdominal pain, diarrhoea, pruritus. High doses are cardiotoxic with prolongation of PR and QT intervals; mefloquine enhances these effects, and sequential use is contraindicated.
- Use—treatment of MDR falciparum malaria.

Antifolates

The antimalarial activity of the biguanides (proguanil) was discovered during the Second World War. Along with the diaminopyrimidines (pyrimethamine), they are referred to as the antifolate drugs and used in combination with other agents for both prophylaxis and treatment.

Proguanil

- A synthetic arylbiguanide. Its metabolite cycloguanil inhibits the erythrocytic stages of all four *Plasmodium* spp. and the hepatic stage of *P. falciparum*. Acts synergistically with atovaquone.
- Resistance arises easily by point mutation in the *DHFR* gene. Worldwide for *P. falciparum*, and reported for *P. vivax* and *P. malariae* in South East Asia.
- Pharmacology—>90% oral absorption; 75% protein-bound; concentrated in erythrocytes; 20% metabolized by the CYP450 enzyme system to cycloguanil (active metabolite). Non-metabolizers occur in Japan and Kenya, leading to resistance; 60% excreted in the urine.
- Adverse effects—GI and renal effects at high doses (>600mg/day).
- Use—antimalarial prophylaxis (with chloroquine); treatment and prophylaxis of drug-resistant falciparum malaria (with atovaquone).

Pyrimethamine

- A synthetic diaminopyrimidine. Active against *Plasmodium* spp., *T. gondii*, and *P. jiroveci*.
- Available as a single agent or in combination with sulfadoxine (not considered combination therapy, as components act on enzymes in the same pathway), dapsone, or mefloquine and sulfadoxine.
- Resistance is due to point mutations on the *DHFR* gene and is widespread in Africa and Latin America. Sequence variations in *P. falciparum* and mutations in the *pfmdr1* gene may also be important. Sulfadoxine resistance is due to mutations in its target dihydropteroate synthase (DHPS).
- Pharmacology—well absorbed PO. Long plasma half-life (111h). CSF levels 10–25% of plasma levels. Secreted in breast milk and crosses the placenta. Hepatic metabolism.
- Adverse effects—megaloblastic anaemia, leucopenia, thrombocytopenia, pancytopenia. Very large doses in children have caused vomiting, convulsions, respiratory failure, and death. Aggravation of subclinical folate deficiency. Teratogenic in animals.
- Use—treatment of malaria in combination with other drugs; treatment of toxoplasmosis and PCP.

Other agents and combination therapies

Atovaquone

- Atovaquone is a hydroxynaphthoquinone that is more active than standard antimalarials against all stages of *P. falciparum*. It is also active against *Babesia* spp., *T. gondii*, and *P. jiroveci*. It blocks the parasite mitochondrial electron transport chain.

- Malaria resistance emerges rapidly, due to point mutations in the parasite's cytochrome bc_1 gene. It is therefore used in combination with proguanil, with which it has synergistic activity.
- Pharmacology—poor oral absorption, improved when given with meals; 99% protein-bound; poor CSF penetration (<1%). Not metabolized. Elimination half-life 73h.
- Adverse effects—fever, nausea, diarrhoea, and rash.
- Use—prophylaxis and treatment of malaria in combination with proguanil; treatment of PCP (atovaquone alone).

Chlorproguanil–dapsone

- Dapsone (➲ see Antileprotics, pp. 75–7) is a sulfa drug that has been combined with chlorproguanil and developed as an affordable combination treatment for African children.
- Although well tolerated and efficacious, it is associated with a higher frequency of serious haematological toxicity than sulfadoxine–pyrimethamine.
- There are also concerns about the potential emergence of cross-resistance to this combination in areas where resistance to sulfadoxine–pyrimethamine is already high.

Tetracycline and doxycycline

- Tetracycline and doxycycline (➲ see Tetracyclines, pp. 56–8) are both protein synthesis inhibitors. They are well absorbed PO, with elimination half-lives of 8h (tetracycline) and 20h (doxycycline).
- Quinine plus tetracycline has been used for treatment of MDR falciparum malaria in Thailand for years.
- Quinine plus doxycycline is recommended for treatment of falciparum malaria in the UK. Doxycycline is also used in prophylaxis of malaria in regions with chloroquine or mefloquine resistance.
- Main limitations—contraindicated in children and pregnant women; photosensitivity with doxycycline; emergence of parasite resistance to tetracycline in areas where it has been extensively used.

Clindamycin

- Clindamycin (➲ see Lincosamides, pp. 51–2) is a lincosamide antibiotic that also acts on the malaria parasite's apicoplast.
- Although numerous studies of quinine plus clindamycin have shown good efficacy and safety profiles in various populations, it has never been widely used.

Artemisinin and its derivatives

Artemisinin (qinghao) is derived from *Artemisia annua* (sweet wormwood). Chinese herbalists have used it for 2000 years. Most clinically important artemisinins are metabolized to dihydroartemisinin, in which form they have comparable antimalarial activity. They are the most effective group of anti-malarial agents and act against quinine-resistant parasites. Although widely used in the developing world to treat malaria, their use in the developed world is hampered by a lack of availability of good manufacturing practice (GMP) products. Oral use in uncomplicated malaria should always be in combination with another agent.

Mode of action

Unclear. They contain an unusual peroxide bridge, believed to be responsible for its action. This may disrupt redox homeostasis, resulting in the production of reactive oxygen radicals. Blood stages of *Plasmodium* spp. are rapidly killed, including gametocytes (the form infective to mosquitoes), thus leading to reduced transmission. In both uncomplicated and severe infections, they have shown faster fever and parasite clearance times than any other agent (including quinine), and are effective in cerebral malaria.

Resistance

Reduced susceptibility has been reported in Cambodia (2008) and Thailand (2012). This resulted in delayed parasite clearance times and it is thought that this has arisen as a result of oral monotherapy. The WHO has called for the banning of all artemisinin monotherapy worldwide.

Agents

- Artemisinin—the original agent. It has poor bioavailability (improved upon in the semi-synthetic derivatives; ➲ see Artemisinin combination therapies, pp. 118–9). Concentrated in erythrocytes and hydrolysed to dihydroartemisinin. Metabolized by hepatic cytochromes. Peak concentrations after 1–3h. Elimination half-life <30min. Can be given PR. Adverse effects include drug-induced fever, reversible decrease in reticulocytes, and neurotoxicity in animal models. Also active against *T. gondii*, *Leishmania major*, and *Schistosoma mansoni* in experimental models.
- Dihydroartemisinin—the active metabolite of artemisinin. Can be given PO and used in treatment of uncomplicated malaria.
- Artemether and arthether—esters of dihydroartemisinin; preparations are oil-based and can be given PO, PR, or IM. Absorbed slowly and erratically, so not suitable for severely ill patients.
- Artesunate—water-soluble hemisuccinate of dihydroartemisinin that may be given PO, PR, or IV. Widely used in the developing world. It is not licensed in the UK or USA, but available on request from most regional ID units (and the CDC in the USA). It is the drug of choice for severe *P. falciparum* malaria, being superior to quinine in efficacy (mortality 15% versus 24%) and tolerability. Counterfeit artesunate (containing little or no active drug) has been sold in South East Asia since the late 1980s. This threatens successful treatment and may have facilitated the emergence of reduced susceptibility recently observed in Cambodia. Side effects include transient neurological abnormalities (e.g. balance) and neutropenia.

Artemisinin combination therapies

The best treatments for uncomplicated falciparum malaria. They combine a highly effective short-acting artemisinin with a longer-acting agent to protect against resistance, and are rapidly and reliably effective. Resistance in the partner drug limits the use of certain combinations. They are safe and well tolerated, although hypersensitivity may occasionally occur. The partner drug determines the adverse effect profiles. They should not be used in the first trimester of pregnancy (safety not established), unless there is no alternative. They are usually given as a 3-day course in a fixed-dose tablet.

- Artesunate–mefloquine—safe, well tolerated, and highly effective. Used in Thailand, South America, and Africa. Disadvantages include its

price and the pharmacokinetic mismatch of its components. However, in Thailand, resistance to mefloquine has actually decreased since its introduction.
- Artesunate–sulfadoxine–pyrimethamine—initially gave promising results in African children, but subsequent studies have been disappointing.
- Artesunate–amodiaquine—one African multicentre trial showed better overall efficacy than amodiaquine alone, but 6% of patients developed neutropenia. The pharmacokinetic mismatch of the components raises concerns about prolonged exposure of parasites to amodiaquine. There is increasing resistance in eastern and southern Africa.
- Artemether–lumefantrine—first fixed-dose combination of artemisinin derivative and another drug. It has become increasingly available in tropical countries, and is well tolerated and affordable ($1). It has been associated with irreversible hearing loss. Pharmacokinetic mismatch of components necessitates a complex 3-day dosing regimen. Widely available in the UK.
- Dihydroartemisinin–piperaquine—good tolerability, high cure rates in MDR falciparum malaria in Cambodia, Vietnam, and Thailand. The slow elimination of piperaquine determines parasitological efficacy and post-treatment prophylactic effect.

Antiprotozoal drugs

Albendazole

- Binds to tubulin, affecting cytoskeleton function. Active against a variety of helminths and some protozoal infections, including giardiasis, microsporidiosis, intestinal worm infections, trichinosis, cutaneous larva migrans, hydatid disease, neurocysticercosis, and lymphatic filariasis.

Amphotericin

(➲ See Polyenes, pp. 80–1.)
- A polyene antifungal active against a variety of fungi and some protozoa, e.g. *Leishmania* spp., *Naegleria*, and *Hartmanella*. Used in the treatment of leishmaniasis.

Antimony compounds

- Sodium stibogluconate is a pentavalent antimonal compound used in the treatment of leishmaniasis. It is active against amastigotes within macrophages. Different species vary in sensitivity.
- Acquired resistance results in poor response and high resistance rates. Relapse also common in immunosuppressed or HIV patients.
- Pharmacology—given IM or IV, with peak concentrations occurring after 1h. Slow accumulation in the CNS and tissues. Excreted in the urine.
- Adverse effects—cough/vomiting (if infused too quickly), arthralgia, myalgia, bradycardia, abdominal cramps, diarrhoea, rash, pruritus, raised LFTs, raised creatinine, raised amylase.

Atovaquone

(➲ See Antimalarials, pp. 112–3.)
- Antimalarial with activity against other protozoa, e.g. *Babesia* spp., *T. gondii*, and *P. jiroveci*.

Benznidazole

- A synthetic 2-nitroimidazole active against *T. cruzi* (Chagas' disease).
- Pharmacology—well absorbed PO.
- Adverse effects—photosensitivity (50%), anorexia, nausea, vomiting, abdominal pain, disorientation, insomnia, paraesthesiae, polyneuritis, seizures.

Ciprofloxacin

(➔ See Quinolones, pp. 62–4.)

- A fluoroquinolone antibiotic with activity against *Cyclospora cayetanensis* and *Isospora belli*. Used as a second-line treatment option.

Clarithromycin

(➔ See Macrolides, pp. 48–50.)

- A macrolide antibiotic with activity against *T. gondii*. A second-line treatment option.

Clindamycin

(➔ See Lincosamides, pp. 51–2.)

- A lincosamide antibiotic with activity against some protozoa, e.g. *P. falciparum, Babesia* spp., *T. gondii*, and *P. jiroveci*.
- Use—second-line treatment of *P. jiroveci* pneumonia; second-line treatment and secondary prophylaxis of cerebral toxoplasmosis.

Co-trimoxazole

(➔ See Co-trimoxazole, pp. 61–2.)

- A diaminopyrimidine–sulfonamide antibiotic with useful activity against *P. jiroveci* (first line), *T. gondii, C. cayetanensis*, and *I. belli*.

Dapsone

(➔ See Antileprotics, pp. 75–7.)

- Sulfonamide derivative, active against *M. leprae, Plasmodium* spp., *T. gondii*, and *P. jiroveci*. Main use is the treatment and prophylaxis of *P. jiroveci* pneumonia and cerebral toxoplasmosis.

Diloxanide furoate

- Dichloromethylacetamide, active against *Entamoeba histolytica*.
- Resistance—none reported.
- Pharmacology—limited human data. Animal data show rapid oral absorption, hydrolysed in the gut, 75% excreted via kidneys within 24h.
- Adverse effects—nausea, vomiting, abdominal distension, flatulence, pruritus, urticarial.
- Use—treatment of intestinal amoebiasis, eradication of cysts after acute amoebiasis.

Eflornithine

- Inhibits parasite growth by inhibition of ornithine carboxylase (required for cellular replications and differentiation). Active against *Trypanosoma brucei gambiense. In vitro* (not used clinically) activity against *P. falciparum, Leishmania* promastigotes, and *Giardia lamblia*.
- Pharmacology—given IV, plasma half-life 3h, good CNS penetration, rapid renal excretion.

- Adverse effects—osmotic diarrhoea, bone marrow suppression, convulsions, hair loss.
- Use—late-stage *T.b. gambiense* infections. NOT effective in *T.b. rhodesiense* infections. Has been used speculatively in PCP.

Fluconazole

(➔ See Triazoles, pp. 83–4.)

- Antifungal with activity against *Leishmania* spp. Used to treat cutaneous leishmaniasis.

Fumagillin

- Antibiotic derived from *A. fumigatus*. Mechanism of action not clear. Suppresses microsporidial proliferation. A second-line treatment of microsporidiosis.
- Given PO. Adverse effects—neutropenia, decreased platelets.

Furazolidone

(➔ See Nitrofurans, pp. 66–7.)

- A nitrofuran antibiotic, active against a variety of bacteria, *G. lamblia*, and *T. vaginalis*.
- Adverse effects—disulfiram reaction with alcohol. Occasionally, fever, urticaria, hypotension, arthralgia, nausea, vomiting, headache, haemolysis (G6PD deficiency).

Iodoquinol

- An 8-aminoquinoline, active against *E. histolytica* and *Dientamoeba fragilis*.
- Pharmacology—slowly and incompletely absorbed (<10%), hepatic metabolism, and renal excretion.
- Adverse effects—nausea, abdominal cramps, rash, acne, optic neuritis with prolonged courses. Contraindicated if allergic to iodine.
- Use—asymptomatic or mild intestinal (non-invasive) amoebiasis.

Melarsoprol

- An arsenical compound, active against *T. brucei* spp. Prevents trophozoite multiplication by binding thiol groups. Very toxic.
- Resistance—due to reduced uptake by trypanosomes.
- Pharmacology—given IV, rapidly metabolized to melarsen oxide which crosses the blood–brain barrier, biphasic elimination.
- Adverse effects—fever, abdominal pain, vomiting, peripheral neuropathy; 10% risk of post-treatment encephalopathy (may be reduced by prednisolone), 2–4% risk of death secondary to treatment.
- Use—late-stage (CNS) African trypanosomiasis caused by *T.b. gambiense* and *T.b. rhodesiense*.

Mepacrine (quinacrine)

- A synthetic acridine derivative with broad antiprotozoal activity—*Blastocystis hominis, E. histolytica, G. lamblia, Leishmania* spp., *Plasmodium* spp., *T. vaginalis, T. cruzi*. Also active against tapeworms.
- Pharmacology—well absorbed PO, extensive tissue binding, concentrated in leucocytes, 10% daily dose excreted in the urine (turns it yellow).

- Adverse effects—yellow staining of skin, dizziness, headache, vomiting, psychosis, haemolytic anaemia, decreased WCC, decreased platelets, urticaria, fever, rash.
- Use—giardiasis, prophylaxis of malaria, treatment of tapeworm, cutaneous leishmaniasis.

Metronidazole

(➲ See Nitroimidazoles, pp. 64–6.)

- A nitroimidazole antibiotic, active against anaerobic bacteria and protozoa, e.g. *T. vaginalis, G. lamblia, E. histolytica, Balantidium coli, B. hominis*.
- First line for giardiasis, intestinal/extraintestinal amoebiasis, trichomoniasis.

Miltefosine

- Hexadecylphosphocholine, active against *Leishmania* spp., *Trypanosoma* spp., and *E. histolytica*.
- Pharmacology—well absorbed and widely distributed.
- Adverse effects—vomiting, diarrhoea, teratogenic (avoid in pregnancy).
- Use—treatment of leishmaniasis.

Nifurtimox

- A nitrofuran antibiotic, active against a variety of bacteria and *T. cruzi*.
- Adverse effects—GI symptoms (40–70%), CNS symptoms (33%), skin rash, haemolysis (G6PD deficiency).
- Use—treatment of acute *T. cruzi* infection. Little effect in chronic Chagas' disease. Used in combination with eflornithine or melarsoprol for the treatment of African trypanosomiasis due to *T.b. gambiense*.

Nitazoxanide

- A broad-spectrum antiparasitic used in the treatment of diarrhoea due to *Cryptosporidium parvum* in children and giardiasis. Previously used in the treatment of HIV-associated cryptosporidiosis, but of doubtful effectiveness in this context.

Ornidazole

(➲ See Nitroimidazoles, pp. 64–6.)

- A nitroimidazole antibiotic used in the treatment of giardiasis, intestinal/extraintestinal amoebiasis.

Paromomycin

(➲ See Aminoglycosides, pp. 46–8.)

- Aminoglycoside antibiotic, similar to neomycin. Poorly absorbed PO, and used as second line for non-invasive amoebiasis (oral) and for non-severe giardiasis in pregnancy when metronidazole contraindicated. Used TOP for cutaneous leishmaniasis and nitroimidazole-resistant trichomiasis (topical).

Pentamidine isethionate

- A synthetic diamidine, active against *P. falciparum, T. gondii, Leishmania* spp., *Trypanosoma* spp., *Babesia* spp., and *P. jiroveci*.
- Pharmacology—negligible oral absorption, given IV or by nebulizer, hepatic metabolism, 15–20% excreted in the urine. Poor CSF

penetration (<1%). Retained in tissues, e.g. liver, kidneys, adrenals, spleen, and lungs, resulting in long terminal half-life (>12 days).
- Adverse effects—phlebitis, injection site abscess, GI symptoms, hypotension, hypo-/hyperglycaemia, hypocalcaemia, neutropenia, decreased platelets, raised creatinine, raised LFTs, pancreatitis, rash.
- Use—treatment of African trypanosomiasis (early stage), prophylaxis and treatment of PCP, treatment of leishmaniasis (antimony-resistant).

Primaquine

(➔ See Antimalarials, pp. 112–3.)
- A synthetic 8-aminoquinoline, active against hepatic stages of *P. vivax* and *P. ovale, P. jiroveci, Babesia* spp., *Leishmania* spp., and *T. cruzi*.
- Use—treatment of *P. vivax* or *P. ovale* malaria, treatment of PCP (with clindamycin).

Pyrimethamine

(➔ See Antimalarials, pp. 112–3.)
- A synthetic diaminopyrimidine, active against *Plasmodium* spp., *T. gondii*, and *P. jiroveci*.
- Adverse effects—abdominal pains, rash, folate deficiency with longer courses (folinic acid replacement is required).
- Use—treatment of malaria (in combination with sulfadoxine or dapsone), toxoplasmosis (with sulfadiazine), and PCP (with dapsone).

Spiramycin

(➔ See Macrolides, pp. 48–50.)
- A macrolide antibiotic; active against *T. gondii* and an alternative to antifolates, e.g. in pregnancy.

Sulfadiazine

(➔ See Sulfonamides, pp. 58–60.)
- Active against *T. gondii*. Used in combination with pyrimethamine.

Suramin

- A sulfated naphthylamine, active against *T. brucei* spp. and used to treat the early stages of African trypanosomiasis. First line for *T.b. rhodesiense*. Second line for *T.b. gambiense* (in which pentamidine is effective and better tolerated).
- Mode of action—binds to plasma proteins and taken up into trypanosomes by endocytosis. Acts synergistically with nitroimidazoles and eflornithine.
- Resistance—clinical relapse rates of 30–50% reported in East Africa.
- Pharmacology—poor oral absorption, given by slow IV infusion, >99% protein-bound, poor CSF penetration, plasma half-life >40 days, not metabolized, high tissue distribution (liver, kidney, adrenal glands), renal excretion.
- Adverse effects—highly toxic, especially in malnourished patients. Immediate reactions (nausea, vomiting, cardiovascular collapse) can be avoided by slow IV injection. May be followed by fever, urticaria. Anaphylaxis is rare (<1 in 2000). Delayed reactions include exfoliative dermatitis, anaemia, leucopenia, jaundice, and diarrhoea.
- Use—African sleeping sickness (early stage), onchocerciasis.

Tetracycline

(➲ See Tetracyclines, pp. 56–8.)

- A tetracycline antibiotic, active against a variety of bacteria, *Chlamydia, Rickettsia*, spirochaetes, *P. falciparum, B. coli, D. fragilis*.
- Use—treatment and prophylaxis of drug-resistant falciparum malaria, treatment of *B. coli* and *D. fragilis*.

Tinidazole

(➲ See Nitroimidazoles, pp. 64–6.)

- Similar to metronidazole, used for amoebiasis, giardiasis, trichomoniasis.

Antihelminthic drugs

Most antihelminthics were discovered and developed for use in veterinary medicine. Although no new antihelminthics have come to the market in recent years, satisfactory results can be achieved with current drugs. The exceptions to this are the treatment of larval cestodes, disseminated strongyloidiasis, and guinea worm.

Generic properties

- Mode of action—cause degenerative alterations in the tegument and intestinal cells of the worm by inhibiting its polymerization into microtubules. This results in inability to uptake glucose by the larval and adult stages.
- Side effects—the main side effects are GI and neurological symptoms, although allergic/anaphylactic reactions may rarely occur as a result of the death of large numbers of worms.

Benzimidazoles

- Act by binding free β-tubulin, blocking its polymerization and hence inhibiting microtubule-dependent glucose uptake.
- All cause GI side effects and should be avoided in pregnancy.

Albendazole

- Active against *Enterobius vermicularis, Ascaris lumbricoides, Ancylostoma duodenale, Necator americanus, Strongyloides stercoralis, Trichuris trichiura, Trichinella spiralis*, animal hookworms, microfilaria, and *Echinococcus* spp. Also active against *G. lamblia* and microsporidia.
- Pharmacology—well absorbed PO, metabolized to albendazole sulfoxide (active metabolite), half-life 8h, renal excretion.
- Adverse effects—leucopenia and raised LFTs with prolonged use. Rarely, neutropenia, pancytopenia, agranulocytosis, thrombocytopenia.
- Use—intestinal worm infections, trichinosis, cutaneous larva migrans (TOP), hydatid disease (± surgery), neurocysticercosis, lymphatic filariasis (± ivermectin), giardiasis, microsporidiosis.

Mebendazole

- Active against *E. vermicularis, A. lumbricoides, A. duodenale, N. americanus, S. stercoralis*, and *T. trichiura*.
- Pharmacology—poor oral absorption; most of the drug and its metabolites (inactive) are retained in the GI tract and excreted in the faeces, <2% excreted by kidneys.
- Use—intestinal worms, trichinosis.

Flubendazole

- A benzimidazole carbamate used in some countries, instead of albendazole, for treatment of ascariasis. Less well absorbed PO.

Tiabendazole (thiabendazole)

- Active against commonest intestinal nematodes. Poor side effect profile and now primarily used for cutaneous larva migrans (topical for single tracks, PO for multiple).

Triclabendazole

- Drug of choice for the treatment of *Fasciola hepatica* liver infections.

Piperazine

- Active against *E. vermicularis* and *A. lumbricoides*.
- Adverse effects—transient mild GI or neurological symptoms; hypersensitivity. Avoid in epilepsy, liver or kidney disease.

Diethylcarbamazine

- A carbamyl derivative of piperazine used in the treatment of lymphatic filariasis and loiasis (*Loa loa, Brugia malayi, Wuchereria bancrofti, Onchocerca volvulus*).
- Pharmacology—>90% oral absorption, 50% metabolized and excreted in the faeces, 50% excreted unchanged in the urine.
- Adverse effects—usually related to the microfilarial burden and may be due to the release of lipopolysaccharide (LPS) from *Wolbachia* spp., e.g. fever, headache, dizziness, transient worsening of lymphangitis. The Mazotti reaction (itch, ocular and constitutional symptoms) may occur in onchocerciasis.

Ivermectin

- A mixture of two semi-synthetic derivatives of avermectins, antibiotics produced by *Streptomyces avertimilis*. Active against *A. lumbricoides, S. stercoralis, O. volvulus, L. loa*, and *Sarcoptes scabiei*.
- Pharmacology—60% oral absorption, rapidly metabolized by the liver, highest concentrations in the liver and fat, excreted in the faeces.
- Adverse effects—Mazotti reactions, GI symptoms, neurological symptoms. Not recommended in pregnancy/breastfeeding.
- Use—onchocerciasis, non-disseminated strongyloidiasis. May be used for lymphatic filariasis (with albendazole), loa loa, and scabies.

Levamisole

- Active against *A. lumbricoides* and hookworms. Paralyses worms that are then passed out in the faeces.
- An alternative to mebendazole for the treatment of ascariasis.

Praziquantel

- A synthetic pyrazinoquinoline; active against schistosomes (causes paralysis and tegumental damage), larval tapeworms, *Fasciolopsis buski, Metagonimus yokogawi, Heterophyes heterophyes, Nanophyetus salmincola, Clorchis* spp., *Opisthorchis* spp., *Paragonimus* spp., and *F. hepatica* (variable activity).

- Pharmacology—>80% oral absorption, undergoes rapid first-pass metabolism to inactive metabolites, low plasma levels, 90% excreted in the urine by 24h.
- Adverse effects—GI symptoms, mild neurological effects during treatment of schistosomiasis; cerebral inflammation and oedema during treatment of neurocysticercosis; risk of visual impairment with ocular cysticercosis.
- Use—schistosomiasis, tapeworm infections, trematode infections (except *F. hepatica*). Resistance is emerging in schistosomes.

Metrifonate

- An organophosphate compound, active against *Schistosoma haematobium*.
- Superseded by praziquantel and no longer readily available.

Niclosamide

- A synthetic chlorinated nitrosalicylanide, active against *Taenia saginata, Taenia solium, Diphyllobothrium latum, Hymenolepis nana*.
- Pharmacology—level of absorption uncertain, metabolized in the liver, passed in the urine and faeces (stains them yellow).
- Use—the most widely used drug for tapeworm infections. Not effective against larval worms.

Oxamniquine

- A synthetic quinoline methanol, active against *S. mansoni*.
- Pharmacology—well absorbed PO. Can be given IM.
- Adverse effects—dizziness, sleepiness, nausea, and headache.
- Use—second-line treatment of *S. mansoni* infections. Higher doses required in Egypt and southern Africa for partially resistant strains.

Pyrantel

- A pyrimidine derivative; active against *E. vermicularis, A. lumbricoides, A. duodenale*, and *N. americanus*. Induces paralysis, allowing worm expulsion.
- Pharmacology—<5% absorbed PO, metabolized, and excreted the in urine; the rest passes unchanged in the faeces.
- Adverse effects—GI symptoms and neurological effects (rare). Antagonistic with piperazine (do not use together).
- Use—single-dose curative in pinworm, ascariasis, and trichostrongyliasis. Several doses required for hookworm.

Part 2

Infection control

6 Infection control 129

Infection control

Introduction to infection control *130*
Basic epidemiology of infection (1) *135*
Basic epidemiology of infection (2) *137*
Infection control committee *138*
Overview of surveillance *139*
Surveillance of alert organisms *140*
Surveillance of hospital-acquired infection *141*
Nature of risk and its assessment *142*
Management of outbreaks *144*
Handwashing *146*
Patient isolation *150*
Management of risks to health-care workers from patients *151*
Management of risk from sharps *153*
Risk from tissues for transplantation *157*
Infection control on renal dialysis units *158*
Management of risk from virally infected health-care workers *158*
Hazard groups *160*
Containment levels *162*
Universal infection control precautions and barrier nursing *163*
Management of antibiotic-resistant organisms, including MRSA *164*
Control of carbapenemase-producing *Enterobacteriaceae* *167*
Control of tuberculosis in hospitals *168*
Control of Creutzfeldt–Jakob disease and transmissible spongiform encephalopathies *169*
Disinfection *172*
Sterilization *174*
Ventilation in health-care premises *176*
Laundry *179*
Waste *180*
Introduction to prevention of hospital-acquired infection *181*
Infections in intensive care *182*
Surgical site infection *185*
Bloodstream infection—mandatory surveillance *187*
Urinary catheter-associated infection *189*
Ventilator-associated pneumonia *191*
Line-related sepsis *193*
Hospital epidemics of diarrhoea and vomiting *196*
Clostridium difficile infection *198*
Infection control in the community *202*

Introduction to infection control

At any one time, in the UK, ~10% of hospital inpatients are suffering from a nosocomial infection.[1] In total, estimates suggest that 300000 patients a year in England acquire a HCAI as a result of care within the NHS. The top five commonest nosocomial infections are as follows:

- intravascular device-related bacteraemia;
- UTI;
- LRTI;
- surgical wound infection;
- skin infection.

The socio-economic impact, in terms of increased length of stay and financial cost, is immense, as is the personal cost to each individual who acquires an essentially preventable infection. In 2007, MRSA bloodstream infections (BSIs) and CDIs were recorded as the underlying cause of, or a contributory factor in, ~9000 deaths in hospitals and primary care in England.

HCAIs are estimated to cost the NHS ~£1 billion a year. These infections have triggered considerable political interest over recent years, resulting in reorganization of hospital and community infection control services and the publication of numerous documents. A 'zero tolerance' approach has been adopted. It is likely that infection control will maintain its high political profile.

Information which will guide reading of this chapter and provide information on current practice and trials in infection control can be found in Boxes 6.1 to 6.4 and Table 6.1.

Box 6.1 Important definitions in infection control

Infection—the deposition and multiplication of organisms in tissues or on body surfaces, which usually causes adverse effects.

Colonization—organisms are present but cause no host response.

Carrier—an individual who harbours a pathogen without manifesting symptoms, thus acting as a distributor of infection. Typhoid Mary was one of the most famous carriers of all time (➔ see Enteric fever, pp. 649–51).

Nosocomial infection—hospital-/health care-acquired infection that was not present or incubating at the time of admission. Often an arbitrary cut-off of >48h post-admission is used. Nosocomial infections also include infections that only appear after discharge, e.g. post-operative wound infection. It also includes occupational infections amongst health-care staff.

Community infection—infection in the community. Be careful to differentiate between community-onset (may include patients recently discharged from hospitals) and community-acquired (community patients with no history of direct or indirect contact with health care) infections.

Decontamination—a process or treatment that cleanses a medical device, instrument, or environmental surface to remove contaminants such as microorganisms.

Box 6.1 (Contd.)

Disinfection—the destruction of pathogenic and other microorganisms by physical or chemical means. Disinfection is less lethal than sterilization, because it destroys most recognized pathogenic microorganisms, but not necessarily all microbial forms such as bacterial spores (➔ see Disinfection, pp. 172–4).

Sterilization—a physical or chemical procedure that destroys all organisms, including large numbers of resistant bacterial spores (➔ see Sterilization, pp. 174–6).

Box 6.2 Infection control abbreviations used in the UK

- *ACOP*—Approved Code of Practice, e.g. for *Legionella*.
- *CCDC*—Consultant in Communicable Disease Control.
- *CDC*—Centers for Disease Control and Prevention (Atlanta, USA).
- *CDSC*—Communicable Disease Surveillance Centre: now CFI (Centre for Infections).
- COSHH—Control of Substances Hazardous to Health.
- *CQC*—Care Quality Commission.
- *CSSD*—Centre for Surgical Sterilization and Disinfection (also called Theatre Supplies Unit, TSU).
- *DH*—Department of Health.
- *DIPC*—Director of Infection Prevention and Control.
- *ECDC*—European Centre for Disease Prevention and Control (Stockholm, Sweden).
- *EPIC*—Evidence-based Practice in Infection Control.
- *HACCP*—Hazard Analysis Critical Control Points.
- *HAI*—hospital-acquired infection.
- *HBN*—Health Building Note.
- *HCAI*—health care-associated infection.
- *HELICS*—Hospital in Europe Link for Infection Control through Surveillance.
- *HGM*—Health Guidance Memorandum.
- *HICPAC*—Hospital Infection Control Practices Advisory Committee (Atlanta, USA).
- *HII*—High Impact Intervention: from 'Saving Lives' programme.
- *HSE*—Health and Safety Executive.
- *HTM*—health technical memorandum.
- *ICC*—infection control committee.
- *ICD*—infection control doctor.
- *ICN*—infection control nurse.
- *ICT*—infection control team.
- *LACORS*—Local Authorities Coordinators of Regulatory Services.
- *MESS*—MRSA Enhanced Surveillance System.
- *MHRA*—Medicines and Healthcare products Regulatory Agency.
- *PEAT*—Patient Environment Action Team.
- *PPE*—personal protective equipment.

(*Continued*)

Box 6.2 (Contd.)

- *RCA*—root cause analysis.
- *RIDDOR*—Reporting of Injuries, Diseases and Dangerous Occurrences Regulations.
- *SUI*—serious untoward incident.
- *UICP*—universal infection control precautions.
- *UKAP*—UK Advisory Panel for health-care workers infected with blood-borne viruses.

Box 6.3 Current emphasis on infection control

The Health and Social Act came into force in April 2011. This states that 'good infection prevention and control are essential to ensure that people who use health and social care services receive safe and effective care. Effective prevention and control of infection must be part of everyday practice and be applied consistently by everyone'. This code of practice details ten criteria that will be used by the CQC to judge how a registered provider complies with infection control. Registered providers include: primary care, primary dental care, independent sector ambulance workers, and secondary care.

- *High Impact Interventions* were published by the DH, based on the care bundle approach. These are simple evidence-based tools, which reinforce the practical actions that clinical staff need to undertake to significantly reduce HAI. The HIIs focus on:
  - central venous catheter (CVC) care (see Box 6.25);
  - peripheral IV cannula care (see Box 6.27);
  - renal dialysis catheter care;
  - prevention of surgical site infection (see Box 6.24);
  - care for ventilated patients (or tracheostomies, where appropriate);
  - urinary catheter care (see Box 6.26);
  - reducing the risk of *C. difficile* (see Box 6.28);
  - cleaning and decontamination of clinical equipment.

The revised Saving Lives tools include summaries of best practice for antimicrobial prescribing and isolating patients with HAI.

- Important approaches include the following:
  - care bundles—these involve multiple discrete steps in the prevention of infection, and should be implemented and monitored by multidisciplinary teams;
  - a culture of *zero tolerance* and *accountability*, with adequate *administrative support*.

See Institute for Healthcare Improvement, available at: ☞ www.ihi.org.

Box 6.4 Clinical trials in infection control/hospital epidemiology

Historically, there have been few controlled trials in infection control, and the evidence base for many procedures is sparse. Initiatives to rectify this include the formation of ORION (Outbreak Reports and Intervention Studies of Nosocomial Infection) and the publication of a CONSORT (Consolidated Standards of Reporting Trials) equivalent statement, in order to raise the standards of research and publication. The most recent version (the CONSORT 2010 Statement) consists of a 25-item checklist and a participant flow diagram. The full text of the ORION Statement and checklist is available at: www.idrn.org/orion.php. These guidelines have been incorporated, with others, into the EQUATOR Network (*E*nhancing the *QUA*lity and *T*ransparency *O*f health *R*esearch, available at: www.equator-network.org). The emphasis is on transparency to improve the quality of reporting and on the use of appropriate statistical techniques, so that the work is robust enough to influence policy and practice.

Table 6.1 Some of the significant UK documents relating to infection control (published since 2000)

National Audit Office (2000). *The management and control of hospital acquired infection in acute NHS trusts in England*. Available at: www.nao.org.uk/publications/9900/hospital_acquired_infection.aspx.
Pratt RJ, Pellowe C, Loveday HP, *et al.*; Department of Health (England) (2001). The epic project: developing national evidence-based guidelines for preventing healthcare associated infections. Phase I: Guidelines for preventing hospital-acquired infections. *J Hosp Infect* **47**:S3–82. (Epic2 was updated in 2006.)
Department of Health (2002). *Getting ahead of the curve: a strategy for infectious diseases*. Available at: webarchive.nationalarchives.gov.uk/+/dh.gov.uk/en/consultations/closedconsultations/dh_4016942.
Department of Health (2007). *Towards cleaner hospitals and lower rates of infection: a summary of action*. Available at: http://webarchive.nationalarchives.gov.uk/+/www.dh.gov.uk/en/Publicationsandstatistics/Publications/PublicationsPolicyAndGuidance/Browsable/DH_4096315.
Department of Health (2007). *Saving lives: reducing infection, delivering clean and safe care*. Available at: http://webarchive.nationalarchives.gov.uk/+/www.dh.gov.uk/en/Publicationsandstatistics/Publications/PublicationsPolicyAndGuidance/DH_078134.
Department of Health (2006). *The Health Act 2006: code of practice for the prevention and control of healthcare associated infections*. London: Department of Health. (Under the 2006 Health Bill, trusts have a duty of care to comply with this code of practice, which will be overseen by the Health Care Commission. The code is divided into three areas: (1) management, organization, and the environment; (2) clinical care protocols; (3) health-care workers.)

(*Continued*)

Table 6.1 (*Contd.*)

Department of Health (2007). *The decontamination of surgical instruments with special attention to the removal of proteins and inactivation of any contaminating human prions: 2006 report*. Available at: http://webarchive.nationalarchives.gov.uk/20130107105354/http://www.dh.gov.uk/en/Publicationsandstatistics/Publications/PublicationsPolicyAndGuidance/DH_072443.
National Audit Office (2009). *Reducing healthcare associated infections in hospitals in England*. Available at: www.nao.org.uk/publications/0809/reducing_healthcare_associated.aspx.
Public Health England (2010). *Guidance on infection control in schools and other childcare settings*. Available at: https://www.gov.uk/government/uploads/system/uploads/attachment_data/file/353953/Guidance_on_infection_control_in_schools_11_Sept.pdf.
National Institute for Health and Care Excellence (2011). *Healthcare-associated infections: prevention and control*. NICE guidelines PH36. Available at: http://www.nice.org.uk/guidance/ph36.
Public Health England (2011). *Infection control in prisons and places of detention: manual for healthcare workers and other staff*. Available at: https://www.gov.uk/government/uploads/system/uploads/attachment_data/file/329792/Prevention_of_infection_communicable_disease_control_in_prisons_and_places_of_detention.pdf.
Public Health England (2012). *Guidelines for the management of norovirus outbreaks in acute and community health and social care settings*. Available at: https://www.gov.uk/government/uploads/system/uploads/attachment_data/file/322943/Guidance_for_managing_norovirus_outbreaks_in_healthcare_settings.pdf.
Public Health England (2014). *Acute trust toolkit for the early detection, management and control of carbapenemase-producing Enterobacteriaceae*. Available at: https://www.gov.uk/government/uploads/system/uploads/attachment_data/file/329227/Acute_trust_toolkit_for_the_early_detection.pdf.
Department of Health (2013). *Prevention and control of infection in care homes: an information resource*. Available at: www.gov.uk/government/uploads/system/uploads/attachment_data/file/214929/Care-home-resource-18-February-2013.pdf
Public Health England (2013). *Updated guidance on the management and treatment of C. difficile infection*. Available at: https://www.gov.uk/government/uploads/system/uploads/attachment_data/file/321891/Clostridium_difficile_management_and_treatment.pdf.

References to relevant topics in other chapters

- Management of rash contact in pregnancy, pp. 790–1.
- Bioterrorism, pp. 846–8.
- Vancomycin-resistance, pp. 42–3.
- Antimicrobial stewardship, pp. 27–8.
- Glycopeptide resistance in *Staphylococcus aureus*, pp. 239–40.

Reference

1 Plowman R, Graves N, Griffin MA, *et al*. (2001). The rate and cost of hospital-acquired infections occurring in patients admitted to selected specialties of a district general hospital in England and the national burden imposed. *J Hosp Infect*. **47**:198–209.

Further reading

Public health bodies—England (Public Health England ➚ www.gov.uk/phe), Scotland (Health Protection Scotland ➚ www.hps.scot.nhs.uk), and Wales (Public Health Wales ➚ www.wales.nhs.uk/healthprotection) each have devolved public health agencies.
Healthcare Infection Society—➚ www.his.org.uk.
The UK Department of Health website provides information on mandatory surveillance schemes, ➚ www.doh.gov.uk.
Health and Safety Executive—➚ www.hse.gov.uk.
World Health Organization—➚ www.who.int.
Centers for Disease Control and Prevention, Hospital Infection Program—➚ www.cdc.gov/hai.
Infection Prevention Society—➚ www.ips.uk.net.
Care Quality Commission—➚ http://www.cqc.org.uk. This is the independent regulator of all health and adult social care in England.
National Institute for Health and Care Excellence (NICE)—➚ www.nice.org.uk.
Society for Healthcare Epidemiology of America—➚➚ www.shea-online.org.
Medicines and Healthcare products Regulatory Agency—➚ www.mhra.gov.uk.
National electronic Library of Infection—➚ www.neli.org.uk.
European Centre for Disease Prevention and Control—➚ http://ecdc.europa.eu.

Basic epidemiology of infection (1)

In order to introduce effective infection control measures, the basic epidemiology of an infection (route of transmission, host risk factors, etc.) must be considered. The incidence and nature of a HAI (as with any infection) depend on the:

- organism;
- host (patients and staff);
- environment.

The organism

The organisms responsible for common nosocomial infections are listed in Table 6.2. These may be acquired endogenously or exogenously.

Endogenous infection

An infectious agent that is already present in the host causes endogenous infection. The infectious agent is usually part of the normal host flora. Antibiotics and exposure to the hospital environment can change the normal flora of the host and may select for resistant organisms. Risk of infection may be reduced by protecting any potential sites of entry, e.g. intravascular lines.

Exogenous infection

When the infectious agent originates from outside of the host. The pathogen is usually acquired from the environment by various routes, including: airborne, direct contact, or percutaneous routes. Within the hospital setting, environmental infection is usually due to a contaminated item of equipment and can be minimized by implementing the correct decontamination, sterilization, and infection control procedures. Cross-infection (or transmission) refers to infection acquired in hospital from another person, either patients or staff. Risks can be reduced by focusing on measures to interrupt transmission, e.g. handwashing.

Table 6.2 Organisms commonly involved in HAIs

Infection	Organism(s) involved
UTIs	Gram-negative bacteria, e.g. *E. coli, Proteus* spp., *Klebsiella* spp., *Serratia* spp. Gram-positive bacteria less common, e.g. *Enterococcus* spp. Fungi are a rare cause, e.g. *C. albicans*
Respiratory infections (non-ventilated patients)	Bacteria, e.g. *H. influenzae, S. pneumoniae, P. aeruginosa, Enterobacteriaceae* Viruses: respiratory viruses Fungi, e.g. *Aspergillus* spp.
Wounds and skin sepsis	Bacteria, e.g. *S. aureus, S. pyogenes*, anaerobes Uncommon cause—(surgical wounds) Gram-negative organisms. e.g. *E. coli*
BSI	Gram-positive bacteria, e.g. *S. aureus*, including MRSA, *Enterococcus* spp., CoNS Gram-negative bacteria, e.g. *E. coli, Proteus* spp., *Klebsiella* spp., *Serratia* spp., *P. aeruginosa* Fungi, e.g. *Candida* spp.
GI infections	Bacteria, e.g. *C. difficile*
	Viruses, e.g. norovirus

The host

Patient risk factors that result in increased likelihood of acquiring an infection in hospital include:

- severity of the underlying acute illness and patient co-morbidities. Severely ill patients are more vulnerable to acquiring an infection and more likely to have a worse outcome;
- use of medical devices—these breach host defences and provide possible portals of entry for organisms;
- extremes of age—the elderly and very young are at higher risk;
- immunosuppression.

Staff risk factors include:

- immunosuppression, e.g. HIV; pregnancy;
- staff who perform exposure-prone procedures are more likely to be exposed to blood-borne viral infections;
- skin conditions (e.g. eczema) increase prolonged carriage of organisms such as MRSA.

Basic epidemiology of infection (2)

The environment

The hospital environment includes all of the physical surroundings of the hospital patients and staff, i.e. the building, fittings, fixtures, furnishings, equipment, and supplies. The following are important environmental issues in the control of infection:

- environmental cleaning (see Box 6.5);
- environmental disinfection;
- decontamination of equipment;
- building and refurbishment, including air-handling systems;
- clinical waste management;
- pest control;
- food services/food hygiene;
- isolation facilities/ability to cohort patients.

Routes of transmission

The isolation precautions required depend on the likely route of transmission of the organism. The main routes are:

- airborne—this is when the infection usually occurs by the respiratory route, with the agent being carried in aerosols (<5 micrometres in diameter);
- droplet—large droplets carry the infectious agent (>5 micrometres in diameter);
- direct contact—infection occurs through direct contact between the source of infection and the recipient, i.e. person-to-person spread;
- indirect contact—infection occurs through 'indirect contact', i.e. via equipment contaminated with body fluids such as urine, faeces, and wound exudates. This route also includes contact via an environmental source, e.g. an outbreak of gastroenteritis transmitted by food;
- inoculation—infection occurs through direct inoculation, e.g. needlestick injury. Other routes include via blood products (hepatitis A, *Yersinia enterocolitica, Serratia*), total parenteral nutrition (TPN), and other fluids (*Enterobacter, B. cepacia, Bacillus cereus*). Multidose vials should be avoided.

Box 6.5 Hospital cleaning

'Dirty hospitals' are frequently reported by the media, with attention drawn to the lack of investment and poor support for hospital cleaning. Providing a clean and safe environment for health care is a key priority for the NHS and is a core standard in *Standards for better health*. Other publications, such as *Towards cleaner hospitals and lower rates of infection*, have further emphasized this and recognize the role of cleaning in minimizing HAIs by the physical removal of dirt, fomites, dust, and human body fluids. In 2007, the National Patient Safety Agency produced guidelines for cleaning (*The national specifications for cleanliness in the NHS: a framework for setting and measuring performance outcomes*). The results of PEAT (Patient Environment Action Team) assessments are calculated against these specifications.

Infection control committee

The National Audit Office report (July 2004) stated that all NHS trusts are responsible for clarifying and explaining accountabilities, including the role, membership, and responsibilities, of the hospital ICC. Thus, the chief executive and trust board are responsible for ensuring effective arrangements for infection control.

Director of Infection Prevention and Control

In 2003, it became mandatory for every trust to appoint a DIPC, to lead the ICC. This was the first time an infection-related post was created at board level, with direct reporting to the chief executive. Clear competencies of the DIPC have been defined by the DH (2004).

Responsibilities of hospital infection control committee

- Endorsing all infection control policies, procedures, and guidelines.
- Providing advice and support on the implementation of policies.
- Collaborating with the ICT to develop the annual infection control programme and monitor its progress.

Membership of hospital infection control committee

Membership may include the:

- DIPC;
- ICT (➔ see Infection control team below);
- chief executive or representative;
- occupational health physician and nurse;
- senior clinical representatives;
- nurse executive director or representative;
- CCDC.

Infection control team

The ICT should be led by the DIPC and include the infection control doctor(s) and nurse(s). The ICT is mainly accountable to the trust chief executive and trust board. ICT responsibilities include:

- ensuring advice on infection control is available on a 24h basis;
- producing the annual infection control programme, in consultation with the ICC, health professionals, and senior managers. This programme will include surveillance of infection, and an audit of the implementation and compliances with selected policies;
- providing education and training on prevention and control of HAI to all grades of hospital staff.

Management of infection control in the community

The CCDC has a key role to play in collaborating with the ICT on the management of hospital and community outbreaks. They are responsible for advising health authorities and primary care organizations. They provide epidemiological advice and have overall responsibility for the surveillance, prevention, and control of communicable diseases and infections in the community (➔ see Infection control in the community, p. 202).

Overview of surveillance

Definitions

Surveillance comes from the French 'to watch over' and means 'vigilant supervision' or 'ongoing scrutiny'. Langmuir, the founder of the CDC in Atlanta, described surveillance as 'the continued watchfulness over the distribution and trends of diseases through systematic collection, consolidation, and evaluation of data'. Often, in the real world, total accuracy of the data must be sacrificed in favour of the practicability, cost-effectiveness, uniformity, and timeliness in which the information can be collected. An important point to remember is there is no point just collecting interesting data; you need to do something with them—as emphasized by an alternative definition of surveillance: 'information for action'.

Surveillance may be active or passive.

- *Active* surveillance is when special effort is made to collect the data, e.g. investigation of an outbreak or survey of a particular disease.
- *Passive* surveillance uses routine data that have already been collected, e.g. the UK national census.

Aims of surveillance

The main aims of surveillance of hospital infection are to keep infection to a minimum level, and prevent and control outbreaks. Every member of medical and nursing staff and every department have a responsibility to collect relevant data on infection rates and to perform regular audits. The ICT advises on this. In addition, routine surveillance from the laboratory can identify new antibiotic-resistant or 'alert' organisms.

Methods of surveillance employed in HAI usually involve a combination of active and passive surveillance systems. Practice varies within and between hospitals, and is largely dependent on the availability of staff and resources. In practice, a number of surveillance methods are used, as each provides different information. These include:

- department-specific—each department collects data on their patient risk factors and infection rates. This is particularly relevant in areas such as the ICU and surgical wards;
- laboratory-based ward liaison, i.e. the ICN reviews patients with 'significant' microbiology cultures and also visits each ward to discuss all patients with the ward staff/infection control link nurse;
- others, including infection control link nurses, and review of patients on antibiotics with known risk factors or indwelling devices.

Evaluation of a surveillance system

- Define the event to be measured ('case definition').
- Define the population under surveillance.
- List the objectives of the system.
- Define the public health importance of the health event (e.g. number of deaths, case fatality ratio, morbidity, economics, preventability).

Some characteristics of a surveillance system are listed in Box 6.6.

Box 6.6 What makes a good surveillance system?

For surveillance to succeed, it should have the following attributes:
- simple (well-designed reporting forms make all the difference!);
- flexible;
- acceptable to the population studied;
- sensitive;
- representative;
- timely;
- reasonable cost.

The quality of the data provided can be evaluated in terms of:
- sensitivity and specificity;
- predictive value (positive and negative);
- usefulness, in relation to the goals of the surveillance (quality indicators).

It is sometimes more valuable (although usually more difficult) to focus on the outcome (e.g. the number of cases of polio), rather than the process (e.g. the number of polio vaccinations).

Ownership is important—feeding the data back to those who collected it will make them more willing to help again in the future!

Does surveillance work?

There is good evidence that surveillance in hospitals actually reduces infection rates. The SENIC study (the Study on Efficacy of Nosocomial Infection Control) was carried out over two decades ago in the USA.[2] One of the main objectives was to determine whether surveillance and infection control programmes lowered the rate of nosocomial infection. SENIC demonstrated that hospitals with active surveillance and infection control programmes could reduce the incidence of infection by 32%. Another important finding of the SENIC study was the need to close the loop and present data back to the clinicians. Clinical audit was also found to be important.

Reference

2 Haley RW, Morgan WM, Culver DH, *et al.* (1985). Update from the SENIC project. Hospital infection control: recent progress and opportunities under prospective payment. *Am J Infect Control*. **13**:97–108.

Surveillance of alert organisms

This may vary between institutions, but, in most UK hospitals, the ICT should be informed of patients suffering from the following conditions, in order to ensure all staff are aware of infection control precautions:
- infectious diarrhoea (*Campylobacter, Salmonella, Shigella, C. difficile*, rotavirus, norovirus, etc.);
- GAS (*S. pyogenes*);
- GBS (invasive infections in neonatal or maternity units);
- meningococcal disease;
- influenza;

- TB;
- HIV;
- hepatitis A–E;
- severe herpes simplex;
- legionnaires' disease;
- VZV (shingles or chickenpox);
- lice/scabies;
- RSV.

Multiresistant organisms

Practice varies between hospital trusts, but, in general, the following organisms should be reported to the ICT. Often patients' notes and electronic records are 'flagged' if a multiresistant organism has been isolated in the past:

- MRSA;
- VRE;
- penicillin-resistant/non-susceptible *Pneumococcus*;
- multiresistant Gram-negative organisms, e.g. ESBL-producing organisms, carbapenem-resistant *Enterobacteriaceae* (CRE).

Surveillance of hospital-acquired infection

Definition

HAI is an infection that was neither present nor incubating at the time of hospital admission, which normally manifests itself >48h later. The term health care-associated infection (HCAI) encompasses any infection by any infectious agent acquired as a consequence of a person's treatment by the NHS or which is acquired by a health-care worker (HCW) in the course of their NHS duties (Health Act 2006).

Criteria for hospital-acquired infection surveillance schemes

In order to obtain accurate results that can be compared to other hospitals, the following criteria are important:

- agreed definitions of infection;
- accurate denominator data;
- correction of infection rates for risk factors, e.g. pre-existing diseases;
- identification of HAI post-discharge.

Brief history of national surveillance schemes

The Nosocomial Infection National Surveillance Scheme (NINSS), launched in the UK in 1996, was set up to monitor the rate of HAI. Trusts enrolled for 3-month modules and were able to compare their performance to others. This was replaced by mandatory laboratory-based MRSA bacteraemia surveillance in 2001 which has evolved over the last decade to include a number of pathogens (see Table 6.3).

Table 6.3 National surveillance schemes in the UK

Surveillance activity	Date	Notes
S. aureus (including MRSA) bacteraemia	2001	6-monthly reports, now quarterly
Glycopeptide-resistant enterococcal (GRE) bacteraemia	2003	Annual reports initially, now quarterly
CDI	2004	Annual reports initially, now quarterly
Orthopaedic surgical site infection	2004	Annual reports
MESS: MRSA Enhanced Surveillance Scheme—additional details of cases of MRSA bacteraemias	2005	Enhanced surveillance data
MRSA	2011	Quarterly
E. coli bacteraemia	2011	

International surveillance schemes

Most other countries have established surveillance programmes, although data are often not comparable between countries/continents because of variations in definitions and methods.

Nature of risk and its assessment

Risk management is something we do every day in our personal lives—such as when crossing the road—but has recently evolved as an important science in health-care settings. In combination with total quality management (TQM), it aims to integrate and coordinate all quality assessment activities, and focus on the identification and correction of any problems, with the ultimate goal of protecting patients.

Key definitions

- *Risk management*—a systematic process of risk identification, analysis, treatment, and evaluation of potential and actual risks.
- *Hazard versus risk*—a hazard is the potential to cause harm, while a risk is the likelihood of harm (in defined circumstances and usually qualified by some statement of the severity of the harm).
- *Total quality management*—a management strategy aimed at embedding awareness of quality in all organizational processes. For how this applies to the diagnostic laboratory, ➲ see Quality assurance and accreditation, pp. 231–3.
- *Controls assurance*—the need to be seen to be doing our 'reasonable best' to reduce risk by using resources effectively.
- *Clinical governance*—a framework through which NHS organizations are accountable for continually improving the quality of their services and safeguarding high standards of care, by creating an environment in which excellence in clinical care will flourish.

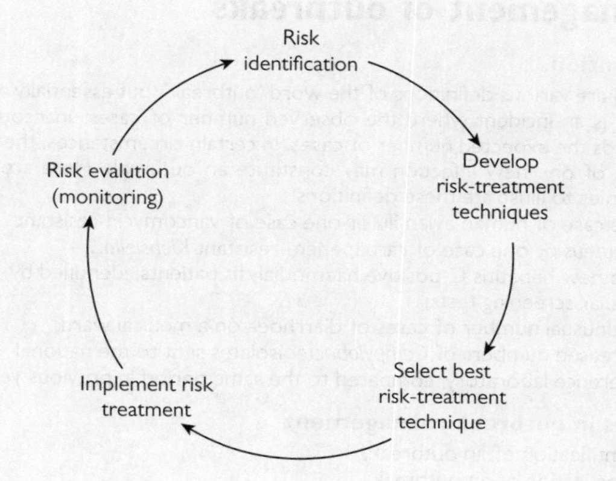

Fig. 6.1 The risk management cycle.

Risk management and economics

Health economics and cost-effectiveness play a big part in risk management. It is particularly important today because of rising health-care costs, governmental cost containment, and adverse claims experience.

Goals of risk management

- Survival of the organization (the NHS).
- Enhanced quality and standard of care.
- Minimization of risk of medical or accidental injuries and losses.
- Improvement of programme effectiveness and efficiency through administrative direction and control.
- Coordination and integration of current policies, functions, programmes, committees, and other aspects relative to the risk management process.
- Avoidance of adverse publicity.
- Minimization of cost of risk transfer (insurance).

The risk management cycle is outlined in Fig. 6.1.

Management of outbreaks

Definition

There are various definitions of the word 'outbreak', but essentially an outbreak is an incident where the observed number of cases unaccountably exceeds the expected number of cases. In certain circumstances, the emergence of one new infection may constitute an outbreak. Here are some examples to illustrate these definitions:

- one case of human avian flu or one case of vancomycin-resistant *S. aureus* or one case of carbapenem-resistant *Klebsiella*;
- two new hepatitis C-positive haemodialysis patients, identified by regular screening tests;
- an unusual number of cases of diarrhoea on a medical ward;
- increased numbers of *Campylobacter* isolates sent to the national reference laboratory, compared to the same period in previous years.

Steps in outbreak management

- Identification of an outbreak.
- Investigation of an outbreak.
- Case definition.
- Describing the outbreak.
- Propose and test hypothesis.
- Control measures and follow-up.
- Communication.

Management of hospital outbreaks

Outbreaks of nosocomial infections must be identified and thoroughly investigated, because of their importance in terms of morbidity and mortality. Also there is a need to identify any breakdown in a process and to prevent spread or future recurrences. The declaration of an outbreak is a decision that should be made by the ICT, in conjunction with senior members of staff from the affected area. The declaration of an outbreak can have a significant impact on patient care, bed pressures, as well as political and financial implications. Before an outbreak is declared, there is often a 'period of increased incidence' (PII).

Period of increased incidence

This situation may result from the transmission of an infecting organism (which would be seen in an outbreak), e.g. norovirus, or may be due to an increase in the number of sporadic cases (the same organism is isolated, but the organisms are found to be unrelated), e.g. CDI where the ribotypes are all different. During a PII, a formal outbreak meeting does not need to be held. However, a full investigation (which does not differ from the investigation performed during an outbreak) should be performed. The main aim is to identify whether there has been a breakdown in infection control and should include:

- review of hand hygiene—review hand hygiene audits, and perform ad hoc audits when necessary. Any deficiencies should be dealt with in real time with educational sessions for staff;

- review ward cleaning—audits are usually performed regularly to review practice. Deficiencies should be addressed, and decisions made regarding enhanced cleaning. Enhanced cleaning can include increased frequency of cleaning of the entire ward or certain areas at greatest risk of causing transmission, e.g. high-touch surfaces, etc.;
- review of ward equipment—the same pieces of equipment have the potential to be used throughout the ward, and they should be properly cleaned and maintained, e.g. commodes. All equipment used in patient areas should be examined;
- review of the environment—determine if there are potential reservoirs in the environment. Remedial building work should be carried out, e.g. repairing cracks in walls, broken ceiling tiles. Rarely environmental screening is required but should be considered;
- review of antibiotic prescribing—antibiotic prescribing can add a selection pressure in favour of the infecting organism.

The PII may become an outbreak. There are often no formal criteria for declaring an outbreak, but it is dependent on a number of factors, including: the pathogenicity of the organism, if the number of cases continues to rise, or if transmission is confirmed. Transmission is usually confirmed once organism-typing results have been obtained. If the organisms are highly related or identical, then a transmission between patients is confirmed, and the cases are highly unlikely to be sporadic. A key strategy for controlling an outbreak or PII is restricting the movement of patients by ward closure, patient isolation, and assessing the risk to contacts.

Ward closure

The decision to close a ward has a significant impact on the functioning of the entire hospital. Most hospitals will experience bed pressures, and the loss of an entire ward due to closure can be devastating. In response to the number of ward closures due to norovirus, the DH produced infection control guidance that allowed bays to be closed, while the remainder of the ward remained open. The principles of this guidance can be useful for managing any outbreak. The decision to close bays or the ward is based on a number of factors, including:

- geographical spread of the patients affected. If the infected cases are clustered within the same bay, then the bay can be closed, and admissions and transfers from this bay restricted. However, if the infected cases are distributed throughout the ward, it is more practical to close the ward than manage >2 bays closed;
- rate of acquisition of new cases. A rapid increase in the number of new cases suggests control will be challenging;
- staff members affected. Staff will interact with numerous patients throughout a ward and also socialize with other members of staff. Therefore, there will be a large number of contacts and potentially infected cases;
- the nature of the ward. Closure of an ICU has enormous implications for patient safety, operating lists, and pressures for the ICU in neighbouring hospitals. Therefore, the decision to close an ICU requires major planning and involvement of senior management;

- the pathogenicity of the organism, e.g. *Legionella*. Any hospital-acquired cases of *Legionella* will often result in the closure of that unit, until water quality can be assessed and the source determined.

Patient isolation and cohorting

Ideally, all infected patients and their contacts should be isolated promptly. This is often impractical due to the lack of side room facilities, and patients who are already symptomatic with the infection should be prioritized for isolation. Contacts should be cohorted into one bay. In a complex outbreak, symptomatic patients may have to be cohorted into one bay, their contacts in another, and unaffected patients in another. When patients are in a cohort, admission to, and discharge from, their bay is restricted. For example, in a bay where contacts are cohorted, no other patients can be admitted to this bay, as there is a risk of exposing an uninfected patient to a potentially infected patient. Likewise, patients can only be transferred out of that bay if they are moving to a side room or being discharged home, or remain asymptomatic beyond the incubation period of the infection to which they were exposed.

Contact tracing

Another key element of controlling an outbreak or PII is identifying contacts of the infected patients. A significant contact is one where the patient has had exposure to the route of transmission of a particular infection and so potentially may be infected, e.g. all patients in a bay where a patient with norovirus has vomited. All patients who are a contact should be observed and appropriately isolated for the incubation period of the illness. If they do not manifest symptoms following the incubation period, then they are highly unlikely to be infected. As part of an outbreak/PII, it is essential to identify and appropriately isolate/cohort all contacts of the index case.

Further reading

Public Health England (2012). *Guidelines for the management of norovirus outbreaks in acute and community health and social care settings*. Available at: ℘ https://www.gov.uk/government/publications/norovirus-managing-outbreaks-in-acute-and-community-health-and-social-care-settings.

Handwashing

The importance of handwashing has been recognized since the nineteenth century when Semmelweiss encouraged medical students in Vienna to wash their hands in chlorinated lime solution on the delivery unit. The maternal mortality rate from puerperal fever in patients attended to by medical students was far lower than those attended to by midwives who did not wash their hands. Today HCW hand hygiene is a topic of global importance. The WHO produced the first global patient safety challenge relating to hand hygiene 'Clean Care is Safer Care'. The goal of Clean Care is Safer Care is to ensure that infection control is acknowledged universally as a solid and essential basis towards patient safety. A fundamental part of this campaign relates to improving hand hygiene amongst HCWs.

- The National Audit Office report (2000) noted a lack of adherence to handwashing procedures (https://www.nao.org.uk/report/the-management-and-control-of-hospital-acquired-infection-in-acute-nhs-trusts-in-england/). Average compliance of HCWs with handwashing is <50%, and technique is often poor and rushed.
- Research has begun to focus on how to change the culture and behaviour on the ward, and improve adherence to policies.
- There is no doubt that good handwashing practice reduces transmission of infections, but, to be effective, all HCWs must comply all of the time.
- The WHO has identified compliance with hand hygiene as a quality indicator for health care.

Skin flora can be divided into two types:

- transient organisms—these are not normally part of the normal flora, and can be picked up from the patient or their environment. Examples include *E. coli, S. aureus, Klebsiella* spp., and *Pseudomonas* spp. They are usually removed by a 'social' handwash (see Box 6.7), with soap and water. 'Hygienic hand disinfection' (see Box 6.8), e.g. with alcohol gel, aims to remove or destroy all transient flora, and there may be a prolonged effect;
- resident organisms—these organisms are usually found deep in the dermis. They do not usually cause infection, except if introduced during invasive procedures, e.g. line insertion or surgical procedures. Examples include CoNS, and aerobic and anaerobic diphtheroids. They are not usually removed by a single handwashing procedure.

Box 6.7 Common handwashing terms

Social handwash

- Cleaning of hands with plain, non-medicated bar or liquid soap and water for the removal of dirt, soil, and various organic substances.

Hygienic handwash

- Cleaning of hands with antimicrobial or medicated soap and water. Most antimicrobial soaps contain a single active agent and are usually available as liquid preparations.

Kampf G, Kramer A (2004). Epidemiologic background of hand hygiene and evaluation of the most important agents for scrubs and rubs. *Clin Microbial Rev* 17:863–93.

Box 6.8 Hygienic hand disinfection

- Normally consists of the application of an alcohol-based hand rub onto dry hands without water.

Surgical scrub

- This procedure aims to remove or destroy all transient flora, and reduce resident flora. There must also be a prolonged effect. Chlorhexidine, povidone–iodine, or alcohol are usually used.

How to wash?

- Using a good handwashing technique (see Fig. 6.2) will clean areas that are often missed (e.g. between the fingers, thumbs, fingertips, areas of the palms, and back of the hands). This should only take 15–30s. Make sure hands are wet before applying soap, and rinse thoroughly before drying. If using a gel, effective decontamination only occurs when the alcohol is rubbed in until the skin is dry.

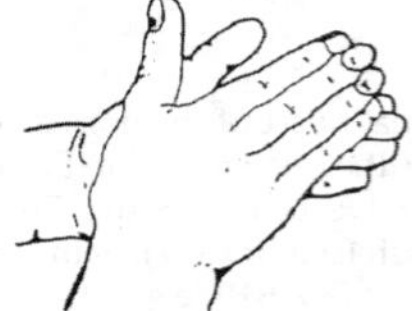

1. Palm to palm

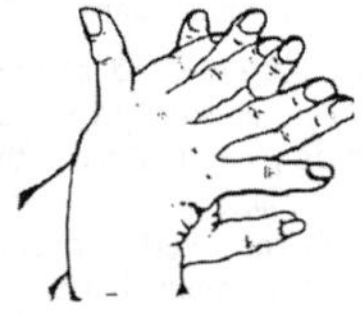

2. Right palm over left dorsum and left palm over right dorsum

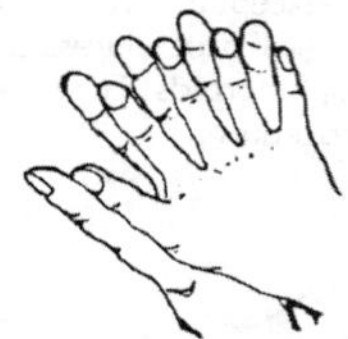

3. Palm to palm fingers interlaced

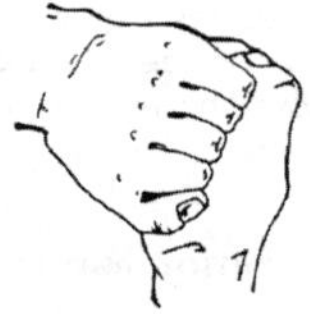

4. Backs of fingers to opposing palms with fingers interlocked

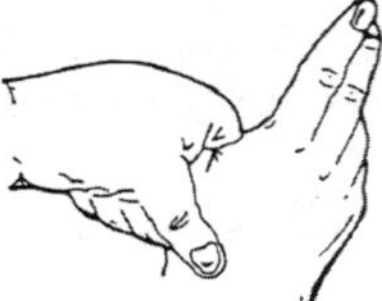

5. Rotational rubbing of right thumb clasped in left palm and vice versa

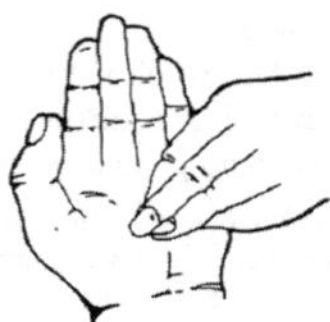

6. Rotational rubbing, backwards and forwards with clasped fingers of right hand in left palm and vice versa

Fig. 6.2 Hand decontamination.

Based on the procedure described by Aycliffe *et al.* in *J Clin Pathol* 1978;**31**:923. Reproduced with permission from BMJ Publishing Group.

When to wash?

- Wash hands after any process that contaminates the skin, and before food preparation, patient contact, or any clinical procedure. Examples include after leaving a source isolation room or before entering a protective isolation room.
- The WHO has produced '5 moments of handwashing'. This is designed to be easy to learn, logical and applicable in a wide range of settings, and to promote a strong sense of ownership.

Measuring compliance with handwashing

The gold standard for measuring compliance with handwashing is direct observation. This may, however, be subject to the Hawthorne effect, in that behaviour tends to improve when an individual is being watched. Alternative methods include devices to electronically monitor the use of soap and handwash dispensers.

What to use?

- In most clinical situations, soap and water, or an alcohol rub, are adequate. The length of time and handwashing technique are more important than which soap is used. There are specifications for sinks in clinical areas. Hand lotions and creams may be used after handwashing to prevent soreness.

Hand care in general

- Nail care—keep nails short and clean. False nails have been the source of HAI, including endocarditis, so should not be worn.
- Jewellery and watches may harbour bacteria and hinder handwashing. Trusts often limit jewellery to a plain wedding band.
- If hands get dry and sore, as often occurs after repeated handwashing, then transient flora may become resident in skin cracks. HCWs should consult occupational health if they are concerned.

Changing the culture

The main factors preventing compliance with hand hygiene are time and system constraints. Many feel that full compliance with complete guidance is unrealistic. Washing with soap and water can take 60–90s; therefore, many institutions have moved to alcohol-based hand rub at the point of care (i.e. at the bedside, rather than at the entrance to the ward). This is easier, takes only 15–20s, is generally microbiologically efficacious, and is better for hands.

Multifaceted approach

Evidence suggests a multipronged approach is the only way to bring about change. For example, key parameters in compliance with alcohol-based hand rubs include education of HCWs, monitoring and feedback to HCWs, good administrative support, and introducing a system change (i.e. putting alcohol gel by each patient).

Cleanyourhands Campaign

The National Patient Safety Agency produced a Cleanyourhands toolkit. The key elements of the campaign were:

- place disinfectant hand rubs near to where staff have patient contact;
- display posters and promotional material where they will influence staff and patients;
- involve patients in improving hand hygiene.

Evaluation of the national Cleanyourhands campaign in 2012 showed that increased procurement of soap was independently linked with reduced CDI, and increased procurement of alcohol hand rub was independently associated with reduced MRSA infection.[3] The Cleanyourhands campaign is no longer active, but the underlying principles are still relevant and used within hospitals.

Reference

3 Stone SP, Fuller C, Savage J, *et al.* (2012). Evaluation of the national Cleanyourhands campaign to reduce *Staphylococcus aureus* bacteraemia and *Clostridium difficile* infection in hospitals in England and Wales by improved hand hygiene: four year, prospective, ecological, interrupted time series study. *BMJ*. **344**:e3005.

Patient isolation

The use of universal infection control precautions should minimize the need for isolation of most patients. In practice, isolation depends on a risk assessment for each patient, and the side rooms/facilities available in each trust. Always act on the patient's clinical presentation, and do not wait for laboratory results to be available, as it may be too late. Involve your ICT early, and consult the DH guidance for further advice (see Box 6.9).

Effective isolation relies on all staff following the necessary procedures, to make sure that none of the transmission barriers are breached. The simplest solution is to use single rooms, but, in an outbreak, multi-bedded bays, or even whole wards, may be used.

Box 6.9 Isolating patients with HAI

Guidance and summary of best practice on isolating patients with HCAI have been published by the DH. These aim to provide all health-care providers with a framework to review and improve isolation practices, and reduce the risk of the spread of infections, thus resulting in a reduction in the total number of infections, and provide safer clinical care of an individual with an infection.

Recommendations cover the following:

1. single room nursing;
2. cohort nursing;
3. management of the patient once isolated:
    - hand hygiene and personal protective equipment (PPE);
    - cleaning and decontamination;
    - movement of the patient.

Patients are isolated for two reasons:

- *source isolation*—to minimize the chance of infecting other patients, e.g. patient with open TB. The air inside the isolation room should be at negative pressure (exhaust-ventilated), compared to the corridor. Patients with highly contagious infections, such as viral haemorrhagic fevers (VHFs), ideally should be nursed in a high-security isolation unit;
- *protective isolation*—to minimize that patient becomes infected, e.g. to protect susceptible or immunosuppressed patients. The air inside the isolation room should be at positive pressure (pressure-ventilated), compared to the corridor. In some critical situations, such as BMT units, where airborne contamination with fungal spores is a problem, the efficiency of air filtration may be increased and laminar flow maintained as a barrier around the patient.

Source isolation

The following measures apply to patients in source isolation.

- Limit transport to other departments (e.g. X-ray) to essential investigations only.
- If a patient does need to go to another department, brief the porters and other staff what precautions are necessary.
- Do not transfer the patient to another ward or health-care institution without discussion with the ICT.
- If the patient is well enough, consider sending them home.
- Keep staff caring for infected patients to a minimum. Try not to let these staff work elsewhere in the hospital.
- After death of an infected patient, maintain infection control precautions, and consult your trust policy for dealing with the body.

Management of risks to health-care workers from patients

Practices are in place to reduce the risk of HCWs acquiring infections from their patients. However, HCWs (including laboratory staff) do become infected at work, with organisms ranging from the relatively benign norovirus to life-threatening conditions. Infection control procedures for patients infected with HIV, hepatitis B, or hepatitis C may be considered together, because routes of acquisition are similar. The main risk of transmission is from the accidental inoculation of blood (➔ see Management of risk from sharps, pp. 153–7). Clearly, it is impossible to identify all carriers of blood-borne viruses, so universal infection control precautions (UICP) (➔ see Universal infection control precautions and barrier nursing, pp. 163–4) are required for all patients.

Infectivity of body fluids from patients with HIV and hepatitis B

The following fluids are potentially infectious:

- blood, CSF, peritoneal fluid, pleural fluid, pericardial fluid, synovial fluid, amniotic fluid, breast milk, semen, vaginal secretions, saliva in the context of dentistry.

NB. The following are *not* regarded as infectious, unless visibly contaminated with blood: faeces, nasal secretions, saliva (except in dentistry), sputum, sweat, tears, urine, and vomit.

Care of patients with HIV or hepatitis B or C

Patients known to be positive for these viruses (or likely to be positive as a result of certain risk factors) should have a risk assessment performed. The risk assessment should fully respect patient confidentiality. The likelihood of exposure of staff or other patients to the patient's blood/body fluids should be considered. Medical and nursing care of infected patients depends on local hospital policy, but here are a few practical suggestions:

- single room isolation—this is only usually required if uncontrolled bleeding or loss of other body fluids is likely, or if the patient has another condition requiring isolation (e.g. diarrhoea, open pulmonary TB, salmonellosis, herpes zoster). On vacation of the room, terminal cleaning is necessary if contamination with blood or body fluids has occurred;
- HBV/HCV-positive patients should not be nursed in close proximity to patients who require haemodialysis/haemofiltration;
- disposal of sharps—if the patient needs single room isolation, sharps must be disposed of in a sharps bin *inside* the room;
- spills—any spills of blood/body fluids should be covered immediately with chlorine-releasing granules or strong (10 000ppm available chlorine) hypochlorite;
- equipment disinfection and sterilization—use single-use/disposable items, whenever possible;
- protective clothing—depends on the likelihood and degree of exposure to the patient's blood and body fluids. Apron and gloves must be worn when dealing with blood or bloodstained body fluids. Masks and protective eyewear are required, wherever there is a possibility of aerosolization/splashing;
- linen from patients in isolation or contaminated with blood or body fluids should be regarded as 'infected linen' (➔ see Laundry, p. 179);
- toilet/bathroom facilities—patients may use the ward facilities, except if there is bleeding (or risk of bleeding) when toilet/bathroom facilities must be reserved for this patient only (or use a commode);
- crockery—disposable crockery is rarely required. If there is excessive bleeding from the mouth, the patient can retain their own crockery and cutlery, which they or the nursing staff wash up;
- waste—clinical waste and disposable items must be placed in yellow bags (➔ see Waste, pp. 180–1), with double-bagging if leakage of body fluids is possible;
- specimen transport—label specimens and accompanying forms with 'Danger of Infection' stickers.

Other infections acquired by health-care workers from patients

Many infections may be transmitted to hospital staff, but the following are recognized more frequently or have more significant consequences:

- viral gastroenteritis;
- *N. meningitidis*—HCWs who intubate the patient or perform mouth-to-mouth resuscitation;

Box 6.10 Education in infection control procedures works!
During the severe acute respiratory syndrome (SARS) epidemic (2004), the proportion of infected HCWs varied from 20% to 60% of cases worldwide, with notable differences between hospitals. The better the education in infection control, the lower the risk of acquiring the infection (McDonald LC, Simor AE, Su IJ, *et al.* (2004). SARS in healthcare facilities, Toronto and Taiwan. *Emerg Infect Dis* **10**:777–81).

- MTB;
- varicella-zoster;
- influenza;
- others, including pertussis, diphtheria, rabies, VHFs.

Box 6.10 shows an example of education in infection control working effectively.

Further reading

Health and Safety Executive. *Sharps injuries*. Available at: www.hse.gov.uk/healthservices/needlesticks.

Health and Safety Executive. *Advisory Committee on Dangerous Pathogens Protection against blood-borne infections in the workplace: HIV and hepatitis*. Available at: http://www.hse.gov.uk/biosafety/diseases/bbv.pdf.

Joint Working Party of the Hospital Infection Society and the Surgical Infection Study Group (1992). Risks to surgeons and patients from HIV and hepatitis: guidelines on precautions and management of exposure to blood or body fluids. *BMJ* **305**:1337–43.

Management of risk from sharps

By following UICPs, all HCWs can minimize risks of infection associated with blood and body fluids. The main risk associated with needlestick and other sharps injuries is transmission of blood-borne viruses; with a significant inoculation of blood through a hollow-bore needle, the rate of transmission to the recipient is as follows:

- ~30% if the donor is HBsAg-positive (the risk is as high as 30% if the patient is HBeAg-positive, while it decreases to 3% if HBeAb-positive);
- ~3% if the donor is hepatitis C antibody-positive;
- ~0.3% if the donor is HIV-positive.

There is also the risk of emerging or unknown agents.

Prevention of sharps injuries

The National Audit Office report (2000) noted poor practice in sharps disposal. Good clinical practice is important in preventing needlestick injuries, e.g.:

- handle needles and other sharps carefully;
- never re-sheathe needles;
- staff using needles or other sharps are responsible for their safe disposal;
- use sharps bins as indicated.

Action in event of sharps injury

- Immediate first aid—encourage bleeding of the area; wash with soap under running water, and cover with waterproof dressing. If eye splash, irrigate well with running water. If splash into mouth, do not swallow, and rinse out the mouth several times with cold water.
- Report the incident to the senior person in that area. Complete an incident form/accident book.
- Contact occupational health or another expert about hospital guidelines (e.g. microbiology/ID physician).
- Risk assessment—consider the hazard (potential to cause harm) and risk (likelihood that harm will occur), based on the injury, the source, and the recipient (see Box 6.11).

Box 6.11 Risk assessment

Consider the injury, the source, and the recipient.

- Injury:
  - extent and depth of injury;
  - size and type of needle;
  - visible contamination with blood;
  - site.
- Source (usually the patient undergoing the procedure but may be unknown):
  - hepatitis B and C, HIV status (if known);
  - viral load/stage of illness if HIV-positive.
- Recipient:
  - hepatitis B vaccine status/antibody level;
  - any conditions that may affect treatment, e.g. pregnancy.

Management of a 'needlestick' injury

(See Table 6.4.)

- Always seek expert advice, usually from occupational health, microbiology, or ID.
- Refer the recipient to occupational health/microbiology/ID immediately. They will make a risk assessment of the severity of the injury.
- If this was a significant injury, then a member of the team looking after the donor (but not the recipient of the injury) should counsel the donor. Blood should be requested for HIV, HBsAg, and HCV antibody. For management of sharps injury from an infected donor, see Table 6.5.
- If pre-test counselling is required, involve trained personnel.
- Note that the source patient may decline to be tested, and this will not affect their medical care.
- Provide patient information leaflets, as appropriate.
- General Medical Council (GMC) guidance offers advice on difficult situations, e.g. if there is conflict between the needs of the recipient and the wishes of the source, or if the source patient is unconscious or has died. Decisions about testing an incapacitated patient must take account of the

Table 6.4 Summary flow chart for needlestick injury

- Check basic first aid has been performed.
- Discuss with occupational health/ID/microbiology.
- Risk assessment—significant injury?

No	Yes
• Occupational health referral for routine assessment • Recipient sample for long-term storage (LTS) and anti-HBs if unknown • Encourage HBV vaccination if not done	• Recipient sample for LTS and anti-HBs if unknown • Request source sample for urgent testing for HIV, HBsAg, and HCV, LTS • Unknown source: gather as much information as possible to make a risk assessment
	Further risk assessment: • Known or highly likely to be HIV +ve—URGENT: infection expert will consider PEP • Known or highly likely to be HBV +ve—URGENT: infection expert will consider HBIG and accelerated vaccine/booster, depending on the recipient's anti-HB status/vaccine history • Known or highly likely to be HCV +ve—no immediate intervention. Infection expert will check HCV RNA on source if known anti-HCV +ve donor. Follow up recipient at 6 and 12 weeks (PCR), 12 and 24 weeks (anti-HCV)

Table 6.5 Management of sharps injury from an infected donor

Donor known positive or likely positive	Action
HIV	*URGENT*. Discuss with an infection expert who will consider PEP. The risks associated with PEP versus the risk of acquiring HIV will be explained to the recipient. PEP usually consists of a 3-day starter pack of antiviral therapy, with plans for ongoing counselling/treatment, depending on results. For further information, see Department of Health (2008) *HIV post-exposure prophylaxis: guidance from the UK Chief Medical Officers' Expert Advisory Group on AIDS*, http://webarchive.nationalarchives.gov.uk/20130107105354/http://www.dh.gov.uk/en/PublicationsandStatistics/Publications/PublicationsPolicyandGuidance/DH_088185.
HBV	*URGENT*. Discuss with an infection expert who will consider HBIG and accelerated vaccination or booster(s), as in Table 6.6.
HCV	No immediate intervention. If donor anti-HCV-positive, they will be tested for HCV RNA to determine whether they are viraemic (greater risk)—HCV RNA tested in the recipient by PCR at 6 and 12 weeks, and anti-HCV tested at 12 and 24 weeks. If signs of infection in the recipient, the test will be confirmed, and the patient will be referred for specialist assessment as soon as possible.

current legal framework governing capacity issues and the use of human tissue. Consult local occupational health services and infection experts. Currently, blood should not be tested for blood-borne viruses from an unconscious patient if it is not in the medical interests of that patient.

- If the injury was significant, then blood will be taken from the recipient for storage. The hepatitis B vaccination history of the recipient should be taken, and a course of vaccination or booster dose considered, as appropriate. With a high-risk donor, HIV PEP and/or hepatitis B immune globulin (HBIG) may be considered. Management of exposure to hepatitis B is discussed in Table 6.6.

Reporting

All injuries should be reported to the senior on duty and recorded on an incident form/accident book. If the injury was with a used needle or instrument, advice should be sought from infection experts/occupational health. A review of equipment/procedures should occur, led by a senior member of the department.

Table 6.6 Management of significant exposure to HBV

In addition to percutaneous inoculation (needlestick, scratch, bite, etc.), this may result from contamination of mucous membranes (e.g. spillage into eyes or mouth) or contamination of non-intact skin (open wounds, dermatitis, eczema). For management of HBV exposure in newborn infants and in sexual contacts, see Public Health England (2013, updated September 2014) *The Green Book (Immunisation against infections disease)*, https://www.gov.uk/government/organisations/public-health-england/series/immunisation-against-infectious-disease-the-green-book.

HBV status of person exposed	Significant exposure	
	HBsAg-positive source	Unknown source
One dose or less of HBV vaccine pre-exposure	Accelerated course of HBV vaccine (doses at 0, 1, and 2 months; may need booster dose at 12 months if continuing risk of exposure)	Accelerated course of HBV vaccine (doses at 0, 1, and 2 months; may need booster dose at 12 months if continuing risk of exposure)
	Also give HBIG × 1	
Two doses or more of HBV vaccine pre-exposure (anti-HBs not known)	One dose of HBV vaccine, followed by second dose 1 month later	One dose of HBV vaccine
Known responder to HBV vaccine (anti-HBs >10mIU/mL)	Consider booster dose of HBV vaccine	Consider booster dose of HBV vaccine
Known non-responder to HBV vaccine (anti-HBs <10mIU/mL) 2–4 months post-immunization	HBIG × 1 A second dose of HBIG should be given at 1 month	HBIG × 1 A second dose of HBIG should be given at 1 month
	Consider booster dose of HBV vaccine	Consider booster dose of HBV vaccine

Additional notes regarding management of significant exposure to HIV

Factors known to increase the risk of transmission of HIV

- Deep and penetrating injury.
- Visibly bloodstained device.
- Needle involved has been in the source patient's artery or vein.
- Source has terminal HIV disease/high viral load.

Risk from tissues for transplantation

The number of organs and tissues that can be successfully transplanted is increasing. The current list of organ transplants includes the heart, kidneys, liver, lungs, pancreas, and intestine. Tissues include bones, tendons, cornea, heart valves, veins, and skin. Rejection and infection arising from anti-rejection therapy are the main risks. Haematology and oncology patients who have received BMTs are at particularly high risk of infection. Infection in a transplant recipient may either be transmitted from the donor with the organ or arise due to the immunosuppressed state of the recipient. Certain infectious agents are particularly recognized as causing infections post-transplant. Depending on which organ has been transplanted, different infection agents are commonly implicated at different time periods. Box 6.12 describes typical problems after a renal transplant.

Surveillance of infections amongst tissue donors

A tissue donation and banking programme is operated by NHS Blood and Transplant (NHSBT) Tissue Services. Donations may come from living and/or cadaveric donors, and include surgical bone (mainly femoral heads), tendons, skin, and heart valves. NHSBT also operate the National Bone Marrow Registry and a cord blood bank. All tissue donors (including stem cell and cord blood donors) are routinely tested for HIV, HCV, HBV, human T-cell lymphotropic virus (HTLV), and syphilis infections. The Advisory Committee on the Safety of Blood, Tissues and Organs (SaBTO) has specific guidance on microbiological safety in transplantation.[4] Data concerning rates of infection are collated by the PHE Centre for Infections and NHSBT.

Box 6.12 Example—infections post-renal transplant

Minor infections are common after a kidney transplant. Urine infections affect ~50% of transplant recipients, especially if the patient has reflux nephropathy or diabetes. More serious infections in the first 6 months post-transplant include pneumonia (e.g. PCP, *Pneumococcus*), CMV, chickenpox, BK virus, and disseminated fungal infection. Each transplant unit will have guidelines for prophylaxis, which may include:

- co-trimoxazole (PCP);
- fluconazole (*Candida*);
- isoniazid for those at risk of TB;
- antibiotics (if UTIs are common);
- valganciclovir or valaciclovir if CMV-positive donor into CMV-negative recipient;
- vaccination, e.g. influenza, Pneumovax®.

Surveillance of infections in blood donors

Every blood donation is tested for markers of HIV, HCV, HBV, HTLV, and syphilis, and only used if all tests are negative. If an infection is detected, the donor is invited to return to the blood centre, when they will be told about their test results, asked for a repeat sample, asked to stop donating blood, and referred to a specialist. In addition to ensuring our blood supply is safe, these data improve our understanding of the epidemiology of blood-borne infections. The National Blood Service and PHE manage a series of schemes which monitor infections in blood and tissue donor and transfusion recipients. This benefits patient safety and public health. For details on blood-borne infections in blood donors, see www.phe.gov.uk. Epidemiological data are also available by testing all pregnant women for HIV, HBsAg, and syphilis.

SHOT (Serious Hazards of Transfusion) is a scheme for reporting investigations into infections in transfusion recipients (www.shotuk.org).

Reference

4 Department of Health (2011). *Guidance on the microbiological safety of human organs, tissues and cells used in transplantation.* Available at: https://www.gov.uk/government/publications/guidance-on-the-microbiological-safety-of-human-organs-tissues-and-cells-used-in-transplantation.

Infection control on renal dialysis units

Outbreaks of blood-borne viruses (HBV, HCV, and HIV) are a well-recognized hazard for patients and staff on haemodialysis units. Adoption of universal precautions has resulted in a fall in the incidence of HBV and HCV in dialysis units over the last 30 years. However, increasing numbers of patients on haemodialysis, increasing numbers of immigrants, and increased foreign travel of dialysis patients may increase future risk. Other blood-borne viruses (hepatitis G; GB virus type C) are higher in dialysis patients, compared to the general population, but their clinical significance is uncertain.

The UK Renal Association has produced NICE-accredited guidelines (2009) on the prevention of spread of blood-borne viruses in the renal unit, including issues of surveillance, segregation, and immunization (see www.renal.org/guidelines).

Management of risk from virally infected health-care workers

Virally infected staff are usually managed by the occupational health department. Please note that up-to-date guidance from the DH should be consulted. The information provided in this section is a guide.

Hepatitis B-infected health-care workers

- Health Service Guidelines HSG (93)40: *Protecting health care workers and patients from hepatitis*. This guidance recommends that *HBV carriers who are e antigen-positive must not carry out procedures* where there is a risk that injury to themselves will result in their blood contaminating a patient's open tissues (i.e. should not perform exposure-prone procedures (EPPs)).

- Health Service Circular (HSC) 2000/020: *Hepatitis B infected health workers.* This circular recommends testing *HBV-infected HCWs who are HBeAg-negative* and perform EPPs. Those with higher viral loads (>1000 genome equivalents (geq)/mL) should have their working practices restricted.
- HCWs on antiviral therapy who are HBeAg-negative and who have pre-treatment HBV DNA levels between 10^3 and 10^5 geq/mL could be allowed to perform EPP on antiviral therapy if their viral load is suppressed below 10^3 geq/mL and monitored regularly.[5]

Hepatitis C-infected health-care workers

- Health Service Circular HSC 2002/010: *Hepatitis C infected health care workers* (and associated guidance). This circular builds upon previous advice from the Advisory Group on Hepatitis and recommends that HCWs who know they are carrying HCV (i.e. are HCV RNA-positive) should not perform EPPs. HCWs who have responded successfully to HCV treatment should be allowed to resume EPPs. Successful response to treatment is defined as HCV RNA-negative 6 months after cessation of treatment. Testing of HCWs for HCV RNA should be done in laboratories where the assay has a minimum sensitivity of 50IU/mL.

HIV-infected health-care workers

The risk of a HCW infecting a patient during an EPP is very low. Worldwide, there are only three reported cases of HCW transmission to patients. These transmissions occurred during high-risk procedures, and the HCWs were not on ART. In the UK, between 1988 and 2008, 39 incidents of potential HIV transmission from a HCW to a patient occurred. Over 10 000 patients were tested, and no cases of HCW transmission to patients were found. PHE guidance (2014) *The management of HIV infected healthcare workers performing exposure prone procedures* recommends:

- all HCWs who undertake EPPs should be tested for HIV antibody;
- HIV-infected HCWs can perform EPPs if they are on effective ART and have a plasma viral load of <200 copies/mL;
- HIV-infected HCWs undertaking EPPs must have the plasma viral load monitored every 3 months. If the viral load is >1000 copies, the HCW must stop performing EPPs immediately;
- patient notification exercises following patient exposure to blood/bodily fluids from HIV-infected HCWs, in general, would only be done if the HCW had a viral load of >1000 copies/mL and on treatment. However, all exposure incidents should be risk-assessed locally;
- patients who are exposed to blood from an infected HCW would only be considered for PEP and HIV testing if the viral load was >200 copies/mL. Otherwise, no action is taken.

Further advice is shown in Box 6.13.

Box 6.13 Further advice from UK Advisory Panel for Healthcare Workers Infected with Bloodborne Viruses (UKAP)

- Although this was originally set up to consider individual cases of HIV-infected HCWs, the UKAP now considers other blood-borne viruses, in particular hepatitis B and C. They can provide advice for specific situations, as well as general policies, and can be contacted at ukap@phe.gov.uk.

Reference

5 Department of Health (2007). *Hepatitis B infected healthcare workers and antiviral therapy*. Available at: http://webarchive.nationalarchives.gov.uk/20130107105354/ http:/www.dh.gov.uk/en/Publicationsandstatistics/Publications/PublicationsPolicyAndGuidance/DH_073164.

Hazard groups

In 1995, the Advisory Committee on Dangerous Pathogens (ACDP) (www.hse.gov.uk/aboutus/meetings/committees/acdp/) classified all microorganisms into hazard groups 1–4, based on their hazard and containment level (CL) (see Table 6.7). The framework is based on their pathogenic potential, route of transmission, epidemiological consequences of escape, and host susceptibility. The hazard groups 1–4 are thus handled at different CLs in the laboratory, defined by Control of Substances Hazardous to Health (COSHH). ACDP category 3 organisms are listed in Box 6.14. For the complete approved list of biological agents for all categories, see www.hse.gov.uk/pubns/misc208.pdf.

Table 6.7 ACDP hazard groups 1–4

Hazard group	CL (see Containment levels, pp. 162–3)	Examples
Group 1 Unlikely to cause human disease	CL1	CoNS
Group 2 May cause human disease May be a hazard to laboratory workers Unlikely to spread in the community Treatment or prophylaxis available	CL2	*S. aureus* *S. enterica* serotype Enteritidis *L. pneumophila* Influenza, norovirus
Group 2+ organisms		*N. meningitidis*, *Legionella*
Group 3 May cause severe human disease Serious hazard to laboratory workers May spread in the community Treatment or prophylaxis available	CL3	See full list in Box 6.14 Examples include: *S. enterica* serotype Typhi (*S.* Typhi); MTB; *Brucella* spp.; HIV; hepatitis B, C, D Prion diseases
Group 4 Severe disease Serious hazard to laboratory workers High risk of spread in the community No treatment or prophylaxis		Haemorrhagic fevers, e.g. Ebola, Lassa fever Note that this group only contains viruses, not bacteria

Box 6.14 List of ACDP category 3 organisms

- Bacteria:
  - *Bacillus anthracis*;
  - *Burkholderia mallei*;
  - *Burkholderia pseudomallei*;
  - *Chlamydophila psittaci* (avian strains);
  - *Coxiella burnetii*;
  - *Ehrlichia sennetsu* (*Rickettsia sennetsu*);
  - *E. coli*, verocytotoxigenic strains (e.g. O157:H7 or O103);
  - *Francisella tularensis* (type A), not type B;
  - *S.* Typhi *S.* Paratyphi *A, B, C*;
  - MTB;
  - *Mycobacterium* (certain species);
  - *Brucella*;
  - *Rickettsia* spp.;
  - *S. dysenteriae* type 1;
  - *Yersinia pestis*.
- Viruses (certain viruses from the following groups):
  - HIV and other retroviruses;
  - hepatitis B, C, D, E;
  - arenaviridae;
  - bunyaviridae;
  - hantaviruses;
  - phleboviruses;
  - nairoviruses;
  - caliciviruses;
  - togaviruses;
  - flaviviruses, e.g. dengue;
  - tick-borne virus group;
  - poxviruses;
  - rhabdoviruses, e.g. rabies;
  - SARS coronavirus.
- Parasites (certain parasites from the following groups):
  - *Echinococcus* spp.;
  - *Leishmania* spp.;
  - *P. falciparum*;
  - *Naegleria fowleri*;
  - *T. solium*;
  - *T. cruzi* and *T.b. rhodesiense*.
- Fungi:
  - *B. dermatidis*;
  - *C. immitis*;
  - *P. brasiliensis*;
  - *H. capsulatum*;
  - *P. marneffei*;
  - *Cladophialophora bantiana*.
- Others:
  - Creutzfeldt–Jakob disease (CJD) and variant CJD (vCJD);
  - Kuru;
  - Gerstmann–Sträussler–Scheinker disease (GSS) and other transmissible spongiform encephalopathies (TSEs).

Containment levels

The CL refers to the physical requirements necessary for working with organisms of different pathogenicity and includes guidance about the facilities, working environment, and safety equipment and procedures (e.g. staff training). There are four different levels (CL1–CL4), and the CL of an organism usually corresponds with its categorization, e.g. all group 3 organisms must be handled at CL3. Guidance from the ACDP with detailed technical information, especially regarding CL2 and CL3, is available on the Health and Safety Executive website (www.hse.gov.uk). This includes the legal requirements in the provision of COSHH, with particular attention to how these influence laboratory design, construction, and operation.

Summary of requirements

Containment level 1 (CL1), i.e. low individual and community risk

- No special facilities, equipment, or procedures are required. Standard well-designed laboratory facilities and basic safe laboratory practices suffice.
- Handwashing facilities must be provided.
- Disinfectants must be properly used.

Containment level 2 (CL2), i.e. moderate individual risk, limited community risk

- The laboratory should be separated from other activities, biohazard sign, room surfaces impervious and readily cleanable.
- Equipment should include an autoclave, certified high-efficiency particulate air (HEPA)-filtered class I or II biological safety cabinet for organism manipulations, and PPE to include laboratory coats worn only in the laboratory.
- All contaminated material should be properly decontaminated.

Containment level 3 (CL3), i.e. high individual risk, low community risk

- Specialized design and construction of laboratories, with controlled-access double-door entry and body shower. All wall penetrations must be sealed. Ventilation system design must ensure that air pressure is negative to surrounding areas at all times, with no recirculation of air; air should be exhausted through a dedicated exhaust or HEPA filtration system. Minimum furnishings, all readily cleanable and sterilizable (fumigation). Laboratory windows sealed and unbreakable. Backup power available.
- Equipment must include an autoclave, certified HEPA-filtered class II biological safety cabinet for organism manipulations, and a dedicated handwashing sink with foot, knee, or automatic controls, located near the exit. PPE should include solid front laboratory clothing worn only in the laboratory, head covers and dedicated footwear, gloves, and appropriate respiratory protection, depending on the infectious agents in use.
- All activities involving infectious materials to be conducted in biological safety cabinets or other appropriate combinations of personal protective and physical containment devices.

- Laboratory staff must be fully trained in the handling of pathogenic and other hazardous material, use of safety equipment, disposal techniques, handling of contaminated waste, and emergency response. Standard operating procedures must be provided and posted within the laboratory, outlining operational protocols, waste disposal, disinfection procedures, and emergency response. The facility must have a medical surveillance programme appropriate to the agents used.

Containment level 4 (CL4), i.e. high individual risk, high community risk

- CL4 is the highest level of containment and represents an isolated unit that is completely self-contained to function independently. Facilities are highly specialized and secure, with an air lock for entry and exit, class III biological safety cabinets or positive pressure-ventilated suits, and a separate ventilation system with full controls to contain contamination.
- Only fully trained and authorized personnel may enter the CL4 containment laboratory. On exit from the area, personnel will shower and re-dress in street clothing. All manipulations with agents must be performed in class III biological safety cabinets or in conjunction with one-piece, positive pressure-ventilated suits.

Universal infection control precautions and barrier nursing

UICP involve following simple infection control precautions for *all* patients. It is difficult to tell which patients are infected and which are not, so all patients should be regarded as 'potentially infected'. Adherence to UICP for all patients should minimize the transmission of HIV, hepatitis B and C, and other infectious agents. It also eliminates confusion amongst staff as to which patients are to be treated as 'infected', and should also prevent any breach of confidentiality.

Main components of universal infection control precautions

- Handwashing (➲ see Handwashing, pp. 146–50).
- Protective clothing.
- Gloves and aprons should be worn if the episode of patient contact involves blood or body fluids, but the risk of splashing is low. If the risk of splashing is high, a waterproof gown, mask, and eye protection should also be worn.
- Disposal of linen and waste (➲ see Laundry, p. 179; ➲ Waste, pp. 180–1).
- Broken skin:
  - clinical staff should cover all skin lesions with a waterproof dressing.
- Sharps (➲ see Management of risk from sharps, pp. 153–7; see Box 6.15):
  - never re-sheathe, bend, or break a needle or any other sharp;
  - dispose of all sharps as a single unit, in a suitable sharps bin;
  - never attempt to retrieve anything from a sharps bin;
  - only fill a sharps bin to full, and secure the lid before disposing of it according to local policy.

Box 6.15 Preventing the risk of microbial contamination from *Saving lives: high-impact intervention no. 1. Central venous catheter care bundle* (2007)

The elements of the care process listed below form the basis of reducing the risk of bacterial contamination. This underpins all other HIIs and should be recorded at the time of the procedure. The three elements are as follows.

Hand hygiene

- Decontaminate hands before and after each patient contact.
- Use correct hand hygiene procedure.
- PPE.
- Wear examination gloves if there is risk of exposure to body fluids.
- Gloves are single-use items.
- Gowns, aprons, and eye/face protection may be indicated if there is a risk of splashing with blood or body fluids.

Aseptic technique

- Gown, gloves, and drapes, as indicated, should be used for the insertion of invasive devices.

Sharps

- Safe disposal of sharps.
- Sharps container available at point of use.
- No disassembling of needle and syringe.
- Sharps should not be passed from hand to hand.
- The container should not be overfilled.

- Spills:
    - any spill of blood or other body fluids that contains blood should be treated with chlorine-releasing granules and left in place for 2min. Afterwards, this should be cleared up with paper towels, wearing gloves and aprons. The area should then be washed with hot water and detergent;
    - if granules are not available, a solution of hypochlorite diluted to 10 000 ppm (1%) should be used in the same way;
    - any spill of urine should be dealt with immediately using hot water and detergent.

Management of antibiotic-resistant organisms, including MRSA

In the section ➔ Control of outbreaks of antibiotic-resistant organisms below, management of antibiotic-resistant organisms will be discussed at the population level. For treatment of individuals, see MRSA, VISA, and Gram-negative bacteria, including CRE (see Boxes 6.16 and 6.17).

Box 6.16 MRSA treatment of nasal/extranasal colonization

- Likely to be beneficial:
  - mupirocin nasal ointment.
- Unknown effectiveness:
  - antiseptic body washes;
  - chlorhexidine–neomycin nasal cream;
  - mupirocin nasal ointment for 5 days (compared with >5 days);
  - systemic antimicrobials.
- Unlikely to be beneficial:
  - tea tree preparations.

Box 6.17 Treatment of MRSA—infection of any body site

- Trade-off between benefits and harms:
  - linezolid (compared with glycopeptides);
  - glycopeptides, compared with linezolid, quinupristin-dalfopristin, or trimethoprim–sulfamethoxazole.
- Unknown effectiveness:
  - azithromycin, clarithromycin, erythromycin;
  - ciprofloxacin, levofloxacin, moxifloxacin;
  - clindamycin;
  - daptomycin;
  - doxycycline, minocycline, oxytetracycline;
  - fusidic acid;
  - quinupristin–dalfopristin;
  - rifampicin;
  - trimethoprim.

Control of outbreaks of antibiotic-resistant organisms

The main steps in controlling an outbreak of antibiotic-resistant organisms are as follows.

- Identify reservoirs of resistant organisms:
  - colonized and infected patients;
  - environmental contamination.
- Halt transmission:
  - improve handwashing and asepsis;
  - isolate colonized and infected patients;
  - eliminate any common source, and disinfect the environment;
  - separate susceptible from infected and colonized patients;
  - consider closing the unit to new admissions.
- Modify host risk:
  - discontinue compromising factors, if possible;
  - control antibiotic use (consider rotation, restriction, or discontinuing antibiotics).

Control of endemic antibiotic resistance

- Appropriate use of antibiotics—this should include optimal choice of agent, the dose, and its duration, based on defined antibiotic policies for both treatment and prophylaxis. The use of topical antibiotics should be limited.
- Infection control—institute guidelines for intensive infection control procedures, and provide adequate facilities and resources, especially for handwashing, barrier precautions (isolation), and environmental control measures.
- Improve antimicrobial prescribing practices through educational and administrative methods.
- Monitor local antibiotic resistance rates, and ensure antimicrobial guidelines are up-to-date.

UK MRSA prevention guidelines

(See Table 6.8.)

In 2009/2010, the UK DH introduced mandatory screening of all elective and emergency hospital admissions, with the aim of preventing MRSA infections. It was subsequently noted that settings without universal screening (e.g. Wales) also saw marked falls in MRSA infection, and the NOW study was commissioned.[6] This demonstrated poor compliance with screening and big falls in MRSA prevalence (often <1%) that meant compliance was unlikely to be cost-effective. At current prevalence levels, it is considered cost-effective to screen only high-risk specialties. Cost-effectiveness increases with increasing prevalence.

Table 6.8 UK guidelines for management of MRSA

Publication	Reference	Notes
Implementation of modified admission MRSA screening guidance for NHS (2014)	Department of Health expert advisory committee on Antimicrobial Resistance and Healthcare Associated Infection (2014)	Outlining a more focused 'cost-effective' MRSA screening policy, reflecting the overall decline in MRSA
UK standards for microbiology investigations: investigation of specimens for screening for MRSA	Public Health England (2014)	Reliable detection of MRSA colonization
Guidelines for the control and prevention of meticillin-resistant *Staphylococcus aureus* (MRSA) in healthcare facilities	Coia JE, Duckworth GJ, Edwards DI, *et al.* (2006). *J Hosp Infect* **63** Suppl 1:S1–44	Infection control guidance and strategies for preventing spread of MRSA or infection with MRSA

Reference

6 Fuller C, Robotham J, Savage J, *et al.* (2013). The national one week prevalence audit of universal meticillin-resistant Staphylococcus aureus (MRSA) admission screening 2012. *PLoS One*. **8**:e74219.

Control of carbapenemase-producing *Enterobacteriaceae*

The UK has seen a rapid increase in the incidence of infection and colonization by MDR carbapenemase-producing organisms. Organisms expressing this resistance mechanism are highly resistant and extremely difficult to treat. PHE published *Carbapenemase-producing Enterobacteriaceae: early detection, management and control toolkit for acute trusts* (Dec 2013). The key to controlling the spread is through early detection and prompt isolation. The major risk factors for colonization are:

- admission to a health-care facility abroad in the last 12 months. The range of countries at risk is extremely broad, from Malta to Taiwan;
- previously colonized or infected with a carbapenemase-producing organism;
- admission to a UK hospital where spread of carbapenemase-producing *Enterobacteriaceae* (CPE) has been a problem (Manchester, London).

If a patient falls into an at-risk group, they must be isolated immediately and screened, and there must be strict adherence to standard infection control precautions.

Screening

Do not wait for screening results before isolating a patient. Screening is done using a rectal swab, and, for an effective screen, faeces must be visible on the swab. Contacts should only be screened when the index case is confirmed.

Infection control precautions

Isolate the patient in an en suite side room. Standard precautions must be strictly adhered to. However, if during patient contact there is the potential that the staff member's uniform will come into contact with a patient, long-sleeved disposable aprons must be used. Enhanced cleaning of the environment must take place, focusing on high-touch surfaces.

Decolonization

There is currently no evidence to attempt skin or gut decolonization.

Environmental cleaning

Following discharge, the isolation room must be deep cleaned.

Rescreening

There are limited data relating to how long humans remain colonized with CPE. Therefore, how long to consider a patient is colonized and when to rescreen are matters for debate. All trusts should produce their own infection control guidance relating to the management of patients colonized with CPE.

Further reading

Public Health England (2013). *Carbapenemase-producing Enterobacteriaceae: early detection, management and control toolkit for acute trusts*. Available at: https://www.gov.uk/government/uploads/system/uploads/attachment_data/file/329227/Acute_trust_toolkit_for_the_early_detection.pdf.

Control of tuberculosis in hospitals

While most TB infections are acquired in the community, the risk of health care-associated TB remains for patients and HCWs. Most health care-acquired TB cases result from delayed diagnosis of TB, inadequate treatment of latent TB, and lack of isolation facilities. An understanding of the routes of transmission is fundamental to preventing the spread of infection. TB is primarily transmitted by the inhalation of small droplets. An important distinction to make in the risk assessment of a patient suspected of having TB is whether they have open pulmonary TB or non-pulmonary TB.

- *Open pulmonary TB*—patients who have 'smear'-positive sputum, i.e. sputum microscopy has detected acid-fast bacilli (AFB) in the sample. These patients are at high risk of transmitting the infection and must be isolated. Smear-negative patients (three sputum samples, spontaneously produced on 3 separate days, which are all smear-negative) are not considered infectious and do not need isolation.
- *Non-pulmonary TB*—TB infection at any other site, e.g. renal TB. Non-pulmonary TB is at low risk of transmission, and these patients can be nursed in the open bay. However, if they have a procedure that may aerosolize the organism, e.g. irrigation of an infected wound, washout of the abscess, then they must be isolated during the procedure, and appropriate respiratory precautions must be used.

The successful control and prevention of TB in hospitals may be achieved through three main approaches:[7]

- administrative—early investigation and diagnosis of those suspected to have TB. All patients suspected of having pulmonary TB must be isolated promptly, while appropriate investigations are carried out;
- environment/engineering—patient isolation and the extent of the precautions are dependent on whether the patient is at risk of MDR- or XDR-TB. All patients suspected of having TB must be risk-assessed and isolated appropriately, pending culture results:
    - low risk of MDR/XDR-TB—can be nursed in a standard side room under normal atmospheric pressure. Respiratory precautions only to be used during aerosol-generating procedures. Following 2 weeks of appropriate treatment, this patient is considered low risk and can be moved out of isolation. However, they remain at a low risk of infectivity and therefore must not be moved into the same bay as an immunocompromised patient, e.g. HIV, oncology patient;
    - high risk of MDR/XDR-TB—risk factors include: history of prior treatment or treatment failure, known contact, birth in a country with a high incidence, HIV co-infection, residence in London, male, age 25–44. If considered high risk, this patient group must be isolated in a negative pressure side room throughout their admission. All contacts with the patient must involve PPE and appropriate respiratory precautions, regardless of whether they are of an aerosol-generating nature or not. Smear-positive material can be rapidly assessed for rifampicin resistance genes by PCR to aid diagnosis.

- personal respiratory protection—barrier nursing, gowns, filtered masks ('duck masks' or FFP3). In the UK, filtered masks are only indicated for patients with suspected/proven MDR-TB and XDR-TB or for aerosol-generating procedures (e.g. bronchoscopy). All masks must be correctly fitted. For further information, see NICE clinical guidelines (2011).

Transmission of tuberculosis from patients

DH guidance includes the importance of being able to identify patients with infectious/potentially infectious TB or who have drug-resistant TB, and facilitate access to, and ensure staff are aware of, the appropriate isolation facilities and infection control precautions to be taken.

Transmission of tuberculosis from health-care workers

When a HCW develops TB, this may lead to expensive, time-consuming, large-scale contact investigations to determine the extent of transmission and prevent further spread. The incidence of acute and latent TB is higher amongst foreign-born HCWs. Difficulties arise in the interpretation of TSTs in this group. Management of HCWs with TB is usually shared by occupational health, infection control, and the clinical teams. For advice about screening all new NHS employees who will have contact with patients or their samples, see NICE clinical guidelines (2011).

Reference

7 Humphreys H (2008). Control and prevention of healthcare-associated tuberculosis: the role of respiratory isolation and personal respiratory protection. *J Hosp Infect.* **69**:91–2.

Further reading

National Institute for Health and Care Excellence (2011). *Tuberculosis: clinical diagnosis and management of tuberculosis, and measures for its prevention and control.* NICE clinical guideline 117. Available at: https://www.nice.org.uk/guidance/cg117.

Control of Creutzfeldt–Jakob disease and transmissible spongiform encephalopathies

The TSEs include CJD (which may be sporadic, familial, iatrogenic, or vCJD), variably protease-sensitive prionopathy, and GSS (see Gerstmann–Sträussler–Scheinker syndrome, p. 468). The prion proteins associated with TSEs are unusually resistant to inactivation by heat and chemicals, so special decontamination procedures are required. Cases of iatrogenic CJD have been transmitted by contaminated pituitary-derived hormones, dura mater grafts, neurosurgical instruments, corneal transplantation, organ transplantation, and blood transfusion. Current challenges faced are in the early detection and diagnosis of vCJD, therapy and support for those affected, and improved understanding of transmission risks.

Variant CJD/new variant CJD

This emerged in the late 1990s and has a distinct clinical presentation (➔ see Creutzfeldt–Jakob disease (CJD) and variant CJD, pp. 466–7), tending to infect a younger age group than classical CJD. The number of new cases of vCJD is falling, but the total number of predicted cases is a topic of debate. In vCJD, prion proteins have been detected in systemic lymphoid tissue before the patient is symptomatic, and the infectious agents are more resistant to inactivation than previously observed. Therefore the greatest risk of cross-infection comes from potential contamination and subsequent failure to remove the prions from clinical equipment. Thus, there are widespread consequences in infection control procedures such as traceability of endoscopes and quarantining of surgical instruments. The quarantining of equipment can have significant financial implications for the hospital.

Risk assessments

All patients admitted for surgery should have a risk assessment performed. The infection control measures are dependent on the risk status of the patient and the nature of the surgery. Patients at increased risk of CJD or vCJD include:

- those who are symptomatic with a neurological condition that is consistent with CJD;
- individuals who have had one or more blood relatives affected by CJD or who have been shown by genetic testing to be at risk;
- those who have received blood products, organs, or tissues from someone who developed vCJD, or they have donated blood and the recipient subsequently developed CJD;
- those who received hormones derived from human pituitary tissue;
- those who have received >300 blood products since 1990.

Patients who fall into one or more of these groups are at risk. The risk of the surgery should then be stratified. This is effectively dependent on whether the surgery involves at-risk tissue.

Medium- to high-risk surgery involves tissues, including:

- neural—brain, spinal cord, and cranial nerves, including olfactory epithelium;
- ocular—posterior eye, retina;
- endocrine—pituitary gland.

Classification of risk and outcomes

If the patient is considered to be at risk and the surgery involves medium- to high-risk tissue, the options are:

- quarantine the equipment for re-use exclusively in the same patient;
- use single-use equipment;
- destroy the equipment.

If the surgery involves an at-risk patient and low-risk tissue, then no special equipment processing is required.

Prevention of transmission of CJD

Always consult trust policy, and involve the ICT. Some general principles are advised for the processing of instruments (see Box 6.18) and in blood transfusion (see Box 6.19), in order to minimize transmission of CJD. Guidance for care of symptomatic or at-risk patients is detailed in Box 6.20. There have been four cases of blood transfusion-associated CJD in the UK. The blood products were all donated when the donor was in the preclinical stage of the disease, and none were leucodepleted. There is no evidence of any UK clinical case of vCJD being linked to a blood transfusion given after 1999. All clinical specimens from known, suspected, or at-risk patients should be handled at CL3 in the microbiology laboratory, as the agent of CJD is in hazard group 3.

Box 6.18 Precautions regarding processing of instruments exposed to low-risk tissue to minimize transmission of CJD

- Staff should practise universal precautions.
- Clean all surgical instruments to remove organic matter before sterilization.
- Consider using single-use instruments, whenever possible. Never reprocess single-use kits—throw them away immediately. Use single-use kits for all lumbar punctures (LPs).
- High-vacuum porous-load autoclaving at 134–137°C for 18min for six cycles can reduce infectivity.
- The following methods are ineffective for prions: autoclaving at 134°C for 3min; alcohol; ethylene oxide; glutaraldehyde; formalin.
- Record the unique identification number of all flexible endoscopes every time they are used, and ensure all instruments are traceable through the audit trail.
- Research in mice has suggested that dental tissue may be infective; thus, instruments used for root canal work should be single-use.

Box 6.19 Precautions regarding blood transfusion to minimize transmission of CJD

- Blood donors who have themselves received a blood transfusion or tissue donation are now excluded (2005).
- Leucodeplete all blood donations—this will reduce infectivity but not eliminate it.
- Plasma for use in those <16 years old is purchased outside the UK.
- Note that screening tests are being developed to detect the prion protein in blood products, but none are currently in use.

Box 6.20 Care of symptomatic or at-risk patients

All patients should be subject to universal precautions. There is no evidence to suggest CJD is spread from person to person by close contact. Patients known to have CJD do not require special nursing precautions or special precautions for management of sharps injuries, exposure to blood and body fluids, used and infected linen, and the disposal of clinical waste. However, particular care must be taken to adhere to trust policy for the following:

- collection, labelling, and transport of clinical specimens—use 'Danger of Infection' stickers, and provide adequate clinical information for laboratory staff to undertake a risk assessment;
- CNS and lymphoid tissue biopsies—these procedures should be performed by experienced staff using disposable equipment. Gloves, goggles, and aprons should be worn, and any contaminated objects should be incinerated.

Further reading

Advisory Committee on Dangerous Pathogens Spongiform Encephalopathy Advisory Committee (2015). *Transmissible spongiform encephalopathy agents: safe working and the prevention of infection.* Available at: https://www.gov.uk/government/uploads/system/uploads/attachment_data/file/260961/report.pdf.

Public Health England (2015). *Infection prevention and control of CJD and variant CJD in healthcare and community settings.* Available at: https://www.gov.uk/government/uploads/system/uploads/attachment_data/file/427854/Infection_controlv3.0.pdf.

Disinfection

Disinfection is the process of killing of microorganisms by physical or chemical means, to render the object 'safe'. It does not imply complete inactivation of all viruses or removal of bacterial spores (as occurs in sterilization).

A disinfectant is defined as a chemical used to destroy microorganisms. These agents only act on surfaces (environmental surfaces, equipment, or body surfaces) and do not penetrate layers of dirt or grease. Thus, disinfection is not a substitute for cleaning. Disinfectants do not usually have a persistent effect.

Use of disinfectants

The environmental use of disinfectants should be restricted to accidental spills or build-up of infected material in areas where this may be a hazard to patients or HCWs.

Different disinfectants have different properties; many are corrosive and toxic, and the speed of action is highly variable. Others, if used correctly, can kill all microorganisms (i.e. sterilize), but most are highly selective and only kill a limited range of organisms. They fall into two main groups (see Table 6.9):

- environmental disinfectants—often too toxic for use on skin; may require protective clothing. Hypochlorite is most commonly used;

Table 6.9 Environmental and skin disinfectants

Class	Examples	Use	Notes
Environmental disinfectants			
Hypochlorite (bleach)	Hypochlorite powder, e.g. Titan® sanitizer; detergent hypochlorite (liquid or tablet), e.g. Domestos®, Presept®	Best general-purpose disinfectant available. However, not suitable for particularly dirty situations. Generally use a solution of 1000 ppm (parts/mL) available chlorine, but increase concentration to 1 ppm if need to destroy hepatitis viruses (e.g. dialysis units). Use hypochlorite granules for spillage of body fluids, except urine	Sodium hypochlorite acts by the release of chlorine on contact with organic matter, so rapidly destroys all bacteria and viruses. However, some agents are unstable, and disinfecting properties may be lost by the rapid release of chlorine on contact with blood, faeces, or textiles. Strong solutions are corrosive to aluminium and other metals
Phenolics	Black fluids, e.g. 'Jeyes® fluid'; white fluids, e.g. 'Izal®'; clear phenolics, e.g. 'Stericol®'	Not for routine environmental cleansing or disinfection; used in laboratory and post-mortem rooms	Derived from coal tar, and in common use in hospitals for over a century. Reasonable in visibly dirty situations. However, many bacteria and viruses are resistant, and prolonged exposure is needed for effective action. Also toxic, so handle with special precautions
Chloroxylenols	'Dettol®'	Household disinfectant	Said to combine some of the properties of the phenolics with hypochlorites. Less effective at killing Gram-negatives than the phenolics, and expensive
Skin disinfectants			
Alcohols	Ethyl alcohol (available as industrial methylated spirit (IMS)); isopropyl alcohol (e.g. 'Mediswabs')	Often used as a base for other skin disinfectants, e.g.iodine or chlorhexidine	Ethyl alcohol (70%) effectively kills organisms on the skin, but this effect ceases after evaporation. Isopropyl alcohol evaporates less rapidly but is thought to be less effective against some viruses

(*Continued*)

Table 6.9 (*Contd.*)

Class	Examples	Use	Notes
Iodine	Huge variety of products, e.g. Betadine®	Surgical scrubs, shampoos, etc.	Iodine dissolved in 70% alcohol is less popular, as it is messy and may be an irritant
Chlorhexidine	Hibitane®, Hibiscrub®	Surgical scrubs, popular disinfectant in hospitals and laboratories	Often marketed with other disinfecting agents and in alcoholic or aqueous solution. Some hospital organisms show resistance to it, but this is not a problem when using the alcoholic solution
Quaternary ammonium compounds (QACs)	Cetrimide	Trauma wounds and other special situations, not used in routine wound cleaning	Ineffective against some hospital organisms, e.g. *Pseudomonas* spp.

- skin disinfectants (also called antiseptics)—often have limited range of action so are inappropriate for environmental disinfection, and usually relatively expensive. Chlorhexidine is the preferred agent. Alternatives are alcohol (inferior) and iodine (irritant).

Other disinfectants may be used to sterilize instruments, but heat treatment is usually preferred (➔ see Sterilization, pp. 174–6).

Selection of a disinfectant

Considerations include:
- which organisms do you want to destroy?
- what is the construction of the object to be disinfected?
- does the object need cleaning first?
- when an agent has been chosen, what concentration of disinfectant is required?

Sterilization

Sterilization is the process by which transmissible agents are killed or eliminated. This includes fungi, bacteria, viruses, and spores, but not prions. There are two main types of sterilization:
- physical sterilization—this includes heat sterilization and radiation (e.g. electron beams, X-rays, γ rays);
- chemical sterilization—this includes *ethylene oxide, ozone, chlorine bleach, glutaraldehyde, formaldehyde, hydrogen peroxide*, and *peracetic acid*.

Cleaning of instruments

Whichever sterilization process is deemed most appropriate, thorough cleaning is essential; otherwise, any dirt or biological matter may shield any organisms present. Physical scrubbing with detergent and water is recommended. Cool water is needed to clean organic matter from instruments, as warm or hot water may cause coagulation of organic debris. Alternative cleaning methods include ultrasound or pulsed air.

Physical sterilization: heat

This can be either dry heat or moist heat sterilization.

- Dry heat sterilization uses hot air that is free (or almost free) from water vapour, so any moisture plays no role in the process of sterilization. Methods include the hot air oven, radiation, and microwave. The dry heat coagulates proteins in any organism and causes oxidative free radical damage and drying of cells.
- Moist heat (steam under pressure) sterilization uses hot air heavily laden with water vapour. Moist heat destroys microorganisms by the irreversible denaturation of enzymes and structural proteins. Water vapour has a very high penetrating property and also causes damage through the formation of oxidative free radicals. Methods include autoclaving, pressure cooking, pasteurization of milk, boiling, and steam sterilizing (steam at *atmospheric pressure* for 90min).

Autoclaves—steam sterilization using autoclaves is commonly used in hospitals and provides an inexpensive means of sterilizing large numbers of surgical instruments. To achieve sterility, a holding time of >15min at 121°C, or 3min at 134°C, is required. Liquids and instruments packed in cloth may take longer to reach the specified temperature so usually need more time. Autoclave treatment inactivates all bacteria, fungi, viruses, and spores. Certain prions may be eradicated by autoclaving at 121–132°C for 60min or 134°C for >18min, but this process is not 100% reliable for CJD (see Box 6.18). Monitoring an autoclave cycle is important and involves recording temperature and pressure over time. To ensure adequate conditions have been met, most hospitals use indicator tape which changes colour. Bioindicators (e.g. based on the spores of *Bacillus stearothermophilus*) are also used to independently confirm autoclave performance. These indicators should be positioned to ensure that steam penetrates the most difficult places. Note that autoclaving is often used to sterilize medical waste prior to disposal.

Chemical sterilization

Chemical sterilization is generally used when heat methods are inappropriate, e.g. for sterilizing heat-sensitive materials such as plastics, paper, biological materials, fibre optics, and electronics. Options include:

- ethylene oxide (EO) sterilization is very common, particularly for disposable medical devices. Sterilization is usually carried out between 30°C and 60°C for objects that are sensitive to higher temperatures, e.g. plastics and optics. EO gas penetrates well and is highly effective, killing all viruses, bacteria, fungi, and spores. However, it is highly flammable, takes longer than any heat treatment, and produces toxic residues. *Bacillus subtilis* spores are used as a rapid biological indicator for EO sterilizers;

- ozone is used to sterilize water and air in industrial settings, and as a surface disinfectant. It can oxidize most organic matter but may be impractical, because it is toxic and unstable and must be produced on site;
- chlorine bleach will kill bacteria, fungi, viruses, and most spores. Household bleach (5.25% sodium hypochlorite) is usually diluted to 1/10 before use. To kill MTB, it should only be diluted 1/5, and, to inactivate prions, it should be 1/2.5 (1 part bleach and 1.5 parts water). For full sterilization, bleach should be allowed to react for 20min. It is highly corrosive (including some stainless steel surgical instruments);
- glutaraldehyde and formaldehyde are volatile liquids, which are only effective if the immersion time is long enough. It can take up to 12h to kill all spores in a clear liquid with glutaraldehyde, and even longer with formaldehyde. Both liquids are toxic if inhaled or if they come into contact with skin. Glutaraldehyde is expensive and has a shelf life of <2 weeks. Formaldehyde is cheaper but much more volatile (in fact, it may be used as a gaseous sterilizing agent);
- ortho-phthalaldehyde has many advantages over glutaraldehyde—shows better mycobactericidal activity, kills glutaraldehyde-resistant spores, is more stable, less volatile, less irritating, and acts faster. However, it is more expensive, and stains skin and proteins grey;
- hydrogen peroxide is a non-toxic chemical at low concentrations and leaves no residue. It can be used to sterilize endoscopes, either in low-temperature plasma sterilization chambers or mixed with formic acid. It can also be used at a concentration of 30–35% under low pressure conditions in the dry sterilization process (DSP). This process achieves bacterial reduction of 10^{-6}–10^{-8} in ~6s, and the surface temperature is increased only 10–15°C;
- guidelines on the decontamination of endoscopes are available at:
  - 🖱 https://www.brit-thoracic.org.uk/guidelines-and-quality-standards/bronchoscopy-diagnostic-flexible-bronchoscopy-in-adults-guideline;
  - 🖱 www.bsg.org.uk/clinical-guidance/endoscopy/guidelines-for-decontamination-of-equipment-for-gastrointestinal-endoscopy.html.

Ventilation in health-care premises

Definitions of different ventilation systems

Positive-pressure ventilation

Positive-pressure isolation rooms are used to prevent the entry of micro-organisms, if patients are susceptible to infections. The air is filtered before entering a sealed room, with a HEPA filter, and air is pumped into the room at a greater rate than it is expelled. This forces air out of the isolation room, keeping the room free of microorganisms. There is usually an anteroom to facilitate the donning of protective clothing and airflows of at least 12 air changes/hour.

Negative-pressure ventilation

Negative-pressure isolation rooms are used to prevent pathogens (e.g. TB) from an infected patient infecting other patients or HCWs in the hospital. It is usually a sealed room, except for a small gap under the door, through which air enters. Direction of airflow can be confirmed by a smoke test (hold a smoke tube ~5cm in front of the bottom of the door, and, if the room is at negative pressure, the smoke will travel under the door and into the room).

HEPA filter

HEPA filters can remove almost all airborne particles of 0.3 micrometres in diameter, e.g. *Aspergillus* spores.

Plenum ventilation

This is the most frequently used system in general-purpose operating theatres. Atmospheric air is filtered in two stages:

- coarse filter to remove dust and debris;
- bacterial filter of ~2 micrometres in pore size, with 95% efficiency, is used inside the inlet grill.

Some air may recirculate within the suite. An exhaust system removes the air to the outside. There are ~20 air changes/hour.

Laminar flow

Laminar flow is used in orthopaedic theatres to reduce the number of microorganisms present. This is of particular value in preventing prosthetic joint infections (PJIs). A continuous flow of filtered air recirculates under positive pressure into the operating field, and any air contaminants generated under surgery are removed from the site. There are ~300 air changes/hour, which should result in <10 cfu/m^3. Different systems include introduction of air horizontally or vertically, in an enclosed, semi-enclosed, or open manner.

Operating theatres

Health Technical Memorandum (HTM) 2025 (specialist ventilation in health-care premises) has been revised as HTM 03-01 (part A covers design and validation, and part B covers operational management and performance ventilation). This is a new set of standard schemes for ventilation of conventional and ultraclean ventilation (UCV) operating theatres. There are four main sections:

- management policy—management responsibilities/legal issues;
- design requirements;
- validation/verification—commissioning (i.e. when a new theatre is built or after major constructional changes), performance tests, handover;
- operative management—day-to-day issues such as minimum standards, maintaining performance, routine maintenance, etc.

For a discussion of practices in operating theatres, see Box 6.21.

Box 6.21 Rituals and behaviours in operating theatres

All operating theatres should have their own up-to-date infection control policy. This should include standard precautions for every invasive procedure and outline the need for an additional risk assessment for each patient, to see if other specific precautions are required. There are many 'rituals and behaviours' that have crept into 'standard practice' in many operating theatres—some of which are beneficial, some are harmful. The standard of evidence varies, but a few practical pointers are listed below. For further discussion, see Woodhead *et al.*[9]

- Patients' clothes—it may not be necessary to change, e.g. for cataract surgery. Jewellery only needs to be removed (for infection control purposes) if near the site of operation.
- Shaving should be avoided. Depilatory cream the day before surgery is preferable, or clippers in the anaesthetic room immediately preop.
- Hand hygiene—scrubbing brushes should not be used on the skin.
- Drapes—there is no evidence for adhesives around the edge of wounds.
- Gloves—needle puncture is not an indication to change gloves; if necessary, a second pair should be worn on top.
- Masks—there is no good evidence that masks reduce infection rates; however, they are recommended to protect the surgeon. The scrub team should wear masks and hats for implants, and the mask should be changed for each procedure. Non-scrubbed staff in plenum ventilated theatres do not require masks or hats.
- Linen—should be waterproof and disposable (European standard).

Air sampling

Microbiological tests are needed to complement the physical monitoring systems, although few studies have demonstrated a link between microbiological air quality and wound infections. For details of performing air sampling and testing infection control rooms, see Walker *et al.*,[8] and, for operating theatres, see *Health Technical Memorandum 03-01: specialized ventilation for healthcare premises* (UK DH). Separate guidance is given for empty and in-use theatres.

- If an empty theatre fails the air sampling tests, check the technique, and repeat sampling. If it fails again, discuss the findings with the ICT, engineers, or other experts. Consider testing the particle penetration of filters and/or the air velocity.
- If an in-use theatre fails the air sampling tests, check the technique, and repeat sampling when the theatre is empty.

References

8 Walker JT, Hoffman P, Bennett AM, *et al.* (2007). Hospital and community acquired infection and the built environment—design and testing of infection control rooms. *J Hosp Infect.* **65** Suppl 2:43–9.

9 Woodhead K, Taylor EW, Bannister G, Chesworth T, Hoffman P, Humphreys H (2002). Behaviours and rituals in the operating theatre. A report from the Hospital Infection Society Working Party on Infection Control in Operating Theatres. *J Hosp Infect.* **51**:241–55.

Laundry

Hospital linen should be processed, so it is not an infection risk to future users. The laundry should remove evidence of previous use, including organisms, but cannot be expected to kill bacterial spores. NHS Executive guidance (HSG(95)18) differentiates used (soiled or fouled) and infected linen, and describes a framework to reduce risk to all staff concerned (porters, laundry staff, etc.), as is shown in Table 6.10. Washing temperature requirements vary between countries. In the UK, the temperature of the cycle should reach 65°C for at least 10min or 71°C for at least 3min. Heat-labile laundry that would be damaged at high temperatures can be washed at 40°C with sodium hypochlorite to give a final concentration of 150 ppm available chlorine to the final rinse. Monitoring of critical points is important under hazard analysis and critical control point (HACCP). These include temperature and exposure times, treatment of rinse water (if potentially contaminated), in-use detergent concentrations, and drying temperatures.

Curtains should be laundered as follows:

- if visibly soiled;
- after an outbreak of viral gastroenteritis, as part of the terminal clean;
- if they are around the bed of a patient who has been barrier-nursed (e.g. with MRSA, *C. difficile*), they should be washed on patient discharge;
- routinely (3 months minimum).

Table 6.10 Categories of linen

Linen category	Definition	Bag colour
Soiled	All used linen that is not fouled or infected	White nylon bag
Fouled	Contaminated with any bodily fluid	White or clear plastic bag, then white linen outer bag Treat as potentially infected, so wear gloves and aprons when handling it
Infected	Linen from patient with, or suspected to have, infection with enteric organism, e.g. diarrhoea and/or vomiting, *Campylobacter*, viral gastroenteritis, *Salmonella, Shigella*, hepatitis A, etc.	Red alginate bag, then red nylon outer bag, labelled with point of origin
	Blood-stained linen from patient with HIV/hepatitis B or C	
	Linen visibly contaminated with sputum from patient with open TB	

Waste

Disposal of waste is subject to strict legislation set out by the DH, Department of the Environment, the Health and Safety Commission Advisory Group, and the amended European Communities Framework Directive on Waste. This legislation places a duty of care on anyone handling clinical waste, including porters and incineration staff. Thus, hospital guidelines apply not only to clinical areas, but throughout the hospital. There is a move towards a unified approach for disposal of infectious and medicinal waste, and to operate the same category codes throughout Europe.

Apart from the direct environmental benefits achieved by the compliant management of health-care waste, the 2013 guidance[10] presents opportunities for introducing cost savings, safer working practices, and reducing carbon emissions related to managing waste.

Clinical waste

Clinical waste is always incinerated and is defined as follows:

- all human tissue and body fluids and related items (e.g. dressings, incontinence pads, stoma bags, and urine containers);
- sharps and contaminated sharp items, e.g. glass;
- certain pharmaceutical products and their containers;
- potentially infected laboratory waste.

Table 6.11 summarizes other types of waste, the national colour-coded system, and recommendations for disposal.

Table 6.11 National colour-coded system for waste disposal containers

Type of waste	Container	Notes
Clinical waste	Yellow plastic bags (orange/red in some hospitals)	Make sure bags are only two-thirds full. Tie them securely, and label each bag with ward of origin, before sending for incineration. If there is a chance that body fluids may leak from a single yellow bag, then use double-bagging
Non-clinical waste	Black plastic bags	
Sharps	Yellow rigid plastic boxes	Do not overfill these boxes. Never re-sheathe needles or separate needles from a syringe, unless using an approved safe method. Put IV giving sets into these boxes too
Glass (larger items)	Black dustbins	
CSSD	Brown bags marked CSSD	
Confidential or cytotoxic waste	Local policies apply	

CSSD, Centre for Surgical Sterilization and Disinfection.

Reference

10 Department of Health (2013). *Health technical memorandum 07-01: safe management of health-care waste*. Available at: https://www.gov.uk/government/uploads/system/uploads/attachment_data/file/167976/HTM_07-01_Final.pdf.

Introduction to prevention of hospital-acquired infection

Results from the 2011 HAI point prevalence survey, conducted in England by the Health Protection Agency (HPA, now PHE), show that 6.4% (a reduction from 8.2% in 2006) of hospital inpatients had a HAI during their stay.[11] Patients on ICUs are at increased risk, and estimates suggest that 15–40% of patients will have at least one HAI. The impact varies from increased length of stay and discomfort to prolonged and permanent disability, and, in some cases, death. The estimated cost to the NHS in 2004 was £1 billion annually.[12]

It is estimated that around 15% of HAIs are preventable through better application of 'good practice'.[13] It is difficult to calculate the costs of introducing prevention methods on a trust basis, but all research so far suggests that it is cheaper to focus on prevention, rather than pay for costs of treating HAI. The National Audit Office report noted that a reduction in HAI by 15% could save £150 million.[12]

Prevention is everyone's business ... not just the infection control team!

There is clearly a need to change the culture and staff behaviour. Currently, this has been highlighted as one of the biggest obstacles. Evidence suggests that a variety of approaches are required, so that the individual HCW accepts personal responsibility. Training and education must be continual, and constant reminders, e.g. poster campaigns, handwashing publicity, and infection awareness days, are effective. Named individuals acting as liaison representatives and role models in each specialty are beneficial. Feedback of infection rates at ward/team level is vital to engage staff, encourage a sense of ownership, and encourage continual review of practice.

Focus points on prevention

- Education and training for health-care staff, especially doctors.
- Better compliance with hand hygiene, care of indwelling lines, catheter care, and aseptic technique.
- Good antibiotic prescribing.
- Hospital cleanliness.
- Consultation with the ICT on wider issues, e.g. new-build projects.

References

11 Health Protection Agency (2012). *English national point prevalence survey on healthcare-associated infections and antimicrobial use, 2011*. Available at: https://www.gov.uk/government/uploads/system/uploads/attachment_data/file/331871/English_National_Point_Prevalence_Survey_on_Healthcare_associated_Infections_and_Antimicrobial_Use_2011.pdf.

12 National Audit Office (2004). *Improving patient care by reducing the risk of hospital acquired infection: A progress report*. Available at: https://www.nao.org.uk/wp-content/uploads/2004/07/0304876.pdf.
13 National Audit Office (2000). *The management and control of hospital acquired infection in acute NHS trusts in England*. Available at: https://www.nao.org.uk/wp-content/uploads/2000/02/9900230.pdf.

Infections in intensive care

Nosocomial infections complicate 25–40% of all ICU admissions. Although ICUs represent <5% of hospital beds, nosocomial infections in the ICU consume a significant amount of hospital resources.

Patients on the ICU are exposed to more broad-spectrum antibiotics (up to 60% of all patients on the ICU are on antibiotics) and medical devices, and more procedures than those on normal hospital wards. Hand hygiene, barrier precautions, cohorting of personnel, and antibiotic policies are particularly important in controlling infection (see Box 6.22).

Organisms

- The causal organism(s) isolated depend on the length of ICU stay (see Table 6.12).
- Recent shift from a preponderance of Gram-negative infections to Gram-positives, probably due to increased line and device-associated infections.
- Increasing prevalence of *Candida* infections, including non-albicans, which may be more drug-resistant.
- More infections with antibiotic-resistant organisms—MRSA, VRE, multi-resistant Gram-negative species such as *E. coli*, *Klebsiella* spp., *Serratia* spp., *Acinetobacter* spp., *S. maltophilia*, *Enterobacter* spp.

Box 6.22 Studies of HAIs on the ICU

- The European Prevalence of Infection in Intensive Care (EPIC) study (1992) was a 1-day point prevalence study looking at >10 000 patients from 17 countries on all ICUs, except paediatrics and coronary care units.[14] The infection data were linked to the patients' APACHE (Acute Physiology and Chronic Health Evaluation) score and 6-week outcome, presence of lines, specific interventions, and demographics. Overall, 45% of patients had some sort of infection, and 20% had at least one infection acquired on the ICU. The commonest were pneumonia (47%), LRTI (18%), UTI (18%), bacteraemia (12%), and wound infection (7%). Organisms were split 50/50 Gram-positive and Gram-negative, the commonest being *S. aureus*, *P. aeruginosa*, CoNS, and *Enterococcus*.
- The Study on the Efficacy of Nosocomial Infection Control (SENIC) looked at the relative change in nosocomial infection over a 5-year period.[15] Overall, when infection control measures were introduced, nosocomial infections were reduced by 32%.

Table 6.12 Organisms isolated depend on the length of ICU stay

Early infection (≤4 days)	Late infection (>4 days)
S. pneumoniae	*Enterobacter* spp.
H. influenzae	*Serratia* spp.
Enterobacteriaceae	*P. aeruginosa*
S. aureus—MSSA	*Acinetobacter* spp.
Streptococcus spp.	*S. aureus*—MRSA
Anaerobes	*Enterococcus* spp.
	Fungi

MRSA, meticillin-resistant *S. aureus*; MSSA, meticillin-sensitive *S. aureus*.

Patients

- Increasing population of immunosuppressed patients, e.g. HIV, BMT, solid organ transplant patients.
- Increasing use of devices, e.g. lines, balloon pumps, pacing wires, endotracheal tubes.
- More invasive procedures, e.g. ventilator, drains.

ICU environment

- Isolating patients with resistant organisms is the aim. As a minimum, there should be at least one side room for every six beds. There should also be sufficient space around each bed (20m^2), wash handbasins between every other bed, adequate ventilation, and sufficient storage space and utility space.

How to minimize infections on the ICU

- Follow evidence-based guidelines and policies.
- Good infection control measures, e.g. handwashing.
- Good 'antibiotic control', e.g. specific policy based on local knowledge.
- Close liaison with infection services, pharmacy, engineers, estates, etc.
- Feed back results of surveillance of resistant organisms.

Selective decontamination of the digestive tract

This is a prophylactic technique, which remains controversial. It aims to eradicate aerobic GNRs from the oropharynx and consists of four components:

- oral antimicrobial applied TOP to the mouth four times daily (qds);
- a liquid suspension containing the same antimicrobials given via NG tube;
- IV antimicrobials for 3 days;
- stringent infection control measures.

A systematic review and meta-analysis of >50 RCTs showed that SDD resulted in a significant decrease in levels of overall BSIs, Gram-negative BSIs, and overall mortality, but had no effect on Gram-positive BSIs.[16] There are concerns, however, about the generation of resistant organisms and the risk of CDI.

Department of Health guidance: infection prevention and control in adult critical care

This contains recommendations for reducing the risk of infection through best practice and sustaining this reduction.

- Sustainable reductions in HCAI require the engagement and active involvement of all staff working in the ICU, supported by the ICT and clinical champions.
- No single action will produce effective infection prevention and control practice. This is achieved by sustained and close adherence to best practice by every member of the ICU team.
- All individuals who come into contact with ICU patients have a responsibility to ensure effective infection prevention and control afforded to them.

Infections in neonatal intensive care

Neonates often have indwelling devices, invasive procedures, and high exposure to antibiotics—and are more vulnerable to infection due to their immature skin and immune systems. More than 10% of neonates develop a neonatal ICU (NICU)-acquired infection,[17] with the commonest sites being the bloodstream (~50%), lower respiratory tract, ear, nose, and throat (ENT), and urinary tract. The commonest organisms are CoNS and enterococci. Many of the principles surrounding the prevention of infection apply to neonatal and special care baby units. In addition, there have been particular issues such as the need to wash babies with sterile water after the outbreaks due to pseudomonal contamination of wash handbasin water taps (see Box 6.23).

Box 6.23 *Pseudomonas* in taps in NICUs

After outbreaks in neonatal units in Wales (2010) and Northern Ireland (2011/2012), during which many babies suffered from invasive pseudomonal infections and some died, there have been huge efforts to reduce the risk to vulnerable babies. The DH published a review of the scientific evidence behind the contamination of hospital water supplies and outlets with *Pseudomonads*, which was followed by new infection control advice and technical guidance. These documents remind everyone to maintain high standards of infection control, and gives advice on best practice to prevent *P. aeruginosa* in specialist care units and how to manage the risks. This includes only using the handwash station for handwashing, flushing taps regularly, and establishing a Water Safety group (Department of Health (2012). *Pseudomonas aeruginosa bacteria preventing and controlling contamination*. Available at: www.gov.uk/government/publications/pseudomonas-aeruginosa-bacteria-preventing-and-controlling-contamination; Department of Health (2012). *Technical guidance issued for healthcare providers on managing Pseudomonas*. Available at: www.dh.gov.uk/health/2012/03/technical-guidance-pseudomonas/).

References

14 Vincent JL, Bihari DJ, Suter PM, *et al.* (1995). The prevalence of nosocomial infection in intensive care units in Europe. Results of the European Prevalence of Infection in Intensive Care (EPIC) Study. EPIC International Advisory Committee. *JAMA*. **274**:639–44.
15 Haley RW, Morgan WM, Culver DH, *et al.* (1985). Update from the SENIC project. Hospital infection control: recent progress and opportunities under prospective payment. *Am J Infect Control*. **13**:97–108.
16 Silvestri L, van Saene HK, Milanese M, Gregori D, Gullo A (2007). Selective decontamination of the digestive tract reduces bacterial bloodstream infection and mortality in critically ill patients. Systematic review of randomized, controlled trials. *J Hosp Infect*. **65**:187–203.
17 Sohn AH, Garrett DO, Sinkowitz-Cochran RL, *et al.*; Pediatric Prevention Network (2001). Prevalence of nosocomial infections in neonatal intensive care unit patients: Results from the first national point-prevalence survey. *J Pediatr*. **139**:821–7.

Surgical site infection

Introduction

Surgical site infections (SSIs) are seen in at least 5% of patients undergoing a surgical procedure. They range from a minor wound discharge through to osteomyelitis. SSIs make up almost 20% of all HAIs, and cause significant morbidity, increased length of stay, and increased costs. Most infections are endogenous (i.e. result from contamination of the incision by the patient's own microbes during surgery). The other route of acquisition is exogenous from the environment or other people. Factors associated with SSIs have been well defined (see Table 6.13), and multiple guidelines and recommendations have been published to aim to prevent SSIs from occurring. This includes the HII as part of the DH Saving Lives Programme (see Box 6.24).

Table 6.13 Factors associated with SSI[18]

Patient-related	Procedure-related
Colonization with *S. aureus*	Antimicrobial prophylaxis
Corticosteroid use	Duration of procedure
Diabetes mellitus	Duration of surgical scrub
Extremes of age	Foreign material
Immunosuppression	Sterilization of instruments
Longer hospital stay	Operating room ventilation
Malnutrition	Preoperative shaving
Obesity	Preoperative skin preparation
Remote infection	Skin antisepsis
Smoking	

Box 6.24 Care Bundle for Preventing SSI: 'Saving Lives' High Impact Intervention No. 4

Preoperative

MRSA screening—follow trust policy. The care bundle recommends screening all patients undergoing implant and cardiothoracic surgery and neurosurgery, and considering other patients according to local policy, e.g. orthopaedic, vascular.

- MRSA decontamination—see recommendations on Healthcare Infection Society website (www.his.org.uk);
- hair removal—use a clipper with a disposable head. Shaving with a razor is not recommended.

Perioperative

- Prophylactic antimicrobial—where indicated, at correct timing, with appropriate agent. Remember repeat dosing in longer procedures.
- Glucose control—maintaining blood glucose <11mmol/L has been shown to reduce wound infections in diabetic patients.
- Normothermia—maintaining a body temperature above 36°C in the perioperative period has been shown to reduce infection rates.

National surveillance of surgical site infection

Mandatory reporting of SSIs in orthopaedic surgery has shown that rates are highest in hip hemiarthroplasty—partly due to the increased risk of infection in these patients and also due to increased detection of infection, as the patients tend to have a long hospital stay. Most of the SSIs reported affect the superficial layers of the wound, but ~25% involve deeper tissues. Annual reports are published by PHE.

Non-pharmacological measures for reducing surgical site infection

- Appropriate hair removal.[18]
- Appropriate operating room air exchanges.
- Appropriate surgical attire.
- Glycaemic control.
- Maintenance of good oxygenation.
- Limit in-and-out traffic.
- Maintain normothermia.
- Proper preparation of the surgical field.

Rates of surgical infection in different types of operation are shown in Table 6.14.

Table 6.14 Rates of surgical infection in different types of operation

Type of operation	Average infected wounds in 100* operations
Knee joint replacement	<1
Hip joint replacement	1
Abdominal hysterectomy	2
Vascular surgery	2
Coronary artery bypass graft	5
Large bowel (gut) surgery	9

*Detected while patients are in hospital or at readmission following the operation.

Data source: HPA. Healthcare-Associated Infections and Antimicrobial Resistance: 2009/10.

Other useful resources

- MRSA guidelines on the Healthcare Infection Society website (www.his.org.uk/resources-guidelines).
- The Health Technology Assessment programme; Drug and Therapeutics Bulletins and the Scottish Intercollegiate Guidelines Network (SIGN), all referenced in Saving Lives High Impact Intervention No. 4.
- American Healthcare Infection Control Practices Advisory Committee (HICPAC) guidelines for prevention of SSI (1999).[18]
- NICE guidelines: prevention and treatment of surgical site infection, October 2008. www.nice.org.uk/guidance/CG74.

Reference

18 Mangram AJ, Horan TC, Pearson ML, Silver LC, Jarvis WR (1999). Guideline for Prevention of Surgical Site Infection, 1999. Centers for Disease Control and Prevention (CDC) Hospital Infection Control Practices Advisory Committee. *Am J Infect Control*. **27**:97–132.

Bloodstream infection—mandatory surveillance

Definitions

Primary bacteraemia is commonly defined as organisms cultured from the blood, without a documented distal source of infection, but including those resulting from an IV or arterial line infection. Over 95% of BSI on ICUs are primary bacteraemias, most of which are line-related.[19] The 2011 point prevalence survey found that 64% of patients who had a BSI had a vascular access device (peripheral or central) *in situ* for the 48h prior to the onset of infection.[20] Secondary bacteraemia is when organisms are cultured from the blood and are related to a documented focus of infection, e.g. infected leg ulcer.

Catheter-related bloodstream infections

Peripheral venous catheters (PVCs) are more commonly used for vascular access, but the risk of BSI is low (➔ see Line-related sepsis, pp. 193–6).

BSIs are more commonly associated with CVC insertion and are a significant cause of morbidity. Estimates suggest that up to 6000 patients a year in England may acquire a catheter-related BSI (CR-BSI). In 2000, the National Audit Office estimated the additional cost of a BSI to be over £6000 per patient.

Prevention of catheter-related bloodstream infections

The combination of a CVC insertion guideline and a monitoring tool has been shown to significantly reduce the incidence of CR-BSI in an ICU (see Box 6.25).[21] Coated catheters and antibiotic-containing locks are helpful (➔ see Antibiotic-containing locks, p. 196).

For further discussion of line-related sepsis, including the care of peripheral lines and visual infusion phlebitis (VIP) score, see ➔ Line-related sepsis, pp. 193–6.

Department of Health Guidance—Taking blood cultures: a summary of best practice

These recommendations aim to ensure that blood cultures are taken for the correct indication at the correct time using the correct technique. See 'Saving Lives' document for details.[22]

- Only take blood cultures (BCs) when there is a clinical need—ideally before antibiotics are started. Document the date, time, site, and indications. Do not take 'routine' cultures.
- Competence—only by trained staff.

Box 6.25 'Saving Lives' High Impact Intervention No. 1: central venous catheter care

On insertion

- Catheter type—single lumen, unless indicated otherwise for patient care; consider antimicrobial-impregnated line if 1–3 weeks duration likely and high risk of BSI.
- Insertion site—subclavian or internal jugular.
- Use alcoholic chlorhexidine gluconate for skin preparation, and allow to dry.
- Prevent microbial contamination—hand hygiene, aseptic technique.
- Sterile, transparent, semi-permeable dressing.

Continuing care

- Full documentation.
- Regular observation of line insertion site—at least daily.
- Catheter site care—intact, clean dressing.
- Catheter access.
- Aseptic techniques when accessing catheter ports.
- No routine catheter replacement.

- Always make a fresh stab—never take from peripheral lines or sites, or immediately above them. If a central line is present, time to positivity of paired peripheral and central BCs may aid diagnosis.
- Thoroughly disinfect the skin before inserting the needle.
- Once disinfected, do not touch the skin again (no touch technique).
- Disinfect the bottle cap before transferring the sample.

Other useful resources

- American Healthcare Infection Control Practices Advisory Committee (HICPAC) guidelines (2002).
- EPIC guidelines—available through the PHE website.

References

19 Richards MJ, Edwards JR, Culver DH, Gaynes RP (1999). Nosocomial infections in medical intensive care units in the United States. National Nosocomial Infections Surveillance System. *Crit Care Med*. **27**:887–92.

20 Health Protection Agency (2012). *English national point prevalence survey on healthcare associated infections and antimicrobial use, 2011*. Available at: https://www.gov.uk/government/uploads/system/uploads/attachment_data/file/331871/English_National_Point_Prevalence_Survey_on_Healthcare_associated_Infections_and_Antimicrobial_Use_2011.pdf.

21 Berenholtz SM, Pronovost PJ, Lipsett PA, *et al* (2004). Eliminating catheter-related bloodstream infections in the intensive care unit. *Crit Care Med*. **32**:2014–20.

22 Department of Health (2011). *Taking blood cultures: a summary of best practice*. Available at: http://webarchive.nationalarchives.gov.uk/20120118164404/hcai.dh.gov.uk/files/2011/03/Document_Blood_culture_FINAL_100826.pdf.

Urinary catheter-associated infection

UTIs are one of the largest groups of HAIs, accounting for 23% of all HAIs.[23] The presence of a urinary catheter and the length of time it is in place are contributory factors. Estimates from the National Audit Office report (2000) put the extra financial cost of urinary infections at >£1100 per patient.[24] This report also suggested that revised urinary catheter management policies could reduce the number of UTIs. The DH 'Saving Lives' programme includes a care bundle for insertion and ongoing care of urinary catheters (see Box 6.26).

Risk factors

- Presence of urinary catheter/convene.
- Duration of catheter.
- Advanced age/diabetes/immunosuppression.

Prevention

Before inserting a urinary catheter

- Is it really necessary? Review the indication for inserting a catheter in this particular patient at this particular time. Only use an indwelling urethral catheter after considering alternative options (penile sheath, incontinence pads). Suprapubic catheters, commonly used for acute retention, have a lower risk of infection.

Box 6.26 Urinary catheter care bundle: High Impact Intervention No. 6

At insertion

- Assess need for catheterization—avoid if possible.
- Clean the urethral meatus prior to catheter insertion.
- Sterile, closed drainage systems are recommended.
- Correct hand hygiene, aseptic technique, and PPE.

Continuing care

- Sterile sampling of urine—perform aseptically via designated catheter port.
- Drainage bag position—above floor, but below bladder level to prevent reflux or contamination.
- Examination gloves—should be worn to manipulate a catheter, preceded and followed by hand decontamination.
- Correct hand hygiene.
- Clean the catheter site regularly.
- Remove the catheter as soon as possible.

- Choose the correct catheter type, catheter size, and drainage system. By selecting the optimum equipment, the risk of infection from recatheterization can be reduced. Use the smallest catheter possible which allows adequate drainage, and make sure the length is appropriate for male/female patients. In general, a catheter with a 10mL balloon capacity should be used, except for specific urology cases.
- Document the date of insertion, and the type and size of catheter.

Insertion of the catheter

- Use sterile equipment and an aseptic technique. Clean the urethral meatus prior to insertion, using soap and water (antiseptic preparations are not necessary). Using a sterile lubricant in both male and female patients should reduce urethral trauma, thus decreasing the risk of infection.
- Antibiotic prophylaxis is *NOT* indicated in most patients. However, in some individual cases, it may be beneficial, e.g. recent culture-positive midstream urine (MSU).

Ongoing management of a catheterized patient

- Review the need for the catheter daily. Remove it as soon as possible.
- Empty the urinary drainage system frequently, to ensure adequate flow and prevent reflux. Use a separate container for each patient, and avoid contact between the drainage tap and container. The drainage bag should only be changed when necessary, according to the manufacturer's instructions.
- Management of the drainage bag requires universal precautions. Wash your hands, and wear a new pair of gloves before manipulating the catheter. Always position the drainage bag below the level of the bladder (to prevent backflow). If this is not possible, e.g. when the

patient is being moved, clamp the drainage tube, and ensure that the clamp is removed as soon as dependent drainage can be resumed.
- Clean the catheter urethral meatus junction daily with soap and water. Do not use antiseptic creams, as these may increase infection. Advise the patient to have a shower, rather than a bath.
- Maintain the connection between the urinary catheter and the drainage system, and only break it for good clinical reasons.
- Only flush a drainage bag if there is a clear indication (e.g. after some surgical procedures, or to manage obstructive problems).
- Do not change a catheter routinely—assess each patient's needs.
- Record ongoing management in the care plan/nursing notes.

Obtaining a urine sample from a catheterized patient

Clean the sampling port with an alcohol swab, then use sterile equipment and an aseptic no-touch technique. If there is no sampling port available, send a sample from the drainage bag (and label it as such).

Other useful resources

- EPIC guidelines for urinary catheter management, including insertion and management of short-term indwelling urinary catheters in acute care (available through the PHE website).

References

23 Emmerson AM, Enstone JE, Griffin M, Kelsey MC, Smyth ET (1996). The Second National Prevalence Survey of infection in hospitals—overview of the results. *J Hosp Infect.* **32**:175–90.

24 National Audit Office (2000). *The management and control of hospital acquired infection in acute NHS trusts in England.* Available at: https://www.nao.org.uk/wp-content/uploads/2000/02/9900230.pdf.

Ventilator-associated pneumonia

Hospital-acquired pneumonia

Respiratory infections are one of the largest contributors to HAIs in England.[25] ~1% of hospital inpatients suffer from hospital-acquired pneumonia (HAP), which results in increased length of stay (7–9 days), increased morbidity, and increased health complications. The causes of HAP are divided into those causing early-onset (<5 days after admission) and late-onset (>5 days) infections (see Table 6.15). For more detail, see the BSAC's 2009 *Guidelines for the management of hospital-acquired pneumonia in the UK* (bsac.org.uk/standards). See also Hospital-acquired pneumonia, pp. 617–8.

Ventilator-associated pneumonia

Pneumonia occurring during mechanical ventilation is the commonest infection in ICUs, and a leading cause of death. In the European Prevalence of Infection in Intensive Care study, VAP contributed to 45% of all infections in ICUs in Europe. Its incidence can vary between 9% and 68% in mechanically ventilated patients. VAP may be due to micro-aspiration of oropharyngeal secretions, aspiration of gastric contents, inhalation of infected aerosols, haematogenous spread from a distant site, and direct inoculation from staff

Table 6.15 Microbiology of hospital-acquired pneumonia

Early onset <5 days	Late onset >5 days	Others based on specific risks
S. pneumoniae	*P. aeruginosa*	Anaerobic bacteria
H. influenzae	*Enterobacter* spp.	*L. pneumophila*
S. aureus	*Acinetobacter* spp.	Viruses: influenza A and B; RSV
Enterobacter spp.	*Klebsiella* spp.	Fungi
	S. marcescens	
	E. coli	
	Other GNRs	
	S. aureus/MRSA	

(cross-infection). Predisposing factors include impaired conscious level, presence of endotracheal or NG tubes, replacement of normal flora due to prior antibiotic treatment, and severely ill and immunocompromised patients. About 50% is defined as early VAP, i.e. within the first 5 days. VAP has significant consequences at the individual and population level:

- increased duration of ventilation;
- increased length of ICU stay and hospital stay;
- increased cost (estimated at almost US $12 000 per patient);
- possible increased mortality.

Emphasis here is on prevention of VAP; for further discussion of pathogenesis, clinical features, diagnosis, and treatment of VAP, see ➲ Ventilator-associated pneumonia, pp. 618–9.

Prevention of ventilator-associated pneumonia

Recommendations to prevent VAP in the ICU include:

- appropriate disinfection and care of tubing, ventilators, and humidifiers to limit contamination—passive humidification and closed suction have not been shown to reduce the incidence of VAP;
- no routine changes of ventilator tubing (have not been shown to reduce incidence and may be harmful);
- avoid antacids and H_2 blockers;
- sterile tracheal suctioning;
- nurse in head-up position;
- SDD—controversial (➲ see Selective decontamination of the digestive tract, p. 183).

The *Ventilator Care Bundle* was initially introduced as part of the 100 000 Lives Campaign in the USA. Its success in preventing VAP depends on all five individual steps of the bundle being performed. These five steps are:

- elevation of head of bed to 30–45°;
- daily 'sedation vacations' or gradually lightening the use of sedatives;
- daily assessment of readiness to extubate or wean from the ventilator;
- peptic ulcer prophylaxis;
- deep venous thrombosis (DVT) prophylaxis.

Additional elements, from 'Saving Lives' HII No. 5

- Appropriate humidification of inspired gas (to prevent inspissation of secretions).
- Tubing management—only replace when visibly soiled or mechanically malfunctioning.
- Continuing care—suctioning of respiratory secretions; wear gloves, and decontaminate hands before and after the suction procedure.

Impact of ventilator care bundle

There have been many studies on the impact of introducing ventilator bundles on ICUs, with positive outcomes overall. One year after introducing a ventilator bundle to a general ICU in the UK, the mean ICU length of stay and the mean number of ventilator days were reduced.[26] Other benefits associated with reduced VAP include better patient outcome, shorter hospital stay, lower costs, and improved staff morale.

Other useful resources

- Centers for Disease Control and Prevention guidelines—*Mortality Morbidity Weekly Report* 2004;**53**:1–36 (available at: www.cdc.gov)
- Canadian Critical Care Society guidelines (*Ann Intern Med* 2004;**141**:305–13).
- American Healthcare Infection Control Practices Advisory Committee (HICPAC) guidelines (2003).

References

25 Emmerson AM, Enstone JE, Griffin M, Kelsey MC, Smyth ET (1996). The Second National Prevalence Survey of infection in hospitals—overview of the results. *J Hosp Infect*. **32**:175–90.
26 Cruden E, Boyce C, Woodham H, Bray B (2005). An evaluation of the impact of the ventilator care bundle. *Nurse Unit Care*. **10**:242–6.

Line-related sepsis

Intravascular devices may be complicated by local infections (e.g. phlebitis) or systemic infections (e.g. BSI, endocarditis, osteomyelitis). The commonest organisms that cause line-related sepsis are CoNS, *S. aureus* (including MRSA), enterococci, *Enterobacteriaceae*, *Pseudomonas* spp., and *Candida* spp. Infection may arise in numerous ways. Usually lines become contaminated by the patient's skin flora at the insertion site, or by the introduction of other organisms via the cannula hub or injection port.

Always consider whether a line is absolutely necessary, or whether an alternative route of administration may suffice (e.g. NG, PR, s/c). Review the continued need for a line daily.

Peripheral venous catheters

PVCs or 'venflons' are used most frequently for vascular access. Although they have a low risk of systemic complications, the overall total morbidity is high, because they are so widely used. Almost all systemic infections are preceded by a visible phlebitis, which should act as a trigger for their removal (see Table 6.16). The care bundle approach for minimizing peripheral line infections is summarized in Box 6.27.

Table 6.16 Visual infusion phlebitis (VIP) score

Score	Description
0	Site looks healthy
1	Mild pain or redness near site
2	Two of the following evident at site: redness, pain, swelling
3	All of the following evident: redness, pain along cannula site, swelling
4	All of the following evident and extensive: redness, pain along path of cannula, swelling, palpable venous cord
5	All of the following evident and extensive: redness, pain along path of cannula, swelling, palpable venous cord, and pyrexia

Box 6.27 Peripheral line care: High Impact Intervention No. 2

On insertion

- Asepsis—prevent microbial contamination by correct hand hygiene and PPE.
- Skin preparation—use (2%) alcoholic chlorhexidine gluconate; allow to dry for maximal effect.
- Dressing—a sterile, semi-permeable, transparent dressing to allow observation of insertion site.
- Documentation—date and site of insertion recorded in notes.

Continuing care

- Continuing clinical indication—ensure all lines and associated devices are still indicated. If there is no indication, then the lines or devices should be removed.
- Line insertion site—regular observation for signs of infection, at least daily.
- Dressing—an intact, dry, adherent transparent dressing is present.
- Line access—use aseptic techniques, and swab ports or hub with alcohol prior to accessing the line or administering fluids or injections.
- Administration set replacement—immediately after administration of blood, blood products, or lipid feeds. Replace all other fluid sets after 72h.
- Routine line replacement—replace in a new site after 72h, or earlier if indicated clinically.

➔ See Bloodstream infection—mandatory surveillance, pp. 187–9, and for 'Saving Lives' High Impact Intervention No. 1: central venous catheter care, see Box 6.25.

Central vascular catheters

CVCs (non-tunnelled) or 'central lines' have the highest rates of CR-BSI. These are harder to prevent than PVC infections. There have been several advances in the diagnosis, prevention, and management of CVCs (see High Impact Intervention No.1; see Box 6.25).[27]

Risk factors

Risk factors associated with line infection include:

- patient characteristics—age, underlying illness, immunosuppression etc.;
- catheter characteristics—material, type, size, coating/impregnation;
- infusate and dressing type;
- experience of person inserting the line, site preparation, anatomical insertion site, and duration of insertion;
- standard of daily line care.

Minimizing line infections

- Hand decontamination—wash hands thoroughly first (➲ see Handwashing, pp. 146–50).
- Aseptic technique—maintain a strict non-touch aseptic technique when manipulating any part of the line or cannula.
- Cannula selection—choose the smallest possible lumen for the fluid to be infused; use a single-lumen CVC, unless multiple ports are required; consider antimicrobial-impregnated or coated CVCs if a line is needed for >3 days. Peripherally inserted central catheter (PICC) lines may be considered for patients anticipated to need vascular access for a longer time period.
- Insertion site—for PVCs, look on the distal arm, away from previous sites and joint areas. For non-tunnelled CVCs, consider each case carefully, as the choice of site is important in minimizing infection. The subclavian has the lowest risk of infection.
- Skin preparation—for PVCs, use a 70% alcohol swab; for CVCs, use alcoholic chlorhexidine gluconate.
- Dressing—a transparent film or sterile gauze is ideal. Write the date of insertion on the dressing. Always replace the dressing after inspecting the insertion site, or if it becomes damp, loosened, or soiled.
- Observation—at least daily, or whenever the line is manipulated. The VIP score may be useful (see Table 6.16).[28] It is the responsibility of the person completing the VIP score to act on the results of a cannula assessment. In general, a cannula should be removed if the score is 2 or greater.
- Catheter removal—replace any lines inserted as an emergency within 24h. Remove any catheter after 72h (PVC) or 7 days (CVC) or if there are signs of infection, e.g. VIP score ≥2. It is the responsibility of the medical staff to review the need for a cannula on a daily basis and to remove it if it is no longer necessary.
- Training and audit play an integral part.

Antimicrobial-coated or impregnated catheters

There has been increased interest in using antimicrobial-coated or impregnated catheters. Agents include antiseptics (e.g. chlorhexidine and silver sulfadiazine, silver, quaternary ammonium compounds) or antibiotics (e.g. minocycline and rifampicin). Ideally, compounds should be active on internal and external surfaces, and mainly target Gram-positive organisms. Evidence supports their use, but some trials were poorly designed, and cost-effectiveness has been queried. Follow your hospital guidelines. One approach is to use coated or impregnated catheters if the line is likely to be in place for >3 days.

Antibiotic-containing locks

A meta-analysis has shown that vancomycin lock solutions in high-risk patients being treated with long-term central intravascular devices reduce the risk of BSI.[29] There may be concerns regarding increasing resistance, e.g. VRE.

Other useful resources

- American Healthcare Infection Control Practices Advisory Committee (HICPAC) guidelines (2002).
- EPIC guidelines (available through the PHE website).

References

27 Raad I, Hanne H, Maki D (2007). Intravascular catheter-related infections: advances in diagnosis, prevention, and management. *Lancet Infect Dis*. **7**:645–57.
28 Jackson A (1998). Infection control—a battle in vein: infusion phlebitis. *Nurs Times*. **94**:68, 71.
29 Safdar N, Maki DG (2006). Use of vancomycin-containing lock or flush solutions for prevention of bloodstream infection associated with central venous access devices: a meta-analysis of prospective, randomized trials. *Clin Infect Dis*. **43**:474–84.

Hospital epidemics of diarrhoea and vomiting

Most outbreaks of diarrhoea and vomiting in hospitals are caused by viruses (norovirus/small round structured virus (SRSV)/winter vomiting virus). However, remember to exclude other important causes, such as *C. difficile*, *Salmonella* spp., and *Shigella* spp., although these bacteria predominantly cause diarrhoea, rather than vomiting.

Enteric precautions

In cases of viral diarrhoea, these precautions apply from when the diarrhoea first starts until 48h after symptoms have settled. If an alternative cause for the diarrhoea is found, enteric precautions are required for different lengths of time, so seek advice from the ICT.

- As soon as the diarrhoea starts, move patients to single rooms, if available. Do not wait for the stool culture/PCR result to come back. Ideally, each patient with diarrhoea or vomiting should have their own toilet, commode, or bedpan. If isolation is not feasible, clean equipment after use with a detergent hypochlorite solution (1000ppm).
- Clean the bed space from which the patient has moved with a detergent hypochlorite solution (1000ppm).
- Staff and visitors should wear gloves and aprons when entering the room.

Visiting may be restricted to exceptional circumstances, if a bay/ward is closed due to norovirus.

- Careful handwashing is vital, after each contact with the patient. Use soap and water, followed by alcohol gel.
- Mask may be considered only if there is a risk of droplets or aerosol generation.

- Prompt decontamination of soiling and spillages should take place. The area should be cleaned with a neutral detergent and hot water, followed by 0.1% hypochlorite (1000ppm available chlorine).
- Some products have been developed which both clean and disinfect at the same time.
- Aerosols from vomiting are an important route of transmission in viral gastroenteritis.
- During an outbreak, clean all toilets on the ward with a disinfectant hypochlorite solution (1000ppm) at least twice a day. Pay particular attention to toilet flush handles, toilet seats, and door handles.
- Dispose of used linen as infected laundry.
- No special treatment is needed for washing crockery or cutlery.

Hospital outbreaks of diarrhoea and vomiting

Patients

- Involve the ICT, and consider holding an outbreak meeting. Notify the ICT of any new cases immediately.
- Patients may need to be cohort-nursed in bays, if there is a lack of side rooms.
- For each patient, send one stool sample for virology, culture, and *C. difficile* toxin.
- Involve the PHE regional laboratory. Patients must be asymptomatic for 48h, before they can be transferred to another health-care setting or nursing home.
- Patients who have not yet developed symptoms should not be transferred elsewhere without consulting the ICT, as they may be incubating the infection.
- Patients may be sent home at any time, even if they still have symptoms.

Staff

- Staff should pay particular attention to handwashing.
- No food or drink should be consumed in clinical areas.
- If symptoms develop, staff should stop work immediately and inform the line manager/occupational health/infection control, as appropriate to their institution. They can return to work 48h after symptoms have settled.
- Nursing staff must not work in any other clinical area without consulting the ICT.
- Key areas of the ward should be cleaned at least twice daily with a neutral detergent and hot water, followed by disinfection with hypochlorite solution at 1000ppm available chlorine. This includes the environment around symptomatic patients, the toilets/commodes/bedpans, bathrooms and showers, and the sluice (especially the macerator/bedpan washer).
- Terminal cleaning/environmental decontamination is important.

Further reading

Public Health England (2012). *Guidelines for the management of norovirus outbreaks in acute and community health and social care settings*. Available at: www.hpa.org.uk/webc/HPAwebFile/HPAweb_C/1317131639453.

Clostridium difficile infection

C. difficile was originally defined as the cause of antibiotic-associated colitis in 1978 and continues to have a significant impact on patient morbidity and mortality. On average, patients with *C. difficile*-associated diarrhoea (CDAD) have an increased length of stay of 21 days, with all the consequent costs. The political profile is high, with compulsory reporting of *C. difficile* rates by acute trusts. For epidemiology, clinical features, pathogenesis, diagnosis, and management of CDI, ➲ see *Clostridium difficile* diarrhoea, pp. 654–6.

Diagnosis

Diagnosis of CDI is controversial—there are many laboratory methods, compounded by two reference methods. In 2012, the HPA published the results of a large prospective observational diagnostic study to determine the best testing strategy for *C. difficile*, so that patients could be appropriately categorized.[30] There are three main categories of laboratory tests:

- glutamate dehydrogenase (GDH) enzyme-linked immunoassay (EIA) which detects whether the organism is present in the gut. Some trusts may use a GDH PCR or nucleic acid amplification test (NAAT) that are approved alternative tests;
- toxin EIA detects whether the organism is producing toxin. Toxin production is a classic feature of CDI;
- toxin gene NAAT or PCR determines whether the organism has the gene encoding the toxin and therefore has the potential to produce it.

The study found that *C. difficile* toxin EIA was not suitable as a stand-alone test for the diagnosis of CDI. A combination of tests, one of which should detect GDH (EIA or PCR if available) and the other should be a sensitive toxin test, must be used. The results are interpreted as follows.

- If GDH EIA is positive and toxin EIA is positive (positive predictive value of 91.4%), then CDI is highly likely.
- If GDH EIA is positive and toxin EIA is negative, then *C. difficile* is present but not producing toxin. These patients are considered to be 'excretors' or 'carriers' of the organism. Therefore, the diarrhoea may have a cause other than CDI. Many laboratories are employing a third test at this stage and use a toxin gene PCR. If the toxin gene PCR is positive, then this suggests the organism has the potential to produce toxin. If the patient has worsening diarrhea, this may suggest the organism has 'switched on' toxin production, and the patient may now have CDI. However, if the toxin gene PCR is negative, then the organism has no potential to produce toxin; therefore, some laboratories will class this as an overall negative result which will be reflected in the report.
- If GDH EIA is negative and the toxin EIA is negative (negative predictive value of 98.9%), then CDI is very unlikely, and this is effectively a negative result.

Other tests also available include vero-cell culture for cytopathic effect, and examination under fluorescent light after culture on specific agar (cefoxitin cycloserine fructose agar (CCFA) or cefoxitin cycloserine egg yolk (CCEY)).

Policies for testing samples vary; in some hospitals, tests for *C. difficile* must be specifically requested, while elsewhere all unformed stools will be tested. It is usual practice not to repeat the test within 28 days, once a patient has a positive result. In general, three negative results are needed to exclude CDI. If a patient tests positive after 48h of admission, then this is classed as a hospital-acquired case and must be reported to the DH. There are strict targets relating to the number of cases a trust is allowed before they are penalized (financially). The number is determined by the DH, based on the previous year's total.

Typing

Various typing techniques have recently been placed in order of decreasing discriminatory ability. These are (most discriminatory first): multiple loci variable number tandem repeat analysis (MLVA), restriction endonuclease analysis (REA), pulsed-field gel electrophoresis (PFGE), surface layer protein A gene sequence typing (slpAST), PCR ribotyping, multiple locus sequence typing (MLST), and amplified fragment length polymorphism (AFLP).[31] The commonest technique used in the UK is PCR ribotyping, which is coordinated by the *Clostridium difficile* Ribotyping Network (CDRN) Service. Further DNA fingerprinting using MLVA can be carried out to investigate clusters, to identify closely related isolates and probable transmission. Antimicrobial susceptibility testing surveillance (metronidazole and vancomycin) is performed on selected isolates.

Control of infection

CDI is transmitted by clostridial spores, which are shed in large numbers by infected patients and are capable of surviving for long periods in the environment. Enteric precautions should be followed, as outlined in ➲ Hospital epidemics of diarrhoea and vomiting, pp. 196–7.

Box 6.28 Reducing the risk of infection from *C. difficile*: 'Saving Lives' High Impact Intervention No. 7 and 8

- Prudent antibiotic prescribing, as per local policy. Minimize broad-spectrum agents; review prescription daily; include stop dates.
- Hand hygiene—wash hands with soap and water before and after each patient contact.
- Enhanced environmental cleaning—use chlorine-based disinfectants to reduce environmental contamination with *C. difficile* spores, as per local policy. Deep-clean and decontaminate a room after a CDI patient has been discharged.
- Isolation—always use a single room, if available; cohort patient care should be applied if a single room is not available.
- PPE—always use disposable gloves and apron when handling body fluids and when caring for CDI-infected patients.
- Cleaning and decontamination must be thorough and follow best practice for all clinical equipment, and not just that used for patients with CDI. Intervention 8 covers location of cleaning activity, correct hand hygiene and PPE, cleaning and decontamination, and correct documentation.

Box 6.29 SIGHT protocol

S—Suspect that a case may be infective where there is no clear alternative cause for diarrhoea.

I—Isolate the patient, and consult with the ICT, while determining the cause of the diarrhoea.

G—Gloves and aprons must be used for all contacts with the patient and their environment.

H—Handwashing with soap and water should be carried out before and after each contact with the patient and the patient's environment.

T—Test the stool for toxin by sending a specimen immediately.

General guidance on *C. difficile* is contained within the document *Clostridium difficile infection: how to deal with the problem*, published by the DH in 2009. There are ten key recommendations for providers and commissioners aimed at reducing cases. These included use of the SIGHT protocol when managing suspected potentially infectious diarrhoea (see Box 6.29). PHE issued updated management and treatment guidance in 2013, emphasizing the importance of a multidisciplinary team review of all CDI patients.[32]

C. difficile infection

Management of the patient

- Review the individual's antibiotic prescription. Consider stopping antimicrobial agents and PPIs. Seek advice from an infection expert, if in doubt.
- Most trusts recommend metronidazole as first line, as it is cheaper and results in less VRE than using PO vancomycin. However, PO vancomycin may be indicated in cases of severe or persistent disease. There is a suggestion that metronidazole may be less efficacious for ribotype 027. Consult your local trust policy. There is no benefit of adding rifampicin to metronidazole.
- Enteric precautions must continue, until the diarrhoea resolves. Patient isolation can discontinue when they have had 48h without diarrhoea and passed a formed stool. If in doubt, seek advice from the ICT. Note that stool may remain positive for *C. difficile* toxin for a considerable time afterwards, so microbiological clearance and repeat specimens are not required.
- Management of recurrence (which can be as high as 25%) may include probiotics, faecal implants, anion exchange resins to absorb toxins, IV immunoglobulin (IVIG), *Saccharomyces boulardii*, and vancomycin with tapering doses or pulse doses. Fidaxomicin (➔ see Fidaxomicin, pp. 45–6) was reviewed by NICE, which concluded that 'fidaxomicin may have advantages in reducing the rate of recurrence, and that local decision makers should take into account the potential benefits alongside the medical need, the risks of treatment, and the relatively high cost of the antibiotic in comparison with other CDI treatment options'.

- Areas of research/development include tolevamer (a polymer that binds toxin and reduces the recurrence rate), rifaximin, monoclonal antibody, and nitazoxanide (antiparasitic agent).

Prevention of infection

- *C. difficile* spores survive in the environment. Disinfect all furniture and horizontal surfaces with dilute hypochlorite solution (1000ppm). Many trusts are now using hydrogen peroxide vapour to clean side rooms, as the coverage of the gas is much greater than physical surface cleaning. However, there are numerous disadvantages to this system, including the cost, staff training, necessity of room sealing, etc.
- When enteric precautions are discontinued, the curtains around the patient's bed must be laundered.
- Handwashing—by washing with soap and water, the dilutional effect of the water and friction through rubbing the hands may help to remove some of the spores. The only way to reduce transmission is to wear gloves, but overall the environment is more important in transmission.
- Probiotics/yoghurt drink are used in some hospitals to try to prevent *C. difficile*, but firm evidence is lacking.
- *C. difficile* vaccines and anti-toxin immunoglobulins are still in research/development stages.
- There is no evidence that giving 'pre-emptive' metronidazole or vancomycin, when a patient starts broad-spectrum antibiotics, is beneficial.

C. difficile 027

CDI due to ribotype 027 strains (known in the USA as NAP1) is associated with increased severity, requirement for switching from metronidazole to vancomycin, recurrence, and mortality. Ribotype 027 produces more toxin A and B *in vitro* (due to an 18bp deletion in the *tcdC* gene) and also more binary toxin. It is resistant to fluoroquinolones and has higher MICs to metronidazole (but remains sensitive). It emerged in North America in 2002/2003 and then spread to northern Europe, accounting for over half of cases in England referred for ribotyping in 2007/2008. This then fell markedly to 21% in 2009/2010, coinciding with reduced incidence and mortality in the UK overall. Epidemiology of CDI shows large regional variation, and mandatory surveillance, with possible fines for exceeding the targets set by local commissioners, keeps it high on the political agenda.

References

30 Department of Health (2012). *Updated guidance on the diagnosis and reporting of Clostridium difficile*. Available at: https://www.gov.uk/government/publications/updated-guidance-on-the-diagnosis-and-reporting-of-clostridium-difficile.

31 Killgore G, Thompson A, Johnson S, *et al.* (2008). Comparison of seven techniques for typing international epidemic strains of *Clostridium difficile*: restriction endonuclease analysis, pulsed-field gel electrophoresis, PCR-ribotyping, multilocus sequence typing, multilocus variable-number tandem-repeat analysis, amplified fragment length polymorphism, and surface layer protein A gene sequence typing. *J Clin Microbiol*. **46**:431–7.

32 Public Health England (2013). *Updated guidance on the management and treatment of C. difficile infection*. Available at: https://www.gov.uk/government/publications/clostridium-difficile-infection-guidance-on-management-and-treatment.

Infection control in the community

Infection control in the community is defined as the infection control service provided outside acute and major hospitals to those in another care setting such as the community or primary care setting. This covers a wide group, including nursing home residents, prisons, renal patients on home dialysis, and outbreaks of diseases in school and places of work. HCWs, family members, and carers are at risk of acquiring infections when caring for patients in the community. The community ICN may have other remits such as contact tracing for TB.

It is estimated that HAIs cost the NHS ~£1 billion a year, and £56 million of this is estimated to be incurred after patients are discharged from hospital. As more patients continually move between hospitals and the community, particularly the older and more dependent patients, the boundaries between hospital infections and community infections are becoming blurred. In addition, the rapid turnover of patients in acute care settings has resulted in more complex care being delivered in the community, which often involves more indwelling devices. It is envisaged that, in the future, HAI in hospitals and the community will be managed as one.

The clinical guideline *Healthcare-associated infections: prevention and control in primary and community care* was published by NICE in 2012 (CG139). In addition to general guidance on hand decontamination, use of PPE, and disposal of waste and sharps, there is detailed information about long-term urinary catheters, enteral feeding, and vascular access devices.

- *Community C. difficile*—CDI is being increasingly recognized in the community. It is generally defined as patients who are diagnosed with CDI in the community, or within 48h of hospital admission. Not all patients have been in a health-care setting recently, and not all have received antibiotics. For further information, ➲ see *Clostridium difficile* infection, pp. 198–201.
- *Community-acquired MRSA*—this is genetically distinct for hospital-acquired MRSA and is becoming commoner (➲ see Meticillin-resistant *Staphylococcus aureus*, pp. 237–9).

Control of antimicrobial resistance in the community

Many countries have launched campaigns to educate doctors and patients about antibiotic misuse and the threat of drug resistance. In the USA, the 'Get Smart' campaign has been driven by the CDC. There are many similar initiatives in the UK (for further information, ➲ see Antimicrobial stewardship, pp. 27–8). Recommended standards for infection control in the community are detailed in Box 6.30.

Box 6.30 Recommended standards for infection control in the community

- The ICNs should be competent for this role and maintain their competence through appropriate professional development.
- There should be sufficient staffing resource to enable the function to be carried out satisfactorily and in accordance with accepted national standards (e.g. decontamination, infection control).
- There should be sufficient support for the team that undertakes the infection control in the community function for a defined population.
- Primary care trusts must have robust arrangements to fulfil their infection control functions.
- There should be a formally agreed infection control guidance for community health-care settings and other establishments that have particular infection control needs.

(Infection Control in the Community Study, CDSC, 2002)

Part 3

Systematic microbiology

7	Bacteria	207
8	Viruses	365
9	Fungi	469
10	Protozoa	511
11	Helminths	541
12	Ectoparasites	571

Chapter 7
Bacteria

Basic principles of bacteriology 209
Bacterial structure and function 210
Bacterial genetics 212
Bacterial growth and metabolism 214
Bacterial virulence and pathogenicity 216
Microbiological specimens 218
Bacterial culture media 219
Identification of bacteria 221
Biochemical tests 225
Automated diagnostics 228
Molecular organism identification 229
Molecular typing methods 229
Quality assurance and accreditation 231
Overview of Gram-positive cocci 233
Staphylococcus aureus 234
Meticillin-resistant *Staphylococcus aureus* 237
Glycopeptide resistance in *Staphylococcus aureus* 239
Coagulase-negative staphylococci 240
Micrococcus species 242
Rothia mucilaginosus 242
Streptococci—overview 242
Streptococcus pneumoniae 243
Enterococci 245
Streptococcus bovis 247
Viridans streptococci 248
Group A *Streptococcus* 249
Group B *Streptococcus* 252
Other β-haemolytic streptococci 254
Other Gram-positive cocci 254
Overview of Gram-positive rods 256
Bacillus species 257
Bacillus anthracis—ADCP 3 258
Corynebacterium diphtheriae 260
Non-diphtheria corynebacteria 262
Listeria 263
Erysipelothrix rhusiopathiae 265
Rhodococcus equi 266
Arcanobacterium haemolyticum 267
Clostridium botulinum 267
Clostridum tetani 269
Other clostridia 270
Actinomyces 271
Nocardia 272
Actinomadura and *Streptomyces* 273
Gram-negative cocci—overview 274
Neisseria meningitidis 274
Neisseria gonorrhoeae 277
Non-pathogenic *Neisseria* 279
Moraxella 279
Anaerobic Gram-negative cocci 280
Escherichia coli 280
Klebsiella 283
Proteus 284
Enterobacter 285
Citrobacter 286
Serratia 287
Salmonella 288
Shigella 291
Other *Enterobacteriaceae* 292
Overview of Gram-negative rod non-fermenters 293
Glucose non-fermenters 294
Pseudomonas aeruginosa 295
Acinetobacter 297
Stenotrophomonas maltophilia 299
Burkholderia cepacia complex 300
Burkholderia gladioli 302
Burkholderia pseudomallei—ACDP 3 302
Overview of fastidious Gram-negative rods 303
Haemophilus influenzae 303
Other *Haemophilus* species 305

HACEK organisms *306*
Gardnerella *309*
Bordetella *310*
Brucella—ACDP 3 *311*
Yersinia pestis—ACDP 3 *314*
Yersinia enterocolitica *315*
Yersinia pseudotuberculosis *316*
Pasteurella *316*
Francisella—ACDP 3 *317*
Legionella *318*
Capnocytophaga *320*
Vibrios *321*
Vibrio cholerae *321*
Vibrio parahaemolyticus *323*
Vibrio vulnificus *324*
Other *Vibrio* species *324*
Aeromonas *325*
Plesiomonas *326*
Campylobacter *326*
Helicobacter *327*
Bacteroides *329*
Prevotella and *Porphyromonas* *331*
Fusobacterium *332*
Spirochaetes—an overview *333*
Treponema species *335*
Borrelia species *337*
Leptospira species *340*
Overview of *Rickettsia*—ACDP 3 *342*
Rickettsial diseases *344*
Coxiella burnetii—ACDP 3 *346*
Bartonella species *348*
Mycoplasma *350*
Chlamydia *352*
Chlamydia trachomatis *353*
Chlamydophila psittaci *354*
Chlamydophila pneumoniae *355*
Mycobacterium tuberculosis—ACDP 3 *355*
Mycobacterium leprae—ACDP 3 *359*
Non-tuberculous mycobacteria *361*

Basic principles of bacteriology

Taxonomy

Taxonomy is the art of dividing into ordered groups or categories. With respect to bacteria, it refers to two main concepts:

- classification—the division of organisms into related groups, based on similar characteristics. The species is the most definitive level of classification. Organisms may be reclassified from time to time, as new information (e.g. genetic relatedness) becomes available;
- nomenclature—the naming of groups and members of a group. This is governed by the International Committee on Systematics of Prokaryotes (www.the-icsp.org). The most recent revision of the International Code of Nomenclature of Bacteria was published in 1992. Amendments are published in journal form (*The International Journal of Systematic and Evolutionary Microbiology*). The basic rules for naming are outlined in Boxes 7.1 and 7.2.

Identification

Taxonomy is dynamic and, throughout its history, has been dependent on the techniques of identification available—originally phenotypic characteristics, and more recently methods of determining the genetic 'relatedness' (phylogenetics) of a group of organisms, which should hopefully lead to a more stable classification, with fewer revisions in the future. Changes are overseen by the Judicial Commission of the International Union of Microbiological Societies.

- Phenotypic characteristics—cellular morphology, staining (e.g. Gram or acid-fast; see Box 7.3), motility, growth characteristics (speed, requirements, colonial appearance), biochemical characteristics (e.g. acid from specific carbohydrates), serology, analysis of metabolic end-products).
- Phylogenetic identification—nucleic acid hybridization (denaturation of double-stranded DNA (dsDNA) into single strands and assessing their ability to anneal to the single strands of another related organism), 16S rRNA sequence analysis.

For identification purposes, simple phenotypic characteristics continue to be used which often (but not always) correlate with genotypes. These methods of phenotypic characterization have been developed and codified over years to facilitate laboratory identification of organisms (collected in texts such as *Bergey's Manual of Systematic Bacteriology*).

Box 7.1 Microorganism nomenclature rules

- Each organism should have only one correct name. Where >1 exists, the oldest legitimate name takes precedence.
- Confusing names should be abandoned.
- Regardless of origin, all names are in Latin or are latinized.
- The first word (genus) always starts with a capital letter.
- The second word (species) is in small letters.
- The genus and species name are underlined or italicized when printed.

Box 7.2 The naming hierarchy

- Order—names ending -ales.
- Families—names ending -aceae.
- Tribes—names ending -eae.
- Genus.
- Species—a collection of strains sharing common characteristics.
- Strain—a bacterial culture derived from a pure isolate.

Box 7.3 The Gram stain

Named after the Danish bacteriologist who devised it in 1884, the Gram stain remains a useful test—the outcome of which is determined largely by the structure of the cell wall. The procedure is simple:

- Cells are stained with crystal violet.
- Then they are treated with iodine, forming a crystal violet/iodine complex in the cell.
- Next they are washed with an organic solvent (acetone-alcohol).
- Then they are stained with a red counterstain, e.g. safranin.

Gram-positive organisms retain the crystal violet/iodine complex within the cell, because of the thick peptidoglycan cell wall, and appear dark purple. In Gram-negative organisms, the stain is leached from the cell, due to disruption of the lipid-rich outer membrane by the organic solvent, and they appear pink.

Bacterial structure and function

Bacteria are prokaryotic—they have a single chromosome that is not enclosed in a nuclear membrane. They are around 0.2–2 micrometres wide by 1–6 micrometres long and exist in four basic shapes: cocci (spheres), bacilli (rods), spirillia (spirals), and vibrios (comma-shaped).

Cytoplasm

Cytoplasm is a gel containing the enzymes, ions, subcellular organelles, and energy reserves of the organism. Energy and food are stored in membrane-bound granules. Glycogen is the major storage material of enteric bacteria. Ribosomes are the sites of protein synthesis. Bacterial ribosomes are 70S (the 'S' referring to a unit of sedimentation on ultracentrifugation) and are formed from two subunits—30S (which contains 16S RNA) and 50S. Ribosomes are formed from specific ribosomal proteins and rRNA (they account for 80% of total cell RNA). They complex with an mRNA transcript from DNA to form polyribosomes (polysomes). Extrachromosomal DNA is often found within the cytoplasm in the form of plasmids. These are covalently closed dsDNA circles and capable of replication, and are inherited by progeny cells. They may contain genetic information encoding structure or functions relating to bacterial virulence (antibiotic resistance, adhesions, toxins, etc.).

Cytoplasmic membrane

The cytoplasm is surrounded by the cytoplasmic membrane, a phospholipid bilayer into which various proteins are inserted. The membrane is involved in the synthesis and secretion of enzymes and toxins, and active transportation of materials into the cytoplasm.

Bacterial cell wall

This provides rigidity and a physical barrier to the outside world. Peptidoglycan provides strength and is found in all bacterial species, except *Mycoplasma* and *Ureaplasma* spp. It comprises a carbohydrate backbone cross-linked by short peptides. Variations in the peptide linkages are responsible for different cell wall characters (see Box 7.3).

Gram-positive cell walls

These are composed of several layers of peptidoglycan, within which are trapped a variety of proteins, polysaccharides, and teichoic acids (polymers of glycerol or ribitol), which stabilize the cell wall and maintain its association with the cell membrane, as well as have roles in cellular interaction and growth. They are antigenic in some organisms. Certain organisms will possess cell wall structures that confer virulence characteristics, e.g. M protein of GAS.

Gram-negative cell walls

These are thinner, but more complex, than those of Gram-positive organisms. Outside the cytoplasmic membrane is a periplasmic space. The outer part of this is bounded by a single peptidoglycan layer, beyond which lies the outer membrane—a phospholipid bilayer within which lie other large molecules. Lipoproteins link this membrane to the peptidoglycan below. Unique to Gram-negative bacteria are the LPS in the outer membrane. These are key surface antigens and endotoxins of Gram-negative organisms. They are composed of lipid A (principally responsible for the endotoxin activity), attached to a core polysaccharide, with side chains which vary within a species and confer the serological identity (O antigen) of individual strains. Other components of the outer membrane include: porin proteins (allow entry to the periplasmic space from the outside) and non-porin proteins (such as PBPs).

'Acid-fast' cell walls

Mycobacterium spp., *Nocardia* spp., and *Corynebacterium* spp. have a modified Gram-positive cell wall. They have a higher cell wall lipid content which is due to mycolic acids, which can also confer virulence characteristics. Acid-fast organisms are so-called because, once stained with red carbol fuchsin dye, they are resistant to decolorization with acid-alcohol—a property conferred by the cell wall lipids.

Bacterial surface structures

Capsules

Certain bacteria possess a capsule around their cell wall, usually composed of polysaccharide, but polypeptide in some organisms. They are manufactured at the cell membrane. They serve to protect cells from toxins, desiccation, complement proteins, and antibodies, and play a role in adherence (e.g. the glucan capsule of *S. mutans* forms the matrix of dental plaque). Capsules are antigenic and can be used to identify certain organisms (e.g. *H. influenzae* type B), and may be detectable in body fluids.

Flagellae

These are long, thin appendages that are anchored in the cytoplasmic membrane and extend through the cell wall into the surrounding medium; they are responsible for cellular motility. They are usually found on GNRs, but motile Gram-positive organisms also exist. Flagellar number and arrangement vary from single (monotrichous) to multiple over the whole surface (peritrichous). The filament is composed of multiple flagellin proteins which have the capacity to self-assemble. The cell membrane-anchored base rotates as part of an energy-dependent reaction, causing the rigid flagella to rotate. They are antigenic, and several genuses, e.g. *Salmonella* spp., are able to alter the antigenic type of flagella they produce (phase variation) by the differential expression of the genes coding various flagellin proteins.

Fimbriae

These are smaller appendages (~15–20 micrometres in length), composed of fibrillin and found on many Gram-negative bacteria. They form hollow tubes and are involved in attachment to cells or mucosal surfaces (also called adhesins). Different adhesins display different binding properties (e.g. mannose), which are partly responsible for the tissue tropism seen with certain species of bacteria. They are also involved in bacterial conjugation and the exchange of DNA from one cell to another. The term 'pili' is given to the fimbriae used by Gram-negative bacteria for DNA transfer in conjugation.

Bacterial genetics

Bacterial DNA

Bacterial genetic information is encoded in the cell's DNA, of which there are two types:

- chromosomal DNA—prokaryotic organisms have a single, covalently closed, circular chromosome of dsDNA. It lies in a supercoiled state within the cytoplasm, not enclosed, but attached to the bacterial cell membrane at certain points. Individual genes are arranged linearly. In *E. coli*, the chromosome contains around 5 million bp. DNA replication and transcription to mRNA occur continually (unlike eukaryotes);
- extrachromosomal DNA—plasmids are small DNA molecules consisting of circular dsDNA. Replication is autonomous and occurs independently of the host cell. Multiple copies of the same plasmid and many different plasmids can coexist in the same cell. Plasmids pass to daughter cells, and some are capable of transferring to other bacteria of the same (or other) species. They code for many different functions and structures, e.g. antibiotic resistance.

Genetic material can move between plasmids and from plasmid to chromosome (and vice versa) via transposons. These are DNA sequences that can copy themselves to a new site, carrying associated genes with them.

In manufacturing proteins, single-stranded 'messenger' RNA (mRNA) is synthesized from dsDNA during transcription by a DNA-dependent RNA polymerase, using the 'sense' strand of the DNA as a template. The mRNA forms a complex with several ribosomes (a polysome–mRNA complex). The mRNA is translated as transfer RNA (tRNA) molecules bearing the appropriate amino acid, and its 'sense' bases associate with the mRNA 'antisense' bases.

Genetic variation

Genetic variation can occur by mutation or direct gene transfer.

Mutation

This occurs when one or more bases in the DNA sequence changes. It is permanent (barring re-mutation to the original sequence) and will be inherited by any progeny. Such changes may alter the amino acid sequence of the encoded protein or may change the circumstances in which a normal protein is produced (transcription changes). Mutations can be:

- deletion—losing a base will cause a frameshift mutation, changing the amino acids represented by the sequence from the point of mutation onwards. Deletions can involve several bases;
- insertion—additional base or bases will also cause a frameshift;
- substitution—change of a single base to one of the other three changes the amino acid represented by the code.

Gene transfer

This is the main means by which bacteria achieve their rapid genetic variability. There are three mechanisms:

- transformation—the uptake of free bacterial DNA from the surrounding environment into recipient cells. Cells able to take up and incorporate free DNA are termed 'competent'. This state is usually transient, occurring towards the late exponential phase of growth, with the expression of surface receptors for DNA. DNA that enters can only be incorporated into the genome if there are homologous regions with which it can integrate (only DNA from related species is likely to achieve it) and requires the presence of the *recA* gene;
- transduction—the exchange of genes by bacteriophages (or simply 'phages'). Phages are viruses that infect only bacteria. Certain phages integrate their genetic material into the bacterial host DNA. During phage replication, excision of a viral sequence from the host DNA may result in fragments of bacterial DNA becoming enclosed within the viral particle. When this particle infects a new bacterial cell, the DNA fragment recombines into the chromosome of the second bacterium. Transduction may be generalized (random accidental host DNA is transferred) or specialized (specific host genes are transferred, as the phage DNA integrates at specific sites). Phage conversion refers to the phenomenon of phage DNA becoming integrated into the bacterial chromosome and bringing about a change in the bacterial phenotype, e.g. toxin production in *Corynebacterium diphtheriae*. This is due to phage DNA precipitating the expression of otherwise unexpressed bacterial genes;

- conjugation—the only mechanism that requires cell-to-cell interaction, and the major means by which bacteria acquire additional genes. Gram-negative cells achieve this by means of the sex pilus, which is encoded on a specific plasmid (the F plasmid). The pilus establishes contact with another cell and is the tube through which DNA is passed. Some organisms integrate the F plasmid into chromosomal DNA—such cells are termed Hfr (high-frequency recombination) cells. Gram-positive cells achieve conjugation by aggregating in response to the production of pheromones by the donor bacterium.

Bacterial growth and metabolism

Bacterial growth requires, logically enough, materials for the manufacture of cell components and a source of energy.

Materials

Some bacteria can synthesize all they require from simple raw materials. However, most pathogenic bacteria require a ready-made supply of the organic compounds they need for growth. Most of these nutrients diffuse freely across the cell membrane to enter the cell. Some are required at high concentration, and uptake is energy-dependent. Enzymes involved in these processes may be inducible (produced in the presence of the substrate) or constitutive (produced constantly and independent of the substrate).

Carbon

Lithotrophic bacteria are able to use carbon dioxide (CO_2) as the sole source of carbon, and use it as the basis of their organic metabolites. Thus, the only other materials needed are water, inorganic salts, and energy. Organotrophic bacteria require organic carbon such as glucose—thus, their energy source is also used in the synthesis of materials. Different bacterial species can utilize different organic carbon sources, *Pseudomonas* spp. being amongst the most versatile.

Nitrogen

Ammonium ions (NH_4^+) provide the nitrogen required by bacterial cells. This is turned into glutamate and glutamine, which, in turn, are processed into certain amino acids, purines, etc. Certain bacterial species and blue-green algae can make ammonium directly from atmospheric nitrogen—predominantly soil-dwelling organisms, but certain human pathogens, such as *Klebsiella* and *Clostridium* spp., can 'fix' nitrogen in this manner. Other organisms produce their NH_4^+ by nitrate reduction or from deamination of amino acids released from proteins.

Growth factors

Substances, such as B vitamins, minerals, certain amino acids, purine, and pyrimidines, are required by many bacteria, although not all are capable of synthesizing their own. An organism is described as prototrophic for a growth factor if it is capable of synthesizing it and does not require an exogenous source. All bacteria need certain inorganic ions such as magnesium and calcium, and some need zinc and copper, amongst others.

Environmental conditions

As well as (of course) water and CO_2, bacteria have specific optimal environmental requirements for growth, including temperature and pH. Oxygen requirements are discussed in the next section.

Energy

- Bacterial metabolism is a balance between biosynthesis (anabolic) and degradation (catabolic reactions). Catabolic reactions power the biosynthetic processes, as hydrolysis of substances being broken down liberates energy which is captured in the formation of the phosphate bonds of ATP.
- An organism's ability to utilize certain carbohydrates (e.g. sucrose, mannose) and convert them to glucose (the starting point for both aerobic and anaerobic catabolism) for metabolism is a useful feature for characterizing bacteria. Many tests in clinical microbiology detect the acidic end-products of bacterial metabolism in controlled conditions.
- The oxygen requirement of a specific organism reflects the means it uses to meet its energy needs.
- Obligate anaerobes—grow only in conditions of high reducing intensity, and oxygen is toxic.
- Aerotolerant anaerobes—anaerobic metabolism, but not killed by the presence of oxygen.
- Facultative anaerobes—can grow in anaerobic and aerobic conditions.
- Obligate aerobes—need oxygen to grow.
- Microaerophilic organisms—best growth is seen in low oxygen levels; high levels may be inhibitory.
- Aerobes produce a free radical superoxide (O_2^-) which is reduced to oxygen and hydrogen peroxide (H_2O_2). Catalase enzymes convert the latter to water and oxygen.

Anaerobic metabolism

Glucose use in anaerobic conditions is fermentation. This occurs via glycolysis, producing pyruvate and two molecules (net) of ATP per glucose molecule. Pyruvate can then enter several different pathways, producing different end-products (e.g. lactic acid, acetaldehyde, ethanol, etc.)

Aerobic metabolism

Glucose use in aerobic conditions is respiration. Pyruvate forms in glycolysis, as in anaerobic conditions, but then enters the Krebs' cycle. Complete oxidation of glucose by these paths results in 38 molecules (net) of ATP per glucose molecule. The Krebs cycle also produces precursors for several other important cellular components such as purines, pyrimidines, amino acids, and lipids.

Bacterial growth

- Bacterial growth occurs, as the mass of cellular constituents increases. Cell division starts once a critical mass is reached, and occurs by binary fission. In a liquid medium, bacteria display a uniform growth curve.
- Lag phase—the cell synthesizes new enzymes and cofactors, and imports nutrients from the media.

- Increasing growth phase—enzymatic reaction rates approach steady state, and cell growth begins.
- Logarithmic growth phase—cell growth and division are at maximum. This is influenced by temperature, the carbon source, oxygen, nutrient availability, and so on.
- Declining growth phase—nutrients are exhausted, and growth slows.
- Stationary phase—new organisms produced equal those dying.
- Death phase—cells die off.

Bacterial virulence and pathogenicity

Definitions

Pathogenicity is defined as the ability of an organism to cause disease, whereas virulence is the degree of pathogenicity within a group of organisms. Virulence is determined by several factors related to the organism and the host, most particularly the infectivity of the bacteria and the severity of the condition it produces. To be considered to be pathogenic, organisms will have strains of varying degrees of virulence.

Pathogenicity

Infection of the host is the necessary first step—infection does not, however, equate with disease. We are all colonized with many bacteria. These, however, only become disease-causing in certain abnormal situations.

The organism must enter the host and attach to the mucous membrane surfaces. Some go no further than this, and disease is caused by exotoxins (e.g. *V. cholerae*); others penetrate deeper and multiply, causing tissue damage and eventually gaining access to blood and potentially disseminating. Some species, such as mycobacteria, are able to reside within cells, taking up long-term residence within the host. Still others are highly specific in the organs they will infect (e.g. *N. gonorrhoeae*). This may be related to the presence of specific receptors for bacterial attachment, or the presence of nutrients (e.g. *Brucella abortus* has a requirement for erythritol, which is found in the bovine placental tissue and results in localization of infection to this site).

Virulence factors

Adhesins

Bacterial cell surface adhesins adhere to complementary structures on the surface of susceptible cells. These adhesins may be fimbriae (➔ see Bacterial structure and function, pp. 210–2), components of the bacterial capsule (see below), and other cell surface antigens. The adherence process is a prerequisite if a microorganism is to infect a cell.

Aggressins

These substances allow the cell to evade host defence mechanisms. These may act to prevent an initial attack and phagocytosis, or to enable to cell to survive once phagocytosed (with the added benefit that, once settled within a phagocytic cell, they are safe from continued exposure to antibody and complement). They include:

- *capsules*—enable organisms to avoid phagocytosis by preventing interaction with the bacterial cell surface and the phagocytic cell, or by concealing surface antigens. Specific antibodies against the capsular material will opsonize the organism and allow its ingestion. Examples include *S. pneumoniae* and *H. influenzae* type B. Mycobacteria have components in their cell wall that prevent lysosome/phagosome fusion, once ingested;
- *extracellular slime substances*—these are surface proteins or carbohydrates (polysaccharides). Examples include the M protein of GAS (*S. pyogenes*) which impairs complement function, protein A of *S. aureus* which binds IgG by the Fc region, interfering with the phagocytosis of opsonized organisms, and LPS of Gram-negative bacteria which may delay or blunt the acute inflammatory response;
- *enzymes*—some bacteria produce proteases which can hydrolyse and inactivate IgA, aiding mucosal colonization. *L. monocytogenes* secretes enzymes that inhibit destruction by the myeloperoxidase system of phagocytic cells. *S. aureus* produces hyaluronidase, an enzyme that depolymerizes hyaluronic acid (responsible for cell-to-cell adhesion), thereby easing the spread of the organism. GAS produce streptokinases that lyse fibrin clots; *Clostridum perfringens* produces collagenases, contributing to its ability to produce necrotizing skin infection;
- *siderophore*—are molecules produced by most pathogenic bacteria, and they scavenge iron from the host. Iron is required for virulence by several bacteria, and siderophores seem to protect bacteria from the killing effects of human serum;
- *plasmids*—although these are not conventional virulence factors, they may code for a wide range of additional features promoting virulence such as antibiotic resistance, sex pili, and chromosomal mobilization (allowing the transfer of genetic material such as antibiotic resistance, toxin, etc. to other cells).

Toxins

Exotoxins are amongst the most potent biological toxins and are mainly produced by Gram-positive organisms. They are usually heat-labile proteins, and many can be inactivated by proteolytic enzymes or neutralized by specific antibodies. The effects are highly varied, e.g. the clinical manifestations of tetanus, botulism, and diphtheria are all due to toxins. Some toxins are secreted in the active form, whereas others require cleavage to become active, e.g. *C. diphtheriae*.[1]

Endotoxins are only produced by Gram-negative bacteria and consist primarily of LPS. They are heat stable and are only partly neutralized by specific antibodies. They are relatively low toxicity, compared to exotoxins. They cause fever, hypotension, haemorrhage, and disseminated intravascular coagulation (DIC), and stimulate cytokine release from macrophages.

1 Interestingly, only those strains that contain a lysogenic bacteriophage (β-corynephage) are able to produce the toxin. The toxin genes exist on the phage genome.

Microbiological specimens

This is a brief overview of specimen collection. Consult your hospital guidelines, laboratory handbook, and the UK Standards for Microbiology Investigations (SMI) available on the PHE website for full details.

A laboratory will perform different tests on different samples, depending on the site, clinical setting, and nature of the specimen. It is therefore important to consider whether the sample you are planning to send will help answer your clinical question, particularly when sending from a site that is not normally sterile. For example, a skin swab may be useful for screening for MRSA but is unlikely to identify the cause of an abscess. Contrariwise, any growth from an LP is likely to be important. Provide full clinical information, including specific organisms in which you may be interested if they are not routinely included.

Blood cultures

BCs are taken to identify patients with bacteraemia. They usually comprise two bottles (aerobic and anaerobic) in adults, but practice may vary. Single 'paediatric' bottles are available. Haematology patients may have a third FAN (Fastidious Antibiotic Neutralization) bottle. BACTEC and BacT/Alert automated systems provide continual monitoring for growth. Recommendations from the DH aim to keep the BC contamination rate to <3% (➔ see Chapter 6).

Urine samples

Urine samples, including MSU, CCU (clean-catch urine), CSU (catheter specimen of urine), bag urine in infants, SPA (suprapubic aspirate), and nephrostomy fluid, are taken to investigate suspected UTIs. Should be sterile. Laboratory practice varies in terms of which samples have dipstick (➔ see Chapter 17, Introduction, p. 679), microscopy (white cells, red cells, epithelial cells), culture (e.g. chromogenic agar), level of speciation, and antibiotic susceptibilities. Epithelial cells may indicate contamination.

Respiratory samples

Respiratory samples, e.g. sputum, bronchoalveolar lavage (BAL), tracheal aspirate, induced sputum, bronchial washings, nasopharyngeal aspirate (NPA), are taken to investigate a suspected infection, along with samples for virology and serology. Laboratory methods may include Gram stain (rarely performed), routine bacterial culture (plus *Legionella* on BAL), *Pneumocystis* antigen detection/PCR, AFB smear, and culture if indicated. Clinical details are critical, e.g. patients with CF require additional investigations for *Burkholderia*, etc. (➔ see Cystic fibrosis, pp. 623–5).

Tuberculosis samples

TB samples include sputum, urine, bronchial washings, etc., and tissue/biopsy specimens and others, as relevant (CSF, bone marrow, fluids, etc.). Smear may be stained by auramine-phenol or Ziehl–Neelsen (ZN) (➔ see *Mycobacterium tuberculosis*—ACDP 3, pp. 355–9). Lowenstein–Jensen slopes largely replaced by the automated Mycobacteria Growth Indicator Tube (MGIT) system.

Stool samples

Stool samples are usually taken to investigate diarrhoea. Routine culture includes *Salmonella, Shigella, Campylobacter, E.coli* O157. Clinical history important in terms of parasitology, TCBS (thiosulfate citrate bile salts sucrose) plates for *Vibrio*, etc. *C. difficile* testing should be specifically requested.

Biopsies

Biopsies, including tissue, bone, and pus, can come from most body sites. Pus is always preferable to a swab, where possible, because of the higher culture yield, especially for anaerobes. These samples usually have Gram stain and routine bacterial culture, with additional culture and tests as indicated by the clinical picture.

Fluids

Fluids (ascitic, pleural, joint, etc.) should be sterile. Gram stain and culture performed as indicated by the clinical picture. More than 250 white cells in ascitic fluid may indicate spontaneous bacterial peritonitis (SBP).

Swabs

Swabs (wound/ulcer, conjunctiva, ear, nose, throat, vaginal, genital) have different culture plates, dictated by the site and suspected infection. Always thoroughly clean a wound first, to avoid colonizing flora. Culture results need careful interpretation to determine the significance of organisms, and remember that superficial swabs are poor predictors of deep/invasive infection.

Cerebrospinal fluid

CSF will undergo cell count (polymorphs, lymphocytes, red cells) and Gram stain. CSF protein and glucose are usually performed in biochemistry. Gram and special stains, such as ZN, India ink, as indicated by the clinical picture. Antigen tests (e.g. cryptococcal antigen), culture, and PCR are available. CSF samples from neurosurgical shunts require careful interpretation due to colonization.

Intravascular catheter line tips

Intravascular catheter (IVC) line tips—not all laboratories process IVC tips. Using a quantification technique, such as the Maki roll, >15 cfu is regarded as significant.

Serum or EDTA blood samples

Serum or EDTA blood samples are required for serological and molecular tests. Consult your local laboratory guidelines.

Bacterial culture media

Selective media enable certain organisms to grow, while inhibiting other organisms, e.g. adding an antibiotic to an agar will select for organisms which are resistant to that agent.

Differential media help distinguish different organisms growing on the same media by virtue of their different biochemical behaviours. For example, those organisms that can ferment lactose will do so if it is present producing acid. pH indicators in the media (neutral red in the case of MacConkey agar) will indicate a change in pH. There are a number of commercial chromogenic agar available, designed to facilitate rapid identification.

Enriched media contain specific nutrients required by certain organisms, including fastidious ones (i.e. *H. influenzae*).

Specific media include:

- blood agar—an enriched differential media used to demonstrate haemolysis and isolate fastidious organisms. It contains 5–10% sheep or horse blood;
- MacConkey agar—selects for Gram-negatives. Contains bile salts (to inhibit most Gram-positives), crystal violet (inhibits certain Gram-positives), lactose, peptone, and a dye (neutral red) that is turned pink by lactose fermenters. Sorbitol MacConkey (S-MAC) helps differentiate enteropathogenic *E. coli*, such as O157, as most are non-sorbitol fermenters;
- CLED (cystine, lactose, electrolyte-deficient agar) is used to isolate and differentiate Gram-negatives, as it inhibits *Proteus* swarming and can differentiate between lactose fermenters and non-fermenters;
- chocolate agar—enriched with heat-treated blood (40–45°C). Particularly good for isolating *S. pneumoniae* and *H. influenzae*;
- Hektoen enteric (HE) agar—Gram-negative selective used for distinguishing between *Salmonella* and *Shigella*. It contains peptone, as well as other various sugars. *Salmonella/Shigella* cannot use the latter but can use the former, alkalinizing the agar and turning a pH indicator blue. Other enteric bacteria use the latter in preference, producing acidic products, turning the indicator yellow/red. In addition, the presence of thiosulfate produces a black precipitate in the presence of hydrogen sulfide (H_2S)—which *Shigella* does not produce (appears green), but *Salmonella* does (black);
- xylose lysine deoxycholate (XLD)—also facilitates discrimination of *Salmonella* from *Shigella*, utilizing thiosulfate (as under HE agar) and differential use of the sugar xylose (*Shigella* appears red; *Salmonella* red with black centres; coliforms yellow/orange);
- mannitol salt agar (MSA)—a high level of salt (7.5–10%) selects Gram-positives such as staphylococci. The presence of mannitol helps separate *S. aureus* (can ferment mannitol, turning phenol red to yellow) from other staphylococci (small pink/red colonies);
- buffered charcoal yeast extract (BCYE) agar—selects for *L. pneumophila*;
- Thayer–Martin agar or New York City (NYC) agar—used to isolate pathogenic *Neisseria* spp. (*N. gonorrhoeae* and *N. meningitidis*).
- Mueller Hinton agar—contains beef infusion, peptone, and starch, and is used primarily for antibiotic susceptibility testing. It is non-selective and non-differential, and facilitates the diffusion of antibiotic from testing discs;
- cetrimide agar—used for the selective isolation of *P. aeruginosa*;
- Tinsdale agar—contains potassium tellurite, which can isolate *C. diphtheriae*. Löeffler's and Hoyle's tellurite agar are also useful for *C. diphtheriae*;
- Sabouraud agar—used to culture fungi. Its low pH (5.6) inhibits the growth of most bacteria. It contains dextrose and peptones. Chloramphenicol is commonly added for the purpose of inhibiting Gram-negative organisms. The growth of fungal structures facilitates identification.

Identification of bacteria

Identification of bacteria in the diagnostic laboratory is based on phenotypic characteristics such as (see Figs. 7.1 to 7.4):

- microscopic appearance;
- growth requirements;
- colonial morphology;
- haemolysis pattern;
- biochemical tests;
- antimicrobial susceptibility patterns;
- mass spectrometry.

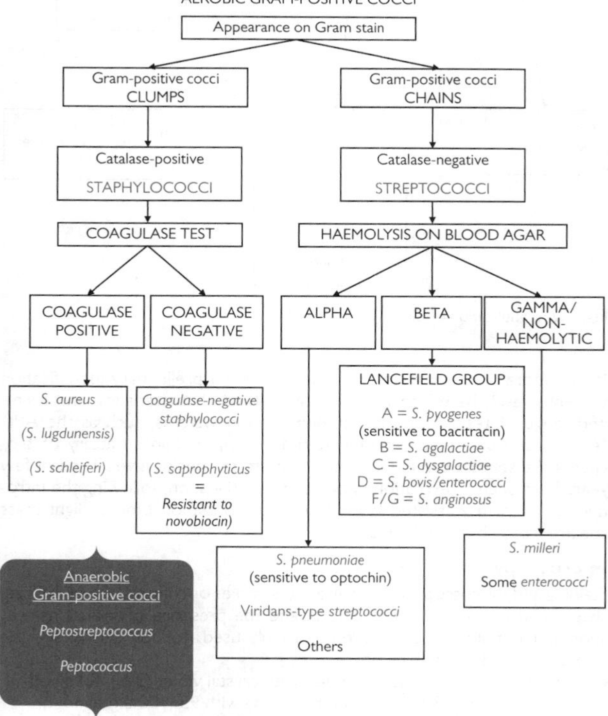

Fig. 7.1 Identification of Gram-positive cocci.

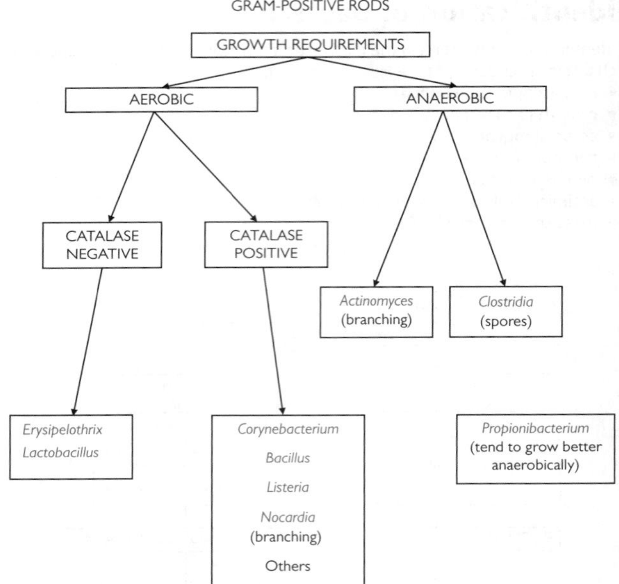

Fig. 7.2 Identification of Gram-positive rods.

Many laboratory technicians are able to make a preliminary identification to genus level, based on clinical data, cultural characteristics, and a limited range of tests. Commercial identification systems, such as the API® (Analytical Profile Index) system (biomérieux), contain a battery of biochemical tests that can identify the organism to species level. The last few years have seen a revolution in bacterial identification, following the introduction of matrix-assisted laser desorption ionization time-of-flight mass spectroscopy (MALDI-TOF).

Microscopy

Staining and microscopic examination of samples or cultures reveal the size, shape, and arrangement of bacteria and the presence of inclusions, e.g. spores. The following stains are commonly used (for full details, see the PHE 2014 UK SMI 'Staining procedures').

- *Gram stain*—a fixed slide is flooded with crystal violet (30s), followed by Lugol's iodine (30s), followed by rinsing with 95–100% ethanol or acetone, followed by counterstaining with 0.1% neutral red, safranin, or carbol fuchsin (2min). Gram-positive organisms stain deep blue/purple, and Gram-negative organisms stain pink/red.

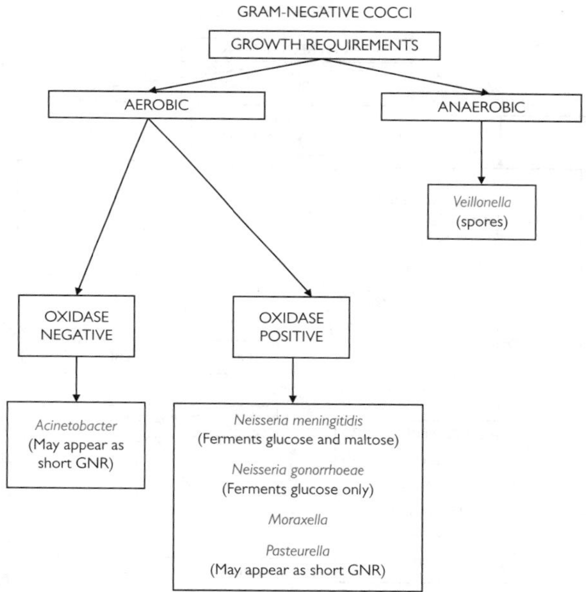

Fig. 7.3 Identification of Gram-negative cocci.

- *Acridine orange stain*—this is used to identify *T. vaginalis* in vaginal specimens. The slide is stained with acridine orange (5–10s), decolorized with alcoholic saline (5–10s), and rinsed with normal saline. Once dry, a drop of saline or distilled water and a coverslip are added, and the slide is examined under fluorescence microscopy. Trophozoites of *T. vaginalis* stain brick red with green nuclei.
- *Auramine stain*—this is used to identify mycobacteria in clinical specimens. It is considered more sensitive than the ZN stain. A heat-fixed slide is flooded with auramine-phenol (1:10) for 10min. It is rinsed with water and then decolorized with 1% acid-alcohol for 3–5min (until no further stain seeps from the film). It is rinsed and stained with 0.1% potassium permanganate for 15s. It is rinsed and allowed to air dry before examination under fluorescence microscopy. AFB appear bright yellow/green against a dark background.
- *ZN stain*—this is used to identify mycobacteria in cultures and provides better morphological detail than an auramine stain. A heat-fixed slide is flooded with strong carbol fuchsin and heated gently until it is just steaming. It is left to cool (3–5min), rinsed with water, and decolorized

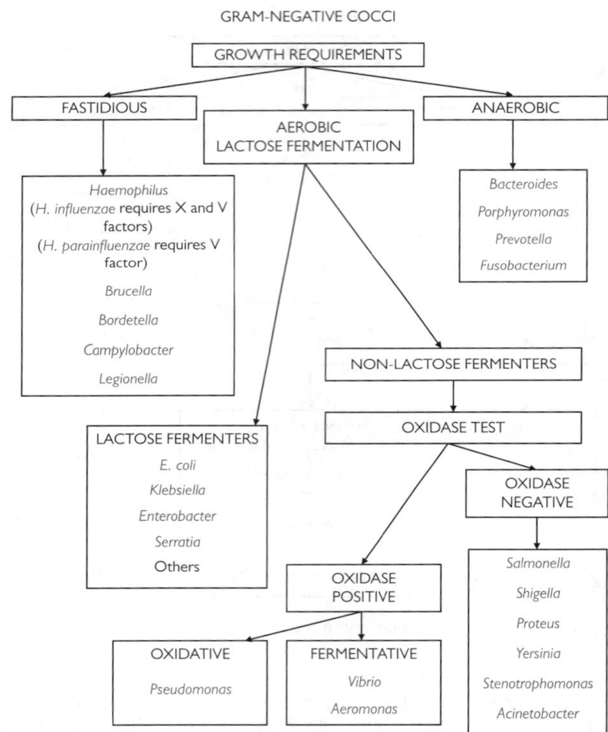

Fig. 7.4 Identification of Gram-negative rods.

with a 3% acid-alcohol solution (5–7min, until the slide is faintly pink). The slide is rinsed with water and counterstained with 1% v/v methylene blue or malachite green (30s). It is allowed to air dry before examination under oil immersion light microscopy. AFB appear red on a blue or green background. A modified ZN stain is used for identification of *Nocardia* spp. and cryptosporidia.

- *Nigrosin (India ink) stain*—this stain is used to identify *C. neoformans* in clinical specimens. A drop of India ink is put on the slide, followed by a drop of the specimen and mixed together. A coverslip is applied, and the slide is examined under light microscopy. *C. neoformans* is identified by a clear zone (capsule) around the organism.

Growth requirements

These can vary considerably and include:

- *atmosphere*—organisms can be divided into categories, according to their atmospheric requirements:
  - strict aerobes grow only in the presence of oxygen;
  - strict anaerobes grow only in the absence of oxygen;
  - facultative organisms grow aerobically or anaerobically;
  - microaerophilic organisms grow best in atmospheres with reduced oxygen concentration (e.g. 5–10% CO_2);
  - capnophilic organisms require additional CO_2 for growth.
- *temperature*—organisms can also be differentiated by their temperature requirements:
  - psychrophilic organisms grow at temperatures of 10–30°C;
  - mesophilic organisms grow at temperatures of 30–40°C;
  - thermophilic organisms grow at temperatures of 50–60°C;
  - most clinically encountered organisms are mesophilic.
- *nutrition*—some organisms grow readily on ordinary nutrient media, whereas others have particular nutritional requirements, e.g. *H. influenzae* requires specific growth factors such as factor X (haemin) and factor V (NAD). Halophilic organisms require high salt concentrations.

Colonial morphology

Bacterial colonies of a single species, when grown on specific media under controlled conditions, are described by their characteristic size, shape, texture, and colour. Colonies may be flat or raised, smooth or irregular, and pigmented (e.g. *P. aeruginosa* is green/blue, or *S. marcescens* is pink) or non-pigmented. Experienced laboratory technicians can often provisionally identify an organism, using colonial appearance alone.

Haemolysis

Some organisms produce haemolysins that cause partial or complete lysis of RBCs in blood-containing media. This haemolysis may be:

- β-haemolytic—a clear zone of complete haemolysis around the colony;
- α-haemolytic—a green zone of incomplete haemolysis;
- non-haemolytic.

This feature is often used in the initial identification of streptococci.

Further information

For information on the identification of bacteria, see the UK SMI, which are a comprehensive referenced collection of recommended algorithms and procedures for clinical microbiology (web search for 'UK SMI').

Biochemical tests

A variety of biochemical tests may be used for the identification of bacteria in the diagnostic laboratory. These may be performed manually but more commonly are done as part of a multi-test commercial kit (e.g. API) or an automated identification system.

Catalase test

Catalase is an enzyme that catalyses the breakdown of H_2O_2 into water and oxygen. Many aerobic and facultatively anaerobic organisms are catalase-positive, whereas streptococci and enterococci are catalase-negative. H_2O_2 solution is drawn up into a capillary tube, and the tip is then touched onto a colony. Vigorous bubbling indicates the presence of catalase. NB. Media containing blood may produce a false-positive result.

Coagulase test

Coagulase is an enzyme that enables breakdown of fibrinogen to fibrin. This test is used to differentiate the staphylococci. Coagulase exists in two forms: bound coagulase/clumping factor (detected by the slide coagulase test) and free coagulase (detected by the tube coagulase test).

Slide coagulase test

A colony is emulsified in a drop of distilled water on a slide. A loop or wire is dipped into plasma and then mixed into the bacterial suspension. A positive test result occurs if agglutination is seen within 10s.

Tube coagulase test

A colony is emulsified in a tube containing plasma and incubated at 37°C for 4h. A visible clot indicates a positive result. If negative at 4h, the tube should be reincubated overnight. NB. MRSA may give a negative result at 4h.

Deoxyribonuclease (DNase) test

DNase is an enzyme that enables the degradation of DNA. This test is used to identify pathogenic staphylococci (e.g. *S. aureus* and *S. schleiferi*) that produce large quantities of extracellular DNase. A colony is streaked onto a DNase plate and incubated at 37°C for 18–24h. The following day, the plate is flooded with hydrochloric acid—unhydrolysed DNA is precipitated, producing a white opacity in the agar. Cultures surrounded by a clear zone (hydrolysed DNA) are DNase-positive. NB. Some strains of MRSA are DNase-negative, and *S. epidermidis* may be weakly positive.

Optochin test

This test is used to differentiate *S. pneumoniae* (optochin-sensitive) from other α-haemolytic streptococci (optochin-resistant). Optochin (ethylhydrocupreine hydrochloride) is a chemical that causes lysis of the cell wall of *S. pneumoniae*. An optochin disc is placed in the centre of the bacterial inoculum and incubated at 37°C in 5% CO_2 for 18–24h. A zone of inhibition of ≥5mm indicates a positive result.

Aesculin hydrolysis test

This test is used to differentiate enterococci (aesculin-positive) from streptococci (aesculin-negative). It tests the ability of the organism to hydrolyse aesculin to aesculetin and glucose in the presence of 10–40% bile. The aesculetin combines with ferric ions in the medium to form a black complex. The organism is inoculated onto a bile aesculin plate or slope, and incubated at 37°C for 24h. Presence of a dark brown or black halo indicates a positive result.

Indole test

The indole test is used to differentiate *Enterobacteriaceae*. It detects the ability of an organism to produce indole from the amino acid tryptophan. A coloured product is obtained when indole is combined with certain aldehydes. There are two methods.

Spot indole test

A piece of filter paper is moistened with the indole reagent, and a colony is smeared onto the surface. A green/blue colour indicates a positive result.

Tube indole test

The organism is emulsified in a peptone broth and incubated at 37°C for 24h. A volume of 0.5mL of Kovac's reagent is added; a pink colour in the top layer indicates a positive result.

ONPG (β-galactosidase) test

This test is used as an aid to differentiate *Enterobacteriaceae*. Two enzymes, permease and β-galactosidase, are required for lactose fermentation. Late lactose fermenters do not possess permease but do have β-galactosidase. Tubes containing *o*-nitrophenyl-β-*D*-galactopyranoside (ONPG) are inoculated with the organism and incubated at 37°C for 24h. If present, β-galactosidase hydrolyses ONPG to produce galactose and *o*-nitrophenol, a yellow compound.

Urease test

This test is used to differentiate urease-positive *Proteus* spp. from the other *Enterobacteriaceae*. Some strains of *Enterobacter* and *Klebsiella* spp. are urease-positive. Inoculate a slope of Christensen's medium with the test organism and at 37°C for 24h. A pink/purple colour indicates a positive result.

Oxidase test

This test determines if an organism has the cytochrome oxidase enzyme and is used as an aid in the differentiation of *Pseudomonas, Neisseria, Moraxella, Campylobacter*, and *Pasteurella* spp. (oxidase-positive). Cytochrome oxidase catalyses the transport of electrons from donor compounds (e.g. NADH) to electron acceptors (usually oxygen). The test reagent *N, N, N', N'-tetra-methyl-p-phenylenediamine dihydrochloride* acts as an artificial electron acceptor for the enzyme oxidase. The oxidized reagent forms the coloured compound indophenol blue.

Further information

For information on the identification of bacteria, see the UK SMI, which are a comprehensive referenced collection of recommended algorithms and procedures for clinical microbiology (web search for 'UK SMI').

Automated diagnostics

Automated identification systems allow rapid identification ± antibiotic susceptibility testing of organisms. Different methodologies have strengths and weaknesses. Selection for use in a diagnostic laboratory depends on factors such as assay throughput, turnaround times, labour, and compatibility with existing systems. The benefits include reduction in labour, faster reporting, and reduced human transcription errors (systems can link directly to laboratory databases). Problems include inoculum preparation (over/under-inoculation or missing a mixed culture), the ability to test only a certain range of organisms (slow-growing, fastidious, or heavily mucoid organisms may need to be processed manually), culture conditions, and data entry. Currently available methods include the following.

VITEK® 2 (biomérieux)

The unknown organism is automatically placed in suspension at an appropriate dilution and inoculated onto a small card that has 64 microwells. Each well contains identification biochemical substrates or antimicrobial dilutions. After inoculation and incubation, the system measures turbidity and colour changes within the card wells. Results are available within 4–24h. There are several caveats to the interpretation of certain organism/antibiotic combinations, but overall the system is accurate, rapid, and safe.

Phoenix™ (Becton Dickinson)

Panels are inoculated manually, thus may require a specific organism dilution for accuracy. It uses colorimetric oxidation–reduction indicator for susceptibility testing, and several fluorometric and colorimetric indicators for identification. Results are available in 4–16h.

MALDI-TOF

MALDI-TOF (matrix-assisted laser desorption/ionization time-of-flight mass spectrometry) is a novel technique used for the identification of bacteria or fungi. The organism is mixed with a suitable matrix material and irradiated with a laser pulse. The resulting hot plume is accelerated in an electric field and enters the flight tube, in which different molecules are separated according to their mass-to-charge ratio, reaching the detector at different times. The mass spectra generated are analysed and compared with stored profiles of known organisms. It is normal practice in a routine laboratory to set a 'cut-off' for acceptable identification. Some species are difficult to distinguish, notably the α-haemolytic streptococci. Mixed cultures can be challenging, and *Shigella* cannot be differentiated from *E. coli*. Despite these limitations, MALDI has been a significant advance in diagnostic bacteriology.

Next-generation sequencing

(➔ See Molecular typing methods, p. 231.) The cost and speed of DNA sequencing are falling rapidly. Although still largely a research tool, it is certain that next-generation sequencing (NGS) will begin to replace traditional culture-based diagnostics for many purposes in the near future.

Molecular organism identification

Real-time or quantitative PCR

Real-time or quantitative PCR (qPCR) is used to amplify and simultaneously quantify a targeted DNA/RNA molecule, as the reaction progresses. The process involves extraction, amplification, and detection. Detection is either by non-specific fluorescent dyes that intercalate with any dsDNA, or by fluororescent marker-labelled DNA probes specific to the reaction concerned. The DNA/RNA quantity is inferred either by reference to a standard control curve (absolute) or relative to an internal control within the reaction (e.g. target is present at four times the quantity of the internal control).

Multiplex PCR

Multiplex PCR allows the detection of multiple PCR targets in a single reaction. Multiplex reactions have been developed for specific clinical syndromes, e.g. respiratory panel for influenza A (H1N1, swine flu), influenza B, RSV, human metapneumovirus, parainfluenza viruses 1–3.

16S rRNA PCR

16S rRNA PCR—16S rRNA is a component of the 30S subunit of the bacterial ribosome. The genes coding it are highly conserved but contain hypervariable genus- or species-specific regions. Thus, 'universal' primers allow gene amplification. This is then sequenced and compared to known sequences for genus/species level identification. Advantages include diagnosis of fastidious or unculturable organisms (e.g. *Tropheryma whipplei*), or identification of a pathogen after antibiotic therapy. 16S rRNA PCR may be negative on a culture-positive specimen—this may be due to low levels of the organism below the detection threshold of the assay or the presence of PCR inhibitors. Certain bacteria can be difficult to identify, because they share most of their 16S sequences (e.g. *E. coli* from *Shigella*, members of the *Streptococcus milleri* complex, *S. pneumoniae* from *Streptococcus oralis*).

18S rRNA PCR

18S rRNA PCR (pan-fungal PCR)—18S rRNA is the eukaryotic homologue of 16S rRNA in prokaryotes. PCR of 18S sequences allows the classification of most *Candida* spp. and many other fungi.

Molecular typing methods

Epidemiological typing of bacteria facilitates infection control investigations and surveillance (i.e. to monitor vaccine effectiveness). Traditional methods are based on phenotypic characteristics, e.g. antibiogram, serotype, phage type. The development of a variety of molecular typing methods has enabled genetic comparison of strains, providing improved discrimination.

Pulsed-field gel electrophoresis

PFGE has been considered the gold standard method for typing bacterial isolates and is still widely used. A highly purified genomic DNA sample is cleaved with a restriction endonuclease that recognizes infrequently occurring restriction sites in the genome of the bacterial species. The resulting restriction fragments can be separated on an agarose gel by 'pulsed-field' electrophoresis, in which the orientation of the electric field across the gel is changed periodically. The separated DNA fragments can be visualized on the gel as bands. Limitations—technically demanding, labour-intensive, time-consuming, may lack the resolution to distinguish bands of nearly identical size, and analysis of results is prone to subjectivity.

Amplified fragment length polymorphism

Genomic DNA is cut with two restriction enzymes, and double-stranded adaptors are ligated to the sticky ends of the restriction fragments. A subset of the fragments are amplified by PCR, using primers complementary to the adaptor sequence, the restriction site sequence, and a number of additional nucleotides from the end of the unknown DNA template. Amplified fragments are separated and visualized on gels. Analysis enables the determination of genetic relatedness amongst bacterial isolates. AFLP is at least as discriminatory as PFGE and is reproducible and portable. However, its major limitations are that it is labour-intensive and expensive.

Random amplification of polymorphic DNA and arbitrarily primed polymerase chain reaction (RAPD PCR)

Random amplification of polymorphic DNA (RAPD) does not require any specific knowledge of the DNA sequence of the target organism. Short arbitrary primers (usually ten bases) are used in a reaction conducted at low, non-stringent annealing temperatures, allowing the hybridization of multiple mismatched sequences. If the distance between two primer binding sites is within 0.1–3kb, an amplicon may be generated. The number and positions of primer binding sites are unique to a particular strain. Amplicons can be analysed by gel or DNA sequencing. RAPD is less discriminatory than PFGE but is widely used, because it is simple, inexpensive, and rapid. The main limit is low intra- and inter-laboratory reproducibility (due to very low annealing temperatures, differences in reagents, protocols, machines).

Repetitive element polymerase chain reaction (rep-PCR)

This method uses primers that hybridize to non-coding intergenic repetitive sequences scattered across the genome. DNA between adjacent repetitive elements is amplified using PCR, and multiple amplicons can be produced. The sizes of these amplicons are then electrophoretically characterized, and the banding patterns are compared to determine the genetic relatedness between the isolates. It is quick, cheap, and discriminatory. Limitations—lacks reproducibility, which may result from variability in reagents and gel electrophoresis systems.

Multilocus variable-number tandem repeat analysis

Bacterial genomes possess many regions with nucleotide repeats. Variable-number tandem repeats (VNTRs) are repeating patterns of one or more nucleotides occurring adjacent to each other (e.g. ATTC ATTC ATTC) and show variations between species. Multilocus variable-number tandem repeat analysis (MLVA) types an organism by differences in the number of tandem repeats at different loci. PCR of the VNTR loci is followed by sizing of the PCR products, allowing calculation of the number of repeats at each locus, creating an MVLA profile.

Single locus sequence typing

Single locus sequence typing (SLST) uses sequence variation within a single gene to distinguish bacterial isolates, e.g. spa typing (*S. aureus* protein A) for *S. aureus*. Not as discriminatory as other methods such as PFGE or multilocus sequence typing (MLST).

Multilocus sequence typing

A total of 450–500bp of 7–8 housekeeping genes are amplified by PCR and sequenced. For each locus, unique sequences (alleles) are assigned arbitrary numbers. Based on the combination of alleles, the sequence type is determined. MLST is unambiguous and reproducible, and has an internationally standardized nomenclature. Allele sequences and sequence typing profiles are available in central databases (℘ pubmlst.org and ℘ www.mlst.net). Main disadvantages of MLST—costly, labour-intensive, and may not be sufficiently discriminatory for outbreak investigations.

Comparative genomic hybridization

A collection of DNA probes attached in an ordered fashion to a solid surface (microarray) is hybridized to DNA extracted from a pathogen. The probes on the array may be PCR amplicons (>200bp) or oligonucleotides (up to 70 mers). Successful hybridization events measured by a scanner. Routine application of this technique is hindered by the high costs of materials and the specialized equipment needed for the tests.

Next-generation sequencing

NGS or whole-genome sequencing (WGS) sequences the genome of organisms much more rapidly and at a much lower cost than traditional sequencing methods. Millions of short sequence reads (35–700bp in length) are produced, and either mapped to a reference genome or assembled to generate the genome. This enables genomic comparison at a nucleotide level and is much more discriminatory than other typing methods. WGS has been used to investigate outbreaks of infections in both hospital and community settings, and rapidly diagnose MDR organisms, e.g. XDR-TB. Cost limits routine clinical use, but this is falling rapidly. It is likely that this technology will replace many of the previously discussed typing methods in the near future.

Quality assurance and accreditation

A TQM system ensures that microbiology laboratories provide a prompt, quality-assured, and clinically appropriate service to its users. This is done through a process of quality planning, which is the part of quality management focused on setting quality objectives and specifying necessary operational processes and related resources to fulfil quality objectives. The main components of a quality management system are:

- written quality objectives consistent with the quality policy;
- a quality manual which is reviewed and updated as required;
- a quality manager responsible for implementation and maintenance of the quality management system;
- document control;
- control of process and quality records, according to current regulations;
- control of clinical material, according to current regulations;
- an annual review of the laboratory's quality management system by the laboratory management.

Quality assurance

The total process whereby the quality of laboratory reports can be guaranteed. A comprehensive quality assurance system includes provision and control of standard operating procedures (SOPs)—education and training, planned maintenance and calibration of equipment, monitoring of turnaround times.

Internal quality control

The processes carried out to check that media, reagents, and equipment are performing within specifications.

Internal quality assurance

Internal quality assurance (IQA) is usually measured by the routine reprocessing of a sample. By assessing two results from the same sample, any discrepancies can be investigated, and, if necessary, practice can be changed to improve the consistency of that particular laboratory test. Part of the laboratory internal quality control (IQC) procedures.

External quality assessment

Provision by an external body of a specimen of known, but undisclosed, content for analysis. External quality assessment (EQA) is not a substitute for other components of the quality system, and, in particular, EQA cannot replace IQC. The National External Quality Assessment Service for Microbiology (NEQAS; ukneqasmicro.org.uk) is organized by PHE. It was established in 1971 and is recognized as a major contributor to quality assurance in clinical diagnostic microbiology. The scheme provides participants with a wide range of specimens and constructive feedback. Participants can monitor the effectiveness of their quality assurance measures, and detect and remedy problems, thus allowing continuing quality improvement.

Laboratory accreditation

Clinical Pathology Accreditation (CPA) UK Ltd was established by various professional organizations, such as the Institute of Biomedical Science (IBMS) and the Royal College of Pathologists, together with the private health sector and the DH. CPA is now a subsidiary of the UK accreditation service (www.ukas.com) and is managing the transition of all CPA-accredited laboratories to the internationally recognized ISO 15189:2012 standard.

Pathology networks

Lord Carter of Coles published his Independent Review of Pathology Services for the DH in 2008. His recommendations suggested that the standard district general hospital with a full range of services would be increasingly unsustainable. He proposed consolidation of acute trust pathology services into managed pathology networks. Arrangements for this 'hub and spoke' model vary by specialty and by region, with some 'spoke' microbiology laboratories retaining 'hot labs' for tests needed within 4h, but many having no on-site microbiology laboratory. Whereas the last few years have seen some service aggregation (e.g. single laboratories for multisite hospital trusts, within London where hospitals are closely located), there has been nothing like the scale of consolidation originally envisioned.

Overview of Gram-positive cocci

Gram-positive cocci are commonly isolated from clinical specimens. They are widely distributed in the environment and are found as commensals of the skin, mucous membranes, and other body sites. Because of their ubiquitous nature, recovery of these organisms from specimens should always be interpreted in the context of the clinical presentation. The two medically most important groups are staphylococci and streptococci.

Classification

The classification of Gram-positive cocci is based on a combination of phenotypic and genotypic characteristics, and has changed over time as a result of genetic sequencing data. The current classification of some medically important Gram-positive cocci is as follows:

- family *Staphylococcaceae*, genus *Staphylococcus*;
- family *Streptococcaceae*, genus *Streptococcus*;
- family *Enterococcaceae*, genus *Enterococcus*;
- family *Leuconostocaceae*, genus *Leuconostoc*;
- family *Micrococcaceae*, genus *Micrococcus* and genus *Rothia*;
- family *Lactobacillaceae*, genus *Pediococcus*;
- family *Aerococcaceae*, genus *Aerococcus* and genus *Abiotrophia*;
- family *Carnobacteriaceae*, genus *Alloiococcus*;
- family *Peptococcaceae*, genus *Peptococcus*;
- family *Peptostreptococcaceae*, genus *Peptostreptococcus*;
- other anaerobic cocci, e.g. genus *Anaerococcus*, genus *Finegoldia*, genus *Parvimonas*, and genus *Peptoniphilus*.

Staphylococci

- Staphylococci are non-motile, non-spore-forming, catalase-positive, Gram-positive cocci.
- They occur as single cells, pairs, tetrads, or grape-like clusters (most common).
- Most species are facultative anaerobes, except *S. aureus* subspecies *anaerobius* and *S. saccharolyticus*, which are anaerobic.
- Staphylococci are normally found on the skin and mucous membranes of animals. In some cases, their location may be very specific, e.g.

S. *capitis* subspecies *capitis* on the scalp or *S. auricularis* in the external auditory canal.
- *S. aureus, S. epidermidis, S. lugdunensis*, and *S. saprophyticus* are the main human pathogens.
- They may be differentiated on the basis of the coagulase test (see Fig. 7.1) into coagulase-positive (e.g. *S. aureus*) and coagulase-negative (CoNS, e.g. *S. epidermidis*).
- In addition, *S. aureus* produces DNase, while other staphylococci are usually DNase-negative.
- There are 30 or so species of CoNS, but it is rarely necessary to identify them at the species level.

Streptococci

- The streptococci are non-sporing, non-motile organisms, and catalase-negative, Gram-positive cocci that grow in pairs and chains.
- Some species are capsulated.
- They are facultative anaerobes and may require enriched media to grow.
- The streptococci are subdivided on the basis of their 'classic' appearance on horse blood agar into α-, β-, and non-haemolytic streptococci.
- The α-haemolytic streptococci (incomplete haemolysis on blood agar, resulting in a greenish tinge) include *S. pneumoniae* (➲ see *Streptococcus pneumoniae*, pp. 243–5) and the viridans streptococci.
- The β-haemolytic streptococci (complete haemolysis/clear zone on blood agar) are grouped on the basis of their Lancefield carbohydrate antigens. The medically important ones are groups A, B, C, F, and G.
- The enterococci (*E. faecalis* and others; ➲ see Enterococci, pp. 245–7) were originally called *Streptococcus faecalis* and often react with group D antisera, but are now a separate genus.
- Non-haemolytic streptococci make up the remainder and include the viridans (*S. mutans, S. salivarius, S. anginosus, S. mitis*, and *S. sanguinis* groups), anaerobic, and nutritionally variant streptococci.
- For a comprehensive review of taxonomic and nomenclature changes of the streptococci, see Facklam (2002).[1]

Other Gram-positive cocci

These include: *Peptococcus, Peptostreptococcus, Leuconostoc, Pedioccoccus, Abiotrophia, Micrococcus*, and *Stomatococcus*.

Reference

1 Facklam R (2002). What happened to the streptococci: overview of taxonomic and nomenclature changes. *Clin Microbiol Rev.* **15**:613–30.

Staphylococcus aureus

S. aureus is a facultatively anaerobic, non-motile, non-spore-forming, catalase-positive, coagulase-positive, Gram-positive coccus. It is a major human pathogen and can cause a wide variety of infections, ranging from superficial skin infections to severe life-threatening conditions, e.g. TSS.

Epidemiology

S. aureus is a skin colonizer and is found in the anterior nares of 10–40% of people. Chronic carriage is associated with an increased risk of infection, e.g. in haemodialysis patients. Nasal carriage has contributed to the persistence and spread of MRSA.

Pathogenesis

S. aureus possesses a wide array of virulence factors, including:

- *ability to form a biofilm*—this is an extracellular polysaccharide network produced by staphylococci (and other organisms) that results in colonization and persistence on prosthetic material. Polysaccharide intracellular adhesin (PIA) is synthesized by the *ica* operon;
- *capsule*—>90% of *S. aureus* isolates have a capsule, with 11 serotypes reported;
- *surface adhesins* (also known as microbial surface components recognizing adhesive matrix molecules, MSCRAMMs)—enables the organism to adhere to host extracellular matrix.These include protein A, clumping factors A and B, collagen-binding protein, fibronectin-binding protein, serine aspartate repeat protein, plasmin-sensitive protein, and surface proteins A to K;
- *techoic and lipotechoic acids*—these are components of the cell wall. Lipotechoic acids trigger release of cytokines by macrophages;
- *peptidoglycan*—is the scaffold for anchoring the MSCRAMMs. It also triggers the release of cytokines. Modification of peptidoglycan synthesis is associated with antimicrobial resistance;
- *haemolysins*—*S. aureus* possesses four haemolysins (α, β, γ, δ);
- *Panton–Valentine leucocidin* (PVL)—this is a haemolysin (induces a pore in the membrane of host leucocytes) encoded by two genes (*lukS* and *lukF*) that are carried on a mobile phage (φSLT). PVL-producing strains are associated with furunculosis, severe haemorrhagic pneumonia, and clusters of MRSA skin infections;
- *exfoliative toxins* (ETs)—ETA and ETB are encoded by the *eta* and *etb* genes, respectively. They cause staphylococcal scalded skin syndrome (SSSS);
- *superantigens*—this group includes TSS toxin (TSST)-1 and staphylococcal enterotoxins (SEs). Enable a non-selective activation of T cells. TSST-1 is associated with TSS, whereas SEs are associated with food poisoning;
- *pathogenicity (genomic) islands*—these are structures that vary in size from 15 to 70kb, and harbour virulence and drug resistance genes, e.g. SaPI1 and SaPI2 carry the gene for TSST-1;
- *resistance islands*—MRSA contains a resistance island called SCC*mec* which confers resistance to meticillin;
- *small colony variants*—slow-growing subpopulations with atypical colony morphology, unusual biochemical characteristics (e.g. coagulase tube test positive only after 18h, thus harder to identify), less susceptible to antibiotics, and implicated in persistent infections. They downregulate genes for metabolism and virulence, while upregulating those for persistence and biofilm formation.

Clinical features

S. aureus can cause a wide spectrum of clinical infections, including:

- skin and soft tissue infections, e.g. impetigo, folliculitis, hidradenitis, mastitis, wound infections, erysipelas, cellulitis, pyomyositis, necrotizing fasciitis;
- bone and joint infections, e.g. septic arthritis, osteomyelitis, discitis;
- systemic infections, e.g. bacteraemia, endocarditis, meningitis;
- prosthetic device-related, e.g. IVC-associated, pacemaker infections, PJIs, etc.;
- toxin-mediated, e.g. scalded skin syndrome, TSS.

Diagnosis

- In some cases, e.g. skin and soft tissue infections, the diagnosis is clinical. In others, appropriate samples, e.g. pus, tissue, or blood, should be taken and submitted to the laboratory for microscopy, culture, and sensitivity (MC&S).
- Gram stain—Gram-positive cocci in clusters.
- Culture on blood agar or liquid media—growth usually occurs within 18–24h. Prolonged incubation detects small colony variants.
- Biochemical tests—catalase-positive, coagulase-positive, DNase-positive.
- Identification—API® Staph, automated methods (i.e. VITEK®, MALDI);
- Typing methods include PFGE, toxin, SCC*mec*, or spa typing;
- Molecular diagnosis, e.g 16S or 23S RNA PCR, or *mecA* gene (for meticillin resistance) and PVL gene PCR.

Treatment

- Treatment depends on the type of infection and drug susceptibility of the organism. Control and removal of any source is vital (e.g. cannula).
- Flucloxacillin PO or IV is used for MSSA isolates.
- Vancomycin or daptomycin IV for suspected *S. aureus* infections where MRSA is a possibility or in penicillin-allergic patients.
- Aminoglycosides exhibit synergism; however, routine combination with flucloxacillin or vancomycin for the treatment of *S. aureus* endocarditis is not recommended. Unlike streptococcal endocarditis, studies have shown little clinical benefit—and an increased incidence of renal dysfunction.
- Other active agents include clindamycin, teicoplanin, and linezolid.
- Duration of treatment depends on the source—7 days for skin and soft tissue infections, and up to 6 weeks for endocarditis. For short-lived bacteraemia with a removable source, e.g. IVC, 2 weeks of treatment is adequate.

Prevention

- Prevention of *S. aureus* infections is based on bacterial decolonization of carriers with local antiseptics, e.g. nasal mupirocin and chlorhexidine soap. This is routinely done for MRSA carriers. MSSA decolonization is performed in some high-risk settings, i.e. dialysis units. There are DH guidelines for the prevention of SSIs. *S. aureus* is the leading cause of such infections.
- Vaccines—a subject of ongoing research, with the aim of reducing bacteraemia rates in those at high risk (e.g. haemodialysis patients). None in use outside of clinical trials.

Meticillin-resistant *Staphylococcus aureus*

MRSA was first detected in 1961, a few months after meticillin was introduced into clinical practice. However, it was not until the 1980s that endemic strains of MRSA with MDR became a global nosocomial problem.

Mechanism of resistance

MRSA strains are resistant to all β-lactams due to alteration in PBP2¢ and consequently the structure of the cell wall. Meticillin resistance is due to the *mecA* gene that codes for the low-affinity PBP2. *mecA* is usually located on an MGE called SCC-*mec* (staphylococcal cassette chromosome). It is believed the *mec* gene was acquired from CoNS—some MRSA strains have also acquired other virulence and resistance genes from CoNS. There are six major SCC-*mec* clones, defined by the class of the *mecA* gene and type of *ccr* (cassette chromosome recombinase) complex. SCC-*mec* types I to III are usually found in health-care settings and are often resistant to additional antbiotics, while types IV and V are commoner in the community, and resistance to non-β-lactam agents is uncommon.

Epidemiology

- Risk factors for MRSA include increasing age, prior antibiotics, indwelling catheters, severe underlying disease, and ICU stay.
- Health care-acquired MRSA (HA-MRSA) rates vary in different parts of the world. During the 1990s, the UK saw an emergence of two epidemic MRSA strains (EMRSA 15 and 16), resulting in a year-on-year increase in MRSA bacteraemias. These strains were also resistant to erythromycin and ciprofloxacin. In 2002, between 25% and 50% of *S. aureus* bacteraemias were due to MRSA in the UK, Ireland, France, Italy, and Portugal. Finland, Denmark, and the Netherlands had very low rates (<5%). The last decade has seen a fall in MRSA rates in the UK to <10% of *S. aureus* bacteraemias in 2013/2014, as a result of good infection control practice and national mandatory surveillance.
- Community-acquired MRSA (CA-MRSA) is a significant issue in the USA, due, in part, to the widespread dissemination of a specific clone USA300. While this has been identified in a number of European countries, it exists only at low levels. Its success in the USA relates to its transmissibility and the presence of other virulence factors such as PVL.

Clinical features

- HA-MRSA (defined as that occurring >48h after hospital admission), community-onset HA-MRSA (that occuring within 12 months of exposure to health care, e.g. dialysis, residence in a care home) causes similar infections to MSSA (➔ see *Staphylococcus aureus*, pp. 234–6). However, patients have higher mortality and longer inpatient stays, and thus cost the health system more than those with MSSA infection.
- CA-MRSA was originally seen in people with a previous history of hospitalization or who were related to HCWs. The emergence of the USA300 clone in the USA was associated with a rise in skin and soft tissue infections in young, healthy individuals. There have also been community outbreaks of CA-MRSA in settings such as sports teams,

day-care centres, prison inmates and guards, and men who have sex with men (MSM). CA-MRSA has evolved from community MSSA, rather than HA-MRSA, and is often sensitive to non-β-lactam antibiotics (e.g. ciprofloxacin) and is PVL toxin-positive.

Laboratory diagnosis of MRSA

- Conventional methods—direct plating onto selective media may produce results within 24h but is of limited sensitivity. Such media include MSA (7% sodium chloride, NaCl), commercial chromogenic products, and Baird–Parker media (isolation rate higher than MSA but contains ciprofloxacin, so only suitable for ciprofloxacin-resistant strains). Enrichment in 2.5% NaCl nutrient broth prior to plating on selective media may increase the diagnostic rate but increases the time for diagnosis. Chromogenic selective MRSA agar is the recommended means if direct plating.
- Molecular detection of the *mecA* gene—commercial systems are available that can detect MRSA directly from screening swabs within 2–3h. Some may fail if there are polymorphisms in the conserved regions of the *SCC-mec* region.
- Detection of a presumptive MRSA strain should be followed by full identification by *S. aureus* and resistance testing. Oxacillin susceptibility disc testing tends to be affected by test conditions; thus, cefoxitin disc testing is considered more reliable (it is also a more potent inducer of *mecA* expression). Criteria for meticillin resistance—oxacillin MIC >2mg/L or meticillin MIC >4mg/L or cefoxitin MIC >4mg/L.
- Isolates with suspected toxin-mediated diseases (e.g. PVL) should be submitted to the Antimicrobial Resistance and Healthcare Associated Infections Reference Unit (AMRHAI), PHE-Microbiology Services, Colindale.
- For full details, web search 'PHE SMI B29'.

Treatment of MRSA

- UK isolates are so far susceptible to glycopeptides (e.g. vancomycin, teicoplanin). There are concerns about an upward 'creep' in vancomycin MIC (attributed to a thicker cell wall), and serum levels should be monitored during therapy, with current practice tending towards a trough of >15mg/L.
- Daptomycin has evidence for its use in complicated skin/soft tissue infections, right-sided endocarditis, and MRSA bacteraemia. It should not be used for pneumonia (it is inhibited by pulmonary surfactant). Daptomycin MIC may increase during therapy, which can lead to microbiologic failure—repeat susceptibility testing is important, if therapy is prolonged and there is evidence of persistent infection.
- There is variable susceptibility to trimethoprim, rifampicin, tetracycline, doxycycline, fusidic acid, aminoglycosides, and nitrofurantoin (treatment of UTIs only). These may provide alternative treatment choices if oral therapy or a second agent is required.
- Other agents active against MRSA include linezolid and quinupristin with dalfopristin. Both may be used to treat MRSA pneumonia.

Infection control issues

The main strategies to control MRSA are screening and decolonization, isolation/cohorting of patients, appropriate hand hygiene by HCWs, and effective cleaning of shared equipment. For more details, ➲ see Management of antibiotic-resistant organisms, including MRSA, pp. 164–6.

Glycopeptide resistance in *Staphylococcus aureus*

Mechanism of resistance

The mechanisms of vancomycin resistance in *S. aureus* are:

- an increase in cell wall turnover that leads to an increase of non-cross-linked *D*-alanyl-*D*-alanine side chains that bind vancomycin outside the cell wall and inhibit binding to target peptides;
- transfer of the enterococcal *vanA* determinant from *Enterococcus* spp. to *S. aureus*.

Intermediate resistance

Strains of *S. aureus* with reduced susceptibility to glycopeptides have been reported in several countries. These organisms have been termed vancomycin-intermediate (VISA) or resistant *S. aureus* (VRSA). The CLSI breakpoints, upon which the definitions are based, were reduced in 2006, in response to reports of treatment failures in infections due to strains with MICs of 2 micrograms/mL:

- susceptible ≤2 micrograms/mL;
- intermediate 4–8 micrograms/mL (VISA);
- resistant ≥16 micrograms/mL (VRSA).

EUCAST recommends reporting all strains with MIC >2 micrograms/mL as resistant on the basis that glycopeptides should not be used to treat such organisms, even at increased doses.

Heteroresistance

A much commoner situation is for a strain to yield a small proportion of daughter cells (1 in 10^5) able to grow in the presence of 8 micrograms/mL of vancomycin. Such heterogeneously resistant strains are called hetero-VISA, and there is considerable debate about their clinical significance.

Vancomycin resistance

The first VISA infection occurred in 1995 in France in a child with leukaemia and catheter-associated MRSA bacteraemia.

The first clinical VRSA infection was reported in the USA in 2002. VRSA (vancomycin MIC >128mg/L, teicoplanin MIC 32mg/L) was isolated from a haemodialysis catheter tip and a chronic foot ulcer of a patient in Michigan. Vancomycin-resistant *E. faecalis* was also isolated from the ulcer, and the transfer of the *vanA* determinant was confirmed by PCR. The first VRSA in Europe was reported from Portugal in May 2013. Once again, a *vanA*-positive vancomycin-resistant *E. faecalis* was co-isolated, suggesting sporadic transfer from one to the other.

Laboratory detection

The detection of glycopeptide resistance in *S. aureus* is problematic, as both VISA and hetero-VISA isolates appear susceptible to vancomycin by routine disc diffusion tests. Furthermore, there have been conflicting recommendations regarding methods of detection. Current advice from the BSAC (September 2013) is as follows.

- A MIC-based method should be used, not disc testing. A control strain should be tested in parallel with each run of test organisms. The acceptable control MIC ranges (mg/L) are ATCC 25923 (vancomycin 0.25–1) and ATCC29213 (vancomycin 0.5–2).
- Laboratories should target testing to invasive or serious infections, or cases of treatment failure. This is supported by the rarity of resistant isolates in the UK (0.2% in BSAC bacteraemia surveillance).

Infection control issues

MRSA is known to be highly transmissible in health-care settings, and it seems reasonable to assume that VISA and VRSA will be likewise highly transmissible. Although infection control experience with VRSA is limited, implementation of rigorous infection control procedures is crucial for containing an outbreak of VRSA in a hospital setting.

Prevention

The appropriate use of antimicrobials, especially vancomycin, is paramount in preventing the continued emergence of VISA and VRSA. Several studies have shown that vancomycin is frequently used for inappropriate reasons. Strategies to reduce inappropriate vancomycin use are essential, e.g. minimize the use of temporary CVCs, diagnostic techniques to avoid prolonged empiric use of vancomycin, prompt removal of *S. aureus*-infected prosthetic devices.

Coagulase-negative staphylococci

CoNS may present as culture contaminants or as true pathogens. Infection is often associated with the presence of prosthetic material, e.g. IVCs, cardiac valves, joint prostheses. Infections are often indolent, but treatment may require removal of the foreign material. These organisms are frequently resistant to multiple antibiotics, which can make therapy difficult.

Epidemiology

CoNS are ubiquitous and are natural inhabitants of the skin. *S. epidermidis* is the commonest species, accounting for 65–90% of all isolates, followed by *S. hominis*. *S. saprophyticus* is a urinary pathogen in young, sexually active women. *S. saccharolyticus* is the only strict anaerobe. Other less frequent species include *S. haemolyticus, S. warneri, S. xylosus, S. cohnii, S. simulans, S. capitis, S. auricularis, S. lugdunensis* (coagulase-positive), and *S. schleiferi* (coagulase-positive).

Pathogenesis

Plasmid DNA is abundant in all species of CoNS, but only a few of the plasmid-encoded genes have been identified. Plasmid-mediated antibiotic resistance to a wide variety of antibiotics is known to occur and may be transferred by conjugation with other organisms. CoNS also produce PIA, resulting in biofilm formation, particularly on prosthetic devices. This biofilm protects the organisms from antibiotics and host defence mechanisms. *S. saprophyticus* produces a number of substances that enable it to attach and invade the uroepithelium.

Clinical features

- Nosocomial device-related bacteraemia (commonest cause).
- Prosthetic valve endocarditis.
- CSF shunt infections.
- Peritoneal dialysis catheter-associated peritonitis.
- UTIs (*S. saprophyticus*).
- Bacteraemia in immunocompromised patients.
- Sternal osteomyelitis (post-cardiothoracic surgery).
- PJIs.
- Vascular graft infections.
- Neonatal nosocomial bacteraemias.
- Endophthalmitis (after surgery or trauma).

Diagnosis

Appropriate samples, e.g. blood, pus, tissues, should be taken and submitted to the laboratory for microbiological examination. The following tests may be performed:

- Gram-positive cocci in clusters, cultures on blood agar or liquid media;
- catalase-positive, DNase test-negative/weakly positive;
- coagulase-negative (exceptions: *S. lugdunensis, S. schleiferi*);
- antimicrobial susceptility testing—*S. saprophyticus* is novobiocin-resistant;
- biochemical tests, e.g. API® Staph, automated methodologies;
- typing, e.g. PFGE;
- molecular diagnosis, e.g 16S or 23S rRNA PCR; *mecA* gene PCR;
- MALDI-TOF.

Treatment

Infections usually require the removal of prosthetic material, if present. CoNS are often resistant to multiple antibiotics; >80% are resistant to meticillin. Most CoNS are sensitive to vancomycin, linezolid, quinupristin/dalfopristin, and daptomycin. Sensitivity to teicoplanin is variable, and a teicoplanin MIC must be checked before using this antibiotic. Note that *S. haemolyticus* frequently demonstrates reduced susceptibility to teicoplanin. *S. saprophyticus* UTIs may be treated with trimethoprim, nitrofurantoin, or a fluoroquinolone.

S. lugdunensis was first described in 1988 and was differentiated from other CoNS via DNA relatedness and a positive slide coagulase (but negative tube coagulase) result. Like other CoNS, it ranges from a harmless skin commensal to a life-threatening pathogen. Unlike other CoNS, it can cause virulent infections similar to *S. aureus*, such as aggressive native valve infective endocarditis (IE), and is susceptible to most antibiotics tested.

Micrococcus species

These are strict aerobes, and *Micrococcus luteus* produces yellow colonies. The Gram-positive cocci are often arranged in tetrads. *Micrococcus* spp. give a positive modified oxidase test, while other *Staphylococcus* spp. (except *S. sciuri, S. lentus*, and *S. vutulus*) are oxidase-negative.

Rothia mucilaginosus

Formerly known as *Micrococcus mucilaginosus* or *Staphylococcus salivarius*, these facultative anaerobe are weakly catalase-positive and are similar to the other CoNS.

Streptococci—overview

For an introduction to streptococci, ➲ see Overview of Gram-positive cocci, pp. 233–4. For classification of streptococci, see Table 7.1.

Table 7.1 Classification of streptococci

Haemolysis	Lancefield group	Species name	Clinical syndromes
α		*S. pneumoniae*	Pneumococcal pneumonia, bacteraemia, meningitis, otitis media, sinusitis
α		Viridans streptococci	Dental caries, endocarditis, abscesses
β	A	*S. pyogenes*	Invasive (necrotizing fasciitis, GAS TSS, bacteraemia, etc.), tonsillitis, skin infections, etc.
β	B	*S. agalactiae*	Neonatal meningitis and bacteraemia
β	C	*S. dysgalactiae* subspecies *dysgalactiae*, *S. dysgalactiae* subspecies *equisimilis*, *S. equi* subspecies *equi*, *S.equi* subspecies *zooepidemicus*	Sore throat, cellulitis
β or χ	D	*S. bovis* and others	*S. bovis* bacteraemia, endocarditis, *S. suis* bacteraemia and meningitis

(*Continued*)

Table 7.1 (*Contd.*)

Haemolysis	Lancefield group	Species name	Clinical syndromes
β	G		Sore throat, bacteraemia, cellulitis
β or χ	A, C, F, G	*S. milleri* (reclassified as *S. constellatus, S. intermedius*, and *S. anginosus*)	Infective endocarditis, abscesses
χ or non	–	Viridans streptococci	Infective endocarditis
Non; anaerobe	–	*Peptostreptococcus*	Abscesses
Genera closely related to streptococci		*Enterococcus, Leuconostoc, Pediococcus, Abiotrophia, Gemella, Aerococcus*	

Streptococcus pneumoniae

S. pneumoniae was first isolated in 1881 by Sternberg in the USA and Louis Pasteur in France. It became recognized as the commonest cause of lobar pneumonia and was given the name pneumococcus. *S. pneumoniae* is an important bacterial pathogen of humans, causing meningitis, sinusitis, otitis media, endocarditis, septic arthritis, peritonitis, and a number of other infections. It is a Gram-positive coccus that grows in pairs (diplococci) or chains. It produces pneumolysin that causes α-haemolysis (green discoloration due to breakdown of Hb) of blood agar.

Epidemiology

- *S. pneumoniae* colonizes the nasopharynx of 5–10% of healthy adults, and 20–40% of healthy children. The rate of colonization is seasonal, with an increase in winter.
- The rate of invasive pneumococcal disease is 15/100 000 persons/year. The incidence is up to 10-fold higher in certain populations, e.g. African-Americans, Alaskans, and Australian aboriginals. Invasive pneumococcal disease is commoner at the extremes of age (age <2 years or >65 years).
- Risk factors for pneumococcal infection include antibody deficiencies, complement deficiency, neutropenia or impaired neutrophil function, asplenia, corticosteroids, malnutrition, alcoholism, chronic diseases (liver, renal, diabetes, asthma, COPD), and overcrowding.
- Antimicrobial resistance is increasing. Penicillin resistance rates are high in certain European countries, e.g. Spain, Portugal, Hungary, Iceland, and in Asia, e.g. Thailand, Hong Kong, Vietnam, and Korea. The major source of resistance is the worldwide geographic spread of a few clones that harbour resistance determinants. Rates of resistance in Europe correlate with the total consumption of β-lactams in that country.

Pathogenesis

A number of virulence factors have been identified:

- capsular polysaccharide >90 serotypes (prevents phagocytosis, activates complement), cell wall polysaccharide (activates complement, cytokines);
- pneumolysin (activates complement and cytokines);
- PspA (blocks deposition of complement, inhibits phagocytosis);
- PspC (inhibits phagocytosis by binding complement factor H);
- PsaA (mediates adherence);
- autolysin (causes release of bacterial components, resulting in trigger of cytokine cascade);
- neuraminidase (possibly mediates adherence).

Antimicrobial resistance

- Penicillin resistance mediated by alterations in PBP2A (low-level resistance) and mutations in PBP2X (high-level resistance). Lower-level β-lactam resistance may be overcome by higher concentrations of the antibiotic. Site of infection determines antimicrobial management.
- Macrolide resistance is mediated by acquisition of the *ermB* (ribosomal methylase) and *mefA* (efflux pump) genes.

Clinical features

S. pneumoniae may cause infection by direct spread of the organism from the nasopharynx to contiguous structures (e.g. middle ear, lungs) or by haematogenous spread (CNS, heart valves, joints). Unusual infections in young people should prompt investigation for HIV. Clinical syndromes include otitis media, sinusitis, exacerbation of chronic bronchitis, pneumonia, meningitis, endocarditis, septic arthritis/osteomyelitis, pericarditis, epidural/cerebral abscess, and skin/soft tissue infection.

Diagnosis

- BC bottles may flag positive, but no organisms are seen on Gram stain due to autolysis of the pneumococcus. The blood may look lysed, and pneumococcal antigen test directly on blood is often positive.
- Grows on routine media—causes α-haemolysis of blood agar. May see central autolysis of colonies (draughtsmen), occasionally mucoid.
- Gram-positive lanceolate diplococci, often with visible capsule.
- Identification—catalase-negative, optochin-sensitive, soluble in 10% bile salts. Commercial identification tests (e.g. API® Strep, latex agglutination tests, serotyping tests) are available. MALDI-TOF identification cannot be relied on for *S. pneumoniae*.
- Penicillin MIC should be determined for invasive isolates.

Treatment

- The original MIC thresholds for determining penicillin resistance were in the setting of meningitis and levels of drug needed in the CSF. Thus, an organism considered resistant for the purposes of meningitis treatment may be susceptible if causing pneumonia.
- Penicillin MIC <0.1mg/L—treat with penicillin or ampicillin.

- Penicillin MIC 0.1–1.0mg/L—treat meningitis with ceftriaxone or cefotaxime. High-dose penicillin or ampicillin is likely to be effective for non-meningeal sites of infection, e.g. pneumonia.
- Penicillin MIC >2.0mg/L—vancomycin ± rifampicin. If non-meningeal site, consider ceftriaxone, high-dose ampicillin, carbapenem, fluoroquinolone.
- Pneumococcal meningitis may benefit from adjunctive corticosteroids.

Prevention

- The 7-valent pneumococcal conjugate vaccine (PCV7) was introduced into the UK childhood immunization schedule in 2006, replaced by a 13-valent product in 2010. Three doses: at age 2 months, 4 months, and 12 months.
- The 23-valent unconjugated polysaccharide vaccine (PPV23) is given to adults of 65 years and 'at-risk' groups, e.g. homozygous sickle-cell disease, asplenia or severe splenic dysfunction, chronic renal disease or nephrotic syndrome, coeliac disease, immunodeficiency or immunosuppression due to disease or treatment, including HIV infection, chronic diseases (cardiac, respiratory, liver, renal), diabetes mellitus, patients with cochlear implants. It is also recommended for those with CSF leak.
- Children at special risk (e.g. sickle, asplenia) should have PCV13, followed by PPV23 after their second birthday (web search 'UK *Green Book* pneumococcal' for full details).
- Prophylaxis—PO penicillin V is recommended for the prevention of pneumococcal disease in asplenic patients, but not for CSF leaks.

Enterococci

Enterococci are environmental organisms that are found in the soil, water, food, and the GI tract of animals. They are Gram-positive cocci that occur singly, in pairs, or in chains, and thus resemble streptococci. Until fairly recently, they were classified amongst the Lancefield group D streptococci. In the 1980s, they were reclassified as a separate genus *Enteroccoccus*, because of different pathogenic, biochemical, and serological profiles. At least 12 different species exist. *E. faecalis* is the commonest clinical isolate (80–90%), followed by *E. faecium* (5–10%). Others include *E. avium, E. casseliflavus, E. durans, E. gallinarum, E. hirae*, and *E. raffinosus*.

Epidemiology

Enterococci are part of the normal gut flora and can cause endogenous or exogenous infections, both in and out of hospital. In the hospital setting, enterococci are readily transmissible between patients and institutions. Risk factors for nosocomial enterococcal infections include GI colonization, severe underlying disease, prolonged hospitalization, prior surgery, renal failure, neutropenia, transplantation, urinary or vascular catheters, ICU admission, and prior antibiotic use.

Pathogenesis

- Enterococci are less intrinsically virulent than organisms such as *S. aureus* and GAS. They do not have classical virulence factors but are able to adhere to heart valves and renal epithelial cells. Several extracellular molecules play an important role in colonization and adherence, e.g. aggregation factor and extracellular surface protein. Other virulence factors include extracellular serine protease, gelatinase, and haemolysins.
- Enterococci are frequently found in cultures of intra-abdominal and pelvic infections—their role in this setting has not been clearly defined.
- Enterococcal bacteraemia carries a high mortality (42–68%), but it is not clear whether this is due to the organism itself or a marker of severe debilitation. However, epidemiological studies have calculated an attributed mortality of 31–37% in patients with enterococcal bacteraemia.
- The intrinsic resistance of enterococci to many antibiotics enables them to survive and multiply in patients receiving broad-spectrum agents, and accounts for their ability to cause nosocomial infections.

Clinical features

UTIs (commonest), bacteraemia and endocarditis, intra-abdominal and pelvic infections, skin and soft tissue infections, meningitis (associated with anatomical defects, trauma, or surgery), respiratory infections (rare), neonatal sepsis, and device-related infections (i.e. prosthetic valve endocarditis, CNS shunt infections).

Diagnosis

- Gram stain—elongated Gram-positive cocci ('cigar-shaped'), often in pairs and short chains.
- Culture—facultative anaerobes that can grow under extreme conditions, e.g. 6.5% NaCl, pH 9.6, temperatures of 10–45°C.
- Biochemical tests—enterococci hydrolyse aesculin and *l*-pyrrolidonyl-β-naphthylamide (PYR).
- Often agglutinate with group D in streptococcal grouping kits.
- Intrinsically resistant to aminoglycosides (low levels), cephalosporins, lincosamides (low level), quinupristin/dalfopristin (*E. faecalis*), co-trimoxazole (*in vivo*).
- All isolates should be tested for susceptibility to ampicillin, gentamicin, vancomycin, teicoplanin, linezolid, quinupristin/dalfopristin, chloramphenicol, and nitrofurantoin (UTIs).

Treatment

- Enterococci are intrinsically resistant to many agents (e.g. cephalosporins, ciprofloxacin) and readily acquire new resistance mechanisms.
- Ampicillin is the usual first-line agent for *E. faecalis* infections, with vancomycin as an alternative. *E. faecium* is usually resistant to ampicillin.
- When bactericidal therapy is needed (e.g. endocarditis, meningitis), combination synergistic therapy of a cell wall agent plus an aminoglycoside should be considered.

- Ciprofloxacin may be active *in vitro* but is not usually recommended clinically (apart from occasionally for UTIs). Newer fluoroquinolones are said to be more active against enterococci, but not against ciprofloxacin-resistant strains.
- For details of vancomycin resistance mechanisms, ➔ see Glycopeptides, pp. 42–4. *E. gallinarum* and *E. casseliflavus* are intrinsically resistant to glycopeptides (pentapeptide terminates *D*-alanine-*D*-serine) (see Box 7.4). High-level resistance to aminoglycosides and vancomycin resistance (VRE) are increasing problems, particularly on renal units.
- VRE bacteraemia has a worse prognosis than vancomycin-sensitive enterococcal bacteraemia, but this may be related to co-morbidity and delay in receiving appropriate antibiotic therapy. Agents which may be active against VRE include linezolid, tigecycline, and daptomycin. Quinupristin/dalfopristin is difficult to obtain in the UK. Linezolid resistance has been detected in enterococci in the UK and is potentially transferable. Choice of agent depends on the source of infection.

Streptococcus bovis

S. bovis bacteraemia and endocarditis are associated with GI disease (primarily colonic malignancy). *S. bovis* biotype 1 (*S. gallolyticus* subspecies *gallolyticus*) bacteraemia has a higher correlation with underlying GI malignancy and endocarditis (71% and 94%, respectively, in one study) than *S. bovis* biotype 2.

Pathogenesis

It is not clear whether *S. bovis* is a marker for malignancy or has an aetiological role. In some cases, *S. bovis* bacteraemia is the only pointer to the GI disease. There are also reports of the malignancy being found up to 2 years after the initial *S. bovis* infection. There seems to be an increase in stool carriage of *S. bovis* in patients with malignancy or pre-malignancy, compared to healthy subjects. Biotype 1 has a type-specific adherence mechanism, which may assist adherence to both cardiac valves and abnormal colonic mucosa.

Clinical features

The main clinical infections due to *S. bovis* are bacteraemia and endocarditis. Occasionally, *S. bovis* causes other infections such UTIs, meningitis, or neonatal sepsis. The GI tract is the usual portal of entry for bacteraemia. Most patients with endocarditis have an underlying valve abnormality or prosthetic valve. They tend to have a subacute course, indistinguishable clinically from endocarditis due to the *Streptococcus viridans* group, but studies suggest *S. bovis* endocarditis has a higher mortality rate (45%), compared to non-*S. bovis* endocarditis (25%). All patients with *S. bovis* bacteraemia should have a comprehensive work-up to exclude colonic malignancy and endocarditis.

Diagnosis

- *S. bovis* may be misidentified as enterococci or viridans streptococci.
- Biochemical tests—*S. bovis* shares a number of properties with enterococci, e.g. they agglutinate with group D antisera, hydrolyse aesculin, and are bile-tolerant. However, they differ from enterococci by growing in 6.5% salt and in the results of the PYR test.
- Identification—the API® Rapid Strep reliably identifies *S. bovis* and differentiates it to the biotype level, which is important for association with malignancy and endocarditis. Generally, *S. bovis* biotype 1 strains produce extracellular glucan from sucrose, hydrolyse starch, and ferment mannitol. *S. bovis* biotype 2 strains are usually negative for these tests. Automated methods, i.e. VITEK® and MALDI-TOF, can reliably identify *S. bovis*. A PCR to differentiate the biotypes has been developed.

Treatment

Penicillin is the treatment of choice for *S. bovis* infections; vancomycin is an alternative in β-lactam-allergic patients.

Viridans streptococci

The viridans streptococci, sometimes known as the oral streptococci, are important in dental caries, endocarditis, bacteraemia, and deep-seated infections (abscesses). They include *S. sanguinis, S. mutans, S. mitis*, and *S. salivarius*. This heterogenous group has been reclassified into five distinct groups, on the basis of 16S rRNA analysis:

- *S. mutans* group—now divided into seven species and collectively known as the 'mutans streptococci'. The commonest are *S. mutans* and *S. sobrinus*;
- *S. sanguinis* group—now divided into *S. sanguinis, S. gordonii, S. parasanguinis*, and *S. crista*;
- *S. milleri* group—now divided into three species: *S. constellatus, S. intermedius*, and *S. anginosus*—called the *S. anginosus* group/group F;
- *S. mitis* group—includes *S. mitis, S. mitior*, and *S. oralis*;
- *S. salivarius* group—includes *S. salivarius* and *S. vestibularis*.

Epidemiology

The viridans streptococci are commensals of the human upper respiratory tract, female genital tract, and GI tract, with large numbers present in the mouth. Each species has its own particular ecological niche.

Pathogenesis

These organisms seem to possess few virulence factors.

- The ability to produce acid, especially by *S. mutans*, is thought to be important in dental caries.
- Production of various carbohydrates, which aid adherence to tooth enamel and gums, is important in colonization.
- Extracellular dextran production is important in the adherence of organisms to heart valves and in resistance to antimicrobial therapy.
- Fibronectin production also mediates adherence to heart valves.

Clinical features

- Endocarditis (common cause in patients with abnormal valves).
- Bacteraemia (may cause severe sepsis in neutropenic patients).
- Meningitis.
- Pneumonia.
- Other infections—abscesses, pericarditis, peritonitis, sialadenitis, odontogenic infections, endophthalmitis.

Diagnosis

- Facultatively anaerobic Gram-positive cocci, catalase-negative.
- Most are α-haemolytic on blood agar; some are non-haemolytic.
- Resistant to optochin and lack bile solubility (unlike pneumococci).
- Unable to grow in 6.5% NaCl (unlike enterococci).
- Can be identified by biochemical tests, API® Strep, or automated methods.

Treatment

- Community-acquired infections are usually sensitive to penicillin—the treatment of choice.
- Other β-lactams, e.g. ceftriaxone, also have good *in vitro* activity against viridans streptococci.
- Nosocomial infections are associated with increased resistance to penicillin and other β-lactams.
- Some strains, e.g. *S. sanguinis* and *S. gordonii*, exhibit tolerance, i.e. they are inhibited at low concentrations of antibiotic, but high levels are required for bactericidal activity.
- Often resistant to aminoglycosides (when traditional breakpoints are applied) but exhibit synergy in combination with β-lactam antibiotics. This principle underlies combination treatment for bacterial endocarditis.
- Vancomycin is used in penicillin-allergic patients and penicillin-resistant infections.

Group A *Streptococcus*

Group A *Streptococcus* (GAS), also known as *S. pyogenes*, is responsible for a variety of conditions—pyogenic (pharyngitis, cellulitis, necrotizing fasciitis), toxin-mediated (scarlet fever), or immunological (glomerulonephritis).

Epidemiology

GAS are upper respiratory tract commensals in 3–5% of adults, and up to 10% of children. Transmission is mainly via droplet spread. Some people develop pharyngitis/tonsillitis; others are asymptomatic, and a handful will become carriers of GAS in the throat. In the 1990s, the number of reports of invasive GAS increased globally, probably due to a re-emergence of more virulent strains. Risk factors for sporadic disease include people >65 years old, those with recent VZV infection, HIV-positive individuals, those with diabetes, heart disease, cancer, and injecting drug use, or those on high-dose steroids. Over time, the epidemiology of GAS infection, in terms of clinical manifestation of disease, has changed, e.g. acute rheumatic fever has become less common, and toxic shock commoner, over the last few decades. The years 2014–2015 have seen an increase in the incidence of scarlet fever cases.

Pathogenesis

GAS possess a number of virulence factors:

- somatic constitutents—hyaluronic capsule (resists phagocytosis), M protein (evasion of phagocytosis inhibits binding of antibody with opsonin), serum opacity factor, lipotechoic acid, fibronectin-binding proteins;
- extracellular products—streptolysin O and S (α-haemolysis on blood agar), DNases A to D, hyaluronidase (facilitates spread through tissues), streptokinase (catalyses plasminogen to plasmin), streptococcal pyrogenic exotoxins (SpeA, SpeB, SpeC, SpeF—superantigens that induce fever), C5a peptidase, streptococcal superantigens (SSA);
- immune-mediated disease, e.g. immune cross-reactions between components of the glomerular basement membrane and cell membranes.

Clinical features

- Pharyngitis—commonest infection. Suppurative complications include tonsillitis, peritonsillar abscess, retropharyngeal abscess, suppurative cervical lymphadenitis, mastoiditis, sinusitis, otitis media.
- Impetigo, erysipelas, cellulitis, necrotizing fasciitis, pyomyositis.
- Scarlet fever—notifiable disease. Pharyngitis associated with scarlatinal rash due to erythrogenic toxin production. Around 90% of cases occur in children under 10 years of age. UK reports of scarlet fever have been increasing since 2013.
- Rheumatic fever—may occur 1–5 weeks after pharyngitis. Migratory arthritis, pancarditis, chorea, rash, and subcutaneous nodules.
- Post-streptococcal glomerulonephritis—may occur after throat infections (commonly M types 12, 1, 25, 4, and 3) and skin infections (commonly M types 49, 52, 53–55, and 57–61).
- Bacteraemia—recent increase in GAS bacteraemia in previously healthy adults. A small proportion of invasive GAS infections start with a respiratory tract infection. Other risk factors—burns, trauma, HIV, injection drug use, alcoholism, immunosuppression, diabetes mellitus, and malignancy.
- Streptococcal TSS—fulminant disease with high mortality is mainly associated with types M1 and 3, but types 12 and 28 are also involved. It involves rapidly progressive symptoms with low blood pressure and multiorgan failure.
- Others—meningitis, osteomyelitis, puerperal sepsis, and septic arthritis.

Diagnosis

- Facultative anaerobic, catalase-negative, Gram-positive cocci, which tend to form long chains when observed on Gram stain. They are non-sporing, non-motile, and usually non-capsulate.
- Culture on blood agar produces smooth, circular colonies 2–3mm in diameter, usually β-haemolytic (large zone), and may be mucoid. Strains that produce haemolysin O, and not haemolysin S, will only demonstrate β-haemolysis when cultured anaerobically. Usually sensitive to bacitracin.
- Serology is used to diagnose immunological complications, e.g rheumatic fever. A rise in anti-streptolysin O titre (ASOT) confirms recent GAS disease. ASOT is reliable in the throat-associated disease, while anti-DNase B is higher and more frequently raised in pyoderma-associated disease.

Treatment

- The treatment of choice is PO phenoxymethylpenicillin (mild infections) or IV benzylpenicillin (severe infections). Pharyngitis is treated for 10 days, invasive disease for at least 14.
- In penicillin-allergic patients, options include azithromycin (comparative clinical and bacteriological response rates to penicillin, but higher GI side effects) or erythromycin. Clindamycin may be used.
- Recent evidence suggests bacteraemia should be treated with IV penicillin and clindamycin. There is no synergy, but clindamycin is associated with a better outcome (perhaps due to protein synthesis inhibition) if the organism is sensitive (penicillin is included empirically, in the event the isolate is clindamycin-resistant).
- Urgent surgical debridement is required in necrotizing fasciitis. May be a role for IVIG in those with invasive infection and shock.

Prevention

- Infection control—GAS can spread from infected patients to close contacts, so isolate patients with invasive disease; use droplet precautions, and involve the ICT early. The available evidence suggests that routine administration of prophylactic antibiotics for close contacts of invasive disease is not justified, but all household contacts should be informed of clinical manifestations of invasive disease and instructed to seek medical attention immediately if they develop any symptoms. Antibiotics are only given to certain 'high-risk' groups (e.g. mother/neonate contact).
- Hospital outbreaks of GAS have been described in the literature. For PHE guidance, see www.gov.uk/streptococcal-infections.
- The main difficulties associated with the development of a GAS vaccine are the widespread diversity of circulating GAS strains and M protein types, the immunological cross-reactivity between epitopes in the M protein and several human tissues, and the lack of a relevant animal model.

Group B *Streptococcus*

Group B streptococci (GBS, *Streptococcus agalactiae*) were first reported as causes of puerperal sepsis in 1938. By the 1970s, GBS had become the main cause of neonatal sepsis in infants aged <3 months.

Epidemiology

- Five to 40% of women are colonized with GBS (genital tract or lower GI tract). Around 25% in UK studies. Colonization of neonates usually occurs via the mother's genital tract. Risk factors—African ethnicity, diabetes.
- *Early-onset neonatal GBS disease* (<7 days)—risk factors include maternal GBS bacteruria, premature rupture of membranes (PROM), delivery <37 weeks, intrapartum fever or amnionitis, and prolonged rupture of membranes. Affects around 1 in 2000 births in the UK and Ireland.
- *Late-onset neonatal GBS disease* (7–90 days)—risk factors include overcrowding, poor hand hygiene, and increased length of stay.
- Over the past 20 years, there has been an increase in invasive GBS disease in non-pregnant adults, most of whom had underlying medical conditions. Risk factors include diabetes, chronic diseases (liver, renal, cardiovascular, pulmonary, GI, urological), neurological impairment, malignancy, HIV, corticosteroids, and splenectomy.

Pathogenesis

Bacterial virulence factors that influence the outcome between exposure and development of colonization/invasive disease include the polysaccharide capsule (in particular, high amounts of sialic acid and type III virulent strains).

Clinical features

- Early-onset neonatal disease (defined as systemic infection in the first 6 days of life; mean age of onset 12h; pneumonia or meningitis) tends to result from vertical transmission *in utero* or at the time of delivery.
- Late-onset neonatal disease (onset 7 days to 3 months of age, mean 24 days, bacteraemia) arises from either horizontal transmission (often nosocomial, due to suboptimal nursery conditions) or horizontal transmission.
- GBS infection in adults and older children, especially those with an underlying disease includes bacteraemia, post-partum infections, pneumonia, endocarditis, meningitis, arthritis, osteomyelitis, otitis media, conjunctivitis, UTI, skin and soft tissue infections, and meningitis.

Diagnosis

- GBS are facultative anaerobic, catalase-negative, Gram-positive cocci. They form chains on Gram stain, and are non-sporing, non-motile, and usually capsulate.
- Culture on blood agar produces smooth, circular colonies of 2–3mm in diameter, usually surrounded by a very small zone of β-haemolysis.

- Selective media containing Todd Hewitt broth and antimicrobials are used to enhance the recovery of GBS.
- Identification—Lancefield group B, resistant to bacitracin, hydrolyse sodium hippurate, do not hydrolyse aesculin, production of CAMP factor (results in synergistic haemolysis with the β-lysin of *S. aureus* on sheep blood agar plate). Identified using API® Strep or via automated methods.
- Typing—GBS may be classified as serotypes I to VIII, based on the basis of capsular polysaccharide and surface protein antigens. Other typing methods—MLST, PFGE.

Treatment

Neonatal infections are usually treated with IV benzylpenicillin. Adults usually receive 10–14 days of IV benzylpenicillin (plus 2 weeks of gentamicin for endocarditis); vancomycin if penicillin-allergic.

Prevention

Routine screening for antenatal carriage is controversial and varies in different countries. Systematic screening is not recommended in the UK for the following reasons.

- The impact of screening on mortality and morbidity is not proven.
- Many screen-positive women may no longer be carriers at the point of treatment or delivery.
- Many thousands of low-risk women would receive IV antibiotics during labour—the consequences of such an expansion in antibiotic use are unknown.
- The incidence of early-onset neonatal GBS disease in the UK (0.5/1000 births) is similar to that seen in the USA (which has a universal screening and treatment programme), despite similar vaginal carriage rates.
- Antenatal antibiotic treatment of GBS carriage, if detected incidentally, is not recommended, as it does not reduce the chance of colonization at the time of delivery.
- Intrapartum prophylaxis should be offered if GBS is detected incidentally during pregnancy and to women with a previous baby with neonatal GBS disease (IV penicillin until delivery, clindamycin if penicillin-allergic) or women with GBS bacteruria. Observe the infant for 24–48h if well and no risk factors (PROM, chorioamnionitis, etc.)
- Newborns with signs of sepsis should be treated with broad-spectrum antibiotics that cover GBS.
- If chorioamnionitis suspected, treat with broad-spectrum antibiotics active against GBS.
- Vaccines—capsular polysaccharide vaccines are under development. One of the difficulties is the existence of a multiplicity of serotypes with different geographical distributions.

For more information, web search 'RCOG green-top guideline 36'.

Other β-haemolytic streptococci

- Group C streptococci—there are four species in this group: *S. dysgalactiae* subspecies *dysgalactiae, S. dysgalactiae* subspecies *equisimilis, S. equi* subspecies *equi, S. equi* subspecies *zooepidemicus*. They are primarily animal pathogens (*S. equi* causes strangles in horses), but *S. equisimilis* and *S. zooepidemicus* can cause a range of infections in humans. The commonest problem in humans is outbreaks of tonsillitis, especially in schools and institutions. Group C streptococci can cause syndromes similar to GAS such as post-partum sepsis, septicaemia, meningitis, pneumonia, and skin and wound infections, but group C infections are usually less severe. Group C streptococci are usually sensitive to penicillin.
- Group F streptococci—formerly known as *S. milleri*, which has a characteristic caramel odour when cultured in the laboratory. *S. milleri* has been reclassified within the viridans streptococci group into *S. constellatus, S. intermedius*, and *S. anginosus* (➔ see Viridans streptococci, pp. 248–9).
- Group G streptococci—these produce infections similar to group A and C streptococci such as sore throat, erysipelas, cellulitis, bone and joint infection, pneumonia, and septicaemia. Occasionally, group G streptococci bacteraemia is associated with underlying malignancy.

Other Gram-positive cocci

Leuconostoc

Leuconostoc are catalase-negative, Gram-positive cocci or coccobacilli, which occasionally cause opportunistic infections. They are usually found on plants and vegetables, or rarely in dairy products and wine. There are only a few case reports of human infections, including bacteraemia (± indwelling line infection), meningitis, and dental abscess.

Note that *Leuconostoc* are intrinsically resistant to glycopeptides (see Box 7.4), because the pentapeptide cell wall precursors terminate in *D*-alanine-*D*-lactate. The usual agent of choice for these infections is penicillin or ampicillin, but they are generally susceptible to most agents with activity against streptococci.

Box 7.4 Gram-positive organisms resistant to glycopeptides

- *Leuconostoc*.
- *Lactobacillus*.
- *Pediococcus*.
- *E. rhusiopathiae*.
- *Nocardia*.
- *S. haemolyticus* (resistant to teicoplanin).
- *E. gallinarum* and *E. casseliflavus*:
  - Both carry VanC which is not transferrable, and are considered intrinsically resistant to vancomycin.

Abiotrophia

Abiotrophia is the new name for the nutritionally variant streptococci (NVS). These organisms have been classified in various ways, but 16S rRNA sequencing defined the new genus *Abiotrophia* to be distinct from the streptococci. NVS are defined by the need for pyridoxal or thiol group supplementation for growth, and thus appear as satellite colonies around bacteria such as *S. aureus*. Gram staining tends to show pleomorphic variable-staining cells. The two main species (*Abiotrophia defectiva* and *Abriotrophia adiacens*) are resistant to optochin and susceptible to vancomycin. Because they grow poorly on solid media, they are easily overlooked if not cultured in broth or subcultured appropriately (e.g. with a *S. aureus* streak or onto selective media).

Abiotrophia are normal flora in the upper respiratory, urogenital, and GI tract, and are clinically important, as they cause ~5% of cases of endocarditis. *Abiotrophia* endocarditis responds less well to antibiotics, and has higher morbidity and mortality, compared to endocarditis due to other streptococci. Correlation of *in vitro* antibiotic susceptibility testing and clinical outcome is a specialist field, and the general recommendation is for long-term combination therapy (e.g. penicillin and gentamicin for 4–6 weeks). Bacteriological failure and relapse rates are high.

Anaerobic Gram-positive cocci

The anaerobic Gram-positive cocci have undergone multiple taxonomic changes. There are currently six genera that may be isolated from humans: *Peptostreptococcus, Peptoniphilus, Parvimonas, Finegoldia, Anaerococcus*, and another group of uncertain taxonomy. The majority of human isolates are *Peptostreptococcus, Peptoniphilus*, and *Anaerococcus*. Less common isolates include *Atopobium parvula, Coprococcus* spp., *Ruminococcus* spp., and *Sarcina* spp.

The anaerobic Gram-positive cocci are part of the normal flora of the mouth, upper respiratory tract, GI tract, vagina, and skin. They can cause abscesses (e.g. brain abscess, often associated with otitis media, mastoiditis, chronic sinusitis, and pleuropulmonary infections), anaerobic pleuropulmonary disease, and bacteraemia (notably due to oropharyngeal, pulmonary, and female genital tract sources). When mixed with other bacteria, they may be involved with serious soft tissue infections such as necrotizing fasciitis. Anaerobic Gram-positive cocci cause osteomyelitis and arthritis at all sites, including bites and cranial infections. Little is known about virulence factors or pathogenesis of infection. Regarding treatment, anaerobic Gram-negative cocci are often mixed with aerobes and other anaerobes on culture plates. Obtaining appropriate specimens may be difficult; culture can be prolonged, and anaerobic sensitivity testing can also be challenging. Usually, a combination of surgery (e.g. drainage/debridement) and antibiotic therapy is required, e.g. metronidazole, penicillin, clindamycin.

Aerococcus

- *Aerococcus viridans* and *Aerococcus urinae* are catalase-negative, Gram-positive cocci. They tend to form tetrads and may resemble staphylococci on Gram stain, but their biochemical and growth characteristics are more characteristic of α-haemolytic streptococci.
- *A. viridans* is generally considered a contaminant on culture but occasionally may be implicated in bacteraemia and endocarditis. It is a low-virulence organism and only causes systemic infections in the immunocompromised. Optimal treatment of such cases is unclear, so consult an infection specialist.
- *A. urinae*, first reported in 1989, has been implicated as a cause of ~0.5% of UTIs. Most patients were elderly with predisposing conditions. It has also been found in patients with urogenic bacteraemia/septicaemia with or without endocarditis. *A. urinae* does not grow on CLED, and is usually susceptible to penicillin and resistant to sulfonamides and aminoglycosides.

Overview of Gram-positive rods

Gram-positive rods can be divided into three groups, based on growth characteristics and/or morphology (see Table 7.2):

- aerobic Gram-positive rods, e.g. *Bacillus, Lactobacillus, Corynebacterium, Arcanobacterium, Listeria, E. rhusiopathiae, Rhodococcus equi*;
- anaerobic Gram-positive rods, e.g *Clostridium, Propionibacterium*;
- branching Gram-positive rods, e.g. *Actinomyces, Nocardia, Actinomadura, Streptomyces*.

Table 7.2 Classification of Gram-positive rods

Group	Examples
Aerobic	*Bacillus* spp.
	Corynebacterium spp.
	Listeria spp.
	E. rhusiopathiae
	R. equi
Anaerobic	*Clostridium* spp.
	Propionobacterium spp.
Branching	*Actinomyces*
	Nocardia spp.
	Actinomadura
	Streptomyces

Bacillus species

Bacillus spp. are environmental saprophytes that are found in water, vegetation, and soil. They are Gram-positive (or Gram-variable) aerobic or facultatively anaerobic, rod-shaped bacilli with rounded or square ends. They form endospores that tolerate extremes of temperature and moisture. The ubiquitous nature of *Bacillus* spp. means that isolation from clinical specimens may represent contamination. Members of the group include:

- *B. anthracis* (➔ see *Bacillus anthracis*—ADCP 3, pp. 258–60);
- *B. cereus*;
- *B. circulans*;
- *B. licheniformis*;
- *B. megaterium*;
- *B. pumilis*;
- *B. sphaericus*;
- *B. subtilis*;
- *B. stearothermophilus*.

Clinical features

- Food poisoning—*B. cereus* is the commonest *Bacillus* causing food poisoning, followed by *B. licheniformis* and *B. pumilis*. Symptoms occur within 24h of ingestion of the preformed toxin in food and usually resolve in 24h. The emetic form presents after 1–5h, with nausea, vomiting, and abdominal cramps. The diarrhoeal form occurs 8–24h after ingestion of food. Production of a heat-labile toxin results in profuse diarrhoea and abdominal cramps (fever and vomiting are rare). Bacteraemia is often associated with the presence of an IVC. *B. cereus* is the commonest isolate, but other species, e.g. *B. licheniformis*, have been reported. Bacteraemia or endocarditis may occur in injecting drug users (IDUs).
- Disseminated infection has been reported in neonates and young children. Neonatal infection is acquired perinatally. Multisystem involvement may occur. Immunocompromise, e.g. neutropenia, is associated with severe, and sometimes fatal, infections.
- CNS infections may occur, following trauma or neurosurgery, or in association with a CSF shunt. Removal of prosthetic material hardware is required. LP may result in *Bacillus* spp. meningitis.
- Eye infections—endophthalmitis may occur, following trauma, eye surgery, or haematogenous dissemination. *B. cereus* is the commonest cause. Keratitis may occur after corneal trauma.
- Soft tissue and muscle infections may occur after injuries or wounds, e.g. road traffic accidents or after orthopaedic surgery.

Diagnosis

Bacillus spp. grow readily on ordinary culture media at environmental temperatures (25–37°C). All species may form spores, but they vary in their colonial morphology, motility, and nutritional requirements. Microscopically, they are large bacteria and are usually Gram-positive (older cultures may be Gram-variable or Gram-negative). Most non-anthracis *Bacillus* spp. are β-haemolytic and motile (unlike *B. anthracis*). They also lack the glutamic acid capsule (thus negative McFadyean's stain). *B. cereus* grows as characteristic blue colonies in PEMBA media.

Treatment

- There is no specific treatment for food poisoning syndromes, and most cases settle in 24h.
- For IVC- or prosthetic device-related infections, removal of the catheter or device is required for cure.
- Most *Bacillus* spp. isolates are susceptible to vancomycin, clindamycin, fluoroquinolones, aminoglycosides, and carbapenems. They are usually penicillin-resistant.
- Serious infections are usually treated with vancomcyin or clindamycin ± an aminoglycoside.

Bacillus anthracis—ACDP 3

The name anthrax is derived from a Greek word for coal and refers to the eschar seen in cutaneous anthrax. Anthrax occurs most commonly in wild and domestic animals in Asia, Africa, South and Central America, and parts of Europe. Humans are rarely infected, and the commonest form of infection is cutaneous anthrax, which is associated with occupational exposure to animal products, e.g. wool, hair, meat, bones, and hides. There have also been outbreaks amongst drug users (2012/2013 in Europe), and cases associated with animal-hide drums. Anthrax was used as an agent of bioterrorism in the USA in 2001 when *B. anthracis* spores were sent in contaminated letters (➲ see Bioterrorism, pp. 846–8).

Pathogenesis

B. anthracis has a number of virulence factors:

- *capsule*—under anaerobic conditions, a polypeptide capsule consisting of poly-*D*-glutamic acid is produced. Synthesis of the capsule is by three enzymes encoded by the *capA*, *capB*, and *capC* genes on the pX-02 plasmid. A fourth protein, encoded by the *dep* gene, catalyses the formation of polyglutamates that inhibit phagocytosis;
- *toxin*—two binary toxins (o)edema factor (EF) and lethal factor (LF) bind a third toxin component protective antigen (PA), before entering the target cell. The three toxin components are also encoded on plasmid pX-01. LF is a zinc-dependent metallopeptidase that inhibits dendritic cell function. EF converts AMP to cyclic AMP (cAMP), resulting in dysregulation of water and ions.

Clinical features

There are four forms of human disease:

- *cutaneous anthrax*—>95% of cases, usually acquired by direct contact with infected animals/animal products. The incubation period is 1–12 days. The initial pruritic papule gradually becomes a vesicular or bullous lesion, surrounded by extensive non-pitting oedema. The central part becomes necrotic and haemorrhagic, and may develop satellite vesicles. Finally, there is a classic black eschar which falls off in 1–2 weeks, unless systemic disease ensues;

- *GI anthrax*—accounts for <5% of cases. Oropharyngeal anthrax presents with fever and neck swelling due to cervical adenopathy and soft tissue oedema after ingestion of contaminated meat. Intestinal anthrax is commoner, and presents with fever, syncope, and malaise, followed by abdominal pain, nausea, and vomiting. Examination shows abdominal distension and a mass in the right iliac fossa or periumbilical area. The third phase is characterized by paroxysmal abdominal pain, ascites, facial flushing, red conjunctivae, and shock;
- *inhalational anthrax*—very rare. Occurs after inhalation of spores. The incubation period is <1 week. It presents as a flu-like illness with non-productive cough, haemorrhagic mediastinal lymphadenopathy, and multilobar pneumonia ± pleural effusions, and bacteraemia. Chest X-ray (CXR) typically shows a widened mediastinum. High mortality rate (45–85%);
- *CNS disease*—very rare. Presents with haemorrhagic meningoencephalitis; 95% mortality.

Diagnosis

- *B. anthracis* is an ACDP category 3 organism.
- Specimens—*B. anthracis* may be isolated from wound swabs (if cutaneous disease); tissue, nasal swabs, and BCs.
- Microscopy—Gram-positive rods in 'box car'- or cigar-shaped chains. The spore is oval-shaped, and central or subterminal. McFadyean's stain shows capsulated, dark, square-ended bacilli in short chains.
- Culture—*B. anthracis* grows readily on ordinary media (optimal incubation temperature 35°C) after 2–5 days' incubation. Colonies are white or grey-white, with a characteristic 'medusa head' appearance. In contrast to most other *Bacillus* spp., *B. anthracis* is non-haemolytic and non-motile. It is penicillin-sensitive, unlike other *Bacillus* spp.
- Identification—*B. anthracis* can be identified by PCR or phage lysis. If *B. anthracis* is suspected, no further identification should be performed—the case should be discussed with the reference laboratory urgently.

Treatment

- Cutaneous anthrax without systemic disease—ciprofloxacin or doxycycline. Duration is 60 days for bioterrorism-related cases and 7–10 days for naturally acquired cases.
- Systemic anthrax with meningitis—ciprofloxacin and meropenem with either linezolid or clindamycin.
- Systemic anthrax without meningitis—ciprofloxacin with either linezolid or clindamycin.
- Monoclonal antibody preparations have been approved by the FDA for use in anthrax treatment.
- For full details, see *Centers for Disease Control and Prevention Expert Panel Meetings on Prevention and Treatment of Anthrax in Adults* (Hendricks and Wright, 2014).

Prevention

Anthrax is a notifiable condition.

- Pre-exposure prophylaxis—human and animal vaccines are available to prevent anthrax. Vaccination is recommended for workers at risk of cutaneous anthrax such as those who work with leather, textiles, or animals. For details, see the UK DH *Green Book*.
- PEP—vaccination is recommended post-exposure to inhalational anthrax. In addition, antibiotic prophylaxis (PO ciprofloxacin or doxycycline) is indicated for PEP of inhalational anthrax.

Corynebacterium diphtheriae

The name for *C. diphtheriae* is derived from the Greek 'korynee' meaning club and 'diphtheria' meaning leather hide (for the leathery pharyngeal membrane it provokes). The organism spreads via nasopharyngeal secretions and can survive for months in dust and contaminated dry fomites. Incidence is highest in young children (>3–6 months old) when protective maternal antibodies wane. Diphtheria is rare in the UK (around ten cases reported in England and Wales each year) but remains a problem in developing countries and the former Russian states. In 2008, an unimmunized boy in London died from *Corynebacterium diphtheriae* var. *mitis*.

Pathogenesis

C. diphtheriae produces a potent exotoxin, the result of the infection with a lysogenic bacteriophage. It consists of two fragments: fragment A (which inhibits polypeptide chain elongation at the ribosome) and fragment B (which helps transport fragment A into the cell). Inhibition of protein synthesis probably accounts for the toxin's necrotic and neurotoxic effects, which are mainly on the heart, nerves, and kidneys. Cell death accounts for the characteristic pharyngeal membrane. It is important to note that other toxigenic *Corynebacterium* strains may cause diphtheria (e.g. *Corynebacterium ulcerans*). Milder infections without toxin production do occur and resemble streptococcal pharyngitis, and the pseudomembrane may not develop. Asymptomatic carriers are important for transmission. Immunity—whether vaccine or natural—does not prevent carriage.

Clinical features

- *Respiratory tract*—asymptomatic upper respiratory tract carriage is common in endemic countries and is an important reservoir of infection. Anterior nasal infection presents with a serosanguinous or seropurulent nasal discharge, often associated with a whitish membrane. Clinical features include fever, malaise, sore throat, pharyngeal injection, and development of a pseudomembrane, which is initially white, then grey with patches of green or black necrosis. Cervical lymphadenopathy may result in a characteristic 'bull neck' and inspiratory stridor.
- *Cardiac disease*—myocarditis occurs after 1–2 weeks, usually as the oropharyngeal disease is improving. Patients should have cardiac monitoring for ST segment changes, heart block, or arrhythmias. Clinical features include dyspnoea, cardiac failure, and circulatory collapse.

- *Neurological disease*—local paralysis of the soft palate and posterior pharynx leads to nasal regurgitation of fluids. Cranial nerve palsies and ciliary muscle paralysis may follow. Peripheral neuritis occurs 10–90 days after onset of pharyngeal disease and presents with motor deficits.
- *Skin infections*—in the countries where public hygiene is poor, cutaneous diphtheria is the predominant presentation, causing chronic non-healing ulcers with grey membranes. Outbreaks have been described in homeless alcoholics in the USA.
- *Invasive disease*—endocarditis, mycotic aneurysms, septic arthritis, and osteomyelitis may be caused by non-toxigenic strains.

Diagnosis

- Culture—nasopharyngeal, throat, or skin swabs should be immediately transported to the laboratory and cultured on suitable culture media (e.g. Löeffler's, Hoyle's tellurite, Tinsdale media). The colonies are black on tellurite media. *C. diphtheriae* shows a halo effect on Tinsdale agar.
- Microscopy—Gram staining of *C. diphtheriae* shows characteristic palisades, resembling Chinese letters. The beaded appearance obtained by Neisser or Albert stains, whereby the volutin/metachromatic granules are dark purple, compared to brown/green counterstain, is characteristic.
- Identification—*C. diphtheriae* is a non-motile, non-sporing, and non-capsulate Gram-positive rod. It is catalase-positive, urease-negative, nitrate-positive, pyrazinamidase-negative, and cystinase-negative. It can be reliably identified with API® Coryne. Isolates should be submitted to the reference laboratory at PHE Colindale for toxigenicity testing. Several methods are available—PCR has replaced the Elek plate or rapid EIA.
- Biotyping—colonial appearance on tellurite and also biochemical tests (e.g. Hiss serum sugars) subdivide *C. diphtheriae* into the biotypes var. *gravis*, *intermedius*, and *mitis*. These biotypes correspond with clinical severity. *Gravis* and *intermedius* (and some *mitis*) biotypes are usually toxigenic. The fourth biotype var. *belfanti* is rare and cannot produce the lethal exotoxin.

Treatment

- Antibiotics—if high clinical suspicion, treat immediately with IV penicillin for 14 days. Alternatives—erythromycin, azithromycin, or clarithromycin. Confirm elimination by nasopharyngeal swab; if cultures are positive, give a further 10 days of antibiotics.
- Anti-toxin may be given at different doses, depending on site severity and patient age (➔ see Guidelines below). First, test the patient with a trial dose to exclude hypersensitivity to horse serum. This can be obtained from the PHE Colindale laboratory.
- Infection control—isolate and barrier-nurse the case. Identify close contacts; take nose and throat swabs, and arrange clinical surveillance for 7 days. Provide prophylactic antibiotics (single dose of benzylpenicillin or 7 days of erythromycin) and booster vaccination for close contacts.
- Diphtheria is a notifiable disease—contact your local health protection unit (HPU).

Prevention

Diphtheria toxoid is part of the triple vaccine DTP (diphtheria, tetanus, polio), given at 2, 3, and 4 months as part of the UK immunization schedule. As a result of vaccination, toxigenic strains lose their selective advantage and become less prevalent, with reduced transmission to unvaccinated individuals. There is no reduction in non-toxigenic carriage. Note that diphtheria can occur in immunized individuals, but disease is less severe.

Guidelines

Bonnet JM, Begg NT (1999). Control of diphtheria: guidance for consultants in communicable disease control. World Health Organization. *Commun Dis Public Health* **2**:242–9.

Public Health England (2015). *Public health control and management of diphtheria (in England and Wales): 2015 guidelines*. Available at: https://www.gov.uk/government/uploads/system/uploads/attachment_data/file/416108/Diphtheria_Guidelines_Final.pdf.

Non-diphtheria corynebacteria

Corynebacteria are also known as coryneforms or diphtheroids. They are environmental organisms found in water and soil, and commensals of the skin and mucous membranes of humans and other animals. In the hospital environment, they may be cultured from surfaces and equipment. Thus, corynebacteria are frequently considered contaminants but may cause severe disease in hospitalized or immunocompromised patients.

Classification

Corynebacteria are classified, according to cell wall composition and biochemical reactions, into the following groups:

- non-lipophilic fermentative, e.g. *C. ulcerans, C. pseudotuberculosis, C. xerosis, C. striatum, C. minutissimum, C. amycolatum, C. glucuronolyticum*;
- non-lipophilic, non-fermentative, e.g. *C. pseudodiptheriticum*;
- lipophilic, e.g. *C. jeikeium, C. urealyticum*.

Clinical features

Infections may be classified into two groups:

- *community-acquired*, e.g. pharyngitis, native valve endocarditis, GU tract infections, periodontal infections;
- *nosocomial*, e.g. IVC-associated bacteraemia, endocarditis, prosthetic device-related infections, SSIs.

Diagnosis

- Microscopy—club-shaped, Gram-positive rods. Cells demonstrate variable size and appearance, from coccoid to bacillary forms, depending on the stage of their life cycle. Corynebacteria typically aggregate to form 'Chinese letter' arrangements when viewed on Gram stain.
- Culture—grow readily on blood agar and BC media. Thioglycolate broth may be used for wound cultures. Special media used for species identification include tryptic soy agar, with or without 1% TWEEN® 80, to assess lipid-enhanced growth.

- Identification—catalase-positive, nitrate-positive, and urease-positive. They can be identified to species level by the API® Coryne system or MALDI-TOF.
- The CAMP test (named after Christie, Atkins, and Munch–Petersen) was used historically. A streak of β-lysin-producing *S. aureus* is plated onto blood agar, with the test strain streaked perpendicular. A positive reaction is seen if CAMP factor (a haemolysin secreted by some corynebacteria) enhances the haemolysis produced by *S. aureus*.
- Susceptibility testing is problematic, but isolates are usually sensitive to vancomycin, teicoplanin, and daptomycin.

Infections caused by various corynebacteria

- *C. ulcerans* is primarily a cause of bovine mastitis. However, it has the potential to produce diphtheria toxin and cause an exudative pharyngitis, indistinguishable from *C. diphtheriae*. Several reported outbreaks of diphtheria have been found to be due to *C. ulcerans*.
- *C. pseudotuberculosis* is an animal pathogen that causes caseous lymphadenitis in sheep. Human disease is rare, but granulomatous lymphadenitis has been seen in farm workers and vets.
- *C. xerosis* is a commensal of the human nasopharynx, conjunctiva, and skin. It may cause invasive disease in the immunocompromised.
- *C. striatum* is a commensal of the skin and mucous membranes. It can rarely cause severe invasive disease in hospitalized patients.
- *C. minutissimum* is a skin commensal which was previously thought to cause erythrasma. Bacteraemia and endocarditis may occur in patients with indwelling catheters or immunocompromise.
- *C. amycolatum* is another skin commensal. There are case reports of invasive disease.
- *C. glucuronolyticum*—normal flora of the GU tract. May cause UTI and prostatitis.
- *C. pseudodiphtheriticum*—normal flora of the upper respiratory tract. Primarily associated with respiratory tract infections in the immunocompromised.
- *C. jeikeium* colonizes the skin of hospitalized patients. It may cause severe nosocomial infections, e.g. bacteraemia, endocarditis, meningitis, CSF shunt infections, PJIs. Risk factors include immunocompromise (malignancy, neutropenia, AIDS), indwelling devices, prolonged hospital stay, broad-spectrum antibiotics, and impaired skin integrity. *C. jeikeium* is resistant to many antibiotics, and vancomycin is the treatment of choice.
- *C. urealyticum* colonizes the skin of hospitalized patients. It causes chronic and recurrent UTIs in the elderly or immunosuppressed.

Listeria

L. monocytogenes is the main pathogen in this genus and affects pregnant women, neonates, the immunocompromised (especially if impaired cell-mediated immunity (CMI)), and the elderly. *L. ivanovii* occasionally causes human infection. Generally, *L. innocua*, *L. welshimeri*, and *L. seeligeri* are non-pathogenic to humans. Up to 5% of healthy adults carry *Listeria* spp. in the gut. *Listeria* infections are rare in the general population but can cause life-threatening bacteraemia and meningoencephalitis in susceptible groups.

Epidemiology

Disease is mainly sporadic but may be part of an epidemic associated with contaminated foodstuffs such as pâté, unpasteurized milk, chicken, or soft cheese. Hospital outbreaks have been reported. Vets or farmers may become infected through direct animal contact. Human–human transmission occurs vertically (i.e. mother–baby). Cross-infection in neonatal units has been reported. Note there was a dramatic rise in non-pregnancy-associated listeriosis between 2001 and 2010 in the UK, especially in those >60 years, reasons for which are unclear.

Pathogenesis

Animal studies have identified listeriolysin O—this is important for bacterial survival after phagocytosis, and its production is related to extracellular iron. In rodents, T lymphocytes are important in protective immunity, rather than antibodies. T cells attract monocytes to the infection, activate them, and destroy the *Listeria*, resulting in granuloma. The organisms themselves show tropism for the brain itself, particularly the brainstem and meninges. In humans, GI disease (e.g. low gastric pH or disrupted normal flora) may help establish *Listeria* infection in the bowel.

Clinical features

- *Pregnancy*—maternal listeriosis is rare before 20 weeks' gestation. After this, infection may be asymptomatic or present with mild symptoms (fever, back pain, sore throat, headache). Fever may result in reduced fetal movements, premature labour, stillbirth, abortion, or early-onset neonatal disease.
- *Neonate*—(i) early neonatal disease occurs <5 days post-delivery, usually presents with septicaemia, and has a mortality of 30–60%; 20–40% of survivors develop long-term sequelae such as lung disease or CNS defects; (ii) late neonatal disease occurs >5 days post-delivery, usually presents as meningitis, and may be hospital-acquired; mortality in late disease is lower (~10%).
- *Adults*—the main syndromes are meningitis, septicaemia, and endocarditis. Rare manifestations include other CNS disease (e.g. encephalitis, cerebritis, CNS abscesses), arthritis, hepatitis, endophthalmitis, continuous ambulatory peritoneal dialysis (CAPD) peritonitis, gastroenteritis, and pneumonia. Risk factors include age, immunosuppression due to steroids, cytotoxic therapy, and HIV. Mortality is high—CNS 20–50%, bacteraemia 5–20%, endocarditis 50%. Up to 75% of survivors of CNS infection have sequelae such as hemiplegia or CNS defects.

Diagnosis

- Microscopy—*Listeria* are short intracellular Gram-positive rods. However, in clinical specimens, they may appear Gram-variable and look like diphtheroids, cocci, or diplococci.
- Note that, in *Listeria* meningitis, a high lymphocyte count in the CSF is not always seen. Gram stain is often negative for organisms, but *Listeria* may be cultured from the CSF ± blood.

- Culture—*Listeria* grow on blood agar, but selective media are available such as those containing aesculin. Colonies are usually β-haemolytic on blood agar and can be mistaken for streptococci or enterococci.
- Identification—*Listeria* are non-sporulating, catalase-positive, aesculin-positive, and oxidase-positive. They show tumbling motility at 25°C and grow optimally at 30–37°C, but better than most bacteria at 4–10°C (refrigeration temperature). *L. monocytogenes, L. ivanovii*, and *L. seeligeri* show enhanced haemolysis in the presence of *S. aureus* (positive CAMP test). Species can also be differentiated by fermentation of *D*-xylose, *L*-rhamnose, and α-methyl-*D*-mannoside, or by API® Listeria/Coryne and MALDI-TOF.
- Typing techniques in current use include phage typing, serotying, PFGE, and multilocus enzyme electrophoresis (MLEE). Serotyping of *L. monocytogenes* with rabbit antisera results in 13 serovars—serovar 4 is the commonest in human infections.

Treatment

IV ampicillin ± gentamicin is the usual regimen for meningitis, with co-trimoxazole or meropenem as an alternative in penicillin-allergic patients. There are no RCTs to establish the most effective drug or duration of therapy. In meningitis, antibiotics are usually given for at least 14 days (21 days in the immunocompromised). Most other clinical syndromes should be treated with ampicillin, with consideration given to adding gentamicin for synergy. Vancomycin may be given for bacteraemia but has been associated with relapse of disease. NB. Cephalosporins should never be used to treat listeriosis due to inherent resistance.

Prevention

Invasive listeriosis is a notifiable condition. Health education and dietary advice to pregnant women, the immunocompromised, and others who are at risk of disease. Co-trimoxazole prophylaxis may prevent *Listeria* infections.

Erysipelothrix rhusiopathiae

E. rhusiopathiae is a thin, pleomorphic, non-sporing, Gram-positive rod. It was first isolated in mice by Robert Koch in 1878 and from swine by Louis Pasteur in 1882. It was identified as a human pathogen in 1909.

Epidemiology

E. rhusiopathiae is found in a variety of animals and invertebrates—the reservoir is thought to be swine—and transmission to humans is by direct contact. Most human cases are associated with occupational exposure, e.g. fishermen, fish handlers, farmers, vets, butchers, abattoir workers.

Clinical features

There are three clinical presentations:

- *erysipeloid*—a localized skin lesion. The organism enters the skin by trauma, and, after an incubation period of 2–7 days, pain and swelling

of the affected digit occur. The lesion is well defined, slightly raised, and violaceous. It spreads peripherally with central fading. Regional lymphadenopathy and lymphangitis may occur;
- *diffuse cutaneous eruption*—this is rare and caused by progression of the primary lesion. Fever, arthralgia, and lymphadenopathy may occur. Recurrence is common;
- *bacteraemia*—this is also rare but frequently associated with endocarditis.

Diagnosis

- *Microscopy*—*E. rhusiopathiae* is a straight to slightly curved Gram-positive rod (1–2.5 micrometres); it decolorizes readily and may appear Gram-negative. Rods may be arranged singly, or in V-shaped pairs, short chains, or non-branching filaments.
- *Culture*—colonial and microscopic appearances vary with the medium, pH, and incubation temperature. Incubation in 5–10% CO_2 improves culture.
- *Identification*—*E. rhusiopathiae* is catalase-negative, oxidase-negative, indole-negative, and Voges–Proskauer- and methyl red-negative.
- *Drug susceptibility*—*E. rhusiopathiae* is usually susceptible to penicillins, cephalosporins, clindamycin, carbapenems, and ciprofloxacin. It is resistant to vancomycin, teicoplanin, sulfonamides, co-trimoxazole, and aminoglycosides.

Treatment

- Penicillin is the treatment of choice.
- Alternatives include ampicillin, cephalosporins, and ciprofloxacin.
- *Erysipelothrix* is intrinsically resistant to vancomycin.

Rhodococcus equi

R. equi (previously known as *Corynebacterium equi*) was identified in 1923 as an animal pathogen causing pneumonia in horses. Since then, it has been found in a wide variety of animals. The first human case was reported in 1967—but, since the 1980s, the increase in immunosuppressed patients (HIV, transplantation, etc.) has been mirrored by an increase in *R. equi* infections.

Clinical features

- Necrotizing pneumonia is the commonest clinical presentation (80%) and is characterized by cavitation on the CXR. BCs are positive in 50% of HIV patients and 25% of solid organ transplant recipients.
- Extrapulmonary infection may affect the brain or present as s/c or organ abscesses. Bacteraemia may also occur, usually associated with IV catheters.

Diagnosis

- *R. equi* is a Gram-positive obligate aerobe that is non-sporing and non-motile.
- Microscopy—it may appear coccoid or bacillary on Gram stain, depending on growth conditions. It can be acid-fast.

- Culture—*R. equi* grows optimally at 30°C and produces salmon-pink colonies. Selective media include colistin nalidixic acid agar (CNA), phenyl ethanol agar (PEA), or ceftazidime novobiocin agar.
- Identification—*R. equi* is catalase-, lipase-, urease-, and phosphatase-positive. It differs from other coryneforms by its lack of ability to ferment carbohydrates or liquefy gelatin. It can be identified using API® Coryne, ribotyping, or RFLP.

Treatment

Optimal treatment has not been determined by clinical trials. *R. equi* is susceptible to vancomycin, erythromycin, fluoroquinolones, rifampicin, carbapenems, and aminoglycosides. Combinations of two or three antimicrobials are usually used, until antimicrobial susceptibility results are available.

Arcanobacterium haemolyticum

Arcanobacterium haemolyticum is a β-haemolytic, catalase-negative, Gram-positive rod which pits the agar when a colony is removed. Identification can be confirmed by API® Coryne. It causes acute pharyngitis (difficult to distinguish from GAS pharyngitis), and has also been associated with infective endocarditis and skin sepsis. It is sensitive to most antibiotics, except co-trimoxazole. Treatment is usually with penicillin or erythromycin.

Clostridium botulinum

C. botulinum is widespread in the soil and environment. It produces one of the most potent toxins known, which causes botulism.

Pathogenesis

Toxins A to G have identical pharmacological effects, despite possessing different antigens. All can cause human disease, but A, B, and E are commonest. Note that type-specific antibody must be given to a patient with suspected botulism (➔ see Clinical features below).

Clinical features

- *Food-borne botulism*—the preformed toxin is ingested from food (hams, sausages, tinned fish, meat, and vegetables, particularly home-preserved, and honey). The food itself may not appear spoiled. Botulinum toxin is absorbed from the human GI tract and blocks the release of acetylcholine mainly in the peripheral nervous system. Initial symptoms include nausea and vomiting, diplopia, and bilateral ptosis (due to oculomotor muscle involvement), followed by progressive descending motor loss with flaccid paralysis. Speech and swallowing become difficult, but the patient maintains consciousness and has normal sensation. Botulism is fatal in 5–10% of cases. Death is usually due to cardiac or respiratory failure.

- *Wound botulism*—causes a similar clinical picture but is due to toxin release secondary to growth of the organism. Outbreaks and ongoing sporadic cases occur in IDUs.
- *Intestinal botulism*—is also due to organism proliferation in the gut and toxin production *in vivo*.
- *Infant botulism*—presents as the 'floppy child syndrome', usually in babies <6 months, as the gut is not yet resistant to colonization.

Diagnosis

If there is a suspected clinical case, involve experts, and always alert laboratory staff, as the toxin is dangerous. Blood (taken prior to the administration of anti-toxin), stool, vomit, and food samples should be tested for the organism and toxin. *C. botulinum* is a motile, strictly anaerobic rod, with optimal growth at 35°C, but some strains are able to grow at as low as 1–5°C. The oval subterminal spores are very hardy—some spores persist, despite boiling at 100°C for several hours. Moist heat at 120°C for 5min usually destroys spores.

Treatment

Involve the ICU, as the patient is likely to need organ support. A polyvalent anti-toxin is available to neutralize unfixed toxin. In food-borne disease, any unabsorbed toxin should be removed from the stomach and GI tract. In wound botulism, give benzylpenicillin and metronidazole, and surgical debridement (reduces organism load and ongoing toxin production). Antibiotics are not recommended for food-borne or intestinal botulism.

Prevention

- Botulinum anti-toxin is effective at reducing the severity of symptoms, if given early in the course of disease. Surgical debridement and antibiotic therapy.
- Avoid home canning. Do not give honey to infants.

Table 7.3 Diseases caused by *Clostridium* spp.

Organism	Clinical syndrome	Toxin production
C. botulinum[a]	Botulism	Neurotoxin
C. tetani[a]	Tetanus	Neurotoxin
C. difficile	Antibiotic-associated diarrhoea/ pseudomembranous colitis	Toxin A and B
C. perfringens[a]	Type A causes gas gangrene	Histiotoxic
C. novyi[a]	Type A causes gas gangrene	Histiotoxic
C. sporogenes	Debate regarding pathogenicity	
C. septicum	Gas gangrene	Histiotoxic
C. histolyticum	Gas gangrene	Histiotoxic
C. sordellii	Gas gangrene	Histiotoxic

[a] Clusters in IDUs in Europe.

Clostridum tetani

C. tetani causes ~10 cases of tetanus/year in the UK. However, this vaccine-preventable disease still causes considerable morbidity and mortality in the developing world. Tetanus is a notifiable disease.

Pathogenesis

Resilient spores survive in soil and the GI tract of horses and other animals. Transmission usually occurs via introduction of spores into open wounds (particularly in IDUs), patients with recent abdominal surgery, patients with ear infections (otogenic tetanus), and neonates after cutting the umbilical cord (tetanus neonatorum). *C. tetani* produces the exotoxins tetanospasmin (powerful neurotoxin which diffuses to the CNS and causes localized or generalized disease) and tetanolysin (oxygen-labile haemolysin).

Clinical features

Localized tetanus involves muscle rigidity and painful spasms near the wound site. The symptoms of generalized tetanus are summarized by ROAST (rigidity, opisthotonus, autonomic dysfunction, spasms, trismus).

Diagnosis

Tetanus is a clinical diagnosis. These microbiological tests support the diagnosis:

- isolation of *C. tetani* from the infection site. *C. tetani* is a motile, obligate anaerobe which classically produces 'drumstick' terminal spores. It is Gram-variable. *C. tetani* produces a thin spreading film on enriched blood agar, due to the motility by peritrichous flagella. If *C. tetani* is suspected, involve the Anaerobe Reference Laboratory;
- presence of tetanus toxin in serum (performed at Colindale Food Safety Laboratory);
- low/no antibody levels to tetanus toxin.

Treatment

Involve the ICU early. Give tetanus immunoglobulin, wound debridement, and antimicrobials, including metronidazole or penicillin. Vaccination with tetanus toxoid following recovery is important to prevent future episodes (see Table 7.4).

Tetanus-prone wound risk factors

- Puncture-type wound.
- Contact with soil or manure.
- Clinical evidence of sepsis.
- Significant degree of devitalized tissue.
- Any wound with delay of >6h before surgical treatment.

Prevention

Tetanus immunization, introduced in the UK in 1961, now involves the combined tetanus/low-dose diphtheria vaccine (Td) (previously single-antigen vaccines (T) were given). Five doses of tetanus toxoid are considered to give lifelong immunity (usually three as DTP as part of childhood immunizations, and two doses of Td later). See the DH *Green Book*.

Table 7.4 Recommendations for vaccination

Immunization status	Clean wound	Tetanus-prone wound	
	Vaccine	Vaccine	Tetanus immunoglobulin
Full, i.e. five doses	No	No	Only if high risk
Primary immunization complete, boosters incomplete but up-to-date	No	No	Only if high risk
Primary immunization incomplete/boosters not up-to-date/never immunized/status unknown or uncertain	Yes—one dose and plan to complete schedule	Yes—one dose and plan to complete schedule	Yes—one dose in a different site

Other clostridia

These anaerobic Gram-positive, spore-forming organisms are responsible for a variety of conditions, many of which involve exotoxin production (see Table 7.3). The rods are pleomorphic, but typically large, straight, or slightly curved, with rounded ends.

- *C. perfringens* causes gas gangrene. It is occasionally isolated from BCs and may be associated with food poisoning (enterotoxin production), endocarditis, or a contaminant. In developing countries, it may cause enteritis necroticans ('pig bel').
- *C. histolyticum* and *C. sordellii* may also cause gas gangrene.
- *C. novyi* gas gangrene is due to *C. novyi* type A (*C. novyi* types B, C, and D are differentiated by toxin permutation and soluble antigen production, and do not cause human disease). Compared to *C. perfringens, C. novyi* bacilli are larger and more pleomorphic. It is a stricter anaerobe and has peritrichous flagella, but motility is inhibited in the presence of oxygen. The oval spores are central or subterminal. There are at least four toxins which possess haemolytic, necrotizing, lethal, lipase, and phospholipase activities. There was a large outbreak amongst IDUs in Scotland in 1999–2000.
- *C. sporogenes* is probably not pathogenic in its own right. It is usually encountered in a mixed wound culture containing accepted pathogens, and may have a role in enhancing local conditions and accelerating an established anaerobic infection.
- *C. septicum* usually lives in the soil, human, or animal gut, and can cause gas gangrene in humans and animals. *C. septicum* bacteraemia is seen with breakdown of gut integrity, e.g. in leukaemia. Gram stain appearance of the organism may be variable, with long, short, and filamentous Gram-positive rods, together with some older Gram-negative cells. Spores start off as swollen Gram-positive 'citron bodies', then tend to be oval, bulging, and either central or subterminal.

C. septicum grows well on ordinary media at 37°C and has numerous peritrichous flagella, hence is actively motile. Colonies are often initially transparent and 'droplet-like', with projecting radiations, then become grey and opaque with time. The α exotoxin has lethal, haemolytic, and necrotizing properties, and can be demonstrated in cultures.
- *C. difficile* (➔ see *Clostridium difficile* infection, pp. 198–201) is a HCAI, subject to mandatory reporting. It can cause CDI and colitis. Clinical features vary, and diagnosis is usually by toxin tests, rather than culture. Infection control measures are paramount to control spread.

Actinomyces

Actinomyces spp. are mouth, gut, and vaginal commensals that may cause the chronic granulomatous infection actinomycosis. The main species of human importance are *A. israelii* and *A. gerencseriae*. Others include *A. meyeri* (isolated from brain abscesses), *A. viscosus* (found in dental caries), and also *A. naeslundii* and *A. odontolyticus*.

Pathogenesis

Actinomycosis is endogenously acquired, and those with dental caries and intrauterine contraceptive devices (IUCDs) are at increased risk. It is unclear why males are affected more than females. Historically, rural farm workers were affected more than those living in towns, purportedly because of poor dental hygiene. Chronic abscesses, tissue destruction, fibrosis, and sinus formation are typical findings. The masses of mycelia in relatively young lesions may be visible as yellow sulphur granules; later on, they form dark brown, hard granules due to calcium phosphate deposition.

Clinical features

Most human cases of actinomycosis are in the cervicofacial area, especially around the jaw. Infection may follow dental procedures. Haematogenous spread to the liver, brain, and other organs is well recognized. In addition to facial disease, clinical presentations include thoracic actinomycosis (due to aspiration of oral *Actinomyces*; characterized by chest wall sinuses and bony erosion of the ribs and spine), appendix or colonic diverticular actinomycosis, pelvic actinomycosis (linked with IUCDs), cerebral actinomycosis, and 'punch actinomycosis' (knuckle infection due to human bite).

Diagnosis

- Histology—tissue biopsies of suspect lesions are stained with fluorescein-conjugated specific antisera, to demonstrate characteristic sulphur granules and mycelia. Any sulphur granules available should be crushed and stained with Gram stain—organisms appear as branching Gram-positive rods. *Nocardia* spp. are morphologically indistinguishable. However, *Actinomyces* are NOT acid-fast, and *Nocardia* are weakly acid-fast.
- Culture—*Actinomyces* often fail to grow aerobically. Growth requires enriched culture (e.g. brain–heart infusion medium or selective media) incubated under micro-aerophilic conditions (i.e. 5–10% CO_2).

Colonies may appear after 3–7 days but may take up to 14. *A. israelii* and *A. gerencseriae* colonies have a 'molar teeth'-shape on agar. Further identification can be confirmed by MALDI-TOF or at a reference laboratory by biochemical tests, fluorescent antisera staining, or gas chromatography of metabolic products of carbohydrate fermentation. Note that sputum often contains oral *Actinomyces*.

Treatment

Surgical involvement is vital, and debridement reduces scarring, deformity, and recurrence rate. Removal of an IUCD is the primary treatment for pelvic disease. Actinomycosis is usually treated with penicillin or ampicillin, for up to 6 months. Broad-spectrum antibiotics, e.g. co-amoxiclav, or ceftriaxone and metronidazole may be needed if there are concomitant pathogens. Despite large doses of antibiotics given for long periods, recurrence is common. The issue seems to be one of tissue penetration, rather than drug resistance.

Nocardia

Nocardia spp. are environmental saprophytes that occasionally cause chronic granulomatous infections in humans and animals. Thirty-three species of *Nocardia* have been shown to cause disease in humans, with members of the *Nocardia asteroides* complex (*N. asteroides sensu stricto, N. farcinica*, and *N. nova*) being the commonest worldwide. Other species isolated from clinical samples include *N. abscessus, N. brasiliensis, N. cyriacigeorgica, N. otitidiscaviarum, N. paucivorans, N. pseudobrasiliensis*, and *N. transvalensis*.

Pathogenesis

Pulmonary nocardiosis is acquired through inhalation of the bacilli. Cutaneous nocardiosis occurs as a result of inoculation injury. Disseminated or CNS nocardiosis occurs following haematogenous spread. Pulmonary and disseminated disease is commoner in immunosuppressed patients.

Clinical features

Pulmonary nocardiosis is commoner in the immunosuppressed and those with pre-existing lung disease, particularly alveolar proteinosis. Presentation and clinical/radiological findings are variable, making the diagnosis difficult. Patients tend to develop multiple lung abscesses. Secondary abscesses, mainly in the brain, occur in approximately one-third of patients with pulmonary nocardiosis. Other clinical presentations include cutaneous disease (e.g. post-trauma) with lymphatic involvement (sporotrichoid), which may progress to a fungating mycetoma.

Diagnosis

- Branching, aerobic Gram-positive rods, weakly acid-fast when decolorized with 1% sulphuric acid (modified ZN stain). Other specialist stains that aid the diagnosis of *Nocardia* include the Gomori methenamine silver method.

- Colonies of *Nocardia* may be coloured (orange/cream/pink), and the surface may be dry or chalky. *Nocardia* can take up to a month to grow on standard media (e.g. Lowenstein–Jensen media, brain–heart infusion agar, and trypticase–soy agar with blood enrichment).
- *Nocardia* organisms can be differentiated from *Actinomyces*, because they are strict aerobes (whereas *Actinomyces* organisms are facultative anaerobes), and *Nocardia* grow over a wide range of temperatures (whereas *Actinomyces* only grow at 35–37°C). *Actinomyces* are not acid-fast.

Treatment

Seek expert advice. Usually a long course (e.g. >3 months in normal hosts, 6 months if immunocompromised) of a sulfonamide ± trimethoprim, e.g. as co-trimoxazole. Alternatives include minocycline, carbapenems, and amikacin. In refractory cases, involve the reference laboratory for sensitivity testing.

Actinomadura and *Streptomyces*

Actinomadura and *Streptomyces* spp. are aerobic filamentous actinomycetes implicated in mycetoma, also known as Madura foot. This is a chronic granulomatous condition that mainly occurs in Africa, Asia, and Central America. The important subspecies are *Actinomadura madurae, Actinomadura pelletieri*, and *Streptomyces somaliensis*.

Mycetoma can be divided into actinomycetoma (bacterial) or eumycetoma (fungal), which has important treatment implications. Other bacterial causes include species of *Madurella, Exophila*, and *Nocardia*.

Diagnosis

Clinically, grains seen within host tissues or in the discharge from sinus tracts are diagnostic of mycetoma. These grains are colonies of the organism, and should be crushed in potassium hydroxide (KOH) and Gram-stained to distinguish between actinomycetoma (Gram-positive filaments) and eumycetoma (septate fungi). These grains should be rinsed in 70% alcohol before culture, to try to eliminate any surface contaminants, and appropriate plates set up at 26°C and 37°C. Macroscopically, grains are often red. *Actinomadura* spp. show many similar properties to *Actinomyces* spp. but strictly *Actinomadura* are not acid-fast when decolorized with 1% sulphuric acid.

Clinical features

Mycetomas usually involve the hand or foot, and arise from traumatic inoculation from soil or plants, usually via thorns or splinters. The chronic granuloma of the skin, s/c tissue, and bone may progress to sinus formation.

Treatment

Seek expert advice, as the regimen depends on the cause, and courses may be up to 9 months. Actinomycetoma tend to respond to therapy better than eumycetoma, which usually requires surgery. A combination of streptomycin with dapsone, rifampicin, co-trimoxazole, or sulfonamides may be used.

Gram-negative cocci—overview

The Gram-negative cocci include a variety of pathogenic and non-pathogenic species (see Table 7.5).

NB. *Acinetobacter* spp. are GNRs that may appear coccoid or bacillary. Unlike *Neisseria* spp., they are oxidase-negative. They are discussed further on ➲ *Acinetobacter*, pp. 297–9.

Table 7.5 Gram-negative cocci

Organism	Microbiology	Syndrome
N. meningitidis	Aerobic, Gram-negative diplococci, oxidase-positive, grow at 37°C on blood and chocolate agar, glucose- and maltose-positive	Meningitis Septicaemia
N. gonorrhoeae	Aerobic, Gram-negative diplococci, oxidase-positive, grow at 37°C on blood and chocolate agar, glucose-positive	Gonorrhoea Septic arthritis Ophthalmia neonatorum
Non-pathogenic Neisseria spp.	Aerobic, Gram-negative diplococci, oxidase-positive, grow at 22°C on nutrient agar	Oral commensals—rarely cause invasive infections
M. catarrhalis	Aerobic, Gram-negative cocci, oxidase-positive, grow at 37°C on blood and chocolate agar	Respiratory pathogen
Anaerobic Gram-negative cocci, e.g. *Veillonella* spp.	Anaerobic, Gram-negative cocci	

Neisseria meningitidis

Vieusseaux first described epidemic cerebrospinal fever in 1805. In 1887, Weichselbaum isolated *N. meningitidis* from CSF. In the late nineteenth century, meningococcal carriage was described. In 1909, different serotypes of *N. meningitidis* were recognized.

Epidemiology

Humans are the only known reservoir of *N. meningitidis*, and ~20% of the population carry the organism in their throat. However, half of these carriage strains are non-capsulate and thus non-pathogenic. During outbreaks, the carrier rate of an epidemic strain may reach 90%. Risk factors for meningococcal disease include:

- lack of bactericidal antibody;
- age—bimodal distribution: 3 months to 3 years and 18–23 years;
- travel to endemic areas, e.g. Africa, Mecca;
- complement deficiencies;
- splenectomy;
- host genetic polymorphisms, e.g. *MBL, TNFA, Fc/RIIa*, and *PAI-1*.

Pathogenesis

To cause infection, the organism must cross the nasopharyngeal mucosa and enter the circulation. The type IV pilus (encoded by *pilC*) is involved in mucosal colonization. The polysaccharide capsule is important in avoiding host immunity (and defines the serogroup of the isolate; see Table 7.6). Various secretion systems help deliver toxins, and IgA protease enhances survival within epithelial cells.

Clinical features

- Acute—meningitis and septicaemia, purulent conjunctivitis (occasionally becomes systemic), monoarthritis, endocarditis, pericarditis, pneumonia.
- Chronic septicaemia with joint and skin involvement is less common.

Diagnosis

- *N. meningitidis* is Hazard group 2. Suspected and known isolates of *N. meningitidis* should always be handled in a safety cabinet.
- CSF examination—in meningitis, the CSF pressure is elevated, and the CSF appears turbid. CSF polymorphs and protein are normally raised, and CSF glucose level is low (normal is >60% of serum level). In very early infection, CSF results may be normal, as the meningeal reaction has not had time to take place.
- Microscopy—Gram-negative intracellular diplococci. Note that, in meningococcal meningitis, CSF usually has a higher yield than BCs. If the Gram stain is negative, a methylene blue stain may pick up scanty meningococci.
- Culture—fastidious, transparent, non-pigmented, non-haemolytic colonies. May be mucoid if capsule production. Oxidase-positive. Identified by API NH, MALDI-TOF, and molecular methods.
- Serogrouping—capsular polysaccharide antigens are identified by slide agglutination test using polyclonal antibodies. There are at least 13 serogroups; the commonest ones are summarized in Table 7.6.
- Serotyping—identification of (PorB) class 2/3 outer membrane protein by a dot-blot enzyme-linked immunosorbent assay (ELISA) using monoclonal antibodies.
- Serosubtyping—identification of (PorA) class 1 outer membrane protein by a dot-blot ELISA using monoclonal antibodies.
- MLST is being evaluated for routine surveillance.
- Meningococcal PCR (send to the meningococcal reference laboratory)—can be performed on CSF, serum, plasma, EDTA blood, or joint fluids.

Microbiology

N. meningitidis produces a capsule which forms the basis of the serogroup typing system. There are now at least 13 serogroups, but the commonest ones are summarized in Table 7.6.

Table 7.6 Major serogroups of *N. meningitidis*

Serogroup	Pattern of disease	Vaccines
A	Epidemic meningitis, associated with different clones	Yes
B	Epidemic strains (and outbreaks). Main serotype in the UK	Meningitis B vaccine licensed in 2013. For introduction into routine schedule in 2015
C	Local outbreaks	MenC vaccine introduced into routine schedule in 1999
W-135	Pilgrims returning from the Hajj	Yes—in high-risk groups
X, Y, Z, 29E, Z′	Rare	

Treatment

- See management of acute bacterial meningitis (➔ see Acute meningitis, p. 718) and septicaemia. Reduced susceptibility to penicillin has resulted in empirical therapy for meningitis being a third-generation cephalosporin (usually ceftriaxone in the UK).
- After treatment, antibiotics—usually ciprofloxacin—should be given for nasopharyngeal eradication, unless ceftriaxone was used for treatment.

Infection control issues

This is a notifiable condition. Droplet infection control precautions are recommended, particularly before the patient has completed 24h of appropriate antibiotic therapy. Public health will arrange chemoprophylaxis—indicated for those who had prolonged close contact in a household-type setting during the 7 days before illness, or transient close contact if exposed to respiratory droplets or secretions around the time of admission. Ciprofloxacin is recommended for all ages and in pregnancy. The advantages of ciprofloxacin over rifampicin (previous choice) are single dose, no interaction with the oral contraceptive pill (OCP), and availability in community pharmacies. The risk of complications is negligible from a single dose. The alternatives (e.g. if ciprofloxacin-allergic) include ceftriaxone. Vaccination may also be offered. For complete guidelines, web search 'PHE meningococcal public health 2012'.

Vaccination

- Group C conjugate vaccine—capsular polysaccharides linked to a carrier protein. Part of the routine UK schedule since 1999. Reported cases fell by 90% in all age groups immunized, and by 66% in other age groups as a result of herd immunity. A booster dose was introduced in 2006, as a result of studies demonstrating waning protection during the second year of life. Similarly, an adolescent booster dose was started in 2013 (for further details, see the PHE website and the DH *Green Book*). Given at 3 months, 12 months, and 14 years of age. Also available combined with *H. influenzae* type B (Hib) vaccine.

- Quadrivalent ACWY vaccine—conjugate and polysaccharide version available. Conjugate is preferred. Recommended for those travelling to areas of risk, including Hajj pilgrimage, parts of Africa, and Asia. See www.nathnac.org.
- Group B protein vaccine—three *N. meningitidis* proteins produced by recombinant technology and a preparation of group B-derived outer membrane vesicles. Shown to be immunogenic and may protect against 88% of MenB strains in the UK. Effectiveness in preventing disease yet to be proven. Licensed. Initially restricted to risk groups (asplenic children, laboratory workers, etc.) due to issues of cost; it entered the routine UK vaccination schedule in 2015. Doses at 2, 4, and 12 months.

Neisseria gonorrhoeae

N. gonorrhoeae only infects humans and causes the sexually transmitted infection (STI) gonorrhoea (see Gonorrhoea, pp. 709–11). This is the second commonest bacterial STI in the UK. Increasing rates of antimicrobial resistance, together with its persistence and association with poor reproductive health outcomes, have made it a major public health concern.

Pathogenicity

Gonococci are divided into four Kellogg types, by colonial appearance, ability to auto-agglutinate, and virulence. Kellogg types T1 and T2 are more virulent and possess many fimbriae, while types T3 and T4 are non-fimbriate and avirulent. In gonococci, the fimbriae are associated with attachment to mucosal surfaces and resistance to killing by phagocytes. Epidemiological typing of gonococci uses both auxotyping (nutritional requirements of arginine, proline, hypoxanthine, uracil, etc.) and monoclonal antibodies against specific proteins.

Clinical features

Gonorrhoea commonly presents as a purulent disease of the urethral mucous membrane and the cervix in females. Secondary local complications (e.g. epididymitis, salpingitis, PID; see Pelvic inflammatory disease, pp. 705–6) and metastatic complications (e.g. arthritis) may occur if the primary infection is inadequately treated. Other manifestations of disease include disseminated gonococcal infection (skin lesions, painful joints, and fever), ophthalmia neonatorum (purulent conjunctivitis of the newborn—a notifiable condition), perihepatic inflammation (Fitz-Hugh–Curtis), and rarely endocarditis or meningitis. Rectal or pharyngeal infection is often asymptomatic and identified through contact tracing. If cultured, gonococcus should always be treated, as it is never a commensal.

Diagnosis

- Microscopy—Gram-negative, intracellular diplococci. This can be done within the GU medicine (GUM) clinic, ensuring prompt treatment of patients.

- Culture—culture remains essential where infection persists after treatment and treatment failure is suspected. Culture is specific, sensitive, and cheap. Urethral swabs from males and endocervical swabs from females should be Gram-stained, and then immediately inoculated onto selective media and placed in enriched CO_2 conditions. Typical Gram stain appearance of *N. gonorrhoeae* (Gram-negative diplococci in association with neutrophils) from urethral/endocervical swabs, together with a consistent clinical presentation, is regarded as adequate for treatment in many cases. However, culture is critical for legal cases and for antimicrobial sensitivity testing. After 24–48h, oxidase-positive colonies appear, and identification can be confirmed by testing for acid production from sugars (API® NH). Identification must be confirmed by two different methods. Selective agars (e.g. NYC or VCAT—containing vancomycin, colistimethate sodium, amphotericin, and trimethoprim) are used. Many laboratories still test for β-lactamase production by the chromogenic cephalosporin (nitrocefin), acidometric, and paper strip methods, although patients are likely to be treated with a third-generation cephalosporin, according to current guidelines.
- NAATs are generally more sensitive (96% in both symptomatic and asymptomatic infections), compared to culture. Males should send first-pass urine, and females a vaginal or endocervical swab. Other specimen types can be tested—NAATs are recommended for asymptomatic individuals (urethral/endocervical) and MSM (rectal/pharyngeal). Positive NAATs from extragenital sites and low-prevalence populations must be confirmed.
- If gonococcus is isolated from a prepubertal girl with vulvovaginitis, it may indicate sexual abuse. A paediatrician should deal with the case sensitively, and senior laboratory staff should be involved. 'Chain of evidence' documentation is required, since evidence may be needed in court.
- Testing for co-infection with *Chlamydia* is recommended, as *Chlamydia trachomatis* commonly accompanies genital gonorrhoea (35% of heterosexual men and 41% of women with gonorrhoea; GRASP 2008).
- For further details, see *United Kingdom national guideline for gonorrhoea testing 2012* (available at: www.bashh.org/documents/4490.pdf).

Treatment

The *UK national guideline for the management of gonorrhoea in adults, 2011* (available at: www.bashh.org/documents/3920.pdf) recommends IM ceftriaxone with PO azithromycin as first-line treatment (azithromycin aims to delay the onset of cephalosporin resistance). Cephalosporins have replaced fluoroquinolones, due to increasing resistance rates. Alternative choices are limited with increasing resistance to penicillin (22% in 2009), tetracyclines (68% in 2009), and azithromycin, and reduced susceptibility to cefixime. Infection with a resistant organism results in an adverse clinical outcome for the patient and results in transmission to other contacts. The 2011 guidelines recommend a test of cure for all cases. A screen for further STIs and contact tracing are indicated in all cases.

Non-pathogenic *Neisseria*

The non-pathogenic *Neisseria* spp. are upper respiratory tract commensals and include: *N. lactamica, N. polysaccharea, N. subflava, N. sicca, N. mucosa, N. flavescens, N. elongata, N. cinerea*, and *N. weaveri*.

Microbiology

N. lactamica and *N. polysaccharea* are the species most commonly isolated from nasopharyngeal swabs during meningococcal surveys. Colonies appear similar to *N. meningitidis*, and they also grow on selective media, unlike the nasopharyngeal commensals. *N. lactamica* is easy to distinguish, as it produces acid from glucose, maltose, and lactose, and gives a positive ONPG test result for β-galactosidase. It is thought that non-pathogenic species have contributed to the acquisition of resistance mechanisms by pathogenic organisms. *Neisseria* spp. are naturally competent for DNA uptake; thus, *N. meningitidis* and *N. gonorrhoeae* have acquired penicillin resistance by picking up the genes from other 'neisserial' flora.

Clinical features

Can occasionally cause invasive diseases such as meningitis, endocarditis, bacteraemia, ocular infections, pericarditis, osteomyelitis, empyema—in such cases, full susceptibility testing should be performed, as penicillin resistance is increasing.

Moraxella

For decades, *M. catarrhalis* was regarded as an upper respiratory tract commensal. However, since the 1970s, it has been recognized as an important and common respiratory tract pathogen.

Microbiology

M. catarrhalis grows well on many media, including blood and chocolate agar. It shows the 'hockey-stick' sign, in that it slides across the agar surface when pushed and can be difficult to pick up onto a loop. *M. catarrhalis* is oxidase-positive, catalase-positive, and DNase-positive, and produces butyrate esterase.

Clinical features

M. catarrhalis causes otitis media, LRTIs in COPD patients, pneumonia (particularly in the elderly), nosocomial respiratory tract infections, sinusitis, and occasionally bacteraemia. Outer membrane proteins (OMPs), lipo-oligosaccharide (LOS), and pili are probably important in pathogenesis.

Treatment

Almost all strains of *M. catarrhalis* produce an inducible β-lactamase. Regardless of the results of ampicillin susceptibility testing, ampicillin should not be used. Suitable agents include co-amoxiclav, cephalosporins, fluoroquinolones, or tetracyclines.

Anaerobic Gram-negative cocci

- *Veillonella* spp. organisms are part of the normal flora of the GI tract of humans and animals. *Veillonella* may be isolated from a variety of clinical conditions, though their role in causing infection is unclear. The commonest species is *Veillonella parvula*, which fluoresces red under ultraviolet (UV) light. *Veillonella* are able to use some of the lactic acid produced by streptococci, lactobacilli, and other bacteria that may induce dental caries. They are associated with supragingival dental plaque and also found as part of the tongue microflora. They are generally regarded as minor components of mixed anaerobic infections.
- *Acidominococcus* spp. and *Megosphora* spp. are other anaerobic Gram-negative cocci found in the human gut. They are considered non-pathogenic.

Escherichia coli

E. coli is the type species of the genus *Escherichia* in the family *Enterobacteriaceae*. It contains a variety of strains, ranging from commensal organisms to highly pathogenic variants. Infections tend to infect the gut and urinary tract, but almost any extraintestinal site may be involved. *E. coli* may be a marker of faecal contamination, e.g. in food and water testing, as it does not otherwise exist outside the animal body.

Pathogenesis

- O and K polysaccharide antigens protect *E. coli* from complement and phagocytic killing, unless antibodies are present. Phagocytosis is usually successful if there are antibodies to K antigens present alone, or to both O and K antigens.
- Haemolysin is more commonly produced by strains causing extraintestinal infections, and is thought to increase virulence.
- The ColV plasmid, harboured by some *E. coli*, encodes an aerobactin-mediated iron uptake system. This is commoner in strains isolated from cases of septicaemia, pyelonephritis, and lower UTIs than in commensal faecal strains.
- Fimbriae—type 1 fimbriae adhere to cells containing mannose residues, possibly contributing to pathogenicity, but their role in UTIs is debated. Other filamentous proteins may cause mannose-resistant haemagglutination, e.g. colonization factor antigens (CFAs) in human enterotoxigenic *E. coli* (ETEC), K88 in pigs. P fimbriae bind specifically to receptors on P blood group antigens of human erythrocytes and uroepithelial cells.
- Other—enteric strains demonstrate specific interactions with the GI mucosa, release toxins, and may harbour plasmid-encoded virulence factors.

Epidemiology

Serotying of *E. coli* is based on O (somatic), H (flagellar), and K (surface/capsular) antigens, as detected in agglutination reactions.

- There are >160 O antigens, and cross-reactions occur between *E. coli* O antigens and O antigens of other species, e.g. *Citrobacter, Salmonella*.
- H antigens are usually monophasic and are determined from cultures on semi-solid agar.
- K antigens traditionally prevented O agglutination (thus, agglutination tests are done on boiled samples). K antigens are acidic polysaccharide capsular antigens, and are divided into groups I and II.

Clinical features

Urinary tract infections

E. coli is the commonest cause of community-acquired uncomplicated UTIs (➲ see Urinary tract infections: introduction, pp. 678–9), and also causes nosocomial UTIs. Clinical manifestations range from urethritis and cystitis to pyelonephritis and sepsis. Many uropathogenic strains originate in the patient's own gut and cause infection by the ascending route. Specific P fimbriae or '*p*ili *a*ssociated with *p*yelonephritis' (known as the PAP pilus), which attach to uroepithelial cells, are important in pathogenesis. These uropathogenic strains may contain additional virulence factors such as haemolysin, ColV plasmids, and resistance to complement-dependent bactericidal effect of serum.

Enteric infections

E. coli is responsible for many cases of diarrhoeal disease, ranging from acute gastroenteritis, particularly in the tropics ('traveller's diarrhoea'; ➲ see Viral gastroenteritis, p. 408), to life-threatening haemorrhagic colitis. The strains involved fall into 4–5 groups, with different pathogenic mechanisms (see Table 7.7).

Bacteraemia

The usual sources of nosocomial *E. coli* bacteraemia are the urogenital, GI, and respiratory tracts, and foreign bodies such as IV lines and endotracheal tubes. The hallmark of cases of Gram-negative bacteraemia is the systemic reaction to LPS or endotoxin, which may be fatal.

Neonatal sepsis

E. coli may cause neonatal meningitis and septicaemia, especially in premature babies. The strains responsible may express the K1 or K5 surface/ capsular antigens, which have enhanced virulence.

Other non-enteric infections

E. coli may cause post-operative wound infections and deep abscesses. Respiratory tract infection is usually opportunistic, often in debilitated patients such as diabetics or alcoholics. Nosocomial pneumonia (± empyema) is usually due to aspiration, rather than haematogenous spread.

Diagnosis

E. coli are usually smooth, colourless colonies on non-selective media and may appear haemolytic on blood agar. Most ferment lactose, appearing yellow on CLED agar (and produce acid and gas in 24–48h), but ~5% are non-lactose fermenters. Usually motile, and those responsible for extraintestinal infections often have a polysaccharide capsule. Usually positive for indole production, ornithine decarboxylase, lysine decarboxylase, and methyl red,

Table 7.7 Clinical features and pathogenic mechanisms of different *E. coli*

Abbreviation	Full name	Clinical features	Pathogenesis
EHEC/VTEC/STEC	Entero-haemorrhagic *E. coli* Verotoxin-producing *E. coli* Shiga toxin-producing *E. coli*	Haemorrhagic colitis/HUS	*Verotoxins* (VT1 and 2), also called shiga-like toxins (SLT1 and 2), are phage-encoded toxins thought to target vascular endothelial cells. The A subunit mediates biological activity, while B subunit is responsible for binding and toxin uptake. Risk of developing HUS depends on the type of shiga toxin, plus host and environmental factors
ETEC	Enterotoxigenic *E. coli*	Traveller's diarrhoea	*ST (heat-stable enterotoxin)* causes increased guanosine monophosphate (GMP), thus altering ion transport, and increased fluid secretion by mucosal cells of small intestine
			LT (heat-labile enterotoxin)—B polypeptide binds to the mucosal surface of the small intestine, allowing the A polypeptide to enter the cell and catalyse adenosine diphosphate ribosylation of the guanine nucleotide component of adenylate cylase, thus increased AMP and increased fluid secretion (as with *V. cholerae*)
			Colonization/adherence factors—see text
EIEC	Enteroinvasive *E. coli*	Disease similar to shigella-like dysentery	
EPEC	Entero-pathogenic *E. coli*	Childhood diarrhoea	
EAEC	Entero-aggregative *E. coli*	Traveller's diarrhoea, especially in Mexico and North Africa	

NB. A novel strain of *E. coli* O104:H4 caused a serious outbreak of bloody diarrhoea/HUS in Germany in 2011. This was an EAEC strain which had acquired shiga toxin Stx2.

and negative for urease, citrate utilization, H_2S production, and Voges–Proskauer test. *E. coli* O157 are usually non-sorbitol fermenters (appear colourless/white on CT-SMAC agar). However, some do ferment sorbitol, so, if high clinical suspicion (e.g. haemolytic uraemic syndrome, HUS), send to the reference laboratory for PCR testing. Remember *E. coli* O157 is an ACDP category 3 organism.

Treatment

The management of *E. coli* depends on the site and severity of the infection. Simple *E. coli* UTIs may respond to trimethoprim or ampicillin. Some hospital-acquired *E. coli* infections are due to multiresistant organisms, and may require treatment with a cephalosporin, fluoroquinolone, aminoglycoside, piperacillin–tazobactam, or carbapenem. Susceptibility data vary geographically (due to prior antibiotic usage), so follow your hospital antibiotic policy. Be guided by antibiotic susceptibility results, and use the narrowest possible targeted therapy. Antibiotics may be harmful in cases of *E. coli* O157.

Klebsiella

Klebsiella spp. are usually harmless colonizers of the human gut. The classification can be confusing, but the main species defined by DNA hybridization studies are *K. pneumoniae* subspecies *aerogenes* (formerly *K. aerogenes*), *K. pneumoniae* subspecies *pneumoniae* (formerly *K. pneumoniae*), and *K. oxytoca*. Other rare respiratory subspecies include *K. pneumoniae* subspecies *ozaenae* and *K. pneumoniae* subspecies *rhinoscleromatis*. Note that some *Klebsiella* have recently been reclassified as *Raoultella*, e.g. *Raoultella ornithinolytica* and *Raoultella terrigena* (➲ see Other *Enterobacteriaceae*, pp. 292–3).

Pathogenesis

Klebsiella that express capsular K antigens are resistant to complement-mediated serum killing. Those with O antigens are resistant to phagocytosis. *Klebsiella* spp. have two iron uptake systems—one uses aerobactin (related to virulence), and the other uses enterochelin (plasmid-encoded).

Epidemiology

There are about 80 K (capsular) antigens recognized overall, and K2, K3, and K21 are common in the UK. There are also five different somatic O antigen types, but these are rarely used for typing. There is an association between the antigenic structure, habitat, and biochemical reactivity, e.g. capsular types 1–6 are commonest in the human respiratory tract. Capsular serotyping, bacteriocin typing, and phage typing are used for epidemiological studies.

Clinical features

Klebsiella infections are rare in the immunocompetent normal host. They tend to cause nosocomial and opportunistic infections (UTIs, pneumonia, other respiratory infections, surgical wound infections, bacteraemia) in those with risk factors (diabetes, COPD, alcoholism). Severe pneumonia with 'redcurrant jelly' sputum and multiple lung abscesses is called Friedlander's pneumonia and has a high mortality.

Diagnosis

Klebsiella spp. are facultatively anaerobic, catalase-positive, and oxidase-negative, and ferment glucose. Organisms are capsular, which may give colonies a mucoid appearance. The capsule is made of glucuronic acid and pyruvic acid. On Gram stain, organisms may look fat and chunky. They are lactose fermenters and are usually fimbriate, but non-motile. They are H_2S- and indole-negative (except *K. oxytoca* which is indole-positive), are Voges–Proskauer-positive, grow in KCN, and can use citrate as a sole carbon source. Different species of *Klebsiella* are usually recognized by different biochemical tests. They can be identified biochemically (API 20E), via MALDI-TOF, or by using automated systems.

Treatment

Most *Klebsiella* spp. are inherently resistant to ampicillin and other penicillins. Many are now multiresistant due to ESBLs and KPCs. Aminoglycoside susceptibility varies between regions. Treat according to local hospital policy and sensitivity data. Carbapenems and fluoroquinolones may be the only options.

Proteus

Proteus mirabilis is most commonly isolated from community UTIs, while *Proteus vulgaris* and *Proteus myxofaciens* tend to cause nosocomial infections. *Proteus* belongs to the tribe *Proteae*.

Pathogenesis

Factors that contribute to the ability of *Proteus* to colonize and infect the urinary tract include:

- production of the enzyme urease which splits urea into ammonium hydroxide. This increases urinary pH and encourages struvite stone formation. These stones act as a nidus for persistent infection and also obstruct urinary flow;
- fimbriae help uroepithelial colonization;
- flagella-dependent motility helps spread in the urinary tract;
- uropathogenic *Proteus* synthesizes several haemolysins.

Clinical features

In addition to urine infections, *Proteus* also causes bacteraemia, wound infections, and respiratory infections in debilitated hospital patients. The human GI tract is the main reservoir of infection for patients who subsequently become infected.

Diagnosis

Proteus organisms rapidly hydrolyse urea. The presence of hundreds of flagellae on each organism makes them extraordinarily motile, which appears as 'swarming' on agar plates, and can produce the Dienes phenomenon (a line of inhibited growth where two strains meet). *Proteus* organisms give positive methyl red reactions, are usually Voges–Proskauer-negative (except some strains of *P. mirabilis*), and can grow in the presence of KCN.

Table 7.8 Biochemical reactions useful to distinguish *Proteus, Providencia,* and *Morganella*

	Proteus mirabilis	*Proteus vulgaris*	*Providencia alcalifaciens*	*Providencia rettgeri*	*Providencia stuartii*	*Morganella morganii*
Ornithine decarboxylase	+	−	−	−	−	+
Gas from glucose	+	+	V	−	−	+
H_2S production	+	V	−	−	−	−
Indole formation	−	+	+	+	+	+
Urease formation	+	+	−	+	−	−

+, most strains positive; −, most strains negative; V, variable.

Adapted from Greenwood et *al. Medical Microbiology; A guide to microbial infections: pathogenesis, immunity, laboratory diagnosis and control*. 15th edition (2000) Churchill Livingstone.

Most *P. mirabilis* strains are indole-negative, while the other subspecies are indole-positive (see Table 7.8).

Phage typing, bacteriocin typing, and serotyping schemes have been developed. The Dienes phenomenon may be exploited for typing—two test organisms are viewed as identical if they show no line of demarcation where the swarming growths meet (after inoculation onto the surface of an agar plate).

Treatment

Antibiotic resistance is increasing, but the indole-negative *P. mirabilis* is generally more sensitive than the indole-positive species (e.g. *P. vulgaris*), which may carry inducible AmpC β-lactamase. Amikacin, new quinolones, and carbapenems may be the only options. Note that *Proteus* is inherently resistant to colistimethate sodium, tetracyclines, and nitrofurantoin.

Enterobacter

The genus *Enterobacter* includes *E. aerogenes, E. cloacae, E. sakazakii, E. taylorae, E. gergoviae, E. asburiae, E. hormaechei, E. cancerogenus*, and *E. agglomerans*. The genus was previously known as *Aerobacter* spp. and belongs to the tribe *Klebsiellae*.

Epidemiology

Enterobacter organisms are common human gut commensals, which rarely cause infection in the immunocompetent host.

Clinical features

E. aerogenes and *E. cloacae* (and occasionally *E. taylorae*) colonize hospital inpatients and cause nosocomial opportunistic infections such as wound infections, burn infections, pneumonia, and UTIs. Risk factors for infection include indwelling lines, frequent courses of antibiotics, a recent invasive procedure, diabetes, and neutropenia. They can often be isolated from diabetic ulcers. *Enterobacter* infections have been associated with IV fluid contamination. *E. sakazakii* has been implicated in severe neonatal meningitis (mortality rate 40–80%), and there have been outbreaks associated with dried infant formula.

Diagnosis

In common with the other *Enterobacteriaceae, Enterobacter* spp. are facultative anaerobes that give a positive catalase result and a negative oxidase result. They ferment glucose (with the production of acid and gas) and also lactose. They do not produce H_2S on triple sugar iron media; they are indole-negative and methyl red-negative; they are Voges–Proskauer-positive, and they can grow in the presence of KCN. They use citrate as a sole carbon source and are ONPG-positive. Unlike *Klebsiella*, they are usually motile and are less likely to be heavily capsulated. The two most important clinical species are *E. aerogenes* (which usually decarboxylates lysine, but not arginine) and *E. cloacae* (usually decarboxylates arginine, but not lysine). *Enterobacter* can be identified by biochemical properties (API® 20E), MALDI-TOF, or automated methods.

Treatment

Enterobacter organisms (except *E. sakazakii*) are usually resistant to first-generation cephalosporins, and readily develop resistance to second- and third-generation cephalosporins due to inducible β-lactamases such as AmpC. Carbapenems are the mainstay of treatment; alternatives include ciprofloxacin and aminoglycosides. *E. sakazakii* tends to be more sensitive to antibiotics overall, and ampicillin and gentamicin in combination are the usual treatment of *E. sakazakii* neonatal meningitis.

Citrobacter

C. koseri (formerly *C. diversus*), *C. freundii*, and occasionally *C. amalonaticus* are associated with nosocomial respiratory and urinary tract infections. Their role as primary pathogens or secondary infections/colonizers is debated. *C. koseri* has also been associated with outbreaks of neonatal meningitis.

Pathogenesis

Animal studies on neonatal meningitis showed that pathogenic strains of *C. koseri* were more virulent and had an extra outer membrane protein, compared to non-pathogenic strains.

Clinical features

The clinical significance of isolation of *Citrobacter* spp. from the urinary and respiratory tracts of debilitated hospital patients is often unclear. When isolated from BCs, it is usually one of a number of species present, and such polymicrobial infections are often associated with a poor clinical outcome (probably due to the patient's general debilitated state, rather than the organism's virulence). However, *Citrobacter* is a recognized cause of endocarditis, and, in neonates, *Citrobacter* organisms (particularly *C. koseri*) can cause severe meningitis and brain abscesses.

Diagnosis

Citrobacter is so named because the organisms can grow on Simmons citrate media. They are usually motile, and methyl red-positive and Voges–Proskauer-negative, and slowly hydrolyse urea. They are usually non-lactose fermenters but may appear as late lactose fermenters. *C. freundii* may be mistaken for *Salmonella*, as it produces H_2S. Note there is considerable cross-reactivity with the O antigens of other *Enterobacteriaceae*.

Treatment

Like many of the other *Enterobacteriaceae* that cause nosocomial infections, *Citrobacter* tend to be multiresistant, so reliance on laboratory antimicrobial susceptibility testing is paramount. *C. freundii* has the inducible AmpC β-lactamase. Plasmid-mediated ESBLs are becoming commoner. Treatment options may include aminoglycosides, antipseudomonal penicillins, carbapenems, and quinolones.

Serratia

There are many named species of *Serratia*, which belong to the tribe *Klebsielleae*. *S. marcescens* is the main one that causes human disease. Infections with *S. liquefaciens*, *S. rubidaea*, and *S. odorifera* are very uncommon.

Epidemiology

Unlike the other *Enterobacteriaceae*, *Serratia* is more likely to colonize the respiratory and urinary tracts of hospital patients (rather than the gut). However, in neonates, the GI tract may be the reservoir for cross-contamination. There have been reports of outbreaks in the USA due to contaminated syringes.

Clinical features

Serratia spp. are opportunistic pathogens, particularly in the health-care setting, and cause respiratory and urinary tract infections, bacteraemias, and skin and wound infections. Patients with IVCs and urinary catheters are at increased risk. *Serratia* infections have been associated with contaminated IV therapy and septic arthritis in patients who have had intra-articular injections. *Serratia* also causes endocarditis and osteomyelitis in injecting drug users (IDUs), and cellulitis in patients on haemodialysis.

Diagnosis

Serratia can be recognized by the production of a characteristic red/deep pink pigment. They are slow or non-lactose fermenters, and usually motile. They have the characteristics of *Enterobacteriaceae*. Like *Enterobacter*, most *Serratia* do not produce H_2S or lactose on triple sugar iron media, are Voges–Proskauer-positive, grow in the presence of KCN, and use citrate as a sole carbon source. *Serratia* can be differentiated from the other *Enterobacteriaceae* by the production of an extracellular DNase.

Treatment

Serratia are often multiresistant to antibiotics. Treat according to local epidemiology, until sensitivity results are available. Options are often limited to amikacin, piperacillin–tazobactam, and carbapenems. Efforts focused on good infection control practice, especially handwashing, are vital in reducing horizontal transmission between patients. Note that *Serratia* organisms are inherently resistant to colistimethate sodium.

Salmonella

Salmonellae belong to the family *Enterobacteriaceae*. There are seven subspecies and over 2400 serovars. The correct nomenclature is *Salmonella enterica*, followed by the serotype (e.g. *Salmonella enterica* serotype Typhimurium). This is commonly abbreviated to S. Typhimurium (serotype not italicized).

Epidemiology

Salmonellae are commensals and pathogens of a wide range of domesticated and wild animals. Some species, e.g. S. Typhi and S. Paratyphi, are well adapted to humans and have no other host. Others are more adapted to animals and rarely affect humans, e.g. S. Arizonae and reptiles. In humans, salmonellae can be divided into those that cause enteric fever (S. Typhi and S. Paratyphi) and the non-typhoidal *Salmonella* spp. (NTS). Salmonellae are usually transmitted by the faeco-oral route.

Pathogenesis

- Infection begins with ingestion of organisms in contaminated food and water.
- Salmonellae express an array of distinct fimbriae that help them to adhere to the intestinal wall.
- They also encode a type III secretion system (T3SS) within *Salmonella* pathogenicity island 1 (SPI-1) that is needed for bacteria-mediated endocytosis and intestinal epithelial evasion.
- A number of SPI-1 translocated proteins (SipA, SipC, SopE, and SopE2) promote membrane ruffling and *Salmonella* invasion.
- Salmonellae are also adapted to survival and replication in the intracellular environment.

Clinical features

- Gastroenteritis (➔ see Infectious diarrhoea, pp. 647–9), enteric fever (➔ see Enteric fever, pp. 649–51), bacteraemia and endovascular infection, localized infections, chronic carrier state.
- *Salmonella* bone and joint infections are seen in patients with underlying haemoglobinopathies.
- Salmonellosis in HIV—20- to 100-fold increased risk. More likely to have severe invasive disease (enterocolitis, bacteraemia, meningitis).

Diagnosis

- *S.* Typhi and *S.* Paratyphi are ACDP category 3 organisms.
- Salmonellae are facultative anaerobic GNRs, which grow readily on routine media. Their growth in specialized media is summarized in Table 7.9. They are motile, oxidase-negative, urease-negative non-lactose fermenters.
- Salmonellae possess LPS somatic (O) heat-stable antigens, and flagellar (H) heat-labile antigens. Usually, the H antigens exhibit diphasic variation, so can exist in phases 1 and 2 (see Table 7.10).
- *S.* Typhi, *S.* Paratyphi C, and some strains of *S.* Dublin and *Citrobacter* produce the Vi polysaccharide capsule, which may mask the O antigens. If only the Vi antiserum is positive, heat the bacterial suspension in boiling water to remove the capsule, and test it again using the same antisera. Rough strains, in which the O antigens are absent, tend to cross-agglutinate with different antisera.

Table 7.9 Appearance of *Salmonella* spp. in different media

Agar	*Salmonella* spp.
MacConkey agar	Non-lactose fermenters appear white
CLED (cysteine, lactose, electrolyte-deficient)	Non-lactose fermenters appear blue
DCA (deoxycholate)	Yellow or colourless, often with a dark centre
XLD agar (xylose lysine deoxycholate)	*Salmonella* appear red, some with black centres
SSA (*Salmonella, Shigella*)	Non-lactose fermenters appear colourless, some with black centres
Hektoen agar	*Salmonella* are blue-green. *S.*Typhimurium and others that reduce sulphur produce a black precipitate
Brilliant green agar	Red-pink colonies surrounded by brilliant red zones
Selenite broth	Growth of *Salmonella* results in a cloudy tube
Tetrathionate broth	Tetrathionate-reducing bacteria (*Salmonella* and *Proteus*) can grow

Table 7.10 Antigenic structure of some *Salmonella* spp.

Serotype	O antigen	H (phase 1)	H (phase 2)
Typhi	9,12 (Vi)	d	–
Paratyphi A	1,2,12	a	–
Paratyphi B	1,4,5,12	b	1,2
Paratyphi C	6,7[Vi]	c	1,5
Typhimurium	1,4,5,12	i	1,2
Enteritidis	1,9,12	g,m	1,7
Virchow	6,7	r	1,2
Hadar	6,8	Z10	e,n,x
Heidelberg	1,4,5,12	r	1,2
Dublin	1,9,12 (Vi)	G,p	–

- Most diagnostic laboratories identify the organism as *Salmonella* by biochemical tests (e.g. API® 20E or shorter panel) or MALDI, and partially determine the antigenic structure with different Poly-O and Poly-H antisera (see Table 7.10). This identifies the causes of enteric fever or invasive serotypes.
- All *Salmonella* should be submitted to a reference laboratory for confirmation of the serotype and further epidemiological investigations, as necessary.
- *Salmonella* isolates are notified to PHE automatically via the CoSurv system.

Treatment

- Enteric fever—the first-line treatment for imported cases of typhoid fever in the UK is ceftriaxone. When susceptibility results are available, options may include ciprofloxacin, azithromycin, ampicillin, or co-trimoxazole. Notifiable condition.
- NTS—gastroenteritis does not usually require treatment, except in the immunosuppressed, neonates, the elderly, and those at risk of bacteraemia. Suitable antibiotics may include—ampicillin, ciprofloxacin, trimethoprim, or chloramphenicol, depending on *in vitro* susceptibility.
- Invasive disease due to NTS (e.g. bacteraemia, meningitis)—always requires therapy. Ceftriaxone penetrates the CSF well so may be used for *Salmonella* meningitis. Source of infection should be investigated.
- Chronic asymptomatic carriers. Management of chronic carriers is debated. Good personal hygiene should prevent spread of disease. In the absence of biliary disease, prolonged antibiotics (e.g. ampicillin, ciprofloxacin) may cure 80% of carriers. Cholecystectomy may be considered for patients with gallstones or chronic cholecystitis, but there is a risk of contiguous spread during surgery.

Shigella

The genus *Shigella* is divided into four species: *S. dysenteriae*, *S. flexneri*, *S. boydii*, and *S. sonnei*, based on serology and biochemical reactions (see Table 7.11). The organisms cause bacillary dysentery by an invasive mechanism identical to enteroinvasive *E. coli* (EIEC). *Shigella* belongs to the tribe *Escherichiaeae*, and DNA hybridization studies show that *E. coli* and *Shigella* are a single genetic species.

Epidemiology

There are ten serotypes of *S. dysenteriae* and 15 serotypes of *S. boydii*. *S. flexneri* can be divided into six serotypes by group- and type-specific antigens, and each serotype can be further subdivided. *S. sonnei* must be typed by other means, such as colicine production or plasmids, as they are serologically homogenous. Most cases of shigellosis in the UK occur in young children, although infection occurs in any age after travel to areas where hygiene is poor. *S. sonnei* is endemic in the UK, while *S. boydii* and *S. dysenteriae*, and most *S. flexneri* infections, originate outside the UK.

Pathogenesis

The infecting dose of *Shigella* is only 10–100 organisms—when one member of a family has acquired the disease, the secondary attack rate is high. Infection can spread rapidly in institutions, especially amongst young children. It is commonly spread by food and water. Laboratory-acquired infection has been reported.

Dysentery results from invasion of the wall of the large bowel, with accompanying inflammation and capillary thrombosis. As the organisms invade and multiply within epithelial cells, cell death results in ulcer formation. Shiga toxin (Stx) inhibits protein synthesis within target cells, by a mechanism similar to ricin toxin production. Some strains also produce an exotoxin, which results in water and electrolyte secretion from the small bowel (similar to cholera toxin), which may result in watery diarrhoea preceding bloody diarrhoea.

Table 7.11 Biochemical reactions of *Shigella*

Shigella spp.	Gas from glucose	ONPG	Indole	Catalase	Acid from		
					Lactose	Mannitol	Dulcitol
dysenteriae 1	–	+	–	–	–	–	–
dysenteriae 2–10	–	V	V	+	–	–	–
flexneri 1–5	–	–	V	+	–	+	–
flexneri 6	V	–	–	+	–	V	V
boydii	–	–	V	+	–	+	V
sonnei	–	+	–	+	(+)	+	–

(+), positive after incubation for ≥48h; ONPG, ortho-nitrophenyl-β-*D*-galactopyranoside; V, variable.

Clinical features

- *S. dysenteriae* usually causes a more severe illness, possibly with marked prostration, paediatric febrile convulsions, toxic megacolon, and HUS.
- *S. flexneri* and *S. boydii* may also cause severe disease, while *S. sonnei* usually causes mild symptoms (see Viral gastroenteritis, p. 408).
- *Shigella* rarely invades elsewhere; metastatic infection is unusual.

Diagnosis

Shigella organisms are non-motile, non-capsulated GNRs. Most appear as non-lactose fermenters after 18–24h incubation on MacConkey or DCA (deoxycholate citrate) agar, but *S. sonnei* is a late lactose fermenter. *Shigella* is urease-, citrate-, and H_2S-negative. *S. dysenteriae* is the only species that cannot ferment mannitol. Suspicious colonies should be confirmed with species-specific antisera, followed by type-specific antisera for all, except *S. sonnei*. *S. dysenteriae* type 1 is an ACDP category 3 organism. Note that MALDI cannot reliably differentiate *Shigella* from *E. coli* due to their close relatedness. *Shigella* isolates are notified to PHE automatically via the CoSurv system.

Treatment

Most cases of *Shigella* are mild and self-limiting, so are treated with oral rehydration therapy, rather than with antibiotics. Antibiotics may be indicated in severe infections, patients at extremes of age, or the immunocompromised. Options include ciprofloxacin, ampicillin, co-trimoxazole, tetracycline, or cephalosporins, according to *in vitro* susceptibility testing. Antibiotics are unlikely to reduce the period of excretion.

Other *Enterobacteriaceae*

- *Hafnia alvei* (formerly an *Enterobacter*)—belongs to the tribe *Klebsielleae*. Found in human and animal faeces, sewage, soil, water, and dairy products. Produces greyish colonies on blood agar and ferments fewer sugars than *Enterobacter*. All *H. alvei* are lysed by a single phage, which does not act on any other *Enterobacteriaceae*. *H. alvei* occasionally causes opportunistic/nosocomial infections, and antibiotic sensitivities are usually similar to those of the *Enterobacter* group.
- *Pantoea agglomerans* (previously known as *Enterobacter agglomerans*)—occasionally causes opportunistic infections in humans (UTIs, bacteraemia, and chest infections) and has contaminated IV fluids in the past. May be isolated from superficial skin swabs and respiratory specimens.
- *Edwardsiella tarda*—infections in humans probably originate from contact with cold-blooded animals. Motile, ferment glucose to produce gas. H_2S-positive, and, as non-lactose fermenters, may be mistaken for *Salmonella* spp. on enteric media. *Edwardsiella* spp. rarely cause disease but are occasionally associated with gastroenteritis, which usually resolves without antibiotics. Reports of bacteraemia, liver abscess, soft tissue infection, and meningitis.

- *Morganella morganii*—member of tribe *Proteeae*. Motile, deaminates phenylalanine rapidly, gives positive methyl red reactions, is usually Voges–Proskauer-negative, and can grow in the presence of KCN. Most are indole-positive and hydrolyse urea rapidly (see Table 7.8). *Morganella* organisms cause HAIs, which are often multiresistant, carrying inducible AmpC, so treatment is usually with carbapenems.
- *Providencia alcalifaciens, Providencia stuartii*, and *Providencia rettgeri*—also tribe *Proteeae*. Motile and deaminate phenylalanine rapidly, positive methyl red reactions, usually Voges–Proskauer-negative and indole-positive, grow in the presence of KCN. Most *P. rettgeri* hydrolyse urea rapidly, while the others are urease-negative (see Table 7.8). *Providencia* causes nosocomial infections in debilitated patients, and treatment is with carbapenems.
- *Raoultella*—oxidase-negative, capsulated, GNRs (formerly designated *Klebsiella*), named after the French bacteriologist Didier Raoult. Unlike most *Klebsiella*, they grow at 10°C, consistent with their recovery from plants, soil, and water. Human infections are rare.
- *Kluyvera*—motile GNRs, oxidase-negative, and ferment *D*-glucose with the production of acid and gas. *K. ascorbata* is a potentially virulent pathogen, isolated from various clinical specimens and reports of UTIs, GI infections, soft tissue infections, and bacteraemia. *K. cryocrescens* is an environmental organism. Usually resistant to penicillins and cephalosporins.
- *Elizabethkingia meningoseptica* or *meningosepticum*—colonies grow slowly and are very pale yellow. Found in fresh and salt water, plants, and soil. Initially recognized as a cause of outbreaks of neonatal meningitis. Linked to nosocomial pneumonia, endocarditis, post-operative bacteraemia, and meningitis in immunocompromised adults. Associated with sepsis and soft tissue infection in the immunocompetent. Isolates are usually multiresistant to antibiotics, and co-trimoxazole/fluoroquinolones may be beneficial. Colistimethate sodium resistance and vancomycin sensitivity/intermediate growth is paradoxical for a Gram-negative bacteria.

Overview of Gram-negative rod non-fermenters

These organisms derive energy from carbohydrates by oxidative (rather than fermentative) metabolism.

Pseudomonads

The pseudomonads are a large and diverse group of aerobic, oxidative GNRs. Most are saprophytes found in soil, water, and moist environments. *P. aeruginosa* is the species most commonly associated with human disease, particularly nosocomial infections. Other opportunistic species of *Pseudomonas* include *P. putida, P. fluorescens* (which has been associated with blood transfusions), and *P. stutzeri*. Organisms recently allocated to new genera include *Burkholderia* (*B. cepacia* and *B. pseudomallei*), *Stenotrophomonas* (*S. maltophilia*), *Comamonas* (➔ see *Delftia acidovorans* below), and *Brevundimonas* (➔ see *Brevundimonas* below).

Delftia acidovorans

Formerly known as *Comamonas acidovorans or Pseudomonas acidovorans*, this rare organism may cause endocarditis in drug users. Confusion arises, as it may grow on *B. cepacia*-selective media and may be resistant to colistimethate sodium and gentamicin.

Brevundimonas

Brevundimonas diminuta and *Brevundimonas vesicularis* are rare and of uncertain clinical significance. There are recent reports of bacteraemia in immunocompromised hosts, treated with piperacillin–tazobactam, amikacin, carbapenems, and tigecycline.

Glucose non-fermenters

This diverse group is taxonomically distinct from the oxidative pseudomonads and the carbohydrate-fermenting *Enterobacteriaceae*. They are mainly opportunistic pathogens and often multiresistant to antibiotics. Identification difficulties arise, because they tend to be biochemically inert.

- *Eikenella corrodens*—oral commensal and cause of endocarditis ('E' in HACEK; ➔ see HACEK organisms, pp. 306–8), meningitis, skin and soft tissue infections (particularly human bites), pneumonia. Facultative anaerobe, requiring incubation in CO_2. The colonies pit ('corrode') the surface of the agar.
- *Flavimonas oryzihabitans*—found in soil, water, and damp environments, and may cause line-associated bacteraemias in the immunocompromised.
- *Flavobacterium*—this group of yellow-pigmented organisms is so genetically diverse that many have been reclassified. *Flavobacterium meningosepticum* is now *Elizabethkingia meningoseptica* (➔ see Other *Enterobacteriaceae*, pp. 292–3). Other flavobacteria now belong to the genus *Sphingobacterium* (➔ see *Sphingobacterium* below).
- *Chryseobacterium*—other than *Chryseobacterium meningosepticum* (➔ see *Elizabethkingia meningoseptica*, p. 293), isolation of these organisms from clinical samples usually reflects colonization.
- *Sphingobacterium*—contains high amounts of sphingophospholipid compounds in cell membrane. Most human isolates of this genus are *Sphingobacterium multivorum* and *Sphingobacterium spiritivorum* which can cause nosocomial infections in various sites. Isolation from respiratory samples from CF patients are of uncertain significance.
- *Shewanella*—*Shewanella putrefaciens* (formerly *Pseudomonas putrefaciens*) is commonly isolated from water and the environment, but rarely causes human disease. It is usually found as part of a polymicrobial infection, typically from cellulitis complicating a leg ulcer or burn.
- *Roseomonas*—known as the 'pink-pigmented coccoid' group. *Roseomonas gilardii* is the commonest species isolated from humans and has been reported to cause community-acquired bacteraemia.
- *Chryseomonas*—infection with the rare *Chryseomonas luteola* is usually associated with peritoneal dialysis catheters or indwelling lines, and may result in peritonitis, endocarditis, bacteraemia, or meningitis.

- *Ochrobactrum*—previously called *Achromobacter, Ochrobactrum anthropi* causes nosocomial opportunistic infections, particularly catheter-related bacteraemia.
- *Oligella*—*Oligella urethralis* (formerly *Moraxella urethralis*) is a GU tract commensal, while *Oligella ureolytica* is usually found in patients with long-term indwelling urinary catheters. They are of low pathogenicity.
- *Alcaligenes*—three clinically relevant species: *Alcaligenes xylosoxidans, Alcaligenes faecalis*, and *Alcaligenes piechaudii*. Found in soil and water, and the GI and respiratory tracts of hospital patients. Nosocomial outbreaks have occurred (generally immunocompromised patients) with a wide range of clinical manifestations. *A. xylosoxidans* is often multiresistant; carbapenems or co-trimoxazole may be required.
- *Agrobacterium*—plant pathogens, usually non-pathogenic to humans, with <50 case reports of human disease in the literature.
- *Sphingomonas paucimobilis*—implicated in nosocomial outbreaks associated with contaminated water. It may be confused with flavobacteria, as it produces a non-diffusible yellow pigment.

Pseudomonas aeruginosa

P. aeruginosa is widespread in soil, water, and other moist environments. Hospitalized patients may be colonized with *P. aeruginosa* at moist sites such as the perineum, ear, and axilla. It is a highly successful opportunistic pathogen, especially in the hospital setting. This success is largely due to its resistance to many antibiotics, ability to adapt to a wide range of physical conditions, and minimal nutritional requirements.

Epidemiology

P. aeruginosa is found almost anywhere in the environment, including surface waters, vegetation, and soil. It usually colonizes hospital and domestic sink traps, taps, and drains. It also colonizes moist areas of human skin, leading to 'toe web rot' in soldiers stationed in swampy areas, and otitis externa in divers in saturation chambers.

Pathogenesis

The broad range of conditions caused by *P. aeruginosa* may be explained by the fact that the pathogen is both invasive and toxigenic. *P. aeruginosa* has low intrinsic virulence in man and animals. Infection occurs when host defences are compromised or the skin/mucous membranes are breached (e.g. neutropenia, burns patients, intensive care patients, indwelling devices), or when a relatively large inoculum is introduced directly into the tissues. The process can be divided into three stages: bacterial attachment/colonization, local invasion, and dissemination/systemic disease. Different virulence factors are produced, depending on the site and nature of the infections, and include:

- exotoxins (exotoxin A and exo-enzyme S) and endotoxins (LPS);
- cytotoxic substances—proteases (elastase and alkaline phosphatase (ALP)), cytotoxin (previously called leukocidin), haemolysins, phospholipases, rhamnolipids, pyocyanin;

- porins;
- pili and fimbriae (important in epithelial adherence, e.g respiratory).

Clinical features

P. aeruginosa causes a wide spectrum of conditions.

- Community-acquired infections are rare, and tend to be mild and superficial. Examples include otitis externa, varicose ulcers, and folliculitis associated with jacuzzis.
- Nosocomial infections with *P. aeruginosa* tend to be more severe and more varied than community infections. *P. aeruginosa* may account for ~10% of all HAIs. Examples include pneumonia, UTIs, surgical wound infections, BSIs, and respiratory infections.
- CF patients (see Box 7.5), burns patients, and mechanically ventilated patients are at particular risk.
- Other conditions associated with *P. aeruginosa* include endocarditis (IDUs and prosthetic valves), eye infections, bone and joint infections, post-operative neurosurgical infections, and ear infections.

Diagnosis

Non-sporing, non-capsulate, motile GNR. Strict aerobe (hence often used in testing anaerobic cabinets) but can grow anaerobically in the presence of nitrate. It grows in many different culture media and produces a characteristic 'freshly cut grass' odour. The typical green-blue colour is due to the diffusible pigments pyocyanin (blue phenazine pigment) and pyoverdin (yellow-green fluorescent pigment; principal siderophore). Other pigments include pyorubrin (red) and pyomelanin (brown). Note that ~10% do not produce detectable pigments, even in pigment-enhancing media. *P. aeruginosa* is oxidase-positive (usually within 10s) and appears relatively inactive in carbohydrate fermentation tests (only glucose is used). It grows best at 37°C and also at 42°C, but not at 4°C. Confusion occasionally arises in differentiating *P. aeruginosa* from other *Pseudomonas* spp. with commercial kits—growth at 42°C; flagella stains and differential sugar fermentation tests may prove useful.

Box 7.5 *P. aeruginosa* in CF patients

P. aeruginosa colonizes up to 80% of CF patients and causes chronic lung infection. Once established, it is refractory to treatment, partly due to the formation of biofilms. Many isolates appear mucoid due to the production of an alginate-like exopolysaccharide capsule (glycocalyx) that resists phagocytosis and contributes to biofilm formation. Isolates may have atypical growth requirements such as appearing auxotrophic for specific amino acids and non-motile. Primary culture plates often show mixed colonial forms that are usually genetically identical. Results for susceptibility testing often vary, and CF clinicians may base their choice on multiple factors, including prior response to treatment. Some strains, such as the Liverpool epidemic strain (LES), are transmissible and may be more aggressive. Typing is available, and CF patients colonized with LES may be segregated to prevent transmission.

For epidemiological studies, serotyping may be useful; four 'O serotypes' account for ~50% of clinical and environmental isolates. PFGE may help discriminate between serotypes. VNTR typing is useful for cross-infection and outbreak investigations, and for surveillance among CF patients.

Treatment

Antipseudomonal agents include ciprofloxacin (the only oral option), ceftazidime, ticarcillin, piperacillin, carbapenems, aminoglycosides (gentamicin, tobramycin, amikacin), polymyxins (colistimethate sodium), and aztreonam. Theoretically, the use of dual therapy should reduce the development of antibiotic resistance and may also have the potential for bacterial synergy, but there is little clinical evidence for this.

Acinetobacter

Historically, a pathogen of tropical climates, *Acinetobacter* spp. are an important cause of nosocomial infections. They accumulate multiple antibiotic resistance mechanisms. Increasing antibiotic-selective pressure and the ability to survive well in the environment (including on curtains and in dust) have contributed to its success as an opportunistic pathogen. There are ~19 genospecies, based on DNA–DNA hybridization studies; seven of these have species names (see Table 7.12).

Epidemiology

Acinetobacter has been an increasingly common nosocomial pathogen since the 1970s, affecting debilitated patients. Infections tend to peak in the summer, and are associated with wars and natural disasters. Nosocomial spread in ICUs is common, and may occur via fomites, the environment, and colonized HCWs. Dramatic multi-hospital outbreaks have occurred. Colonization of British military casualties repatriated to the UK from Iraq and Afghanistan has caused infections and onward transmission to other hospitalized patients. In the UK, there have been outbreaks of two multiresistant clones carrying carbapenem-hydrolysing class D β-lactamases (OXA-23 and OXA-51). These are now widespread.

Table 7.12 Genomic species of *Acinetobacter*

Genospecies	Species name
1	*A. calcoaceticus*
2	*A. baumannii*
4	*A. haemolyticus*
5	*A. junii*
7	*A. johnsonii*
8	*A. lwoffi*
12	*A. radioresistens*
Other	*Acinetobacter* spp. unnamed (>14)

Risk factors

Risk factors include:

- community-acquired infections—alcoholics, smokers, chronic lung disease, diabetes, and living in a tropical, developing country;
- HAIs—ICU, ventilation, urinary catheter, IV lines, length of stay, treatment with broad-spectrum antibiotics, TPN, surgery, wounds.

Pathogenesis

This organism has very few virulence factors, which explains why it only causes opportunistic infections. It occurs naturally as a saprophyte in soil and water, and occasionally colonizes moist human skin. The ability to survive in the environment is probably related to the capsule, the production of bacteriocin, and prolonged viability under dry conditions.

Clinical features

Acinetobacter spp. are able to infect almost every organ system, though it is vital to distinguish true infection from pseudo-infection (e.g. pseudo-bacteraemia due to skin colonization). The commonest site of infection is the respiratory tract where it causes nosocomial pneumonia, particularly VAP, adult CAP, and community-acquired tracheobronchitis and bronchiolitis in children. Other sites include the urinary tract, intracranial (usually post-neurosurgery), soft tissue (burns, wounds, and device-associated cellulitis), eye infections, endocarditis, and bone. Nosocomial bacteraemia is usually associated with the respiratory tract or IV catheters, and has a reported mortality rate of 17–46%. *A. baumannii* bacteraemia tends to be more severe.

Diagnosis

Acinetobacter spp. classically appear as Gram-negative coccobacilli, although they may retain crystal violet so appear Gram-positive. They are generally encapsulated, non-motile organisms, which readily grow on routine media as white, mucoid, oxidase-negative, catalase-positive colonies. Misidentification may arise using API profiles, as they are biochemically relatively unreactive, but acidification of glucose, haemolysis of RBCs, and ability to grow at 44°C are more reliable characteristics.

Treatment

- International surveillance systems (e.g. MYSTIC) have observed increasing resistance. In 2009, 61% of isolates were resistant to ceftazidime, 86% to carbapenems. Carbapenem susceptibility may be discordant (e.g. imipenem-susceptible, meropenem-resistant). Polymyxins (e.g. colistimethate sodium) usually have activity, but resistance occurs. Susceptibility testing should include carbapenems, aminoglycosides (including amikacin), sulbactam, polymyxins, e.g. colistimethate sodium, and tigecycline. There is some evidence to support combination therapy with rifampicin and colistimethate sodium ± carbapenem.
- 'Multidrug resistance' is generally defined as non-susceptibility to at least one agent in three or more antibiotic classes.
- Empirical treatment might include a combination of a cephalosporin or carbapenem with a fluoroquinolone, aminoglycoside, or colistimethate sodium if local resistance rates are high.

- Once susceptibility is known, the usual rules of antibiotic stewardship should apply (i.e. the narrowest-spectrum effective agent)—there are no data to demonstrate that combination therapy reduces the emergence of resistance.
- Inhaled/neb colistimethate sodium may be useful in pneumonia, and intrathecal or intraventricular administration in meningitis caused by highly resistant strains. IV colistimethate sodium achieves low lung and CSF concentrations.
- Involve reference laboratory and infection control team as appropriate.

Prevention

For the full 2006 PHE prevention guidance, web search 'PHE *Acinetobacter* prevention'.

Stenotrophomonas maltophilia

Previously called *Pseudomonas maltophilia* or *Xanthomonas maltophilia*, this organism is a cause of nosocomial infection. It is an opportunistic pathogen of relatively low virulence but has an amazing ability to survive in a wide range of environments. It is inherently resistant to most antibiotics.

Epidemiology

Ubiquitous in the environment, *S. maltophilia* has been isolated from multiple sources in hospitals, including water (tap and distilled), nebulizers, dialysis machines, solutions, IV fluids, thermometers, etc. Transmission of nosocomial infections has been associated with hospital water or contaminated disinfectant solutions. Studies have shown that most outbreaks result from antibiotic-selective pressure (especially the extensive use of carbapenems, to which *S. maltophilia* is intrinsically resistant) and exposure to multiple environmental strains, rather than cross-infection.

Risk factors

Risk factors for nosocomial infections include: intensive care, increased length of stay, treatment with broad-spectrum antibiotics, malignancy (especially if immunosuppressed), instrumentation (e.g. urinary catheter, IV lines, intubation, TPN, CAPD), patients with COPD, and neutropenia.

Pathogenesis

Potential virulence factors include those involved in adherence to plastics, and production of exoenzymes such as elastase and gelatinase.

Clinical features

S. maltophilia can cause a variety of infections, ranging from superficial to deep tissue to disseminated disease. It is most commonly isolated from the respiratory tract, and distinguishing true infection from colonization can be difficult. *S. maltophilia* pneumonia has a high mortality rate, especially when associated with bacteraemia or GI obstruction. Other common sites of *S. maltophilia* infection include skin and soft tissues, intra-abdominal, the urinary tract, the eyes (especially in contact lens wearers), and device-related infections. Endocarditis is also reported.

Diagnosis

A motile, non-lactose-fermenting GNR that grows readily on standard media. It is a strict aerobe. It is often pale yellow on blood agar, with an ammonia-like smell. Most are oxidase-negative, catalase-positive, and DNase-positive, and can hydrolyse aesculin and ONPG. It is the only pseudomonad that gives a positive lysine decarboxylase reaction. Resistance to a carbapenem may be a useful marker. Note that *S. maltophilia* is increasingly isolated from sputum from patients with CF. It grows well on colistimethate sodium-containing media so may be misidentified as *B. cepacia*.

Treatment

Unfortunately, results of antibiotic susceptibility testing correlate poorly with treatment outcome. The drug of choice is co-trimoxazole. Other options to consider include ticarcillin–clavulanic acid, doxycycline, minocycline, newer-generation quinolones, and third-generation cephalosporins. There is clinical evidence that co-trimoxazole and moxifloxacin may be synergistic. Most strains are resistant to aminoglycosides.

Burkholderia cepacia complex

Previously classified as *Pseudomonas cepacia*, these opportunistic pathogens are a particular problem in CF patients. Other risk factors for infection include chronic granulomatous disease and sickle-cell haemoglobinopathies. There are at least 18 different phylogenetically similar, but genomically distinct, species (termed genomovars) in the *B. cepacia* complex. Most important are *B. cepacia, B. multivorans*, and *B. cenocepacia* (genomovars I, II, III, respectively). The prevalence of each varies with geographic region.

Epidemiology

Members of the complex are found in the natural environment and have been isolated from multiple sources in hospitals. Environmental transmission may occur via contact with respiratory equipment, water supplies, or disinfectants. However, transmission between colonized patients to other CF patients is more significant, and patients should be segregated into separate groups (e.g. for outpatient clinics and summer camps). This can be a highly emotive issue. Patient-to-patient transmission is commonest with *B. cenocepacia* but has also been reported for *B. multivorans* and *B. dolosa*. The epidemiology within CF units has changed as a result of segregation—*B. cenocepacia* has declined in many European units, and *B. multivorans* (now commonest) strains acquired by patients are genotypically unrelated, suggesting an environmental source, rather than patient-to-patient transmission.

Pathogenesis

These organisms can survive in a wide range of environments. Virulence factors include adherence to plastics, production of elastase, gelatinase, adhesin (a mucin-binding protein), siderophores, flagella, efflux pumps, haemolysin, exopolysaccharide, quorum-sensing systems, and metalloproteases. Resistance to non-oxidative neutrophil killing may be important.

Clinical features

Genomovars II and III are the commonest causes of *B. cepacia* colonization in CF patients. The three main patterns of infection are:

- chronic asymptomatic carriage;
- progressive deterioration over months, with frequent hospital admissions, recurrent fevers, and weight loss in a similar manner to *P. aeruginosa*;
- necrotizing pneumonia and bacteraemia, associated with rapid deterioration, which is nearly always fatal. Risk factors for this pattern include females with poor lung function and severe CXR changes ('cepacia syndrome')—particularly associated with *B. dolosa, B. multivorans*, and *B. cenocepacia*;
- pre-lung transplant colonization is associated with high post-transplant mortality. This effect is most pronounced with *B. cenocepacia*. A small study suggested 1-year survival of 29%, compared to 89% in those colonized with other genomovars (and 92% in this *cepacia*-free). Death in the early post-transplant period may be characterized by cepacia syndrome. Abscess and empyema are later complications.

In other patients, *Burkholderia* spp. can cause a range of other infections, from superficial to deep tissue to dissemination disease, but these are rare.

Diagnosis

Burkholderia spp. are motile, non-lactose fermenting, aerobic GNRs. Selective media are necessary for culture. MALDI and commercial systems or kits should not be used to identify members of the *B. cepacia* complex. Colistimethate sodium resistance may be a useful indicator. Identification can be difficult and should be confirmed by molecular (genotypic) methods at a reference laboratory because of the implications for the patient and infection control. For further information, see the Cystic Fibrosis Trust 2010 guideline *Laboratory standards for processing microbiological samples from people with cystic fibrosis* (available at ☞ www.cysticfibrosis.org.uk/about-cf/publications).

Treatment

B. cepacia complex members show high rates of resistance to antipseudomonal antibiotics, including colistimethate sodium. Agents, such as co-trimoxazole, chloramphenicol, minocycline, and carbapenems, show good *in vitro* activity against *Burkholderia* spp. However, there are limited clinical data on the best approach to treatment. Clearance of some drugs is increased in the CF population which may make dosing difficult. Use of combination therapy is debated, but, in general, two or more drugs with *in vitro* activity are used. Synergy has not been consistently demonstrated clinically or *in vitro*—the aim is to reduce the development of resistance. Note that all *Burkholderia* spp. are constitutively resistant to colistin, and many become multiresistant on treatment. Commonly used combinations include meropenem with ceftazidime or tobramycin.

Burkholderia gladioli

Formerly known as *Pseudomonas marginata* and closely related to *B. cepacia* complex. Can be distinguished from the other *Burkholderia* microbiologically, because it is oxidase-negative. An opportunistic pathogen in CF and associated with a poor outcome.

Burkholderia pseudomallei—ACDP 3

B. pseudomallei (formerly known as *Pseudomonas pseudomallei*) causes melioidosis, which is endemic in parts of South East Asia, Northern Australia, and the Caribbean. It is a major cause of community-onset septicaemia in North East Thailand.

Epidemiology

In endemic areas, *B. pseudomallei* can be cultured from moist soil, surface water (rice paddies), and the surface of many fruit and vegetables. Rodents carry it.

Pathogenesis

B. pseudomallei can survive and multiply within phagocytes; hence, a long course of antibiotics is recommended, and antibiotics active *in vitro* do not always lead to clinical cure.

Clinical features

B. pseudomallei is usually acquired through inhaling contaminated particles or cutaneously through skin abrasions. It can infect almost any organ. Manifestations range from subclinical infection to pneumonia (may cavitate with profound weight loss, resembling TB), skin ulcers/abscesses, genital infection and prostatitis, bone and joint infection, encephalomyelitis, or overwhelming septicaemia. Parotid infection occurs in children. May present years after exposure, due to the intracellular nature of the organism.

Diagnosis

- *B. pseudomallei* is a Hazard group 3 organism. All specimens should be handled in CL3 if melioidosis is suspected clinically.
- Samples—if case suspected, culture blood, sputum, urine, throat, and rectal swabs, as well as any lesion/pus.
- Gram staining—may show small bipolar GNRs.
- Culture—grows well on blood or Ashdown medium nutrient agar, after 1–2 days. They appear either wrinkled and dry, or mucoid, and, after prolonged incubation, may turn orange. A strict aerobe, and oxidizes glucose and breaks down arginine. The API 20NE reliably identifies most isolates. Characteristically resistant to gentamicin and colistimethate sodium.
- Early involvement of the reference laboratory is recommended for confirmatory tests, e.g. PCR, IgM- and IgG-specific ELISAs, serology (but note there are problems with sensitivity and specificity).

Treatment

Even mild disease should be treated intensively. The first 14 days should be with an IV agent (ceftazidime or a carbapenem) or longer if clinical improvement is slow. This should be followed by at least 3 months' oral therapy to prevent relapse (6 months for bone or neurological infection). Co-trimoxazole is preferred. Co-amoxiclav is an alternative—but less effective. Note that resistance to these oral agents may develop during treatment; seek expert advice.

B. mallei causes glanders, which is a rare disease of horses in Asia, Africa, and the Middle East. It is a Hazard group 3 organism but has not been isolated in the UK since the 1940s. In humans, it causes symptoms similar to melioidosis.

Overview of fastidious Gram-negative rods

These organisms often require specialist supplementation or media for culture. They can be divided by appearance on Gram stain as follows:

- Coccobacilli:
  - *Haemophilus*;
  - HACEK organisms;
  - *Gardnerella*;
  - *Bordetella*;
  - *Brucella*;
  - *Yersinia*;
  - *Pasteurella*;
  - *Francisella*.
- Rods with pointed ends:
  - *Legionella*;
  - *Capnocytophaga*.
- Curved rods:
  - *Vibrio*;
  - *Aeromonas, Plesiomonas*;
  - *Campylobacter*;
  - *Helicobacter*.

Streptobacillus moniliformis causes rat bite fever, as does *Spirillium minor*.

Haemophilus influenzae

H. influenzae is a small, fastidious Gram-negative coccobacillus, belonging to the family *Pasteurellaceae*. It is highly adapted to humans and found in the nasopharynx of 75% of healthy children and adults.

Epidemiology

Polysaccharide encapsulated (serotypes a–f) and non-encapsulated 'non-typeable' strains. Droplet transmission. *H. influenzae* serotype b (Hib) used to be a common cause of invasive infections in children, including meningitis, septic arthritis, and epiglottitis. The annual incidence of invasive Hib disease dropped dramatically after the introduction of the Hib conjugate vaccine in 1993. The lack of a toddler booster saw the incidence rising due to waning immunity and rising cases from 1999. Booster vaccination to those under 4 years old from 2004 saw a reduction in invasive disease across all age groups, as carriage fell.

Pathogenesis

H. influenzae inhabits the upper respiratory tract of humans; 25–80% of healthy people carry non-capsulated organisms, while 5–10% carry capsulated strains (~50% of which are capsular type b). In addition to the polysaccharide capsule that facilitates invasion, virulence factors of capsular type b include fimbriae (involved in attaching to epithelial cells), IgA proteases (aid colonization), and OMPs (involved in invasion). There is evidence that simultaneous viral infection may initiate invasion. Other serotypes and unencapsulated strains are rarely invasive but can cause pneumonia or severe disease in high-risk groups.

Clinical features

- Invasive infections, e.g. meningitis, epiglottitis, bacteraemia with no clear focus, septic arthritis, pneumonia, cellulitis. Mostly caused by capsular type b. Types e and f and non-capsulated strains may also cause serious disease. Infections generally occur between 2 months and 2 years of age, as babies <2 months are protected by maternal antibody.
- Non-invasive infections, e.g. otitis media, sinusitis, endometritis, purulent exacerbations of COPD. These local infections are usually associated with non-capsulated organisms. There may be an underlying abnormality (anatomical or physiological). Intercurrent viral infection may precipitate an infection.

Diagnosis

- Culture—growth in the presence of X (haemin) and V (nicotinamide adenine dinucleotide (phosphate), NAD(P)) factors. X is needed to synthesize certain respiratory enzymes that contain iron (e.g. cytochrome c, cytochrome oxidase, catalase, peroxidase). V is required for oxidation–reduction processes in metabolism. Blood agar (BA) contains both X and V, but *H. influenzae* grows poorly. NAD supplementation improves growth on BA, as will streaking an organism that excretes NAD, e.g. *S. aureus*—this phenomenon is called *satellitism*. *H. influenzae* grows well on chocolate agar, which is made by heating BA at 70–80°C for a few minutes to inactivate the NADase which normally limits utilization of V factor. Growth is also better in CO_2-enriched conditions. Antibiotic susceptibility testing with discs may be unreliable—nitrocefin strips are recommended to test for β-lactamases. Oxidase-positive.
- Antigen detection, e.g. latex agglutination. Beware of cross-reactions with *S. pneumoniae* and *E. coli*. Culture is needed for confirmation. Molecular tests, e.g. PCR, are available.

- Capsule detection—encapsulated strains of *H. influenzae* are responsible for most invasive infections (e.g. meningitis and epiglottitis), while respiratory infections and otitis media are usually associated with non-encapsulated strains. The polysaccharide capsule can be demonstrated by the Quellung reaction with type-specific antisera.
- Antigenic type—there are six antigenic types (a–f). Hib causes the most severe invasive infections.
- Biotypes—there are eight biotypes of *H. influenzae* (I–VIII), based on indole, ornithine decarboxylase, and urease reactions. The commonest are biotypes I–III, and the most invasive (type b) organisms are biotype I.

Treatment

- Severe infection—first line: third-generation cephalosporins, e.g. ceftriaxone. Bactericidal, penetrate the CSF and are clinically effective. Alternatives include co-trimoxazole, ampicillin (but ~20% of UK type b strains produce a β-lactamase), or chloramphenicol.
- Non-invasive infection—PO ampicillin (~20% of UK non-capsulated strains are β-lactamase-positive), co-amoxiclav, or azithromycin.
- BLNAR (β-lactamase-negative ampicillin-resistant) *H. influenzae* are becoming increasingly recognized worldwide. The mechanism of resistance is altered PBPs. β-lactamase is absent phenotypically, but the ampicillin MIC ≥4mg/L. They are usually sensitive to ceftriaxone.

Prevention

- Vaccine—Hib conjugate vaccine (capsular polysaccharide and protein) was introduced in the UK in 1992. Now given at 2, 3, 4, and 12 months. The impact of vaccination far exceeded that predicted, due to the added benefit of herd immunity. Give to unimmunized contacts of index cases. For detailed information about the use of the Hib vaccine, web search 'UK *Green Book* HIB'.
- Chemoprophylaxis—only required if the index case is confirmed or probable and under 10 years of age, or there is a vulnerable individual in the household (ideally within 48h, but up to 4 weeks after index diagnosis). Preferred agent is rifampicin. Reduces carriage and onward transmission. May be considered for close contacts in school outbreaks. For full details, see PHE 2013 guidance *Revised recommendations for the prevention of secondary Haemophilus influenzae type b (Hib) disease*.

Other *Haemophilus* species

Haemophilus spp., other than *H. influenzae*, have been considered rare causes of human disease in the past. However, they may cause infections more commonly than was previously believed. Most are normal flora of the human mouth and upper respiratory tract. They may be associated with infections such as endocarditis, respiratory tract infections, septicaemia, brain abscess, meningitis, and soft tissue infections.

Haemophilus parainfluenzae

H. parainfluenzae is increasingly recognized as a cause of human infection. Clinical infections are similar to those caused by *H. influenzae*, but *H. parainfluenzae* tends to be less virulent. *H. parainfluenzae* has been reported as a cause of pharyngitis, epiglottitis, otitis media, conjunctivitis, dental abscess, pneumonia, empyema, septicaemia, endocarditis, septic arthritis, osteomyelitis, meningitis, abscesses, and urinary and genital tract infections. *H. parainfluenzae* differs from *H. influenza*, in that it is V factor-dependent only.

Haemophilus haemolyticus and *Haemophilus parahaemolyticus*

It is commonly thought that these species rarely cause human disease. However, standard methods do not reliably distinguish *H. haemolyticus* from *H. influenzae*, so it may be commoner than previously considered.

Aggregatibacter aphrophilus

The species *Haemophilus aphrophilus, Haemophilus paraphrophilus*, and *Haemophilus segnis* have been reclassified as a single species *Aggregatibacter aphrophilus*—together with *Actinobacillus actinomycetemcomitans*. Organisms require CO_2 for growth, and are independent of X factor and variably dependent on V factor for growth. They cause a variety of infections, including sinusitis, otitis media, pneumonia, empyema, bacteraemia, endocarditis, septic arthritis, osteomyelitis, meningitis, abscesses, and wound infections

Haemophilus ducreyi

This causes chancroid, an STI, common in Africa and South East Asia. It presents as a painful penile ulcer associated with inguinal lymphadenopathy. Microbiological diagnosis may be made when Gram-negative coccobacilli are isolated from a lymph node aspirate or from ulcer swabs. Microscopy is classically described as a 'shoal of fish' appearance. Treatment options include tetracyclines, erythromycin, and co-amoxiclav.

Haemophilus influenzae biogroup *aegyptius*

H. influenzae biogroup *aegyptius* was previously known as *Haemophilus aegyptius* or the Koch–Weeks bacillus. It is very similar biochemically to *H. influenzae* biotype III but can be differentiated by PCR. It causes Brazilian purpuric fever (conjunctivitis leading to fulminant septicaemia, with a high mortality) and epidemic purulent conjunctivitis. Combination therapy with ampicillin and chloramphenicol is usually recommended.

HACEK organisms

The HACEK organisms (see Box 7.6) are rare causes of endocarditis (➔ see Infective endocarditis, pp. 630–2), which tends to be insidious in onset (mean time to diagnosis ~3 months). Most are part of normal human mouth flora and are occasionally associated with periodontitis and infections elsewhere (e.g. joints). They grow slowly and may need prolonged incubation (14 days) in CO_2 supplementation. High index of suspicion and close liaison with the laboratory are crucial.

Box 7.6 The HACEK organisms

- *Haemophilus influenzae*
- *Haemophilus parainfluenzae*
- *Haemophilus parahaemolyticus*
- *Aggregatibacter aphrophilus*
- *Aggregatibacter segnis*
- *Aggregatibacter actinomycetemcomitans*
- *Cardiobacterium hominis*
- *Eikenella corrodens*
- *Kingella kingae*

Aggregatibacter actinomycetemcomitans

A mouth commensal and major pathogen of the genus *Aggregatibacter*. There are two other *Aggregatibacter* spp.: *A. aphrophilus* (includes *H. aphrophilus* and *H. paraphrophilus*) and *A. segnis* (formerly *H. segnis*).

- Diagnosis—difficult to culture. Fastidious and grows slowly, so BCs should be incubated for at least 14 days. Growth is enhanced by CO_2 supplementation (5–10%). *Aggregatibacter* may form 'granules' in BCs or broth (the media remains clear). On Gram stain, often look coccoid or coccobacillary, resembling *Haemophilus*. Urease-negative, indole-negative, catalase-positive, and reduces nitrate. Do not grow on MacConkey and are biochemically similar to *Pasteurella* spp.
- Pathogenesis—periodontal disease is associated with the ability to invade and multiply within gingival epithelial cells and the production of a leucotoxin that lyses neutrophils. Other potential virulence factors include a bacteriocin, endotoxin, chemotaxis-inhibiting factor, and fibroblast-inhibiting factor.
- Clinical—can cause endocarditis, joint infections, and severe periodontal disease. Has been found (together with some *Haemophilus* spp., fusiforms, and anaerobic streptococci) in actinomycotic lesions.
- Treatment—usually susceptible to third-generation cephalosporins (4 weeks for native, and 6 weeks for prosthetic, valve endocarditis). Periodontitis requires debridement with antibiotic treatment (e.g. tetracyclines).

Cardiobacterium hominis

C. hominis is the only species in the genus. It is normal flora in the human mouth, nose, and throat, and occasionally other mucous membranes and the GI tract. Unlike the other HACEK organisms, it rarely causes diseases other than endocarditis.

- Diagnosis—GNR with a pleomorphic appearance and may be difficult to decolorize during Gram staining. Culture is enhanced in 5–10% CO_2 and high humidity. It grows well on blood agar and chocolate, with slight β-haemolysis, but poorly on MacConkey agar. It is catalase-negative and oxidase-positive. It produces indole (although positivity is weak with many strains), which helps differentiate it from other HACEK organisms.

- Treatment—sensitivity testing is difficult, because of the slow growth, but it is usually susceptible to β-lactams, tetracycline, and chloramphenicol. However, a β-lactamase-producing isolate that was also resistant to cefotaxime has been reported. Hence, the current first-line recommendation of ceftriaxone for HACEK organisms may not be optimal for *C. hominis* endocarditis—an alternative regimen to consider is co-amoxiclav and gentamicin.

Eikenella corrodens

E. corrodens exists as normal mouth and upper respiratory tract flora.

- Diagnosis—facultative anaerobic GNR. Oxidase-positive, catalase-negative, urease-negative, indole-negative, and reduces nitrate to nitrite. About 50% of strains create a depression in the agar ('corroding bacillus'). As with the other HACEK organisms, culture is slow and enhanced in 5–10% CO_2.
- Clinical features—subacute endocarditis, but is more commonly found as part of mixed infections (e.g. human bite wounds, head and neck infections, respiratory tract infections). It often coexists with *Streptococcus* spp. Infections are usually indolent, taking >1 week from time of injury to clinical symptoms of disease. Suppuration is common and may smell like an anaerobic infection.
- Treatment—usually susceptible to the β-lactams, tetracyclines, and fluoroquinolones. It is uniformly resistant to clindamycin, erythromycin, and metronidazole, and often resistant to aminoglycosides.

Kingella kingae

There are four species of *Kingella*, which all colonize the respiratory tract and rarely cause human disease: *K. kingae* (previously known as *Moraxella kingae*), *K. indologenes* (now known as *Suttonella indologenes*), *K. denitrificans*, and *K. oralis*. *K. kingae* is the commonest, and a recent increase in cases is likely to be due to increased awareness of the organism and improved diagnostics.

- Diagnosis—misidentified as *Moraxella* or *Neisseria* in the past. They are short GNRs with tapered ends, which sometimes appear coccoid. They tend to resist decolorization, so may look Gram-positive. *Kingella* is catalase-negative, oxidase-positive, and urease-negative, and ferments glucose. *K. kingae* grows on blood and chocolate agar, but not MacConkey. To increase the chance of recovering *K. kingae* from joint fluid, the fluid should be inoculated into BC bottles, rather than just plated out directly onto agar plates.
- Clinical features—most cases of invasive disease occur in children aged between 6 months and 4 years. *K. kingae* most commonly causes bacteraemia, endocarditis (of native and prosthetic valves), and septic arthritis. *K. indologenes* and *K. denitrificans* also cause endocarditis. *K. oralis* is found in dental plaque, but its relationship with periodontal disease is unknown.
- Treatment—most *Kingella* spp. appear susceptible to penicillins and cephalosporins; however, a β-lactamase-producing isolate of *K. kingae* has been reported. Alternatives include aminoglycosides, co-trimoxazole, tetracyclines, erythromycin, and quinolones.

Gardnerella

Gardnerella vaginalis is found in the female genital tract and is associated with bacterial vaginosis (BV)/non-specific vaginitis (➔ see Bacterial vaginosis, pp. 695–7). It is usually classified with GNRs, although it is normally susceptible to vancomycin. Of interest, electron microscopy (EM) studies have noted the cell wall to be either Gram-negative or Gram-positive, or to show an atypical laminated appearance.

Epidemiology

There is debate whether specific biotypes have been associated with BV. Newly acquired strains of *G. vaginalis* may precipitate BV, rather than overgrowth of previously colonizing biotypes.

Pathogenesis

Adherence of *G. vaginalis* to vaginal and urinary epithelial cells may play a role in the pathogenesis of BV and UTIs. Pili have been seen on *G. vaginalis*, and haemagglutinating activity has been shown. *G. vaginalis* also produces a cytolytic toxin (haemolysin). It is serum-resistant, which may aid survival during bloodstream invasion at childbirth.

Clinical features

- BV—*G. vaginalis* is almost universally present in women with BV, along with mixed anaerobic flora.
- UTI—*G. vaginalis* is isolated from <1% of UTIs and, because of its presence in the female genital tract, could represent vaginal contamination. However, it has been found from suprapubic aspirates, and also in association with renal disease and interstitial cystitis.
- Bacteraemia—this rare event is associated with female genital tract conditions such as chorioamnionitis, post-partum endometritis, and septic abortion. Neonatal infection has also been reported.

Diagnosis

Gardnerella is a facultative anaerobe, which appears as a pleomorphic Gram-variable rod. It is oxidase- and catalase-negative, non-encapsulated, and non-motile. It needs enriched media for growth. It is also urease-, indole-, and nitrate-negative. Note that *G. vaginalis* is susceptible to sodium polyanetholesulfonate (SPS), which is found in most BC bottles, so bacteraemia figures may be underestimated. In clinical practice, BV is diagnosed using the Amsel criteria.

Treatment

G. vaginalis is usually susceptible to penicillin, clindamycin, and vancomycin, and resistant to colistimethate sodium, cefalexin, and tetracyclines. Metronidazole is usually the preferred treatment for BV. See the *UK National Guideline for the management of bacterial vaginosis 2012* (available at ➚ www.bashh.org/documents/4413.pdf).

Bordetella

B. pertussis and *B. parapertussis* cause whooping cough, which is a notifiable disease in England and Wales. The other species only cause human infections under special circumstances—these are *B. bronchiseptica* (causes kennel cough in dogs and snuffles in rabbits), *B. avium* (bird pathogen), *B. hinzii*, *B. holmesii*, and *B. trematum*.

Epidemiology

The organism is spread by droplet infection and is highly infectious. Pertussis has the highest incidence in infants but also occurs in adolescents and adults. Morbidity and mortality are higher in females than males and in those <6 months old. In the UK, pertussis displays 3- to 4-yearly peaks in activity.

Pathogenesis

B. pertussis produces a number of biologically active substances that are thought to play a role in disease:

- surface components, e.g. filamentous haemagglutinin (FHA), pertactin, and fimbriae;
- toxins such as pertussis toxin (PT), adenylate cyclase toxin (ACT), tracheal cytotoxin (TCT), and dermonecrotic toxin (DNT);
- other products, e.g. tracheal colonization factor and BrKA (*Bordetella* resistance to killing).

Clinical features

- Incubation of 7–10 days is followed by a 'catarrhal stage' similar to a viral URTI. Fever is unusual. Cough gradually worsens over 1–2 weeks.
- A 'paroxysmal stage' follows. In children, there may be distinctive whoops, gagging, cyanosis, conjunctival haemorrhage, and vomiting. These are most bothersome at night. Lasts for 2–8 weeks. Symptoms are less severe in vaccinated children and adults in whom prolonged cough may be the only symptom.

Diagnosis

- Microscopy—tiny coccobacilli, occur singly or in pairs. *B. pertussis* and *B. parapertussis* are non-motile.
- Culture—on Bordet–Genou agar, pearly colonies on days 3–4; CCBA agar (charcoal cephalexin), *B. pertussis* produces glistening greyish white colonies, *B. parapertussis* colonies are larger and duller, and become visible sooner. Does not grow on nutrient agar and grows poorly on BA. Culture lacks sensitivity.
- Molecular—PCR for toxin promoter or insertion sequence IS481 (occurs in *B. pertussis*, *B. holmesii*, and some *B. bronchiseptica*). Consider reference laboratory confirmation (per nasal swab or NPA) in cases of compatible respiratory illness in a child <12 months on paediatric intensive care unit (PICU) or paediatric ward.
- Serology—anti-PT IgG antibody levels are determined using an EIA, on paired sera or single samples taken >2 weeks after onset for any individuals with prolonged cough.

Treatment

- Whooping cough is a notifiable condition.
- Recommended for children with clinical pertussis (even in the absence of laboratory diagnosis) or asymptomatic with a positive PCR for the purposes of reducing transmission. Treatment has to be early (within 7 days of symptoms) to decrease severity, thus is of limited help in the paroxysmal phase—it does, however, eliminate carriage. Patients are most contagious in the catarrhal phase and first 2 weeks of cough.
- Adults can be considered for treatment if symptoms are under 2 weeks, or if cough persists after 4 weeks, particularly if they are in one of the priority groups mentioned under the point *Antibiotic prophylaxis* below.
- Usual agents are clarithromycin or azithromycin for 7 days. Co-trimoxazole for 14 days is an alternative.
- Antibiotic prophylaxis—a 2007 Cochrane review concluded there was insufficient evidence to determine the benefit of prophylactic treatment of pertussis contacts. UK guidelines recommend offering prophylaxis to close contacts of an index case if disease onset was within 21 days AND one of the contacts belongs to a priority group—in which case, all close contacts should be offered treatment. Priority groups include those under 1 year who have received <3 doses of pertussis vaccine, pregnant women, HCWs working with infants and pregnant women, and those who work, or share a house, with an infant under 4 months of age (and thus not fully vaccinated). See *HPA guidelines for the public health management of pertussis* (October 2012) and *Information for healthcare workers exposed to whooping cough* (June 2013) on the PHE website.

Vaccine

- Acellular pertussis (aP) vaccine is given in the primary immunization course as DTaP/IPV/Hib, at ages 2, 3, and 4 months. A further booster as dTaP–IPV is given with preschool boosters, as vaccine immunity wanes over time. There were major epidemics of whooping cough in 1977/1979 and 1981/1983, after immunization coverage dropped from >80% to 30%, following a report linking the vaccine to brain damage.
- A national outbreak in the UK in 2011/2012 affected all age groups, including infants <3 months of age. An enhanced surveillance scheme was set up, and pertussis immunization offered to pregnant women to protect infants from birth.

Brucella—ACDP 3

Brucella spp. (see Table 7.13) cause brucellosis (undulant fever, Mediterranean fever, Malta fever) and contagious/infectious abortion in cattle. This zoonosis is transmitted via contaminated or untreated milk and milk derivatives, or direct contact with infected animals or their carcasses. *Brucella* spp. survive well in aerosols and resist drying, so are candidates for agents of bioterrorism (➔ see Bioterrorism, pp. 846–8).

Table 7.13 Main species of *Brucella*—note that the host relationship is not absolute, and man and domestic animals may be susceptible to infections by different species

Brucella spp.	Animal infected	Human manifestations
B. abortus	Cattle; bison and elk in North America	Brucellosis
B. suis	Pigs (swine brucellosis)	Brucellosis
B. melitensis	Goats/sheep	Brucellosis
B. canis	Dogs (mainly beagles in the USA)	Mild disease only
B. ovis	Sheep (Australia and New Zealand)	No evidence this species infects man

Epidemiology

Virtually eliminated from most developed countries, including the UK (animal vaccination, pasteurization, screen/slaughter of infected herds). It remains endemic in Africa, the Middle East, central and South East Asia, South America, and some Mediterranean countries (including Greece, Turkey, Portugal, Spain, Italy, and Southern France). Human–human transmission has been documented but is rare—methods include breast milk, sexual transmission, and congenital disease. Around ten cases occur in the UK annually—almost always acquired abroad. Brucellosis also occurs through occupational exposure of laboratory workers, vets, and slaughterhouse workers. A careful epidemiological patient history is crucial, regarding travel, diet (e.g. unpasteurized dairy produce), and possible exposure.

Pathogenesis

After ingestion (or entry via skin abrasions or inhaling infected dust), the bacteria live in the regional lymph nodes during the incubation period (usually 2–8 weeks). They then enter the circulation and subsequently localize in different parts of the reticulo-endothelial system, forming granulomatous lesions that may result in complications in many organs. *Brucella* organisms surviving within granulomas may cause relapses of acute disease or result in chronic brucellosis.

Clinical features

Brucellosis has a wide variety of clinical presentations. The 'undulant' or wave-like fever rises and falls over weeks in ~90% of untreated patients. Malodorous perspiration is said to be pathognomonic. Localized infection occurs in 30%, osteoarticular most commonly, with epididymo-orchitis in ~6%. Other symptoms include weakness, headaches, depression, myalgia, and body pain. Hepatomegaly and splenomegaly may occur. Sequelae are also variable, and include granulomatous hepatitis, anaemia, leucopenia, thrombocytopenia, meningitis, uveitis, and optic neuritis. Infection in pregnancy is associated with abortion, premature delivery, and intrauterine infection with fetal death.

Diagnosis

- *Brucella* is a hazard group 3 organism. Laboratory exposure is a HSE-reportable clinical incident, requiring RIDDOR reporting and thorough risk assessment of laboratory staff. Guidance on prophylaxis and follow-up of staff can be found via the brucellosis reference laboratory (PHE website ☞ https://www.gov.uk/government/organisations/public-health-england).
- Culture from blood or bone marrow. Marrow culture is the gold standard—most sensitive, especially in chronic disease, and less affected by prior use of antibiotics. Growth can take up to 8 weeks. Coccobacilli or short bacilli. May occur singly, in chains, or in groups. Non-motile, non-sporing, and non-capsulate. Aerobic, and *B. abortus* requires 5–10% CO_2 to grow. The three main species (*B. melitensis, B. abortus, B. suis*) can be differentiated biochemically and by antigenic structure. Each species can be further divided into biotypes—there are >9 biotypes of *B. abortus*, >3 of *B. melitensis*, and >5 of *B. suis*.
- Serology—raised (1:160) or 4-fold rise in antibody titre over 2 weeks in symptomatic patients suggests the diagnosis of active *Brucella*. Difficult to interpret in those from endemic areas or relapsed infection. Demonstration of antibodies: standard agglutination, mercaptoethanol test, Bengal Rose reactions, ELISA. At the reference laboratory, all sera are screened with a *Brucella* antibody assay and specific IgG/IgM enzyme immunoassays. Positive samples then undergo further testing with in-house micro-agglutination and complement fixation.
- Other—histology (e.g. granulomatous hepatitis), radiology (e.g. the 'pedro-pons sign', preferential erosion of antero-superior corner of lumbar vertebrae), PCR (positive within 10 days of infection—not widely available).

Treatment

Drugs must enter macrophages and be active in an acidic environment.

- Uncomplicated—doxycycline 6 weeks, with either 14–21 days' streptomycin OR 6 weeks' rifampicin. Fluoroquinolones (also in combination) have a role in relapsed or resistant disease.
- Focal infection, including articular, neurological—at least 12 weeks' treatment and 3-drug regimes may be required for neurological disease or endocarditis (which also needs surgery).
- Antibody levels may be measured to monitor response to therapy.

Prevention

Good standards of hygiene in the production of raw milk and its products, or pasteurization of all milk, will prevent brucellosis acquired from ingestion of milk. Also avoid contact with infected animals. Vaccination of young cattle helps to protect animals against *B. abortus* but is not completely effective. However, it helps to limit the spread of disease and thus aids eradication. Only by testing all animals, and slaughtering those with positive results, can the disease be truly eradicated.

Yersinia pestis—ACDP 3

Y. pestis causes plague. There are three clinical syndromes: bubonic, pneumonic, and septicaemic (see Table 7.14). Found worldwide, but most cases are reported from developing countries of Africa and Asia. There are ~10 cases annually from rural areas of the USA. The last case acquired in the UK was in 1918.

Pathogenesis

The somatic (heat-stable) and capsular (heat-labile) antigens are important in virulence and immunogenicity. Somatic antigens V and W help resist phagocytosis, and the capsular antigen containing the immunogenic fraction (F1) is antiphagocytic also. Other virulence factors include an LPS endotoxin, the ability to absorb iron as haemin, and temperature-dependent coagulase and fibrinolysin.

Diagnosis

- Culture—short Gram-negative coccobacillus, occurs singly or in pairs (or as chains in fluid culture). Old cultures are pleomorphic and may resemble yeast cells. Non-sporing, non-motile, and often capsulated at 37°C. Methylene blue shows bipolar staining. *Yersinia* spp. grow between 14°C and 37°C, with optimal growth at 27°C. Small, non-haemolytic colonies are seen on blood agar at 24h. Catalase-positive

Table 7.14 Features of the main clinical forms of plague

	Bubonic	Pneumonic	Septicaemic
Transmission	Rat flea bites *Xenopsylla cheopis*	Respiratory aerosols from rat fleas Person-to-person spread in crowded, unhygienic conditions, during epidemics May arise as a complication of bubonic or septicaemic plague	Primary infection Complication of bubonic or pneumonic plague
Diagnostic specimen	Fluid from buboes	Sputum	BC/blood films
Clinical symptoms	Fever, painful buboes, inguinal lymphadenopathy	Cough or haemoptysis ± bubo	Fever, hypotension, no buboes
Incubation period	2–8 days	1–4 days (maximum 6 days)	2–8 days
Mortality if untreated	~60%	High mortality (approaching 100%)	High mortality (approaching 100%)

and oxidase-negative. Although *Y. pestis* grows on MacConkey, it tends to autolyse after 2–3 days. Organisms are citrate-, indole-, and urease-negative. Usually cultured from a bubo aspirate, but may also grow from blood, CSF, or sputum. Cefsulodin, Irgasan, Novobiocin (CIN) agar is selective for *Yersinia* and *Aeromonas* spp ('bull's eye' appearance).
- Direct immunofluorescence is a more rapid diagnostic method.
- Serological tests for yersiniosis (acute and convalescent) include the complement fixation test and haemagglutination of tanned sheep red cells to which F1 capsular antigen has been adsorbed.

Treatment

Early antibiotic therapy for suspected cases (e.g. streptomycin, gentamicin, or doxycycline) reduces the otherwise high mortality to ~10%. Contacts may also be given antibiotic prophylaxis. Patients with pneumonic plague should be isolated until they are sputum smear-negative (usually ~3 days since starting treatment). There is no vaccine currently available. It is a notifiable disease.

Yersinia enterocolitica

Epidemiology and clinical features

- *Y. enterocolitica* resembles *Y. pestis* and *Y. pseudotuberculosis* on culture and morphologically, but differs antigenically and biochemically. The commonest serotypes causing human infection in Europe are 3 and 9. Acquired from eating infected meat or milk. Patients with conditions associated with iron overload (e.g. haemochromatosis) and the immunosuppressed are at increased risk of *Yersinia* infections.
- Usually presents as a febrile illness associated with bloody diarrhoea, and may mimic salmonellosis, shigellosis, or appendicitis. Other presentations include mesenteric lymphadenitis and septicaemia, which may be fatal in the elderly. Secondary complications include erythema nodosum, polyarthritis, peritonitis, Reiter's syndrome, meningitis, osteomyelitis, and hepatic, renal, and splenic abscesses. *Y. enterocolitica* has been cultured from pseudotuberculous lesions in animals.

Treatment

- Gastroenteritis usually resolves without antibiotics. In severe infection, the recommended regimen is doxycycline plus an aminoglycoside. Alternatives—ceftriaxone, co-trimoxazole, and fluoroquinolones. Note resistance to penicillin.
- If the patient is on desferrioxamine, this should be stopped, as it may increase the severity of infection.

Yersinia pseudotuberculosis

Epidemiology and clinical features

- Strains can be differentiated by somatic and flagellar antigens, some of which are shared with *Y. pestis*. Most human infections due to serotype 1.
- Causes a fatal septicaemia in animals and birds. Humans usually acquire the infection from contact with water polluted by infected animals or from eating contaminated vegetables—infection due to direct contact with animals is rare. In humans, yersiniosis ranges from asymptomatic to a fatal typhoid-like illness with fever, purpura, and hepatosplenomegaly. Mesenteric adenitis ± erythema nodosum may mimic appendicitis and tends to infect males aged 5–15 years.

Diagnosis and treatment

- GNR, slightly acid-fast, grows poorly on MacConkey (like *Y. pestis*). Can produce urease and motile at 22°C, unlike *Y. pestis*.
- Shows *in vitro* susceptibility to ciprofloxacin, tetracyclines, aminoglycosides, sulfonamides, and penicillin. Mesenteric adenitis is usually self-limiting.

Pasteurella

The genus *Pasteurella* includes the species *P. multocida, P. haemolytica* (now known as *Mannheimia haemolytica*), *P. canis, P. stomatis*, and *P. pneumotropica. Pasteurella* live in the mouth, and GI and respiratory tracts of many animals (especially dogs and cats) ± humans. *P. multocida*, the most frequent human isolate, usually causes skin and soft tissue infections.

Epidemiology

Fifteen serotypes of *P. multocida* have been identified, based on four capsular antigens and 11 somatic antigens. PFGE can be used to compare strains. Humans acquire infection from animal bites or inhaling air contaminated by infected animals' coughing.

Pathogenesis

In animals, *P. multocida* causes haemorrhagic septicaemia, which is usually fatal. Most virulent *Pasteurella* strains have a polysaccharide capsule, which is antiphagocytic and protects against intracellular killing by neutrophils. Also, some strains produce a leukotoxin, and some bind transferrin.

Clinical features

- *P. multocida* causes skin and soft tissue infections after animal bites, most commonly a localized abscess with cellulitis and lymphadenitis. *P. multocida* has also been associated with URTIs and LRTIs. Other sites of infection are uncommon—these include meningitis post-head injury, bone and joint infections, septicaemia, endocarditis, and intra-abdominal infections.

- *P. haemolytica* is not thought to be pathogenic for humans. It causes pneumonia in sheep and cattle, and septicaemia in lambs, and also infects poultry and domestic animals.
- *P. pneumotropica* may be isolated from the respiratory tract of laboratory animals. There are reports of it causing human infections, e.g. animal bite wound infections, septicaemia, and URTIs.

Diagnosis

P. multocida is a facultative Gram-negative coccobacillus, which appears pleomorphic in culture and does not grow on MacConkey agar. At 37°C, organisms are capsulated, non-sporing, and non-motile. They show bipolar staining with methylene blue. Most are fermentative, and oxidase-positive, catalase-positive, and indole-positive.

Treatment

Penicillin is the mainstay of treatment, and there is a wealth of clinical experience to support this. It is resistant to oral first-generation cephalosporins, flucloxacillin, clindamycin, and erythromycin. It is sensitive *in vitro* to fluoroquinolones, which may be considered in penicillin-allergic patients.

Francisella—ACDP 3

F. tularensis is primarily an animal pathogen (rabbits and hares), which occasionally infects humans as accidental hosts, as a result of contact with infected animals or invertebrate vectors (especially in summer months). Only two of the five subspecies are clinically important: type A (*F. tularensis* subspecies *tularensis*) is highly virulent, and type B (*F. tularensis* subspecies *holarctica*) less virulent. It is a potential agent of bioterrorism (➔ see Bioterrorism, pp. 846–8).

Epidemiology and pathology

Tularaemia is endemic in North America and parts of Europe, Asia, northern Australia, and Japan. Most cases in man are sporadic, though outbreaks have been reported. It may survive for days in moist soil and in water polluted by infected animals, and for years in culture at 10°C. Organisms are killed in 10min after exposure to moist heat at 55°C. There is evidence from animal experiments of intracellular multiplication of *F. tularensis*. The capsule and citrulline ureidase activity contribute to virulence.

Clinical features

Infection (tularaemia) ranges from asymptomatic to septic shock, depending on the virulence of the particular strain, host immune response, route of entry, and degree of systemic involvement. A history with relevant epidemiology is vital. There are two main forms:

- *ulceroglandular*—commonest, patients usually report animal contact—acute-onset fever, headache, and rigors, usually followed by glandular lesions, and skin ulceration may occur (hands/arms after animal exposure, head/neck, trunk, or perineum after tick exposure, e.g. eschar);

- *typhoidal/pulmonary*—follows insect exposure or inhaling infected dust, eating contaminated food or water. Acute-onset fever, headache, and rigors, followed by respiratory or typhoid-like symptoms.

Diagnosis

F. tularensis is a Hazard group 3 organism. It is a small, non-motile, non-sporulating, capsulated Gram-negative coccobacillus, which shows characteristic bipolar staining with carbol fuchsin (10%). It stains poorly with methylene blue. It is a strict aerobe, and culture requires the addition of egg yolk or rabbit spleen to agar. Traditional microbiological methods are being replaced by immunological and molecular tests, including ELISA and immunoblots for antibodies (but tests relying on antibody detection are limited in early clinical stages of disease). If a case is suspected, involve the PHE Reference Unit at Porton Down promptly. It is a notifiable organism.

Treatment

Seek expert advice. Streptomycin or gentamicin are antibiotics of choice, with the addition of chloramphenicol for meningitis. Ciprofloxacin is an oral option for those with mild illness. A 10- to 14-day course is required. Relapse is commoner with tetracycline or chloramphenicol, as they are bacteriostatic for *F. tularensis*. The live vaccine is based on an attenuated strain of *F. tularensis*. PEP with doxycycline or ciprofloxacin may be considered after potential inhalation.

Legionella

This organism is named after the outbreak of pneumonia affecting >180 members of the American Legion at a convention in Philadelphia in 1976. *Legionellaceae* naturally live in water and only incidentally infect humans. This may result in either legionnaires' disease or Pontiac fever. There are 52 different genetically defined species of *Legionella*, of which ~50% infect humans. *L. pneumophila* serogroup 1 is the most pathogenic and accounts for ~95% of human cases.

Epidemiology

Legionella is acquired via inhalation of contaminated aerosolized water (e.g. from spas, showers, air conditioning systems, water storage tanks, nebulizers). Water systems are more likely to be contaminated with *Legionella* if the temperature is outside the recommended range (it should be <20°C or >55°C), if the flow is obstructed, or if biofilms have formed. It is an intracellular organism and can survive in amoebae, within the environment. The incubation period is 2–10 days, and occasionally symptoms may develop up to 3 weeks post-exposure. It is not transmitted person-to-person. Most cases are isolated, but clusters and outbreaks occur.

Pathogenesis

After the infection is established, pneumonic consolidation develops, characterized by proteinaceous fibrinous exudates pouring into the alveoli. The mechanism of distant toxic changes (e.g. confusion, hallucinations, focal neurology) is poorly understood. *Legionella* organisms are engulfed by monocytes and may survive intracellularly for prolonged periods of time.

Clinical features

In addition to the two main clinical syndromes, rare conditions (e.g. prosthetic valve endocarditis, wound infections) have been reported:

- *legionnaires' disease*—rapidly progressive pneumonia characterized by fever, respiratory distress, and confusion. Mortality of >10% in healthy people. May be associated with hyponatraemia. Risk factors include age >50 years, hospital admission, immunosuppression, and smoking. Men are affected more than women;
- *Pontiac fever*—a brief flu-like illness, with a high attack rate but low mortality.

Diagnosis

- *Microscopy/culture*—short rods/coccobacilli may be difficult to see by Gram stain, so fluorescent antibody stains or silver impregnation may help. Grows best on media such as buffered charcoal yeast extract, which contains iron plus cysteine as an essential growth factor. Some strains prefer 2.5–5% CO_2 at 35–36°C. *L. pneumophila* colonies usually appear by day 5, but other species may require 10 days. Colonies may autofluoresce under UV light. Serogroups can be differentiated by slide agglutination or fluorescent antibody tests (FATs), which are available at reference laboratories.
- *Antigen detection*—*Legionella* urinary antigen test (ELISA) only detects serogroup 1 of *L. pneumophila*, thus will be negative in outbreaks caused by other serogroups.
- *Molecular methods*—*Legionella* PCR is available at some reference centres.
- *Antibody detection*—FAT, RMAT (rapid micro-agglutination test), or ELISA. A >4-fold rise or titre 1:256 is usually diagnostic. Remember that antibodies may take >8 days to develop after onset of infection and may persist for months/years post-infection. Some cross-reactivity with *Campylobacter*.

Treatment

- Conventional susceptibility tests in broth and agar are unreliable. Many antibiotics with *in vitro* activity (e.g. β-lactams and aminoglycosides) are ineffective. Macrolides, quinolones, tetracyclines, and rifampicin are effective, as they have good intracellular penetration.
- Preferred—newer macrolides (azithromycin, clarithromycin) and respiratory quinolones (levofloxacin). The latter may bring about more rapid defervescence, but outcomes are similar. Duration 7–10 days.
- Combination therapy may have a role for the treatment of endocarditis.

Control and prevention

Legionnaires' disease is a notifiable condition. Control relies on good design and maintenance of water systems to prevent growth of *Legionella* organisms, and subsequent treatment of the source (e.g. contaminated water systems) if a case occurs (see Box 7.7). The main approaches to control

Box 7.7 *Legionella* guidance

A full list of UK guidance, including water system maintenance, case investigation, and prevention, is available on the PHE website (🔗 www.gov.uk/government/collections/legionnaires-disease-guidance-data-and-analysis).

are physical (heat, UV light, sonication), chemical (inhibiting scale formation, use of biocides to kill amoebae, use of charcoal filters), and plumbing (maintenance, no dead legs in the system, pumps in series, not parallel, no dead spaces in the heaters, regular flushing of the system).

Capnocytophaga

Genus *Capnocytophaga* in the family *Flavobacteriaceae*. Two groups:

- species associated with dog bite infections (and occasionally bites from other animals such as rabbits or cats): *C. canimorsus* and *C. cynodegmi*;
- species found in the human mouth—*C. ochracea, C. gingivalis, C. sputigena, C. haemolytica*, and *C. granulosa*.

Epidemiology

While *C. canimorsus* and *C. cynodegmi* are most commonly associated with bites, occasionally infections occur merely after exposure to dogs. Species found in the human mouth produce a variety of enzymes that help invasion of periodontal tissue (e.g. acid and alkaline phosphotases, aminopeptidases, IgA, proteases, and trypsin-like enzymes).

Clinical features

Amongst animal bite infections, *C. canimorsus* is commoner and more severe than *C. cynodegmi*, with a mortality approaching 30%. Risk factors—asplenic patients, alcoholics, and those on steroids. Asplenic patients with *C. canimorsus* infection may present with shock, disseminated purpuric lesions, and DIC. Fulminant infections may also occur in healthy people, although infections tend to be milder. Meningitis, endocarditis, pneumonia, corneal ulcer, cellulitis, and septic arthritis due to *C. canimorsus* have also been reported.

Species found in the human mouth may be important in localized juvenile periodontitis. May colonize the female genital tract, and associated with intrauterine infection, amnionitis, and neonatal infections in premature babies. Rare presentations—endocarditis, eye infections, and peritonitis.

Diagnosis

- Long, thin, delicate GNRs, typically fusiform, but older cultures often show pleomorphic sizes and shapes. Facultative anaerobes, and grow best with CO_2 enrichment. On blood or chocolate agar, may appear yellowish, with a spreading edge with finger-like projections due to the typical gliding motility. They do not grow on MacConkey agar.
- Differentiation of individual species usually requires reference laboratory assistance. In general, species from the human mouth are oxidase-negative and catalase-negative, while those from animals' mouths are oxidase-positive and catalase-positive.

- *C. canimorsus* is more fastidious than the others and may be difficult to grow from BCs—culture on enriched agar (e.g. heart infusion agar with rabbit or sheep blood) for 14 days in 10% CO_2 may help.

Treatment

Co-amoxiclav is usually recommended. Asplenic patients should be given prophylaxis after a dog bite, pending culture, as the organism may take a while to grow, and mortality is high. Resistance to the β-lactams has been reported in the human mouth species, e.g. *C. haemolytica* and *C. granulosa* are often resistant to β-lactams and aminoglycosides. All species are usually sensitive to clindamycin, erythromycin, tetracyclines, and quinolones.

Vibrios

The genus *Vibrio* (family *Vibrionaceae*) includes over 30 species. The most important ones that result in human infections are *V. cholerae, V. parahaemolyticus*, and *V. vulnificus*. Other species, such as *V. alginolyticus, V. damsela (*now known as *Listonella damsela*), *V. fluvialis, V. hollisae* (now known as *Grimontia hollisae*), and *V. mimicus*, occasionally cause opportunistic infections.

Vibrio cholerae

There are ~20 cases of cholera (➔ see Cholera, pp. 652–3) imported into the UK every year. These are most commonly O1-El Tor. In the mid 1990s, a new serogroup (O139) appeared in the Bay of Bengal—this was the first time a non-O1 serogroup had resulted in epidemic cholera.

Epidemiology

Cholera is prevalent in Central and South America, Africa, and Asia. There are >130 different O (somatic antigen) serogroups of *V. cholerae*. Serogroup O1 (the 'cholera vibrio') causes epidemic cholera, and some strains of non-O1 (the 'non-cholera or non-agglutinable vibrios) can also cause diarrhoea. Serogroup O1 is usually acquired by the faecal–oral route, while non-O1 *V. cholerae* may be associated with consumption of seafood or exposure to saline environments. The two biotypes of serogroup O1 (*El Tor*, which is the commonest, and *classical*) can be distinguished by susceptibility to phage, and the fact that El Tor is haemolytic and resistant to polymyxin B. The subtypes of serogroup O1 are Ogawa (most common), Inaba, and Hikojima (which possesses determinants of both other subtypes).

Pathogenesis

The potent cholera enterotoxin, produced by serogroup O1 and some non-O1 strains, comprises five B (binding) subunits and one A (active) subunit. Insertion of the B subunits into the host cell membrane forms a channel for subunit A to enter the cell. By causing the transfer of ADP ribose from NAD to another protein, adenylate cyclase is irreversibly activated, and cAMP is overproduced. The resulting hypersecretion of chloride ion (Cl^-) and bicarbonate ion (HCO_3^-) causes massive loss of water and electrolytes (rice-water stool). Other features important in pathogenesis of serogroup O1 include production of mucinase and other proteolytic enzymes (which help the organism reach the enterocytes), the motility of the organism, and adhesive haemagglutinins (aid close adherence to enterocyte surface). Non-O1 strains may produce other enterotoxins, cytotoxins, haemolysins, and colonizing factors.

Cholera is transmitted by contaminated food or water, and requires a large infective dose. Humans are the only host. Only a handful of those infected are symptomatic (ratios quoted are 40 asymptomatic carriers to one symptomatic individual for El Tor, and 5:1 for classical), which underscores the need for good hygiene.

Clinical features

V. cholerae usually causes the typical profuse watery diarrhoea of cholera, which may rapidly lead to hypovolaemic shock and death from dehydration. Milder cases are similar to other causes of secretory diarrhoea, and asymptomatic infections also occur. Non-O1 *V. cholerae* usually causes mild, sometimes bloody, diarrhoea, but may occasionally be severe and resemble cholera. Patients exposed to aquatic environments may suffer from wound infections, and bacteraemia and meningitis have been reported.

Diagnosis

During an epidemic, cholera is a clinical diagnosis. Otherwise, diagnosis is based on high clinical suspicion, together with culture or dark-field microscopy of stool (comma-shaped organisms are seen moving around, which ceases when diluted O1 antisera is added). Vibrios are short, curved, or 'comma-shaped' aerobic GNRs, which are motile by a single polar flagellum. They ferment both sucrose and glucose, but not lactose, and reduce nitrate to nitrite. Most are oxidase-positive (test must be performed from non-selective media) and produce indole. The growth characteristics of vibrios are summarized in Table 7.15. *V. cholerae* is non-halophilic (i.e. can grow on media without added salt), provided the necessary electrolytes are present. *V. cholerae* can grow at 42°C (along with *V. parahaemolyticus* and *V. alginolyticus*). Vibrios are tolerant to alkali but have a low tolerance to acid. *V. cholerae* is usually Voges–Proskauer-positive. Vibrios accumulate on the surface of alkaline peptone water. If a loopful is inoculated onto thiosulfate-citrate-bile salts-sucrose agar, *V. cholerae* appear as a yellow sucrose fermenter, which is oxidase-positive. *V. cholerae* is killed by most detergents and by heating at 55°C for 15min. However, it can survive for up to 2 weeks in salt water at ambient temperatures, and also on chitinous shellfish for 2 weeks, even if refrigerated. Where API® methods are used for identification, inoculation with NaCl is required.

Treatment

Cholera is a notifiable condition. Rehydration is key. Antibiotics (e.g. azithromycin, ciprofloxacin) reduce the duration of disease and period of excretion of *V. cholerae* in the stool of infected patients. Antibiotic treatment is not routinely required but should be considered in those with severe illness or during an outbreak. In the UK, a killed oral vaccine is licensed for relief workers and travellers to remote endemic areas. However, the most important preventative strategies are improvement of sanitation and food and water standards.

Table 7.15 Growth characteristics of *Vibrio* spp.

Species	TCBS	Biochemistry	Salt requirement	Growth at 42°C
V. cholerae	Yellow	Oxidase-, nitrate-, lysine-, ONPG-positive	Not halophilic (0–3% NaCl)	Yes
V. parahaemolyticus	Green	Lysine-, indole-positive	Halophilic (3–6% NaCl)	Yes
V. vulnificus	Green (85%), yellow (15%)	Lactose-, lysine-, salicin-positive	Halophilic (3–5% NaCl)	No
V. alginolyticus	Yellow	Lysine-, Voges–Proskauer-positive	Halophilic (3–10% NaCl)	Yes

Vibrio parahaemolyticus

V. parahaemolyticus is ubiquitous in fish and shellfish, and the waters they inhabit. Outbreaks of diarrhoea occur infrequently in the UK.

Epidemiology

V. parahaemolyticus infection is common in South East Asia, particularly Singapore and Japan. However, it also occurs in the UK and USA, particularly during summer months.

Pathogenesis

Kanagawa-positive strains (➔ see Diagnosis below) of *V. parahaemolyticus* adhere to human enterocytes and produce a heat-stable cytotoxin.

Clinical features

V. parahaemolyticus is usually acquired through ingesting seafood and causes acute explosive diarrhoea. Extraintestinal infections arise from handling contaminated seafood or exposure to the aquatic environment, the commonest being wound infections.

Diagnosis

This organism is halophilic (salt-loving), hence will not grow on CLED agar. Clinical strains of *V. parahaemolyticus* usually appear as green, non-sucrose-fermenting colonies on TCBS agar, but isolates from estuary and coastal waters may ferment sucrose. Stool samples should be enriched in alkaline peptone water containing 1% NaCl. The Kanagawa phenomenon refers to haemolysis of human erythrocytes on Wagatsuma's agar by strains of *V. parahaemolyticus* which cause gastroenteritis. Oxidase-positive; where API® methods are used for identification, inoculation with NaCl is required.

Treatment

Rehydration is the main intervention for patients with diarrhoea. Severe infections require treatment with fluoroquinolones, doxycycline, or third-generation cephalosporins. Antibiotics do not shorten the duration of symptoms. Prevention strategies involve good food hygiene standards.

Vibrio vulnificus

V. vulnificus has been called the 'terror of the deep' due to the severe fulminant infection it can cause.

Epidemiology

Infections are commonest in areas with higher water temperatures such as the mid-Atlantic and Gulf Coast states of the USA. Septicaemia arises from eating contaminated raw shellfish, while wound infections are due to injuries sustained in aquatic environments.

Pathogenesis

The polysaccharide capsule helps resist phagocytosis and bactericidal effects of human serum. The association with liver disease (with increased serum iron levels) may be explained by the ability of virulent strains to use transferrin-bound iron. Toxin production is also important.

Clinical features

There are three main infections associated with *V. vulnificus*:

- fulminant septicaemia, followed by cutaneous lesions. This is associated with a high mortality (50%). Immunosuppressed patients are at increased risk, particularly elderly male alcoholics with liver dysfunction;
- wound infection, rapidly progressing to cellulitis, oedema, erythema, and necrosis. Patients may develop septicaemia, and it may be fatal;
- acute mild diarrhoea, usually in those with mild underlying conditions.

Diagnosis

This organism is halophilic (➔ see Diagnosis, p. 323). For further growth characteristics, see Table 7.15. Where API® methods are used for identification, inoculation with NaCl is required.

Treatment

Early treatment with ceftazidime and doxycycline is key.

Other *Vibrio* species

- *V. alginolyticus* is the commonest *Vibrio* organism found in seafood and seawater in the UK. It is a halophilic organism, which will not grow on CLED but grows in 10% NaCl. Colonies are large and yellow (sucrose-fermenting) on TCBS agar, and there is swarming on non-selective media. Causes opportunistic wound infections associated with exposure to seawater, usually self-limiting.
- *V. fluvialis* is phenotypically similar to *Aeromonas hydrophila* (➔ see *Aeromonas*, p. 325). Implicated in outbreaks of diarrhoea; acquired from seafood.
- *V. damsela* (now known as *Listonella damsela*) is a halophilic organism acquired in warm coastal areas. Cause of wound infection.

- *V. hollisae* (now known as *Grimontia hollisae*) has been associated with diarrhoea and bacteraemia in areas of warm seawater in the USA. It is acquired from raw seafood.
- *V. mimicus* is associated with gastroenteritis from eating raw oysters. There are also reports of ear infections. It occurs in environments similar to *V. cholerae*.

Aeromonas

Aeromonas spp. are aquatic organisms. *A. hydrophila*, *A. sobria*, and *A. caviae* are the main species, and *A. salmonicida* is an economically important fish pathogen. The genus *Aeromonas* has undergone a number of taxonomic and nomenclature revisions recently, and has been moved from the family *Vibrionaceae* to the new family *Aeromonadaceae*.

Epidemiology

A cause of diarrhoea and soft tissue infections. Diarrhoea is commoner in the summer months when water concentrations of aeromonads are higher. Outbreaks may occur.

Pathogenesis

Gastroenteritis is the commonest disease associated with *Aeromonas*, but its role is debated. It is capable of producing an enterotoxin, and antibiotics active against *Aeromonas* may improve patient symptoms. It may be that only specific subsets of *Aeromonas* are pathogenic.

Clinical features

Diarrhoea tends to be watery and self-limiting, but is occasionally more severe. Chronic colitis following diarrhoea has been reported. In addition to gastroenteritis, there are reports of *Aeromonas* septicaemia in the immunocompromised, and wound infections in healthy people and those undergoing leech therapy. It should be considered as a cause of soft tissue infection in those with water exposure. There are rare reports of nosocomial bacteraemia, peritonitis, meningitis, and eye and bone and joint infections.

Diagnosis

This facultatively anaerobic GNR is usually β-haemolytic on blood agar and ferments carbohydrates to produce acid and gas. It grows readily on MacConkey agar, and lactose fermentation is variable. Growth on TCBS agar is also variable. It is oxidase-positive, so can be distinguished from the oxidase-negative *Enterobacteriaceae*. Suitable plates for detection of *Aeromonas* from stool include CIN agar or blood agar containing ampicillin. Note that not all laboratories routinely culture stools for *Aeromonas*, and some enteric media actually inhibit its growth.

Treatment

There are no controlled trials, but clinical improvement has been seen with antibiotics that are active *in vitro* such as fluoroquinolones, co-trimoxazole, and aminoglycosides (except streptomycin). Resistance to the carbapenems has been reported due to chromosomal carbapenemases.

Plesiomonas

Plesiomonas shigelloides, the only species in the genus, is associated with outbreaks of gastroenteritis in warm climates. In the literature, it has been known as *Pseudomonas shigelloides*, C27, *Aeromonas shigelloides*, and *Vibrio shigelloides*. The taxonomic status has varied—it is related to *Proteus* but is currently placed in the family *Enterobacteriaceae*.

Epidemiology

P. shigelloides is found in soil and water (mainly fresh water, but also salt water in warm weather). It is usually transmitted to humans via water or food (e.g. shrimp, chicken, and oysters), and also colonizes many animals. Most patients recently travelled abroad.

Pathogenesis

There is no animal model, and no pathogenic mechanism has been identified. Volunteer studies have been largely unsuccessful in causing disease. Hence, it has been difficult to prove a causal relationship.

Clinical features

Symptoms vary from mild self-limiting diarrhoea to mucoid bloody diarrhoea with features of entero-invasive disease. It has occasionally resulted in serious extraintestinal infection such as osteomyelitis, septic arthritis, endophthalmitis, SBP, pancreatic abscess, cellulitis, cholecystitis, and neonatal sepsis with meningitis. Bacteraemia is rare and usually in the immunocompromised.

Diagnosis

This motile, facultatively anaerobic GNR does not ferment lactose. It grows readily at 35°C on most enteric agars, such as MacConkey, but does not grow on TCBS. It appears non-haemolytic and is oxidase-positive. Selective techniques are needed to isolate it from a mixed culture.

Treatment

The role of antibiotics is unclear, and results of studies conflicting. *In vitro*, it is usually sensitive to quinolones, cephalosporins, and carbapenems.

Campylobacter

Campylobacter organisms are spiral-shaped flagellate bacteria belonging to rRNA superfamily VI. *C. jejuni* is the commonest cause of diarrhoea in most developed countries. *C. coli* also causes diarrhoea. *C. fetus* is the type species of the genus and causes abortion in sheep and cows. It occasionally causes septic abortions in humans and bacteraemia/soft tissue infections in the immunocompromised. Some species, including *C. lari* and *C. upsaliensis*, cause diarrhoea in children in developing countries, while species, such as *C. concisus* and *C. rectus*, are associated with periodontal disease.

Pathogenesis

Campylobacter organisms are ingested (faeco-oral transmission), then colonize (and usually invade) the jejunum, ileum, and terminal ileum, occasionally extending to the colon and rectum. Mesenteric lymph node involvement and transient bacteraemia may occur. Histological findings of acute inflammation ± superficial ulceration are the same as in *Salmonella*, *Shigella*, or *Yersinia* infections.

Clinical features

Campylobacter gastroenteritis is variable in terms of symptoms and severity. In severe cases, GI haemorrhage, toxic megacolon, and HUS have been reported. Other complications include meningitis, deep abscesses, cholecystitis, and reactive arthritis. ~25% cases of Guillain–Barré syndrome (GBS) have been documented preceding *Campylobacter* gastroenteritis—the lipo-oligosaccharide cell surface structures act as critical factors in triggering GBS through ganglioside mimicry.

Diagnosis

This small, spiral GNR has a single unsheathed flagellum at one or both poles and is extremely motile. Staining with carbol fuchsin reveals a characteristic 'seagull' appearance. Selective blood-free agar are used (e.g. charcoal-cefoperazone-deoxycholate agar (CCDA) containing charcoal, sodium pyruvate, and ferrous sulfate). It is micro-aerophilic and grows best at 42°C. Like *Helicobacter*, *Campylobacter* organisms undergo coccal transformation under adverse conditions and are biochemically inactive. However, they are oxidase-positive. *C. jejuni* is the only species that hydrolyses hippurate. Typing methods include serotyping (Penner scheme for O antigens, and Lior scheme for heat-labile surface and flagellar antigens), biotyping, phage typing, and newer molecular methods.

Treatment

Rehydration and symptom relief are usually adequate, as *Campylobacter* infection is usually self-limiting in 5–7 days. However, in severe dysenteric disease, erythromycin or ciprofloxacin may be prescribed. Resistant strains, especially *C. coli*, may respond to trimethoprim or co-trimoxazole. Good hygiene standards are important in prevention. Infective organisms may be excreted in the stool for ~3 weeks after resolution of diarrhoea. There is no vaccine.

Helicobacter

The genus *Helicobacter* contains up to 17 species, which colonize the stomach of different animals. *H. pylori* is a spiral-shaped flagellate bacteria belonging to rRNA superfamily VI, which colonizes humans (it is found in ~50% of the world population). *H. pylori* was discovered in 1983 in Australia by Warren and Marshall, who went on to receive the Nobel Prize for Medicine in 2005. Its importance in the pathogenesis of peptic ulcer disease and malignancy soon became clear. *H. cinaedi* and *H. fennelliae* are associated with proctitis in homosexual men.

Pathogenesis

As with other bacteria in rRNA superfamily VI, *H. pylori* is adapted to colonizing mucous membranes (in this case, the gastric mucosa only) by penetrating mucus. The cagA protein is important in virulence. After phosphorylation by tyrosine kinase, cagA is injected into epithelial cells by a type IV secretion system. This alters signal transduction and gene expression in host epithelial cells.

Clinical features

H. pylori is associated with 95% of duodenal and 70% of gastric ulcers. Epidemiological studies have highlighted the association of *H. pylori* and gastric cancer, and WHO classifies *H. pylori* as a group 1 carcinogen.

Diagnosis

This GNR is shaped like a helix and has a tuft of sheathed unipolar flagella. It is strictly micro-aerophilic and requires CO_2 for growth. It is relatively inactive biochemically, except for strong urease production. Under adverse conditions, it undergoes coccal transformation. PHE/British Infection Association (BIA) have produced guidelines on testing and management of *H. pylori*. Options for testing patients are as follows:

- serology—if positive, this indicates the patient has been infected but does not differentiate between active and past infection. Not advised for use in the elderly. High negative predictive value in low prevalence countries;
- biopsy of stomach or duodenum—histology ± urease test ± culture;
- urea breath tests—the patient drinks ^{14}C- or ^{13}C-labelled urea, which is metabolized by *H. pylori*, producing labelled CO_2 that can be detected in the breath. This test is also used to assess effectiveness of treatment but is affected by PPI use;
- rapid urease test (the enzyme urease produced by *H. pylori* catalyses the conversion of urea to ammonia and bicarbonate, which is reflected by a rise in pH)—this is usually performed on a biopsy sample;
- faecal antigen tests—affected by PPI use.

The urea breath test or stool antigen test have greater sensitivity and specificity than serology for diagnosis, and can also be used to confirm eradication. The patient should receive no antibiotics for 4 weeks before the tests, and no PPI for 2 weeks before the tests. Molecular typing of *H. pylori* is more useful than serotyping.

Treatment

NICE has issued clinical guidelines on the investigation and management of dyspepsia (web search 'NICE guidance CG184').[2] Eradication of *H. pylori* in patients testing positive is beneficial in duodenal/gastric ulcers and low-grade MALToma (mucosal-associated lymphoid tissue), but *not* in gastro-oesophageal reflux disease (who should be offered a PPI). Triple therapy consists of a PPI (e.g. omeprazole) and two antibiotics (e.g. amoxicillin, clarithromycin, or metronidazole), and achieves >85% eradication. Clarithromycin or metronidazole should not be given if they have been used for any infection in the previous year. ~10% of patients fail treatment, possibly due to antibiotic resistance (see Box 7.8).

Box 7.8 Antibiotic resistance in *H. pylori*

Antibiotic resistance varies geographically. Metronidazole resistance varies from ~50% in Europe to 90% in developing countries. Clarithromycin resistance is <10% in Europe but may be rising. A recent meta-analysis has shown that pre-treatment clarithromycin resistance may reduce the effectiveness of therapy by 55%. To date, no strains with resistance to amoxicillin or to tetracycline have been detected in the UK. Levofloxacin is being investigated as an alternative antibiotic for resistant strains.

A Cochrane review (2006) of eradication therapy for peptic ulcer disease in *H. pylori*-positive patients found that treatment had a small benefit in initial healing of duodenal ulcers, and a significant benefit in preventing the recurrence of both gastric and duodenal ulcers, once healing had been achieved.[3] Other treatment includes probiotics (which improved eradication rates and reduced adverse events in a recent meta-analysis) and bismuth compounds.

References

2 National Institute for Health and Care Excellence (2014). *Gastro-oesophageal reflux disease and dyspepsia in adults: investigation and management*. NICE clinical guideline 184. Available at: https://www.nice.org.uk/guidance/cg184.

3 Moayyedi P, Soo S, Deeks J, *et al*. (2006). Eradication of Helicobacter pylori for non-ulcer dyspepsia. *Cochrane Database Syst Rev*. 2:CD002096.

Bacteroides

More than 30 genera of anaerobic GNRs are recognized, but human infections are largely restricted to four of these: *Bacteroides, Prevotella, Porphyromonas*, and *Fusobacterium* (see Table 7.16). These organisms are found in the mouth, GI tract, and vagina, and are amongst the most important constituents of 'normal flora'. They may cause a variety of infections in humans, particularly polymicrobial infections and abscesses. *B. fragilis* is the most important species; it is found in the GI tract and is associated with a wide variety of infections.

Pathogenesis

Virulence factors of *Bacteroides* spp. include:

- capsular polysaccharide—inhibits opsonization/phagocytosis, promotes abscess formation, and promotes adherence to epithelial cells;
- pili and fimbriae—promote adherence to epithelial cells and mucus;
- succinic acid—inhibits phagocytosis and intracellular killing;
- enzyme production—contribute to tissue damage and/or promote invasion and spread, e.g heparinase, fibrinolysin, hyaluronidase, neuraminidase;
- synergy between anaerobic and facultative bacteria (see Box 7.9).

Table 7.16 Characteristics of anaerobic Gram-negative rods

Organism	Growth in 20% bile	Pigmented	Fluorescence	Usually resistant to	Usually sensitive to
B. fragilis	Yes	No	No	Penicillin Vancomycin Kanamycin Colistimethate sodium	Erythromycin Rifampicin
Fusobacterium	Variable	No	No	Erythromycin Vancomycin	Colistimethate sodium Penicillin Kanamycin
Prevotella	No	Brown/black	Brick-red	Vancomycin	Rifampicin Colistimethate sodium Penicillin
Porphyromonas	No	Brown/black	Brick-red		Rifampicin Penicillin Vancomycin

Box 7.9 Synergy in anaerobic infections

- Infections involving anaerobes usually contain multiple anaerobic bacteria, as well as facultative anaerobic bacteria.
- Evidence suggests true synergy between anaerobic and facultative bacteria, with formation of abscesses occurring more readily with infections involving both groups of bacteria than either alone.
- Facultative organisms may lower the oxidation–reduction potential in the microenvironment, promoting more favourable conditions for anaerobes.
- Anaerobic bacteria may inhibit phagocytosis of facultative bacteria.
- *B. fragilis* produces β-lactamases in abscess fluid that may protect other normally susceptible bacteria from antimicrobials.

Clinical features

- Intra-abdominal infections—*B. fragilis* is the commonest anaerobic isolate in intra-abdominal abscesses, often polymicrobial infections.
- Diarrhoea—enterotoxin-producing strains have been implicated in diarrhoea in children.
- Bacteraemia—*B. fragilis* is the commonest isolate in anaerobic bacteraemias. The source is usually intra-abdominal and associated with abscesses, malignancy, bowel perforation, or surgery. Septic shock is less common in *B. fragilis* bacteraemia than in bacteraemia caused by aerobic Gram-negative bacilli; this is presumably related to the absence of lipid A in the endotoxin of *B. fragilis*.

- Endocarditis—associated with large vegetations and high frequency of thromboembolic complications.
- Skin and soft tissue infections—often found as part of mixed flora in diabetic and decubitus ulcers. *B. fragilis* has also been isolated from cutaneous abscesses of the lower limbs.
- Bone and joint infections—*B. fragilis* may rarely cause osteomyelitis and septic arthritis.
- CNS infections—anaerobic meningitis is rare, and most laboratories do not culture CSF anaerobically. In the cases of anaerobic meningitis that have been described, *B. fragilis* is the commonest isolate. In contrast, anaerobes are frequently implicated in brain abscesses.

Diagnosis

- *Bacteroides* are non-spore-forming, non-motile anaerobic GNRs.
- On blood agar, *Bacteroides* appear as glistening, non-haemolytic colonies which are aerotolerant.
- Gram stain may reveal pale pink, pleomorphic coccobacilli, with irregular or bipolar staining.
- They can be differentiated from other anaerobic GNRs by growth in 20% bile.
- The MASTRING™ ID (Mast Diagnostics) may be used to identify *B. fragilis* in the laboratory. This is a ring containing six antibiotic discs that is placed on the culture plate and incubated anaerobically at 37°C for up to 3 days. *B. fragilis* is usually sensitive to erythromycin and rifampicin, and usually resistant to penicillin G, vancomycin, kanamycin, and colistimethate sodium. API® 20A or Rapid ID® 32A (biomérieux) can be used.
- Molecular identification and MALDI can also be used.

Treatment

- Drainage of abscesses and debridement of necrotic tissue is the mainstay of treatment for anaerobic infections. However, some abscesses (e.g. brain, liver, and tubo-ovarian) have been managed with antimicrobial therapy alone.
- The choice of antibiotics to treat anaerobic infections is usually empirical, as most of the infections are polymicrobial and require broad-spectrum therapy
- *Bacteroides* is usually sensitive to antimicrobials such as metronidazole, clindamycin, chloramphenicol, carbapenems, cefoxitin, and β-lactam/β-lactamase inhibitor combinations (e.g. co-amoxiclav, piperacillin–tazobactam).

Prevotella and *Porphyromonas*

Prevotella and *Porphyromonas* formerly belonged to the genus *Bacteroides* (➔ see Bacteroides, pp. 329–31) but were reclassified in 1990.

- The genus *Prevotella* includes *P. melaninogenica, P. bivia, P. oralis*, and *P. buccalis*.
- The genus *Porphyromonas* includes *P. gingivalis, P. endodontalis*, and *P. asaccharolytica*.

Pathogenesis

- Virulence in *P. melaninogenica* is associated with the capsular polysaccharide, which inhibits opsonophagocytosis, promotes abscess formation, and also promotes adherence to epithelial cells.
- In *P. gingivalis*, pili and fimbriae aid adherence to epithelial cells and mucus.
- Production of various enzymes may also aid evasion of the host immune response or promote tissue destruction.

Clinical features

Prevotella and *Porphyromonas* contribute to the formation of abscesses and soft tissue infections in various parts of the body. They also cause infections of the oral cavity (such as periodontal and endodontal disease), female genital tract infections, osteomyelitis of the facial bones, and human bite infections.

Diagnosis

- These are non-spore-forming, non-motile, anaerobic Gram-negative bacilli.
- They are usually isolated (along with other anaerobes) from abscesses and soft tissue infections.
- *Prevotella* and *Porphyromonas* may both appear pigmented—usually brown/black.
- Young unpigmented colonies can show brick-red fluorescence under UV light.
- Gram stain reveals small, pale pink coccobacilli.
- *Prevotella* and *Porphyromonas* are both inhibited by 20% bile.
- *Prevotella* are *moderately* saccharolytic, whereas *Porphyromonas* are asaccharolytic.

Treatment

- The mainstay of treatment for anaerobic infections is surgical drainage of abscesses and debridement of necrotic tissue.
- *Prevotella* and *Porphyromonas* are usually sensitive to agents such as metronidazole, clindamycin, chloramphenicol, and cefoxitin. Penicillin resistance is common, but isolates are usually susceptible to co-amoxiclav and other β-lactam/β-lactamase inhibitor combinations.

Fusobacterium

Fusobacterium spp. colonize the mucous membranes of animals and humans, and occasionally cause infections of the oral cavity and head and neck. Clinically, the most important species are:

- *F. nucleatum* (subspecies *nucleatum, polymorphum*, and *fusiforme*);
- *F. necrophorum* (subspecies *necrophorum* and *fundiliforme*).

Epidemiology

Fusobacteria are commensals of the oral cavity. As with other obligate anaerobes, the significance of these organisms is being increasingly recognized. However, *Fusobacterium* infections are relatively rare in the UK.

Pathogenesis

Fusobacterium spp. produce LPS endotoxin which is biologically active. They also produce metabolites that are important to oral spirochaetes.

Clinical features

- *F. necrophorum* causes severe systemic infections such as Lemierre's disease (➔ see Lemierre's syndrome, p. 595), post-anginal sepsis, and necrobacillosis.
- Lemierre's disease is a severe systemic disease which occurs in previously healthy young adults, and usually presents initially as severe sore throat, followed by fever, cervical lymphadenopathy, and unilateral thrombophlebitis of the internal jugular vein. Metastatic infection with spread to the lungs, pleural cavity, bones, or brain may occur. If untreated, the condition leads to death in 7–15 days.
- Other species commonly isolated from oral infections include *F. periodonticum, F. alocis, F. sulci*, and *F. naviforme*.
- Species found in the GI or GU tracts (e.g. *F. mortiferum, F. necrogenes, F. varium*, and *F. gonidiaformans*) may cause intra-abdominal infections, osteomyelitis, ulcers, and skin/soft tissue infections.
- *F. ulcerans* was originally isolated from tropical ulcers but may be found in other sites.

Diagnosis

- *Fusobacterium* are long, thin GNRs with pointed ends ('fusiform') that are often arranged in pairs. They are non-spore-forming and non-motile.
- They may be haemolytic on blood agar and may grow in the presence of 20% bile.
- They can be identified using commercial tests, e.g. MASTRING™ ID (Mast Diagnostics) and the API® 20A or Rapid ID® 32A (biomérieux).
- Molecular techniques (e.g. PCR) have been developed.

Treatment

- The mainstay of treatment for anaerobic infections is surgical drainage of abscesses and debridement of necrotic tissue.
- Lemierre's syndrome and other severe invasive disease is usually treated with a combination of penicillin and metronidazole, for 2–6 weeks.
- Alternatives include clindamycin monotherapy, co-amoxiclav, piperacillin-tazobactam or chloramphenicol.

Spirochaetes—an overview

The spirochaetes are a group of helical organisms sharing many properties with Gram-negative bacteria. The vast majority are non-pathogenic, but a few are important causes of disease in humans (see Table 7.17). There are aerobic and anaerobic species, both free-living and parasitic. Axial filaments, fixed at each end of the organism, run along the outside of the protoplasm within the outer sheath and give the characteristic coiled appearance. These are similar to bacterial flagella and are capable of constricting, warping the cell body and enabling the bacterium to move by rotating it in space.

Table 7.17 Overview of spirochaetes of clinical significance

Genus	Species	Clinical disease	Morphology	Culture	Diagnosis
Treponema	*T. pallidum* subsp. *pallidum*	Syphilis	Appear identical. Thin helical cells 10 x 0.15 micrometres. Visible on dark-field microscopy	Cannot be cultured *in vitro*; remain motile in specific enriched media at 35°C for several days	Direct detection only means in primary syphilis; mainstay is serology; cross-reactivity between species
	T. pallidum subsp. *pertenue*	Yaws			
	T. pallidum subsp. *endemicum*	Endemic syphilis			
	T. carateum	Pinta			
Borrelia	*B. recurrentis*	Louse-borne relapsing fever	Helical; 3–20 x 0.25 micrometres. Can be stained with aniline dyes	Can be cultured, but not practical	Demonstration of spirochaetes in peripheral blood smears; immunological and PCR-based tests available
	B. hermsii and others	Tick-borne relapsing fever			
	B. burgdorferi	Lyme disease		Culture possible from biopsy of rash	Serology; can remain positive for years
Leptospira	*L. interrogans*	Leptospirosis	Motile, 10 x 0.1 micrometres. Stain poorly—visible on dark-field or phase contrast	Specialized media. Allow minimum 6 weeks	Serology; molecular techniques available

Treponema species

Four members of the genus *Treponema* cause human disease: *Treponema pallidum* subspecies *pallidum* (syphilis) and three 'non-venereal' treponematoses.

Microbiology

Morphologically identical, *Treponema* spp. appear as motile, helical rods on dark-field microscopy. They are thin, around 10 micrometres long and 0.15 micrometres wide. They cannot be cultured *in vitro* (unlike the non-pathogenic treponemes) but remain motile in specific enriched media for several days at 35°C. Organisms remain viable after freezing. The organisms all share a significant degree of DNA homology and are very similar antigenically, thus all cause positive serological tests for syphilis.

Epidemiology and clinical features

- *Treponema pallidum* subspecies *pallidum*—the causative agent of syphilis. An increasing incidence in the UK, beginning in the 1960s, plateaued in the mid 90s, but several large outbreaks between 1998 and 2003 saw diagnoses of infectious syphilis in men rise 15-fold. Transmission—sexual contact, direct vascular inoculation (IDU, transfusions), direct cutaneous contact with infectious lesions, or transplacental infection (congenital syphilis; ➔ see Syphilis, pp. 786–7). Interacts with HIV in both acquisition and diagnosis. For clinical features, ➔ see Syphilis, pp. 714–6. For details of treatment, ➔ see Syphilis—management, p. 716.
- *Treponema pallidum* subspecies *pertenue*—the causative agent of yaws, a chronic non-venereal disease endemic in the humid tropics (Central Africa, South America, South East Asia, and parts of the Indian subcontinent). Acquired in childhood through contact with infectious skin lesions. Incubation: 3 weeks. Affects the skin (papular skin lesions which may ulcerate) and bones (periosteitis, dactylitis). Primary stage: lesion at inoculation site; secondary stage: dissemination of treponemes, causing multiple skin lesions; latent stage: usually asymptomatic (most patients remain non-infectiously latent for their lifetime); tertiary stage (<10% patients 5–10 years later): bone, joint, soft tissue deformities.
- *Treponema pallidum* subspecies *endemicum*—the causative agent of non-venereal endemic syphilis or 'bejel'. Endemic in dry subtropical or temperate areas of the Middle East, India, Asia, and parts of Africa. Infection occurs in childhood and is associated with poor standards of hygiene. Transmission: contact with mucosal lesions or contaminated eating utensils/water. Incubation: 10–90 days. Primary lesions (1–6 weeks): patches in mouth, followed by skin lesions resembling the chancres of venereal syphilis; secondary stage (6–9 months): macerated patches on lips and tongue, anogenital hypertrophic condyloma lata, painful osteoperiostitis of long bones; tertiary stage: destruction of cartilage and bone, gummata of skin, bones, and nasopharynx. CNS/CVS (cardiovascular system) disease is very rare.

- *Treponema carateum*—the causative agent of pinta, the most benign of the endemic treponematoses, affecting only the skin. Endemic to South/Central America. Spread by contact with infected skin. Incubation 2–3 weeks. Primary lesion: papule or erythematous plaque on exposed surfaces of the legs, foot, forearm, or hands, which slowly enlarges, becoming pigmented and hyperkeratotic. May be associated with regional lymphadenopathy. Secondary lesions: disseminated lesions of similar appearance, appearing 3–9 months later. Late/tertiary pinta: disfiguring pigmentary changes and atrophic lesions.

General diagnosis

- Direct detection—culture (the gold standard) is expensive and time-consuming, and is used primarily in research. Direct detection of organisms by microscopy (dark-field or immunofluorescence) of material scraped from a lesion is the usual means of diagnosis in primary infection. PCR of such material, CSF, or vitreous fluid may be helpful in some circumstances.
- Serological diagnosis—the mainstay. Serological tests fall into two groups. Both show cross-reactivity amongst the four *Treponema* spp.:
  - non-treponemal tests (e.g. Venereal Disease Research Laboratory (VDRL), rapid plasma reagin (RPR))—detect antibodies (both IgG and IgM) to cardiolipin produced as a response to treponemal infection, and are not specific but are very sensitive. Samples with very high antibody titres may give false-negative results (the 'prozone' phenomenon) in early infection or HIV. Poor sensitivity in late-stage infection. Quantitative with antibody titres tending to decline with time—a phenomenon accelerated by therapy. False positives occur in pregnancy, TB, and endocarditis, amongst others;
  - treponemal tests—use specific treponemal antigens and are consequently more specific. Qualitative. They can detect late-stage infection and remain positive after successful therapy (e.g. *T. pallidum* haemagglutination assay (TPHA), EIA, fluorescent treponemal antibody absorption test (FTA-ABS)).

Diagnosis of syphilis

Traditionally, diagnosis was made by a sensitive non-treponemal screening test, with positive samples followed up using a more specific treponemal assay. Recent guidelines reverse this.[4]

- Specific tests should be performed first line, including EIA IgM if primary syphilis suspected (detected by end of week 2 after infection).
- Perform quantitative non-treponemal tests when treponemal tests are positive—this helps stage disease and indicates the need for treatment. A VDRL/RPR titre >16 and/or positive IgM indicate active disease within appropriate clinical context. Yaws/Pinta may give identical results—it may be appropriate to manage as if they had latent syphilis.
- Tests are often negative in late syphilis, but this does not exclude the need for treatment. Repeat positive tests on a second specimen for confirmation. Discrepant results are repeated using an immunoblot. FTA-ABS is no longer recommended for this purpose.
- Repeat screening in seronegative patients at recent risk of acquiring disease—there is a seronegative window in early primary syphilis (➲ see Syphilis, pp. 714–6).

Treatment

Early syphilis and pinta/yaws/bejel—prolonged antibiotic therapy is required due to the slow dividing rate of *T. pallidum* (averages one doubling *in vivo* per day). Highly sensitive to penicillin and a long-acting depot injection of benzathine benzylpenicillin is the standard therapy. A single dose is sufficient for early infection. Alternative: 15-day course of azithromycin (increasing reports of resistance) or doxycycline. ➲ See p. 716 for further management advice.

Reference

4 Kingston M, French P, Goh B, *et al.*; Syphilis Guidelines Revision Group 2008, Clinical Effectiveness Group. UK National Guidelines on the Management of Syphilis 2008. *Int J STD AIDS*. **19**:729–40.

Borrelia **species**

Relapsing fever

Relapsing fever is caused by several *Borrelia* spp. transmitted by arthropods, characterized by recurring episodes of fever. Two distinct clinical forms were recognized as far back as ancient Greece: epidemic louse-borne and endemic tick-borne relapsing fever. The presentation of abrupt fever, muscle aches, and joint pains with crisis, remission, and then relapse are similar for both, but the periodicity tends to be characteristic (e.g. 5.5 days for louse-borne versus 3.1 days for tick-borne). The recurrent nature is thought to be due to antigenic variation of the spirochaetal OMPs.

Epidemiology

- Tick-borne relapsing fever is worldwide and transmitted by soft-bodied *Ornithodoros* ticks. Most tick species carry distinctive borreliae. Epidemiology depends on the local vector, e.g. *Ornithodoros hermsi* is the commonest vector in California and Canada and lives in dead trees and on rodents and transmits *Borrelia hermsii*. Infection is passed down the tick generations, thus disease tends to be endemic.
- Louse-borne relapsing fever has occurred in Africa, the Middle East, and Asia. Human body louse inhabits only humans, and *Borrelia recurrentis* is not transmitted vertically within lice, thus is maintained by passage from louse to human and then back to another louse, which remains infective for its entire life. Therefore, infection is associated with poverty and overcrowding, and disease tends to be epidemic.

Clinical features

Incubation and symptoms are similar in both conditions. Three to 8 days after exposure, there is abrupt-onset fever, headache, myalgia, arthralgia, chills, weakness, anorexia, epistaxis, cough/haemoptysis, and weight loss. Examination findings include hypotension, hepatosplenomegaly, lymphadenopathy, nuchal rigidity, jaundice, photophobia, injected conjunctiva, and iritis.

- Tick-borne disease—the primary episode lasts 3–6 days and is followed by a critical episode that may cause fatal shock. The first relapse occurs 7–10 days later. Subsequent relapses are less severe. The average number of relapses experienced is three but can be as many as ten.
- Louse-borne disease—there are fewer relapses than with tick-borne infection, and hepatic or splenic involvement is commoner as are neurological manifestations (coma, hemiplegia, meningitis, seizures).

Diagnosis

Culture is possible, but not practical, and serology is not diagnostically helpful. Five % of patients have a positive VDRL. Most useful is demonstration of spirochaetes in peripheral blood smears (and other body fluids—marrow aspirates, CSF). Unlike the other spirochaetes, borreliae stain well with acid aniline dyes such as Giemsa. They are most likely to be found during febrile episodes when the sensitivity of blood smears is around 70% for louse-borne fever (less for tick). Multiple thick and thin smears may need to be examined. Immunological and PCR-based tests are available. Other laboratory findings include deranged clotting tests and elevated LFTs.

Treatment

- Tick-borne relapsing fever—tetracycline is the drug of choice, given for 7–14 days. Other: doxycycline 7 days, erythromycin 10 days.
- Louse-borne relapsing fever—a single dose of doxycycline (preferred), tetracycline, erythromycin, or benzylpenicillin.
- Jarisch–Herxheimer reactions can occur (usually within the first 2h after antibiotic administration), particularly in louse-borne relapsing fever. Features—sweating, tachycardia, hypertension, followed by profound hypotension. It can be fatal and appears to be mediated partly by tumour necrosis factor (TNF)-α. Pre-administration of steroids does not appear to limit the reaction significantly. Anti-TNF-α antibodies may help.

Lyme disease

Caused by infection with, and the host immune response to, *B. burgdorferi*. Acquired by the bite of *Ixodes* (hard) ticks, and co-infection with other tick-borne organisms can occur (e.g. babesiosis).

Epidemiology

Ticks acquire and spread infection through feeding on infected animals (particularly deer). A tick must be attached for 2–3 days to pass on infection. Only small numbers of bacteria are present in the tick until it feeds. Eighty-five per cent of human infections occur while the tick is in the nymph stage (spring to summer), and 15% in the adult stage (autumn). Cases are commonest in children aged 5–9 years and adults aged 60–69 years. Only 40% give a definite history of tick bite. Cases occur across Europe, China, Japan, Australia, and parts of the USA. It is relatively rare in the UK, most cases occurring in the south (New Forest and Salisbury Plain), East Anglia, Cumbria, and Scottish highlands.

Clinical manifestations

Clinical features may be a result of direct bacterial infection (particularly in the early stages of disease) or a consequence of an immune response leading to symptoms in many organs (e.g. arthritis). They differ with the strain of *Borrelia* involved. Less than 10% of those in endemic areas with no history of symptoms are seropositive. Features may be seen in three overlapping stages:

- *early localized*—around 7 days after a tick bite, patients may develop erythema chronicum migrans (EM), an expanding painless annular skin lesion centred on the bite, with or without local lymphadenopathy. It is probably a result of the inflammatory response to the organism in the skin. Multiple lesions can occur, following a single bite. Lasts 2–3 weeks untreated. Lymphocytoma is a rare local blue/red nodule or plaque on the ear, nipple, or scrotum. It may be mistaken for cutaneous lymphoma;

- *early disseminated*—weeks/months after the bite, patients develop constitutional symptoms, malaise, generalized lymphadenopathy, hepatitis, arthritis (50%—initially intermittent and migratory, it may evolve into chronic monoarticular arthritis in 10%), neurological features (15%—meningitis, meningoencephalitis, cranial nerve lesions, and neuropathy), cardiac features (10%—atrioventricular (AV) block, pericarditis, CCF);
- *late persistent* (but can occur within the first year)—arthritis (usually knee with synovitis/effusion), neurological (including focal deficits, fatigue, and neuropsychiatric problems). Acrodermatitis chronica atrophicans (ACA) is a decoloration of the skin of the extremities (similar in appearance to peripheral vascular disease), mostly associated with *Borrelia afzelii*.

Microbiology

Three members of the *B. burgdorferi sensu lato* complex cause Lyme disease: *B. garinii* and *B. afzelii* in Asia, and *B. burgdoferi sensu stricto* in North America. *B. garinii* and *B. afzelii* are the commonest European clinical isolates. These differences account for the variation in clinical manifestations across the world (*B. garinii* associated with neurological disease, *B. afzelii* with ACA, *B. burgdorferi sensu stricto* with joint symptoms).

Diagnosis

Laboratory support is not required for a clear clinical diagnosis of EM but should be sought for all later manifestations. Treat unvalidated investigations offered by commercial 'Lyme specialty' laboratories with caution.

- Direct detection—culture is possible from EM biopsy, but requires specialist media and takes 2–6 weeks. PCR may be useful on CSF in acute neuroborreliosis (10–30% sensitivity), tissue from ACA (>90% sensitivity) or lymphocytoma (80% sensitivity), and synovial fluid in refractory arthritis.
- Serology—most patients are seropositive within 2–4 weeks. Guidelines recommend a 2-stage approach: a sensitive EIA, followed by immunoblot (Western) of those with reactive or equivocal results. EIA may give false positives in the presence of other spirochaetes (syphilis), glandular fever, and autoimmune disease. IgM immunoblots are also prone to false positives—reserve for those with acute presentations and high probability of disease. Specific response is sensitive but develops late (30% positive in the acute phase, 70% at 2–4 weeks, 90% at 4–6 weeks). Prompt antibiotic therapy may prevent a good antibody response. Some patients remain positive for years, thus active and inactive infection cannot be distinguished. Interpret tests with caution in those without a travel history or presentation consistent with Lyme disease. Do not test those with no symptoms, even with a history of tick bite. Serology is nearly always positive in late neuroborreliosis, ACA, and arthritis.

- Lumbar puncture—for cell count and serology in those patients with neurology if the diagnosis is not obvious.

Treatment

- Early-stage skin manifestations, arthritis, or Bell's palsy—doxycycline or amoxicillin PO for 14–21 days. If arthritis persists, repeat the course, or consider IV ceftriaxone for 14–21 days. Azithromycin is a third-line agent and associated with treatment failures.
- Late or neurological disease—ACA, 21–28 days of doxycycline; isolated meningitis, 14–21 days of doxycycline; encephalitis/myelitis, 14 days of IV ceftriaxone; third-degree heart block, 14–21 days of IV ceftriaxone; late neuroborreliosis, 14–28 days of IV ceftriaxone.

Prevention

- Patients probably remain at risk of reinfection after treatment.
- Practice tick avoidance, and promptly remove any attached ticks.
- Doxycycline prophylaxis (single dose) is practised in the USA for those within 3 days of a bite from a tick that has been attached for >36h in an endemic area. European guidance is less categorical, as tick infection rates are lower, *Borrelia* spp. less pathogenic, and the window for treatment less reliable.

'Seronegative chronic Lyme disease' should be considered rare, with only two case reports of seronegative ACA and no reliable reports of seronegative late-stage neuroborreliosis. 'Post-Lyme syndrome' refers to non-specific symptoms for >6 months after effective treatment. Physicians should ensure alternative diagnoses have not been missed (e.g. multiple sclerosis, malignancy, etc.). Prolonged antibiotic courses have not been shown to be effective.

Further reading

British Infection Association (2011). The epidemiology, prevention, investigation and treatment of Lyme borreliosis in United Kingdom patients: a position statement by the British Infection Association. *J Infect* **62**:329–38.

Leptospira species

Leptospira are motile, obligately aerobic spirochaetes. They stain poorly but can be visualized on dark-field or phase contrast microscopy. Two species are identified: *Leptospira interrogans* (includes all human pathogens) and *Leptospira biflexa* (a saprophytic species). *L. interrogans* has >200 serotypes, and antigenically related organisms are grouped into serovars (a synonym for serotype) for classification. Recent DNA analysis does not correlate well with serological classification. The 'type' strain is *L. interrogans* serovar *icterohaemorrhagiae*, and the type disease leptospirosis.

Leptospirosis

A biphasic disease with initial septicaemia and a secondary phase characterized by immune phenomena (vasculitis, aseptic meningitis). Weil's disease is a severe form characterized by jaundice and acute renal failure.

Epidemiology

Leptospira are found worldwide. The primary reservoirs of most leptospiral serovars are wild mammals. These continually reinfect domestic populations, and at least 160 mammalian species are affected. The organism has been recovered from rats, pigs, dogs, cats, and cattle, amongst others, but rarely causes disease in these hosts. Rodents are the most important reservoir, and rats the commonest worldwide source. There are associations between particular animals and serovars (e.g. *L. interrogans* serovar *icterohaemorrhagiae* and rats). Humans are incidental hosts, and onwards transmission is rare. Transmission occurs when people come into contact with infected animal urine, e.g. canoeing, swimming in lakes and rivers, farming. It is primarily a disease of tropical and subtropical regions, and infection in temperate regions is uncommon.

Pathogenesis

After gaining entry via the skin or mucous membranes, the organism replicates in blood and tissue. Leptospiraemia particularly affects the liver and kidney, causing centrilobular necrosis and jaundice, or intersititial nephritis and tubular necrosis, respectively. Renal failure may occur, exacerbated by hypovolaemia. Other organs affected include muscle (oedema and focal necrosis), capillaries (vasculitis), and the eye (chronic uveitis).

Clinical features

- Incubation 7–12 days. The majority of patients (90%) develop mild disease without jaundice; 5–10% develop the severe form (Weil's).
- First phase ('septicaemic')—organism can be cultured from blood, CSF, and most tissues. Lasts 4–7 days. Characterized by a flu-like illness, cough, haemoptysis, rash, meningism, and headache. One to 3 days of improvement follows. Patients may become afebrile.
- Second stage ('immune' or 'leptospiruric phase')—antibodies may be detected, and the organism isolated from urine. Features are due to the immunological response to infection and may last up to a month. Disease may be anicteric (in which death is rare) or icteric. Aseptic meningitis is the most important feature of anicteric disease and is seen in 50% of cases. Icteric disease is characterized by jaundice, hepatosplenomegaly, nausea/vomiting, anorexia, and diarrhoea/constipation. Organisms can be isolated from blood <48h after jaundice onset. Weil's disease is characterized by jaundice, renal failure, hepatic necrosis, lung disease, and bleeding. It starts at the end of stage one.
- Other features—uveitis (<10%—can occur <1 year after initial illness), subconjunctival haemorrhage (92% of patients), renal impairment (uraemia, haematuria, oliguria), and pulmonary (haemorrhage, acute respiratory distress syndrome (ARDS)).
- Overall mortality is 10%; up to 40% in those with hepatorenal involvement.

Diagnosis

- Direct examination—dark-field examination of blood, CSF, or urine may demonstrate *Leptospira*, but there is a high false-positive rate (misinterpretation of fibrils, red cell fragments). It is not recommended.
- Culture—there has been little change in culture techniques over the years. It is difficult and insensitive, and requires several weeks of

incubation. Specialized culture media are required (e.g. Ellinghausen-McCullough-Johnson-Harris (EMJH) which contains 1% bovine serum albumin and TWEEN® 80, a fatty acid source). They should be inoculated within 24h of specimen collection (either blood or CSF in heparin or sodium oxalate). Leptospiral culture can be established by subculture of routine BC samples. Organisms can be isolated from blood and CSF in the first week of illness in 50% of cases. In the second phase of illness, they can be found only in the urine where they may be isolated for up to 1 month. Cultures can be reported as negative after 6–12 weeks.

- Molecular techniques—quantitative PCR assays to detect leptospiral DNA have been developed. They are sensitive, can distinguish different species, and allow early diagnosis, and organisms can be detected after antibiotic therapy has been initiated.
- Serology—the mainstay of diagnosis. Commercial tests using genus-specific antigens are used to screen sera, and positive reactions confirmed in a reference laboratory using the micro-agglutination test (MAT) with live *Leptospira* (killed have lower sensitivity). The MAT detects agglutinating antibodies in patient serum and is relatively serovar-specific, so a large number of antigens must be tested. Interlaboratory variation is high. A positive MAT is considered to be a 4-fold increase in antibody titre, or a switch from seronegative to a titre of 1/100 or over. Early samples tend to cross-react; convalescent samples are more specific and diagnostic. EIA for IgM is useful for diagnosing current infection, but cross-reactions occur.

Treatment

- Mild disease—doxycycline (preferred as also effective for rickettsial disease which may be confused with leptospirosis), amoxicillin PO for 5–7 days.
- Severe disease—penicillin G, ceftriaxone IV for 5–7 days.
- Children or pregnant women can be treated with amoxicillin or ceftriaxone. Azithromycin is an alternative in severe allergy.
- Prophylaxis—doxycycline reduces morbidity and mortality in endemic areas, but has no impact on infection rates, as measured by seroconversion. It is likely to be useful in cases of accidental laboratory exposure or military and adventure travel. Animal vaccines are available against specific serovars.

Overview of *Rickettsia*—ACDP 3

Microbiology

Rickettsiae are fastidious, obligate intracellular Gram-negative coccobacilli (0.3 micrometres by 1–2 micrometres). They survive only briefly outside a host (unlike *Coxiella*, with whom they were previously classified) and are maintained in a cycle involving mammal reservoirs and arthropod vectors. Isolation is usually only performed in reference laboratories.

Epidemiology

Zoonotic reservoirs are varied and include wild rodents, dogs, and livestock. Humans are incidental hosts, with the exception of louse-borne typhus where humans are the main reservoir. *Rickettsia rickettsii, Rickettsia typhi, Rickettsia tsutsugamushi*, and *Rickettsia akari* can exist as vector commensals. *Rickettsia prowazekii*, however, kills its human body louse vector within 3 weeks. For geographical distribution, see Table 7.18.

Table 7.18 Overview of rickettsial disease

	Species	Syndrome	Vector (geography)	Clinical features
Spotted fever group	*R. rickettsii*	Rocky Mountain spotted fever	*Ixodid* ticks (Western hemisphere)	Incubation ~7 days. Fever, headache, myalgia, eschar, rash. Multisystem involvement; 20% untreated mortality
	R. conorii	Mediterranean spotted fever	*Ixodid* ticks (Mediterranean, Africa, and India)	Incubation ~5 days. Eschar and local lymphadenopathy. Rash. Mild
	R. africae	African tick bite fever	Tick (sub-Saharan Africa, East Caribbean)	5–7 days. Mild illness, minimal rash, eschar with lymphadenopathy
	R. akari	Rickettsial pox	Mite (USA, Africa, Korea, and Russian Federation)	Incubation ~7 days. As for *R. conorii* plus vesicular rash resembling chickenpox
Typhus group	*R. prowazekii*	Epidemic typhus	Body louse (South America, Africa, Asia)	Incubation ~10 days. Fever, headache, neurological, and GI symptoms. Rash. 20–50% untreated mortality
		Brill–Zinsser disease	Nil—recurrence years after primary attack	Similar, milder illness than epidemic typhus, developing years after recovery—in West was seen in East European immigrants after World War II. Lasts around 2 weeks
	R. typhi	Murine (endemic) typhus	Flea (worldwide where human/rat coexist)	Similar to epidemic typhus, but much milder
	R. tsutsugamushi	Scrub typhus[a]	Mite (South Pacific, Asia, Australia)	Eschar common. Similar to epidemic typhus

[a]So-called 'scrub' typhus, as the vector is harboured in scrub vegetation. The chigger mites stay within several metres of where they hatch and are transovarially infected. Infection therefore occurs in very focused rural 'mite islands'.

Diagnosis

- Usually based upon clinical features and epidemiological history. The presence of a typical rash or eschar suggests the diagnosis.
- Culture—usually only performed in reference laboratories. Blood or biopsy tissue from skin lesions should be frozen at −70°C. Organisms may be isolated in small laboratory animals or in embryonated eggs. Highly infectious if aerosolized—fatal laboratory-acquired infections have occurred.
- Detection of antigen—direct immunofluorescence of skin lesions in spotted fevers (rash or eschar) can identify organisms. Sensitivity is around 70%, with specificity approaching 100%. Organisms are most likely to be in a blood vessel near the centre of the lesion—the biopsy should include this to increase chances. Availability is limited. PCR assays are available but rarely used outside of research centres.
- Serology—not useful acutely, but the main means of confirming diagnosis. Antibodies first appear around days 7–10 after infection. A 4-fold rise on a convalescent sample is required for diagnosis, but a single titre over 1:64 is very suggestive of infection (sensitivity 95%). Most tests cannot distinguish between spotted fever group species.
  - Micro-immunofluorescence is the most sensitive/specific test—it requires trained personnel and a fluorescence microscope.
  - Latex agglutination tests are available for Rocky Mountain spotted fever (RMSF). A single positive test is considered diagnostic. Rarely produce positive reactions in convalescence.
  - Complement fixation and the Weil–Felix[2] test are neither sufficiently sensitive nor specific.

Rickettsial diseases

Rickettsiae replicate within the cytoplasm of infected endothelial and smooth muscle cells of capillaries and small arteries. They cause a necrotizing vasculitis, with consequent protean manifestations. The classic triad of fever, headache, and rash, with the appropriate travel and exposure history, should alert to the possible diagnosis. An eschar (black, ulcerated lesion) may develop at the bite site. Severity varies greatly with species—any organ can be involved.

Spotted fevers

Rocky Mountain spotted fever

- Clinical features—the most virulent spotted fever, with 20% mortality if untreated. Fever, myalgia, and headache follow a 2- to 14-day incubation. GI involvement may suggest an acute surgical abdomen. Maculopapular rash (90% cases, more likely to be spotless in the elderly or black) appears around days 3–5, often starting at the hands, and may become petechial or necrotic. Gangrene in 4%. Severe multisystem

2 In 1915, in Poland, Weil and Felix found that serum from patients with typhus agglutinated certain strains of *P. vulgaris*. It has been the mainstay of diagnosis for many years.

involvement is common, including lung (pneumonia, effusions, oedema), nervous system (meningitis, focal deficits, e.g. deafness), and renal impairment. Thrombocytopenia and DIC can occur. Death at around 10 days, sooner in fulminant cases (more frequently in black males with G6PD deficiency).

- Treatment—tetracycline, chloramphenicol (preferred in pregnancy), or doxycycline for 7 days, continuing for 2 days after the patient becomes afebrile. It is recommended that doxycycline is used, even in children with suspected RMSF, given the life-threatening nature of the disease. No demonstrated benefit from steroid therapy.

Other spotted fevers

- Mediterranean spotted fever (boutonneuse fever) is a much milder disease; 5–7 days after inoculation, patients develop an eschar, with local tender lymphadenopathy and a generalized maculopapular rash with abrupt onset of fever and headache. Mortality is rare, but disease severity varies with the specific strain. Severe disease is more likely in those with diabetes, cardiac disease, and G6PD deficiency, and the elderly.
- African tick bite fever (*R. africae*) causes a mild clinical illness (fever, headache, myalgia), eschars, regional lymphadenopathy with scant or absent rash. May be a common cause of fever in returning travellers.
- Rickettsial pox (*R. akari*, transmitted by house mouse mite) outbreaks typically occur after mouse extermination programmes result in starving mites that seek an alternative source of blood. Presentation is similar to Mediterranean spotted fever, with the addition of a vesicular rash that resembles chickenpox.

Treatment of all of these fevers is with doxycycline 100mg bd for 5–7 days.

Typhus group

Epidemic typhus

- In recent decades, epidemic typhus has been reported in Burundi, Rwanda, Ethiopia, the highlands of Algeria, and a few remote regions of mountainous South and Central America.
- Clinical features—unusual in that humans are the reservoir,[3] and outbreaks are thus commonest in conditions of crowding, especially winter and war. The louse feeds on an infected person, and bites and defecates on the next, and infected faeces (which may remain infectious for as long as 100 days) are scratched into the bite.
  - Acute disease—after 1-week incubation, abrupt onset of headache and fever is followed by maculopapular rash at day 5. This involves the entire body within days. Neurological features (confusion, drowsiness, coma) are common, as is multisystem involvement (DIC, jaundice, myocarditis, pulmonary infiltrates). Mortality is 20–50% untreated—low in children, high in the elderly.

3 Although *R. prowazekii* infection has been demonstrated amongst flying squirrels in the USA, with the squirrel flea and louse as vectors.

  - Brill–Zinsser disease—a recrudescence years after the initial episode. Usually a mild illness. Abrupt onset with fever, headache, malaise, and often rash. Patients are often elderly, and symptoms may be attributed to pre-exisiting ailments.
- Prevention—delousing, doxycycline prophylaxis for HCWs in affected areas.
- Treatment—as for RMSF. Early therapy nearly eliminates fatal illness.

Murine typhus
- Clinical features—longer incubation (up to 2 weeks), and patients rarely recall flea exposure. Fever, headache, and myalgia are followed by rash in 50%. Some may develop multisystem features, but this is less common than with epidemic louse-borne typhus. Mortality is <1%, higher in the elderly and those with G6PD deficiency.
- Treatment—spontaneous recovery usually occurs within 2 weeks if untreated. Antibiotic treatment is as for RMSF.

Scrub typhus
- Clinical features—not as severe as epidemic typhus. An individual is inoculated by the bite of the chigger mite, and develops abrupt fever and headache 6–18 days later. Usually tender lymph nodes and an eschar at the inoculation point. Severity varies widely—neurological features can occur. Untreated mortality varies—up to 30%. Many serotypes (unlike the other organisms), so people may become infected again.
- Treatment—as for RMSF, but resistance to doxycycline and chloramphenicol has been seen in Northern Thailand. Treatment may need to be prolonged to avoid relapse (2 weeks). Azithromycin may be an alternative.

Coxiella burnetii—ACDP 3

Q fever (as in 'Query') is the name coined by the medical officer in Queensland, Australia, who first investigated the outbreak of febrile illness that hit 20 employees of a Brisbane meat works.

Microbiology

C. burnetii is morphologically similar to the rickettsiae but, with a variety of genetic and physiological differences, is now classified separately (more closely related to *Legionella*). It is a significantly hardier organism and may be transmitted by aerosol or infected milk. It can form spores and is able to survive outside a host for some time—over 40 months in skimmed milk at room temperature. It grows in the phagosomes of infected cells, rather than the cytoplasm (as other *Rickettsia*)—appreciating the more acidic environment the phagosome affords. A characteristic feature is its antigenic 'phase' variation. If isolated from humans/animals, it is highly infectious and expresses phase I antigens. However, once subcultured within cells, its capsule LPS antigens change (phase II), and it is not infectious. This shift allows differentiation of acute and chronic Q fever.

Epidemiology

Found around the world, and a zoonosis, the organism is usually acquired from occupational exposure to cattle or sheep but can be caught from many different animals—exposure to parturient cats is an important risk factor. Acquisition from unpasteurized dairy products has occurred, and person-to-person spread is possible but unusual. It exists in a tick reservoir, but this is thought to be an insignificant route of direct human infection—it is likely they infect those animals from which man may acquire it. Infected ungulates are usually asymptomatic, although abortion/stillbirth may result. Organisms from a heavily infected placenta may be found in the soil for 6 months, and the air for 2 weeks after parturition. The largest outbreak yet described took place in the Netherlands in 2009 where it was previously unknown. It is a common cause of fever in armed forces personnel returning from Iraq and Afghanistan. Other risk factors—those living downwind from farms or contaminated manure, abattoir workers, vets.

Clinical features

- Incubation—humans are infected by inhalation (occasionally ingestion). Rare cases have occurred by transplacental transmission, intradermally, and via blood transfusions. Organisms proliferate in the lungs, and bacteraemia follows. Up to 50% of cases may be asymptomatic. Presentation is 2–5 weeks after infection.
- Acute Q fever—ranges from a self-limiting febrile illness (commonest), a prolonged fever of unknown origin (FUO) with granulomatous hepatitis, to a pneumonia. The pneumonia may be an incidental finding, as part of an FUO or a severe atypical pneumonia, with dry cough, fever, fatigue, pleuritic chest pain, pleural effusion, and diarrhoea. It may be rapidly progressive, resembling legionnaires' disease. Hepatomegaly and rashes are common. Acute Q fever can be complicated by behavioural disturbances, GBS, myo-/pericarditis, arthritis, glomerulonephritis, severe headache, and aseptic meningitis, amongst others. Autoantibodies are often found (anti-mitochondria, smooth muscle). Mortality is around 1% and associated with myocarditis. Acquisition during pregnancy increases the risk of obstetric complications.
- Chronic Q fever—defined as infection lasting >6 months. Occurs in 1–5% of cases and may present years later. The commonest manifestation is culture-negative endocarditis. It usually occurs in those with pre-existing valve damage (<40% of such patients with acute Q fever develop endocarditis, unless treated promptly). Thus, patients diagnosed with Q fever should have valvular disease excluded. Hepatitis, osteomyelitis, vascular graft infection, and neurological infection are also recognized. Immunocompromised and pregnant hosts are at higher risk of chronic disease.

Diagnosis

- Culture—difficult and hazardous for laboratory staff; a category 3 organism.
- Serology—the organism has two biological phases. Antibodies to phase II are produced first. Phase I antibodies appear weeks later. If antibodies to both phases are present simultaneously, chronic infection (specifically

endocarditis) should be considered. Cross-reactions occur with *Bartonella* infection. Immunofluorescence is the most widely used test. Seroconversion may be detected 7–15 days after symptom onset, and 90% have detectable antibodies by day 21. A high phase II titre indicates acute infection, whereas a high phase I titre suggests chronic infection—particularly, it remains high 6 months after treatment completion. Those at high risk of chronic disease (valve abnormalities, immunodeficiency, pregnancy) should undergo serial serological testing for at least 6 months.
- Molecular—PCR tests exist but are not in widespread use outside of specialist reference labs.

Treatment
- Pneumonia—infection is nearly always self-limiting. Even without therapy, people begin to recover at around 2 weeks. However, treatment is indicated in all cases to reduce the chance of chronic disease—doxycycline, or chloramphenicol for 2–3 weeks. Long-term co-trimoxazole is an alternative during pregnancy. Patients should have an echocardiogram to exclude valve abnormalities. If normal, they should have serological follow-up testing at 3 and 6 months to ensure resolution.
- Valve abnormalities—those with acute Q fever who are found to have an underlying valve disease should be considered for prophylaxis (12 months of hydroxychloroquine with doxycycline), even in the absence of endocarditis, given the high risk of its development.
- Endocarditis—combination antibiotic therapy for a prolonged period (minimum 18 months; lifelong has been mooted in some cases), e.g. tetracycline with rifampicin, doxycycline with hydroxychloroquine. Valve replacement may be required.
- Consider Q fever in the diagnosis of culture-negative endocarditis.

Bartonella species

Microbiology
Bartonellae are Gram-negative intracellular organisms belonging to the genus *Bartonella*, closely related to *Brucella*, based on 16S rRNA analysis. Most species causing human infection are associated with mammalian reservoirs that may experience chronic asymptomatic infection.

Clinical syndromes
- Bartonellosis (*Bartonella bacilliformis*)—a biphasic disease transmitted by *Phlebotomus* sandflies. Endemic to Andean regions (Peru, Colombia, Ecuador).
  - Oroya fever—3–12 weeks after inoculation. Mild or severe (fever, headache, confusion, acute anaemia due to erythrocyte invasion). Complications: abdominal pain, thrombocytopenia, seizures, dyspnoea, hepatic/GI dysfunction, angina; 40% untreated mortality. Treatment: chloramphenicol plus a β-lactam for 14 days. Risk of

opportunistic infections in survivors (e.g. *Salmonella*, toxoplasmosis). Asymptomatic bacteraemia with *B. bacilliformis* occurs in 15% of survivors.

- Verruga peruana is a late-stage manifestation, usually experienced by populations native to the Andes. Crops of skin lesions appear weeks to months after an untreated acute infection. Initially miliary, they become nodular, then 'mulaire' (red round lesions, 5mm in diameter). Occur on mucosal surfaces and internally. Histology demonstrates neovascular proliferation with occasional organisms.

- Cat-scratch disease (*Bartonella henselae*)—commonest cause of lymphadenopathy in children/young adolescents; 3–10 days after inoculation, a papule or pustule may be visible at the site. Most present at 2–3 weeks with the onset of regional lymphadenopathy and fever. Rarely, headache, sore throat, and skin rash. Lymph nodes settle over 2–4 months, even without treatment. Complications (commoner in the immunocompromised): encephalopathy, retinitis, bone/skin involvement, granulomatous hepatitis. Conjunctival exposure may present as Parinaud's oculoglandular syndrome (ocular granuloma/conjunctivitis, preauricular lymphadenopathy). Other atypical presentations: FUO, osteomyelitis, hepatic/splenic granulomas. Diagnosis is based on history. Biopsy may be necessary to exclude lymphoma. Blood or tissue culture should be attempted in cases of FUO, neuroretinitis, or encephalitis after cat exposure, especially if immunocompromised. Treatment: mild, 5 days of azithromycin; disseminated, 14 days of rifampicin plus azithromycin; neuroretinitis, 4–6 weeks of doxycycline or azithromycin plus rifampicin.
- *Bacillary angiomatosis* (BA)—unusual vascular proliferation caused by *B. henselae* or *Bartonella quintana* infection. Usually occurs in the immunocompromised, mostly HIV patients with CD4 $<100/\text{mm}^3$, but also transplant patients and those on chemotherapy. Lesions begin as small papules that grow into round red/purple nodules that can ulcerate. May also appear as flat, hyperpigmented plaques. Occur in the skin, liver, spleen, bone, mucosal surfaces, heart, CNS, and bone marrow. Pathogenesis: the organism's outer membrane adhesin binds to endothelial cells, and induces endothelial proliferation and new vessel formation. Numerous organisms are visible in lesions stained with Warthin–Starry silver stain. Diagnosis: lesion biopsy. All patients should be treated: 6–8 weeks of erythromycin or doxycycline for cutaneous disease, longer if recurrence occurs. Skin lesions may be excised. Without therapy, systemic infection (fever, abdominal pain, anorexia) can occur.
- *Bacterial peliosis* (BP)—characterized by blood-filled cystic lesions scattered throughout a visceral organ. Cases involving the liver (peliosis hepatis) and spleen present with weight loss, diarrhoea, abdominal pain, nausea, fever, hepatosplenomegaly, and elevated liver enzymes. Caused by *B. henselae* or *B. quintana* (less common, affecting bone). Most patients also have BA and previous cat exposure.
- *Fever, bacteraemia, endocarditis* (*B. quintana*)—acquired by scratching infected louse faeces into skin lesions. Epidemics occur in conditions of overcrowding and poor sanitation (e.g. soldiers in World War I—'trench

fever'). Bacteraemia has been described in homeless alcoholics. Incubation is 3–40 days, followed by a relapsing fever with headache, rash, and splenomegaly. Recognized cause of culture-negative endocarditis in those with HIV and immunocompetent alcoholics. *B. henselae* bacteraemia occurs in the immunocompetent as well as those with HIV. Diagnosis is by culture, or PCR/serology if culture-negative. Treatment: 4–6 weeks of macrolides and tetracyclines. Endocarditis may need surgery and very prolonged antibiotic courses.

Diagnosis

- Direct examination—Giemsa-stained blood films may detect *B. bacilliformis* in areas of endemic Oroya fever (large number of organisms). Not useful in the detection of *B. henselae* or *B. quintana*, due to the low level of blood-borne organisms. May be visible by silver staining of lesions in BA or BP and in lymph nodes in early cat-scratch disease.
- *Culture*—may fail to trigger CO_2 detection systems; *B. henselae* grows on chocolate agar, with characteristic white, dry, cauliflower-like colonies. These become visible 5–14 days after incubation at 37°C in 5% CO_2. On Gram stain, they are small, curved bacilli 2 micrometres by 0.5 micrometres, and display twitching motility when mounted in a saline drop. They are non-reactive for many standard biochemical tests. Colonies with the appropriate morphological characteristics can have their identity confirmed by cellular fatty acid analysis, immunofluorescence antibody, or using commercial enzymatic substrate kits.
- *Molecular*—PCR or DNA hybridization techniques can be used to speciate isolates. Direct detection of *Bartonella* organisms in pus or tissue is possible using PCR with wide-ranging sensitivity, depending on the technique and sample.
- *Serology*—EIA or immunofluorescence kits may be used to demonstrate anti-*Bartonella* antibodies in culture-negative endocarditis, those with cat-scratch disease, or HIV-associated aseptic meningitis, etc. There is substantial cross-reactivity between *B. henselae* and *B. quintana*, as well as with certain *Chlamydia* spp.

Mycoplasma

Microbiology

Amongst the smallest free-living organisms (0.2 micrometres in diameter) and lack a cell wall (bound only by a trilaminar membrane). Possess a small genome with limited biosynthetic capabilities. Require enriched media for growth. The term '*Mycoplasma*' refers to a member of the class *Mollicutes*, thus encompassing the genera *Mycoplasma* and *Ureaplasma*. Many species have been isolated, but only four are significant human pathogens, a property attributed to tip organelles that interact with host cells.

Mycoplasma pneumoniae

Common cause of respiratory tract infection all year round (peaking in winter), affecting all ages, but with most disease between 5 years to young adulthood. Droplet transmission. Organism attaches to respiratory epithelial cells and multiplies locally producing H_2O_2, resulting in epithelial damage. Incubation is for 2–3 weeks, and presentation is usually insidious, e.g. flu-like, wheeze (especially in children), intractable cough. Less than 10% develop pneumonia (commonest cause of 'atypical'). Multiple lobes may be involved, but without consolidation; effusions in 20%. Disease is usually self-limited, resolving over 3–10 days without antibiotics. CXR abnormalities may take 6 weeks to clear. Antibiotic therapy (e.g. erythromycin) speeds resolution but rarely eradicates the organisms—recurrences can occur. Antibodies produced against *M. pneumoniae* cross-react with brain cells and erythrocytes (cold agglutinins). Immunity is not long-lasting. Complications (many immune-mediated): pleuritis, pneumothorax, lung abscess, haemolytic anaemia (cold agglutinins), thrombocytopenia, arthritis, rashes (e.g. erythema nodosum and multiforme), myocarditis, GBS, transverse myelitis, acute disseminated encephalomyelitis. Meningoencephalitis is thought to be due to direct invasion. Immunodeficiency predisposes to severe disease.

Ureaplasma urealyticum and *Mycoplasma hominis*

Part of the commensal flora in male and female urogenital tracts. Sexually transmitted, the rate is related to sexual activity and is much lower amongst women using barrier contraception. They are associated with GU infections, including non-gonococcal urethritis, epididymitis (rare), endometritis, chorioamnionitis, PID, pyelonephritis, and neonatal bacteraemia/abscesses. Additionally, they are statistically linked with prematurity, low birthweight, and infertility, and—in the case of *U. urealyticum*—colonization of the respiratory tract is linked to the development of chronic lung disease of the newborn. Both may be isolated from blood cultures in women with post-partum fever (10% of cases), and may cause septic arthritis and s/c abscesses in those with immunodeficiency. Sternal wound infections with *M. hominis* have occurred in heart and lung transplant patients.

Other *Mycoplasma* organisms

Mycoplasma genitalium is a cause of non-gonococcal urethritis and may also have a role in respiratory tract disease. *Mycoplasma fermentans, Mycoplasma penetrans*, and *Mycoplasma pirum* have been isolated in those with HIV and are unusual in their ability to actively invade cells. Certain organisms found in animal hosts have caused human disease if sufficient exposure and predisposing co-morbidity (e.g. *Mycoplasma arginini, Mycoplasma canis*—in dogs).

Diagnosis

- Direct detection—indirect fluorescent antibody tests to detect *M. hominis* in genital samples have been developed (not widely used).
- Culture—specimens should be inoculated to culture media as soon as possible. Several media are used—most are diphasic (media with agar overlayed by media without agar). All species grow at 35–37°C

but differ in their optimal pH, atmospheric conditions, and substrate utilization.

- *M. pneumoniae*—rarely attempted, as requires up to 4 weeks. Growth is indicated by pH change. Positives are subcultured to agar, and colonies should then be visible after a week. Identity is confirmed by serological methods or enzyme substrate tests.
- Genital *Mycoplasma* samples are inoculated into broth and onto agar, and should be kept for 8 days (although *M. genitalium* and *M. fermentans* can take longer and are not routinely looked for). Broths that exhibit a change in colour are plated to the appropriate agar. Plates are examined by microscope each day for colonies. Selective plates and colonial morphology are usually sufficient to allow identification. Antisera are available to confirm *M. hominis*.

- Molecular—PCR techniques are available and are perhaps most useful in acute respiratory illness. Not yet in widespread use.
- Serology—*M. pneumoniae* complement fixation tests detect early IgM, and IgG to a lesser extent. EIAs are surplanting them, being more sensitive than culture in detecting acute infection (sensitivity 97.8%). A 4-fold rise between acute and convalescent (14 days) samples is diagnostic of recent infection.

Treatment

- *M. pneumoniae* is sensitive to a wide range of agents—tetracyclines, quinolones, or macrolides (resistance emerging, e.g. Japan, China), e.g. azithromycin for 5 days, doxycycline for 7–14 days.
- *M. hominis* is usually resistant to macrolides. Some genital *Mycoplasma* isolates have been found to be tetracycline-resistant and carry the *tetM* resistance determinant (also found in other genital tract organisms, e.g. GBS). Doxycycline considered first line. Fluoroquinolones usually active. Clindamycin may be appropriate in neonates.
- *U. urealyticum*—usually resistant to clindamycin and less susceptible to quinolones. Doxycycline first line. Erythromycin or azithromycin are effective.

Chlamydia

Small obligate intracellular (unable to produce ATP) Gram-negative organisms. Outside a host cell, they are tiny (300nm in diameter), inactive 'elementary' bodies. They infect cells by receptor-mediated endocytosis, inhibit lysosome fusion, and reside in a membrane-protected 'inclusion' body where they grow (800nm in diameter). Three species produce human disease. The family *Chlamydiaceae* was reorganized in 1999 on the basis of genetic similarities. *C. trachomatis* remains in the genus *Chlamydia*, but *psittaci* and *pneumoniae* were moved to a new genus *Chlamydophila*. They differ antigenically in host preference and antibiotic susceptibility.

Chlamydia trachomatis

Clinical features

There are 15 different serovars causing distinctive clinical syndromes. Natural infection confers only short-lived protection against reinfection.

- *Lymphogranuloma venereum* (LGV) (serovar L1, L2, L3)—endemic in Africa, India, South East Asia, South America, and the Caribbean. Sexually transmitted. The organism enters through skin abrasions and causes a small papule or ulcer (primary lesion) on genital mucosa or nearby skin 3–30 days after infection. It heals rapidly, and, weeks later, the patient develops secondary symptoms: lymphadenopathy (usually inguinal/femoral), fever, headache, myalgias, proctitis (particularly in MSM, and may resemble IBD), and occasionally meningitis. Nodes may coalesce, forming abscesses and buboes.
- *Trachoma* (serovar A, B1, B2, C)—chronic follicular keratoconjunctivitis that leads to corneal scarring and is the most common cause of preventable blindness in the developing world (500 million affected, around 9 million blind). First infection acquired in childhood. Resolves, but multiple reinfections, and the consequent host response results in conjunctival scarring and corneal damage. The inner surface of the eyelid scars and inturning eyelashes further abrade the cornea (see Box 7.10).
- *Inclusion conjunctivitis* (serovars D to K)—sexually transmitted eye infection of adults (of whom slightly over half have concurrent genital tract infection) and a cause of neonatal conjunctivitis (probably from the mother's genital tract, but can occur even if delivered by Caesarean section—5 days to 6 weeks after delivery). No corneal scarring.
- *Neonatal pneumonia* (serovars D to K)—most acquired from the mother's genital tract. Seen in 10–20% of infants born to infected mothers. Usually symptomatic by 8 weeks with nasal congestion, cough, etc., and only moderately ill.
- *STIs* (serovars D to K)—epididymitis (along with *N. gonorrhoeae*, the common cause in the under 35s), urethritis, proctitis (usually asymptomatic), salpingitis, cervicitis with consequent PID and infertility. Reactive arthritis/Reiter's syndrome may follow. Perihepatitis (Fitz-Hugh–Curtis syndrome) is an inflammation of the liver capsule and adjacent peritoneum seen in the setting of PID, presenting with right upper quadrant pain.

Box 7.10 WHO grading of trachoma

- Trachomatous inflammation follicular—5+ follicles in upper tarsal conjunctiva.
- Trachomatous inflammation intense—pronounced tarsal conjunctival inflammation obscuring at least half of deep tarsal vessels.
- Trachomatous conjunctival scarring—scars on tarsal conjunctiva.
- Trachomatous trichiasis—1+ eyelash rubs on eyeball.
- Corneal opacity—opacity obscuring part of pupil margin.

Diagnosis

Trachoma may be diagnosed on clinical grounds. Other clinical presentations require laboratory identification for a definitive diagnosis. The majority of genital STIs are asymptomatic.

- NAAT—the test of choice, performed on vaginal swabs (best), male first-catch urine, rectal or conjunctival swabs. PCR, transcription-mediated amplification (TMA), and strand displacement amplification techniques are all sensitive (80–99%, depending on assay and sample) and specific (>98%).
- Immunoassay rapid testing—rapid tests based on monoclonal antibody binding of chlamydial antigens from patient-collected samples have been developed, allowing same-day results.
- Direct detection—microscopy of certain Giemsa-stained clinical specimens (particularly neonatal conjunctivitis) may allow direct visualization if there are sufficient bacterial inclusion bodies in the cytoplasm. Monoclonal antibodies and immunofluorescence increase sensitivity.
- Culture—research tool only, as being obligate intracellular organisms, the techniques for culturing are similar to those used in virus culture.
- Serology—most useful for epidemiological studies.

Treatment

- Trachoma—transmission is by flies or eye-to-hand in endemic areas, thus hygiene is important for control (rates fall quickly with socio-economic improvement). Systemic therapy (erythromycin or doxycycline) is effective in areas of low transmission (where reinfection is less frequent). Eyelid surgery can prevent further mechanical damage. In endemic areas, treatment is best delivered over an entire region (reduces reinfection). WHO guidelines recommend mass treatment if the prevalence of active trachoma amongst 1–9 year olds in a region is over 10%.
- LGV—aspirate buboes. Doxycycline for 3 weeks.
- Genital and ocular infections in adults—single-dose azithromycin, or doxycyline for 7 days. Longer courses of amoxicillin may be effective in pregnant women. Remember that gonococcal infection may coexist.
- Neonatal infections—erythromycin PO for 14 days for conjunctivitis (topical therapy will not eliminate carriage) and pneumonia. Prenatal screening of mothers and treating those infected with *Chlamydia* is 90% effective in preventing infants from acquiring infection.

Chlamydophila psittaci

C. psittaci infects many kinds of birds, thus the classic term for infection caused by this bacteria 'psittacosis' (derived from the Greek word for parrot) is not so accurate a description as 'ornithosis'. It is an occupational disease of zoo workers, petshop workers, and poultry farmers. Human-to-human transmission occurs but is very rare. Infection is primarily acquired by inhalation of organisms from aerosolized avian excreta or respiratory secretions from sick birds (mouth-to-beak resuscitation has been implicated in acquisition). Transient exposure is sufficient (e.g. petshop customers, gardening), and cases have occurred following exposure to other infected animals (e.g. dogs, sheep). The disease is found worldwide. Incubation is 5–14 days, and presentation is with fever, chills, malaise, cough, headache, breathlessness, mild pharyngitis, and epistaxis. Less commonly, nausea, vomiting, and jaundice may be seen. Examination may demonstrate the features of an atypical pneumonia. Other features: bradycardia, peri-/myocarditis, culture-negative endocarditis, splenomegaly, meningitis, encephalitis, GBS, rashes, acute glomerulonephritis, severe respiratory failure, sepsis, shock. Relapses can occur. Infection in pregnancy may be life-threatening. Diagnosis: serology, micro-immunofluorescent antibody (MIF) test is sensitive and specific for *C. psittaci*. A 4-fold rise in titre or high IgM titre is considered diagnostic. Complement fixation tests are more widely available but cannot differentiate between chlamydial species. Culture is avoided due to the risks to laboratory staff. PCR-based tests are available. Treatment: tetracycline or doxycycline for 2–3 weeks (reduces the risk of relapse). Erythromycin may be used in children and pregnant women.

Chlamydophila pneumoniae

The cause of 3–10% of CAP cases amongst adults. Adolescents tend to experience mild pneumonia/bronchitis. Older adults can experience more severe disease. Fifty per cent of young adults have serological evidence of previous infection. Unlike *C. psittaci*, human-to-human transmission by respiratory secretions is the norm. In most populations, infection is commoner in males (may reflect cigarette use). Incubation is 3–4 weeks, and symptoms of a URTI are followed by bronchitis or pneumonia 1–4 weeks later. Most infections are mild or asymptomatic. Other features: hoarse voice, non-productive cough, headache. Fever is often absent. Extrapulmonary features: meningoencephalitis, GBS, myocarditis, reactive arthritis. Symptoms can be very prolonged, even with treatment. Diagnosis: serology, preferably MIF. A definite case requires a 4-fold rise in titre—single elevated IgG titres may be seen in the uninfected elderly as a consequence of repeated infections. Antibody tests may be negative in the early weeks after infection—it can take as long as 8 weeks for a significant IgG response to develop after primary infection. Other tests: PCR, direct immunofluorescence, and immunoassay cell culture tests. Treatment: doxycycline or erythromycin for 10–14 days. Response is often slow.

Mycobacterium tuberculosis—ACDP 3

The MTB complex comprises several species, including *M. tuberculosis*, *M. bovis*, *M. africanum*, *M. microti*, and *M. caprae*. The term tuberculosis (TB) describes a broad range of clinical diseases caused by MTB (and less commonly *M. bovis*). For treatment of TB disease, ➲ see Antituberculous agents, pp. 71–5.

Epidemiology

MTB is estimated to infect one-third of the world's population and is the second most frequent infectious cause of death worldwide after HIV. There are around 8 million new cases of active TB every year, causing around 1.7 million deaths. Most cases occur in the developing world. In the developed world, despite a general downward trend, there has been an increase in incidence in certain groups, e.g. immigrants from high-prevalence countries and HIV-infected patients. Infection is acquired by inhalation of infectious droplet nuclei or occasionally skin inoculation. The resurgence of TB in Africa has been fuelled by HIV, which increases the risk of developing all forms of TB. The emergence of MDR- (resistance to at least isoniazid and rifampicin) and XDR- (resistance to rifampicin, isoniazid, a quinolone, and an injectable agent) TB has further complicated management and is discussed further elsewhere (➲ see Second line, p. 73–4).

Microbiology

Mycobacteria are aerobic, non-sporing, non-motile, weakly Gram-positive bacilli, characterized by their cell envelope, of which mycolic acid is a key component. It is this that enables it to resist destaining with acid-alcohol after staining with aniline dyes hence acid-fast bacilli (AFB). MTB is slow-growing, with a generation time of >24h in laboratory media. At least 3–4 weeks are needed to grow the organism on solid media in most cases. Liquid culture systems are faster, with BACTEC detecting the growth of MTB in as little as 8 days with smear-positive specimens. Once grown, identification is by morphology/biochemical properties or nucleic acid detection.

Immunology and pathogenesis

Inhaled infectious droplets lodge in the alveoli. They may either be cleared by the innate immune system or establish infection. Such infection may be immediately active (primary disease) or latent, and/or activate many years later, determined by the interplay between the organism and host cell-mediated immune response. Disease occurs in 10% of otherwise healthy infected people, half within the first 3 years after infection.

- Primary infection—inhaled TB bacilli multiply in alveolar macrophages that, in turn, produce cytokines (TNF-α, platelet-derived growth factor, transforming growth factor-β, fibroblast growth factor), attracting neutrophils and other phagocytic cells. These form a nodule or 'tubercle' (granulomatous in histology). This will enlarge if infection is progressive, and bacilli may reach regional lymph nodes. A tubercle plus regional lymphadenopathy is termed the Ghon complex. Bacilli proliferate until an effective cell-mediated immune response is mounted. If this is ineffective, progressive lung disease and dissemination may occur.
- Reactivation—otherwise healthy individuals with latent TB infection have a 5–10% chance of reactivating and developing active disease over their lifetime. The chance is much higher in those with co-morbidities associated with immunosuppression (e.g. diabetes, malignancy), and rates with advanced HIV are ~10% a year. Disease is more likely to be localized than that seen with primary infection.

Clinical features

Pulmonary TB is the commonest presentation. TB may also disseminate (miliary TB) or affect almost any other organ (extrapulmonary TB): pleural cavity, pericardium, lymph nodes, GI tract and peritoneum, GU tract, skin, bones and joints, and CNS (➔ see Tuberculous meningitis, pp. 726–7).

Diagnosis

- Diagnosis is based on a combination of compatible clinical syndrome, supportive radiological investigations, and detection of AFB or culture of MTB from clinical specimens. The gold standard for diagnosis is culture.
- Samples of sputum or tissue are liquefied, decontaminated (to prevent overgrowth of media by bacteria), neutralized, and centrifuged, and the deposit inoculated into solid or liquid media. Sterile site samples, e.g. CSF, do not need decontamination, and loss of viability may occur.
- Acid-fast stains:
  - Ziehl–Neelsen stain (carbol fuchsin stain, decolorize with acid-alcohol, counterstain with methylene blue). A sputum specimen needs at least 10 000 cfu/mL to give a positive smear. The Kinyoun stain is similar, but modified to make heating unnecessary;
  - auramine stain (fluorochrome phenolic auramine or auramine–rhodamine stain, acid-alcohol decolorization, potassium permanganate counterstain). Up to ten times more sensitive than ZN, and advances in fluoroscopic lighting (e.g. long-life LEDs) are making the technology more suitable for resource-poor settings.
- Nucleic acid detection tests allow rapid diagnosis of MTB in clinical specimens, detecting as few as 1–10 organisms/mL (e.g. AMPLICOR® Mycobacterium Tuberculosis Test). They cannot replace smear, culture, and phenotypic drug sensitivity testing. Testing of AFB smear-positive sputum is 95% sensitive and 98% specific (compared to culture); smear-negative is around 80% sensitive and 95% specific. Results must be interpreted within the context of the clinical scenario. The Xpert® MTB/RIF assay is an automated PCR system that can identify TB and rifampicin resistance from clinical specimens (including sputum, pus, CSF). Sensitivity for detecting TB is >98% on smear-positive sputa, 75–90% if smear-negative. Detection of rifampicin resistance (rpoB gene) is >97% sensitive and >98% specific. Results can be available within 2h. The WHO has recommended the system, in place of smear microscopy, for the diagnosis of drug-resistant TB or TB in HIV-infected patients.
- Culture methods can detect as few as ten organisms per mL. Media are classically egg- (Lowenstein–Jensen, better growth), agar- (Middlebrook 7H10, better speed and allows colony morphology examination), or liquid- (Middlebrook 7H12) based. Growth in liquid media is faster (<8 days for smear-positive sputum) than in solid (3–8 weeks). Specimens are generally inoculated into both solid (e.g. an LJ slope) and liquid media system. This provides a backup, should liquid culture fail. Commercial liquid culture systems include BACTEC™ and MGIT™.
- Identification is usually done at reference laboratory level, once a mycobacterium has been isolated. Techniques include high-pressure

liquid chromatography (HPLC) of mycolic acids, DNA sequencing of 16S rRNA, PCR restriction enzyme assay, and DNA probe hybridization (LiPA® MYCOBACTERIA, Innogenetics). Typing can be performed for epidemiological purposes, e.g. MIRU VNTR.

- Drug susceptibility testing—phenotypic testing takes >3 weeks, depending on growth speed. Rapid tests include:
  - microscopic observation drug susceptibility—media with and without antibiotics are inoculated with the patient specimen and examined for growth. Concerns regarding biosafety;
  - nucleic acid amplification to identify known drug resistance mutations. Line probe assays (e.g. Hain Genotype MTBDRplus) are recommended by the WHO for rapid screening for MDR-TB in low- or middle-income settings. They can be performed on positive cultures or smear-positive sputum. DNA is extracted from the specimen, multiplex PCR used to amplify those regions of the genome associated with known resistance mutations, and reverse hybridization performed in which single-stranded amplicons bind to specific probes attached to test strips which can be read visually.
- Tuberculin skin test—purified protein derivative (PPD) is a standardized protein precipitate of tuberculin. The Mantoux test is performed by intracutaneous injection of five tuberculin units of PPD in 0.1mL of solution. The reaction diameter is read after 48–72h (induration, NOT erythema which may be larger). Specifics of interpretation vary with guidelines. In the UK, <6mm is negative; 6–14mm is positive but could be due to bacillus Calmette–Guérin (BCG) vaccination or exposure to NTM; 15mm or greater is strongly positive and suggestive of TB infection or disease. False-negative reactions occur in up to 20% of patients with TB and in HIV-infected patients. Delayed reactivity (>10mm induration after 6 days) may occur in certain populations, e.g. Indochinese immigrants. Sensitivity and specificity vary with the specific cut-offs chosen, but overall 97% specific for latent TB amongst the non-BCG-vaccinated (around 60% in vaccinated populations) and 80% sensitive.
- Interferon gamma release assays or 'IGRA' (T-SPOT®, QuantiFERON®-TB Gold) detect T cells responsive to antigens specific to MTB (e.g. ESAT-6, CFP-10, thus avoiding issues of BCG cross-reactivity). They are used for the diagnosis of latent TB and cannot distinguish this from active infection. A negative result does not rule out active TB. Specificity >95% for the diagnosis of latent TB; sensitivity is around 90% for T-SPOT®, and 80% for QuantiFERON®. Sensitivity remains high in children <3 years and in HIV co-infection. In the UK, TST is first-line for screening, with follow-up IGRA, if necessary, unless HIV-positive or immunocompromised when IGRA (alone or with TST) is recommended.

Prevention

- Vaccination—BCG is a live attenuated vaccine derived from *M. bovis*. It is given to infants and children in high-prevalence areas and results in a 60–80% reduction in the incidence of TB. It should only be given to infants <12 weeks or children who are TST-negative. Although it does not prevent infection, BCG vaccination reduces the risk of disseminated

disease in children. BCG is contraindicated in HIV-infected individuals. Vaccination can occasionally cause disseminated BCG infection, usually in immunosuppressed patients. Intravesical BCG (used to treat bladder cancer) can cause liver or lung granulomas, psoas abscess, or osteomyelitis. Trials of novel vaccine candidates are ongoing.
- Treatment of latent disease—the aim of testing people for latent TB infection is to find those at higher risk of developing active disease who would therefore benefit from preventative therapy. There is no point testing those in whom treatment would not be considered. Risk groups include those likely to have recently acquired infection (e.g. tested as part of contact tracing; the risk of TB disease is highest in the first 2–3 years), HCWs, and the immunosuppressed (e.g. anti-TNF therapy). For detailed indications, see the 2016 UK NICE guidance (➔ p. 628). The usual regimen is isoniazid for 6 months, or rifampicin and isoniazid for 3 months. The risk of isoniazid hepatotoxicity increases with age (<1% <35 years, >5% in the over 65s); thus, testing is not indicated in older people with moderate/slightly increased risk for reactivation.

Mycobacterium leprae—ACDP 3

Leprosy or Hansen's disease is caused by infection with *M. leprae*, an obligate intracellular parasite whose only natural hosts are humans and armadillos. Experimental infections can be induced in the mouse footpad. The clinical manifestations of leprosy include skin lesions, deformities, and peripheral neuropathy, making it one of the most socially stigmatizing diseases. Leprosy exhibits a spectrum of clinical features, ranging from lepromatous (multibacillary) to tuberculoid (paucibacillary) forms.

Epidemiology

The WHO began an ambitious leprosy elimination programme (defined as <1 case per 10 000 in endemic countries) in the 1990s. Multidrug treatment was made available free to all patients, and the number of new cases has fallen from 763 000 in 2001 to 232 857 in 2012. Only a couple of endemic countries still have to achieve the 'elimination' threshold. The greatest number of new cases in 2011 occurred in India, Brazil, and Indonesia. Leprosy is associated with poverty and rural residence, but not HIV infection. Distribution in endemic countries is non-homogeneous, suggesting that genetic factors may play a role in disease expression. The mode of transmission is unclear but thought to be human-to-human, or via nasal droplet infection or direct inoculation into the skin. Incubation is long, with an average of 5–7 years (range 2–40 years), and peak onset is in young adults.

Microbiology

M. leprae is an AFB with a dense lipid capsule outside the cell wall, best visualized by a modified Fite stain (it may be decolorized by the ZN stain). It grows best at temperatures 27–33°C, consistent with its preference for cooler areas of the body. It multiplies very slowly (doubling time 12–13 days) and, as an obligate intracellular organism, cannot be cultured in artificial media. Experimental infection of the mouse footpad can be used to assess antimicrobial susceptibility.

Clinical features

Disease ranges from 'tuberculoid' (or paucibacillary) with few organisms and a robust cell-mediated immune response to 'lepromatous' (or multi-bacillary) with weaker immune response, higher number of organisms, and greater infectivity. Clinical manifestations are largely confined to the skin, upper respiratory tract, and peripheral nerves. Most serious sequelae are a result of peripheral nerve damage, resulting in deformities (e.g. ulnar, median, peroneal nerve palsies), loss of peripheral parts of digits, and plantar ulceration.

- *Lepromatous leprosy*—characterized by numerous skin nodules, plaques, and a thickened dermis that typically occur in cool areas of the body, e.g. earlobes and feet. No apparent resistance, with poor cell-mediated immune response. Involvement of the nasal mucosa results in congestion, epistaxis, and rarely septal collapse ('saddle nose'). May also cause loss of eyebrows and eyelashes, trichiasis, corneal scarring, uveitis, lagophthalmos, testicular dysfunction, and amyloidosis.
- *Tuberculoid leprosy*—characterized by hypopigmented, anaesthetic skin plaques, and asymmetric peripheral nerve involvement. It is typically paucibacillary (non-infectious) and associated with a good cell-mediated immune response.
- *Borderline leprosy*—the majority of patients, with manifestations intermediate between the two polar forms.
- *Reversal reactions ('type 1 reaction')*—an abrupt increase in inflammation within previously quiescent skin lesions, new skin lesions, neuritis, and fever in borderline leprosy patients either before (downgrading reaction) or after (reversal reaction) starting therapy. If the neuritis is not treated promptly, irreversible nerve damage may occur.
- *Erythema nodosum leprosum ('type 2 reaction')*—affects >50% of lepromatous and borderline leprosy patients after initiation of therapy. Clinical features include painful nodules (usually on extensor surfaces, may pustulate or ulcerate), neuritis, fever, malaise, anorexia, uveitis, lymphadenitis, orchitis, anaemia, leucocytosis, and glomerulonephritis.

Diagnosis

- Biopsy—full-thickness skin biopsies should be taken from skin plaques or nodules in lepromatous patients and from the periphery of lesions in tuberculoid patients. Nerve biopsies may result in loss of function and should only be performed if diagnostic uncertainty justifies the risk.
- Mycobacterial cultures—should be performed on biopsy material to exclude cutaneous TB.
- PCR—assays are available and, performed on biopsies, have a sensitivity of >90% in lepromatous, and 34% in tuberculoid, disease.
- A firm diagnosis of leprosy requires the presence of a characteristic peripheral nerve abnormality or the demonstration of AFB in skin biopsies or split skin smears. In atypical cases, two of the following three criteria are required: a clinically compatible skin lesion, dermal granuloma on skin biopsy, hypoaesthesia within the lesion.

Treatment

Treatment requires combination therapy with two or more agents, e.g. dapsone, clofazimine, and rifampicin. Ethionamide, prothionamide, and certain aminoglycosides have also been used. Newer agents, such as minocycline, clarithromycin, fluoroquinolones, look promising. For treatment regimens, ➲ see Antileprotics, pp. 75–7. Drug resistance is uncommon. Relapses occur (usually within 5–10 years) but are rare (around 1%) and more likely if treatment is not completed.

Prevention

Household contacts of cases should be monitored annually for evidence of disease, but drug prophylaxis is not justified. BCG vaccination offers some protection (single dose around 50% protective).

Non-tuberculous mycobacteria

This group of organisms comprises about 50 species of mycobacteria, excluding those in the MTB complex and *M. leprae*. Other names for NTM include atypical mycobacteria, opportunistic mycobacteria, or mycobacteria other than tuberculosis (MOTT).

Classification

NTM were previously classified according to growth rate, colonial morphology, and pigmentation (Runyon classification). This has been superseded by molecular methods but nonetheless remains useful to separate NTM into three groups:

- *rapidly growing mycobacteria* (≤7 days incubation), e.g. *M. fortuitum* complex, *M. chelonae/abscessus* group, *M. mucogenicum*, and *M. smegmatis*;
- *slow-growing mycobacteria* (>7 days incubation), e.g. MAC, *M. kansasii, M. xenopi, M. simiae, M. szulgai, M. scrofulaceum, M. malmoense, M. terrae/nonchromogenicum* complex, *M. haemophilum*, and *M. genavense*;
- *intermediately growing mycobacteria* (7–10 days), e.g. *M. marinum, M. gordonae*.

Clinical features

The NTM can cause a wide spectrum of diseases (see Table 7.19).

Diagnosis

Because the signs and symptoms of NTM lung disease are often variable and non-specific, diagnosis requires multiple positive respiratory cultures. Diagnosis of NTM infections at other sites requires positive cultures from pus, tissue biopsies, or blood cultures.

- Microscopy—the acid-fast stains used for identifying MTB (➲ see Diagnosis, pp. 357–8) also work well for identifying NTM.
- Culture—appropriate culture media include Middlebrook 7H10 or 7H11 agar or BACTEC® broth. Samples from skin and soft tissue infections need to be plated at 28–30°C, as well as at 35–37°C, as some species

Table 7.19 Clinical syndromes caused by NTM

Syndrome	Commonest causes
Chronic bronchopulmonary disease (adults, CF patients)	MAC, *M. kansasii, M. abscessus*
Cervical lymphadenitis (children)	MAC
Skin and soft tissue infections	*M. fortuitum* group, *M. chelonae, M. abscessus, M. marinum, M. ulcerans*
Bone and joint infections	*M. marinum*, MAC, *M. kansasii, M. fortuitum* group, *M. abscessus, M. chelonae*
Disseminated infection (HIV-positive)	*M. avium, M. kansasii*
Disseminated infection (HIV-negative)	*M. abscessus, M. chelonae*
Catheter-related infections	*M. fortuitum, M. abscessus, M. chelonae*

only grow at low temperatures, e.g. *M. chelonae, M. haemophilum*, and *M. marinum. M. xenopi* grows best at 42°C. Other species have special growth requirements, e.g. *M. genavense* (BACTEC® broth for 6–8 weeks) and *M. haemophilum* (iron supplementation).

- Identification—although traditional biochemical and other standard tests may be performed, identification of NTM increasingly uses rapid molecular methods such as HPLC of mycolic acids, PCR–RFLP analysis of the heat-shock protein gene, genetic probes for mycobacterial RNA and 16S ribosomal DNA sequencing.
- Drug susceptibility testing—various methods are used, including agar disc elution, broth microdilution, E-test, and BACTEC® radiometric detection. However, the clinical utility for susceptibility results is not as well established for many NTM as it is for TB. Rapid growers, in particular, tend to be resistant to classic TB medications.
  - MAC—no value in testing sensitivity for any drug other than the macrolides (clarithromycin, azithromycin). No proven link between *in vitro* susceptibility and clinical response for other drugs.
  - *M. malmoense, M. xenopi*—there is no correlation between *in vitro* susceptibility and *in vivo* response.
- Strain comparison—for epidemiological studies, standard biochemical identification and susceptibility testing have been superseded by molecular methods.

Treatment

Treatment may be medical, surgical, or a combination of the two. The choice of drugs and duration of treatment depend on the causative organism, site of infection, and patient's HIV status. Treatment is summarized in Table 7.20.

Table 7.20 Treatment of atypical mycobacterial infections

Causative organism	British Thoracic Society (BTS) guidelines[a]	American Thoracic Society (ATS) guidelines[b]	Comments
M. avium complex (MAC), normal host	Pulmonary: rifampicin + ethambutol + isoniazid for 24 months	Clarithromcyin (or azithromycin) + rifabutin (or rifampicin) + ethambutol (until culture negative for 1 year)	May add streptomycin for initial 2–3 months for severe disease; extrapulmonary disease: surgical excision
MAC, immunocompromised	Rifabutin + ethambutol + clarithromcyin (or azithromycin)	Clarithromycin (or azithromycin) + ethambutol + rifabutin. Amikacin or streptomycin initially for severe disease	Primary prophylaxis if CD4 count <50/mm3. Lifelong treatment required
M. abscessus	Rifampicin + ethambutol ± clarithromycin	Amikacin + cefoxitin for severe disease. Newer macrolides	Surgical excision
M. chelonae	Pulmonary: rifampicin + ethambutol + clarithromycin; extrapulmonary: ciprofloxacin + aminoglycoside or imipenem ± clarithromycin	Tobramycin + cefoxitin or imipenem for severe disease. Clarithromycin or clofazimine PO	Surgical excision
M. fortuitum	Pulmonary: rifampicin + ethambutol + clarithromycin; extrapulmonary: ciprofloxacin + aminoglycoside or imipenem ± clarithromycin	Pulmonary: two agents (macrolides, quinolones, doxycyline, minocycline); extrapulmonary: amikacin + cefoxitin or imipenem	Optimal regimen not defined; surgical excision
M. haemophilum	Pulmonary: rifampicin + ethambutol + clarithromycin	Ciprofloxacin + rifabutin + clarithromycin	Optimal regimen not defined; surgical excision
M. kansasii	Pulmonary: rifampicin + ethambutol (9 months)	Isoniazid + rifabutin + ethambutol (18 months, with 12 months smear-negative)	

(Continued)

Table 7.20 (*Contd.*)

Causative organism	British Thoracic Society (BTS) guidelines[a]	American Thoracic Society (ATS) guidelines[b]	Comments
M. malmoense	Pulmonary: rifampicin + ethambutol ± isoniazid (24 months)	Rifampicin + isoniazid + ethambutol ± quinolones and macrolides	Extrapulmonary: excision
M. marinum	Rifampicin + ethambutol or co-trimoxazole or tetracycline	Clarithromycin or minocycline or doxycycline or co-trimoxazole or rifampicin + ethambutol (± 3 months)	Surgical excision
M. scrofulaceum		Clarithromycin + clofazimine ± ethambutol	Chemotherapy rarely indicated; surgical excision
M. ulcerans	Rifampicin + ethambutol + clarithromycin	Rifampicin + amikacin or ethambutol ± co-trimoxazole (4–6 weeks)	Surgical excision and skin grafting
M. xenopi	Pulmonary: rifampicin + ethambutol ± isoniazid for 24 months	Macrolide + rifamycin + ethambutol ± streptomycin	Extrapulmonary: excision

a British Thoracic Society (BTS) guidelines. *Thorax* 2000;**55**:210–18.

b American Thoracic Society (ATS) guidelines. *Am J Respir Crit Care Med* 2007;**175**:367–416.

Chapter 8

Viruses

Basic principles of virology *366*
Viral replication *367*
Viral pathogenesis *368*
Overview of viruses *370*
Influenza—introduction *375*
Influenza—clinical features and diagnosis *377*
Influenza—treatment/prevention *378*
Parainfluenza *380*
Respiratory syncytial virus *381*
Coronaviruses *383*
Metapneumovirus *384*
Measles *384*
Mumps *387*
Rubella *389*
Parvovirus B19 *390*
Herpesviruses *392*
Human herpesvirus type 6 *393*
Human herpesvirus type 7 *394*
Human herpesvirus type 8 *394*
Herpes simplex *396*
Varicella-zoster virus *399*
Infectious mononucleosis *402*
Epstein–Barr virus *402*
Viral gastroenteritis *408*
Rotavirus *409*
Norovirus *410*
Astroviruses *411*
Hepatitis A virus *411*
Hepatitis B virus *413*
Hepatitis D virus *417*
Hepatitis C virus *418*
Hepatitis E virus *421*
Hepatitis viruses *423*
HIV virology and immunology *425*
HIV laboratory tests *427*
Enterovirus (including Coxsackie) *430*
Lymphocytic choriomeningitis virus (LCMV) *432*
Alphaviruses *433*
Bunyaviridae *435*
Adenovirus *436*
Human papillomavirus *439*
Polyomaviruses *442*
Poxviruses *444*
Poliovirus *445*
Human T-cell lymphotropic virus *449*
Flaviviruses *451*
Yellow fever *455*
Dengue *457*
Viral haemorrhagic fevers *459*
Filoviruses *461*
Arenaviruses (Lassa fever) *462*
Rabies virus *463*
Prion diseases *465*

Basic principles of virology

Classification

Viruses are classified on the basis of a number of criteria. These include:

- type of nucleic acid (DNA, RNA) and strand number (single, double);
- conformation of the nuclear material (linear, circular, etc.);
- whether the genetic information is positive or negative sense;
- nucleocapsid symmetry;
- presence or absence of an envelope;
- their antigenic or genetic similarity.

They are grouped into orders, families, subfamilies, and genera. There are no consistent rules governing the naming of individual viruses. Some are named according to the disease they produce (poxvirus), others by acronyms (papovavirus—papilloma polyma vacuolating virus), some by appearance (coronavirus), and still others after the location in which they were first identified (Marburg). They may rarely be called after their discoverers (Epstein–Barr). Official names should be Latinized and printed in italic.

Properties and structure

Viruses are small (20–150nm in diameter) protein packages, containing genetic material (DNA or RNA); some also contain enzymes. Viruses depend on living cells for their existence, genome expression, and replication. They have colonized most life forms, including bacteria, plants, insects, and animals. The viral particle is composed of structural proteins. A capsid (protein coat) protects the nucleic acid contents and facilitates viral entry to a host cell. It is composed of many capsomeres (protein subunits). The term nucleocapsid refers to the capsid and viral nucleic acid. Certain viruses contain enzymes (e.g. RT in HIV). Some viral capsids have an outer envelope (derived from the plasma membrane of the infected cell from which it was released), into which are embedded protein spikes. Beneath the envelope, some viruses may have a stabilizing membrane protein. The entire particle is referred to as a virion.

Nucleocapsids may take several geometric forms:

- helical (like a spiral staircase)—the nucleic acid forms the central core, with the nucleocapsid proteins forming the steps, e.g. single-stranded RNA (ssRNA) viruses such as influenza and rabies. These viruses are enveloped, the envelope itself resting on the underlying membrane protein shell;
- icosahedral (20 triangular faces with 12 corners), e.g. all human DNA viruses—each capsomere may itself be made of several peptides. DNA herpesviruses have an icosahedral structure and are additionally surrounded by a lipid envelope;
- complex—these viruses do not fall into neat structural categories and often have large genomes, e.g. poxvirus.

Viral genomes

The genetic material may be DNA or RNA (RNA viruses tend to have smaller genomes). Nucleic acid conformation varies widely between viral families (double-stranded, single-stranded, linear, circular, etc.). Genomes vary widely in size but are limited by the space available in the virion. Bacteria may have several thousand genes, but even the largest viruses have <200 genes, and the smallest perhaps only four (such viruses may produce >1 protein from the same gene by means of RNA splicing or frameshifting). Viruses evolve rapidly due to the high number of genome duplications undergone in short spaces of time. RNA viruses have high error rates, with genomes diverging by as much as 2% in the course of a year—1 million times the rate of eukaryotic cell DNA genomes. Many mutations are non-functional but some will allow the virus to evade host immune responses and medical therapies.

The genome encodes both structural and non-structural (NS) proteins (enzymes required for viral expression and replication). The manner in which expression occurs depends on the nature of the nucleic acid:

- DNA viruses make RNA copies of the relevant segments of their DNA to direct protein synthesis—they may use host enzymes to achieve this or rarely carry them within the virion;
- positive-sense RNA viruses produce mRNA directly;
- negative-sense RNA viruses possess enzymes that produce positive-strand copies that are used as mRNA;
- retroviruses produce DNA from their RNA. This is integrated into the host's chromosomal DNA, transcription then taking place in broadly the same way as host mRNA is made from host DNA.

Viral replication

The manner in which a virus infects a cell varies but generally involves the interaction of a viral protein and host cell receptor (proteins, glycoproteins, or glycolipids intended for other functions and simply exploited by the virus), precipitating internalization. Once in the cell, the virus uncoats (sheds its protein shell) and frees the nucleic acid, at least partially. It needs to achieve two things: the production of its enzymes and structural proteins, and replication of the viral genome.

Transcription

The manner in which mRNA is produced depends on the nature of the genome. Ribosomes translate the viral mRNAs. Proteins may be produced in phases—'early' proteins may be involved in DNA synthesis or act as transcriptional activators to speed viral expression over host proteins; 'late' proteins are produced from mRNA transcribed from newly synthesized viral nucleic acid and tend to be structural. Some viruses produce a single long polypeptide which is then cleaved by proteases into individual proteins. Proteins often undergo post-translational processes such as glycosylation.

Viral genome replication

RNA viruses produce an RNA polymerase, either packaged with the virion (negative-sense viruses) or manufactured upon infection (positive-sense viruses). This rapidly produces RNA copies for incorporation into the viral particles. Genetic variation may arise by two mechanisms:

- mutations can occur due to errors in replication and the absence of proofreading activity in enzymes such as RNA replicase and RT. DNA viruses replicate their genomes in the host nucleus where the necessary host enzymes can be exploited. The exceptions are the poxviruses which carry DNA polymerases with them and are thus capable of working entirely in the cytoplasm;
- recombination of genetic material can occur either within a genome or between two viruses of the same kind if the host cell is co-infected with both viruses. RNA viruses are also capable of gene reassortment which, although not a true mutation, may result in progeny with a quite different phenotype from parental strains, e.g. influenza pandemics may be a consequence of reassortment between human, avian, and swine flu.

Viral assembly

This may occur predominantly in the nucleus (e.g. adenovirus) or in the cytoplasm (e.g. poliovirus). Viral release then occurs by budding from the cell surface (e.g. measles), lysis of the cell (e.g. polio), or cell-to-cell spread. Some, such as HIV, may require a phase of post-release maturation. Overall, a complete viral life cycle typically takes 6–8h, with the potential to produce thousands of viruses from each infected cell.

Viral pathogenesis

The effect of viral infection on the host ranges from asymptomatic infection to devastating disease with a wide variety of clinical manifestations. Viral species vary in pathogenicity, and different strains of the same species may vary in virulence.

Entry

Viruses enter the body through the skin (usually via some degree of trauma) or via mucous membranes (where they adsorb directly to epithelial cells, in which they undergo primary replication). Resulting infections may be localized (e.g. papillomavirus and warts, conjunctivitis) or generalized, in which case pathology is not necessarily focused at the organ initially infected (e.g. enteroviruses are spread faeco-orally, yet cause encephalitis). Transmission may also occur vertically (mother to child) and iatrogenically (organ transplants, blood transfusions, etc.).

Cytopathic effect

Viruses may disrupt the function of the cells they infect. This may result in inhibition of host–cell protein manufacture and lead to the death of the cell, lysis, and the release of virion. Alternatively, they may precipitate cell fusion, forming multinucleated giant cells or syncytia (e.g. RSV). Others may form inclusion bodies within the cell (eosinophilic or basophilic staining areas within the cell, representing aggregations of virions, sites of viral synthesis, or degenerative change). These inclusions can occur within the cytoplasm or nucleus.

Extent of infection

Some viral infections remain confined to tissues at, or continuous with, the site of entry. They may form focal lesions (e.g. skin and papillomavirus) or affect large areas of specific mucous membranes (e.g. viral gastroenteritis), and tend to have short incubation periods. Other viruses produce generalized infections, an initial phase of local replication near to the site of entry, being followed by haematogenous spread (primary viraemia) to regional lymph nodes. This allows infection of large reticulo-endothelial organs, resulting in secondary viraemia. The virus may travel free in the blood or within infected blood cells. It travels to organs distant from the site of entry and may infect specific organs preferentially. Such infections tend to have longer incubation periods.

Target organs

Symptoms depend on the target organ:

- skin—rashes are a common feature of viral infections and may be due to virus replication in the skin (vesicular rashes of herpes simplex and varicella-zoster), the killing of infected cells (measles), or more general features of infection (DIC, thrombocytopenia);
- respiratory tract—the lung may be involved in local infections (e.g. influenza) but can also be involved in generalized viral infections (e.g. chickenpox or measles pneumonitis);
- liver—the hepatitis viruses (hepatitis A to E) are tropic for the liver, which may also be affected as part of a more generalized infection (e.g. EBV, CMV);
- CNS—the CNS can be invaded either as a result of viral passage along nerves (e.g. rabies) or by haematogenous spread (e.g. polio).

Illness duration

Viral illness may be acute or chronic.

- Acute viral illnesses present within a relatively short period of time. Most such infections are mild, with a quick spontaneous recovery, e.g. chickenpox, measles, mumps, rubella. Some may have delayed serious features after an apparent recovery (e.g. encephalitis), or cause a rapid decline and possible death (e.g. rabies, VHFs).
- Chronic or persistent infections require the survival of viral DNA within the host cell, either integrated within the host DNA or in episomal form separate from it. They may be latent with no apparent illness or virus, but with occasional periods of reactivation (e.g. herpes simplex, varicella-zoster), or chronic with continuous production of infectious virus (hepatitis B, hepatitis C, HIV).

Transformation

Some viruses have the potential to induce malignant change. For example, EBV is associated with Burkitt's lymphoma, nasopharyngeal carcinoma, primary cerebral lymphoma, and post-transplant lymphoproliferative disorder (PTLD).

Overview of viruses

See Table 8.1.

Table 8.1 Summary of viruses and common clinical syndromes

Group	Virus	Consider in the differential of …								
		Respiratory	Rash	Hepatic	Muscular	Diarrhoea	Encephalitis	Meningitis	Shock	Other
DNA viruses										
Adenoviridae	Adenovirus (➔ pp. 436–8)	•••				•••	••	••		Cystitis, conjunctivitis
Herpesviridae	HSV-1 and -2 (➔ pp. 396–9)	•	•••				••(1)	••(2)		Genital, eye, dissemination
	EBV (➔ pp. 402–5)	•	•	•	•••		•	•		
	VZV (➔ pp. 399–402)	•	•••	•			•	•		
	CMV (➔ pp. 405–8)	•	•	••	••	•	•	•		Congenital
	HHV-6 and -7 (➔ pp. 393–4, p. 394)		••							Fever alone
	HHV-8 (➔ pp. 394–6)		•							Kaposi's sarcoma
Poxviridae (also smallpox) (➔ pp. 444–5)	Molluscum		•••							
	Orf		•••							
	Monkeypox		•••							

Parvoviridae	Parvovirus B19 (➔ pp. 390–2)		●●●					Arthropathy, aplastic anaemia, congenital
Papovaviridae	HPV (➔ pp. 439–41)							Warts, epithelial tumours of skin
	Polyomavirus (➔ pp. 442–3)		●●					
Hepadnaviridae	Hepatitis B (➔ pp. 413–17)			●●●				Progressive focal neurodeficits
RNA viruses								
Orthomyx-oviridae	Influenza (➔ pp. 375–6)	●●●			●	●		
Paramyxoviridae	Parainfluenza (➔ p. 380)	●●●						
	Mumps (➔ pp. 387–8)					●●	●	Parotitis, epididymo-orchitis, GBS
	Measles (➔ pp. 384–6)	●●	●●●			●	●	SSPE
	RSV (➔ pp. 381–2)/ metapneumovirus (➔ p. 384)	●●●						

(Continued)

Table 8.1 (*Contd.*)

Group	Virus	Consider in the differential of …								
		Respiratory	Rash	Hepatic	Muscular	Diarrhoea	Encephalitis	Meningitis	Shock	Other
Coronaviridae	Coronavirus (➔ pp. 383–4)	●●●				●●				
Picornaviridae	Poliovirus (➔ pp. 445–8)						●			Paralysis, myocarditis
	Non-polio enteroviruses (➔ pp. 430–2)	●●	●●				●●●	●●●		Myopericarditis, conjunctivitis
	Hepatitis A virus (➔ pp. 411–12)			●●●						
	Rhinovirus (➔ pp. 590–1)	●●●								
Reoviridae	Rotavirus (➔ pp. 409–10)					●●●				
Retroviridae	HTLV-1 and -2 (➔ pp. 449–50)									Spastic paraparesis, leukaemia/ lymphoma
	HIV-1 and -2[a] (➔ pp. 425–7)		●●●				●			Immuno-deficiency

Togaviridae (➔ pp. 433–5)	Rubella (➔ pp. 389–90)	•	•••				Congenital
	Alphaviruses (➔ pp. 433–5)		•••		•••		Arthralgia
Flaviviridae	Yellow fever (➔ pp. 455–6)		••	•••	•	•	Haemorrhage
	Dengue (➔ pp. 457–8)		••	••	•	•••	Haemorrhage
	Hepatitis C (➔ pp. 418–21)			•••			
	Japanese encephalitis (➔ pp. 451–4)				•••		
Bunyaviridae (also Rift Valley fever)	Hantavirus (➔ pp. 435–6)	•				•••	Haemorrhage, renal failure
	CCHF (➔ pp. 435–6)					•••	Haemorrhage
	California encephalitis (➔ pp. 435–6)				•••		

(*Continued*)

Table 8.1 (*Contd.*)

Group	Virus	Consider in the differential of …								
		Respiratory	Rash	Hepatic	Muscular	Diarrhoea	Encephalitis	Meningitis	Shock	Other
Arenaviridae	Lassa (→ pp. 462–3)					●●	●	●	●●●	Haemorrhage
	LCMV (→ p. 432)		●●●				●●	●●		Congenital
Filoviridae	Marburg, Ebola (→ pp. 451–4)		●●						●●●	Haemorrhage
Rhabdoviridae	Rabies (→ pp. 463–5)						●●●			
Other	Astrovirus and calicivirus (→ pp. 410–1)					●●●				

●●● very frequently seen; ●● commonly seen; ● occasionally seen.

'Congenital' indicates viruses with the potential to cause significant sequelae if infecting the developing fetus.

CCHF, Congo–Crimean haemorrhagic fever; CMV, cytomegalovirus; EBV, Epstein–Barr virus; GBS, Guillain–Barré syndrome; HHV, human herpesvirus; HIV, human immunodeficiency virus; HPV, human papillomavirus; HSV, herpes simplex virus; HTLV, human T-cell lymphotropic virus; LCMV, lymphocytic choriomeningitis virus; RSV, respiratory syncytial virus; SSPE, subacute sclerosing panencephalitis; VZV, varicella-zoster virus.

[a] HIV may, of course, present in a multitude of ways; however, the commoner presentations of primary HIV infection (as opposed to a subsequent opportunistic infection) are rash and encephalitis.

Influenza—introduction

One of the commonest infectious diseases of man, primarily causing epidemics of URTI. Global pandemics may follow dramatic antigenic changes—21 million died in the 1918–1919 pandemic.

The virus

Members of family *Orthomyxoviridae*. Negative-sense ssRNA viruses.
The three distinct influenza viruses are:

- influenza A—cause of the typical influenza syndrome and pandemics;
- influenza B—similar clinically but does not cause pandemics;
- influenza C—afebrile, common cold-like syndrome; does not occur in epidemics.

All have host cell-derived envelopes, embedded with glycoproteins important to viral entry and exit. These have haemagglutinin (HA) or neuraminidase (NA) activities, which are key antigenic components. At least 17 HA and ten NA variants have been identified in influenza A viruses. EM appearance of the viral particles is variable—spherical to filamentous. Viruses are named by their type, place of initial isolation, strain, year, and antigenic subtype, e.g. A/Victoria/3/75/H3N2.

Pathogenesis

- The virus enters respiratory epithelial cells and replicates, and progeny are released—the cell dies. Viral shedding may start within 24h of infection—illness follows 24h later.
- There is diffuse inflammation of the trachea and bronchi, with an ulcerative, necrotizing tracheobronchitis in severe cases. Primary viral pneumonia is uncommon but is severe when it occurs. Bacterial superinfection is common, facilitated by damage to the mucociliary escalator, and virus-induced defects in lymphocyte and leucocyte function. Viral levels fall rapidly after 48h of illness, becoming undetectable by 5–10 days.
- Antigenic variation—alteration of viral antigenic structure allows the production of variants, to which there may be little or no herd immunity. This variation involves changes in the HA and NA glycoproteins and takes place by two mechanisms:
    - antigenic drift—relatively minor changes that occur every year or so through a gradual accumulation of amino acid changes. There is a selective pressure for those changes which are less well recognized by the host antibody, and these viruses begin to predominate;
    - antigenic shift—major antigenic change that may herald flu pandemics due to lack of population immunity. Type A viruses are able to infect a variety of species (humans, pigs, horses, birds), and, if genes from different viruses recombine, entirely new strains result. Occasional avian flu strains arise with bird-to-human infectivity, but minimal human-to-human transmission (e.g. H5N1, H7N9), a consequence of differences in the binding preference demonstrated by viral HA molecules. Human viruses prefer sialic acid (2–6) galactose, conveniently found on epithelial cells of the upper respiratory tract.

Avian HA tends to prefer sialic acid (2–3) galactose, found in humans only deep on the terminal bronchi and alveoli. Recombination events may happen in a third party easily infected by viruses from both birds and humans, e.g. pig. The H1N1 'swine' flu virus is thought to be a result of the recombination of two swine, one human and one avian flu strain within a pig. Pandemics often arise in Asia where humans, pigs, and birds live in close proximity. Other pandemics may have been caused by direct viral adaptation to humans (1918 pandemic probably due to a pig virus).

Epidemiology

- Outbreaks are associated with excess rates of pneumonia and influenza-related illness and mortality, peaking in the winter and varying with the viral type responsible. Not all influenza-related deaths present as pneumonia.
- Seasonal flu attack rates are highest in the young, mortality is highest in the elderly; both are increased in those with pre-existing medical problems, e.g. cardiovascular/pulmonary/liver/renal impairment, or immunodeficiency.
- Person-to-person transmission occurs by dispersion in small-particle aerosols. The virus is present in large quantities in the secretions of infected people. One individual can infect a large number of others, contributing to the explosive nature of outbreaks. Outbreaks can occur in an epidemic or pandemic fashion:
    - *epidemics* are confined to a single location, e.g. town/country, and occur almost exclusively in winter. They start abruptly with cases seen initially in children and then adults, peak within 3 weeks, and last around 6 weeks. Different strains may circulate simultaneously;
    - *pandemics* are severe outbreaks caused by type A viruses that spread worldwide. Associated with the emergence of a new virus, to which the population has no significant immunity, and characterized by rapid transmission, often out of the usual patterns of seasonality and with high levels of mortality amongst healthy young adults. The capacity of the influenza virus to continue to cause human disease on such a scale is a function of frequent antigenic changes. In the early years after a pandemic, disease is clinically severe, becoming milder as herd immunity improves.
- The H1N1 'swine flu' pandemic of 2009/2010 spread rapidly throughout the world. Rates of infection were highest in those <25 years old and, unlike seasonal flu, low in those over 65, perhaps due to pre-existing immunity against antigenically similar viruses circulating before 1957. Secondary attack rates were probably similar to those of seasonal flu, but rates of hospitalization and mortality were higher, especially amongst the pregnant and immunosuppressed. Unlike the seasonal H1N1 circulating at the time, <99% of pandemic H1N1 strains were susceptible to oseltamivir. Pandemic H1N1 replaced the previous seasonal H1N1 strain and is now essentially 'seasonal'.

Influenza—clinical features and diagnosis

Clinical features

- Uncomplicated disease—1- to 2-day incubation is followed by an abrupt onset of symptoms. Fever, chills, headache, malaise, myalgia, eye pain, anorexia, dry cough, sore throat, and nasal discharge. After around day 3, respiratory features dominate, as fever and other systemic features settle. Convalescence may take 2 or more weeks. Elderly patients may present with fever and confusion and few respiratory features. Attack rates are highest in children, who may present with croup.
- Complicated influenza—risk factors for complicated disease outside of pandemics include pregnancy, age >65 years, chronic cardiac/lung/renal/liver disease, diabetes, immunosuppression, and morbid obesity. Primary viral pneumonia presents with rapidly worsening cough, breathlessness, and hypoxia (resembles ARDS). Mortality is high. Secondary bacterial pneumonia develops shortly after an initial period of improvement, following the influenza syndrome. Pathogens: *S. pneumoniae*, *H. influenzae*, and less commonly *S. aureus*. Other respiratory complications: croup, COPD, and CF exacerbations. Non-respiratory complications: myositis, myo-/pericarditis, encephalitis, GBS.
- Immunocompromised patients may be at risk of severe disease. Includes those receiving chemo-/radiotherapy, BMT recipients receiving immunosuppressive drugs within the last year, those on high-dose steroids, and HIV patients with CD4 <15% of total lymphocytes. Viral shedding may be prolonged in these groups.

Diagnosis

The diagnosis of influenza can be made, with some confidence, on clinical criteria alone during an outbreak—85% accuracy in some studies. Laboratory diagnosis is important outside of outbreaks or in the institutional setting.

- Rapid antigen detection—commercial immunoassays that detect flu A and B nucleoprotein antigens. Can be performed in 15min, but sensitivity is low (around 60%), compared to PCR, especially if performed after 48h of illness when viral shedding rapidly declines.
- Reverse transcriptase PCR (RT-PCR)—sensitive and specific, with relatively rapid results and the ability to differentiate between types/subtypes. Detects low quantities of viral RNA in nasal/throat swabs, and BAL and NPA specimens.
- Viral culture—virus isolated from sputum or swabs, cultured in cell lines, and detected within 3–5 days by its cytopathic effect. Now used only in public health surveillance.
- Serology—paired samples (10–20 days apart); samples showing a 4-fold rise in antibody titre can be considered diagnostic. Not useful in clinical decision-making.

Influenza—treatment/prevention

Treatment

(See Table 8.2.)

- Antiviral agents may be used in secondary care for any patient in whom they are clinically indicated if influenza is confirmed or suspected. In primary care, they may be used once the DH has issued notice that influenza is circulating. NICE and PHE issue treatment guidelines for the UK.
- Treatment and prophylaxis is with the NA inhibitors (oseltamivir, zanamivir, and peramivir; ➲ see Antivirals for influenza, pp. 94–6). The amantadines are no longer recommended.
- Resistance to oseltamivir was becoming common (>90% of tested strains) in seasonal H1N1 flu prior to the 2009 H1N1 pandemic. The pandemic strain replaced the previous seasonal strain, and resistance is now unusual. It has been noted to arise in severely immunocompromised patients who have received oseltamivir (for treatment or prophylaxis). These strains have generally remained sensitive to zanamivir, and treatment guidelines reflect this.
- If treatment is indicated, do not wait for laboratory confirmation. It should commence within 48h of onset of symptoms but may reduce the risk of severe illness if given up to 5 days after symptom onset.
- If a patient is unable to take inhaled zanamivir, aqueous zanamivir can be given by inhalation (unlicensed). IV zanamivir should be used if the patient is on the ICU.
- If oseltamivir-resistant virus is suspected, or a patient does not respond to therapy within 5 days, treat with zanamivir, and test for resistance.
- General measures—adequate hydration, antipyretics (not aspirin in children), and decongestants.
- The rapidly progressive nature of secondary bacterial infections argues for early presumptive use of antibiotics where suggested by the clinical scenario.
- A 2014 Cochrane review suggested that, while NA inhibitors are effective as prophylaxis and shorten symptom duration by an average of half a day, they have no impact on hospital admission or the development of pneumonia (Jefferson T, Jones MA, Doshi P, *et al.* (2014). Neuraminidase inhibitors for preventing and treating influenza in healthy adults and children. *Cochrane Database Syst Rev* 4:CD008965).

Table 8.2 Influenza treatment recommendations

Uncomplicated, previously healthy	No treatment. Oseltamivir only if physician believes serious risk of complications
Uncomplicated, at-risk groups, including pregnancy	Oseltamivir PO 5 days, within 48h or later at clinical discretion. Zanamivir as second line or if higher risk of oseltamivir resistance (e.g. H1N1)
Complicated (needs hospital admission, hypoxic, lung infiltrate, CNS involvement, etc.)	Oseltamivir PO/NG, zanamivir as second line or if higher risk of oseltamivir resistance (e.g. H1N1)

Prevention

Vaccines

- Inactivated vaccines are the main control measure. In 2012, the Joint Committee on Vaccination and Immunisation recommended vaccination should be offered to all children aged between 2 and 16. The UK DH recommends annual vaccination for:
  - >65 years old;
  - all people aged 6 months or older in a clinical risk group (chronic respiratory disease, e.g. COPD, chronic heart disease, chronic kidney disease, chronic liver disease, diabetes, immunosuppressed people, asplenia, pregnancy (any stage), morbid obesity). See *Green Book* for a comprehensive list;
  - all children aged between 2 and 16 not in clinical risk groups. This extension was implemented in a phased manner (2013 onwards).
- Vaccination should also be offered to: household contacts of immunocompromised people, HCWs, others as clinical judgement suggests (e.g. other chronic illness, long-term care home residents, etc.).
- Vaccines are prepared each year and are usually trivalent, containing two type A (H1N1, N3N2), and one type B, strains. Strains are collected continuously across the world, and those to be included in the year's vaccine chosen by educated guess. It takes 6–9 months to produce a vaccine once its components are decided.
- Two doses are required in children under 9 years who have not been previously vaccinated. Otherwise, a single dose is sufficient, usually given in October. The main contraindication to vaccination is hypersensitivity to hens' eggs.
- Protection is around 70% and lasts for 1 year. Diminished responses are seen in organ transplant recipients receiving immunosuppressive therapy. Protection is reduced in the elderly.

Antiviral agents

- Vaccination does not preclude PEP, when indicated. Prophylaxis should be given only if the last potential flu contact was within 36h (zanamivir) to 48h (oseltamivir), unless recommended by an appropriate specialist.
- If exposure was to suspected/confirmed oseltamivir-resistant virus, prophylaxis is with zanamivir inhaled (INH).
- Previously healthy (excluding pregnant women)—no prophylaxis.
- At risk of complicated flu (including pregnant women)—oseltamivir PO for 10 days.
- Severely immunocompromised (excluding children under 5)—zanamivir INH od for 10 days. If unable to administer, then oseltamivir as above.
- Children <5 years in at-risk groups—oseltamivir for 10 days.

Further reading

Public Health England (2015). *PHE guidance on use of antiviral agents for the treatment and prophylaxis of seasonal influenza (2015–16)*. Available at: https://www.gov.uk/government/uploads/system/uploads/attachment_data/file/457735/PHE_guidance_antivirals_influenza_2015_to_2016.pdf.

Public Health England (2015). *Influenza: the green book, chapter 19*. Available at: https://www.gov.uk/government/publications/influenza-the-green-book-chapter-19.

Parainfluenza

A group of viruses causing respiratory illnesses, from upper respiratory tract symptoms in healthy children to severe pneumonia in the immunosuppressed.

The viruses

- *Paramyxoviridae* and members of either genus *Respirovirus* (parainfluenza types 1 and 3) or *Rubulavirus* (types 2, 4A, and 4B).
- Negative-sense ssRNA viruses with host cell-derived envelope.

Epidemiology

- Ten per cent of adult acute respiratory illness and 60% of childhood croup cases with demonstrated cause are due to parainfluenza. Extensive spread within families. Nosocomial/residential care outbreaks occur.
- Parainfluenza type 3 is the most frequently isolated member and, like RSV, is commonly seen in the first 6 months of life. It is endemic and may be isolated throughout the year, peaking in spring. Types 1 and 2 occur in autumn, often alternating each year. Type 4 is rarely isolated.

Pathogenesis

- Transmission is by droplet spread. Replication occurs in respiratory epithelial cells, peaking 2–5 days after infection. Types 1 and 2 usually infect the larynx and upper trachea (croup), and type 3 the distal airway (bronchiolitis, pneumonia).
- Reinfection may occur and tends to cause milder upper airway disease, probably representing waning of immunity—antigenic variation is not progressive (unlike influenza virus). Mucosal immunity is most important for resisting infection. CD8 T cells are important in viral clearance.

Clinical features

- Healthy individuals—children: upper respiratory tract illness (those under 5 years), otitis media, croup, bronchiolitis (infants under 6 months); adults: URTI.
- Immunocompromised—severe disease in recipients of BMT or lung transplants in all age groups. May cause pneumonia with high rates of mortality. Other immunodeficiencies are associated with prolonged viral shedding.

Diagnosis

- Viral isolation by tissue culture and immunofluorescence is the gold standard, but PCR-based tests have higher sensitivity and are more widely available. Nasal washings have a higher sensitivity than nasal swabs.
- Paired serology can confirm a diagnosis but is unhelpful clinically.

Treatment

- No specific antiviral therapy. No proven benefit with immunoglobulin. Reduce immunosuppression where relevant.
- Some advocate inhaled steroids for the clinical treatment of croup.
- No vaccine is currently available.

Respiratory syncytial virus

RSV is a major cause of LRTI in young children.

The virus

- A member of the *Paramyxoviridae* family. An ssRNA virus with host cell-derived envelope. Two antigen groups (A and B), which differ in envelope proteins and non-structural protein-1. Several strains from both groups may circulate in the same outbreak.

Epidemiology

- RSV infection has been found worldwide. In temperate parts, outbreaks are annual, occurring in the winter months. Mild outbreaks may be followed by more severe outbreaks the next year.
- The major cause of childhood pneumonia/bronchiolitis (90% of children admitted with an LRTI in the peak of an epidemic); 95% of children are seropositive by age 2 years. Naturally acquired immunity to RSV is incomplete, and, while healthy adults will have mild symptoms, it is an important cause of severe respiratory illness in the elderly and immunosuppressed.
- Boys and those under 2 years experience the most severe illness—severity is also affected by socio-economic factors.
- An important nosocomial infection. May survive <24h in patient secretions deposited on non-porous surfaces, and around an hour on porous surfaces (tissues, fabric, skin).

Pathogenesis

- Transmission is by inoculation of the nasopharynx or the eye with secretions or fomites. Incubation of 2–8 days. Infants often have evidence of pneumonia as well as bronchiolitis.
- Lymphocytic infiltration of the areas around the bronchioles with wall and tissue oedema is followed by proliferation and necrosis of the bronchiolar epithelium: bronchiolitis. Sloughed epithelium and mucus block small airway lumens, leading to air trapping and hyperinflation. Air absorbed distally to obstructed airways leads to areas of atelectasis.
- Disease is due to the vulnerability of the small airways of the very young to inflammation and obstruction (resistance to airflow being inversely related to the cube of the radius), and possibly immunopathology (severe disease was seen in children vaccinated with an experimental inactivated vaccine in the 1960s).

Clinical features

- Young children—pneumonia and bronchiolitis (➔ see Bronchiolitis, pp. 609–11) are the commonest manifestations in infants. Tracheobronchitis and croup are less common. All may occur in association with fever and otitis media (RSV is present in 75% of middle ear effusions from children with respiratory infection). Rarely asymptomatic. Those with LRTI may have a preceding URTI with nasal congestion and pharyngitis. Cough and fever are common in young children. Clinical findings include wheeze and crepitations.

Many infants have both pneumonia and bronchiolitis. CXR changes are few, regardless of severity. Hypoxia may be profound. Duration of illness is 7–21 days. Acute complications: apnoea, secondary bacterial infection. RSV may be a contributing factor to sudden infant death syndrome. Long-term studies suggest those hospitalized with RSV LRTI may have a higher rate of later reactive airway disease.

- Older children and adults—a severe 'common cold' with nasal congestion, cough, fever, earache (in children); <50% of infected older people develop pneumonia (particularly those in residential homes); 2–6% of hospitalized adults with pneumonia have RSV. Secondary infections cause URTI or tracheobronchitis.
- Severe disease—young infants, the premature, and those with underlying disease (congenital and cardiopulmonary disease, e.g. CF) are at risk of severe RSV; <66% of deaths occur in those with underlying disease. Prematurity is a risk into the third year of life. Immunodeficient patients (including those with transplants and on chemotherapy) have extensive pulmonary infiltration and prolonged viral shedding.

Diagnosis

- Clinical diagnosis can be made, with some confidence, in children during an outbreak. Serology is only useful epidemiologically.
- An NPA is the best sample for laboratory diagnosis. Viral culture is the standard (characterized by the typical syncytial appearance, and the cytopathic effect at around days 3–7), but antigen capture techniques and PCR (usually part of a respiratory multiplex) are faster and more widely available.

Treatment

- General—oxygen, fluids, respiratory support. Bronchodilators may help wheeze in some children but are not routinely recommended. No specific benefit from steroids or antibiotics.
- Nebulized ribavirin—not routinely recommended in infants/children with acute bronchiolitis. Some studies suggest a benefit on chronic respiratory symptoms, but there is insufficient evidence to support its use for this purpose. May have a role in the treatment of immunosuppressed adult BMT recipients and immunosuppressed children with severe disease.

Prevention

- Infection control—vital in hospitalized cases. Handwashing, eye–nose goggles, and glove use reduce nosocomial infections. Infected patients should be isolated or cohorted, especially on wards with high-risk patients.
- Immunotherapy—active immunization is not available. Palivizumab (RSV monoclonal antibody) reduces morbidity in infants <12 months old at risk of severe RSV (extreme prematurity, acyanotic heart disease, congenital lung disease, immunodeficiency). Administered to such infants once a month during outbreaks, it reduces disease severity and hospital admissions for respiratory illness.

Coronaviruses

Enveloped viruses of the family *Nidovirus*. Large positive-sense ssRNA genome that replicates using a set of nested mRNAs ('nido' for 'nest'). The name derives from Latin 'corona' (crown), reflecting the EM appearance of the viral spike protein that populates the surface of the virus and determines its host tropism.

Classic community-acquired coronavirus

Found worldwide. In temperate climates, human coronavirus (HCoV) respiratory infections tend to occur in winter. Spread is by aerosol or contact with infected secretions. Immunity is acquired, but reinfection common (either by waning immunity or antigenic variation). Outbreaks occur in hospitals and residential care homes. Presentations may be:

- respiratory—HCoV account for <20% of all adult acute URTIs and may cause acute otitis media in children. They have been isolated from infants with pneumonia and associated with wheeze in children, and may trigger asthma attacks in adults and children. In the elderly, they cause flu-like illnesses, pneumonia, and acute exacerbations of bronchitis;
- enteric—there is an association between the presence of coronavirus particles on stool EM and diarrhoea in infants or necrotizing enterocolitis in neonates;
- diagnosis is rarely helpful, as treatment is supportive. RT-PCR tests are available.

Severe Acute Respiratory Syndrome (SARS) coronavirus

SARS was recognized in China in November 2002 and had spread to affect 29 countries across the world by February 2003. The epidemic had died out by July 2003; 8096 cases were reported, with a fatality rate of 11% (43% in those over 60 years of age). Between July 2003 and May 2004, there were four small and rapidly contained outbreaks of SARS, three of which were associated with laboratory releases and the fourth thought to be due to an animal source. The cause was a novel coronavirus. Animals are thought to be the main reservoir. Transmission is by droplets and contact with contaminated surfaces—nosocomial transmission was common in the early stages of the outbreak. The virus is present in stool and may cause diarrhoea.

- Clinical features—incubation is 2–10 days. A 3- to 7-day febrile prodrome follows, notable for the absence of upper respiratory symptoms. The respiratory phase typically starts with a dry cough, progressing to breathlessness and progressive pulmonary infiltrates on CXR.
- Diagnosis—during the outbreak, RT-PCR was performed but sensitivity appeared limited (<70% positive on NPAs in week 2 of illness). No systematic study was performed to validate tests. Serological testing by ELISA at 3 weeks appeared most sensitive.
- Treatment—no specific therapy. Care is supportive. Patient isolation and infection control precautions were key to the control of the 2002/3 outbreak. This was greatly facilitated by the relatively long prodrome that enabled patients to be identified and isolated before they became infectious.

Middle East Respiratory Syndrome (MERS) coronavirus

This betacoronavirus, closely related to several bat coronaviruses was identified in 2012 from a man admitted to hospital in Saudi Arabia with pneumonia and renal failure. Shortly after his admission, an identical virus was identified in Qatar in a patient with similar features who had travelled to Saudi Arabia. Cases followed across the Middle East and were reported in five other countries amongst patients returning from the Middle East. The UK, France, Italy, and Tunisia reported limited human-to-human transmission to close contacts of the index cases. The case fatality rate was reported as 60%.

- Clinical features—incubation around 5 days (but <10 days). Symptoms range from none (positive RT-PCR tests were found in several asymptomatic close contacts), mild respiratory illness, to severe pneumonia requiring ventilation or extracorporeal membrane oxygenation. Other symptoms: pericarditis, renal failure, DIC, diarrhoea. Those with underlying medical problems seem at greater risk of severe disease.
- Diagnosis—RT-PCR testing of lower respiratory tract specimens is most sensitive. Testing multiple specimens taken at different times from different sites increases the likelihood of detecting virus. Guidance should be sought from national public health authorities regarding who to test, based upon contemporary epidemiology.
- Treatment is supportive, and infection control paramount.

Metapneumovirus

Identified in 2001 as a cause of respiratory tract disease in Dutch children. Like RSV and parainfluenza virus, it is a member of the family *Paramyxoviridae*. Transmission is by droplet spread, and outbreaks are seasonal (late winter, early spring in Europe and the USA). Clinical features are indistinguishable from those caused by RSV, and it is a cause of respiratory tract disease in both children and adults worldwide; 98–100% of people are seropositive by age 10 years; it is a significant pathogen in LRTIs of children and is implicated in nosocomial spread of infection in hospital wards. Symptoms are identical to those of RSV in children (mild URTI to severe cough, bronchiolitis, and pneumonia) and older adults (cough, fever, respiratory distress). Diagnosis is by PCR of respiratory secretions or serology. There is as yet no specific treatment. Ribavirin, which has a role in the treatment of RSV, is active *in vitro* and in mice, but its efficacy in humans is not known.

Measles

An acute highly infectious disease of children, characterized by cough, coryza, fever, and rash. Humans are the only natural host.

The virus

- A member of the family *Paramyxoviridae*, genus *Morbillivirus*; ssRNA, enveloped virus; covered with short surface projections: haemagglutinin (H) and fusion (F) glycoproteins.

Epidemiology

- Found in every country in the world. Without vaccination, epidemics lasting 3–4 months would occur every 2–5 years.
- Airborne, spread by contact with aerosolized respiratory secretions, and one of the most communicable of the infectious diseases. Sensitive to light and drying, but can remain infective in droplets for some hours.
- Patients are most infectious during the late prodromal phase when coughing is at its peak. Immunity after infection is lifelong.

Pathogenesis

- The virus invades the respiratory epithelium, and local multiplication leads to viraemia and leucocyte infection. Reticulo-endothelial cells become infected, and their necrosis leads to secondary viraemia. The major infected blood cell is the monocyte.
- Tissues that become infected include the thymus, spleen, lymph node, liver, skin, and lung. Secondary viraemia leads to infection of the entire respiratory mucosa, with consequent cough and coryza. Croup, bronchiolitis, and pneumonia may also occur.
- Koplik's spots and rash appear a few days after respiratory symptoms—may represent host hypersensitivity to the virus.

Clinical features

- Incubation is 2 weeks (longer in adults than children). A prodromal phase (coinciding with secondary viraemia) of malaise, fever, anorexia, conjunctivitis, and cough is followed by Koplik's spots (blue-grey spots with a red base, classically found on the buccal mucosa opposite the second molars), then rash. Patients feel most unwell around day 2 of the rash. From late prodrome to resolution of fever and rash is around 7–10 days. Rash begins on the face and proceeds down, involving the palms and soles last. Erythematous and maculopapular, and may become confluent. It lasts around 5 days and may desquamate as it heals.
- Complications—bacterial superinfection (pneumonia and otitis media); acute encephalitis (1 in 2000 and probably due to host hypersensitivity to virus), characterized by fever recurrence, headache, seizures, and consciousness changes during convalescence; subacute sclerosing panencephalitis (SSPE)—chronic degenerative neurological condition, occurring years after measles, due to persistent CNS infection with measles virus, despite a vigorous host immune response; spontaneous abortion and premature labour—unlike rubella, there is no association with fetal malformations, but the disease can be more severe in pregnancy, and infants can acquire it. Infants born to mothers with active infection should be given immunoglobulin at birth.
- Prior to vaccination, measles was a common cause of viral meningitis and remains so in unvaccinated populations, usually occurring with a rash.
- Special conditions:
    - modified measles—a very mild form of the disease seen in people with some degree of passive immunity, e.g. those receiving immunoglobulin or babies under 1 year;

- atypical measles—seen in those who received early killed measles vaccines and are later infected by wild-type virus. The rash is atypical and may resemble Henoch–Schönlein purpura (HSP), varicella, spotted fever, or a drug eruption. High fever, peripheral oedema, pulmonary infiltrates, and effusions may occur. The disease is more severe, has a longer course, and is thought to be due to hypersensitivity to the virus in a partially immune host. It is rare now, but those who have received only killed vaccine should be offered live vaccine;
- immunocompromised patients (including the malnourished) may experience severe disease, e.g. primary viral giant cell pneumonia, encephalitis, SSPE-like encephalitis. They may not develop a rash, making diagnosis difficult. Immunocompromised people should be passively immunized following exposure, even if previously vaccinated.

Diagnosis

Diagnosis can usually be made clinically. Laboratory confirmation is useful in atypical cases or the immunocompromised. Suspected and confirmed cases should be reported to public health.

- Other—immunofluorescence microscopy of cells in secretions, RT-PCR.
- Virus isolation—possible in renal cell lines, growth slow. Useful in the immunodeficient where antibody responses may be minimal.
- Serology—a 4-fold increase in measles antibody titre between acute and convalescent specimens is diagnostic. IgM is detectable from day 3 after rash onset, and IgG from days 7–14.

Treatment

- Supportive therapy and treatment of bacterial superinfection.
- Vitamin A 100 000-200 000IU PO has been shown to reduce disease severity amongst children in developing countries. It may have benefit in developed countries in those with, or at risk of, complications. It should be avoided at or after immunization when it appears to reduce seroconversion.

Prevention

- Measles vaccine is given as part of MMR (measles, mumps, rubella) at 12 months and preschool. It can be given earlier in at-risk populations, but responses are suppressed, and an additional dose should be given later.
- The UK saw an increase in measles cases in 2012/2013 amongst 10–16 year olds. Over 2000 cases were reported, of which 20% required hospitalization. This was probably a result of those who missed vaccination in the late 1990s/2000s, as a result of concern (now discredited) over a possible link between MMR and autism. Vaccine coverage fell to <80%. A catch-up programme for 10–16 year olds was announced in 2013.
- Passive immunization with immunoglobulin is recommended for those exposed susceptible people at risk of severe or fatal measles—it must be given within 6 days of exposure to be effective. Such groups include children with defects in cell-mediated immunity, those with HIV or malignant disease, and unvaccinated pregnant women. Details are available on the PHE website (under 'Immunoglobulin' in 'Infections A-Z').

Mumps

Mumps is an acute generalized viral infection of children and adolescents, causing swelling and tenderness of the salivary glands, and rarely epididymo-orchitis. More severe manifestations are commoner in older patients. The name may derive from the English verb 'to mump'—to be sulky.

The virus

- A member of the *Paramyxoviridae* family; ssRNA virus; irregular, spherically shaped virion (average diameter 200nm); the nucleocapsid is enclosed by a three-layer envelope.
- The nucleocapsid contains the S (soluble) antigen, to which antibodies may be detected early in infection.
- Glycoproteins on the surface have HA, NA, and cell fusion activity, and include the V (viral) antigen detected in late infection by complement fixation.

Epidemiology

- Endemic throughout the world. Prior to vaccination, epidemics took place every 2–5 years, with 90% of cases occurring in those under 15 years.
- In the USA, one-third of cases occur in those over 15 years. UK incidence has been increasing amongst those born between 1981 and 1989 who missed routine MMR (first introduced in 1988) and are now at university. In 2004, there was a dramatic increase of cases in England and Wales amongst those born before 1987, many of whom had received just one dose of MMR in the 1998 'catch-up' campaign.
- Passive immunity makes infection uncommon in children under 1 year.

Pathogenesis

- Transmitted by droplet spread or direct contact. Most infectious just before parotitis.
- During incubation, the virus proliferates in the upper respiratory tract, with consequent viraemia and localization to glandular and neural tissue.
- Parotid glands show interstitial oedema and serofibrinous exudate with mononuclear cell infiltration. Cases of orchitis are similar with the addition of interstitial haemorrhage, polymorphonuclear infiltration, and areas of local infarction due to vascular compromise.

Clinical features

- Incubation is 2–4 weeks. A 24h non-specific prodrome of fever, headache, and anorexia is followed by earache and ipsilateral parotid tenderness. The gland swells over 2–3 days and is associated with severe pain. Swelling can lift the earlobe up and outward. The other side follows within a couple of days in 75% of cases. Patients experience difficulty in pronunciation and mastication. Once swelling has peaked, recovery is rapid—within a week. Complications of parotitis (e.g. sialectasis) are rare. Other salivary glands may be involved.
- CNS involvement—the commonest extraglandular manifestation in children. *Meningitis* is seen in <10% of those with parotitis, although

<50% of cases of mumps meningitis show no evidence of glandular disease. Onset is 4–7 days after glandular symptoms but can occur 1 week before or 2 weeks later. Male > female. Symptoms resolve 3–10 days later, and recovery is complete with no sequelae. CSF findings—typical of viral meningitis (➲ see Viral meningitis, pp. 722–4); hypoglycorrhachia (low CSF glucose) is seen in up to 30% of cases, more than in other viral meningitides. *Encephalitis* is seen in 1 in 6000 and takes two forms: early onset which represents direct neuron damage due to viral invasion, and a larger late-onset (7–10 days) group representing a post-infectious demyelinating process. Recovery takes around 2 weeks, and sequelae (e.g. psychomotor retardation) and death (around 1.4% of cases) may be seen. *Other* neurological manifestations include transient deafness, permanent deafness (1 in 20 000), ataxia, facial palsy, transverse myelitis, and GBS.

- Presternal pitting oedema and tongue swelling (thought to be due to lymphatic obstruction by swollen regional glands) (6%).
- Epididymo-orchitis—the commonest extraglandular manifestation in adults, seen in 20–30% of post-pubertal males with mumps (one in six cases bilateral). Rare before puberty. May be the only manifestation of mumps. Abrupt onset with fever, and a warm, swollen (up to four times normal), tender testicle with erythema of the overlying skin. Fever resolves at 5 days with gonadal symptoms following. Some degree of atrophy may be seen in 50%, once recovered. Infertility is rare.
- Other: oophoritis (5% of post-pubertal women with mumps—impaired fertility and premature menopause have been reported but are rare), migratory polyarthritis, pancreatitis, myocarditis, nephritis, thyroiditis, mastitis, and hepatitis.

Diagnosis

- Diagnosis is usually clinical. Laboratory confirmation is required for epidemiological purposes or when disease is atypical.
- Serum amylase is elevated in parotitis or pancreatitis (isoenzyme analysis is required to differentiate the source).
- Serology—serum IgM antibody testing should be performed as soon as disease is suspected. It remains positive for <4 weeks but may be negative in 50% of the previously immunized with acute infection. A convalescent sample 2–3 weeks after the first demonstrating a 4-fold or greater increase in IgG titre is diagnostic.
- Viral culture—present in saliva from 2 days before symptom onset to 5 days after. May be present in CSF up to 6 days after onset.
- PCR-based tests are available.

Treatment

- Symptom control—antipyretics and fluids if persistent vomiting.
- No benefit in steroid use has been demonstrated.
- Anecdotal evidence that IFN-α speeds resolution of orchitis.

Prevention

Vaccination is >95% effective, and takes place at 12 months and preschool as part of MMR.

Rubella

An acute, mild, exanthematous viral infection of children and adults, resembling mild measles, but with the potential to cause fetal infection and birth defects.

The virus

- A member of the family *Togaviridae*, in the genus *Rubivirus*.
- Spherical in shape, with a diameter of 60nm. Relatively unstable.

Epidemiology

- Unlike measles, rubella is only moderately contagious. Prior to vaccination, incidence was highest in the spring amongst children aged 5–9 years.
- Once termed 'third disease', measles and scarlet fever being the first and second exanthematous infections in childhood.
- After infection or vaccination, most people develop lifelong protection against disease. Reinfection occurs (the majority asymptomatic), as demonstrated by rises in antibody titre in previously vaccinated people.
- There have been rare cases of congenital rubella acquired through the reinfection of a vaccinated mother.

Pathogenesis

- Spread is by droplets; patients are at their most contagious when the rash is erupting, and the virus may be shed from 10 days before to 2 weeks after its appearance.
- Rash may be immune-mediated—it appears as immunity develops and viral titres fall.
- Primary viraemia follows infection of the respiratory epithelium; secondary viraemia occurs a few days later, once the first wave of infected leucocytes release virions.
- Infants with congenital rubella shed large quantities of virus for many months.

Clinical features

- Incubation is 12–23 days. Post-natal rubella is a mild infection. Many cases are subclinical. Adults may experience a prodrome of malaise, fever, and anorexia. The main symptoms are lymphadenopathy (cervical and posterior auricular) and a maculopapular rash (starting on the face and moving down) that may be accompanied by coryza and conjunctivitis, and last 3–5 days. Splenomegaly can occur.
- Complications are uncommon—arthritis affecting the wrists, fingers, and knees and resolving over a month may be seen, as the rash appears (women > men); haemorrhagic manifestations occur in 1 in 3000 (children > adults) and may be due to thrombocytopenia, as well as vascular damage; encephalitis occurs in 1 in 5000 (adults > children), with a mortality of up to 50%.
- Congenital rubella—can be catastrophic in early pregnancy, leading to fetal death, premature delivery, and many congenital defects. Rare since the introduction of vaccination. The younger the fetus when infected,

the more severe the illness. In the first 2 months of gestation, there is an up to 85% chance of being affected by either multiple defects or spontaneous abortion. In the third month, there is around a 30% chance of developing a single defect (e.g. deafness), dropping to 10% in the fourth month and nil after 20 weeks. Temporary defects include low birthweight, low platelets, hepatosplenomegaly, hepatitis, meningitis, and jaundice. Permanent defects include hearing loss, cardiac abnormalities, microcephaly, inguinal hernia, cataract, and glaucoma. Developmental defects may become apparent as the infant grows, e.g. myopia, mental retardation, diabetes, behavioural and language disorders.

Diagnosis

- Its mild nature makes clinical diagnosis difficult.
- Serology—positive IgM on a single sample or a 4-fold rise in IgG in paired sera is diagnostic. IgM may be positive in cases of reinfection. Serological diagnosis of congenital rubella in neonates may necessitate the analysis of several samples over time to determine whether antibody titres are falling (maternal antibody) or rising (recent infection). Detection of rubella IgM in a newborn's serum indicates infection.
- Intrauterine diagnosis has been made by placental biopsy and by cordocentesis with detection by PCR.

Treatment

- No treatment is indicated in most cases of post-natal rubella.
- Immunoglobulin was once given to exposed susceptible pregnant women—however, it does not prevent viraemia, despite suppressing symptoms, and is not recommended.
- All women of childbearing age should be vaccinated before pregnancy.

Prevention

Vaccination achieves a seroconversion rate of 95%. Women should not become pregnant in the 3 months following vaccination.

Parvovirus B19

Parvovirus B19 has a wide variety of clinical manifestations, depending on the state of the host: 'slapped cheek' ('fifth') disease in children, aplastic crisis in those with underlying haemolytic disorders. The virus was found in 1974, while evaluating assays for HBsAg—sample 19 in panel B gave a 'false positive', and EM revealed the guilty virus.

The virus

- A member of the family *Parvoviridae*, genus *Erythrovirus* (so-called because replication occurs only in human erythrocyte precursors). B19 is the only known human pathogenic parvovirus. They are non-enveloped and extremely resistant to physical inactivation.

Epidemiology

- Infection common in childhood—50% are IgG-positive by 15 years, and 90% antibody-positive by 90 years. Infected children pass the virus on to uninfected members of their family. Patients are infectious from 24 to 48h before the viral prodrome until rash appearance.
- In temperate climates, infection is commonest from late winter to early summer. Rates peak every 3–4 years. Prevalence higher in Africa.
- Infection may be passed vertically, by respiratory secretions, or from blood and blood products (standard thermal treatments and solvent detergents are not completely effective), although viraemia is rare.

Pathogenesis

- Parvovirus B19 infects erythroid progenitors and erythroblasts. The receptor it uses to infect cells—P antigen—is found on megakaryocytes, endothelial cells, fetal myocardial cells, and erythroid precursors. Those who lack P antigen on their erythrocytes are resistant to infection.
- Causes a self-limiting (4–8 days) halt in red cell manufacture, as infected cells are destroyed. This may be unnoticed in those with normal erythroid turnover. Falls of 2–6g/dL are not uncommon in those with high turnover (e.g. haemoglobinopathies); aplastic anaemia may result.
- The infected fetus may have severe manifestations (anaemia, myocarditis, heart failure), due to high red cell turnover and the immature immune response. These effects are reduced by the third trimester.
- Rash and arthralgia associated with some forms of the disease are probably immune complex-related.

Clinical features

- Twenty per cent of infections are asymptomatic.
- Erythema infectiosum (EI)—the commonest manifestation; 5–7 days of fever, coryza, and mild nausea/diarrhoea is followed by classic 'slapped cheek' rash (fiery, red eruption with surrounding pallor). A second erythematous maculopapular rash may follow on the trunk and limbs 1–2 days later, fading to produce a lacy appearance. Adults have milder manifestations. Pruritus (especially soles of the feet) can occur.
- Arthropathy—seen in adults, women > men. Symmetric, mainly small joints of hands/feet. Lasts 1–3 weeks; may persist or recur for months.
- Transient aplastic crisis (TAC)—abrupt cessation of erythropoiesis with absent erythroid precursors in the bone marrow. Described in a wide range of haemolytic conditions: sickle-cell (nearly 90% of TAC episodes), thalassaemia, pyruvate kinase deficiency, autoimmune haemolytic anaemia. It has also been seen after haemorrhage, in iron deficiency anaemia, and in those who are otherwise well (deficiencies in other blood lineages may occur). Patients can be severely ill: dyspnoea, confusion, cardiac failure. Does not appear to cause true, permanent aplastic anaemia.
- Pure red cell aplasia (PRCA)—anaemia in the immunosuppressed (HIV, congenital immunodeficiency, patients undergoing transplantation). Administration of immunoglobulin may be beneficial.
- Virus-associated haemophagocytic syndrome—usually healthy patients with cytopenia; characterized by histiocytic hyperplasia and haemophagocytosis. Self-limiting.

- Fetal infection—10–15% of non-immune hydrops fetalis. Where maternal infection occurs, fetal loss averages 9% and occurs within the first 20 weeks of pregnancy. There is no evidence of long-term abnormality in those who survive.
- Other manifestations—encephalitis, myocarditis, hepatitis, vasculitis, erythema multiforme, glomerulonephritis, idiopathic thrombocytopenia purpura (ITP), HSP.
- Chronic infection with anaemia may occur in the immunosuppressed.

Diagnosis

- IgM detection—90% of cases positive by the time of the rash in EI or by day 3 of TAC. IgM remains detectable for up to 3 months. IgG is detectable by day 7 of illness and remains detectable for life. It is not useful in diagnosing acute infection or in attributing manifestations such as chronic arthropathy to B19.
- Virus nucleic acid detection tests (DNA hybridization, PCR)—sensitive but, in immunocompetent people, viral DNA can only be detected for 2–4 days.
- Immunocompromised people with chronic infection do not mount an immune response, and diagnosis relies on detecting DNA by PCR.
- Fetal infection can be confirmed by amniotic fluid sampling, and investigations should include maternal B19 serology.

Treatment

- General measures, e.g. non-steroidal anti-inflammatory drugs (NSAIDs) for arthritis, transfusions for TAC.
- Immunosuppressed patients with chronic infection may benefit from temporary cessation of immunosuppression and IVIG. If disease recurs, they may require repeated courses. Some HIV-infected patients will resolve chronic B19 infection with the initiation of ART.
- Intrauterine blood transfusions may help some cases of hydrops. For details of management of B19 in pregnancy, ➲ see Patients presenting with a non-vesicular rash, p. 792.

Prevention

Unlike 'slapped cheek' patients, those with TAC and PRCA are infectious at presentation and should be separated from high-risk contacts (glove and gown, own room, mask, etc.) for 7 days or for the duration of the illness. Pregnant HCWs should not care for such patients.

Herpesviruses

Enveloped, dsDNA viruses. Similar morphologically but differ clinically and biologically. Three groups:

- alpha-herpesviruses (HSV-1, HSV-2, and VZV);
- beta-herpesviruses (CMV, human herpesvirus (HHV)-6 and HHV-7, Simian herpes B);
- gamma-herpesviruses (EBV and HHV-8).

Human herpesvirus type 6

A lymphotropic virus and the single commonest cause of hospital visits in infants with fever. The cause of roseola (also known as sixth disease or exanthem subitum).

The virus

- A herpesvirus, originally called B-lymphotropic virus, now shown to grow in many different cell types (T cells, macrophages, etc.).
- Two subtypes (A and B), which differ in their epidemiology and growth.

Epidemiology

- Seroprevalence varies, but most industrialized nations report rates of 75–95%. Nearly all humans infected by age 2 years, probably by maternal saliva.
- Most isolates from healthy people are HHV-6B. Both 6A and 6B have been identified in the chronically unwell or immunosuppressed.

Pathogenesis

- Incubation is 5–15d. Primary infection is via the oropharynx. Regional lymph nodes and mononuclear cells (especially CD4 T cells) are subsequently infected, and the virus spreads throughout the body, leading to significant impairment of immune function.
- Like other herpesviruses, it causes an initial infection and lifelong latency (integrating into the human genome), and has the potential for clinical reactivation, especially in hosts who are immunocompromised. Asymptomatic carriers may excrete the virus for months.
- Specific mechanisms for host immune evasion facilitate persistent infection.

Clinical features

- Infantile fever—fever without rash is the commonest manifestation and may be accompanied by periorbital oedema. Ten per cent of cases in one series of acute febrile illnesses were attributed to HHV-6. Benign febrile convulsions may occur and are more frequent than fever alone explains—perhaps due to viral replication within the CNS.
- Exanthem subitum (sixth disease)—an illness of infants and young children. Three to 5 days of fever and upper respiratory tract symptoms are followed by the development of rose-pink papules that are mildly elevated and non-pruritic, and blanch on pressure. Rash lasts around 2 days and may be associated with malaise, vomiting, diarrhoea, cough, pharyngitis, and lymphadenopathy. Most infants are asymptomatic.
- Encephalitis—can occur alone or as a complication of exanthem subitum. Virus frequently detected in the CNS, even in absence of symptoms.
- Immunocompromised hosts—as with other herpesviruses, immune suppression permits replication, with the potential for clinical illness. It should be considered in the differential of fever in children with cancer (including lymphoma). Pneumonitis, colitis, encephalitis, marrow suppression, graft failure, and GVHD in BMT recipients have all been attributed to it, but often in the presence of other pathogens (such as CMV) with better established pathological pedigrees.
- Other—infectious mononucleosis, hepatitis, chronic fatigue syndrome (causality unproven).

Diagnosis

- Exanthem subitum does not need specific investigation or treatment due to its self-limiting nature. Diagnosis should be confirmed in those patients who are recipients of organ transplants or patients with immunodeficiency, encephalitis, or hepatitis.
- Serology—rarely helpful, as nearly everyone is positive by age 2 years. IgM assays are not good indicators of acute infection; paired sera are required. CMV antibodies may cross-react with HHV-6.
- Viral culture—it is very unusual to detect it in the healthy, and high rates of recovery in the immunocompromised, regardless of presentation, negate its usefulness as a diagnostic tool.
- PCR—tests are available. Qualitative detection is of limited use, as it may be present latently and does not indicate causality. Quantification of cell-free virus in serum, CSF, etc. may be more useful.

Treatment

- Most cases are self-limiting and need no treatment.
- Similar antiviral sensitivity pattern to CMV—foscarnet is active against HHV-6A and -6B; ganciclovir is active against HHV-6B (some reports of relative resistance in HHV-6A), and aciclovir is inactive. There are no controlled trials.

Human herpesvirus type 7

Epidemiology

- First demonstrated in 1990 from peripheral blood mononuclear cells of a healthy adult. Its role in human disease is yet to be defined.
- Infects nearly all humans by age 5 years. A commensal inhabitant of saliva.
- Homology to HHV-6 is limited but confused earlier serological studies.

Pathogenesis

- Very similar to HHV-6; it is a lymphotropic virus that infects $CD4^+$ T cells and encodes genes allowing it to evade the immune system.

Clinical features

- Generally asymptomatic. Probably causes similar fever and rash syndromes to HHV-6.
- It may be a cofactor for symptomatic CMV disease in renal transplant recipients.

Human herpesvirus type 8

A herpesvirus associated with several human neoplasms, including Kaposi's sarcoma (KS), primary effusion lymphoma, and Castleman's disease.

The virus

A gamma-herpesvirus (like EBV), first identified in KS tissue from patients infected with HIV.

Epidemiology

- 'Classic' KS was first recognized in the 1870s amongst those of Mediterranean and Eastern European descent. Later a more aggressive 'endemic' form was recognized across black populations of East Africa. In the 1980s, clusters of KS amongst homosexual men contributed to the recognition of HIV. It has also been seen in renal transplant recipients. HHV-8 has been identified in lesions from all forms of KS.
- Reported seroprevalence amongst healthy US adults ranges from 2% to 30%, and 25–90% in homosexual HIV-positive men without KS. In Africa, seropositivity increases with age, reaching 49% in those over 50 years.
- Over 95% of HIV-associated KS cases are in homosexual men, in whom it is up to 15 times commoner than in those acquiring HIV non-sexually.
- Epidemiological studies suggest a sexual route of HHV-8 transmission, but other means of transmission are not clear. HHV-8 DNA has been detected in the semen and saliva of HIV-infected patients with KS, and not healthy controls.

Pathogenesis

- In the healthy host, T cells and natural killer (NK) cells play a key role in controlling HHV-8. It infects a wide variety of cell types, including endothelial and epithelial cells. Like EBV, it exists in latent and lytic phases.
- Encodes cell cycle regulatory proteins and cytokine homologues which probably contribute to the pathogenesis of KS and other malignancies.
- KS lesions consist of inflammatory, endothelial, and red blood cells.

Clinical features

- Primary infection—may be associated with a fever/rash in children, and new-onset lymphadenopathy has been described in HIV-negative MSM undergoing HHV-8 seroconversion. Fever, splenomegaly, pancytopenia, and rapid-onset KS have been described in immunocompromised patients.
- KS—four epidemiological types (classic, endemic, HIV-associated, transplant-associated). Lesions are vascular, often nodular (0.5–2cm in diameter), and appear on skin, mucous membrane, or viscera (lung and biliary tract particularly). Violaceous or brown/black in pigmented skin. Visceral disease may involve any organ (e.g. GI—can bleed, pulmonary—effusions). Lymphoedema may follow regional lymph node infiltration. Endemic KS is slow-growing and has little prognostic significance. In AIDS patients with KS, the health impact of the lesions is generally of less importance than opportunistic infections.
- Primary effusion lymphoma (PEL)—an aggressive B-cell lymphoma seen in AIDS patients, with a predilection for body cavities. Presents as lymphomatous effusions, arising predominantly in the pleural, pericardial, or peritoneal cavities.
- Castleman's disease—an uncommon lymphoproliferative disorder, first described in the 1950s. Localized (unicentric, UCD) forms are benign and may be cured by surgical excision. Multicentric Castleman's disease (MCD) is associated with HIV, and is aggressive and often fatal.

HHV-8 is associated with <50% of HIV-negative MCD and 100% of HIV-positive MCD.

- Other—inconclusive claims have been made of HHV-8 isolation in some skin cancers and certain cases of multiple myeloma, idiopathic pulmonary hypertension, and sarcoidosis.

Diagnosis

Diagnosis of KS can usually be made clinically, but biopsy can confirm. Lesion biopsy is required for the diagnosis of PEL and Castleman's disease. PCR for HHV-8, while available, is of little benefit in the diagnosis of KS (viraemia is not universal). In contrast, it may have a role in the management of patients with MCD—patients with active disease are viraemic, and HHV-8 quantification can be used to track response to treatment. Serology is of limited clinical utility.

Treatment

- As yet, no role for specific HHV-8 antiviral therapy. Ganciclovir, cidofovir, and nelfinavir, amongst others, all have *in vitro* activity.
- KS:
  - forty per cent of transplant-associated KS will respond to reduction of immunosuppression alone. This risks graft rejection, and an alternative is to switch immunosuppressive therapy to sirolimus, which has antiangiogenic effects against KS;
  - HIV-positive patients require ART. Isolated KS lesions can be observed. Individual lesions of cosmetic impact can be irradiated, or intralesional vinblastine administered. Other indications for treatment include lymphoedema, bulky lesions in the oropharynx, and pulmonary disease. Extensive disease may be treated with chemotherapy (liposomal anthracycline such as doxorubicin). Those who progress on therapy should receive second-line therapy (paclitaxel, etoposide, IFN-α). Life-threatening disease may require combination chemotherapy. Experimental therapy includes monoclonal antibodies against vascular endothelial growth factor.
- PEL—HIV-positive patients should receive ART and chemotherapy. Even with treatment, mean overall survival is 6 months. Where possible, non-HIV-related cases should have any immunosuppressive therapy reduced.
- Castleman's disease—UCD, excision of lesions is curative; MCD, rituximab (anti-CD20 monoclonal antibody) is emerging as the treatment of choice, combined with combination chemotherapy if disease is aggressive.

Herpes simplex

HSV infects a wide variety of cells and is cytopathic to those in which it completes a full replication cycle, with the exception of certain neuronal cells. In these, it may establish latent infection. Reactivation of the viral genome can occur, resulting in the production and release of viral particles with infection of adjacent cells. Its genome encodes around 80 gene products; sequence homology between HSV-1 and -2 is around 50%

Epidemiology

- HSV exists worldwide; humans are the only known natural reservoir.
- Nearly all adults have antibodies to HSV-1 by their 40s—prevalence is highest in lower socio-economic groups.
- HSV-2 antibodies correlate with sexual activity—that of either the individual or their partners—appearing in puberty and being closely related to the number of partners and the presence of a history of STIs.
- HSV-2 seroprevalence is around 22% in the USA (slightly higher in women than men), a little lower than this in the UK, and, in general, higher in developing countries.
- Half of HSV-2 seroconversions are subclinical, more in those who have previously been infected with HSV-1. Symptomatic reactivation is common.
- Infection with one viral type confers partial immunity to the other.

Pathogenesis

- Infection occurs via close contact with an individual who is shedding virus peripherally. The virus enters through mucosal surfaces or skin breaks, and replicates locally, often with no clinical manifestations.
- Viral progeny infect neurons and travel via the axon to the nerve ganglion (e.g. HSV-1 to the trigeminal, HSV-2 to the sacral nerve root ganglion) where a second phase of replication takes place; the virus then spreads peripherally along sensory nerves, accounting for the large areas that may be involved in clinical disease. After primary disease resolution, infectious HSV cannot be detected, but viral DNA may be found in up to half of ganglion cells.
- Reactivation mechanisms are not clear—viral subtype, route of infection, and host factors all contribute. Individuals infected with HSV-1 both orally and genitally experience reactivation more frequently orally. On the other hand, HSV-2 local reactivation is 8–10 times more frequent if acquired genitally.
- Individuals with impaired cellular immunity (transplant recipients, patients with AIDS) may develop severe, possibly disseminated and life-threatening, disease.

Clinical features

- Clinical manifestations are various, influenced by the site of infection, viral type, host age, and immune status. First infections tend to be more severe than reactivation, with more systemic features, longer symptom duration, and a higher rate of complications. Both viral subtypes can cause genital and orofacial infection.
- Cutaneous manifestations (➔ see Viral skin infections, pp. 768–70).
- Visceral infection—viraemia usually results in multiple organ involvement, but single organs may be affected. Severe disseminated disease is rare but occurs at increased frequency in women in the third trimester of pregnancy (➔ see Herpes simplex, pp. 788–9).
  - HSV oesophagitis—may follow disease extension from the pharynx or by viral reactivation via the vagal nerve. Ulceration usually involves

the distal oesophagus with retrosternal chest pain and dysphagia. Disease may resemble invasive *Candida* infection.
- Pneumonitis—rare. Tends to occur in the severely immunosuppressed; mortality exceeds 80%.

- Encephalitis—>95% of cases caused by HSV-1, incidence peaking in those aged 5–30 years and those over 50 years old. Higher rates in the immunocompromised. Primary infection may cause encephalitis in children and young adults, but most older adults have evidence of previous infection with disease resulting from reactivation or reinfection with exogenous virus. Onset is usually acute (may be insidious) with a prodrome of headache, behavioural change, and fever. Other symptoms: focal neurological signs (classically temporal lobe), seizures, and coma. Diagnosis is by CSF PCR (98–99% sensitive; false negatives have occurred within the first 72h of symptoms—consider repeating lumbar puncture and PCR if history good). Electroencephalography (EEG) and computerized tomography (CT) may demonstrate characteristic focal features but can be normal early in illness. Magnetic resonance imaging (MRI) is more sensitive. Brain biopsy for culture and histology is rarely indicated.
- Meningitis—more commonly caused by HSV-2. Cases may complicate genital herpes (women > men), with symptoms following genital lesions by 3–10 days. It is usually benign in the immunocompetent, lasting 2–4 days and resolving over 3 days. CSF findings: raised white cells (majority lymphocytes, polymorphonuclear cells in early infection), glucose usually over 50% of blood levels, but hypoglycorrhachia occurs, raised protein; PCR for HSV DNA is the most sensitive means of diagnosis.
- Other neurological features—sacral radiculopathy, autonomic nerve dysfunction (hyperaesthesia/anaesthesia of the lower back and sacral area, constipation, urinary retention, transient impotence resolving over 4–8 weeks), transverse myelitis—decreased tendon reflexes and reduced muscle strength in lower extremities, autonomic features.

Diagnosis

- Herpetic ulcerations resemble those of other causes. Laboratory diagnosis is important to guide therapy where there is doubt.
- Histology—may demonstrate giant cells or intranuclear inclusions. Direct fluorescent antibody testing is highly specific.
- Viral culture allows identification within 48h; not widely available.
- PCR to detect HSV DNA—very sensitive, particularly with samples from late-stage lesions and CSF in CNS infections.
- Serology—useful in the identification of asymptomatic carriers.

Treatment

- Aciclovir PO shortens the duration of primary attacks of cutaneous, oral, and genital herpes. It is less effective against recurrent disease but may be given prophylactically where recurrences are very frequent and in the immunocompromised. Valaciclovir PO has better oral bioavailability and is indicated for treatment of primary HSV infections.

It is also used in treatment/suppression of recurrent infections in immunocompromised or HIV-positive patients.

- Severe and disseminated HSV infection—IV therapy.
- Encephalitis—antiviral therapy (IV aciclovir for 14–21 days) should be given to suspected cases of HSV encephalitis until the diagnosis can be confirmed; it reduces mortality from 70% to around 25%. In patients with low probability of HSV encephalitis (normal imaging, normal CSF, normal mental state), a negative PCR from the CSF taken after 72h of symptoms reduces the likelihood of disease to <1%.

Varicella-zoster virus

VZV causes two distinct diseases: a primary infection—chickenpox (varicella), and shingles (herpes zoster)—and the localized recurrence.

The virus

- A dsDNA virus around 200nm in diameter and a member of the *Herpesviridae* family. The lipid-containing envelope is studded with glycoprotein spikes that are the primary markers for humoral and cell-mediated immunity.
- Spreads between cells by direct contact and may be isolated in many human cell lines.

Epidemiology

- Acquired via the respiratory tract. Humans are the only known reservoir, and >90% of people are seropositive by 20 years of age.
- Infection is common in childhood (90% of cases in those under 13 years), peaking in late winter and early spring. Secondary attack rates in susceptible siblings within a household are around 80%.
- Patients are infectious for 48h before rash appearance, and 4–5 days after vesicles crust over.
- After infection, the virus becomes latent within the dorsal root ganglia.
- Reactivation, causing shingles, occurs in 20% of the population. All ages are affected; highest incidence in the elderly and immunocompromised.
- Mortality—under 2 per 100 000 for children, increasing 15-fold for adults.

Pathogenesis

- After infection and local replication, patients become viraemic.
- Viral replication in the skin precipitates degenerative changes of epithelial cells with ballooning and the appearance of multinucleated giant cells and eosinophilic intranuclear inclusions.
- Vesicles contain a cloudy fluid (leucocytes, fibrin, and degenerate cells) and either rupture, releasing infectious virus, or slowly resolve.
- Necrosis and haemorrhage may occur in the upper part of the dermis.
- Histological findings of the skin are similar in chickenpox and shingles.

Clinical features

Chickenpox

- Incubation is 10–14 days. A 1- to 2-day febrile prodrome may be followed by constitutional symptoms (malaise, itch, anorexia) and rash.
- Rash begins as maculopapules (<5mm across), progressing to vesicles that quickly pustulate, forming scabs which fall off 1–2 weeks later.
- Lesions appear in successive crops over 2–4 days, starting on the trunk and face and spreading centripetally. May rarely involve the mucosa of the oropharynx and vagina.
- Complications—secondary bacterial infection of lesions usually with Gram-positive organisms (including streptococcal toxic shock), acute cerebellar ataxia (1 in 4000 children under 15 years, onset 7–21 days after rash and resolves over 2–4 weeks), encephalitis (0.2% cases, characterized by depressed consciousness, fever, vomiting, and seizures, and may be life-threatening in adults; recovery over 2 weeks; 5–20% experience progressive deterioration and die), cerebral angiitis (after herpes zoster ophthalmicus), meningitis, transverse myelitis, pneumonitis (1 in 400 adult VZV cases), myocarditis, bleeding, and hepatitis.
- Immunocompromised—children (especially those with leukaemia) may have more lesions, often haemorrhagic, taking up to three times longer to heal; increased risk of visceral involvement (lung, liver, CNS); increased risk of severe infection in BMT recipients, especially those receiving anti-thymocyte globulin or experiencing GVHD—almost half have cutaneous or visceral dissemination.
- Pregnancy—high risk of pneumonitis, especially if a smoker and after 20 weeks' gestation. Risk of neonatal infection if maternal disease is between 5 days before and 2 days after delivery, with mortality <30% without treatment. For PEP, ➔ see Preventing neonatal varicella, p. 795.

Herpes zoster

- Unilateral vesicular eruption in a dermatomal distribution (most commonly thoracic and lumbar), often preceded by 2–3 days of pain in the affected area. Maculopapular lesions evolve into vesicles, with new crops forming over 3–5 days. Resolution may take 2–4 weeks.
- Other manifestations—eyelids (first or second branch of the trigeminal); keratitis (herpes zoster ophthalmicus—sight-threatening and requires ophthalmic referral); intraoral—palate, tonsillar fossa, tongue (maxillary or mandibular branch of trigeminal nerve); Ramsay–Hunt syndrome—pain and vesicles in the external auditory meatus, ipsilateral facial palsy, loss of taste to the anterior two-thirds of the tongue (geniculate ganglion); encephalitis; granulomatous cerebral angiitis (after zoster ophthalmicus); paralysis (anterior horn cell involvement).
- Immunocompromised patients—disease is more severe with prolonged lesion formation and recovery with higher risk of cutaneous dissemination and visceral involvement. Rarely fatal. Those with HIV have an increased incidence of complications such as retinitis, acute retinal necrosis, chronic progressive encephalitis, chronic zoster.
- Post-herpetic neuralgia—uncommon in young people but occurs in up to 50% of those over 50 years old.

Diagnosis

- Usually made clinically, but laboratory confirmation useful in atypical rash or in presentations without skin manifestations (e.g. encephalitis, disseminated disease).
- Serology—IgG antibodies to VZV indicates prior infection and the presence of immunity. Some commercial ELISAs may lack sensitivity to detect the lower levels of IgG in older people who have not been recently re-exposed to varicella.
- PCR—testing of vesicular fluid and CSF is rapid and specific. Testing of blood may be helpful in transplant patients with possible visceral disease. PCR has largely replaced viral culture for diagnostic purposes.

Treatment

Chickenpox

- General measures—prevent secondary infection of lesions, antihistamines for itch to reduce scratching, paracetamol for fever.
- Aciclovir—a 7-day PO course started within 24h of onset reduces the duration and severity of illness. Not recommended for routine use in immunocompetent children <12 years, as the clinical impact is modest. Limited trial data supporting the use of valaciclovir in chickenpox.
    - Adults—treat if it can be started <24h. No benefit after this.
    - Children—consider treating those >12 years of age, those on intermittent steroid therapy (PO or INH), secondary household cases (which tend to be more severe), and those with a history of chronic skin or heart/lung disorders.
    - Those with complications, dissemination, or immunosuppression—treat with IV aciclovir, regardless of the time since symptom onset. Good evidence for its safety after 20 weeks' gestation.

Shingles

- General measures (as discussed under ➔ Chickenpox above), ophthalmic referral if eye involvement.
- Oral antiviral therapy (aciclovir, valaciclovir) is recommended for those presenting within 72h of symptoms, or longer if lesions are still appearing. Benefits are greatest in those >50 years, but treatment can be considered for younger patients. Treatment is for 7 days.
- All immunocompromised patients should be treated without delay, even if after 72h. IV treatment may be necessary.
- There is no evidence supporting the routine use of steroids.
- Post-herpetic neuralgia is unusual beyond 4 weeks, but such cases can be difficult to treat. They usually resolve over 6–24 months. Therapies include tricyclics, counter-irritants, and gabapentin.

Prevention

- Vaccine—varicella vaccination (a live attenuated preparation) is recommended for non-immune HCWs and healthy household contacts of immunocompromised patients (e.g. siblings of a leukaemic child). The shingles vaccine (Zostavax®) contains live attenuated virus, with a significantly higher titre than the varicella vaccine. It reduces the incidence of shingles by 51% and reduces post-herpetic neuralgia by 66%

in those aged 60–69 years. It is recommended for those aged over 70 years, the age at which its cost-effectiveness is greatest.
- Varicella-zoster immune globulin (VZIG) does not prevent infection but reduces disease severity. Most effective if given within 72h. Indicated for seronegative patients with a contact history who are at increased risk of complications: those with defects in cell-mediated immunity; those on significant doses of steroids; those who have received BMT, radiotherapy, or chemotherapy within the last 6 months; organ transplant recipients on immunosuppression; pregnant women; infants whose mothers develop chickenpox (but not zoster) between 1 week before and 1 week after delivery, or infants who are exposed to chickenpox/zoster within the first week of life and whose mothers have no history of prior infection or are seronegative.

Infectious mononucleosis

Infectious mononucleosis is a syndrome of sore throat, fever, and lymphadenopathy, with atypical lymphocytosis; 80–90% of cases are due to EBV, which is generally associated with a positive heterophile antibody test. Most of the remainder are caused by CMV. Young adults and adolescents are most frequently affected. Other conditions that should be considered include viral hepatitis, acute toxoplasmosis, rubella, streptococcal throat, primary HIV, and diphtheria.

Epstein–Barr virus

A human herpesvirus, the cause of heterophile-positive infectious mononucleosis and associated with African Burkitt's lymphoma.

The virus

- Enveloped hexagonal nucleocapsids containing dsDNA which encodes around 80 proteins.
- The virus is easily cultivated in human B cells and nasopharyngeal epithelial cells. The cell surface receptor for the virus is the receptor for C3d complement protein.
- Early after infection, Epstein–Barr nuclear antigens (EBNAs) are detectable in cell nuclei. Viral DNA may become incorporated into host DNA in transformed cells, but most remain in a circular, non-integrated form.
- The virus remains latent in most infected cells.

Epidemiology

- Worldwide. Infection acquired earlier in tropical countries than industrialized countries. By adulthood, 90–95% of most populations are antibody-positive.
- In the UK, 50% seroconvert before the age of 5 years, with a second wave in teenage years—the group in whom clinical manifestations are commonest. Infection does not occur in epidemics, and the virus is of relatively low transmissibility. Spread is by intimate contact.

- Incidence is the same for men and women (but female peak age-specific incidence occurs 2 years earlier) but is 30 times higher in the white population than the black population, reflecting the higher rate of early primary infection in the black population.

Pathogenesis

- The virus infects epithelial cells and susceptible B lymphocytes. Incubation is 30–50 days, less in young children. It can persist in the oropharynx of those who have recovered from infectious mononucleosis <18 months.
- EBV-related infectious mononucleosis prompts the synthesis of antibodies against viral antigen and unrelated antigens such as those found on sheep, horse, and beef red cells (heterophile antibodies), and less frequently platelets, neutrophils, and ampicillin.
- In early illness, there is a mononuclear lymphocytosis—most cells bear T-cell markers. The immune response includes both T cells and NK cells. Atypical lymphocytosis resolves by recovery—the virus is, however, not eliminated from the host.

Clinical features

- Infection usually asymptomatic in young children (perhaps mild changes in LFTs). When there are symptoms, they are more likely to experience rash, neutropenia, or pneumonia than adults; 50% of cases in adolescence are asymptomatic. Typical case: triad of fever, sore throat, and lymphadenopathy (symmetric involvement of cervical, axillary, and sometimes inguinal nodes) which may be abrupt or follow a 1- to 2-week prodrome of anorexia and malaise; 5% develop a rash (macular, urticarial, petechial, or erythema multiforme-like); 90–100% develop a pruritic maculopapular rash if given ampicillin (may appear after stopping the drug).
- Examination—pharyngitis (exudative in 33%, with palatal petechiae in 25–60%), hepatomegaly, splenomegaly (50% cases—maximal at day 8, resolving over 10 days), periorbital oedema, and lymphadenopathy. Tonsillar enlargement can be so great as to threaten the airway. Abdominal pain, particularly in the left upper quadrant, may be related to hepatomegaly or splenic enlargement, which may be rapid. There is a danger of splenic rupture with minor trauma or even spontaneously.
- Fever resolves over 10–14 days. Recovery from fatigue can take longer, with good days interspersed with periods of symptom recrudescence.
- Complications—death is unusual but may follow neurological complications, airway obstruction, or splenic rupture.
    - Haematological—thrombocytopenia (50%), autoimmune haemolytic anaemia (0.5–3% cases with 70% having cold agglutinins; haemolysis apparent days 7–14 and recovers over 6 weeks; corticosteroids may help), splenic rupture (0.2%, usually in the second or third week of illness and may be abrupt or insidious following rapid increase to 2–3 times the normal size; usually associated with left upper quadrant and shoulder pain; 50% of cases have associated trauma, therefore recommend patients to avoid contact sports), lymphoproliferative disorders (haemophagocytic lymphohistiocytosis, PTLD).

- Neurological—encephalitis, cerebellitis, meningitis (may find atypical lymphocytes in CSF), Guillain–Barré, optic neuritis, Bell's palsy; 85% of cases with neurological features recover completely.
- Other—hepatitis (90%, jaundice in only 5%), renal (interstitial nephritis), cardiac (pericarditis, myocarditis), lung (rarely pneumonia).

EBV associations with other diseases

- Neoplastic disorders—Burkitt's lymphoma (tumour from >95% of African cases contains EBV genome; malaria appears to be a cofactor), nasopharyngeal carcinoma, HIV-associated non-Hodgkin's lymphoma, Hodgkin's lymphoma, and both polyclonal B- and T-cell lymphomas.
- Infection in immunocompromised children—several congenital immunodeficiencies are associated with the development of EBV-associated lymphoproliferative disorders. X-linked immunoproliferative syndrome has a particular association with acute fatal infectious mononucleosis with hepatic necrosis and pancytopenia.
- EBV and HIV—EBV is associated with polyclonal B-cell lymphomas seen in AIDS patients and is the cause of oral hairy leukoplakia. In children, it is associated with smooth muscle tumours.

Diagnosis

General findings

- Haematological—peripheral lymphocytosis representing activated T cells responding to virus-induced B-cell proliferation (peaks days 7–21, with lymphocytes/monocytes accounting for 70% of the total WCC of 20–50 000 leucocytes/mm^3), atypical lymphocytes (about 3% of cells—large, vacuolated, basophilic, eccentric lobulated nucleus—also seen in CMV, rubella, mumps, drug reactions, amongst others), neutropenia (60–70% of cases), thrombocytopenia (50% but bleeding is rare).
- Biochemical—LFT abnormalities (90% of cases), mild elevation of bilirubin (45%), low-level cryoglobulins (IgG and IgM) in 90% of cases.

Specific tests

- Heterophile antibodies—EBV-infected B cells produce polyclonal IgM antibodies. Some of these (heterophile antibodies) agglutinate the RBCs of other species. Such antibodies may be present in the sera of some healthy patients and those with lymphoma. Pre-incubation with guinea pig cells removes these. Antibody titre is reported as the highest serum dilution at which sheep or horse (more sensitive) red cells are agglutinated; 40% of patients are positive by week 1, and 80% by week 3, of illness. Delayed appearance may be associated with prolonged convalescence. A test remains positive for up to 1 year. The Paul–Bunnell test measures agglutination of sheep RBCs by patient sera; the Monospot test measures the agglutination of formalinized horse RBCs after pre-absorption of sera with guinea pig cells. Commercial Monospot tests have a slightly greater sensitivity than the classic tube test.
- EBV-specific antibodies—positive antiviral capsid antigen (VCA) IgM and negative EBNA (expressed only as the virus establishes latency)

is a sensitive and specific indicator of acute infection. Positive VCA-IgG, positive EBNA, and negative VCA-IgM (remains positive for 4–12 weeks) suggest infection between 3 and 12 months ago. VCA-IgG and EBNA remain positive for life.
- PCR for EBV—role in the management of transplant recipients with EBV-related lymphoproliferative disorders. Not recommended in immunocompetent patients.

Treatment

- The majority of cases are self-limiting and do not require specific therapy. The virus is poorly transmitted, and isolation is unnecessary. The level of activity a patient undertakes depends on symptom severity. Some may require bed rest. Patients should not participate in contact sports or heavy lifting for between 3 weeks and 2 months.
- Admit to hospital those patients with evidence of splenic rupture, airway compromise, dehydration, significant thrombocytopenia, or haemolytic anaemia, and other major complications.
- Corticosteroids may be indicated in cases of severe thrombocytopenia, haemolytic anaemia, impending airway obstruction, and CNS or cardiac involvement. Response is usually rapid, and doses can be tailed off over 1–2 weeks.
- Antiviral drugs—no evidence of benefit in acute EBV infection. Unsurprising as ongoing viral replication is less important than host immune responses in the symptomatic phase. It has been shown to reduce oral hairy leukoplakia in HIV-positive patients and to induce temporary remission of a polyclonal B-cell lymphoma in renal transplant recipients.
- Surgical interventions are necessary for splenic rupture, and a tracheotomy may be indicated in some cases of airway obstruction.
- General malaise can persist for up to 3 months or more. The reasons behind prolonged recovery are not clear. Haematological and hepatic complications settle over 2–3 months. Adults with neurological complications may be left with residual deficits.

Cytomegalovirus

A herpesvirus—the largest virus to infect humans—found across the world and the cause of a wide spectrum of clinical syndromes from congenital disease to pneumonia.

The virus

- A dsDNA virus encoding around 230 proteins, many of which are directly involved in downregulating the host immune response (e.g. preventing class I human leucocyte antigen (HLA) molecule transport to the surface).
- The genome is surrounded by a nucleoprotein core, which, in turn, is covered by matrix proteins and a lipid envelope.
- Infects by endocytosis. CMV replication takes place in the nucleus of the cell, resulting in large nuclear inclusions useful in diagnosing infection.

- After acute infection, CMV persists in a non-replicating form, reactivating with immunosuppression or illness. A third of secondary infections may represent reinfection with a new exogenous CMV strain.

Clinical features

- *Mononucleosis*—primary infection in a young adult produces an infectious mononucleosis picture (fever, sore throat, lymphadenopathy). The heterophile agglutinin test is negative. Lymphadenopathy and sore throat are milder than with EBV. CMV disease tends to have more systemic features. The virus is acquired by intimate contact and typically by transfusion. Complications: interstitial pneumonia (seen in BMT patients in whom there is a high mortality, despite antiviral therapy; rare occurrence in healthy people in whom therapy is not required), hepatitis (common and mild in the immunocompetent), GBS (CMV is the precipitant of around 10% of GBS cases), meningoencephalitis, myocarditis, thrombocytopenia, and haemolytic anaemia (common in children with congenital CMV), rash (usually mild—can be associated with ampicillin).
- *Patients with AIDS*—co-infection with CMV is seen in over 90% of homosexual men with HIV-1, and there is an increased risk of serious CMV disease once CD4 cells fall below 100/mm^3. Early ART has seen the incidence of end-organ CMV disease fall by over 80%. Retinitis is the commonest manifestation (➔ see Uveitis, pp. 753–4), once seen in one-third of HIV-infected patients. Polyradiculopathy is the commonest CNS manifestation of CMV, characterized by ascending weakness in the legs, and loss of bowel and bladder control. GI manifestations include oesophageal erosions, colitis (fever and diarrhoea which can be complicated by perforation or partial obstruction due to lesions resembling KS), pancreatitis, and cholecystitis. Characteristic inclusion bodies may be seen on biopsy.
- *Immunosuppressive therapy*—agents, such as cyclophosphamide and azathioprine, are sufficient in themselves to reactivate CMV—corticosteroids, insufficient alone, act synergistically with these agents. Ciclosporin increases CMV disease only in combination with steroids.
- *Transplant recipients*—immunosuppressive regimes render such people prone to severe CMV. It is the commonest pathogen isolated after solid organ transplantation. Some cases represent reactivation of latent infection; many are acquired from the transplanted organ or transfused blood. The severity of the end-organ disease caused by CMV reflects the degree of immunosuppression. The most important source of infection is the transplanted organ or transfused blood:
  - bone marrow—before the use of prophylactic regimes, CMV-seropositive allogeneic BMT recipients had ~80% chance of reactivation, of which a third developed end-organ disease, e.g. FUO, interstitial pneumonitis (fever, dry cough, and dyspnoea, usually within the first 4 months—poor outcomes), enteritis, retinitis, hepatitis, marrow suppression;

- liver—CMV infection, particularly CMV hepatitis, is a leading cause of morbidity in the first 3 months following transplantation. It may lead to liver failure and repeat transplantation. Biopsy is required to distinguish it from graft rejection, a complication with the opposite management strategy. Prolonged IV ganciclovir at the time of transplantation may reduce the incidence in seronegative recipients;
- kidney—the rate of CMV infection of seronegative recipients following transplantation of a kidney from a seropositive donor is over 80%; such primary infections tend to be more symptomatic than reactivation secondary to immunosuppression. Primary infections may present with 'CMV syndrome': fever, leucopenia, atypical lymphocytes, lymphocytosis, hepatosplenomegaly, myalgia, arthralgia. CMV pneumonia is less severe than with BMT—ganciclovir therapy can be lifesaving. Significant CMV hepatitis is rare.

- *Congenital infection*—intrauterine CMV infection is less common than perinatal infection and tends to be seen in infants born to primiparous mothers experiencing primary CMV infection during pregnancy (around 30% of primary maternal infections are estimated to transmit to the fetus; rates are highest in late pregnancy when cervical CMV levels are higher). It may be a cause of intrauterine death. Around 5–20% of newborns are symptomatic at birth (small for age, hepatosplenomegaly, petechial rash, multiple organ involvement, ocular abnormalities, hearing loss, microcephaly, and cerebral calcification); another 15% develop delayed progressive hearing loss. Diagnosis is best made by the confirmation of infant viruria within the first week of life. Congenital infection has been reported in infants born to CMV-immune mothers. Perinatal infection follows acquisition from virus carried in the cervix or breast milk. Symptoms include sepsis, pneumonitis, mild CMV mononucleosis, and hearing loss.

Diagnosis

- It is important to distinguish CMV infection from CMV disease. CMV may be detectable by PCR but does not necessarily prove CMV disease. Histological changes may confirm this (e.g. enteritis), and, in some settings (e.g. BMT), viral PCR titres give an idea of the probability of CMV disease.
- Serology—rarely useful acutely. The presence of IgM (remains raised for months) or an increase in IgG titre indicates recent infection.
- Culture—slow (<4 weeks) and rarely performed. Isolation of virus does not necessarily indicate active disease.
- Antigenaemia—tagged monoclonal antibodies are used to detect CMV proteins. Largely superseded by nucleic acid detection tests.
- Nucleic acid detection—PCR, DNA probes, and nucleic acid sequence-based amplification assays are available. Their use is best established in immunocompromised hosts. The same test should be used if monitoring changes within a patient—results are not comparable between assays.
- Biopsy of infected tissue may reveal the distinctive appearance of CMV-infected cells (e.g. inclusion bodies).

Treatment and prevention

- Infection in immunocompetent individuals does not require treatment.
- Ganciclovir, foscarnet, and cidofovir (➔ see Antivirals for cytomegalovirus, pp. 92–4) inhibit the CMV DNA polymerase and are effective at treating CMV end-organ disease in the immunocompromised. AIDS-related retinitis responds to PO valganciclovir. Those with sight-threatening lesions should be considered for intravitreal or IV ganciclovir. Intravitreal treatment should be accompanied by PO valganciclovir. Induction therapy should last at least 3 weeks. Those not on HAART should be initiated, and maintenance valganciclovir continued until CD4 >100 and expert review confirms that retinitis is quiescent. Relapse may occasionally occur in those with CD4 counts above 100.
- Serious CMV disease may be prevented after BMT and solid-organ transplantation with antiviral therapy. Both pre-emptive (initiation of therapy to those with evidence of viral replication in the absence of symptoms) and prophylactic (therapy to all those with positive CMV serology) strategies have shown benefit. Because of the risk of drug toxicity, many centres reserve prophylactic therapy for those most at risk (e.g. CMV-positive donors and CMV-negative recipients).

Drug resistance

For antiviral activity, ganciclovir requires phosphorylation by both viral and cellular enzymes. Resistance may be conferred by mutations in either the viral enzyme responsible for phosphorylating the pro-drug or the CMV DNA polymerase, or both. Mutations in both these regions may render a virus resistant to both ganciclovir and cidofovir. Cross-resistance between ganciclovir and foscarnet has not been observed. Foscarnet resistance has been reported.

Viral gastroenteritis

Viruses account for over half of diarrhoeal episodes in infants and young children, particularly in poorer, overcrowded parts of the world where viral diarrhoea and dehydration account for millions of deaths each year. Acute viral gastroenteritis is seen in three settings:

- sporadic gastroenteritis of infants (usually rotavirus, sometimes adenovirus; ➔ see Adenovirus, pp. 436–8);
- epidemic gastroenteritis occurring in semi-closed communities (families, institutions, ships) or as a result of classic water/food-borne infection (mostly caliciviruses; ➔ see Norovirus, pp. 410–1);
- sporadic acute gastroenteritis of adults (caliciviruses, rotaviruses, astroviruses; ➔ see Astroviruses, p. 411, adenoviruses).

All are transmitted faeco-orally, but droplet spread and food contamination can also occur. Asymptomatic infection is common. Diagnostic tests are used primarily for the purpose of identifying the cause of an outbreak, rather than an individual case—patients have usually recovered.

Rotavirus

Outnumbers other viral causes of diarrhoea by 4:1, causing around 50% of those cases requiring hospitalization in the developed world. The cause of an estimated 500 000 deaths worldwide.

The virus

- From the family *Reoviridae*, genus *Rotavirus*. Three antigenically distinguishable groups (A to C) cause human disease. Virtually all outbreaks worldwide are caused by group A organisms.
- On EM, they have a wheel-like appearance (Latin '*rota*'). They have no envelope—just an outer capsid and core.

Epidemiology

- Found worldwide. Infectious dose very small—100 organisms or even less. Transmission is faeco-oral (contaminated food or water, direct contact, or inhalation of aerosol from vomit or faeces), and virus is shed for up to a week after symptom onset. Many strains are avirulent.
- Almost all children are infected within the first 3 years of life. There appears to be no difference in exposure risk in low-income countries (unlike bacterial causes of diarrhoea). Antibody to virus is acquired by 80–100% of the population by age 3 years.
- Highest incidence is between 6 months (maternal antibody wanes) and 24 months old. Severe disease may still occur in younger and older children; however, those under 2 months are more resistant to disease.
- Infection is seasonal in temperate countries (peaking in winter), with attack rates around 20–30% for a child's first two seasons. Susceptibility continues throughout life—50% of parents experience infection if they have an infected infant.

Pathogenesis

- Viral capsid protein vp4 binds glycolipids on the surface of villous epithelial cells lining the small intestine, leading to virus entry.
- Diarrhoea is induced through several mechanisms—certain strains have non-structural proteins that act as enterotoxins, causing diarrhoea directly; loss of villus tip cells decreases absorptive capacity, and a decrease in intestinal disaccharidases can cause osmotic diarrhoea. Rotavirus-induced lactase deficiency lasts up to 2 weeks.

Clinical features

- Incubation 1–2 days. Infants/young children experience fever, vomiting (duration 2–3 days), and watery (bloodless) diarrhoea (duration 4–5 days).
- More severe cases may have prolonged symptoms and develop an isotonic dehydration, requiring hospital treatment. No clear evidence that rotavirus causes any other syndrome. Children with immunodeficiency can develop a gastroenteritis lasting many weeks.
- Asymptomatic viral shedding occurs.

Diagnosis

- EM is rarely used. Rapid diagnostic tests with high levels of specificity (albeit less sensitive) include ELISA and latex agglutination kits.
- Other techniques—electrophoresis (no false positives and allows the identification of strain-identical infections), PCR (allows serotyping).

Treatment

- For more information on the management of diarrhoea, ➲ see Infectious diarrhoea, pp. 647–9.
- Fluid replacement is fundamental. Should be administered orally in mild and moderate cases. Feeding early in illness (within 24h) promotes enterocyte regeneration and reduces gut permeability. Fruit juices and soft drinks should be avoided. Milk can be given to infants, lactose-free, carbohydrate-rich foods to older children.
- There is no role for antibiotics, antimotility drugs, etc.

Prevention

- Prevention by hygiene alone is difficult. Asymptomatic shedding is common. They are relatively resistant to common handwashing agents and can survive for some time on hard surfaces and in water.
- For management of hospital outbreaks, ➲ see Hospital epidemics of diarrhoea and vomiting, pp. 196–7.
- There are currently two oral vaccines available, and their use has been associated with a 60% fall in death rates due to diarrhoea. The WHO recommends their addition to the immunization schedules of those regions in which their efficiency has been demonstrated. They have been in use in the USA since 2006, and were added to the UK schedule for 2013 (two doses at 2 and 3 months of age).

Norovirus

- A genus of diverse ssRNA viruses from the family *Calciviridae* ('calci' deriving from the cup-like indentations in the surface of the virus—Latin '*calyx*'). All are considered to be strains of a single species, Norwalk virus—first isolated in 1972.
- Associated with point-source outbreaks amongst adults (particularly in closed settings such as ships, hospitals, and the military) and common causes of diarrhoea in children worldwide. In the UK, outbreaks are common in winter ('winter vomiting').
- Incubation is 24–48h; symptoms last 2–3 days. Vomiting is a dominant feature in most affected people. Very infectious, with high secondary attack rates. Pathological changes are similar to those seen in rotavirus infection.
- Vehicles for infection include water, food that has come into contact with contaminated water, and even contact with lakes or pools with which an infected individual has been in contact. They are relatively resistant to inactivation by chlorine and can survive days on contaminated fabrics. Outbreaks last 1–2 weeks, but recurrent episodes on ships are common, despite efforts to disinfect the ship between

cruises. Disease is self-limiting—IV fluid replacement may be indicated in rare instances of severe dehydration.
- Antibody may be detected in up to 90% of older children and adults. Resistance to a specific virus lasts a maximum of 2–3 years, and there is little, if any, cross-protection against infection by other strains.

Astroviruses

- RNA viruses, members of the family *Astroviridae*, and important causes of gastroenteritis in children and adults. The name is derived from its 5- or 6-pointed star appearance when examined by EM.
- Cause diarrhoea in schools, day-care institutions, and hospitals; usually in children under 3 years of age. Asymptomatic infection is common, and they appear to be less pathogenic in adults than norovirus.
- Incubation is 3–4 days, with symptoms lasting up to 5 days. Diarrhoea, malaise, and nausea are dominant—vomiting less so. Disease is self-limited, and treatment directed at maintaining hydration.

Hepatitis A virus

Hepatitis A virus (HAV) is an enterically transmitted picornavirus. Outbreaks of infectious hepatitis have been recognized for centuries, but it was first demonstrated in the stool of infected volunteers in 1973.

The virus

HAV is a 27–28nm spherical, non-enveloped virus. Purification of the virus yields three distinct types of particle: mature virions, empty capsids or particles with an incomplete genome, and less stable particles with a more open structure. The HAV genome is a single-stranded, positive-sense, linear RNA of 7474 nucleotides. As with other picornaviruses, the coding region is divided into three parts: P1 (encoding the four capsid proteins VP1–4), P2, and P3 (encoding seven non-structural proteins). Four genotypes have been identified; all belong to the same serotype. Viral infection of hepatocytes is not cytopathic, but the cytotoxic T-cell response results in cell death.

Epidemiology

HAV has a worldwide distribution. It is associated with overcrowding and poor sanitation, and is endemic in the developing world where it is an infection of childhood. In the UK, improved hygiene has seen the incidence fall in children, resulting in greater susceptibility in adults. The decade from 1999 to 2009 saw laboratory-confirmed cases fall from 1342 to 352 in England and Wales. Recent outbreaks in the UK have occurred among MSM, IDUs, and homeless people using hostels. Other risk groups include: children and staff in childcare facilities, patients and staff in mental health institutions, and travellers to endemic areas (Indian subcontinent, Far East, Eastern Europe). Transmission is faeco–oral. Community outbreaks have occurred as a result of water or food contamination.

Clinical features

Incubation is 15–50 days (average 30 days).

- *Subclinical infection*—common in children (>90% if <5 years of age).
- *Acute hepatitis*—this occurs more frequently with increasing age. An abrupt prodrome of fever, headache, malaise, anorexia, vomiting, and right upper quadrant pain is followed <7 days after by dark urine, pruritus, and pale stools. Occasionally, diarrhoea, cough, coryzal symptoms, or arthralgia may occur (commoner in children). Physical findings: jaundice, hepatomegaly, splenomegaly (5–15%). People feel better once jaundice appears, which peaks within 14 days.
- *Complications*—include prolonged cholestasis, relapsing disease, fulminant hepatitis (rare, commoner in older patients), extrahepatic disease, and triggering of autoimmune chronic active hepatitis.

Diagnosis

- LFTs are elevated, with very high aspartate transaminase (AST) and ALT levels. Bilirubin and ALP are usually only mildly elevated.
- Serology—detection of anti-HAV IgM confirms the diagnosis and remains positive for 3–6 months. It is present at the onset of symptoms. Anti-HAV IgG becomes positive at 2–3 months and persists for life.

Treatment

- Acute hepatitis—symptomatic (avoid paracetamol and alcohol); 85% have full clinical/biochemical recovery by 3 months, and nearly all by 6 months.
- Fulminant hepatitis—patients should be treated with supportive therapy and referred for consideration of liver transplantation. Fatalities are commoner with advancing age and in those with hepatitis C co-infection.

Prevention

- Pre-exposure prophylaxis—best done by vaccination. Several inactivated HAV vaccines exist, and these have largely superseded the use of immunoglobulin. Two doses of HAV vaccine are given, at 0 and 6–12 months, and provide protection for at least 10 years. Indications for immunization include: travellers to endemic areas, homosexuals, IDUs, those with chronic liver disease, haemophiliacs, regular recipients of blood products, high-risk employment (e.g. laboratory workers, residential centre staff, sewage workers), and military personnel.
- PEP—prior to vaccination, human normal immunoglobulin (HNIG) was used for prevention, particularly for travellers to endemic regions. It is now used for PEP if protection is required in a shorter time than that provided by vaccination. Current guidance recommends vaccination of unvaccinated close contacts of cases of hepatitis A with onset of jaundice within 1 week. If the interval is longer, HNIG is used (followed by vaccination if exposure risk is ongoing). Full details are available in the *Green Book* (web search 'UK immunisation Green Book').

Hepatitis B virus

HBV is a DNA virus that causes acute and chronic viral hepatitis in humans. It has a diameter of 42nm, with an outer envelope that contains HBsAg proteins, glycoproteins, and cellular lipid. HBsAg proteins may also be released from HBV-infected cells as small spherical particles or filamentous forms. Beneath the envelope is the internal core or nucleocapsid, which contains hepatitis B core antigen (HBcAg). The third antigen HBeAg is a truncated form of the major core polypeptide. It is released from infected liver cells in which HBV is replicating. HBV has one of the smallest viral genomes, consisting of a 3200bp circular DNA molecule. There are eight genotypes (A–H). The genome has four long open reading frames (ORFs):

- C (core or nucleocapsid) gene, encodes HBcAg and HBeAg. Mutations in the pre-core region result in HBV mutants that lack HBeAg;
- S (surface or envelope) gene, which includes the pre-S1, pre-S2, and s regions; encodes HBsAg;
- P (pol or polymerase) gene, encompasses 3/4 of the viral genome and overlaps part of the C gene, the S gene, and part of the X gene. It encodes a polypeptide with DNA polymerase and ribonuclease H activity;
- X gene, encodes a polypeptide, with several functions.

Epidemiology

HBV infection is a global public health problem, with an estimated 400 million people chronically infected and ~1 million deaths per year. Prevalence ranges from 0.1–2% in low-prevalence countries (e.g. the USA, Western Europe) to 10–20% in parts of China and sub-Saharan Africa. This variation largely reflects differences in the age at which infection occurs, as the risk of chronicity is greatest in the very young (90% for perinatal infections), compared to adults (5% become chronic). HBV may be transmitted vertically/perinatally (especially in high-prevalence areas), sexually, by contaminated transfusion, by IV drug use, by needlestick injury, and horizontally (especially between children in intermediate-prevalence areas). Perinatal transmission rates reach 90% in HBeAg-positive mothers—the majority occur at or after birth (neonatal vaccination is 95% protective).

Clinical features

- Acute hepatitis—incubation 1–4 months. Seventy per cent of patients are asymptomatic; 30% develop acute hepatitis. Symptoms include malaise, nausea, abdominal pain, and jaundice. These settle over 1–3 months, but fatigue may persist. Fulminant hepatic failure occurs in 0.1–0.5% of acute infections and is thought to be immunologically mediated, rather than directly due to the virus. Severe cases of acute disease should be considered for antiviral therapy.
- Chronic hepatitis—follows 5–10% of adult acute infections. May be asymptomatic for many years. Exacerbations of infection may occur, mimicking acute hepatitis or presenting as liver failure. Extrahepatic manifestations (probably immune complex-mediated): serum sickness, polyarteritis nodosa, and membranous (less commonly

membranoproliferative) glomerulonephritis, with most cases seen in children (presents as nephrotic syndrome). Three phases:

- replicative immune-tolerant phase (perinatal infections only)—high levels of virus (HBeAg-positive) but no hepatitis, normal ALT, and a largely normal liver;
- replicative immune clearance—HBeAg seroconversion may occur, often associated with biochemical exacerbations (due to an increase in immune lysis of infected hepatocytes) which may be misinterpreted as acute hepatitis B. Severe exacerbations may warrant antiviral therapy. Some patients fail to achieve sustained seroconversion ('abortive immune clearance');
- inactive carrier state in which liver disease is in remission and patients are HBeAg-negative, anti-HBe-positive, ALT usually normal, although some cases may still have histologically active liver disease. Several normal ALTs and HBV viral loads over 12 months are required to confirm someone is inactive due to the fluctuating nature of disease. Some patients have moderate HBV replication and active liver disease but remain HBeAg-negative—they have variants that cannot produce HBeAg due to pre-core or core promoter mutations. Such patients tend to be older with more advanced liver disease and fluctuations in HBV DNA and ALT.

- A few patients with chronic HBV infection may show delayed clearance of HBsAg (around 0.5–2% patients per year). Some remain HBV DNA-positive.
- Complications of chronic HBV—end-stage liver disease (15–40% of cases), hepatocellular carcinoma (HCC). Disease progression is associated with HBeAg positivity, high DNA levels, those with prolonged replicative phase, alcohol, and co-infection with HCV or hepatitis D virus (HDV).

Diagnosis

Diagnosis is made serologically (see Table 8.3).

- HBsAg—appears 1–10 weeks after acute infection, prior to symptoms. Those who clear infection become negative after 4–6 months. Positivity beyond this time indicates chronic HBV. Its disappearance is followed by the development of anti-HBs antibody. A few patients may be positive for HBsAg and anti-HBs, suggesting that the antibody cannot neutralize the virus and patients are therefore carriers.
- HBcAg—an intracellular antigen and not detectable in serum. Anti-HBc is predominantly IgM in early infection and may be the only indicator of infection in the window between HBsAg loss and anti-HBs production. It may remain for a couple of years, and titres can rise during flares, which may lead to the mistaken diagnosis of acute infection. Isolated anti-HBc may be seen in two other situations: many years after recovery from acute HBV (anti-HBs fallen to undetectable levels), many years after chronic HBV (HBsAg fallen to undetectable levels). HBV DNA may be detected in the liver of these patients.

Table 8.3 Diagnosis of hepatitis B virus

	HBsAg	Anti-HBs	HBeAg	Anti-HBe	Anti-HBc IgM	Anti-HBc IgG	HBV DNA
Acute infection	✓		✓				+++
Window					✓		+
Prior infection		✓				✓	
Vaccinated		✓					
Chronic (high infectivity)	✓		✓			✓	+++
Chronic (low infectivity)	✓			✓		✓	±
Pre-core mutant	✓			✓		✓	++

- HBeAg—a secretory protein and marker of HBV replication and infectivity. Associated with high levels of HBV DNA. HBeAg seroconversion to anti-HBe may be delayed for years in patients with chronic HBV. When it occurs, it is usually associated with a decrease in DNA and reduction in liver inflammation. Pre-core mutants (➲ see Hepatitis B virus, pp. 413–7), however, may have active liver disease in the absence of HBeAg.
- HBV DNA assays—real-time PCR techniques allow quantification of HBV DNA. This is useful in determining whether a patient will benefit from therapy, as high levels are associated with cirrhosis and its complications. DNA may remain detectable in the serum after recovery from acute infection, suggesting 'clearance' is more about 'control' by the immune system. This contrasts with patients who become HBeAg-negative during nucleoside/nucleotide therapy who generally have undetectable DNA by PCR. Rare cases of occult HBV (detectable DNA, but negative HBsAg, and even absent anti-HBc) have been described—this may be due to mutations leading to altered expression or structure of HBsAg.
- Other investigations: LFTs, gamma-glutamyl transferase (GGT), clotting, screening for other blood-borne viruses and haemochromatosis, liver biopsy (disease severity).
- Liver biopsy is especially important in those who do not meet treatment criteria but have high HBV DNA, as they may benefit from treatment if the disease is histologically active. A normal ALT does not predict mild findings in someone with active viral replication.

Treatment

- General—avoid alcohol; safe sexual practices; hepatitis A vaccination (low-prevalence areas); avoid occupations that may spread HBV (e.g. surgery, dentistry); HBV immunization of household contacts; surveillance for HCC and oesophageal varices.
- Antiviral therapy—a summary follows. For full guidance, see *European Association for the Study of the Liver clinical practice guidelines: management of chronic hepatitis B 2012, revised version.*[1]
  - HBeAg-positive—treat compensated cirrhosis and HBV DNA >2000IU/mL or decompensated cirrhosis with detectable HBV DNA. Otherwise treat if HBV DNA >20 000IU/mL and ALT >2× upper limit of normal (ULN) in those without cirrhosis. Delay for 3–6 months in newly diagnosed patients, as they may spontaneously seroconvert. Observe those with chronic hepatitis with ALT <2× ULN, unless they experience recurrent hepatitis flares or have advanced histological findings. Those with normal ALT are relatively unlikely to seroconvert. Those with higher ALTs are the most likely to respond to therapy. Treatment endpoint is HBeAg seroconversion. Once this occurs and HBV DNA is undetectable, treatment continues for at least 12 months. Fifty per cent seroconvert by 5 years.
  - HBeAg-negative—treat if chronic hepatitis diagnosed (ALT >2× ULN and HBV DNA >2000IU/mL), as remission is rare. Treatment is prolonged. IFN, entecavir, or tenofovir are preferred, as they achieve rapid viral suppression with low rates of resistance acquisition. Endpoint not clearly established, and treatment may need to continue for many years. Virological relapse is common on cessation, but HBV DNA levels are often low with normal ALT.
  - Consider treatment in those with acute liver failure, those with complications of cirrhosis, to prevent reactivation of chronic HBV during chemotherapy or immunosuppression, and in those with very severe or protracted acute HBV (progression to chronic disease occurs in <5%, so general treatment is not recommended).
  - Lifelong treatment is recommended for those with compensated cirrhosis (to prevent liver failure and HCC) and decompensated cirrhosis;
- Choosing the regime (for more details of drugs, ➲ see Antivirals for hepatitis B, pp. 97–9).
  - Resistance and poor potency limit lamivudine and adefovir, respectively. Largely superseded by newer agents.
  - Telbivudine is a potent inhibitor of HBV replication, but a low barrier to resistance emergence renders it non-ideal as first-line therapy in those with high viraemia or for long-term therapy.
  - IFN cannot be used in decompensated cirrhosis. Favoured in younger patients. Courses are finite (5–24 months). Patients with HBV genotype A are more likely to seroconvert.
  - Tenofovir is potent and active against lamivudine-resistant virus. Resistance is rare with up to 5 years treatment.

- Entecavir is potent with low rates of resistance. Favoured in primary treatment, rather than in those with lamivudine resistance. May have a role in those with decompensated cirrhosis, as rapid viral suppression. Agent of choice in those with renal impairment.
- There is a move to combination therapy (as with HCV and HIV). Most trials to date have been with lamivudine plus another agent, and trials with the newer agents are ongoing.

Prevention

Strategies include education, screening of blood products, immunization (e.g. HCWs, MSM, close family contacts of an infected individual, those regularly receiving blood products, haemodialysis recipients), and post-exposure vaccination (sexual contacts, needlestick recipients, neonates born to infected mothers). Hepatitis B immunoglobulin should be given to neonates born to HBsAg-positive mothers (unless anti-HBe positive) and unvaccinated needlestick recipients from HBsAg-positive donors.

Reference

1 European Association for the Study of the Liver (2012). *EASL clinical practice guidelines: management of chronic hepatitis B 2012, revised version*. Available at: www.easl.eu/_clinical-practice-guideline.

Hepatitis D virus

Hepatitis delta virus (HDV) is a defective virus whose replication requires HBV. Hence those with HDV are always co-infected with HBV. Virions of HDV consist of a core of delta antigen and single-stranded circular RNA enclosed in an envelope provided by HBV (with HBsAg). It is currently classified into eight genotypes. Most patients with delta antigen in the liver have anti-delta antibodies in their serum. HDV superinfection usually results in the suppression of HBV replication by mechanisms as yet unknown (HBsAg and HBV DNA levels drop).

Epidemiology

- It is thought that 5% of chronic HBV carriers worldwide may be infected with HDV. However, the prevalence of HDV in HBV carriers varies around the world—it is endemic in Mediterranean countries (around 10% in Italy) and the Far East (90% in the Pacific islands, 5% in Japan), but largely confined to at-risk groups in other Western countries.
- There is a higher incidence of HDV infection in HBsAg-positive patients with acute and chronic hepatitis, compared with asymptomatic carriers.

Clinical features

- Symptoms range from asymptomatic to fulminant liver failure (rare, but still ten times commoner than in other viral hepatitis). Clinical features seem to cluster in geographical areas that may relate to the prevailing genotype in that area, e.g. Western countries see higher rates of fulminant disease that may relate to genotype 1 (predominates in the West).

- Simultaneous co-infection with HBV/HDV—causes acute hepatitis indistinguishable from classical acute hepatitis B (although perhaps with higher rates of liver failure, particularly in IDUs). It is thought around 5% of people develop chronic HDV.
- HDV superinfection of a carrier of HBV—may cause liver flare (may present as severe acute hepatitis if HBV is undiagnosed). Up to 80% of people become chronically infected.
- In the longer term, HDV seems to exacerbate the pre-existing liver disease due to HBV, with potentially rapid progression of cirrhosis (within 2 years).

Diagnosis

- First, diagnose HBV—HDV cannot exist without it. Consider HDV in those with acute HBV if they have HDV risk factors or experience particularly severe hepatitis, and in those with established HBV with severe liver flare.
- HDV antibodies—appear late (4 weeks) and may vanish after resolution of acute infection. Present in high titres in chronic infection.
- HDV RNA—can be detected in serum by hybridization or RT-PCR assays. Used to assay for eradication after treatment of HBV.
- Differentiating between HBV/HDV co-infection and HDV superinfection relies on the detection of high levels of IgM anti-HBc (in those co-infected).

Hepatitis C virus

The virus

HCV is a spherical, enveloped RNA flavivirus. Its genome is a positive ssRNA molecule, encoding a polyprotein that is processed into at least ten proteins: core protein (C), envelope proteins (E1 and E2), NS2a, and six non-structural proteins (NS2, NS3, NS4a, NS4b, NS5a, NS5b). At least seven major genotypes (genotypes 1–7) exist, and these may be further grouped into subtypes (e.g. 1a, 1b, 1c). Different subtypes predominate in different geographical locations. The high replication rate and absence of proofreading by NS5b polymerase result in the rapid accumulation of mutations (multiple quasi-species exist at any one time).

Epidemiology

HCV infects an estimated 170 million people worldwide. In developed countries, HCV prevalence is low (0.5–2%), apart from in IDUs. In certain geographic areas, HCV is commoner, e.g. Egypt, Japan, Italy, and may be related to reuse of needles for injection, acupuncture, or folk remedies. Transmission routes: transfusion, injecting drug use, nosocomial (needle-sticks, dialysis, inadequate sterilization of colonoscopes). Sexual transmission or mother-to-child transmission is rare.

Natural history and pathogenesis

Fifteen per cent of acutely infected people clear the virus in 3–24 months after infection; 85% develop chronic infection. HCV-specific cytotoxic T-lymphocyte responses play an important role in suppressing HCV RNA levels. There is a broad humoral response to HCV epitopes, but these are not sufficient to clear the virus. Infection results in hepatic inflammation, steatosis, and ultimately hepatic fibrosis and HCC (estimated risk 5–25% after 10–20 years). Factors associated with cirrhosis include alcohol, HBV or HIV co-infection, HLA B54, HCV genotype 1b, HCV quasi-species complexity, and high levels of HCV viraemia.

Clinical features

- *Acute hepatitis C*—75% of infections are anicteric. Symptomatic infection is similar to acute HAV and HBV, but with lower transaminases. Presents 7–8 weeks (range 2–26) after exposure. If diagnosed early, treatment is appropriate.
- *Fulminant hepatitis C*—is unusual in Western countries. Commoner in those with HBV co-infection. Occurs in 40–60% of cases in Japan.
- *Chronic hepatitis C*—85% of patients. Associated with fatigue, malaise, and reduced quality of life indices. ALT levels fluctuate independently of symptoms, whereas HCV RNA levels remain fairly constant. Eventually progresses to cirrhosis, decompensated liver disease, and HCC.
- *Extrahepatic manifestations*—essential mixed cryoglobulinaemia, membranoproliferative glomerulonephritis, sporadic porphyria cutanea tarda, Mooren's corneal ulcers, Sjögren's syndrome, lichen planus, pulmonary fibrosis, thyroid hormone abnormalities.

Diagnosis

- Serology—detection of antibody to recombinant HCV peptides. Third-generation EIAs have a sensitivity of ~97% and can detect HCV antibody within 6–8 weeks. The positive predictive value is ~95%, but much lower in low-prevalence populations such as blood donors; thus, confirmatory testing by HCV RNA detection is essential. Immunocompromised patients (including HIV) may have false-negative serology.
- HCV RNA—detectable within days to 2 months after exposure (varies with inoculum size). Serial measurements performed during treatment are best done with the same product. Qualitative tests can detect <50IU/mL HCV RNA (e.g. Roche AMPLICOR® HCV detection) and are used to confirm diagnosis and achievement of a sustained virological response (SVR)—➔ see pp. 420–1. Quantitative tests report a viral titre and are used to assess response to treatment. New real-time PCR assays detect <10–15IU/mL and may be sensitive enough for both purposes.
- Genotype testing—essential before treatment. The line probe assay reports the genotype and subtype. Only the former is used in planning therapy at present.
- Liver disease severity—assess prior to therapy. It is important to identify those with cirrhosis, as prognosis and treatment selection are altered. Fibrosis can be assessed non-invasively (elastography), with liver biopsy reserved for those cases in which there is uncertainty or

multiple aetiologies. Baseline histology may be useful in decision-making regarding ongoing treatment in those who later experience adverse effects. Sampling variability may lead to underdiagnosis of cirrhosis. Elastography (e.g. FibroScan®) uses ultrasound to assess hepatic tissue stiffness as a proxy of fibrosis. It assesses a larger area than that sampled by biopsy and may be more representative of the whole liver.
- Acute hepatitis C—diagnosis is confirmed by newly positive HCV RNA PCR and conversion to HCV antibody-positive within 12 weeks. In the absence of a documented initial negative test, distinguishing acute from chronic is problematic. Circumstantial evidence, clinical features, timing of aminotransferase changes, and presence of liver fibrosis may help.
- Chronic hepatitis C—positive ELISAs should be confirmed with a HCV RNA test. High-risk patients with negative PCRs should be retested a few months later, in case of false-negative results.

Treatment

The aim is to achieve a 'sustained virological response' (SVR, the absence of HCV RNA by PCR at 6 months after finishing treatment). An SVR is associated with 98–100% chance of being RNA-negative in the longer term and reduces all-cause mortality. Treatment has been revolutionized by direct-acting antivirals such as sofosbuvir. Response is affected by the genotype, race, baseline viral load, and certain host genetics (e.g. IL-28B polymorphisms). Regimen selection depends on the genotype, duration, side effect profile, stage of liver disease/fibrosis, and drug interactions. Cirrhotic patients achieving an SVR should continue to be monitored, as they remain at risk of HCC. Full details are available in the European Association for the Study of the Liver (EASL) guidelines.[2]

- General measures—symptom management, psychological support, screening for complications of cirrhosis, test for HBV, counselling on risk to contacts, lifestyle (alcohol, drug use), etc.
- Who to treat—consider in all patients with compensated or decompensated chronic liver disease, prioritizing those with significant fibrosis or cirrhosis. Priority groups include: decompensated cirrhosis (IFN-free regime), those with HIV co-infection, pre-/post-liver transplant, significant extrahepatic manifestations (e.g. vasculitis), and those at high risk of onward transmission (IDUs, haemodialysis). Patients with no or mild disease can have the timing of therapy individualized.
- Contraindications to treatment—ribavirin/PEG-IFN: those with major uncontrolled depression, untreated thyroid disease, autoimmune hepatitis (and other conditions exacerbated by the drugs), kidney, heart, or lung transplant. Protease inhibitors: an array of drug interactions and side effects that need to be taken into account.
- Decompensated cirrhosis—the primary treatment is liver transplantation. Such patients should only be treated at specialist centres.
- Treatment regimes—see EASL 2015 guidelines for full details.[2]
  - Genotype 1—six treatment options, four of which are IFN-free, e.g. weekly PEG-IFN, daily ribavirin and sofosbuvir for 12 weeks; ledipasvir/sofosbuvir for 12 weeks. Alternatives include triple

therapy with PEG-IFN, ribavirin, and a PI (boceprevir or telaprevir). DAA-containing regimes achieve an SVR of >90%.
- Genotype 2—first line is sofosbuvir and ribavirin for 12 weeks, which achieves SVRs of 97% in treatment-naïve patients without cirrhosis. If unavailable, dual therapy with PEG-IFN and ribavirin 400mg bd for 24 weeks achieves an SVR rate of ~80%.
- Genotype 3—less responsive to sofosbuvir than genotype 2; improved by extending course if treatment-naïve; thus, first line is sofosbuvir with ribavirin for 24 weeks (SVR of 87–95%). Treatment-experienced patients with cirrhosis achieve an SVR of 60% with this regime—PEG-IFN, ribavirin, and sofosbuvir for 12 weeks is favoured. Alternative: sofosbuvir and daclatasvir daily for 12 weeks (24 if cirrhotic).
- Genotype 4—IFN-containing regimes are as for genotype 1 treatment. IFN-free regimes include sofosbuvir with ledipasvir or simepravir or daclatasvir (plus ribavirin if cirrhotic).
- Genotypes 5 (found predominantly in South Africa) and 6 (South East Asia, South China, Hong Kong)—weekly PEG-IFN, daily ribavirin and sofosbuvir for 12 weeks. Sofosbuvir with ledipasvir or daclatasvir are IFN-free alternatives. IFN and ribavirin alone, if sofosbuvir not available.

- Acute hepatitis C—if spontaneous clearance does not occur within 12 weeks of suspected inoculation, or the chance of chronic infection is high (e.g. acquired via transfusion), treatment should be offered. All genotypes are currently treated with PEG-IFN, usually with ribavirin, for 12–24 weeks. SVRs of 80% are reported.

Prevention

No vaccine currently exists. Transmission reduction is by screening of blood, improving adherence to universal infection control precautions, and needle exchange programmes. Average seroconversion after sharps injury from HCV-positive source is 1.8%. Recipients should be screened for sero-conversion and referred for treatment, as indicated.

Reference

2 European Association for the Study of the Liver (2015). *EASL recommendations on treatment of hepatitis C 2015*. Available at: ꩜ www.easl.eu/_clinical-practice-guideline.

Hepatitis E virus

Hepatitis E virus (HEV) is an enterically transmitted member of the family *Hepeviridae*. It is the commonest cause of acute hepatitis in certain parts of Asia and is becoming commoner in the UK. Infection with hepatitis E may be asymptomatic or range in severity from mild to fulminant hepatitis; the latter is commoner in pregnant women and older men.

The virus

- An icosahedral, non-enveloped ssRNA virus (30–32nm in diameter).
- The genome is 7.2kb in length, encoding three ORFs—ORF1 encodes non-structural proteins; ORF2 encodes the capsid; ORF3 encodes an immunogenic protein of unknown function.
- There are four genotypes—1 and 2 appear to be confined to humans; 3 and 4 infect humans and animals (pigs in the case of 3). Genotype 3 may cause milder disease.

Epidemiology

- Epidemiology is similar to that of hepatitis A, if somewhat less readily transmitted with a narrower distribution. The highest incidence is in Africa, Asia, Central America, and the Middle East. It is increasingly recognized in industrialized nations.
- Hosts—HEV has a wide host range and has been shown experimentally to infect New and Old World monkeys, swine, rodents, and sheep. In the UK, the reservoir is thought to be pigs (85% are anti-HEV-positive).
- Transmission—most epidemics of HEV have been waterborne, some food-borne, and infection may follow blood transfusion in endemic areas. Cases in Japan, Germany, and France have been attributed to the consumption of undercooked deer, boar, and pig meat. Zoonotic transmission, e.g. from swine, may occur, as evidenced by high seroprevalence amongst those with occupational exposure to animals. Person-to-person transmission (e.g. within a household) appears uncommon. Perinatal transmission has been reported, and severe neonatal disease can occur.
- Seroprevalence—the presence of anti-HEV antibodies is 15–60% in endemic countries, and higher than expected in non-endemic regions (overall US rate reported at 21%, higher in those consuming organ meat). In the UK, over 70% of cases are indigenously acquired (a case control study implicated processed pork products). In both the UK and USA, most cases are due to genotype 3 which may not manifest clinically. HEV seroprevalence is low in infants and children. Peak incidence in 15–35 year olds (men more commonly infected).

Pathogenesis

The incubation period is 2–8 weeks. The duration of infectivity is at least 1 week before to 2–5 weeks after symptom onset. Viraemia may be prolonged (45–112 days). The replicative pathway is not fully understood, as HEV does not replicate well in cell culture. The histological changes are characteristic: hepatocyte 'ballooning', cytoplasmic cholestasis, focal cytolytic necrosis, and 'pseudoglandular' alteration.

Clinical features

Infection may be asymptomatic or range in severity from mild to fulminant hepatitis. Acute HEV is clinically indistinguishable from other causes of viral hepatitis (although relatively more severe than HAV), with fever, nausea, vomiting, jaundice, and abdominal tenderness. Cholestasis may be prolonged; arthralgia and urticarial rash may occur. Fulminant hepatitis is commoner in the third trimester of pregnancy and older men, and carries a high mortality (up to 20%); this accounts for the overall fatality rate of 0.5–3%. Outcome can be poor in those with chronic liver disease. Chronic HEV infection occurs amongst organ transplant recipients, appearing to be related to impaired HEV-specific T-cell responses.

Diagnosis

- Serology—specific IgM and IgG responses occur early in the infection, usually by the onset of clinical illness. These can be detected using commercial tests based on ELISA or Western blot assays. Anti-HEV IgM can be detected in up to 90% of cases 1–4 weeks after acute infection. This response wanes, so that, by 3 months, anti-HEV IgM is only detectable in 50% of patients. Anti-HEV IgG is detectable 2–4 weeks after onset of illness; a single high titre or rising titres suggest recent infection.
- HEV is detectable by RT-PCR in blood and stool. Viraemia is usually short-lived but may persist up to 4 months—it is a more sensitive means of diagnosis than serology. In stool, it appears around 1 week before illness onset, remaining until 2 weeks after.

Treatment

There is no specific therapy, and treatment is supportive. Patients who develop liver failure should be referred for transplantation. Immunosuppressed patients with chronic infection may respond to reductions in immunosuppressive therapy. Case reports suggest a role for ribavirin.

Prevention

Improved sanitation is likely to be important in the control of an infection that is predominantly spread by the faeco-oral route. Travellers to endemic areas should avoid water of unknown purity, uncooked shellfish, etc. Pork should be cooked properly to prevent possible zoonotic transmission. Several HEV vaccines are under development.

Hepatitis viruses

Acute viral hepatitis is characterized by a necro-inflammatory response in the liver. It can be caused by a number of viruses and may be mimicked by many other infectious diseases and non-infectious causes. It is usually a self-limiting disease, but can progress to fulminant hepatitis (rare, but 1–20% mortality) or chronic liver disease (depending on the cause). A flow chart for the investigation of acute hepatitis is given in Fig. 8.1.

Hepatitis viruses

Over the past 30 years, at least five primarily hepatotropic viruses have been identified:

- hepatitis A virus (➔ see Hepatitis A virus, pp. 411–2);
- hepatitis B virus (➔ see Hepatitis B virus, pp. 413–7);
- hepatitis C virus (➔ see Hepatitis C virus, pp. 418–21);
- hepatitis D virus (➔ see Hepatitis D virus, pp. 417–8);
- hepatitis E virus (➔ see Hepatitis E virus, pp. 421–3).

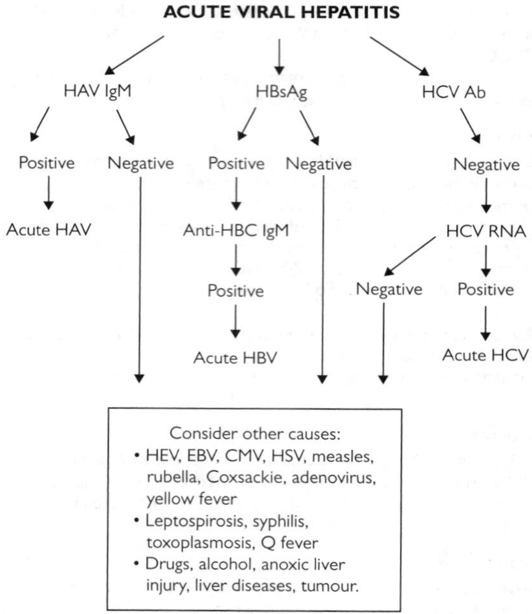

Fig. 8.1 Investigation of acute hepatitis.

Novel hepatitis viruses

Further efforts to identify novel viruses have led to the discovery of other candidate viruses, the significance of which are debated.

Hepatitis G

Two closely related flaviviruses, hepatitis G virus and GB virus type C (GBV-C), have been identified relatively recently. They are spread by the parenteral route and sexual intercourse, and, to a lesser extent, from mother to child. Seroprevalence is high, and the distribution global. It does not appear to be pathogenic in humans.

Other viruses

Many other viruses can induce hepatitis as one feature of a wider clinical syndrome. These include:

- EBV (➔ see Epstein–Barr virus, pp. 402–5);
- CMV (➔ see Cytomegalovirus, pp. 405–8);
- HSV (➔ see Herpes simplex, pp. 396–9);
- measles virus (➔ see Measles, pp. 384–6);

- rubella virus (➔ see Rubella, pp. 389–90);
- Coxsackie B virus (➔ see Enterovirus, pp. 430–2);
- adenovirus (➔ see Adenovirus, pp. 436–8);
- yellow fever virus (➔ see Yellow fever, pp. 455–6).

Differential diagnosis

Other non-viral infectious diseases may cause acute hepatitis:
- leptospirosis (➔ see *Leptospira* species, pp. 340–2);
- syphilis (➔ see Syphilis, pp. 714–6);
- toxoplasmosis (➔ see *Toxoplasma gondii*, pp. 517–20);
- Q fever (➔ see *Coxiella burnetii*—ACDP 3, pp. 346–8).

Finally, non-infectious causes may also mimic viral hepatitis:
- drug-induced hepatitis;
- anoxic liver injury;
- alcoholic hepatitis;
- cholestatic liver disease;
- Wilson's disease;
- Budd–Chiari syndrome;
- liver tumours.

HIV virology and immunology

HIV is an enveloped RNA virus belonging to the retrovirus family.

Types and subtypes

- HIV-1 accounts for the majority of infections worldwide (estimated 32 million). Divided into four groups (M, N, O, P), of which M ('main', the pandemic strain) is the commonest and, in turn, divided into 11 subtypes or clades, designated A–K. The majority of infections in Europe and North America are caused by clade B. Clades A, C, and D dominate in Africa. Group O ('outlier') strains circulate in parts of West Africa, and N ('non-M/O') accounts for a few strains in Cameroon. Group P was identified in Cameroon in 2009 and is closely related to the simian immunodeficiency virus (SIV). In addition, 'circulating recombinant forms' (CRFs) are derived from two or more viruses of different subtypes; CRFs are given a code, e.g. CRF01_AE (a combination of clade A and E viruses). Sequence analysis suggests HIV clades M and N arose from SIV circulating within distinct West African chimpanzee communities.
- HIV-2 occurs primarily in West Africa (1–2 million of infections worldwide). It is less readily transmissible than HIV-1, and is associated with lower viral loads, higher CD4 counts, and slower disease progression. Treatment is more complex, as it is not susceptible to NNRTIs or fusion inhibitors (➔ see Non-nucleoside reverse transcriptase inhibitors, pp. 106–8); the protease has natural polymorphisms, rendering it resistant to certain PIs (➔ see HIV protease inhibitors, pp. 108–9), and the effectiveness of CCR5 antagonists is unclear, as HIV-2 may use other co-receptors more effectively than HIV-1. Probably originally a zoonosis, transmitted from West Africa sooty mangabey monkeys to humans. Dual HIV-1/2 infection can occur.

Virus structure

- The HIV-1 virion is composed of (see Fig. 8.2):
    - viral envelope, constructed from host cell membrane, into which are inserted HIV-1 envelope proteins (e.g. gp41 and gp120) and host proteins (e.g. major histocompatibility complex (MHC) class II molecules);
    - matrix, predominantly protein p17;
    - core, containing viral RNA associated with protein p7, the enzymes reverse transcriptase, protease, and integrase, and the major structural proteins p6 and p24.
- The genomic structure of HIV consists of *gag-pol-env* genes flanked by two complete viral long tandem repeats (LTRs):
    - *gag* gene products—p24, p17, p7, p6, p2, p1;
    - *pol* gene products—protease, reverse transcriptase, and integrase;
    - *env* gene products—gp120, gp 41.
- The virus also encodes several other genes of diverse function, e.g. *vif, vpr, tat, rev, vpu, nef* (HIV-1 only), and *vpx* (HIV-2 only).

Virus life cycle

- Infection is initiated by binding of the envelope protein gp120 to CD4 molecules found on some T cells, macrophages, and dendritic (e.g. on mucosal surfaces) and microglial cells. Binding is also mediated by a second receptor, usually CCR5 or CXCR4.
- Fusion of the viral envelope with the host cell membrane results in release of the viral core into the cytoplasm. Viral complementary DNA (cDNA) is produced by reverse transcription and integrated into the

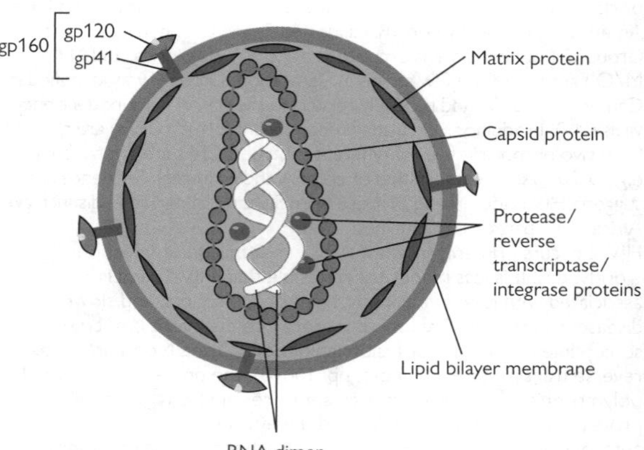

Fig. 8.2 HIV-1 virus structure.

host genome to form proviral DNA. In the presence of appropriate host cell stimulation, the viral 5′ LTR produces viral mRNA transcripts.
- New virions are released from the host cell membrane by budding and infect other CD4-positive cells.

Immunology

HIV infection is associated with a wide array of immune dysfunction.
- Infected cells reach the lymph nodes and plasma. HIV RNA levels rise rapidly, paralleled by a massive CD4 T-cell depletion, particularly in the GI compartment.
- As $CD8^+$ T cells rebound, plasma RNA levels fall, and any 'seroconversion' symptoms settle. HIV RNA levels stabilize at a 'set point' by 6 months after infection. A variable period of time later, HIV RNA levels rise, and CD4 T cells fall once again, with consequent pathology.
- Cells of the monocyte–macrophage lineage serve as a reservoir of infection, are central to the pathogenesis of HIV-associated CNS disease, and contribute to impaired host defences against intracellular pathogens, e.g. MTB.
- As well as suppression, HIV infection causes immune dysregulation with B-cell hyperactivation, hypergammaglobulinaemia, and abnormalities of neutrophil function (predispose to *Candida* infections) and NK cells.

For clinical manifestations of HIV, ➔ see pp. 825–40, and for drug treatment of HIV, ➔ see pp. 101–10.

HIV laboratory tests

HIV may be diagnosed by: serology, detection of viral antigens (p24, gp120, gp41), detection of viral RNA/DNA, or culture.

HIV serology

- Antibodies to gp41 and p24 are the first to appear, following infection. IgG arises at 6–12 weeks in most patients, and 95% by 6 months. IgM assays are not used due to poor sensitivity.
- The standard test consists of a screening EIA, followed by a confirmatory Western blot; sensitivity of 99.5% and specificity of 99.9% in patients with established disease (>3 months after transmission).
- The 'window period' between infection and detectable antibody has shrunk, as testing has improved. Third-generation antibody tests have reduced it to 3–6 weeks. Fourth-generation tests incorporate antigen testing within the assay, shrinking it further.
- False-negative tests may be a result of: 'window period', seroreversion (in advanced disease; establishing the patient on therapy will result in a positive test), 'atypical host response', agammaglobulinaemia, non-M type (P can only be detected by PCR) or HIV-2 infection, and technical error. False-negative rates vary with population prevalence—from <0.001% in low-seroprevalence groups (e.g. blood donors) to 0.3% in high-seroprevalence groups.

- False-positive results occur in 0.0004–0.0007%. Causes include autoantibodies, HIV vaccine trial recipients, and technical error.
- Indeterminate tests—consider HIV RNA testing and repeat serology at 3 months. An at-risk patient is likely to be seroconverting. Low-risk patients are unlikely to have HIV, and, if RNA is undetectable, it is highly unlikely this is because the level is below the detection threshold (which is theoretically possible in at-risk patients).
- Rapid testing is increasingly available. Cheap, can be performed on saliva, results available in minutes; >99% sensitive, but studies suggest specificity can be as low as 96% in some populations; confirmatory testing is important.
- HIV-2—most assays detect HIV-2 but cannot distinguish it from HIV-1. Supplemental testing may be required, depending on the product used. HIV-1 Western blots may be positive (cross-reactivity or HIV-1 co-infection), indeterminate, or negative. In the latter two scenarios, if HIV-1 RNA is negative, do a HIV-2 Western blot or PCR.

Combined antibody–antigen testing

- Fourth-generation assays detecting both antibody and p24 antigen. They further shorten the window period (if only by a few days). Sensitivity and specificity are >99%.

Viral detection

- Diagnosis—not approved for this purpose but useful for when serology is likely to be misleading, e.g. early HIV infection (prior to seroconversion), agammaglobulinaemia, and neonatal HIV infection.
- Management—testing is done at baseline and then every 3–4 months. The target of therapy is undetectable viral load. The time to viral nadir depends on pre-treatment viral load, potency of the regimen, adherence, pharmacology, and resistance. An expected response is a reduction in viral load by 1 $\log_{10}$ copies/mL at 1 week. Failure to achieve a reduction in viral load of 1 $\log_{10}$ copies/mL at 4 weeks suggests non-adherence, inadequate drug exposure, or pre-existing resistance. Failure to achieve a reduction in viral load of 1 $\log_{10}$ copies/mL at 8 weeks constitutes virological failure (USA guidelines).
- Biological variations—viral RNA levels rise during acute illness, vaccination, and HSV infection. Patients should not be tested within a month of such events. Most assays allow a variation of 0.5 $\log_{10}$ between tests—such changes are unlikely to represent clinically significant treatment success/failure.
- *HIV-1 real-time RT-PCR*, e.g. COBAS® AmpliPrep/COBAS® TaqMan® HIV-1 Test—highly sensitive tests with a broad dynamic range (40–10 million copies/mL). Previously two different assays were required for low and high viraemia (standard and ultrasensitive AMPLICOR® RT-PCR detecting 400–750 000 and 50–100 000 copies, respectively). There is inter-test variability—it is important to use the same assay when tracking RNA changes.
- *Nucleic acid sequence-based amplification (NASBA)*, e.g. NucliSens® HIV RNA QT—large, dynamic range. Its nucleic acid extraction method removes certain inhibitory substances, allowing testing of various body fluids (e.g. CSF, semen) and heparinized blood (not compatible with RT-PCR).

- *Branched-chain DNA*, e.g. Versant® HIV-1 RNA, with a range of 75–500 000 copies/mL
- *HIV-1 DNA PCR*—qualitatively detects cell-associated proviral DNA. The primary test for diagnosis of HIV-1 in infants born to infected mothers and in children under 18 months (maternal antibody confuses serological testing). Positive even in those on ART (when plasma viral RNA is suppressed). Sensitive (>99%) but may miss very recent (e.g. perinatal) infection. Some assays less sensitive for non-clade B virus.

CD4 T-lymphocyte count

- The CD4 count is used to assess prognosis for progression to AIDS, formulate the differential diagnosis in a symptomatic patient, and guide therapeutic decisions.
- The standard method involves flow cytometry. This relies on fresh cells and is expensive. An alternative system (TRAx CD4 Test Kit) uses EIA technology and may be more suitable for resource-limited settings.
- The normal mean is 800–1050 cells/mm^3 (range 500–1400 cells/mm^3). There is considerable analytical variability in CD4 test results, e.g. the 95% confidence interval for a true count of 200 cells/mm^3 is 118–337 cells/mm^3. CD4 counts may also be influenced by seasonal and diurnal variations, intercurrent illnesses, and corticosteroids.
- The CD4 count is usually tested every 3–6 months in untreated patients, and every 2–4 months in patients on treatment. The CD4 count typically increases by ≥50 cells/mm^3 at 4–8 weeks after viral suppression with antiretrovirals, and then 50–100 cells/mm^3 per year thereafter. Factors that correlate with a good response include a high baseline viral load and a low baseline CD4 count.

Resistance testing

- The prevalence of ≥1 major resistance mutation in treatment-naïve patients varies from <0.5% in some African countries to 40% in high-risk Western population groups (http://hivdb.stanford.edu/surveillance/map/).
- Drug resistance testing is recommended in all new diagnoses, drug-naïve patients about to start therapy, and treatment-experienced patients experiencing virologic failure, and in pregnancy (to facilitate treatment optimization to reduce transmission risk).
- Limitations of resistance testing: sufficient viral load (>500–1000 copies/mL); will miss resistance exhibited by variants comprising <5–20% of the circulating viral population, as well as any virus in sequestered havens, e.g. CNS, latent CD4 cells, genital tract.
- Genotypic assays—detect the presence of known mutations associated with resistance. Reverse transcriptase, protease, and integrase genes are amplified. The amplicons generated from the dominant species are sequenced. Mutations for each gene are reported using a letter–number–letter standard, e.g. K103N. Assays for fusion inhibitors and CCR5 inhibitors are becoming available. They will obviously not detect novel mutations, and interpretation may be difficult if there are many mutations present. See hivdb.stanford.edu for more information on interpretation. Genotypic testing cannot detect variants representing <20% of viral quasi-species. Techniques capable of detecting these

low-frequency isolates include point mutation assays, clone sequencing, and ultradeep sequencing.
- Phenotypic assays—measures the ability of HIV to replicate at different concentrations of tested drugs *in vitro*, in a manner analogous to bacteriological sensitivity testing. Recombinant viral assays involve insertion of reverse transcriptase and protease genes from a patient's strain into a laboratory clone. This and a wild-type reference strain are used to infect a cell line, and replication at various drug concentrations is compared. Results are reported as IC_{50} for the test strain relative to the reference strain. Threshold interpretation is not always straightforward—the gold standard would ideally be based on virological outcome, but this is difficult to define and assess with multidrug regimens. Phenotypic resistance testing is more expensive and time-consuming than genotypic testing, but useful in treatment-experienced patents.
- Tropism assays—85% of treatment-naïve patients will have a virus that uses CCR5 as its co-receptor. This falls to 50% amongst treatment-experienced patients with late disease, reflecting a switch to the use of CXCR4. Testing for viral tropism is important when considering the use of a CCR5 antagonist (e.g. maraviroc). Phenotypic assays are recommended in the USA, and genotypic assays (inferring tropism from the gp120 V3 sequence) in the UK.

Enterovirus (including Coxsackie)

The human enteroviruses and parechoviruses are genera within the family *Picornaviridae* ('pico', very small). The genus *Enterovirus* includes polio, Coxsackie A and B, and the echoviruses. Here we consider the non-polio enteroviruses, the cause of many syndromes, including childhood fever–rash, meningitis, myocarditis, and even neonatal sepsis. For polio, ➔ see Poliovirus, pp. 445–8.

The viruses

- Small RNA viruses, most identified in stool during polio research. Historically divided into subgroups: polioviruses, group A and B Coxsackie viruses, and echoviruses (enteric cytopathic human orphan viruses). New enteroviruses are now simply numbered sequentially.
- Some clinical syndromes are caused by many enteroviral types (e.g. rashes and meningitis). Others are associated with specific enteroviruses (e.g. Coxsackie B and pericarditis).

Epidemiology

- Found worldwide throughout the year, but, in temperate climates, infections peak in the summer and autumn months.
- Seventy-five per cent of cases occur in those under 15 years old, with attack rates highest in those under 1 year. Over 90% of non-polio enteroviral infections are asymptomatic or cause only a mild febrile illness.

Pathogenesis

- Infection may take place via the respiratory tract but is mainly faeco-oral.
- Viral replication occurs in the respiratory and GI epithelium, passing to regional lymph nodes. Patients become viraemic (usually undetectable).
- Most clear the infection and experience no symptoms. A minority experience further viral replication at distant reticulo-endothelial sites and a secondary viraemia that coincides with their non-specific illness. This major viraemia sees dissemination to other organs, e.g. the CNS.
- Humoral immunity is the main host defence—people with an isolated cell-mediated immune deficiency are not predisposed to severe enteroviral illness. The virus is shed in faeces for weeks after symptom resolution.

Clinical features

- *Aseptic meningitis*—manifestations of enteroviral meningitis vary with host age and (particularly humoral) immune state:
  - *neonates*—fever, vomiting, rash, anorexia, upper respiratory tract symptoms, and altered mental state. Meningeal signs are uncommon, and presentation is usually non-specific. Severe meningoencephalitis is a rare manifestation (death rate of 10%) and may be associated with hepatic necrosis, myocarditis, and necrotizing enterocolitis;
  - *older children and adults*—severe disease is rare. Commonly manifests as sudden fever (may be biphasic, with a gap as long as 2–10 days), nuchal rigidity, headache, photophobia, and non-specific features (e.g. vomiting, anorexia, diarrhoea, upper respiratory tract symptoms). Those with humoral immune deficiency can develop chronic meningoencephalitis that may last for years and is often ultimately fatal. There may be general features of enteroviral infection (e.g. pharyngitis), as well as those specific to the infecting enterovirus (characteristic rashes, pericarditis). In uncomplicated disease, the illness usually lasts a week. Sequelae are rare in those beyond the neonatal period.
- Other neurological syndromes:
  - *encephalitis*—lethargy, drowsiness, seizures, paresis, coma. Features can be focal (particularly with Coxsackie A infection): focal motor seizures, cerebellar ataxia, hemichorea;
  - *paralysis*—sporadic flaccid paralysis has been seen with Coxsackie A7 and enterovirus 71, amongst others. It is less severe than that seen with polio, and rarely permanent. GBS is associated with certain Coxsackie A and echovirus types. Other neurological manifestations include transverse myelitis and opsoclonus–myoclonus.
- *Other manifestations of enteroviral disease*—rashes: herpangina, hand, foot, and mouth disease; respiratory: URTI, epidemic pleurodynia (spasmodic rib pain and fever); cardiac: myopericarditis (➲ see Myocarditis, pp. 636–8); ophthalmological: acute haemorrhagic conjunctivitis (➲ see Conjunctivitis, pp. 749–51).

Diagnosis

- See referenced sections for diagnosis of non-neurological disease.
- CSF—clear, and pressure is usually normal/slightly raised. WCC raised: initially neutrophils, but lymphocytes dominate within 6–48h of symptoms. Higher counts are associated with a greater likelihood of viral identification. A slight rise in CSF protein and depression in CSF glucose may be seen. Viral identification by culture is not sensitive (around 30%) due to the low viral titre in CSF. RT-PCR is more sensitive (60–90%) and over 94% specific for enteroviral meningitis.
- Concomitant testing from sites other than the CSF may aid diagnosis; however, the virus is shed from some parts of the body for several weeks after infection has resolved, and, during viral seasons, enterovirus is produced by 7.5% of healthy controls.

Treatment

- Exclude bacterial aetiology of suspected meningitis. Otherwise treatment rests on symptom relief.
- Immunocompromised people (e.g. B-cell deficiency) with persistent enteroviral infection may benefit from immunoglobulin.
- Antiviral agents are in development—one of those, pleconaril, interferes with the viral capsid protein, altering attachment and uncoating. However, its benefits in enteroviral meningitis appear modest at best.

Lymphocytic choriomeningitis virus (LCMV)

- An ssRNA virus (family *Arenaviridae*), a human zoonosis found worldwide. Rodents are its primary host in whom it causes asymptomatic infection. Human cases are rare, and one-third of such infections are subclinical; 50% of clinical infections have neurological involvement.
- Infection is by inhalation or consumption of infected excreta, and it typically causes a febrile, self-limiting, biphasic disease. Individuals exposed to rodents (living conditions, pet handlers, laboratory personnel) are at risk for the infection. Transmission of infection during organ transplantation has occurred.
- Primary viraemia leads to CNS infection and a non-specific febrile illness with rash and lymphadenopathy. Secondary viraemia follows a few days later and is associated with meningitis/meningoencephalitis. Clinical course is benign, with <1% of cases fatal.
- It is a significant teratogen. Acquired congenitally, it produces similar abnormalities to congenital CMV; 35% of congenital infections are thought to lead to fetal loss; 84% of surviving infants have neurodevelopmental sequelae (e.g. cerebral palsy, seizures, mental retardation, visual problems, hydrocephalus).

Alphaviruses

Along with the genus *Rubivirus* (containing just rubella; ➔ see Rubella, pp. 389–90), a member of the family *Togaviridae*. Virions are lipid-enveloped, containing 11–12kb positive-stranded RNA.

Epidemiology

- All medically significant alphaviruses are vector-borne (they were once called the group A arboviruses). 'New World' viruses predominantly cause encephalitis and circulate in North and South America. 'Old World' viruses cause predominantly fever, rash, and arthropathy. See Table 8.4. Geographic spread is determined by the distribution of their vectors.
- Only some of the many viruses identified are known to cause human disease or cause only a rare and mild 'fever–arthropathy'.
- Some are maintained in an animal–vector cycle (e.g. eastern equine encephalitis (EEE): birds–mosquito), with a third-party vector transmitting to other animals (e.g. horses) or man. Animal infections may precede human—animal health surveillance can warn of human outbreaks.
- Humans can develop a viraemia significant enough to infect mosquitoes with some agents (Venezuelan equine encephalitis, VEE), but not others (EEE).

Pathogenesis

- Incubation 1–12 days. Bite of an infected mosquito deposits virus in the subcutaneous tissues. VEE has been acquired by aerosol in the laboratory.
- Non-neurotropic agents cause viraemia, skin lesions (lymphocytic perivascular cuffing and red cell leak from capillaries), and arthralgia. Virus persists in synovial macrophages, with host response leading to an inflammatory arthritis.
- Neurotropic viruses cause viraemia and fever in early infection, indicating replication in non-neural tissues. Infection of capillary endothelial cells is thought to allow subsequent CNS invasion. Acute encephalitis follows, and lesions may be seen throughout the brain and spinal cord. Transplacental spread can occur with VEE and Western equine encephalitis (WEE).

Clinical features

- Encephalitis—headache, high fever, chills, nausea, and vomiting. Respiratory symptoms may be seen with WEE. In cases with CNS involvement (<1% adults, 4% children), confusion and somnolence follow within a few days. Seizures are commoner in the young. Infants may develop bulging fontanelles. CSF protein and lymphocyte counts are high. Sequelae (70% infants after EEE, 30% WEE): mental retardation, behaviour change, paralysis. Case fatality rate: <1% overall, 20% encephalitis cases.
- Fever, rash, arthritis—rapid-onset fever (up to 40°C) and chills—may last several days, remit, then recur (saddleback fever chart). Rash usually appears on day 1 (can be late)—a face and neck flush evolves to maculopapular lesions on the trunk, limbs, face, and palms/soles, and may be pruritic. Arthralgia lasts a week to a few months, is polyarticular, and affects small joints that may be swollen. Other features: headache, photophobia, and sore throat. Long-term joint problems may be associated with HLA B27.

Diagnosis

- History—the epidemiology of each disease is fairly specific (see Table 8.4).
- Acute and convalescent serology, but of limited use in those living in endemic areas.

Table 8.4 Clinical syndromes caused by alphaviruses

Name	Location	Vector	Features
'New World': cause predominantly encephalitis			
Eastern equine encephalitis	Eastern and Gulf Coast USA, southern Canada, and northern South America	Enzootic vector: *Culiseta melanura*, breeds in freshwater swamps and feeds on birds (which become infected but may be asymptomatic). Vectors to human: *Aedes* and others	Summer disease of horses, children, and the elderly. Rare, but case fatality over 50%
Western equine encephalitis	North and South America	*Culex tarsalis*	Summertime disease of horses and humans—highest incidence in infants
Venezuelan equine encephalitis	South and Central America	Many different mosquito species	Rainy season; human disease follows horse by 1–2 weeks. Most severe in children
'Old World': cause predominantly fever, rash, and polyarthritis			
Chikungunya	Africa and Asia	*Aedes stegomyia* and *Aedes aegypti*	Sporadic outbreaks (90% population seropositive in sub-Saharan Africa)
O'nyong-nyong	Africa	*Anopheles*	
Mayaro	South America, Caribbean	*Haemagogus* and others	Fever and rash
Sindbis	Africa, Scandinavia, CIS, Asia	*Culex* maintains a bird cycle; several species infect man	Outbreaks occur at times of rainfall and flooding
Ross River	Australia, Oceania		Epidemic polyarthritis. Joint symptoms can last up to 3 years after infection

Treatment and prevention

- No specific therapy.
- Prevention depends on vector control and mosquito avoidance.
- Animal vaccines exist for EEE, WEE, and VEE—in limited non-commercial human use.

Bunyaviridae

The virus

Four genera: *Bunyavirus, Phlebovirus, Nairovirus,* and *Hantavirus*. They are spherical, enveloped viruses containing three negative-sense RNA segments coding for around six proteins.

Epidemiology

- *California encephalitis (CE) viruses*—CE is the commonest childhood CNS infection in the USA. La Crosse virus is the main cause. The virus is maintained in the mosquito vector population by transovarial transmission, and each summer the infected mosquito mass increases, as they feed on viraemic squirrels, foxes, etc.
- *Rift Valley fever (RVF)*—maintained in sub-Saharan Africa by transovarial transmission in some *Aedes* spp. Infected eggs in the soil remain viable for years, hatching in heavy rains. Sheep and cattle amplify infection.
- *Congo–Crimean haemorrhagic fever (CCHF)*—tick transmission and may also be acquired through contact with infected animals which may be asymptomatic (cattle and sheep). Found in parts of Africa, Asia, Eastern Europe, and the Middle East. Person-to-person spread may occur in acute infection.
- *Hantaviruses*—each viral species has a principal rodent host. The rodents become chronically infected and excrete virus in urine and saliva for months. Infection is acquired through animal bites or aerosols of virus-contaminated urine or faeces. Person-to-person spread is rare.

Clinical features

- *CE*—most human infections are asymptomatic. Incubation 3–7 days, then fever, encephalitis, or meningoencephalitis. Severity ranges from mild viral meningitis to a severe disease similar to herpes encephalitis. Aphasia, ataxia, paralysis, and convulsions (50% of cases) can occur. CT usually normal; MRI may aid diagnosis; EEG usually abnormal; 90% of La Crosse virus cases occur in those under 15 years old. Mortality in acute disease around 1%. Sequelae include EEG abnormalities (75% at 1–5 years), epilepsy (10%), and emotional lability (10%).
- *RVF*—a febrile illness; 10% experience retinitis and vasculitis that can cause a permanent loss of vision; 1% develop fulminant disease after 3–6 days of fever, with haemorrhage and hepatitis—half of these patients die. There are rare cases of severe encephalitis.
- *CCHF*—short incubation (3–5 days) leads to pre-haemorrhagic phase (fever, headache, myalgia), and then 3–5 days later haemorrhagic manifestations (shock, DIC, bleeding, thrombocytopenia). Convalescence 10–20 days after onset. Mortality 20–50%.

- *Hantavirus*:
  - haemorrhagic fever with renal syndrome—caused by 'Old World' viruses. Incubation 5–40 days, then fever, thrombocytopenia, and acute renal failure (interstitial nephritis). In the severe form (Hantaan virus), a toxic phase (headache, back pain, fever, blurred vision, erythematous rash, and petechiae) may be followed by severe shock. Those surviving can have prolonged renal insufficiency (oliguria, electrolyte and acid–base abnormalities, then polyuria), bleeding, and pneumonitis. Mortality is 5% with Hantaan infection—one-third in the shock phase, two-thirds in the renal phase. The milder form (Puumala virus) is fatal in <1% of clinical cases;
  - Hantavirus pulmonary syndrome—caused by 'New World' viruses. A 4- to 5-day febrile prodrome is followed by pulmonary oedema and shock. If hypoxia and shock are well managed, the vascular leak resolves in a few days. Thrombocytopenia may be seen.

Diagnosis

- Diagnosis of CE and Hantavirus infection is serological. Patients are IgM-positive by the time they are symptomatic in primary infection. PCR tests are not widely available, and viral RNA disappears from circulation early on in disease. Viral isolation from the CSF in CE is rare.
- CCHF and RVF viruses are readily cultured from blood of infected patients, and PCR or antigen detection by ELISA may be useful in severe cases, but the aerosol infection risk limits its usefulness. Antibodies can be detected at 5–14 days, coinciding with clinical improvement.

Treatment and prevention

- There are no vaccines in general use, and prevention is by public health measures to reduce vector numbers and personal avoidance.
- Ribavirin has been used effectively in treating Hantavirus infection and CCHF. Treatment is 10 days. Evidence suggests it has a role in the therapy of RVF.
- Supportive measures—anticonvulsants, fluids, circulatory/renal support.

Adenovirus

A cause of acute infections of the respiratory tract, and less commonly the conjunctivae, and GI and GU tracts.

The virus

- DNA virus of around 70nm in diameter, with a complex outer capsid consisting of 252 subunits forming a 20-sided icosahedron.
- The three different types of subunits (hexons, pentons, and fibres) differ immunologically—some antigenic sites common to all adenoviruses, others type-specific.
- There are around 50 human serotypes, some of which are associated with specific clinical syndromes. Similar viruses found in some animals.

Epidemiology

- Worldwide—different geographical areas see different syndromes associated with different serotypes. Transmission: respiratory, faeco-oral, fomites. Can survive long periods on surfaces. Day-care centre and household outbreaks are common.
- Most people have serological evidence of infection by age 10 years; 75% of childhood febrile illness may be attributable to adenovirus in developed settings.
- Infecting serotype and consequent disease are related to age. Types 1, 2, 5, and 6 are commoner in young children (cause URTI); types 3, 4, 7, and 14 in young adults (URTI and LRTI); types 8 and 19 cause adult eye infections.

Pathogenesis

- Generally causes lytic infection of epithelial cells, resulting in cell death with the release of up to 1 million progeny (up to 5% are infective).
- Latent/chronic infection can be demonstrated in lymphoid cells (e.g. tonsils) where only small numbers of virus are released.
- Oncogenic transformation is demonstrated experimentally in animals and tissue culture. Viral DNA integrates with host DNA. No infectious virus produced.

Clinical features

- Respiratory infection—incubation is around 4–5 days, and illness takes the form of mild pharyngitis/tracheitis (cough, fever, sore throat, and rhinorrhoea) or, less commonly in infants, bronchiolitis and atypical pneumonia (serotype 7). Type 14 has been associated with severe pneumonia in young adults. Most cases improve over 3–5 days.
- Pharyngoconjunctival fever (serotypes 3, 7)—a syndrome occurring in outbreaks amongst children and characterized by acute onset of conjunctivitis, pharyngitis, fever, and adenitis. Initially affecting one eye, the other usually becomes involved. Symptoms last 3–5 days; bacterial superinfection is uncommon, and there is no permanent eye damage. Respiratory involvement rarely progresses to the lungs. Contaminated swimming areas have been implicated in some outbreaks.
- Epidemic keratoconjunctivitis (serotypes 8, 19, 37)—a slow-onset, usually bilateral, conjunctivitis, seen in adults and acquired through such routes as contaminated hand towels and ophthalmic solutions. Incubation is 4–24 days; conjunctivitis lasts up to 4 weeks, with subsequent development of keratitis. The cornea may be involved for several months. Secondary spread to household contacts in 10% of cases.
- Haemorrhagic cystitis (types 7, 11, 21)—seen in children (male > female) and causes around 3 days of macroscopic haematuria; the means of infection is unclear. It is also seen in children and adults undergoing BMT.

- Infantile diarrhoea (serotypes 40, 41)—a common cause of watery diarrhoea and fever, lasting up to 2 weeks. Distinct causative serotypes. Certain of the common 'respiratory adenoviruses' may be associated with intussusception. Viral secretion may continue for months after a primary infection; thus, its detection does not confirm causality.
- Intussusception (serotypes 1, 2, 3, 5)—adenovirus was isolated in over 40% of intussusception cases in one series.
- Encephalitis/meningoencephalitis (serotypes 7, 1, 6, 12)—pneumonia is often an associated finding. Chronic meningoencephalitis occurs in patients with hypogammaglobulinaemia.
- The immunosuppressed—those undergoing BMT or solid organ transplant are at increased risk of adenoviral infection, both of the organ system transplanted and disseminated disease (e.g. lung, gut, CNS). Dissemination is commonest in children but occurs in adults and has a high mortality. Adenovirus may be detected in those with AIDS (particularly in the urine or GI tract), and diseases, such as colitis, parotitis, and encephalitis, have been attributed to it. The significance is not clear, as most patients are asymptomatic.
- Other—fatal dissemination in neonates, pericarditis, congenital abnormalities.

Diagnosis

- Culture—it is easy to culture the virus from respiratory specimens, stool, urine, and conjunctival scrapings. All serotypes, except 40 and 41, produce typical cytopathic changes in human epithelial monolayers at 2–7 days. Isolated virus can be grouped and serotyped.
- Antigen detection—indirect immunofluorescence allows detection of the virus quickly and cheaply, and correlates well with culture. Insufficiently sensitive in the immunocompromised.
- PCR—sensitive and specific, and can be performed on a variety of specimens (CSF, fixed tissues, blood). Difficult to interpret a positive result from the upper respiratory tract or stool, as this may represent viral shedding, rather than symptomatic infection.
- Serology—infection is demonstrated by a 4-fold rise in antibodies between acute and convalescent samples. ELISA is group-specific, while viral neutralization assays are serotype-specific.

Treatment and prevention

- Most infections are self-limiting, and there is no proven benefit of antiviral treatments. Anecdotal reports suggest a beneficial role for cidofovir in treating severe disease in the immunocompromised. Ganciclovir has limited *in vitro* activity against adenovirus.
- Effective vaccines have been developed—they have been used in the US military—but they are not generally available.

Human papillomavirus

A group of viruses producing epithelial tumours of the skin and mucous membranes, and associated with genital tract malignancies.

The virus

- Non-enveloped dsDNA viruses of the genus *Papillomavirus* of the family *Papovaviridae*. Certain viral proteins have transforming properties that contribute to the development of malignancy.
- Serotypes differ in the body site they tend to infect (see Table 8.5). Over 100 human papillomavirus (HPV) types have been identified, of which over 40 infect the anogenital area. Worldwide prevalence of HPV amongst women is 10%.

Pathogenesis

- All types of squamous epithelium may be infected by HPV. Warts develop around 3 months (range 6 weeks to 2 years) after inoculation.
- Infects the basal cells of the stratum germinativum, with replication and viral assembly taking place as basal cells mature and move to the surface. Virions are shed, along with dead keratinocytes.
- Warts and condylomata are associated with proliferation of epidermal layers, resulting in acanthosis and hyperkeratosis. Some infected cells may develop characteristic perinuclear vacuolation—koilocytosis.
- HPV DNA may be found in normal-looking cells, accounting for recurrence after treatment for warts. Excessive proliferation of the basal layer is a pre-malignant feature. DNA is extrachromosomal in benign disease but usually integrated in malignancy.
- Disease occurs at increased frequency and severity in those with immunodeficiencies or HIV or those receiving immunosuppressive therapy. May be more severe in pregnancy.
- Genotypes vary in their cancer association (cervical, anal, penile, oropharyngeal); 70% of worldwide cervical cancer is associated with HPV 16 and 18.

Table 8.5 The clinical spectra of HPV disease

Clinical manifestation	Commonest HPV types
Cutaneous warts	1, 2, 3, 10
Warts in meat and fish handlers	7, 2
Epidermolysis verruciformis	2, 3, 10, 5, 8, 9, 12, 14, 15, 17
Condylomata acuminata	6, 11
Low-grade intraepithelial neoplasia	6, 11
High-grade intraepithelial neoplasia and cervical carcinoma	16, 18
Recurrent respiratory papillomatosis	6, 11

Clinical features

- *Cutaneous warts*—groups at risk of developing warts include butchers and fish handlers (minor trauma facilitates infection). Close personal contact may be important in transmission. Resolve in 90% by 5 years. Very rarely progress to verrucous carcinoma.
  - Common warts (71%) occur frequently amongst school-aged children, with a well-defined, exophytic appearance. Commonly found on the back of the hands, between fingers, and on palms and soles. May coalesce.
  - Plantar (and palmar) warts (34%) are commonest amongst adolescents/young adults. Appear as raised bundles of fibres—often painful.
  - Planar warts (4%) are irregular, slightly elevated papules. Seen in childhood.
- *Epidermodysplasia verruciformis*—a rare genetic condition characterized by the appearance of disseminated cutaneous warts in early life (under 10 years old), with a high incidence of malignant transformation (one-third of patients in young adulthood). Associated with a relatively specific group of HPV types. Vary in appearance.
- *Anogenital warts*—the commonest viral sexually transmitted infection (STI) in the UK, with highest rates in women aged 16–19 years, and men aged 20–24 years. Increased in those with many partners or those not using barrier contraception. Around 66% of those having sex with an individual with warts will develop them within 3 months. Young children may develop genital warts from hand contact with non-genital lesions—their presence should, however, prompt the consideration of abuse. Seventy-five per cent of patients with anogenital warts are asymptomatic, with the remainder experiencing itching, burning, and tenderness. Appearance: exophytic papules, which may be sessile or pedunculated, small (<1mm), or coalesce into large plaques.
  - Men—the commonest affected area in uncircumcised is the preputial cavity (85%); in the circumcised, the penile shaft is more commonly involved. Other sites: urethral meatus, distal urethra, perianal (especially MSM). Increased risk of anal cancer if history of anal warts.
  - Women—mostly affected over the posterior introitus, labia, and clitoris. The application of 3% acetic acid may whiten vulval lesions. The presence of external genital warts should prompt the consideration of cervical HPV and cervical intraepithelial neoplasia (CIN). Genital warts may spontaneously remit (~10% of cases over 4 months). Lesions can become very large, particularly during pregnancy or when immunosuppressed. They may cause local destruction, enter the spectrum of CIN, or rarely transform into invasive squamous cell carcinoma. CIN has a variable outcome, depending on the HPV type and grade of tumour (grade 1: 60% regress, 1% become invasive; grade 3: 33% regress, 12% progress).

- *Recurrent respiratory papillomatosis*—disease of the larynx and airways existing in two forms: juvenile- and adult-onset. Juvenile infection is probably acquired intrapartum. Median age at onset is 3 years, patients presenting with hoarseness or an altered cry. Disease may spread to the trachea and lungs, resulting in obstruction, stridor, infection, and respiratory compromise. May require surgical excision. Adult disease is associated with a high number of sexual partners and oral–genital contact. Presentation is less aggressive, with rare malignant transformation.
- *Other*—conjunctival papillomas, epidermoid cysts, co-infection with EBV in oral hairy leukoplakia in HIV-infected patients.

Diagnosis

- Diagnosis is usually made from clinical examination, assisted by use of the colposcope and 3% acetic acid.
- Biopsy may be indicated to confirm diagnosis (➲ see Genital warts, pp. 699–701). HPV antigen detection and PCR-based tests are available.

Prevention

- Vaccination—two subunit vaccines are available, made from the major protein of the viral coat or capsid, one quadrivalent (Gardasil® serotypes 16, 18, 6, and 11) and one bivalent (Cervarix® types 16 and 18). Given as three doses over 4–5 months. Both are over 99% effective at preventing pre-cancerous lesions associated with HPV 16 and 18, and protection appears to be maintained for at least 7 years. Gardasil® offers additional protection against genital warts caused by types 6 and 11. Vaccination should take place prior to becoming sexually active. The UK vaccinates girls at age 12 years. It initially chose Cervarix® for its programme in 2008, switching to Gardasil® in 2012.
- Barrier contraception may reduce HPV transmission during intercourse.
- Cervical smears are essential in detecting pre-malignant changes, even if vaccinated (➲ see Genital warts, pp. 699–701).

Treatment

- *Cutaneous warts*—most cutaneous warts undergo spontaneous resolution. The two main treatment modalities for hand warts: daily salicylic acid-based preparations or cryotherapy 3-weekly—both achieve cure in up to 70% of cases. Salicylic acid cures around 80% of deep plantar warts, but only 50% of mosaic plantar warts. Other modalities exist: curettage, cryotherapy, and electrosurgery.
- *Anogenital warts*—treatments include the use of local caustic agents (e.g. podophyllum or trichloroacetic acid), cryotherapy, electrosurgery, surgical excision, and immune therapies such as imiquimod (a toll-like receptor 7 agonist) or IFN, both the latter applied TOP and acting through stimulation of local cytokine production.
- *Epidermodysplasia verruciformis*—lesions should be carefully observed, and malignant lesions treated rapidly.
- *Recurrent respiratory papillomatosis*—endoscopic cryotherapy or laser surgery. There may be roles for interferon alfa and cidofovir.

Polyomaviruses

While polyomavirus infection is common and asymptomatic in the majority, they are important causes of disease in the immunosuppressed.

The virus

- Members of the family *Papovaviridae* (small, non-enveloped viruses with dsDNA genomes). Two genera: *Polyomavirus* and *Papillomavirus*.
- Polyomaviruses are found in humans, monkeys, and mice, and are relatively species-specific. There are two key human polyomaviruses BK and JC (named with the initials of the patient in whom each was first identified). JC virus (JCV) is associated with PML, and BK virus (BKV) with post-renal transplant nephritis and ureteral stenosis. They have around 75% nucleotide homology.
- Merkel cell polyomavirus has been recently identified and may be causally linked to the development of Merkel cell carcinoma.

Epidemiology

- Sixty to 80% of European adults have antibodies to JCV, BKV, or both—BKV infection probably occurs at around age 4 years, and JCV infection at age 10 years. No evidence of perinatal infection. Faeco-oral and respiratory transmission has been suggested.
- JCV is detectable by PCR in the urine of asymptomatic immunosuppressed patients and, less commonly, healthy adults.
- Both viruses have been linked to the development of tumours (particularly brain), but a causal relationship has not been proven.
- PML used to be seen only in older patients with haematological malignancy or receiving steroid therapy—now over half of the deaths associated with PML occur in those with HIV infection.

Pathogenesis

- Primary JC and BK viraemia probably leads to the establishment of latent infection in the kidney. Immunosuppression allows viral reactivation and replication, leading to viruria.
- The virus infects peripheral blood mononuclear cells, and it is by this means they probably travel to, and infect, the CNS.
- Not known whether PML follows reactivation of latent JCV in the CNS or new CNS infection following reactivation of renal JCV. The virus probably directly infects oligodendrocytes, leading to demyelination.

Clinical features

Primary infection is usually asymptomatic, but children may experience mild upper respiratory tract symptoms.

- *BKV and JCV viruria*—uncommon in those without immune impairment:
  - pregnant women—JCV/BKV is found in <3% of pregnant women in the last trimester, ceasing rapidly post-partum. Probably represents reactivation (due to immunosuppression or hormonal change);
  - renal transplant recipients—BK viruria is seen in 10–45% of patients after transplantation, representing both reactivation and primary infection of the recipient from a previously infected kidney. Most

cases occur in the first 3 months after surgery and are asymptomatic. Some cases of BKV infection lead to graft nephropathy, and it has been associated with ureteric stenosis;
    - BMT recipients—BKV viruria occurs in <50% of patients, most <2 months after the procedure and probably due to reactivation; Associated with the development of haemorrhagic cystitis.
    - other immunodeficiencies—BKV viruria with renal complications has been reported in cases of other causes of immunodeficiency.
- *PML*—caused by JCV. Presentation is similar in both those with HIV and those with other immunodeficiencies: rapidly progressive focal neurological deficits, including hemiparesis, visual field defects, aphasia, ataxia, and cognitive impairment. Late features include cortical blindness, quadriparesis, dementia, and coma. Abnormalities occur predominantly in cerebral white matter and, less commonly, in the cerebellum and brainstem. Spinal cord involvement is rare. Death usually occurs within 6 months of diagnosis, although some experience a 2- to 3-year fluctuating course.

Diagnosis

Serology is unhelpful, given the high seroprevalence, so diagnosis relies on virus detection and pathological findings. Viral culture is difficult, as both JCV and BKV are very slow-growing.

- Viruria—cytological examination is useful for the detection of viruria, although a normal appearance does not exclude infection; infected cells have large nuclei with a large basophilic intranuclear inclusion. These changes can be confused with those caused by other viral infections, e.g. CMV, adenovirus. PCR detects the virus but is positive in a proportion of health controls and the elderly.
- Plasma PCR—results correlate with, and predict the risk of, BKV-associated nephropathy.
- PML and JCV—brain biopsy allows definitive diagnosis, demonstrating multiple asymmetric foci of demyelination, cytopathic changes apparent in oligodendrocytes, and EM revealing viral particles within their nuclei. Fluorescent antibody staining allows identification of JCV. CT scan appearance may be less dramatic than the severity of the clinical findings suggests—hypodense, non-enhancing white matter lesions. MRI is more sensitive. PCR of CSF to identify JCV DNA should only be used in combination with imaging and clinical findings—sensitivity is variable, depending on the technique, and may be positive in immunosuppressed patients without PML.

Treatment

- The majority of patients with BKV and JCV are asymptomatic and do not require treatment.
- PML patients with HIV may demonstrate marked improvement with the introduction of ART.
- BKV-induced nephropathy may respond to the reduction of immunosuppression. Several drugs with *in vitro* antiviral activity have been used, but clinical efficacy has not yet been conclusively proven (quinolone antibiotics, IVIG, leflunomide, cidofovir).

Poxviruses

The largest of all virus groups, and, unlike most other DNA viruses, replication occurs in the infected cell's cytoplasm, rather than within the nucleus.

The viruses

- Large, asymmetric virions containing dsDNA and enzymes enabling cytoplasmic replication.
- Extremely resistant to chemical and physical inactivation, and remain infective for months at room temperature, or years if frozen.

For viruses and their respective hosts, see Table 8.6.

Vaccinia

- Derived from cowpox in the early nineteenth century by person-to-person transmission. Now has no natural host. Jenner observed in 1798 that inoculating people with pustular material from cowpox gave protection from smallpox, inventing 'vaccination'. Routine vaccination for smallpox has been discontinued.
- Vaccinia continues to have a role amongst military personnel, as a vaccine vector for other infections, and in immunotherapy. Protection is almost 100% for 1–3 years, with disease-attenuating protection for <20 years.
- Complications of vaccination include fever, regional lymphadenopathy, post-infectious encephalitis (1–2 weeks later), and skin eruptions.

Variola (smallpox)

- Unlike vaccinia, variola infects only humans, and occasionally monkeys.
- Two main viral strains: the virulent variola major (mortality 20–50%) and the milder variola minor (mortality <1%).

Table 8.6 Genera of *Poxviridae* with example species

Genera	Viruses	Normal host
Orthopoxvirus	Vaccinia	Man, derived from cowpox
	Variola	Man, (monkeys)
	Monkeypox	Monkeys, (man)
Avipoxvirus	Fowlpox	Chickens
Capripoxvirus	Sheep-pox	Sheep
Leporipoxvirus	Myxoma	Rabbit
Parapoxvirus	Bovine papular stomatitis virus	Cow, (man 'milker's nodule')
	Pseudocowpox virus	Cattle, (man)
	Orf	Sheep and goats, (man)
Suipoxvirus	Swinepox	Pigs
Molluscipoxvirus	Molluscum contagiosum	Man
Yatapoxvirus	Tanapox	Monkeys, (man—resembles monkeypox)

- Rapid diagnosis can be made using PCR, EM, or gel diffusion techniques on vesicular fluid. It no longer exists in nature (last case: Somalia, 1977).
- Incubation is <12 days, then a 2-day prodrome is followed by a rash (maculopapules, vesicles to pustules and scabs). In fulminant disease, death can occur before the rash. Today only two laboratories in the world are known to have isolates of variola.

Monkeypox

- Causes vesicular illness in monkeys, similar to smallpox. Sporadic cases of human infection occur in endemic areas (rainforests of Western and Central Africa), and some imported cases have been seen in the USA.
- Rash resembles smallpox and is contagious to other humans. A 1996/1997 outbreak in the Congo had a fatality rate of 1.5%.

Parapoxviruses

- Found worldwide. Native to a variety of animals, and some members are capable of infecting humans. Can persist within herds for long periods.
- Orf (sheep and goats) and pseudocowpox (cattle) cause lesions in the mouth and skin, and passage to humans is acquired by direct contact with the animal or contaminated objects. Lesions in humans are milder (vesicle to pustules) with prolonged incubation and can last for weeks.
- Diagnosis is from vesicular material, examined by PCR, EM, or culture.

Molluscum contagiosum

- The only poxvirus specific for humans in the post-smallpox era. Found worldwide and spread by close human contact.
- Causes small, firm, umbilicated papules on exposed epithelial (children) or genital areas (adults). Usually resolve spontaneously but can persist for months, in the context of immunosuppression, or become generalized in atopic patients.
- A common disease of childhood, and in adolescents as a result of sexual transmission or contact sports. It is an opportunistic pathogen in AIDS patients—can cause generalized infection, with large atypical lesions resembling basal cell carcinomas.
- Diagnosis is clinical but may be confirmed, if necessary, by histology, as lesions can resemble those of other conditions, including cryptococcosis and histoplasmosis.
- Management is by local therapy (cryotherapy, excision, podophyllotoxin, etc.) and improving immunological function. Severe cases associated with immunocompromise may respond to interferon alfa or cidofovir.

Poliovirus

The virus

- Group C human enterovirus and member of the family *Picornaviridae*.
- Three serotypes—infection by one confers protective immunity only to that type, with little heterologous protection. Prior to widespread vaccination, paralytic disease was caused largely by type 1.

- Transmission—faeco-oral; pharyngeal in epidemics. Wild-type and/or vaccine-strain virus may circulate in a population, depending on regional vaccine use and the level of endemic wild-type viral transmission.
- Humans are the only natural host (infections can be achieved experimentally in primates). Wild-type strains vary widely in neurovirulence.

Epidemiology

- Polio was largely sporadic in the nineteenth century, affecting mostly children <5 years. By 1950, developing world infections were epidemic in nature, most cases in children aged 5–9 years (one-third in those over 15 years). This was attributed to rising standards of hygiene, delaying inapparent infections that previously took place in childhood and conferred widespread immunity. The resulting pool of older, susceptible individuals facilitated epidemics—the higher rate of paralytic disease due to the loss of protective maternal antibody.
- Rates fell dramatically after vaccine introduction. The last naturally occurring UK case was in 1984. Of the 41 cases notified between 1984 and 2009, 30 were vaccine-associated and six imported, and wild-type virus was not detected in the remainder.
- The Global Polio Eradication Initiative has seen the number of countries in which polio transmission has never been interrupted fall from >125 (1988) to two (Afghanistan, Pakistan), although many countries remain vulnerable and at risk of outbreaks (e.g. Nigeria, Ethiopia, Iraq, Somalia, and South Sudan, amongst others).

Pathogenesis

- The virus enters through the GI tract and replicates in the gut and adjacent lymphoid tissue. Reaches susceptible reticulo-endothelial tissue via the bloodstream.
- Asymptomatic cases stop at this point. Type-specific antibodies are formed. Otherwise, replication and viraemia occur (the 'minor illness').
- The CNS is probably infected by retrograde axonal transport from muscle to nerve to cord. Neurons throughout the grey matter are affected, especially those within the anterior horn of the spinal cord and the motor nuclei of the medulla and pons. Distribution of lesions is similar in all cases—it is their severity that determines clinical disease.

Clinical features

- Incubation—9–12 days from acquisition to prodrome ('minor illness'—2–3 days of fever, headache, sore throat, anorexia, vomiting, abdominal pain), and 11–17 days until the onset of paralysis ('major illness').
- Manifestations:
  - inapparent—95% of cases are asymptomatic;
  - abortive—4–8% of infections experience just the prodrome;
  - non-paralytic polio—severe, abortive, with signs of viral meningitis;
  - spinal paralytic polio—frank paralysis occurs in 0.1% of infections. Children experience the classic biphasic illness—the 2- to 3-day minor illness coincides with viraemia and is followed by

2–5 asymptomatic days before the abrupt onset of the major illness. Headache, fever, malaise, vomiting, neck stiffness, and muscle pains are followed after 1–2 days by flaccid weakness and paralysis of anything, from a single muscle to quadriplegia (very rare in infants). Initially, hyperactive reflexes become absent. Paralysis is asymmetric, with proximal involvement more severe than distal, and the legs more commonly involved than the arms. Bladder paralysis usually accompanies the legs. Occasional cases progress from onset of weakness to quadriplegia and bulbar involvement within hours—more commonly progression is over 2–3 days, halting when the patient becomes afebrile. Sensory loss is rare (consider GBS);

  - bulbar paralytic polio—paralysis of those muscle groups innervated by the cranial nerves, resulting in dysphagia, nasal speech, and dyspnoea. Seen in 5–35% of paralytic cases. Medullary circulatory and respiratory centres may become involved. Mixed bulbar and spinal involvement is common;
  - polioencephalitis—an uncommon form occurring mainly in infants. Confusion, disturbed consciousness, and seizures with spastic paralysis (upper motor neuron involvement).

- Prognosis—prior to vaccination, mortality of paralytic disease was 5–10%, rising to 20–60% with bulbar involvement. Two-thirds with paralytic disease have a degree of permanent weakness on recovery, and complete recovery is rare with severe paralysis, particularly if requiring ventilation. Those surviving bulbar disease show the best recovery, with significant improvement by 10 days and ultimately usually attaining normal function. Most reversible muscle paralysis in spinal disease will have resolved by 1 month, with some improvement up to 9 months.
- Post-poliomyelitis syndrome—20–30% of previously paralysed patients experience a new onset of weakness, pain, and atrophy in previously affected muscle groups 25–35 years after acute illness. This is thought to be due to attrition of motor units in innervated muscle that is already less innervated due to the initial disease.
- Risk factors for paralysis—prepubertal male, pregnancy, B-cell deficiency (increases the risk of oral polio vaccine (OPV)-associated disease), strenuous exercise within first 3 days of major illness, IM injections (paralysis localizes to the limb injected or injured within 2–4 weeks before infection), the tonsillectomized (eight times the risk of those with tonsils).
- Complications—respiratory compromise (diaphragmatic and intercostal muscle paralysis, upper airway obstruction, respiratory centre impairment), myocarditis, GI haemorrhage, ileus, complications of paralysis.
- Differential—other enteroviruses, West Nile, Guillain–Barré, herpes zoster, rabies, botulism, diphtheria, cord lesions, neuropathies, myopathies.

Diagnosis

- CSF—viral identification by PCR or culture (less sensitive) is gold standard.
- Throat—the virus may be detected in the first week of illness.
- Faeces—may be detected for several weeks. In areas of low incidence, it is important to identify the viral strain (wild-type or vaccine-related), as the presence of vaccine-virus is not uncommon in the healthy and does not conclusively prove the aetiology.
- Serology—paired sera; cannot distinguish wild-type from vaccine.

Treatment

- No specific antiviral therapy. Management is supportive.
- Bed rest is essential in the acute phase to reduce the extension of paralysis.
- Avoid IM injections.
- Ventilatory assistance is required once vital capacity falls to <50%. Tracheal intubation is indicated in severe cases of bulbar paralysis.
- Physiotherapy can start once the progression of paralysis has ceased.
- Multidisciplinary management of long-term physical sequelae.

Vaccination

- Inactivated polio vaccine (IPV)—developed by Salk and introduced in the UK in 1956. The preparations now used contain all three serotypes and have seroconversion rates equal to OPV. Neutralizing antibodies are found in 100% of people after the third dose. Recipients develop little or no secretory antibody and are thus capable of asymptomatic infection and shedding to unimmunized contacts.
- OPV—developed by Sabin in 1963. It is trivalent—four doses are required to achieve seroconversion to all three serotypes. Non-immune recipients shed virus in faeces for up to 6 weeks. OPV promotes antibody formation in the gut (providing local protection against viral entry) and boosts community immunity (recently vaccinated children excrete virus which may be acquired by their contacts). Those in tropical countries who receive all the recommended doses may fail to seroconvert for all three serotypes, possibly related to the prevalence of diarrhoeal disease and vaccine formulation. Around one dose in every 2.6 million results in vaccine-virus-related disease—both in receivers (usually those under 4 months of age, 7–21 days after administration) and their contacts (usually young adults, 20–29 days after administration); 22% of reported cases occur in those with humoral immunodeficiency. The syndrome is similar to naturally occurring disease but is more protracted.
- For this reason, endemic countries tend to use OPV for primary immunization (low cost, ease of administration), whereas countries without polio (including the UK and USA) use IPV.

Human T-cell lymphotropic virus

HTLV-1 and -2 are retroviruses. HTLV-1 is associated with certain forms of adult T-cell leukaemia/lymphoma and neurological disease. HTLV-2 has not yet been definitively linked to a specific disorder.

The virus

- Spherical virions; 65% nucleotide homology between HTLV-1 and -2.
- Non-human primates are thought to be the natural reservoir of HTLVs.
- Unlike the lentiviruses (retroviruses such as HIV) which have a cytopathic effect, HTLV transforms T cells, immortalizing them. Around 0.1–1% of PBMCs carry viral DNA in the host genome in the asymptomatic, rising to 30% in disease.
- HTLV-1 isolates show a high degree of similarity (92–97%) across the world (unlike HIV-1). Small variations seem to reflect the geographical origin—it has been classified into five clades.
- HTLV-2 has three subtypes: 2a (IDUs in North America), 2b (indigenous groups of Central/South America), and 2c (urban Brazil).

Epidemiology

- HTLV-1 is widely scattered. Endemic in some regions and widespread in immigrants from these areas; parts of the Caribbean, Central/West Africa, Melanesia, the Middle East, India, and parts of South America. Estimated 10–20 million of infected people worldwide.
- HTLV-2 is found largely amongst IDUs and their sexual contacts, as well as some Native American populations.
- Transmission occurs sexually (mostly male to female, risk increased in the presence of genital ulceration), via blood products (those with cellular components, not plasma derivatives—the infectious titre in plasma is extremely low), or from mother to child (breastfeeding being the predominant route; 15–20% of breastfed children of HTLV-positive mothers acquire it). Most infections are lifelong and asymptomatic.

Clinical features

- *Adult T-cell leukaemia/lymphoma (ATL)*—proliferative disorder of mature $CD4^+CD25^+$ T cells. Integration of the provirus into the cellular genome is monoclonal (T cells originate from a single transformed cell), and the virus appears to be latent in neoplastic cells. One to 4% lifetime risk of a HTLV-1 carrier developing it. Clinical features: lymphadenopathy, hypercalcaemia, lytic bone lesions, skin lesions (nodules through to erythroderma), and hepatosplenomegaly. Patients can be immunocompromised, and opportunistic infections are common (*S. stercoralis* in Japan). Classified into four types:
    - smouldering ATL—5% of cases. Normal cell count, but 5% or more abnormal T-cell morphology with skin lesions and can last for years;
    - chronic ATL—20% of cases. Raised cell count, with organomegaly, skin or pulmonary involvement, but no effusions, or bone or CNS involvement. Median survival: 24 months;

  - lymphomatous ATL—around 20% of cases. Lymphadenopathy, hepatosplenomegaly, skin lesions. Normal cell counts. Median survival: 10 months;
  - acute ATL—around half of cases. Presents as leukaemia or high-grade non-Hodgkin's lymphoma. Median survival: 6.2 months.
- *HTLV-1-associated myelopathy (tropical spastic paraparesis)*—a chronic progressive demyelinating disease affecting the spinal cord and white matter of the CNS; 5% lifetime incidence in HTLV-1 carriers; onset typically at >30 years of age. Features: gait disturbance, leg weakness/stiffness with moderate to severe spasticity, back pain, bladder/bowel dysfunction, variable degrees of sensory loss. Progression varies—some have long periods of only mild difficulty walking; others become bed-bound over a median of 21 years. Unlike ATL, infected lymphocytes are polyclonal and may cause disease indirectly by activating autoimmune T cells or by infecting CNS glial cells, precipitating a cytotoxic response.
- Other disease associations:
  - HTLV-1—arthropathies, uveitis, polymyositis, infectious dermatitis, Sjögren's syndrome, and possibly mycosis fungoides;
  - HTLV-2—unconfirmed associations with rare haematological malignancies and neurodegenerative disorders.

Diagnosis

- ELISA-based tests are used to screen for HTLV. Positives are confirmed using more sensitive techniques to distinguish HTLV-1 and -2 (e.g. PCR).
- ATL—diagnosis is by histology (blood cell appearance, skin lesion biopsy), cytogenetics, immunophenotyping, and confirming the monoclonal integration of proviral DNA into malignant cells.
- HTLV-1-associated myelopathy—MRI may show lesions; CSF may reveal atypical lymphocytes.

Treatment

Adult T-cell leukaemia/lymphoma

- Combination chemotherapy. Side effects may outweigh benefits in indolent disease. Durable remissions are rare, with most relapsing within 12 months. Intensive (more toxic) chemotherapy regimes give higher initial response rates, but with significant morbidity and similar overall 3-year survival.
- Allogeneic stem cell transplantation may benefit those in whom remission is achieved.
- Zidovudine, in combination with IFN-α, was reported to induce remission in 26% of patients in one series.
- Monoclonal antibodies (coupled to yttrium-90) against the IL-2R chain (expressed by ATL cells) have been reported as effective in some patients.

HTLV-1-associated myelopathy

- No effective treatment. Danazol has been reported to improve gait and bladder function. Corticosteroids, plasmapheresis, cyclophosphamide, and interferon alfa may produce transient responses.

Flaviviruses

The family *Flaviviridae* includes the genus *Flavivirus*, along with the genus *Pestivirus* and the hepatitis C-like viruses. Although genetically similar, there is no known antigenic relationship between these genera. The group derives its name from yellow fever (the type species—*flavus* being Latin for 'yellow'). The genus *Flavivirus* has around 70 members, 30 of which are known to cause human disease. Most are arthropod-borne or zoonotic viruses. Here we consider those members for which encephalitis is the defining clinical feature. Dengue and yellow fever itself are covered in ➲ Dengue, pp. 457–8 and ➲ Yellow fever, pp. 455–6, respectively.

Viral structure

- Positive-sense ssRNA contained within a nucleocapsid. Spherical virions, 50nm in diameter, with an outer lipid envelope packed with the membrane (M) and envelope (E—involved in cell attachment and containing several epitopes involved in viral neutralization) glycoproteins.
- Cross-neutralization assays allow flaviviruses to be classified into one of eight antigenic groups, the most important of which are the JE complex (Japanese encephalitis (JE), St Louis encephalitis, West Nile virus, Murray Valley encephalitis virus), dengue complex, tick-borne virus complex (Central European encephalitis, Russian Spring–Summer encephalitis, Kyasanur Forest disease).

Pathogenesis

- Incubation 4–28 days (usually 7). One in 250 infections are symptomatic.
- Old age is the most significant risk factor for severe disease.
- The virus replicates locally. Brief viraemia (rarely recovered from blood), followed by CNS invasion. CNS spread occurs cell-to-cell, with meningeal inflammation, cerebral oedema, and encephalitis (particularly temporal, thalamus, brainstem, and anterior spinal cord). Far Eastern tick-borne encephalitis may result in changes resembling polio, with damage to motor neurons in the brainstem, and cervical and upper lumbar cord.

Viruses causing encephalitis

Diagnosis

- Relies on serology. Viral isolation is rarely useful with neurotropic flaviviruses, as isolation from blood is only likely in the first week (before the onset of neurological features). Isolation from CSF is possible in early fulminant disease, and it may be isolated from tissue samples (brain, spleen, etc.) in some cases. PCR of acute-phase serum may allow early diagnosis but is frequently negative in later disease, as viraemia is short-lived.
- ELISA for IgM against the virus is positive in CSF (<90% cases) and serum (<70% cases) by the time of admission to hospital and, in the majority of cases, by day 10 of illness. Tests can remain positive for months, and, in areas where several flaviviruses circulate, it can be

difficult to distinguish acute from previous infection and between different flaviviruses. Vaccination history and the potential for cross-reaction with other flaviviral antibodies should be borne in mind—particularly in areas in which several flaviviruses are circulating. Reference laboratories may provide more specific neutralization assays capable of greater type specificity.

Japanese encephalitis

- *Epidemiology*—found throughout Asia (Pakistan to Eastern Russia) and responsible for up to 65% of hospitalized encephalitis cases in areas of high endemicity. Outbreaks have occurred in Northern Australia and the Pacific islands. Widespread childhood immunization in China, Japan, and Korea has resulted in a large fall in incidence. Transmitted by *Culex* mosquitoes, with viral amplification occurring in pigs and aquatic birds. Humans are incidental hosts. Conditions for mosquito breeding are most favourable in rural areas (e.g. rice paddies) where the risk of infection is highest. Most infections are subclinical and occur in childhood (2–10 years of age); thus, 80% of young adults are immune in endemic areas. Regions with high vaccine uptake see most infections in the elderly.
- *Clinical features*—infection is symptomatic in <1% of cases. Severe encephalitis (25% fatality, even with intensive care facilities). Main findings at presentation: high fever and altered consciousness (personality change to coma). Early symptoms: lethargy, fever, headache, abdominal pain, vomiting. Over a few days progress to: agitation, delirium, motor abnormalities (facial paralysis, dysconjugate gaze, convulsions, hemiparesis, focal weakness, flaccid and spastic paralysis, ataxia, tremor, choreoathetosis, and other extrapyramidal signs), neck stiffness, coma (some needing ventilatory support). Severe cases may be quickly fatal. Milder cases see improvements after 1 week. Neurological recovery can take weeks to years, with one-third having residual problems at 5 years, and psychological sequelae in over 50% of children. Secondary complications include infections and pressure sores. Abortion may be precipitated where infection is acquired in the first or second trimester.
- *Laboratory findings*—leucocytosis, hyponatraemia, raised CSF lymphocytes, normal/slightly raised CSF protein; EEG shows diffuse delta waves (occasionally seizure activity); CT/MRI may show cerebral oedema and abnormalities in the brainstem, cerebellum, and spinal cord.
- *Treatment and prevention*—no specific therapy. Anecdotal reports of benefit from interferon alfa and ribavirin were not borne out by controlled trials. JE vaccines are available—three doses of an inactivated vaccine over 4 weeks is around 90% effective. Side effects include angio-oedema and urticaria, and there have been reports of encephalomyelitis. Because of the low risk of acquiring JE while travelling, it is not recommended routinely. A live vaccine is available only in China.

St Louis encephalitis

- *Epidemiology*—outbreaks have occurred throughout the USA and in parts of Canada and Mexico; sporadic cases occur further afield, including South America and parts of the Caribbean. Transmitted in an enzootic cycle (birds) by different *Culex* spp. in different geographical areas; human infection is incidental. Eastern USA sees periodic regional outbreaks in late summer, usually in urban areas where polluted water provides mosquito-breeding areas. Vectors are most active in the evening. Incidence of infection is highest in men and the homeless. In Western USA, infection occurs at low levels all year, often associated with irrigated areas. An estimated 1 in 300 infections result in clinical illness, with the risk greatest in the elderly and lowest in children (1:800).
- *Clinical features*—incubation 4–21 days. Three broad syndromes: febrile illness, aseptic meningitis, and fatal encephalitis. Most severe and fatal cases occur in adults and the elderly. Early symptoms: malaise, fever, headache, myalgia, and upper respiratory and abdominal symptoms. After several days: lethargy, confusion, tremor, ataxia and other cerebellar signs, vomiting and diarrhoea, generalized weakness, meningism (children), tremor (eyelids, lips, extremities), cranial nerve palsies. Most patients do not progress to coma, and convulsions are rare. Overall fatality 8% (20% of cases in those over 60 years). Children often have residual deficits but show late recovery. Adults may have residual neurological and psychological disturbance for some months.
- *Laboratory findings*—leucocytosis, hyponatraemia (syndrome of inappropriate antidiuretic hormone secretion, SIADH), proteinuria, raised CSF pressure in one-third of cases, raised CSF protein in two-thirds; EEG shows generalized slowing with delta waves.
- *Treatment and prevention*—no specific treatment. A pilot study indicated interferon alfa might reduce the incidence of persistent quadriplegia. A randomized trial is needed. Bird and mosquito surveillance may allow outbreak prediction and the early use of insecticides in at-risk areas, with public health education to reduce mosquito exposure.

Tick-borne encephalitis

- *Epidemiology*—*Ixodes* tick-borne viruses causing encephalitis include central European encephalitis (CEE) (principally in Austria and surrounding countries, but also Scandinavia and other parts of Europe), Russian spring–summer encephalitis (RSSE) (Eastern Russia, Korea, China, Japan), louping ill (Britain—an occupational disease of vets and butchers), the Siberian subtype (Vasilchenko virus), and Powassan virus (North America). Incidence is highly variable within countries at risk (e.g. RSSE occurs primarily in sylvatic locations). Viruses are transmitted between ticks and vertebrates, and passed vertically to tick offspring. Human infections are incidental and in central Europe tend to occur from April to November. Most cases occur in adults 20–50 years of age. Infection has been acquired by the consumption of unpasteurized milk from infected animals (CEE) and through handling infected meat (louping ill, CEE).

- *Clinical features*—incubation 7–14 days, but up to a month; 1 in 250 of CEE infections are symptomatic, and, of those, 5–30% develop neurological features. Illness is biphasic (initial phase may not be reported). Early features: fever, headache, malaise, vomiting. Symptoms resolve at 1 week. Those who develop the second neurological phase do so after a 2- to 10-day remission, after which fever, headache, and vomiting return. Neurological features: aseptic meningitis, encephalitis, myelitis (particularly shoulder girdle and upper limb paralysis which may be permanent), autonomic and bladder disturbances, bulbar involvement; 1% of cases are fatal (mostly elderly); 40% experience sequelae (ataxia, psychological disturbance). RSSE tends to be monophasic and more severe with seizures, coma, brainstem involvement, and serious neurological sequelae much commoner. Powassan virus produces a severe disease that may resemble herpes encephalitis. NB: a history of tick bite is only given in half of cases. Neuroborreliosis should be considered—both as a differential and because ticks and patients may be dually infected.
- *Laboratory findings*—early-phase leucopenia, late-phase leucocytosis, moderate CSF lymphocytosis.
- *Treatment and prevention*—treatment is supportive. Passive immunization with tick-borne encephalitis immunoglobulin has been tried, but there is a significant risk of exacerbating the disease. Inactivated vaccines are available and are widely used in areas at risk. Local control through the use of acaricides to reduce tick numbers is effective, but not practical, over large areas.

Other

- *West Nile fever*—the leading cause of epidemic viral encephalitis in the USA. Related to JE. Symptoms seen in 20–40% of infections. Presentations: a self-limiting febrile illness and arthropathy (very much like dengue), meningitis (especially children), encephalitis (especially adults), flaccid paralysis or mixed. Elderly people are at increased risk of severe disease, including hepatitis, pancreatitis, and myocarditis. Severe neurological disease leads to death in 5% of cases. It is transmitted between *Culex* mosquitoes and birds, and is the most widespread of the arboviruses (Africa, Europe, Asia, America, the Middle East). While a role for IFN-α and ribavirin has been suggested, there are no controlled trials supporting efficacy and anecdotal evidence of harm with the latter.
- *Murray Valley encephalitis*—related to West Nile and found in Australia and Papua New Guinea. Causes encephalitis with coma, limb paralysis, and respiratory depression in severe cases.
- *Kyasanur Forest disease and Omsk haemorrhagic fever*—related viruses transmitted by ticks and found only in the Kyasanur Forest of India and parts of Siberia, respectively. A 3- to 8-day incubation is followed by the abrupt onset of fever, headache, and photophobia, with hepatosplenomegaly and petechiae. Gum, GI tract, and pulmonary haemorrhage can occur, with renal failure in severe cases. Symptoms then remit for up to 3 weeks before the onset of a neurological syndrome. Case fatality: Kyasanur 5–10%, Omsk 3%.

Yellow fever

The type species of the genus *Flavivirus* (➔ see Flaviviruses, pp. 451–4).

Epidemiology

- Originated in Africa. Probably introduced into the Americas by mosquito-infested slave-trading ships. Now found in areas of sub-Saharan Africa and South America, but has not been documented in Asia.
- Two patterns of transmission occur:
  - urban (epidemic)—occurs in Africa and represents human-to-human transmission by *Aedes aegypti* mosquitoes. Outbreaks tend to be large due to the high density of both vector and human, combined with low vaccine coverage;
  - jungle (enzootic)—infection maintained in monkeys, transmission occurring via *Haemagogus* (South America) and *Aedes* (Africa) mosquitoes. Human cases occur when susceptible individuals are bitten by infected mosquitoes (e.g. forestry workers). Viraemic individuals may precipitate urban transmission cycles on returning home.
- African epidemic attack rates can be high (30 people in 1000, estimated >100 000 cases a year), with death rates of 20–50%. Declining epidemics reflect changes in viral activity and human immunity (natural and vaccination). In South America, a few hundred cases are reported each year, and urban outbreaks are unusual.
- Person-to-person transmission is theoretically possible in any area where the vector exists (including Southern USA).

Pathogenesis

- The virus is inoculated by mosquitoes and replicates in local lymph nodes, spreading via the bloodstream to other lymphoid sites and tissues.
- Viraemia peaks around days 5–6, corresponding with an increase in inflammatory cytokine production and the onset of symptoms.
- Widespread haemorrhages develop on mucosal surfaces, the skin, and other organs. Gastric erosions may precipitate haematemesis, and there can be extensive hepatocellular damage with lobular necrosis. Renal impairment may be secondary (pre-renal) or due directly to viral infection. Neurological impairment is usually due to oedema and haemorrhage, rather than encephalitis. Other features may include coagulation deficiency, myocarditis, and systemic inflammatory response syndrome (SIRS).

Clinical features

- Incubation—3–6 days. Mosquitoes may become infected if biting within the first 3–5 days of illness.
- Symptoms—range from asymptomatic to a haemorrhagic fever. Commonly biphasic, starting with abrupt-onset headache, fever, and myalgia lasting 3–4 days. Most people recover at this point. After a few hours'/days' respite, severe cases go on to a second phase of high fever, back pain, nausea, vomiting, abdominal pain, and drowsiness, before experiencing jaundice, hepatitis, and bleeding. Haematemesis, melaena, epistaxis, and petechial

and purpuric rashes may occur. Patients may become oliguric and uraemic. Other: myocarditis, arrhythmias, shock, metabolic acidosis, acute tubular necrosis, confusion, seizures, and unconsciousness.
- Laboratory findings—leucopenia in the early stages, thrombocytopenia, coagulation abnormalities, very high transaminases (AST may be more than ALT if myocarditis), normal or slightly raised ALP, uraemia, metabolic acidosis, albuminuria (a characteristic feature of yellow fever hepatitis), and raised CSF protein.
- Prognosis—those who survive the critical period commonly get bacterial pneumonia or sepsis. Hepatic recovery is good—chronic hepatitis is not a feature. Death rate in severe cases of haemorrhagic fever can be as high as 50%.

Diagnosis

- Severe yellow fever resembles other VHFs circulating in Africa and South America, so laboratory confirmation is required for conclusive diagnosis.
- Viral detection—frequently possible, as patients present while still viraemic, allowing the detection of viral antigens or virus culture. PCR-based assays are becoming more widely available. Viral cell culture is possible.
- Serology—in primary infections, IgM detection by ELISA is over 95% sensitive on serum samples taken 7–10 days after illness onset. In secondary infections, positive assays for IgG and IgM can be 100% sensitive at 5 days. Paired serum samples showing a 4-fold rise in titre confirm the diagnosis. Cross-reactivity is problematic in those who have been exposed to several flaviviruses. Neutralization assays are most specific but are only offered in specialized laboratories. Complement fixation assays can distinguish between the flavivirus complexes but rise at only 4–6 weeks after onset. ELISA rapid tests are available.

Treatment and prevention

- Treatment is supportive—fluid balance, management of coagulopathy and renal insufficiency, reducing the risk of GI bleeding, etc.
- In some areas of the world, it may be necessary to exclude the patient from mosquitoes to prevent onward transmission.
- The 17D vaccine is highly effective, and a single dose produces long-term protection in 95% of people. Travellers to at-risk countries should receive the vaccine every 10 years, although a single dose may provide lifelong protection. It is recommended for routine use in 35 African countries, but uptake is low.
- The vaccine should only be given to travellers entering an area of genuine risk. Vaccine complications include encephalitis (0.8 per 100 000), of which infants are at higher risk (it is contraindicated in those <4 months of age), and yellow fever vaccine-associated viscerotropic disease (0.4 per 100 000), a syndrome resembling yellow fever itself with a high fatality rate (63%). Risks factors include old age and thymus disease (e.g. myasthenia, thymoma). The estimated risk of death in an unvaccinated traveller to an endemic area is 1 in 5000.
- Vector reduction is difficult and expensive, but has been achieved in some areas.
- In South America, surveys to identify dead monkeys can warn of an increased risk to humans.

Dengue

A flavivirus (➔ see Flaviviruses, pp. 451–4) and arbovirus transmitted by *Aedes* mosquitoes (particularly *A. aegypti* and, to a lesser extent, *A. albopictus, A. polynesiensis*) causing fever (dengue fever, DF) that may be complicated by fluid leak, shock, and haemorrhage (dengue haemorrhagic fever, DHF).

Epidemiology

- Four distinct serotypes. Infection with one provides brief (<6 months) cross-protection to all four, after which immunity remains to the infecting serotype only. Later secondary infection with one of the other three is then associated with an increased risk of severe disease (DHF).
- Worldwide outbreaks of dengue began at the start of the twentieth century. 'Breakbone fever' was recorded in Australia in 1897. After the Second World War, transmission of multiple serotypes greatly increased in South East Asia—with a consequent increase in cases of DHF.
- Dengue occurs in regions of the tropics in which its vector is found: South East Asia, parts of South/Central America, and parts of sub-Saharan Africa. DHF can be endemic where >1 viral type circulates.
- It takes 2 weeks for a mosquito to become infective after feeding on a viraemic individual. *Aedes* are day-biting and easily disturbed, and a single mosquito can infect an entire household. They breed in open water (domestic containers, puddles, etc.); thus, urban transmission can be very intense.
- Around 3 billion people live in areas at risk of dengue, with 100 million cases per year of DF and 500 000 cases of dengue shock. Transmission occurs in two broad patterns:
  - epidemic—a single viral strain enters a region with sufficient susceptible hosts, causing an epidemic. Attack rates <50%. This was the pattern prior to the Second World War and remains so in island nations and pockets of Africa and South America;
  - hyperendemic—multiple serotypes circulate throughout the year, increasing in the rainy season. Incidence varies year to year, as host immunity changes and new viral strains emerge. In some regions, 5–10% of the population are infected annually.

Pathogenesis

- The virus disseminates in the blood within 2–3 days of an infected bite. Patients are viraemic for 4–5 days. Malaise reflects the cytokine response.
- Some patients, usually those previously infected, develop a severe immunopathological response (DHF), thought to be due to antibody-dependent enhancement; heterologous antibody is non-neutralizing and enhances viral uptake, increasing the infected cell mass. The consequently exaggerated inflammatory response includes vasoactive cytokines that contribute to fluid leak. Structural damage to blood vessels is not a feature (unlike Ebola).
- It is rare for individuals to have >2 episodes of dengue.

Clinical features

- DF—asymptomatic in up to 80% of infants and children (often difficult to distinguish from other causes of fever). Tends to be more severe in adults; 4–7 days' incubation, followed by abrupt fever, headache, muscle pain, and rash (macular erythema with petechiae on extensor surfaces), with rapid progression to prostration, and back and abdominal pain. Defervescence occurs after 2–7 days—it may settle and recur (saddleback fever pattern). Recovery may be followed by prolonged fatigue and occasionally depression. Other features: minor mucosal bleeding (severe in some cases, e.g. pre-existing peptic ulcer), subcapsular splenic bleeds, hepatitis, neurological features (may represent the effects of cerebral oedema or viral encephalitis).
- DHF (dengue shock syndrome)—the early features are identical to mild disease. Severe symptoms tend to occur at defervescence (when, notably, the viral load is falling rapidly), with reduced perfusion, central cyanosis, sweating, and other signs of shock. Platelets fall; petechiae develop, with spontaneous bruising and bleeding from mucosal surfaces. Fluid leak occurs (increase in haematocrit, pleural effusions, and ascites). The duration of illness is 7–10 days, and, with support in the critical period (fluid therapy, etc.), mortality is under 1%. Without support, death rates can reach 50%. Complications: encephalopathy, hepatic failure, renal failure, dual infections (Gram-negative sepsis, parasitic disease).

Diagnosis

- Clinical—DF is not easily distinguished from other causes of childhood febrile disease, and, even in cases of shock, DHF may resemble yellow fever. Leucopenia, low platelets, and abnormal LFTs are common.
- Viral detection—tests for viral RNA or NS1 antigen are available and more sensitive than serology in the early stages of illness. Useful in the first 3 days of illness or if IgM is negative on a sample in the first 6 days.
- Serology—less specific than PCR due to cross-reactivity between different flaviviruses. Neutralization assays allow different dengue serotypes to be distinguished in primary infection. Acute infection can only be confirmed by demonstrating a rise in acute/convalescent titre, e.g. IgM antibody capture (MAC)-ELISA for IgM (more specific to dengue complex)—detectable by day 6 of illness and persists for 30–90 days.

Treatment and prevention

- Supportive treatment—antipyretics, oral rehydration, close observation of fluid status with appropriate interventions (IV fluids, circulatory support); avoid invasive procedures.
- The WHO algorithm for classifying, monitoring, and identifying severe disease (e.g. 20% increase in haematocrit, narrowed pulse pressure, etc.) and guiding fluid replacement has been responsible for large falls in mortality.[3]
- Prevention—there are several experimental vaccines, but none in widespread use. Vector control is effective, but expensive, and rarely practical in the regions that most need it.

Reference

3 World Health Organization (2009). *Dengue guidelines for diagnosis, treatment, prevention and control*. Geneva: World Health Organization.

Viral haemorrhagic fevers

VHFs are severe, potentially life-threatening illnesses caused by members of several viral families (see Table 8.7). Most patients are not severely unwell when they present, and VHF should be considered as a cause of fever/rash/sore throat in patients who have visited at-risk areas within the last 21 days—*but* remember malaria is a much more likely diagnosis. Here we consider the filoviruses and arenaviruses. Certain bunyaviruses (➔ see *Bunyaviridae*, pp. 435–6) and flaviviruses (➔ see Flaviviruses, pp. 451–4) may cause similar presentations.

Table 8.7 Viral families causing viral haemorrhagic fevers

Virus	Source or vector	Distribution
Arenaviridae		
Junin (Argentine haemorrhagic fever)	Rodent	Agricultural areas of northern Buenos Aires province
Machupo (Bolivian haemorrhagic fever)	Rodent	North Eastern Bolivian savannah
Guanarito (Venezuelan haemorrhagic fever)	Rodent	Cleared forest areas of Venezuela
Lassa	Rodent	West Africa
Bunyaviridae		
Congo–Crimean haemorrhagic fever	Tick or contact with infected animals	CIS, the Middle East, Africa
Hantavirus (haemorrhagic fever with renal syndrome)	Rodent	Parts of China, Asia, Russia, and Europe
Rift Valley fever	Mosquito	Sub-Saharan Africa
Filoviridae		
Ebola	Unknown	DRC, Sudan, and Côte d'Ivoire
Marburg	Unknown	Uganda, Western Kenya
Flaviviridae		
Yellow fever	Human or monkey, via mosquito	South America, sub-Saharan Africa
Dengue	Human via mosquito	Asia, sub-Saharan Africa, South America
Omsk haemorrhagic fever	Tick	Siberia
Kyansanur Forest disease	Tick	Kyansanur Forest, India
Togaviridae		
Chikungunya	Mosquito	Africa and Asia

Management of suspected viral haemorrhagic fever

The following is drawn from guidance issued by the UK DH ACDP.[4] Refer to the full document at ℛ https://www.gov.uk/government/organisations/public-health-england.

- *Presentation*—early features are mild and non-specific: fever, cough, headache, sore throat, nausea, vomiting, weakness, and abdominal and chest pains. Severe features present later: haemorrhage, encephalopathy, hepatitis, shock. Patients are infectious after developing symptoms.
- *Differential diagnosis*—malaria should be excluded as soon as possible. Also consider typhoid fever, dengue, and rickettsial infection.
- *Infection control*—strict infection control precautions aim to prevent secondary infection of other patients, and hospital and laboratory staff. Onward transmission to other people requires contact with the patient or infected secretions—aerosol transmission is not thought to be a significant means of infection. Medical and laboratory staff should be meticulous in taking blood, handling fluids, disposing of excreta, and performing invasive procedures. Gloves, water-repellent aprons, face visors, and masks should be used. Sharps and other contaminated equipment should be disposed of extremely carefully. Recovering patients may excrete virus in the urine for weeks.
- *Risk assessment*—patients are classified as 'possibility' and 'high possibility' of VHF. Those with febrile illness who have cared for/had contact with body fluids from a suspected VHF case are automatically considered 'high possibility'. Those with fever who have returned from a VHF-endemic area within 21 days should be assessed as follows:
  - have they lived/worked in rural conditions where Lassa is endemic?
  - have they travelled to any area with a current VHF outbreak?
  - have they had tick exposure in an area endemic for CCHF?
  - have they visited caves or mines in a VHF-endemic area?
  - is fever persisting after 72 hours of antimalarials and antibiotics?
- If the answer to all these is 'no', they are considered to have 'possible VHF' and should be isolated and urgently screened for malaria. If they have bruising/bleeding, expert advice should be sought. If malaria negative and fever continues, an urgent VHF screen should be performed. If the answer to any of these questions is 'yes', they are considered 'high possibility of VHF', should be screened for malaria and VHF, and expert advice sought. If bruising/bleeding or VHF screen is positive, they should be transferred to a high-security medical facility.
- *Sample processing*—samples from a 'possible' case can be treated as normal. Samples from a 'high possibility' case should have urgent malaria and VHF screens sent. Routine tests can be performed locally at CL 2 with additional precautions. The laboratory must be informed of all specimens before receipt, so they can be segregated and processed separately with dedicated equipment. Such tests should be kept to a minimum.
- *VHF screen*—in the UK, these tests are performed by HPA Porton. A 24h service is provided, offering 24h molecular testing for VHF. Results are usually available within 6h of sample receipt. After seeking local/regional input, cases can be discussed with the service on 0844 778 8990.

Reference

4 Advisory Committee on Dangerous Pathogens (2015). *Management of Hazard Group 4 viral haemorrhagic fevers and similar human infectious diseases of high consequence*. Available at: https://www.gov.uk/government/uploads/system/uploads/attachment_data/file/478114/VHF_guidance_updated_7_Sept_15.pdf.

Filoviruses

Named after their characteristic filament-like morphology, filoviruses are elongated structures, 80nm across and 800–1000nm long. Genetic material is negative-sense ssRNA. The two agents identified (Ebola and Marburg) show no serological cross-reactivity. Details of their natural history remain elusive. Viral particles are stable and highly infective.

Epidemiology

- Outbreaks emerge abruptly. Source may be traced to a single human or primate index case, but no further.
- Exact routes of transmission unknown. Infection acquired parenterally has a high mortality, but most infections probably occur through skin or mucous membrane contact with infected bodily fluids. Aerosol transmission has taken place, with devastating consequences amongst HCWs (following medical procedures), sexual transmission, burial ceremonies and contaminated surfaces and materials are important.
- Marburg virus—identified in 1967 when African green monkeys brought from Uganda to Germany developed a haemorrhagic illness subsequently transmitted to humans (seven deaths amongst 31 cases). Primary cases associated with close contact with monkey blood or cell culture, and secondary cases with human blood exposure. Cases have occurred in Western Kenya and Zimbabwe. Mortality is around 25%.
- Ebola—identified in 1976. Five subtypes identified: Zaire, Sudan, Côte d'Ivoire, Bundibugyo, and Reston. The latter appears to be maintained in an animal reservoir in the Philippines and was first identified after an outbreak amongst macaques imported from there to the USA. Early Ebola outbreaks were exacerbated through the use of infected needles. Without precautions, rates of infection of household contacts can reach 17%. Case fatality rates range from 30% (Bundibugyo) to over 80% (Zaire subtype). See WHO Fact Sheet No. 103 for details of the large and complex West African Ebola outbreak in 2014/15.

Clinical features

- Incubation 5–10 days. Abrupt onset of fever, myalgia, and headache. Nausea, vomiting, abdominal pain, diarrhoea, and chest pain follow. Petechiae, haemorrhages, and spontaneous bruising occur, as disease progresses. A maculopapular rash can develop around the fifth day.
- In week 2, patients either become afebrile and improve, or develop shock and multiorgan dysfunction with DIC, and renal and liver failure.
- Convalescence is prolonged. The virus is detectable in semen/urine for weeks.

Diagnosis

- Clinical clues—travel to at-risk areas or contact with monkeys, maculopapular rash (not seen with other VHFs).
- Rapid ELISA and RT-PCR-based tests are available. These are performed only by specialist laboratories.

Treatment and prevention

- There are no specific treatments—management is supportive.
- Prevention—early recognition, patient isolation, and barrier nursing.
- Clinical trials of Ebola vaccines are underway.

Arenaviruses (Lassa fever)

A family of ssRNA viruses. All are parasites of rodents, each virus showing specificity for a single rodent species. Here we consider Lassa fever. Other members include lymphocytic choriomeningitis virus (➔ see p. 432; a cause of fever and meningitis) and the *Tacaribe* complex of viruses (causes of VHF in South America).

Epidemiology

- Found in West Africa. The multimammate rat hosts are chronically infected and show no evidence of disease. Humans are infected through contact with excreta.
- Unlike other arenaviruses, person-to-person transmission of Lassa can occur. Endemic transmission occurs throughout the year, with nosocomial outbreaks (where aerosol and parenteral transmission have been implicated) in the dry season.

Clinical features

- Incubation 7–12 days. Most infections in Africa are mild, with severe disease in <10% of cases—mortality in this group can be as high as 25%.
- Symptoms—fever, chest pain, back and abdominal pain, cough, vomiting, diarrhoea, sore throat, conjunctivitis, facial oedema, and CNS features (encephalitis, meningism).
- Severe cases in the second week—shock, fluid leak (facial and pulmonary oedema, ascites, pleural effusions), mild haemorrhages from mucosal surfaces. Pregnancies in maternal infections frequently abort—high maternal mortality.
- Late complications in less severe cases—cranial nerve deafness (up to one-third of hospitalized cases), pericarditis, uveitis, and orchitis.

Diagnosis

- Viral detection—culture from blood, throat swabs, and urine is possible within the first 7–10 days.
- Serology—IgM detection is rapid and sensitive, around 75% of patients being positive on admission in Sierra Leone in one study.

Treatment and prevention

- No vaccine available.
- Ribavirin therapy initiated before day 7 reduces mortality significantly (from 55% to 5% in one study) but improves survival at all stages of illness.

- Contacts should be monitored for development of illness, with early presumptive use of ribavirin if fever develops.
- Nosocomial transmission can be reduced through barrier nursing and isolation, wherever possible (person-to-person spread by aerosol appears to occur).
- Rodent control is rarely practical in the countries affected.
- PEP with ribavirin may have a role after a known high-risk exposure (e.g. mucous membrane contamination by blood from a known case).

Rabies virus

Present throughout history, rabies (Latin 'madness') virus produces near uniformly fatal encephalitis.

The virus

- Negative-sense ssRNA virus, a member of the family *Rhabdoviridae*, genus *Lyssavirus*. Virions are bullet-shaped (180nm long by 75nm wide).
- The genus has six members—classic rabies is serotype 1. The other five rarely cause human disease (e.g. European bat lyssavirus 2 caused the death of a bat handler in Scotland in 2003).

Epidemiology

- Worldwide, with the exception of Antarctica and certain islands; 25 000–61,000 deaths each year, most in Asia and mostly rural.
- Many mammals maintain and transmit rabies; dogs account for 54% of animal cases; also foxes, raccoons, and bats (4%). Other susceptible animal species develop disease and do not transmit (camels, horses).
- Epidemiology of human disease reflects the pattern of animal infection. In developing regions, most human cases are acquired through dog bites. Developed nations have largely eliminated disease from domestic animals—most human infections follow exposure to rabid wild animals. Cases have followed corneal and solid organ transplantation.
- Animal rabies has been increasing in the USA, generally in raccoons. Two to three fatal human cases are reported in the USA each year. In the UK, the last locally acquired human case of *classical* rabies occurred in 1902. There have been 25 rabies deaths in the UK since 1946—all were imported, and none received PEP.

Pathogenesis

- The virus enters through a break in the skin or across mucosal surfaces, attaching to muscle and nerve cells. Replicates within muscle cells.
- Antirabies immunoglobulin and vaccine can prevent spread at this stage—once the peripheral nerve is entered, it cannot be stopped.
- Nerve innervating the muscle is infected first. Replication continues in peripheral neurons, as viral particles migrate along the axon by retrograde axoplasmic flow (50–100mm/day), unlike HSV which uses microtubular transport systems and therefore infects faster.
- On reaching the cord, the rabies virus spreads throughout the CNS, reaching the rest of the body (e.g. saliva) via peripheral nerves.

- The mechanism of CNS damage is uncertain. It may interfere with neurotransmission or act in an excitotoxic manner. The post-mortem brain in furious rabies is characteristic of encephalitis with Negri bodies (round eosinophilic cytoplasmic inclusions). These are concentrated in hippocampal pyramidal cells but may be found in cortical neurons. Paralytic rabies affects the spinal cord (inflammation and necrosis) and may cause segmental demyelination. Myocarditis can occur.

Clinical features

- Risk of acquiring rabies is related to the size of the inoculum (e.g. multiple bites, bite directly on the skin versus through clothing) and the location of the bite (greater risk with the face, compared to extremities).
- Incubation—days to years; most develop symptoms within 3 months.
- Initial symptoms—fever, headache, malaise, vomiting, with altered sensation at the bite site, subtle personality changes. May see myo-oedema (localized contraction of the muscle when struck with a tendon hammer, disappearing over a few seconds).
- Acute neurological disease develops 4–10 days later. Coma follows after 2–14 days. Patients die an average of 18 days after symptom onset. Two main clinical presentations:
  - furious (encephalitic) rabies (80% of cases)—anxiety, biting, hydrophobia (an exaggerated respiratory tract irritant reflex), delirium, agitation, seizures, hyperventilation, pituitary dysfunction (e.g. diabetes insipidus), cardiac arrhythmias, autonomic dysfunction (pupillary dilatation, salivation, priapism);
  - paralytic rabies (20% of cases)—the spinal cord and brainstem are predominantly affected, and patients develop an ascending paralysis that may resemble GBS or a symmetrical quadriparesis. Meningeal signs may develop, then confusion and coma.

Diagnosis

- Incubation—no tests are useful; assess risk of exposure to a potentially rabid animal, and promptly initiate prophylactic treatment.
- Symptomatic—the standard is direct fluorescent antibody staining of a skin biopsy taken from the nape of the neck; the virus localizes in hair follicles (50% positive in the first week of illness). PCR of biopsies is 98% sensitive/specific, PCR of saliva nearly 100% if three samples tested.

Treatment and prevention

- Prevention—reducing disease in animal populations is central to the control of human disease. Vaccination of cats and dogs is a legal requirement in many countries, and vaccination of wild animals is effective in regions that can maintain it.
- Pre-exposure vaccination—generally offered to those in high-risk occupations or travelling to at-risk countries with limited access to medical facilities. Three IM or intradermal injections on days 0, 7, and 21. Booster dose every 2–3 years, based on serology (if titre low).

- Post-exposure treatment (PET)—wound care by thorough washing with 20% soap solution and irrigation with a virucidal agent (e.g. iodine) may reduce the risk of rabies by as much as 90%. Local advice should be sought regarding the risk of rabies. Observe the animal for 10 days if apparently healthy—it should undergo pathological examination if its behaviour changes. PET should be started immediately, if thought necessary. It has a good record and appears safe in pregnancy. Immunocompromised patients may not respond sufficiently to vaccination and should have antibody titres checked at 2–4 weeks.
  - *If not previously vaccinated*, rabies immunoglobulin is infiltrated around the wound, with any remaining dose given IM at an anatomical site distant from that of vaccine administration. Vaccine then given IM deltoid on days 0, 3, 7, 14, and 30.
  - *If previously vaccinated*, immunoglobulin should not be given, and vaccine should be given IM deltoid on days 0 and 3.
- Treatment after symptom onset—generally, treatment initiated after symptom onset is of no benefit. The 'Milwaukee' protocol involves induction of coma with ketamine and midazolam, high-dose ribavirin, and amantadine.[5] There are case reports of its success, but also of its failure. There is no role for vaccine or immunoglobulin.

Reference

5 Willoughby RE, Tieves KS, Hoffman GM, *et al.* (2005). Survival after treatment of rabies with induction of coma. *New Engl J Med.* **352**:2508–14.

Prion diseases

Prions (proteinaceous infectious particle) are small infectious pathogens responsible for a number of transmissible neurodegenerative diseases. They contain protein and are resistant to procedures that modify or hydrolyse nucleic acid, but are fairly sensitive to procedures that digest or denature protein. The five human diseases all have certain properties in common:

- pathologic manifestations confined largely to the CNS;
- long incubation times (kuru up to 30 years);
- progressive and fatal;
- similar neuropathological features (astrocytosis with little inflammatory response and usually small vacuoles—the spongiform change);
- accumulation of an abnormal (PrPSc) form of a host protein (PrPc). They have very different biological properties—PrPc is sensitive to protease degradation and exists predominantly on the cell surface in an α-helix form; PrPSc is resistant to protease degradation and is found predominantly intracellularly with a β-sheet secondary structure. The normal function of PrPc is unknown. It appears that the presence of PrPSc (derived from an exogenous source or formed endogenously in familial diseases) triggers conformational change in PrPc (analogous to crystallization), producing PrPSc in an exponential manner.

Creutzfeldt–Jakob disease (CJD) and variant CJD

- *Familial CJD*—autosomal dominant disorder with variable penetrance. Mean age of onset is around 65 years and the longest clinical course. Several mutations in the gene encoding prion protein have been identified in familial CJD, and some have associations with particular disease phenotypes (e.g. age of onset, rate of progression). Prion gene mutations are very rarely found in cases of sporadic CJD.
- *Sporadic CJD* (sCJD, around 90% instances)—incidence 1 per million worldwide. Age of onset 57–62 years. Cases have occurred in older teenagers. Early onset should prompt the consideration of iatrogenic sources of infection: cadaveric growth hormone and gonadotropin, dural grafts, corneal transplants, liver transplants, and contaminated neurosurgical instruments. The illness duration is around 4–8 months. Presents with rapidly progressive dementia and myoclonus. Around a third experience visual or cerebellar features in early stages. Myoclonus can be aggravated if the patient is startled. Two-thirds of patients eventually develop extrapyramidal signs; 40–80% develop corticospinal tract signs such as hyper-reflexia and spasticity; visual features include cortical blindness and agnosia. Seizures, sensory signs, cranial nerve lesions, and autonomic dysfunction may occur but are uncommon.
- *New variant CJD* (vCJD)—distinct from sCJD, affecting younger patients (mean age 29 years), with a longer illness (14 months) and a distinct clinical presentation. vCJD is attributed to consumption of cattle infected with bovine spongiform encephalopathy (BSE). A large outbreak of BSE in the UK in the 1980s/1990s was attributed to cattle feed made from scrapie-infected sheep carcasses. It peaked in 1992, 4 years after the introduction of a ban on ruminant feed. Five million animals were slaughtered, in the effort to halt the epidemic. By July 2012, 176 human cases of definite or probable vCJD had been reported in the UK—all died. Cases peaked in 2000 (27 diagnoses) and have now fallen to around one diagnosis per year. There have been four cases of vCJD infection associated with blood transfusion (none since 2006). Symptoms are sensory (pain and paraesthesiae of face, hands, feet, and legs) and psychiatric (depression, delusions—until dementia obscures). Unlike sCJD, there is prominent cerebellar involvement and widespread PrPSc-positive amyloid plaques throughout the cerebellum and cerebrum.
- *Diagnosis*—routine tests, including standard CSF examination, are rarely helpful. Other causes of dementia and encephalopathy should be excluded (e.g. syphilis, HIV, nutritional, metabolic).
  - Imaging—MRI may pick up abnormalities associated with CJD and certain findings specific to vCJD, but scans can be normal.
  - EEG—between 70% and 95% of patients ultimately develop a typical pattern of slow background waves interrupted by generalized, bilaterally synchronous, biphasic or triphasic periodic sharp wave complexes. They are said to be 91% specific for sCJD and are not seen in vCJD.

  - CSF protein markers—protein 14-3-3 (92% sensitive, 80% specific in sCJD, but only 50% and 91%, respectively, in vCJD), tau protein (best sensitivity and specificity for vCJD). Elevations may be seen in HSV encephalitis, metabolic encephalopathies, and cerebral metastases.
  - Tonsil biopsy—patients with vCJD (but not sporadic) may have detectable PrPSc in follicular dendritic cells within lymphoid germinal centres. This is highly sensitive and specific for vCJD.
  - The gold standard remains examination of brain material: spongiform change, neuronal loss, reactive gliosis, and little inflammatory response. PrPSc can be identified by Western blot of material obtained at autopsy or biopsy.
- *Treatment*—all prion diseases are invariably fatal, and there is no effective therapy. Symptom progression has apparently slowed in individual patients treated with pentosan polysulfate.
- *Prevention*—people at increased risk of CJD (e.g. recipients of blood or organs from a donor who went on to develop it, those treated with human growth hormone before 1985) should not donate blood or tissue and alert medical staff if they need to undergo any procedures. See Box 8.1; full details are available in the CJD section of https://www.gov.uk/government/organisations/public-health-england.

Kuru

Originally endemic within a specific tribal group of Papua New Guinea, epidemiological studies suggested it was transmitted through ritual cannibalism, and there have been no further cases since the practice was abandoned. A prodromal phase of headache and arthralgia is followed by progressive neurological decline (ataxia, tremor, choreoathetosis, myoclonus) and dementia. Cranial nerve abnormalities, weakness, and sensory loss occur late in the disease, if at all. Laboratory tests are unhelpful, and EEG does not share the characteristic features of those seen in some cases of CJD. The pathologically distinct feature of kuru is the presence of PrPSc plaques, predominantly in the cerebellum (similar, but not identical, to those seen in vCJD).

Box 8.1 Transmission of prion diseases

(See ➲ pp. 169–72) Kuru, CJD, and BSE have been transmitted to primates via the oral route. Repeated oral inoculations are more effective than single doses. There is no evidence that ingestion is a means of transmission for sCJD, GSS, or FFI. The highest concentrations of infectious material are to be found in the brain, spinal cord, and eye, with material also present in the CSF, lymphoreticular organs, lung, and kidney. Iatrogenic transmission appears to require direct inoculation, implantation, or transplantation of infectious material. In terms of HCWs' protection, universal precautions are adequate, and care should be taken to identify and safely dispose of material that may carry an infection risk. There are specific guidelines for the performing of autopsies in suspected cases of CJD. For guidance, use *Minimise transmission risk of CJD and vCJD in healthcare settings*, published by the UK ACDP TSE Risk Management Subgroup (available via the PHE website).

Gerstmann–Sträussler–Scheinker syndrome

A rare prion disease (<10 cases/100 million people per year), predominantly familial in nature. It is inherited in an autosomal dominant fashion, with nearly complete penetrance. The key feature is spinocerebellar degeneration, with dementia developing at a mean age of around 43–48 years. Average illness duration is 5 years. It is associated with several prion protein gene mutations, which may contribute to the clinical heterogeneity—some families have prominent dementia; and others have extrapyramidal signs, for example. Within a family, the same mutation can produce a varied phenotype. Laboratory tests are helpful only insofar as they may allow the exclusion of other diagnoses. Definitive diagnosis requires the examination of the brain, which shows the finding typical of prion disease, together with plaques similar to those of kuru and vCJD. These plaques may have an atypical distribution, resembling that of Alzheimer's disease. In the past, some cases may have been diagnosed as Alzheimer's disease.

Fatal familial insomnia

Fatal familial insomnia (FFI) is a prion disease showing autosomal dominant inheritance and presenting in middle age or above (range 35–61 years) with insomnia, autonomic dysfunction, and motor abnormalities (ataxia, myoclonus, etc.). Patients can experience hallucinations, confusion, and memory problems, but dementia is rare. Some patients develop endocrine disturbance (increased cortisol, loss of circadian pattern of growth hormone secretion). Average disease duration is 13 months. Neuropathology (neuronal loss, gliosis) is focused in thalamic nuclei, with changes seen occasionally in the cerebellar and cerebral cortices. Spongiform change is rare. PrPSc concentrations are the lowest of the prion diseases. Changes may be seen in EEG and sleep studies.

Chapter 9

Fungi

Overview of fungi 470
Candida species 472
Superficial *Candida* infections 475
Invasive *Candida* infections 476
Treatment of *Candida* 478
Malassezia infections 478
Other yeasts 479
Cryptococcus 480
Pneumocystis jiroveci 482
Aspergillus 484
Mucormycosis 489
Eumycetoma 491
Dermatophytes 492
Other moulds 494
Sporothrix schenckii 495
Chromomycosis 497
Histoplasma capsulatum—ACDP 3 498
Blastomyces dermatitidis—ACDP 3 503
Coccidioides immitis—ACDP 3 505
Paracoccidioides brasiliensis—ACDP 3 508
Penicillium marneffei—ACDP 3 509

Overview of fungi

Fungi are aerobic eukaryotes with limited anaerobic capabilities. They have chitinous cell walls and ergosterol-containing plasma membranes (human cell walls contain cholesterol). They may grow as yeasts (single-celled, reproduce by budding), moulds (form multicellular hyphae which grow by branching and extension), or both—dimorphic, growing as yeasts *in vivo* and at 37°C *in vitro*, but as moulds at 25°C.

Reproduction

Fungal reproduction may be sexual or asexual. Virtually all fungi can produce asexual spores by mitosis. Sexual spores are formed by the fusion of two haploid nuclei, followed by meiotic division of the diploid nucleus. Certain fungi can only sexually reproduce with other colonies of a different compatible mating type (e.g. *Histoplasma* spp.).

Pathogenesis

Fungal infections may be cutaneous (e.g. dermatophyte infection), subcutaneous (e.g. following traumatic inoculation—sporotrichosis), or systemic (see Table 9.1). Systemic mycoses usually follow inhalation-acquired primary lung infection but may be caused by normal flora in an immunocompromised host (e.g. *C. albicans*). Disease may be a consequence of toxin production (e.g. aflatoxin) or the host immune response to an infecting agent. Organism characteristics facilitating infection include: good growth at 37°C, the production of substances such as keratinases by dermatophytes (digest keratin in skin, hair, nails), the ability to change form (exist in nature as moulds but take on yeast forms in a host, allowing them to spread and become pathogenic), and the ability to adhere to surfaces (e.g. *C. albicans*), antiphagocytic capsules (*C. neoformans*) or persist following phagocytosis, allowing dissemination via macrophages. Generally, hosts have a high level of innate immunity to fungi—most infections are mild and self-limiting. This resistance derives from the fatty acid content of the skin, pH of the skin, mucosal surfaces and body fluids, epithelial turnover, competition with the normal bacterial flora, transferrin, and cilia of respiratory tract. Cell-mediated immunity (CMI) is important in controlling fungal infection. Humoral responses play a part, but patients with defects in CMI experience more severe fungal infections than those with humoral defects.

Epidemiology

- Host factors—immunocompromise leads to a general increase in opportunistic fungal infections. Certain conditions predispose to specific organisms: diabetic ketoacidosis and rhinocerebral mucormycosis, AIDS and histoplasmosis, antibiotics and candidal vaginitis.
- Environment affects the pattern of fungal disease. Some are worldwide but seen mostly in individuals whose lifestyles place them at risk of exposure (e.g. a gardener experiencing s/c inoculation of *S. schenckii* through minor trauma). Others are more likely to be seen in people living in, or visiting, specific regions (e.g. *C. immitis* in the desert of south-western USA).

Table 9.1 Overview of common fungi causing human disease

Phylum	Organism	Syndrome				Comment
		D	O	SC	SU	
Basidiomycota	**Yeasts**					
	Cryptococcus neoformans	–	–			Mild lung granuloma in healthy
	Trichosporon beigelii		–		–	May disseminate
	Rhodotorula spp.		–			
	Malassezia furfur		–		–	Pityriasis versicolor
Ascomycota	*Candida* spp.		–		–	
	Pneumocystis jiroveci (was *carinii*)		–			
	Dimorphic fungi					
	Histoplasma capsulatum	–				Histoplasmosis
	Blastomyces dermatitidis	–				Blastomycosis
	Sporothrix schenkii	–	–	–		Acquired by local trauma. Rare dissemination
	Coccidioides immitis, *Paracoccidioides brasilensis*	–				In the Americas
	Penicillium spp.		–			Disseminate in immunosuppressed
	Moulds					
	Aspergillus spp.	–	–	–		Allergic, localized and invasive disease
	Epidermophyton spp., *Trichophyton* spp., *Microsporum* spp.				–	Dermatophytes—infect skin, hair, and nails
	Fusarium spp.		–	–		Disseminate in immunosuppressed
	Pseudallescheria boydii		–	–		Mycetoma. May also infect any organ or disseminate
	Madurella spp., *Acremonium* spp., *Exophilia* spp., etc.			–		Mycetoma
Zygomycota	*Mucor* spp., *Rhizopus* spp.	–	–			Rare invasion, e.g. mucormycosis

D, disseminated infection; O, opportunistic infection; SC, subcutaneous infection; SU, superficial infection.

Candida species

A yeast and the commonest cause of fungal infection. *C. albicans* is responsible for 90% of cases of infection and for 40–50% of cases of fungaemia. Non-albicans species are increasingly associated with invasive candidiasis and tend to be more resistant to certain antifungal drugs. *Candida* in a blood culture should never be viewed as a contaminant—look for a source.

Mycology and epidemiology

- Small ovoid cells that reproduce by budding. Both sexual and asexual forms exist. Of the over 150 *Candida* spp., only nine are frequent human pathogens—*C. glabrata* and *C. albicans* account for ~70–80% of cases of invasive candidiasis. The others are: *C. guilliermondii, C. krusei, C. parapsilosis, C. tropicalis, C. pseudotropicalis, C. lusitaniae*, and *C. dubliniensis*.
- *C. albicans* is ubiquitous and may be found in soil, food, and hospital environments. They are normal commensals of humans (skin, sputum, GI tract, female genital tract, etc.). The vast majority of human infections are of endogenous origin.
- *C. krusei* is found in many environmental sites. It is fluconazole-resistant and often found colonizing patients receiving fluconazole prophylaxis.
- *C. parapsilosis* (adheres well to synthetic materials) and *C. tropicalis* are now commoner causes of IV catheter infections and endocarditis than *C. albicans*.
- *C. glabrata* infections of ICU patients are associated with a low survival rate. *Candida* spp. are uncommon laboratory contaminants.

Pathogenesis

The rise of *Candida* spp. infection relates to the increase in medical interventions: the use of antibiotics (suppressing normal bacterial flora and permitting the proliferation of *Candida* organisms), IV catheters (providing a route of entry) or prosthetic implants, and GI tract surgery. Immune suppression mediated by disease (e.g. HIV) or therapies, such as steroids, are also associated with increased rates of infection. The immune response to *Candida* infection is mediated by humoral and cellular mechanisms (cf. patients with AIDS who demonstrate high susceptibility to cutaneous infection). *Candida* spp. virulence factors include surface molecules that permit organism adherence to other structures (human cells, extracellular matrix, prosthetic devices), acid proteases, and the ability to convert to a hyphal form.

General points on diagnosis

- Many patients will require early treatment in the absence of a conclusive microbiological diagnosis. Those at risk (e.g. the neutropenic) who remain febrile, despite broad-spectrum antibiotic therapy, should be suspected of having systemic candidiasis. Therapy should be started early and empirically in such patients. Always consider positive culture results from sterile sites to be significant. *Candida* may contaminate BCs, but treatment is usually indicated, as distinguishing contamination from infection is very difficult. BCs are positive in 50–60% of cases of disseminated disease. Serology is rarely useful.

- *Culture*—strict aerobes that grow well when present in biopsy specimens. Unfortunately, BCs in proven candidaemia are positive in only around 60% of cases (usually within 48–96h). Yeast forms (Gram-positive) and hyphae may be found on microscopy of clinical specimens (facilitated by 10% KOH). Appear as smooth, white colonies on agar. Presumptive identification of *C. albicans* is possible by inoculating organisms from a colony into a small tube of serum—germ tubes should form within 90min, which tend not to be seen with the other species (relatively high rates of false positives and false negatives). Accurate speciation relies on physiological characteristics (e.g. fermentation, nitrate utilization) and can be demonstrated on commercial indicator agar preparations (ChromAgar™) and with multiparameter kits.
- *Fungal antigen detection assays*—are useful adjuncts in the diagnosis and monitoring of invasive fungal infection:
  - 1-3 beta-*D*-glucan—a cell wall component in a wide variety of fungi, except *Cryptococcus* and the zygomycetes. It is a broad-spectrum assay that detects *Aspergillus, Candida, Fusarium, Acremonium*, and *Saccharomyces* spp. The commercial blood assay (Glucatell®) has a sensitivity of 75–100% and a specificity of 88–100% for candidaemia. Its negative predictive value is useful, but the positive predictive value is limited by the ubiquitous nature of glucan (e.g. positive due to exposure to the cellulose in certain haemodialysis membranes, or surgical gauze);
  - *Candida* mannan assay—sensitivity ranges from 31% to 90% (less for non-albicans species).
- *Sensitivity testing*—*in vitro* susceptibility testing can help guide the treatment of candidiasis to a greater extent than for the other fungi. Testing is not always available locally. Knowledge of the infecting species is highly predictive of likely susceptibility and can be used to guide therapy. Susceptibility testing is important in managing deep infections of non-albicans species, particularly if the patient has been previously treated with an azole. *C. albicans* is rarely resistant to azoles, whereas certain non-albicans species may show intrinsic resistance to these and certain other antifungal agents (see Table 9.2).

Table 9.2 Treatment of *Candida* infections

Presentation	First-line treatment	Duration	Comment
Candidaemia in non-neutropenic adults	Flucon or echino (alternative LFAmB or voricon)	14 days after first negative BC and resolution of symptoms	Remove intravascular catheters. Eye exam. Echino if moderate/ severe or recent azole exposure
Candidaemia in neutropenic adults	Echino or LFAmB. (alternative flucon or voricon)	Duration uncertain, but at least 14–21 days after first negative BC, resolution of symptoms, and resolved neutropenia	Flucon only in those without previous exposure with mild illness. Voricon if mould coverage desirable. IVC removal advised

(*Continued*)

Table 9.2 (*Contd.*)

Presentation	First-line treatment	Duration	Comment
Suspected candidaemia in neutropenia	LFAmB, caspo, or voricon (alternative flucon if no prior exposure)	Uncertain	Consider antifungals in neutropenia after 4 days of fever unresponsive to antibiotics
Chronic disseminated candidiasis	Flucon if stable, LFAmB in unwell (alternative echino)	Until resolution or calcification of radiological lesions (usually months)	Flucon may be given after 1–2 weeks of AmB therapy if stable or improved
Candidal cystitis	Flucon (alternative AmB-d or 5-FC). Modify once culture results available	2 weeks	Remove/replace stents/catheters. High-risk patients should be treated as disseminated, even if asymptomatic
Pyelonephritis	Flucon (alternative AmB-d with/ without 5-FC)	2 weeks	If suspected dissemination, treat as such
Endocarditis	LFAmB with/ without 5-FC (alternative echino). Flucon step down if sensitive	Variable, depending on surgical outcome	Valve replacement is nearly always necessary. Long-term suppression with flucon if this is not possible
Meningitis	LFAmB with/ without 5-FC	Several weeks	Flucon follow on therapy
Endophthalmitis	AmB-d with 5-FC (alternative flucon or LFAmB)	At least 6 weeks, as determined by repeated eye exam	Vitrectomy is usually necessary if vitritis present
Oropharyngeal candidiasis	Clo or nystatin or flucon PO (alternative itracon, voricon, or AmB oral suspension)	7–14 days after clinical improvement	Topical for mild, flucon for moderate/ severe
Oesophageal candidiasis	Flucon PO (alternative echino, AmB-d, itracon, voricon)	14–12 days	IV therapy may be required in severe cases

AmB-d, amphotericin B deoxycholate; caspo, caspofungin; clo, clotrimazole; echino, an echinocandin; 5-FC, 5-flucytosine; flucon, fluconazole; itracon, itraconazole; LFAmB, liposomal amphotericin B; voricon, voriconazole.

Superficial *Candida* infections

For details of the cutaneous manifestations of candidal infection,  see Fungal skin infections—candida, p. 766.

Mucous membrane infection

Thrush

A form of oral candidiasis characterized by white, creamy patches on the tongue and oral mucosa. Scraping removes the lesions, leaving a sore bleeding surface. Diagnosis can be confirmed using a KOH smear or Gram stain to demonstrate hyphae and yeast forms. Other manifestations include acute atrophic candidiasis (affecting the tongue), chronic atrophic candidiasis (associated with denture use), angular cheilitis (not caused solely by *Candida*), and *Candida* leukoplakia (white plaques affecting the cheek, lips, and tongue; may be pre-cancerous). Oral thrush is associated with the use of inhaled steroids (often resolves spontaneously, even without reduction in steroid use, or with topical therapy), malignancy, and AIDS. Treatment is usually topical (systemic where this fails). Prophylaxis with fluconazole has been effective in the prevention of oral *Candida* infections in cancer and AIDS patients, but remains controversial. It is no longer routinely recommended in AIDS patients, due to the development of resistance. It does reduce the rate of clinical candidiasis in patients undergoing immunosuppressive therapy.

Candida oesophagitis

The majority of cases are associated with HIV or the treatment of malignant disease of the haematopoietic or lymphatic systems. May occur in the absence of oral disease. Symptoms include dysphagia, retrosternal chest pain, nausea, and vomiting. Symptoms may be mild, even in extensive disease. Diagnosis is made by endoscopy and biopsy. In practice, diagnosis is often made presumptively in those with AIDS or malignancy, on the basis of oral thrush and symptoms of oesophagitis. Extensive disease may result in intraluminal protrusions and partial obstruction. Perforation is rare. Severely immunocompromised patients may be co-infected with CMV or HSV. Fluconazole has been demonstrated to have greater efficacy than ketoconazole in AIDS patients with *Candida* oesophagitis.

Gastrointestinal candidiasis

Usually associated with malignant disease, the commonest manifestation being focal invasion of benign stomach ulcers. Diffuse gastric mucosal involvement is rare. Small and large bowel infection also occurs with white plaques, erosions, pseudomembrane, and ulceration visible on endoscopy.

Vulvovaginitis

Candida is the commonest cause of vaginitis, and 75% of women have at least one episode in their lives. Predisposing factors include diabetes, antibiotic therapy, and pregnancy. Oedema and vulval pruritus may be accompanied by discharge that may be scanty or thick. Secondary infection of perineal skin and the urethra can occur.

Invasive *Candida* infections

Candidaemia/candidiasis

Patients at risk of dissemination include those with malignancy (particularly acute leukaemia), burns patients, and those with complicated post-operative courses (e.g. organ transplants, GI tract surgery). Multiple organs tend to be affected. The pathological features are small abscesses and diffuse microabscesses with a granulomatous reaction. While it *may* represent colonization of a venous catheter, *Candida* in a BC should be treated with antifungals, and the patient examined carefully for manifestations of disseminated disease. Incidence is rising with the increased number of susceptible patients and use of indwelling catheters. Presentation varies from mild fever to severe sepsis, and it can spread haematogenously to multiple organs. Always check for endocarditis and eye involvement (chorioretinitis or vitritis in ~25%), and consider other sites: skin (pustules/nodules), renal/muscle abscess, prosthetic vascular devices, CNS. Disease may be more extensive than symptoms suggest. Management always involves removal of lines or prosthetic material. BCs are positive in <60% of those with proven candidaemia, and diagnosis is often made very late or at post-mortem. Tests for *Candida* antigen have a high rate of false-negative results—diagnosis is largely clinical. Cultures should be repeated several times, and catheters removed or replaced (but not by passing the new one over a wire at the site of the old). Speciation and isolate sensitivity should be confirmed. Therapy should be continued for at least 2 weeks after the first negative BC.

CNS candidiasis

May infect both brain substance and meninges. Around 50% of *Candida* meningitis cases occur in the context of disseminated disease. Meningitis may present non-specifically or with features typical of meningism. Parenchymal infection takes the form of scattered multiple microabscesses and can have extremely variable clinical presentations. Infection may follow trauma, neurosurgery, or colonization of a ventricular shunt. CSF may show lymphocytosis, with low glucose, but these findings are not consistent. Organisms are visible on Gram stain in 40% of cases. The mortality rate is very high without therapy. Complications: hydrocephalus.

Cardiac candidiasis

Candida endocarditis usually affects the aortic and mitral valves. Associations include valve disease, chemotherapy, implantation of prosthetic heart valves, prolonged use of IVCs, heroin addiction (*C. parapsilosis* the commonest cause), and pre-existing bacterial endocarditis. Around 50% of cases follow cardiac surgery (associated with the length of the post-operative course reflecting the use of IV lines and antibiotics). Most cases present within the first 2 months post-operatively; <40% of cases are caused by non-albicans species; >70% of patients have positive BCs. Prior to antifungal therapy, mortality was 90%. Combined prolonged (6–10 weeks) medical and early surgical treatment has brought this to around 45%. There is a high risk of relapse. Patients should be followed up for at least 2 years post-operatively. It may be appropriate to use long-term suppressive therapy, e.g. fluconazole. Other cardiac manifestations: myocardial microabscesses, pericarditis.

Urinary tract infection

Probably follows extension of vaginitis in women or acquired by sexual contact with a woman with candidal vaginitis in men. There is frequently a history of recent antibiotic use. Candiduria is a common finding (particularly in those with urinary catheters) and does not equal renal tract infection. *Candida* cystitis is associated with prolonged catheterization. Bladder perforation occurs in severe cases. Renal infection may occur haematogenously or, less commonly, by retrograde spread (particularly in association with renal tract obstruction or diabetes), causing papillary necrosis, fungal balls, and perinephric abscesses. Surgery may be required to remove fungal balls. Prosthetic material within the tract should be removed. Asymptomatic candiduria should be treated in renal transplant patients, the neutropenic, low-birthweight infants, and those undergoing urinary tract interventions (e.g. nephrostomy).

Bone and joint infection

Candida osteomyelitis may affect the vertebrae and discs, wrist, femur, scapula, humerus, and costochondral junctions. BCs are usually negative. Diagnosis is by aspiration of the affected area. Most cases follow haematogenous spread but may occur secondary to spread from the skin. Surgery may be required. Septic arthritis due to *Candida* occurs in the context of dissemination, trauma, surgery, and intra-articular injection of steroids. It may be a complication of AIDS and rheumatoid arthritis. *C. albicans* is the commonest cause in the context of disseminated infection. Non-albicans species are commoner when infection is local.

Intra-abdominal infection

Peritonitis may complicate peritoneal dialysis (PD), GI perforation, and surgery. Infection tends to remain localized—dissemination is extremely rare in cases associated with PD, and around 25% in cases secondary to GI perforation. Other GI organs that can be affected include the gall bladder, spleen, liver, and pancreas. Hepatosplenic infection occurs in the severely immunocompromised. *Candida* peritonitis due to PD can be treated by local instillation of amphotericin B (can be painful) or fluconazole. Catheter removal may be indicated. *Candida* from long-standing post-operative drains may represent colonization—its presence does not equal infection, and treatment is not always required. Its identification from CT-/ultrasound scan (USS)-guided biopsy or ascites from an undrained abdomen suggests infection that must be treated. The failure rate for treatment of liver and spleen infection is high.

Candidiasis of the biliary tract may require drainage.

Other

- Respiratory tract candidiasis—may cause a diffuse infiltrate, following haematogenous spread (resembling heart failure or PCP in the early stages), or a bronchopneumonia due to local inoculation from the bronchial tree. While *Candida* is frequently recovered from BAL in ICU patients, it is an extremely rare cause of pneumonia in those with otherwise normal immune systems. Definitive diagnosis depends on biopsy.
- Ocular infection—➔ see Uveitis, pp. 753–4.

Treatment of *Candida*

Key points

(See reference 1.)

- Remove infected IV lines, and replace infected valves, if possible.
- Non-albicans species are often fluconazole-resistant, while remaining sensitive to newer azoles and echinocandins. Thus, knowledge of the infecting species is predictive of likely susceptibility.
    - *C. albicans* is generally sensitive to fluconazole. Resistance may occur in the immunosuppressed with prolonged fluconazole exposure.
    - *C. glabrata* is less susceptible to azoles (increased drug efflux) and amphotericin (use higher doses). Cross-resistance amongst all azoles is common. Echinocandins generally remain effective.
    - *C. krusei* is intrinsically resistant to fluconazole (due to altered P450 isoenzyme) and less susceptible to voriconazole and amphotericin (use higher doses). It remains sensitive to the echinocandins.
    - *C. lusitaniae* is susceptible to azoles but uniquely amongst *Candida* spp., frequently resistant to amphotericin.
    - *C. parapsilosis* remains susceptible to most antifungals, but the MICs with all the echinocandins are higher than with other species.
- Amphotericin is first line in most disseminated and deep organ infection—*especially* if there is a risk of fluconazole resistance. Most strains are sensitive, and lipid formulations are less nephrotoxic. Used in combination with flucytosine for invasive disease (e.g. meningitis).
- Susceptibility testing is important in managing deep infections of non-albicans species, particularly with previous azole exposure.
- Azoles are a useful continuation therapy for *C. albicans* infections initially controlled with other agents.

Reference

1 Pappas PG, Kauffman CA, Andes D, *et al.*; Infectious Diseases Society of America (2009). Clinical practice guidelines for the management of candidiasis: 2009 update by the Infectious Diseases Society of America. *Clin Infect Dis.* **48**:503–35.

Malassezia infections

Lipophilic yeasts (grow in the presence of certain fatty acids), oval or round in shape, and normal commensals of the skin that they colonize in late childhood. They are a cause of skin infections and IVC sepsis (e.g. newborns receiving lipid infusions).

Pityriasis versicolor

Superficial skin infection characterized by hypopigmented lesions usually confined to the trunk and proximal limbs. Usually caused by *Malassezia globosa* or *Malassezia furfur*.

- *Pathogenesis*—clinical infection is usually associated with yeasts transforming to hyphal forms from their round/oval appearance. Although seen at greater frequency in those with Cushing's syndrome, there is no clear association with T-cell suppression. Commoner in the tropics and may be precipitated by sun exposure. A carboxylic acid produced by the yeast may lead to the depigmentation.

- *Clinical features*—non-itchy macules develop on the trunk and proximal limbs, and may be hypo- or hyperpigmented. They can coalesce, forming scaly plaques.
- *Diagnosis*—direct microscopy of the lesions will reveal yeasts and hyphae. They may fluoresce under UV light. Organisms are best seen in skin scrapings after ink and KOH staining.
- *Treatment*—some lesions resolve spontaneously. Otherwise, topical treatment for 2 weeks with an azole, terbinafine cream, selenium lotion, or 20% sodium thiosulfate is usually effective. Severe cases may require a course of oral azole.

Malassezia folliculitis

Topical therapy may be effective. Systemic treatment is often necessary. Three clinical presentations:

- itchy papules/pustules on the back and upper chest, sometimes appearing after sun exposure;
- multiple small papules across the back and chest in patients with seborrhoeic dermatitis. Lesions may display erythema and scaling;
- multiple pustules across the trunk and face in patients with HIV.

Seborrhoeic dermatitis

The cause is not known, but *Malassezia* has been implicated in its pathogenesis. There is no evidence that direct invasion precipitates the appearance of seborrhoeic dermatitis, but most cases resolve with a course of azole.

Catheter sepsis

Infections are treated with catheter removal and treatment with either amphotericin or an azole (if found to be sensitive). There have been reports of successful treatment with catheter removal alone, as well as with antifungal treatment alone.

Other yeasts

Trichosporon species

Trichosporon beigelii can be part of the commensal flora of humans. It can cause invasive infections in the immunocompromised and has also been identified in prosthetic valve infections. Trichosporonosis is an acute, febrile infection with dissemination to multiple organs. The means of acquisition is not clear. Diagnosis is by biopsy and culture. BCs tend to be positive late in the course of illness. Amphotericin has been used in treatment.

Rhodotorula species

A cause of disseminated infections in immunocompromised patients, usually acquired through IVC infection following BMT.

Cryptococcus

An encapsulated yeast-like organism that reproduces by budding.[2] The cell is round or ovoid (4–6 micrometres in diameter), and surrounded by a capsule of variable size. There are four capsular serotypes (A to D). Genotypic differences have led to reclassification: *C. neoformans* belong to A and D (var. *grubii* and var. *neoformans*, respectively) and cause infections in the immunodeficient. B and C are now considered a separate species (*C. gattii*) and are more likely to cause infections in the immunocompetent.

Epidemiology

C. neoformans is a ubiquitous environmental saprophyte found worldwide. It has been isolated from pigeon droppings, and contaminated soil and fruit. Infections caused by *C. gattii* are largely restricted to tropical and subtropical areas and has been cultured from eucalyptus trees. Infection occurs by inhalation of aerosolized organisms, but there is no evidence of person-to-person transmission or laboratory-acquired infection. Rare routes of transmission include organ transplantation from infected donors or cutaneous inoculation. There is no evidence of zoonotic transmission. Cryptococcosis occurs more commonly in patients with defects in T cell-mediated immunity: AIDS (80–90% of cryptococcal infections, CD4 <100 cells/mm^3), prolonged glucocorticoid treatment, post-transplantation (peak period 4–6 weeks), malignancy, and sarcoidosis.

Pathogenesis

A number of potential virulence factors have been identified: capsular polysaccharide, melanin/mannitol production, and a lack of soluble anti-cryptococcal factors in CSF. The inflammatory response to infection is variable. The characteristic lesion consists of cystic clusters of fungi spread throughout the brain, with no inflammatory response. Less commonly, focal inflammatory lesions (cryptococcomas) are found. In severe infections, the leptomeninges are thickened with distension of the subarachnoid by a white gelatinous material (capsular polysaccharide).

Clinical features

- Cryptococcal meningitis—acute or chronic, and symptoms may be mild and non-specific. Fever and neck stiffness may be minimal or absent. Papilloedema (30%), cranial nerve palsies (20%), blindness. Seizures occur late. Differential diagnosis: other mycoses, TB meningitis, viral meningoencephalitides, meningeal metastases.
- Pulmonary cryptococcosis—asymptomatic or dyspnoea, cough, chest pain. Physical signs are unusual. May be rapidly progressive in AIDS. Differential: tumour, PCP, pulmonary TB, histoplasmosis.
- Other sites—skin lesions, bone lesions, oral lesions, vulvar lesions, post-transplant pyelonephritis, prostatic cryptococcosis.

Laboratory diagnosis

- *CSF*—elevated opening pressure (>500mm CSF), low glucose, high protein, high WCC (>20/mm^3, lymphocyte predominance). CSF abnormalities may be minimal in AIDS. Check cryptococcal antigen.

- *India ink smear*—India ink or nigrosin staining of the CSF deposit shows a capsule, double cell wall, and refractile inclusions in the cytoplasm in 20–50% of HIV-negative cases and in around 75% of AIDS patients.
- *Fungal culture*—samples include CSF, sputum, and urine. Grows on Sabouraud agar within 3–7 days. Smooth, convex, yellow/tan colonies on solid media or brown on birdseed agar (melanin production). Unlike other yeasts, it does not produce pseudomycelia on cornmeal or Tween agar. Confirmation is by detection of phenol oxidase activity (solely produced by *Cryptococcus*), sugar fermentation, or molecular tests.
- *Cryptococcal antigen test*—latex agglutination tests have sensitivities of ≥90% and can be performed on CSF or serum. False-positive tests occur, but titres are usually ≤1:8 (may result from infection with *T. beigelii* and *Capnocytophaga*).
- *Histopathology*—methenamine silver or periodic acid–Schiff (PAS) staining shows a yeast-like organism with narrow-based buds. Mayer's mucicarmine stain stains the capsule rose red.

Treatment

- *Meningitis*—antifungal therapy, combined with aggressive management of raised intracranial pressure (ICP), is associated with better outcomes. Those with raised ICP at diagnosis, or developing symptoms suggestive of it, should have daily LPs to reduce the pressure to <20cm CSF or 50% of the opening pressure. Those requiring LPs after 4 weeks probably need a shunt.
  - *Induction*: amphotericin and flucytosine. Rapidly fungicidal. Continue for 2 weeks (4–6 weeks if using amphotericin alone, in non-HIV/non-transplant hosts or cryptococcomas). Some authorities recommend repeat LP after induction, to ensure sterilization of CSF.
  - *Consolidation*: high-dose fluconazole (400mg daily) for 8–10 weeks.
  - *Maintenance therapy*: fluconazole (200mg daily) for at least a year in patients with ongoing risk (e.g. low CD4). Consider monitoring cryptococcal antigen until CD4 >200 cells/mm^3.
  - Selected AIDS patients with mild, asymptomatic CNS cryptococcosis have been treated successfully with a long course of high-dose PO fluconazole (<1g/day) and flucytosine—however, many have significant problems with drug side effects (GI and bone marrow toxicity).
- *Pulmonary disease*—mild to moderate infections in the immunocompetent can be treated with PO fluconazole alone. Those with severe disease or multiorgan involvement should be treated as for meningitis. Surgical excision may be curative.

Prognosis

Prognosis depends on the severity of the illness at presentation and the nature of any underlying disease. Relapse is rare in those HIV patients who respond to treatment, continue suppressive therapy, and experience improved immune function on ART. Note that immune reconstitution inflammatory syndrome (IRIS) may occur in the early weeks of ART. Steroids may be indicated in severe cases.

Pneumocystis jiroveci

For many years, *Pneumocystis carinii* was thought to be a protozoan, but rRNA analysis suggests that it is more closely related to fungi. The human-derived organism was renamed *Pneumocystis jiroveci*, whereas the rat-derived organism remains *Pneumocystis carinii*. The first cases of pneumonitis in humans were recognized in malnourished European children during the Second World War.

Microbiology

P. jiroveci is an unusual fungus, lacking ergosterol in its cell wall and therefore not susceptible to certain antifungals. It is extremely difficult to culture *in vitro*, so biochemical and metabolic studies of the organism have been limited. Three developmental stages exist: the trophic form, the sporocyte, and the spores.

Epidemiology

P. jiroveci is ubiquitous in the environment and has a worldwide distribution. Acquisition is by the airborne route. It was originally believed that primary infection occurred in childhood, with the organism persisting in a latent state. It is now thought that frequent clearance and reinfection is more likely. Cluster outbreaks have occurred in hospitals, suggesting person-to-person transmission is commoner than previously thought. Risk factors for disease include:

- debilitated infants and those with severe protein malnutrition;
- primary/acquired immunodeficiency, e.g. HIV with CD4 <200 cell/mm^3;
- immunosuppressive drugs (e.g. glucocorticoids)—especially in organ transplantation or malignancy.

Pathogenesis

Once inhaled, the trophic form attaches to the alveolar type I cell and undergoes proliferation. Impaired humoral and T cell-mediated immunity contribute to its uncontrolled proliferation. The host immune response results in the production of inflammatory cytokines (e.g. TNF-α and IL-1), which contribute to lung damage. The principal histological finding is a foamy eosinophilic alveolar exudate. There may be hyaline membrane formation, interstitial fibrosis, and oedema.

Clinical features

- *Pneumonia*—HIV patients tend to experience insidious onset of fever, dyspnoea, non-productive cough, and reduced exercise tolerance over days/weeks. There may be sputum production, haemoptysis, or chest pain. Non-HIV cases are more likely to present with fulminant respiratory failure that may occur following a *decrease* in immunosuppression. Examination reveals tachypnoea, tachycardia, exercise-induced hypoxia, and crackles (in <30% of adults). Infants may be cyanosed with respiratory distress. CXR may show diffuse bilateral interstitial ground-glass infiltrates, but lobar or nodular changes can occur.

- *Extrapulmonary disease*—this occurs mainly in the context of advanced HIV infection and is rare. The most commonly affected sites are the lymph nodes, spleen, liver, bone marrow, GI tract, eyes, thyroid, adrenal glands, and kidneys. Clinical findings may vary from incidental findings at autopsy to severe progressive disease.

Laboratory diagnosis

- Microscopy—*P. jiroveci* is rarely found in expectorated sputum; induced is much more sensitive (50–90%). BAL increases the diagnostic rate to >90% in HIV cases, especially if multiple lobes are sampled or the procedure is directed to the sites of radiographic involvement. Yield is lower in non-HIV cases and in those receiving aerosolized pentamidine (decreased organism burden). Transbronchial biopsy may provide further information but is associated with complications. Open lung biopsy may be helpful. A variety of stains have been used to identify *P. jiroveci*, e.g. methenamine silver, Wright Giemsa. Commercial immunofluorescence tests and immunohistochemistry are more sensitive but expensive.
- Molecular diagnostics—PCR amplification and detection of *P. jiroveci* DNA has proved highly sensitive and reasonably specific. It is of particular use in non-HIV infected cases. However, the detection of a PCR product in a clinical specimen may represent subclinical infection.
- Antigen detection—beta-*D*-glucan is present in all fungal cell walls so, while not specific for PCP, may have a role in diagnostic evaluation.

Treatment

The treatment of choice is high-dose co-trimoxazole (120mg/kg/day in four divided doses) for 14–21 days. Side effects: skin rash, fever, cytopenias, vomiting, hepatitis, pancreatitis, nephritis, hyperkalaemia, acidosis, CNS symptoms. Alternatives: atovaquone (mild/moderate disease), clindamycin with primaquine (test for G6PD), IV pentamidine. Adjunctive corticosteroids are recommended for HIV-positive patients with PO_2 of <70mmHg, and should be considered in hypoxic non-HIV patients (less data on their efficacy). Start ART within 2 weeks if HIV-positive.

Prognosis

Untreated PCP in immunocompromised patients is fatal. Poor prognostic factors include hypoxia (PaO_2 <7kPa), high alveolar–arterial oxygen gradient (>45mmHg), and extensive pulmonary infiltrates. Short-term mortality (1–3 months) in HIV-infected patients has fallen to 10–20%, whereas the mortality in HIV-negative patients remains 30–50%. Patients who recover are at risk of developing recurrent episodes or pneumothoraces.

Prevention

- *HIV-infected patients*—primary prophylaxis with co-trimoxazole is recommended in HIV-infected patients with a CD4 count <200 cells/mm^3. Secondary prophylaxis is recommended for life but may be discontinued in patients with CD4 count consistently >200 cells/mm^3. Alternative regimens: dapsone ± pyrimethamine + folinic acid or IV pentamidine isethionate.

- *HIV-negative patients*—chemoprophylaxis should be considered in all patients with predisposing conditions (see above). Co-trimoxazole is the agent of choice, as there is limited clinical experience in HIV-negative individuals with other regimens.

Further reading

Briel M, Bucher HC, Boscacci R, Furrer H (2006). Adjunctive corticosteroids for *Pneumocystis jiroveci* pneumonia in patients with HIV-infection. *Cochrane Database Syst Rev.* **3**:CD006150.

Aspergillus

A mould capable of causing a wide range of disease in both healthy and immunocompromised individuals.

Mycology

- Many species cause invasive disease in humans. The most frequently identified are *Aspergillus fumigatus* (around 90%), *Aspergillus flavus*, and *Aspergillus niger*.
- Pathogenic species grow better on routine mycological media at 37°C than non-pathogenic, most of which cannot grow at this temperature. Colonies become apparent at 36–90h. Sporulation (required for speciation) occurs up to 2 days later, longer with less common species.
- Identification of common species is by microscopic and colonial appearance. Detailed identification requires more specialized methods.
- Microscopy of pathological specimens may reveal hyphae (best seen on silver stains), but sporulation is not often seen (save in specimens taken from air-containing areas such as the lung); thus, the organism cannot be distinguished from other pathogenic moulds by this means.

Epidemiology

Found worldwide, favouring decomposing vegetable material (e.g. potted plants, spices, farms). Molecular techniques have demonstrated that colonized individuals and those with aspergilloma tend to pick up several different genotypes over time. Most invasive infections are caused by a single genotype.

Pathogenesis

- Disease spectrum is wide. Time from exposure to disease in invasive aspergillosis ranges from 36h to months. Disease may follow infection by organisms that have already colonized an individual (e.g. in neutropenia).
- Many factors influence disease form and severity—organism growth rate (*A. fumigatus* being the fastest), spore size (*A. fumigatus*' small spores allow them to pass deep into the lung), the hydrophobic coat of conidia (protection from host defence), the ability to adhere to epithelial surfaces (achieved by *A. fumigatus* much more effectively than other species), enzyme/toxin production (e.g. aflatoxin produced by *A. flavus*).
- Host defences include lung macrophages (capable of ingesting and killing conidia), T lymphocytes (appear to be important in chronic and allergic disease), complement proteins, and neutrophils (damage hyphae). Corticosteroids impair macrophage and neutrophil killing.

Clinical features

Non-invasive disease

- Superficial—cutaneous infections are rare (usually neutropenic patients or burns). Commoner is otomycosis—growth of *A. niger* in those with chronic otitis externa which may cause itch and discomfort. Cleaning and topical therapy with 3% amphotericin or clotrimazole are curative.
- Allergic bronchopulmonary aspergillosis (ABPA) occurs in those with asthma or CF and hypersensitivity to airway colonization by *Aspergillus*. Presents with worsening asthma or lung function. Patients may have an eosinophilic pneumonia or airway sputum impaction. Blood tests may reveal eosinophilia early in disease. Oral corticosteroids can help exacerbations, and inhaled steroids may prevent episodes from occurring. PO itraconazole may help those requiring long-term steroids. *Aspergillus* may also cause allergic sinusitis, best managed by aeration of the affected sinus.
- Aspergilloma—pulmonary aspergilloma follows *Aspergillus* colonization of pre-existing cavities or cysts left from TB, sarcoidosis, or PCP. TB cavities 2cm or larger have a 15–25% risk of developing an aspergilloma. Some patients are asymptomatic; most have productive cough, haemoptysis, weight loss, wheeze, and clubbing. Culture of sputum may reveal the organism, and IgG precipitins may be detected in serum. Radiological imaging demonstrates the hyphal mass as a cavity surrounded by a rim of air. Complications: massive haemoptysis (may be fatal—consider embolization or surgery), spread of infection to pleurae or vertebrae, dissemination. Aspergilloma must be distinguished from chronic invasive disease requiring systemic therapy. Treatment: 10% of cases resolve spontaneously; surgical resection has a role in the treatment of isolated lesions in those with good lung function; amphotericin has been injected into cavities, with some effect; PO itraconazole provides symptomatic relief. Sinus aspergilloma may develop in the ethmoid or maxillary cavities. Surgical drainage is usually sufficient in those with no evidence of mucosal involvement. Medical therapy should be used in combination with surgery in those with invasive disease or involvement of the frontal or sphenoid sinus.
- Eye—*Aspergillus* keratitis (less commonly endophthalmitis) may occur following ocular trauma or haematogenously (e.g. IDU, endocarditis). Early recognition and treatment are essential for a good outcome. Corneal smears may reveal hyphae, and cultures are usually positive. Keratitis may be treated with TOP amphotericin (27% response when given hourly). Superficial infections may be treated with TOP clotrimazole. PO itraconazole is effective in up to 75% of cases. Surgery is required where medical therapy fails or where there is the threat of ocular perforation or the formation of a descemetocele (a herniation of the posterior limiting layer of the cornea). Vitrectomy may be required to establish the diagnosis, and intraoperative examination of the specimen for hyphae allows immediate administration of intravitreal amphotericin. Systemic therapy is also recommended.

Invasive disease

Uncommon, occurring most frequently in the setting of iatrogenic immunosuppression (haematological malignancy, transplantation).

- Invasive pulmonary disease—over 80% of patients with invasive disease have pulmonary infection. The immunocompromised tend to experience few symptoms but progress rapidly, whereas the less immune-impaired have more symptoms with a slowly progressive, chronic course.
  - Acute invasive pulmonary aspergillosis—early stages: dry cough and a mild fever (25% have no symptoms); later: pleuritic chest pain, haemoptysis, breathlessness in those with bilateral disease who can become hypoxic. May resemble pulmonary embolism (PE) or mucormycosis. CXR changes can be non-specific (consolidation, cavities, wedge-shaped lesions, lower lobe shadowing) or absent (10% of cases). High-resolution CT images aid prompt diagnosis: early disease—nodules with the 'halo' sign (a zone of ground-glass attenuation surrounding a nodule or mass); in later disease, with neutrophil recovery, these may cavitate, producing the 'air-crescent' sign. Focal or nodular disease has a better prognosis than diffuse or bilateral infection. In focal disease, the danger is that of massive haemoptysis that may occur with no warning.
  - Chronic invasive pulmonary aspergillosis—less frequent than acute. Predisposing conditions: AIDS, alcoholism, diabetes mellitus, chronic granulomatous diseases, corticosteroid therapy for chronic pulmonary diseases. Some patients have no identifiable predisposing factors. Presentation: weeks of chronic productive cough. Other symptoms: haemoptysis, fever, weight loss. Infection may extend to the chest wall, spine, or brachial plexus. CXR shows cavitation and consolidation. May resemble aspergilloma (previous images demonstrating the presence of a pre-existing cavity may help distinguish). Definitive diagnosis is by positive culture of a biopsy specimen. Patients usually have strongly positive serum *Aspergillus* antibodies (with the possible exception of AIDS patients).
- Airways—commoner in lung transplant and AIDS patients. *Aspergillus* tracheobronchitis varies from mild inflammation to severe ulcerative disease; 80% experience symptoms (cough, fever, breathlessness, pain, haemoptysis), which become more severe with progression. Complications: stridor, tracheal perforation, dissemination, airway occlusion, death. Diagnosis by bronchoscopy. CXR usually normal in early disease.
- Sinus—invasive *Aspergillus* sinusitis can be acute or chronic:
  - acute—fever, cough, nosebleeding, headaches, discharge, sinus discomfort. Decreased blood flow to the affected nasal areas results in loss of sensation and ultimately ulceration. Infection may extend to the palate, orbit, and brain. CT or MRI identifies the extent of disease. Culture or hyphal identification within tissue confirms diagnosis;
  - chronic—most have no identifiable immunocompromise. Early symptoms: nasal congestion, discharge, loss of smell, headache.

Clinically indistinguishable from other causes of sinusitis. As disease extends, proptosis, loss of vision, ocular pain, and features of stroke may develop. Radiological features are similar to those of acute disease. Obtaining a positive culture may require multiple samples.

- Brain—10–20% of cases of disseminated disease develop cerebral aspergillosis. It is rare in the immunocompetent when it is usually secondary to neurosurgery. Severely immunocompromised individuals have a non-specific presentation with confusion and seizures, and death following a few days later. Less severely immune-impaired patients tend to have headache and focal neurological features. Fever may occur. Meningitis is rare. Contrast CT appearances are of infarction or of a ring-enhancing abscess with oedema. Lesions may be deep and surgically inaccessible. Diagnosis rests on culture and microscopy of a biopsy or aspiration sample. This may not be possible, and diagnosis can be made presumptively in those with invasive disease elsewhere and typical radiological appearances.
- Other—endocarditis (BCs usually negative, and valve replacement is necessary to achieve cure), pericardial, intestinal, oesophageal, renal, vascular graft, bone.

Diagnosis in invasive disease

- Radiology—perform CT assessment of the lungs and sinuses or MRI of the brain within 24h if clinical suspicion of invasive aspergillosis.
- Airway disease—bronchoscopic biopsy is rarely positive in focal lung disease. A needle biopsy or surgical resection (superior to open biopsy) is appropriate for peripheral pulmonary lesions. Focal lesions near the great vessels should prompt urgent resection (risk of massive haemoptysis). Positive BAL cultures support the diagnosis in the context of at-risk patients with suggestive radiological features. Antigen tests can be performed on BAL fluid.
- Histology—organisms may be observed, but several filamentous fungi have similar appearances, and culture is important for confirmation.
- Antibody testing—*Aspergillus* precipitin antibodies, while useful in diagnosing ABPA and aspergilloma, have no role in invasive disease.
- Serum antigen tests—the galactomannan (a fungal exoantigen released by all pathogenic *Aspergillus* spp. during growth) assay has moderate accuracy for diagnosis of invasive aspergillosis in immunocompromised patients. It is best used in the setting of suspected disease (in which the higher prevalence leads to better positive predictive value). Sensitivity/specificity for proven invasive disease in those with haematological malignancy or haematopoietic cell transplantation is 71%/89%. Less useful in solid organ transplant recipients and paediatric patients with primary immunodeficiencies. May become positive a week before clinical disease is manifest. NB. Sensitivity is reduced if the patient is receiving mould-active antifungals; false positives may follow absorption of galactomannan from the gut (e.g. mucositis) or the administration of Tazocin®; other fungi produce galactomannan (*Fusarium, Histoplasma* spp.). The 1-3 beta-*D*-glucan test has a high negative predictive value that may help exclude invasive disease in adults (➔ see *Candida* species, pp. 472–3).

- A diagnostic approach—appropriate imaging, non-invasive tests (sputum, galactomannan testing). If positive in the correct clinical context, this may be sufficient for therapy. Otherwise, BAL if relevant (with sample for galactomannan), lung biopsy if safe and technically feasible. Culture from sterile sample or culture with histology demonstrating invasion provides definitive diagnosis. However, culture is insensitive. Treatment should not be withheld from those at risk with suggestive features.

Treatment

(See reference 2.)

- Primary prophylaxis (e.g. with voriconazole) is effective in at-risk groups, but the specific patients who might benefit remain ill-defined.
- Invasive aspergillosis is fatal in virtually all cases, if untreated. Good outcomes require aggressive diagnosis in risk groups, early presumptive treatment, early changes in treatment if response is poor, and early surgical resection of lung lesions located near the hilum/ great vessels. Evaluating the response takes longer in those with less immunocompromise.
- Invasive aspergillosis—voriconazole is the treatment of choice. Alternative: liposomal amphotericin. If invasive mould infection suspected, but the organism is not confirmed, empirical treatment with amphotericin is preferred, as it is also active against mucormycosis (intrinsically resistant to voriconazole). Consider measuring voriconazole levels; standard dosing results in low levels in some patients. Duration: generally continued until all symptoms and signs have resolved; longer (many months) in those with persistent immune deficits. Consider secondary prophylaxis in those at risk of relapse (e.g. those continuing to receive chemotherapy). Caspofungin may be used in combination therapy if there is no response to first-line treatment. Be aware of interactions between azole drugs and chemotherapeutic agents. *A. terreus* is less susceptible to amphotericin. Some *A. fumigatus* isolates have increased MICs for azoles.
- Acute invasive sinusitis—first-line treatment is amphotericin. Itraconazole is not as effective for this form of disease.
- Chronic invasive sinusitis—surgical debridement and prolonged medical therapy. Relapse is common.
- Cerebral disease—surgery is useful only for diagnosis, unless the lesion is superficial and isolated. Otherwise, antifungal therapy is key.
- Surgery—indicated for focal invasive pulmonary disease, persisting lung shadows prior to BMT or aggressive chemotherapy, significant haemoptysis, or lesions near to great vessels and airways.
- See IDSA guidelines for full treatment guidelines.[3]

References

2 The Aspergillus Website. Available at: www.aspergillus.org.uk.

3 Walsh TJ, Anaissie EJ, Denning DW, *et al.*; Infectious Diseases Society of America (2008). Treatment of aspergillosis: clinical practice guidelines of the Infectious Diseases Society of America. *Clin Infect Dis*. **46**:327–60.

Mucormycosis

Mucormycosis is a clinical syndrome caused by a number of fungal species belonging to the order *Mucorales* (class *Zygomycetes*).

Mycology

Spores form and grow rapidly in the mould form in both tissues and the environment. Common species causing mucormycosis include *Rhizopus*, *Rhizomucor*, and *Mucor*. Microscopy allows a degree of speciation, and the hyphae of *Mucorales* are sufficiently different (broad and irregularly branched) to allow them to be distinguished from *Aspergillus* (narrow and regularly branched).

Epidemiology

All members of the order are widespread in decaying matter. As testament to their ubiquitous nature, they have been isolated from wooden tongue depressors, and infection has resulted from their use as splints in neonates. Clinical disease is limited largely to the immunocompromised, transplant patients, those with diabetes mellitus, and trauma patients. Infection may be rhinocerebral, respiratory, cutaneous, disseminated, or localized to specific organs.

Pathogenesis

Infection is acquired via the respiratory tract or in primary cutaneous infection via the inoculation of spores into skin abrasions. Spore germination follows in hosts whose immune response is deficient. Macrophages and neutrophils are important in preventing growth, and normal human serum is fungistatic. Invasive disease is favoured by hyperglycaemia and acidosis, and in patients receiving desferrioxamine (an agent which enhances fungal growth experimentally). Cases are not as significantly raised in those with AIDS as might otherwise be expected. Hyphae invade tissues, penetrate blood vessel walls, and may grow along the vessel, contributing to thrombosis and necrosis.

Clinical features

- Rhinocerebral disease—a disease of the immunosuppressed, seen in diabetic patients (particularly if acidotic) and neutropenic leukaemia patients on antibiotics. Almost invariably fatal, causing septic necrosis and infarction of the tissues of the nasopharynx and orbit. Patients develop facial pain or headache with fever, and may have orbital cellulitis, with proptosis and conjunctival swelling, evolving cranial nerve defects, and black, crusty material apparent in the nasopharynx. Fungal invasion of vessels may lead to retinal artery thrombosis and visual impairment. Other complications: ptosis/pupil dilatation (secondary to cranial nerve lesions), cerebral abscess, cavernous sinus/internal carotid artery thrombosis. X-ray of the sinuses may show mucosal thickening, and fluid and bone destruction may be apparent on CT. Endoscopic evaluation of the sinuses should be performed to assess appearance and obtain tissue. Features may recur after apparently successful therapy—patients should be monitored.

- Pulmonary disease—usually secondary to neutropenia and seen in BMT or leukaemia patients receiving chemotherapy. Symptoms are initially mild: fever, mild shortness of breath, and cough. With progression, haemoptysis may develop, and erosion of a blood vessel can cause severe pulmonary haemorrhage. CXR may show infiltration, consolidation, and cavities. Infection may start in one lung segment but often disseminates in the late stages (e.g. multiple lung area, spleen, kidney). Diabetics may develop a milder chronic form of pulmonary infection.
- Cutaneous disease—outbreaks have been associated with colonized bandages. The appearance is of cellulitis, but, if unrecognized, the organism penetrates deeper into the skin, and necrosis may follow vascular invasion. Dissemination may follow. May take the appearance of a chronic ulcer. Cases have occurred with minor trauma (e.g. gardeners), major trauma, burns, insect bites, and dissemination from a distant site.
- GI disease—seen in those suffering from malnutrition, although cases have occurred in renal transplant recipients. Any part of the tract may be infected, and it is rapidly fatal. Symptoms include abdominal pain, fever, nausea, and vomiting.
- CNS disease—rare and usually due to direct invasion from infected sinuses. Cases have occurred in leukaemia patients with no obvious route of acquisition and as a result of open head trauma. Presentation is with decreasing levels of consciousness and multiple focal neurological deficits.
- Other—endocarditis, osteomyelitis, renal infection, allergic sinusitis.

Diagnosis

- Clinical suspicion should be raised by the presence of vascular invasion and tissue necrosis that may manifest as black eschars and discharge. These are markers of advanced disease, and the earlier the diagnosis the better the outcome. Lesions may be apparent only on the nasal mucosa and palate.
- Diagnosis rests on identifying the organism in tissue biopsy. Swabs are insufficient. There is usually an associated neutrophilic infiltrate, and tissue necrosis may follow blood vessel invasion with an inflammatory vasculitis. Organisms rarely appear in BCs. The differential includes *Aspergillus* infection, rapidly progressive orbital tumour, cavernous sinus thrombosis, PE, and acute leukaemia.

Treatment

- Good outcomes rest on early diagnosis and correction of any predisposing factors, e.g. acidosis, hyperglycaemia, immunosuppression. Overall mortality is around 50%.
- Invasive disease—high-dose amphotericin B in combination with aggressive surgical debridement of necrotic tissue. Reconstructive surgery may be necessary once recovered. Duration: until clinical resolution (usually several weeks/months). Posaconazole has been used in salvage or for oral step-down therapy. The other azoles are ineffective.
- Primary cutaneous disease—local debridement and TOP amphotericin. Treatment duration should be guided by response.

Eumycetoma

Mycetoma is a chronic, slow-growing, destructive infection, usually involving the hands or feet and characterized by the spread of the infecting organism from its subcutaneous site of implantation to adjacent structures. Serous discharges contain small grains of organism colonies.

- Actinomycetoma—caused by filamentous branching bacteria.
- Eumycetoma—caused by fungi.

Epidemiology

Found in tropical regions—most commonly in India, Mexico, parts of sub-Saharan Africa, and Yemen, amongst others. Rare in temperate areas but may be seen in south-western USA. Causative organism varies with geography: *Madurella mycetomatis* accounts for most cases worldwide; *Madurella grisea* is a common cause in South America; *Pseudallescheria boydii* in the USA; *Leptosphaeria senegalensis* and *Leptosphaeria tompkinsii* are common causes in West Africa. Geographic distribution of the causative agents is related to local climate (e.g. rainfall).

Pathogenesis

Soil fungi enter tissues of the foot or hand after local trauma. Infection spreads along tissue planes, destroying connective tissue and bone. Multiple sinuses and tracts form between the surface, each other, and deep abscesses. Inflammation and scarring lead to enlargement and disfigurement of the infected area. Histologically, the appearance is of a suppurative granuloma with grains embedded in abscesses. Grain appearance is often characteristic of the specific organism.

Clinical features

Seen most frequently in men aged 20–40 years, often farmers and rural labourers. The foot is the most commonly affected area; other regions include the hand, leg, arm, head, thigh, and even the back (carrying contaminated sacks). Early manifestation is a small, painless nodule. This quickly increases in size (faster in actinomycetoma) and ruptures, forming a sinus. Additional nodules appear in adjacent areas, as some areas heal. The cycle of swelling, discharge, and scarring leads to a swollen mass of deformed tissue with multiple discharging fistulae. Lymphatic spread to regional nodes may occur. Cortex of bone may be invaded. Osteolytic lesions can be seen on X-ray. Pathological fractures are less common than would be expected. Constitutional symptoms are rare. Fever implies secondary bacterial infection.

Diagnosis

The appearance is fairly typical: indurated swelling, deformity with multiple sinus tracts draining grainy pus. Grains may be black, white, yellow, red, or pink, depending on the causative organism, e.g. white to yellow grains with *Acremonium* spp., *Aspergillus nidulans*, *A. flavus*, *Cylindrocarpon cyanescens*, *P. boydii*, and *Fusarium* spp.; black grains with *Corynespora cassiicola*, *Curvularia* spp., and *M. mycetomatis*. They can be difficult to spot in tissue sections. Tissue Gram stain can detect the fine branching hyphae of actinomycetoma, but other stains are better for the detection of eumycetoma grains (e.g. PAS stain). A good idea of the causative organism can be drawn from grain characteristics. They can be cultured for more exact diagnosis—biopsy specimens are best to avoid contamination. Serological diagnosis is possible in some centres.

Treatment

Mycetoma at all stages is usually amenable to medical therapy. Surgery usually leads to recurrence or mutilation that is more severe than that pre-existing. Treatment success depends on identification of the causative organism. All cases of actinomycetoma are treated with a combination of streptomycin sulfate and a second agent determined by the causal species (e.g. dapsone for *A. madurae*). Eumycetoma caused by fungi is treated with azoles, usually itraconazole, ketoconazole, or voriconazole (preferred for *P. boydii*). Fluconazole cannot be used due to intrinsic resistance. Treatment continues in all cases for at least 12 months, longer with extensive bone involvement. There is a role for surgery in combination with effective medical treatment, e.g. for bulk reduction.

Dermatophytes

A group of fungi capable of invading the dead keratin of skin, hair, and nails, causing dermatophytosis (tinea). Also known as 'ringworm', several species infect humans and belong to the genera *Epidermophyton, Microsporum*, and *Trichophyton*. Clinical classification is by the body area involved: tinea capitis (scalp hair and the commonest in children), corporis (trunk and limbs), manuum and pedis (palms and soles, and the commonest overall worldwide), cruris (groin), barbae (beard area and neck), faciale (face), unguium (nail—also known as onychomycosis and affecting 2.7–4.7% of adults in the UK).

Mycology

- May be anthropophilic, zoophilic (causing incidental human infection), or geophilic (found primarily in soil and infrequent causes of human infection outside certain specific tropical regions). All favour humid or moist skin. Cases occur worldwide, but incidence is highest in hot, humid regions.
- The commonest anthropophilic species is *Trichophyton rubrum*, a common cause of tinea pedis or tinea cruris in temperate regions, and tinea corporis in the tropics. Spread is through contact with infected desquamated skin scales, e.g. through sharing common washing facilities.
- *Epidermophyton floccosum* may cause tinea cruris and foot infections, either sporadically or in outbreaks in institutions.
- *Trichophyton concentricum* is a cause of tinea corporis in remote parts of the humid tropics, often affecting infants shortly after birth.
- Some species have specific geographical distributions: *Trichophyton tonsurans* is the main cause of tinea capitis in the UK and USA, and *Trichophyton violaceum* in India.

Pathogenesis

Infection is transmitted by hardy arthrospores formed by dermatophyte hyphae. Direct contact between individual people is not necessary. Fungal cells adhere to keratinocytes where they germinate and invade. Host susceptibility to infection appears to be influenced by genetic factors, local moisture, and CMI. Risk factors: moist conditions, communal baths, athletic activities leading to abrasions (wrestling, judo, etc.), atopy, genetic predisposition, impaired CMI (e.g. Cushing's disease, AIDS—may lead to severe infection, e.g. extensive disease, abscess, dissemination).

Clinical features

The key feature is an annular scaling patch, with a raised margin showing a degree of inflammation, the centre usually less inflamed than the edge. The precise appearance varies with the affected site, the fungal species involved, and the host immune response. Inappropriate application of topical steroids may lead to an infection showing none of the classical signs. Differential diagnosis: seborrhoeic dermatitis, psoriasis, eczema, erysipelas, impetigo.

- Tinea capitis—a disease of childhood (medium chain-length fatty acids in sebum inhibit growth in post-pubertal adults). Found worldwide. Endemic infections affecting a large number of children tend to be caused by anthropophilic organisms, and sporadic cases by zoophilic fungi. Those infections in which the arthrospores are found on the hair surface are termed ectothrix infections, and those in which the spores develop within the hair, endothrix infections. Clinical findings: scalp scaling and hair loss; may resemble dandruff. In ectothrix infections, the hair tends to break a few millimetres above the skin, in contrast to endothrix infections where the hair breaks at the skin surface. Inflammation is variable and may be severe with pustules and an exudative crust. Untreated, it usually remits spontaneously after puberty.
- Tinea corporis ('ringworm')—several causes. Anthropophilic species produce only mild inflammation and consequently a less well-defined skin lesion (e.g. *T. rubrum*), whereas zoophilic species produce more inflamed lesions that may contain pustules (e.g. *Microsporum canis*). Tinea barbae affects only the beard area with scaly plaques, pustules, and vesicles. Tinea imbricata is a variant caused by *T. concentricum*, characterized by a rash composed of concentric rings of scales. It is endemic in parts of South East Asia, the South Pacific, Central America, and South America.
- Tinea pedis—seen in children and young adults, and usually due to infection with *T. rubrum* or *Trichophyton mentagrophytes*. Toe-web fissures, maceration, scaling of soles, erythema, vesicles/pustules, bullae. 'Athlete's foot' is typical, but infection with other organisms may produce a similar appearance.
- Tinea cruris—*T. rubrum* or *E. floccosum*. Erythematous lesions with central clearing and raised borders in the groin and, less commonly, the scrotum. Usually seen in young men.
- Tinea unguium (onychomycosis)—often associated with infection of adjacent skin. Nail usually invaded from the distal and lateral aspects with onycholysis (separation of the nail from the nail bed), thick,

discoloured (white, yellow, brown, black), dystrophic nails. Commoner with increasing age. Causes: *Scopulariopsis brevicaulis, Acremonium* spp., *Fusarium* spp.

Diagnosis

Skin scrapings, nail specimens, or plucked hairs are treated with KOH and examined by direct microscopy. Samples should be taken from the edge of the lesion. Look for hyphae and arthrospores around the hair shaft. Fungal cultures may be performed (culture on Sabouraud agar containing antibiotics and antifungal agents to selectively suppress the growth of environmental fungi—growth may take at least 2 weeks). Examination of the lesions under UV light may help in the diagnosis of tinea capitis—hairs infected with *Microsporum audouinii* and *M. canis* fluoresce yellow-green, those infected with *Trichophyton schoenleinii* dull green. It is important to identify the organism causing scalp infection—the presence of an anthropophilic species should prompt screening of classmates and the family of affected children. Zoophilic infections rarely spread from child to child.

Treatment

- Tinea capitis—topical therapy ineffective. Oral treatment with griseofulvin, terbinafine, or itraconazole.
- Tinea pedis, corporis, and cruris—TOP ketoconazole 2%, miconazole 2%, or clotrimazole 1% rubbed into the affected area daily for 2–6 weeks. Extensive or unresponsive disease may need systemic therapy.
- Infections confined to the palms/soles may respond to keratolytic agents such as Whitfield's ointment (compound benzoic acid ointment BP).
- Nail infections—topicals rarely work. Terbinafine PO is first line (70–80% cure for fingernails after 6 weeks and toenails after 12 weeks' treatment). Well tolerated, but there is a low risk of hepatic injury (1 in 70 000). Check baseline LFTs. Itraconazole an alternative.

Other moulds

Pseudallescheria boydii

Found in soil and fresh water throughout the world. The asexual form is called *Scedosporium apiospermum*. It causes two distinct diseases: mycetoma (➔ see Eumycetoma, pp. 491–2) and pseudallescheriasis (all other infections). Pseudallescheriasis may affect the lung, bone, joints, and the CNS, skin, and soft tissue. Infection may be acquired by inhalation or through skin trauma. Weeks or months may pass between a local fungal inoculation and the development of symptoms.

- Immunocompetent—subacute/chronic infection, e.g. osteoarticular. Cerebral abscesses have occurred as a result of near drowning in pond water (probably due to spread from infected paranasal sinuses).
- Immunocompromised—acute and severe, including invasive pulmonary disease reminiscent of pulmonary aspergillosis. Cerebral abscesses may develop in association with lung infection.

- There have been cases of indolent meningitis caused by *P. boydii*. Isolation of the organism from sterile sites is diagnostic. It is rarely cultured from blood. Effective antifungal therapy has not been established. Resistance to amphotericin B has been reported. Successful treatment regimes have utilized both surgical debridement and voriconazole.

Scedosporium prolificans

An uncommon cause of human infection, with several dozen cases reported worldwide. Immunocompetent patients experience focal disease, usually osteoarticular. Immunocompromised patients may develop disseminated infection. Fungaemia, skin lesions, myalgia, pulmonary infiltrates, and cerebral lesions have all been reported. Diagnosis is made by culture. The organism is intrinsically resistant to most antifungals. Most therapy successes have involved debridement. Disseminated disease carries a high mortality.

Fusarium species

Found in soil and, in the healthy, causes disease only rarely, usually through traumatic inoculation. *Fusarium* spp. may cause endophthalmitis, skin infection, musculoskeletal infections, and mycetoma. May disseminate in the immunocompromised. Systemic fusariosis occurs most commonly in patients with acute leukaemia and prolonged neutropenia, and those undergoing BMT. Presentation is with fever and myalgia unresponsive to antibiotics. Skin lesions are seen in up to 80% of cases, often starting as macules and progressing to necrotic papules. Infection may progress rapidly to death in the severely neutropenic. Once neutrophils recover, infection is more subacute and progresses slowly, or is controlled and cured. Diagnosis is by culture. Unlike aspergillosis, BCs are often positive (50% cases). High-dose amphotericin is the drug of choice. Overall mortality ranges from 50% to 80%, and survival is nearly always associated with recovery from neutropenia.

Dark-walled fungi

Phaeohyphomycosis is a loose term designating infection with moulds with dark walls in culture, but not always in tissue. These organisms are a cause of brain abscess (e.g. *Cladophialophora bantiana*), allergic fungal sinusitis (e.g. *Bipolaris, Exserohilum*), and cutaneous disease.

Sporothrix schenckii

A dimorphic fungus and the cause of sporotrichosis. May take the form of cutaneous infection, granulomatous pneumonitis, or disseminated disease.

Mycology

- Dimorphic. Demonstrating the temperature-dependent conversion is a useful means of identification. Hyphal colonies are initially white and later turn brown/black, as they produce pigment.

Epidemiology

- Found across the world—most human infections occur in tropical and subtropical parts of the Americas.
- Animal-to-human transmission has been described. Human-to-human is rare.
- Identified in soil, plants, straw, and wood, and outbreaks have occurred in association with exposure to mine timbers, hay, thorned plants, etc.

Clinical features

- Cutaneous sporotrichosis—fungus is inoculated into the skin at sites of minor trauma, with disease usually arising in cooler body areas such as distal extremities. There are no systemic symptoms. Lesions may take the form of either a fixed plaque, which does not spread and may spontaneously resolve, or painless, smooth or verrucous, erythematous papulonodular lesions (0.5–4cm in diameter) which often ulcerate and can be followed by secondary lesions along the line of proximal lymphatics.
- Extracutaneous sporotrichosis—*osteoarticular* is commonest, involving the extremities, e.g. elbow, knee, hand, foot. Most present with primary involvement of a single joint (swollen, painful, with an effusion and possibly a sinus tract). Other joints may become involved without therapy. There are few systemic features. Repeated joint aspiration and culture or synovial biopsy may be necessary to make a diagnosis. *Pulmonary sporotrichosis*—one-third of patients are alcoholic, one-third have a pre-existing illness (e.g. diabetes, sarcoidosis), and one-third are healthy. They may be asymptomatic, but productive cough, fever, and weight loss are common, as are raised inflammatory markers. CXR reveals cavitation with or without hilar lymphadenopathy and effusions. Sputum Gram stain and culture are usually diagnostic, but long-term follow-up with repeated cultures may be necessary for diagnosis. Untreated disease leads to progressive respiratory decline. *Other*—meningitis (CSF: high lymphocytes, high protein, low glucose), endophthalmitis, sinuses, kidney, testes.
- Multifocal extracutaneous sporotrichosis—in healthy people, lesions tend to be single-site. Multifocal disease with systemic features is usually seen in those with immunosuppression. Untreated infection is fatal.
- Patients with HIV—those with low CD4 counts are at greater risk of widespread ulcerative skin lesions and systemic dissemination. Presentation may be with arthritis and resemble seronegative arthropathies such as Reiter's syndrome. Visceral involvement occurs: meningitis, lung abscess, liver and spleen, endophthalmitis, bone marrow, sinus invasion, etc.

Diagnosis

- Culture—success may require multiple samples taken from affected sites at different times. A positive BC indicates multifocal disease. Although culture of skin lesion fluid may be positive, biopsy is best.
- Histology—a pyogranulomatous response is usually apparent and, in the presence of yeast forms, can be diagnostic. Again, multiple samples may be necessary. Yeast may be cigar or oval in shape.

Differential diagnosis

- Cutaneous disease—fixed lesions: bacterial pyoderma, foreign body granuloma, dermatophyte infections, cutaneous TB, and other granulomatous conditions; lymphocutaneous lesions: nocardiosis, leishmaniasis, mycobacterial infections (e.g. *M. chelonae, M. marinum*).
- Osteoarticular disease—TB, gout, rheumatoid arthritis.
- Pulmonary disease—TB and other mycobacteria, histoplasmosis, coccidioidomycosis.

Treatment

- Cutaneous disease—itraconazole or saturated potassium iodide (5–10 drops PO tds, increased slowly to 40 drops per dose; side effects include anorexia, diarrhoea, and parotid gland enlargement). Treatment course is usually 6–12 weeks. Prognosis is good. There have been cases described in which simply warming the lesion has been curative, reflecting the organism's temperature sensitivity.
- Osteoarticular disease—itraconazole is used as initial therapy. Amphotericin is curative in two-thirds. Duration is at least 12 months. Relapse is common, and functional outcomes often poor.
- Pulmonary disease—prior to cavitation, amphotericin may be effective. Advanced disease requires surgical resection of cavities and a course of lipid-formulation amphotericin. PO itraconazole can be used as step-down therapy. Total duration is at least 12 months.
- Meningitis—varying response to amphotericin, and some advocate combination therapy with 5-flucytosine. Step down to itraconazole, once initial therapy complete. At least 12 months' treatment required.
- Immunocompromised patients may require lifelong itraconazole therapy for multifocal extracutaneous disease.

Further reading

Kauffman CA, Bustamante B, Chapman SW, Pappas PG; Infectious Diseases Society of America (2007). Clinical practice guidelines for the management of sporotrichosis: 2007 update by the Infectious Diseases Society of America. *Clin Infect Dis*. **45**:1255–65.

Chromomycosis

A localized chronic fungal infection of cutaneous and subcutaneous tissue, caused by several species and producing verrucous lesions.

Mycology

- Several different species cause chromomycosis—all take the appearance of dark brown cells, occurring singly or in small clusters. Culture colonies are dark with a grey/green or brown/black surface.
- Agents grow slowly, and culture may take 6 weeks.
- Organisms include *Fonsecaea pedrosoi* (the most commonly isolated agent), *Fonsecaea compacta, Phialophora verrucosa, Cladosporium carrionii* (common in Australia, South Africa, and Venezuela).

Epidemiology

- Occurs worldwide but commonest in tropical/subtropical areas amongst barefoot workers.
- Found in soil, decaying vegetation, etc., and inoculated into the skin by minor trauma; thus, feet and legs are the most commonly affected areas.

Clinical features

- Lesions can appear a long time after inoculation.
- Primary lesion usually a small pink papule that may itch and is followed (possibly many months later) by crops of either warty, violaceous nodules or firm tumours. These tend to enlarge and form groups with ulceration and dark haemopurulent material on the surface. Satellite lesions may occur.
- Some people develop annular, papular lesions with active edges and healing in the centre which can become scarred or form keloid. Fibrosis and oedema of the affected limb may occur in severe cases.
- Complications: secondary infection, lymphoedema (elephantiasis), fistula formation, haematogenous spread (rare), squamous carcinoma in long-standing lesions, late recurrence (years later sometimes).
- Differential diagnosis—blastomycosis, yaws, tertiary syphilis, leishmaniasis, mycetoma, sporotrichosis, *M. marinum*, leprosy.

Diagnosis

- All forms of disease produce characteristic sclerotic bodies which may be identified on biopsy along with pyogranulomata and microabscesses. Microscopy of exudates may reveal hyphal strands.
- Culture is necessary to confirm identity and may take 6 weeks.

Treatment

- Early small lesions—surgical excision or cryotherapy is effective.
- Late disease—most cases present late with large lesions. Local heat and several antifungals have been reported as effective, e.g. itraconazole. Treatment duration may last well over a year. It has been used in combination with flucytosine in cases of relapse.

Histoplasma capsulatum—ACDP 3

A dimorphic fungus and emerging infection in parts of the Americas.

The organism

- A member of the class *Ascomycetes*. Recognized as a fungus in the 1930s, leading to the re-evaluation of many TB cases in the USA whose diagnosis had been made on CXR alone.
- *H. capsulatum* contains between four and seven chromosomes. Restriction fragment length polymorphism (RFLP) of certain genes permits strains to be placed in one of six groups that correlate with virulence and geographical location.
- Mating types exist: (+) and (−). These are found in equal ratio in soil, but the (−) predominates in clinical isolates.

- It is dimorphic—the mycelial phase grows at ambient temperatures, the yeast phase at 37°C. The mycelial phase exists in two forms: macroconidia (<15 micrometres) and microconidia (<5 micrometres; the infective form being small enough to reach terminal bronchioles).

Epidemiology

- Found throughout the world, but commonest in warm, humid environments, e.g. southern USA (estimated 500 000 cases a year). It is associated with the presence of bat and bird guano. Birds do not carry the organism—bats can and shed it in their droppings.
- Infection tends to occur when soil disruption (e.g. excavation) releases fungal elements that are then inhaled.
- Disease develops in men more often than women (4:1), which may reflect the association of chronic pulmonary disease with smoking (previously commoner in men).

Pathogenesis

- Microconidia settle in terminal airways, are phagocytosed by neutrophils and macrophages, and then switch to the yeast phase over hours/days. They migrate to the local lymph nodes and beyond. The resulting inflammatory response produces caseating or non-caseating granulomas, consisting of fungal elements, mononuclear cells, T cells, and calcium deposits. Excessive granuloma formation may be followed by fibrosis.
- Macrophages are the key mediator of resistance to *H. capsulatum*. T cells (CD4+ in particular) are important in acquired immune defence—B cells and antibodies have little role in resistance. CD4 cells seem to be vital for the activation of mononuclear phagocytes through cytokine release. CMI limits, but does not eliminate, infection—infected people contain dormant organisms for years. These pose a risk only if the individual subsequently becomes immunosuppressed.

Clinical features

Pulmonary histoplasmosis

- Acute primary infection—incubation is 1 week to a few months. Most patients are asymptomatic. Around 10% become very unwell. Severity affected by inoculum size, age (the young and the old), underlying disease, and presence of immunodeficiency. Symptoms: high fever, headache, dry cough, substernal chest pain, malaise, weakness, arthralgias, erythema nodosum, and erythema multiforme. Examination: added respiratory sounds, hepatosplenomegaly (rare). CXR: hilar lymphadenopathy and patchy pneumonitis which may calcify with time (differential includes sarcoidosis, haematological malignancy, and TB). Most symptoms settle by day 10 but may persist in those with a large initial inoculum. Laboratory tests are non-specific. Diagnosis is by antibody/antigen testing and/or BAL (diagnostic in 40%).
- Cavitary (chronic) pulmonary histoplasmosis—seen in men over 50 years with existing lung disease (e.g. COPD). Symptoms: low-grade fever, cough, weight loss, night sweats, and chest pain. Any existing pulmonary impairment may be exacerbated. CXR: cavitating lesions,

mostly in the upper lobes (90%) near a bulla. Resolves spontaneously in up to 60%. Diagnosis by serology and sputum/BAL culture. Avoid biopsy due to the potential for complications in this patient group. Healing leads to fibrosis with consequent respiratory impairment. Recurs in 20%. Death is rare.

- Complications—histoplasmoma: a mass lesion resembling a fibroma and a rare complication of primary infection. Usually located in the lung. Enlarges slowly over years, forming a calcified mass. Mediastinal granuloma: granulomatous inflammation in response to infection leads to massive enlargement of the mediastinal lymph nodes (up to 10cm) that may cause airway impingement. Fibrotic tissue formed during healing can distort airways (leading to pneumonia and bronchiectasis), the oesophagus, or the superior vena cava. Large nodes may penetrate the airways, creating sinuses or fistulae to the pericardium or oesophagus. Rarely, mediastinal fibrosis can develop, affecting all structures within the mediastinum. Diagnosis is by histology and antibody testing, as there are rarely any viable organisms. Pericarditis: seen in 5–10% of patients and probably an immune response to adjacent infected lymph nodes. Ocular histoplasmosis (uveitis or panophthalmitis) occurs rarely.

Progressive disseminated histoplasmosis

Occurs in 1 in 2000 acute infections. Risk factors: age, immunosuppression (AIDS, primary immunodeficiency, steroids, TNF-α inhibitors, etc.). Most cases probably represent reactivation of quiescent fungi, although progressive disseminated histoplasmosis (PDH) may result from primary infection or reinfection with a large inoculum. Diagnosis is made through a combination of antigen tests (urine, serum, CSF, BAL), histology, antibody tests, and culture. Urinary antigen is positive in 95% of immunocompromised patients. Serum antibody tests are positive in 90% of immunocompetent patients.

- Acute PDH—associated with a fulminant course and seen in children and the immunosuppressed (HIV and haematological malignancies). Symptoms: abrupt onset of fever, cough, weight loss, and diarrhoea. Children: chest features dominate; also hepatosplenomegaly, cervical lymphadenopathy, mouth ulcers, jaundice, anaemia (90%), and low platelets and WCC. CXR may show enlarged hilar lymph nodes and patchy pneumonitis. Untreated mortality is 100%, and, prior to antifungal therapy, children died around 6 weeks after symptom onset as a result of DIC, haemorrhage, or secondary infections. Adults with HIV: before antiretrovirals, up to 25% of AIDS patients in an endemic area could develop infection. Findings: hepatosplenomegaly, lymphadenopathy, cutaneous signs (rash, bruising, petechiae), anaemia, low platelets. Rarer manifestations: colonic masses, perianal ulcers, meningitis, encephalitis. Untreated fatality is 100%; with therapy, 80% survive. The rare severe form, reactive haemophagocytic syndrome, is often fatal despite therapy.
- Subacute PDH—symptoms are prolonged. Hepatosplenomegaly is common, but fever, weight loss, and laboratory abnormalities are less pronounced. Infective lesions may occur in the GI tract (ulceration),

CNS (chronic meningitis, cerebritis, and mass lesions), adrenal glands (affected in 80%, but overt Addison's seen in only 10%), and vascular structures (endocarditis and infection of aortic aneurysms). CSF in chronic meningitis shows lymphocytosis, elevated protein, and low glucose. Basilar meninges are badly affected, and hydrocephalus may develop.

- Chronic PDH—seen exclusively in adults. It is distinguished from subacute disease by the mild chronic nature of the symptoms. Malaise and lethargy are the key complaints. Fever is less common. The commonest physical finding is painless mouth ulceration (may appear malignant). Yeasts and macrophages can be identified on biopsy from the centre of the lesion.

African histoplasmosis

H. capsulatum var. *duboisii* is found in Africa along with var. *capsulatum*. Infection has a distinct clinical presentation, with skin and bone being the most frequently affected organs (perhaps reflecting cutaneous inoculation). Patients develop ulcers, nodules, and rashes that may resemble psoriasis. Osteolytic lesions develop in the skull, ribs, and vertebrae. Infection can become disseminated and affect multiple organs, resembling infection with *C. immitis* (perhaps due to the larger size of the var. *duboisii* yeast form, compared to var. *capsulatum*).

Diagnosis

- Culture—isolation of *H. capsulatum* is the only sure way to confirm a diagnosis of histoplasmosis. Sensitivity varies: 10–15% for sputum from patients with acute pulmonary histoplasmosis, 60–90% from patients with cavitatory disease, 65% from CSF with meningitis. Rates higher with repeated sampling. Specimens are cultured for 6 weeks at 30°C in brain–heart infusion agar with blood, antibiotics, and cycloheximide; 90% of positives grow fungus by day 7. In endocarditis, BCs are often negative; heart valves are frequently positive. The organism is rarely found in pleural or pericardial fluid—best grown from the pleura or pericardium.
- Antigen detection—galactomannan assays performed on urine or serum are positive in 90% of patients with progressive disseminated disease, and 20% of those with acute pulmonary histoplasmosis. May also be performed on BAL samples. Useful for detecting relapses in those with PDH and more sensitive than serology. It is sensitive and fairly specific in the diagnosis of meningitis from CSF samples. Cross-reactivity with *Blastomyces* and *Coccidioides* spp. causes false-positive results.
- Serology—use only in those with a compatible clinical presentation. False negatives in 50% of immunosuppressed patients. Complement fixation tests are more sensitive, but less specific, than immunodiffusion. One to 5% of healthy people living in endemic areas have positive serology.
  - Complement fixation—a 4-fold rise or titre of 1:32 suggests active infection (75% of patients 6 weeks after inoculation). Rising titres in the previously treated imply relapse. Less than 15% false-positive rate due to other fungi (coccidiomycosis, blastomycosis), TB, sarcoidosis.

 - Immunodiffusion test detects antibodies to the H and M fungal glycoproteins in patient sera. Anti-M antigen is detected in 80% of cases but does not distinguish active disease from previous infection. The presence of anti-H antigen suggests active infection but is not sensitive.
- Histology—rapid identification of fungus from tissues and body fluids. It may be positive in up to 40% of blood smears from patients with acute PDH.
- PCR—assays are rapid and specific, but sensitivity is currently poor.

Treatment

- Acute pulmonary histoplasmosis—most cases do not require treatment. Moderate illness and those with symptoms after 4 weeks can be treated with itraconazole (6–12 weeks). Give liposomal amphotericin for the first 2 weeks of therapy in severe disease, and consider steroids.
- Mediastinal granuloma—if symptoms, treat as above. Amphotericin may be preferable if rapid resolution of symptoms is required.
- Mediastinal fibrosis—antifungal therapy is not recommended. Surgery is often difficult, and fibrosis may recur. Obstructed vessels can be stented.
- Histoplasmoma—surgical excision if enlarging; 2–3 months' therapy with an azole may be beneficial afterwards.
- Cavitary pulmonary histoplasmosis—treatment should be given to those with progressive infiltrates, thick-walled cavities, or persistent cavities impairing respiratory function. Itraconazole 400mg daily for 6 months leads to improvement in up to 85% of patients. Amphotericin should be used in the immunosuppressed or if disease progresses on therapy. Relapse is seen in up to 20%, and surgical resection may be necessary.
- Acute PDH—life-threatening PDH should be treated with early liposomal amphotericin. Most patients show significant improvement in the first week. Mild disease can be treated with a 12-month course of itraconazole. Patients with AIDS and those on long-term immunosuppressive therapy should receive lifelong itraconazole.
- Subacute and chronic PDH—itraconazole 400mg daily gives a 90% success rate. Alternative: amphotericin.
- Meningitis—treatment is with liposomal amphotericin for 4–6 weeks, followed by 12 months of itraconazole (poor CNS penetration). Assess with weekly LPs. Relapses are common. Around 50% are cured (more in the immunocompetent, less in the immunocompromised).
- Endocarditis—amphotericin and surgical removal of the infected valve.
- Pericarditis—may be seen after acute PDH. The pericardium is rarely infected. Bed rest, NSAIDs, and possibly steroids (beware of exacerbating active histoplasmosis lesions) usually suffice. Cardiac tamponade is uncommon.
- See IDSA guidelines for further details on the treatment of histoplasmosis.[4]

Prevention

There is no vaccine available at present. Prevention rests on educating those who work in areas where there is a risk of acquiring infection, e.g. workers in buildings and other environments that have served as bat habitation. In HIV-infected patients who have had histoplasmosis, secondary prophylaxis is given until the CD4 count is consistently above 200 cells/mm^3.

Reference

4 Wheat LJ, Freifeld AG, Kleiman MB, *et al.*; Infectious Diseases Society of America (2007). Clinical practice guidelines for the management of patients with histoplasmosis: 2007 update by the Infectious Diseases Society of America. *Clin Infect Dis*. **45**:807–25.

Blastomyces dermatitidis—ACDP 3

A dimorphic fungus and cause of systemic pyogranulomatous disease.

Mycology

Grows in the mycelial form at room temperature and as a yeast at 37°C. The mycelial form grows on plates by 3 weeks and produces the infectious conidia (2–10 micrometres in diameter). Yeast cells are multinucleate with thick cell walls and have a similar appearance *in vitro* as in clinical specimens. *B. dermatitidis* is the asexual stage of *Ajellomyces dermatitidis*, the sexual form which requires opposite mating types for reproduction.

Epidemiology

Limited information, as there is no sensitive skin test. Endemic areas: south-eastern USA, parts of South America, the Middle East, and India. African strains are serologically distinct from American. Favours decaying wood material in moist areas. Symptomatic disease occurs in <50% of infections.

Pathogenesis

Infection is acquired via the lungs. Conidia are inhaled and convert to the yeast phase. A non-caseating granulomatous response usually follows, although respiratory disease may not be apparent. The organism may disseminate to other sites. The histology of cutaneous disease is distinct, producing pseudoepitheliomatous hyperplasia with microabscesses. In appearance, it may resemble other skin lesions (e.g. squamous cell carcinoma). Mucosal involvement of the mouth and larynx may take a similar appearance. Protection from infection is mediated primarily by natural resistance (e.g. alveolar macrophages—rates are not greatly increased in those with immunocompromise) and cellular immunity (antibodies confer no protection).

Clinical features

Almost any organ can become infected. Some patients present with an acute pneumonia, but most experience a more chronic course.

- Acute infection—following exposure, there is an incubation period of 4–6 weeks before the development of non-specific flu-like symptoms: fever, arthralgia, and cough (initially non-productive but may later produce purulent sputum). CXR may demonstrate an area of consolidation. There have been reports of spontaneous resolution of such acute pneumonias.
- Chronic pulmonary infection—chronic pneumonia with productive cough, pleuritic chest pain, haemoptysis, weight loss, and low-grade fever. CXR may show infiltrates, mass lesions (which may resemble malignancy), and cavities, but effusions are rare. Miliary disease or diffuse pneumonitis is unusual—both have a high mortality.

- Skin—commonest extrapulmonary manifestation, seen in up to 80% of cases. May occur in the absence of respiratory features. Lesions may be verrucous or ulcerative—both may occur in the same patient. Verrucous lesions resemble squamous cell carcinoma. Where there is discharge, microscopy may reveal yeast forms. Subcutaneous nodules represent cold abscesses and are usually seen in acutely ill patients with severe pulmonary or extrapulmonary disease at another site.
- Bone and joint—long bones, vertebrae, and ribs. Extension may lead to arthritis. Organisms are seen in synovial aspirates.
- GU tract—around 25% of men have GU involvement, usually of the prostate.
- CNS—uncommon in the normal host. More likely (e.g. as abscess or meningitis) in patients with AIDS who develop blastomycosis.
- The immunocompromised—an unusual opportunistic pathogen in HIV patients. Disease is more severe and more likely to be fatal in those with late-stage AIDS. CNS infection is seen in 40% of cases. Similar severity is seen in patients with immunocompromise due to steroid therapy and chemotherapy. Up to 40% of cases are fatal. Treat suspected cases early—most deaths occur within a few weeks. Relapse is common if immunodeficiency remains, and long-term suppression should be considered.

Diagnosis

- Microscopy of secretions—the characteristic yeast cell may be seen in a wet preparation of sputum or pus. Body fluids, such as urine or pleural fluid, should be centrifuged, and the sediment examined. BAL may be useful in patients who are not producing sputum. When organisms are sparse, they may be more easily identified on Papanicolaou preparations.
- Histology—visualized by Gomori's methenamine silver and PAS stains.
- Culture—material should be inoculated on Sabouraud or more enriched agar and incubated at 30°C. The mycelial form is not diagnostic, and ideally conversion to yeast at 37°C should be demonstrated. This is not always possible, and nucleic acid probes can confirm identification.
- Serology—complement fixation, immunodiffusion, and ELISA-based tests are available, but sensitivity and specificity vary widely. A negative test does not rule out disease, and a positive does not, on its own, warrant therapy (cross-reactivity with endemic mycoses)—rather it should fuel the hunt for the organism.
- Antigen detection—a commercial assay is available, but its modest specificity (79%) limits its utility.

Treatment

All patients should receive therapy. A small number of cases do resolve spontaneously, but these cannot be predicted at presentation. Surgery has a role in the drainage of large abscesses and the resection of necrotic bone tissue, in combination with medical therapy.

- Mild to moderate pulmonary/disseminated disease—itraconazole for 6 months (12 in osteoarticular). Relapses do occur, and patients should be followed up for 2 years.

- Severe pulmonary/disseminated and the immunosuppressed—liposomal amphotericin 1–2 weeks, then itraconazole ~12 months. Relapse is commoner in those with immunocompromise.
- CNS disease—liposomal amphotericin for 4–6 weeks, then PO azole for 1 year. Voriconazole may be best (good activity and CNS penetration), but limited data.
- See IDSA guidelines for full details on management of blastomycosis.[5]

Reference

5 Chapman SW, Dismukes WE, Proia LA, *et al.*; Infectious Diseases Society of America (2008). Clinical practice guidelines for the management of blastomycosis: 2008 update by the Infectious Diseases Society of America. *Clin Infect Dis*. **46**:1801–12.

Coccidioides immitis—ACDP 3

A dimorphic fungus found in certain regions of the Western hemisphere and a cause of respiratory illness.

Mycology

May exist as a mycelium or a spherule (a structure unique to this organism). The mycelial form is seen on routine laboratory agar and in soil. Mature cells can develop a hydrophobic outer layer that renders them capable of prolonged survival (arthroconidia). Once airborne, these may be inhaled and deposited in the lungs where they begin to multiply. The resultant spherule consists of a thin wall containing many endospores. This wall eventually ruptures, allowing the spread of endospores.

Epidemiology

Endemic to certain regions of the Western hemisphere with an arid climate, hot summers, and alkaline soil (e.g. regions of southern USA, Mexico, Central America, parts of South America). Arthroconidia transport (e.g. in dust storms) has resulted in infections in non-endemic areas. Infections tend to occur when the soil is dry towards the end of summer. The organism is most easily isolated after the winter rains. The number of new infections varies greatly year to year; 30% of people living in the endemic regions of the USA show evidence of prior exposure.

Pathogenesis

Most infections follow inhalation of arthroconidia. There are rare cases of cutaneous infection (which tend to resolve without treatment). Inflammation follows its conversion to a spherule. The resulting pulmonary lesion consists of neutrophils and eosinophils and, if infection becomes chronic, granulomas with lymphocytes and multinucleated giant cells. Both acute and chronic lesions may be found at different sites in the same individual. Control of infection relies on the T-cell response, and those with deficient T-cell immunity are at risk of severe disease. The innate immune response appears to be important against arthroconidia and endospores.

Clinical features

Up to two-thirds of infections produce only mild or subclinical disease, and, of those producing respiratory symptoms, most follow a self-limiting course. Complications may occur up to 2 years later and do not correlate with the severity of the original infection.

- Early respiratory infection—symptoms develop 1–3 weeks after exposure: cough, pleuritic chest pain, breathlessness, and fever. Onset is usually slow but can be abrupt. Inhalation of a large number of arthroconidia may result in early symptoms. Weight loss and migratory arthritis can occur, and some develop skin rashes, ranging from a fine papular rash early in illness to erythema multiforme and nodosum (particularly in women). Laboratory tests may reveal peripheral blood eosinophilia and raised inflammatory markers. Around 50% of patients have CXR changes: effusions, infiltrates, hilar lymphadenopathy, and cavities. Most infections resolve without complications over several weeks. There are rare cases of severe diffuse coccidioidal pneumonia (due either to massive exposure or haematogenous seeding), leading to respiratory failure and septic shock with a high mortality. One-third of coccidioidal infections in HIV-positive patients (typically those with CD4 <100 cells/mm^3) present in this manner.
- Pulmonary nodules and cavities—4% of lung infections result in a nodule that may reach up to 5cm in diameter. Although usually asymptomatic, a biopsy may be necessary to distinguish it from a neoplastic lesion. Nodules may liquefy and drain via a bronchus to form a cavity. Cavities are usually peripheral, and, although half close within 2 years, some may cause pain, cough, and haemoptysis, as well as provide a focus for the development of mycetoma. Peripheral cavities can rupture, causing a pyopneumothorax.
- Chronic fibrocavity pneumonia—associated with diabetes or pre-existing lung fibrosis; some people develop chronic fibrotic pneumonia with widespread pulmonary infiltrates and cavities involving >1 lobe. Patients may experience night sweats and weight loss.
- Dissemination—rare (0.5% of cases overall). Those with immunodeficiency (solid organ transplants, late-stage HIV infection, high-dose steroids, Hodgkin's disease) are at greater risk. Many with disseminated disease do not develop respiratory features and have normal CXRs. Sites of dissemination: skin (causing maculopapular lesions, verrucous ulcers, and abscesses with a predilection for the nasolabial fold), joints (knee, hand, wrist, feet), bone (particularly the vertebrae—which may progress to develop a paraspinous abscess), and meningitis—the most serious manifestation. Meningitis develops a few weeks to a few months after initial infection and is usually fatal within 2 years of diagnosis. CSF findings: elevated pressure, raised protein, low glucose, raised eosinophils. The basilar meninges are usually involved, and hydrocephalus is a common complication in children.

Diagnosis

- Clinical features of coccidioidal infection are not specific, and laboratory tests are required to establish diagnosis. Travel history is vital—exposure can be subtle (e.g. changing planes within an endemic area). Complications are usually apparent within 2 years of exposure, but infection may have occurred many years previously in the immunodeficient. Most diagnoses are made serologically, with culture in severe cases.
- Isolation of the organism—definitive diagnosis is by culture of, or identifying fungal elements within, clinical specimens (e.g. biopsy, sputum). *Coccidioides* spp. are never normal flora. Stains, such as silver, PAS, or haematoxylin and eosin (H&E) will reveal spherules. *C. immitis* grows on standard microbiological media in aerobic conditions and typically takes the form of a white mould at around 1 week. At this point, it is highly infectious. Unlike the spherule, the mycelial form is not unique, and reference laboratories make identification either antigenically or by the detection of specific rRNA.
- Serology—most patients are not very symptomatic, and diagnosis is by serology. Serology is important in the diagnosis of coccidioidal meningitis, as CSF is usually culture-negative. Tests are highly specific, and even borderline positive results should be treated seriously. Antibodies may only become detectable weeks/months after illness onset, and negative tests do not exclude infection. The tube precipitin (TP) antibody (IgM) test detects a fungal cell wall polysaccharide and is positive in 90% of patients by the third week of illness; complement fixing antibodies (predominantly IgG) are detected later and for longer than TP antibodies, and their presence in CSF is important in the diagnosis of coccidioidal meningitis; ELISA tests for IgG and IgM are highly sensitive and specific on both CSF and serum; immunodiffusion tests are the most specific assays. Some laboratories screen with ELISA and confirm with immunodiffusion. CF/immunodiffusion tests can be reported qualitatively, allowing assessment of treatment response.
- Antigen detection—a urinary antigen test is available. Sensitivity is 71%, thus best used as part of a wider diagnostic strategy.
- Skin testing—for delayed-type hypersensitivity to coccidioidal antigens, is useful epidemiologically, but limited as a diagnostic tool.

Treatment

- Uncomplicated primary disease—newly diagnosed patients should be assessed for the extent of disease and factors that increase the risk of dissemination or future complications. If otherwise well, those with mild disease do not need therapy but should be followed up for a year.
- Consider treatment with an azole antifungal for 3–6 months in those with:
  - moderate/severe pulmonary infection—weight loss of over 10%, night sweats for 3 or more weeks, infiltrates that are either bilateral or involve more than half of a lung, persistent hilar lymphadenopathy, symptoms persisting for over 2 months;

- risk of dissemination—the immunosuppressed, pregnant women;
- severe pulmonary disease, e.g. pre-existing lung fibrosis;
- amphotericin is the preferred agent in cases of severe pulmonary disease or those who are deteriorating. Surgery may be required in some patients (e.g. cavities that do not resolve). Debridement and drainage of infected sites are essential in extensive bone infection, and, in cases of vertebral infection, stabilization may be required.

- Persistent fibrocavitary pneumonia—treatment is usually started with PO azoles. Up to 60% respond with improved symptoms and CXR. Those who do not may respond to amphotericin.
- Meningitis—treat initially with fluconazole (response rate of 70%). Voriconazole may be an alternative. Consider intrathecal amphotericin if no response or in the first trimester of pregnancy. Hydrocephalus may require shunting. Cerebral abscesses may need draining.
- Other forms of dissemination can usually be treated with PO azoles, except in those who are showing rapid deterioration or have infection in critical places when amphotericin is preferred. Treatment is continued for at least a year, and for 6 months beyond the end of recovery. Relapses occur in one-third. Lifelong suppressive therapy may be required.
- See IDSA guidelines for further details on the management of cocciodioidomycosis.[6]

Reference

6 Galgiani JN, Ampel NM, Blair JE, *et al.*; Infectious Diseases Society of America (2005). Coccidioidomycosis. *Clin Infect Dis*. **41**:1217–23.

Paracoccidioides brasiliensis—ACDP 3

A cause of chronic progressive systemic mycosis in South America.

Mycology

P. brasiliensis is a dimorphic fungus (at 37°C a yeast, below 28°C a mycelium). At 37°C, colonies take around 10 days to appear and have a creamy, soft appearance. Mould-form colonies take up to a month to develop.

Epidemiology

Limited to South America from Argentina to Mexico, causing infections in forest regions with high year-round humidity and mild temperatures. Brazil has the highest number of reported cases. It has been isolated from soil. Human infection is probably acquired by inhalation. Most cases occur in men over 30 years of age. Agricultural workers, smokers, and alcoholics are at greater risk.

Clinical features

Most primary cases are subclinical. The organism can remain dormant for prolonged periods, disease becoming apparent only in states of debilitation or immunosuppression. Causes subacute severe disease in the young and chronic disease in adults, in whom it has a better prognosis with therapy.

- Lung—breathlessness, and CXR may reveal nodular infiltrates which are often bilateral. Lesions concentrated in the mid and lower zones; apices are usually clear. Cavities, fibrosis, emphysema, and right ventricular hypertrophy become more likely, as disease becomes chronic.
- Mouth and upper respiratory mucosa—ulcerated lesions of the mouth, lip, gums, tongue, and palate. Other features: tooth loss, dysphonia, nasal lesions.
- Cutaneous lesions—warty, ulcerated lesions over legs and orifices.
- Other—lymphadenopathy (sometimes with fistulae), diminished adrenal function, spleen, liver, gut, vascular system, bone, CNS.

Diagnosis

- Microscopy with KOH—reveals the organism (identified by its distinctive multiple budding) in >90% of cases where sputum or exudates are available.
- Biopsy—often diagnostic. Histology shows granuloma with multinucleated giant cells that may contain fungi. Ulcerated lesions may show a pyogenic reaction, and skin lesions may have intraepithelial microabscesses.
- Culture—on Sabouraud-dextrose agar (keep for 6 weeks).
- Serology—immunodiffusion is most reliable. Remains positive after successful treatment. Complement fixation tests (CFTs) cross-react with *H. capsulatum*.

Treatment

- Mild/moderate—itraconazole PO for 6–12 months.
- Severe—amphotericin or co-trimoxazole IV. Voriconazole may be an alternative. Switch to an oral agent once improved (20–40 days). Duration may need to be >2 years if co-trimoxazole is used or CNS involvement.
- Relapse may occur in <5% of those with chronic disease treated with itraconazole, and <25% of those treated with co-trimoxazole. Immunocompromised patients are at particular risk. Serological testing and radiological follow-up may guide decisions on duration.

Penicillium marneffei—ACDP 3

A thermally dimorphic fungus that may cause severe disseminated infection.

Epidemiology

Limited to South East Asia and southern China. Humans and bamboo rats are the only known hosts. The exact route of transmission is unknown but is thought to be inhalation or rarely inoculation. Infection is commonly seen in young adults with HIV (fourth commonest opportunistic infection in Thai patients). Cases are seen in immunocompetent children and adults. Occupational exposure to soil is a risk factor.

Clinical features

Occurs late in HIV infection (CD4 count <100 cells/mm^3). Patients present with around 1 month of fever, weight loss, and skin lesions (pustules, papules, ulcers, or abscesses of the face, upper trunk, or extremities). Pharyngeal and palatal lesions are common in those with HIV. Most have anaemia and weight loss, with around half presenting with fungaemia or lymphadenopathy. Hepatomegaly, splenomegaly, haemoptysis (secondary to cavitating lung lesions), joint infections, and pericarditis may occur. The diagnosis should be considered in those with immunocompromise and history of travel to an affected area. Disease may present many years after travel.

Diagnosis

- Histology—a presumptive diagnosis may be made on smear (skin lesion, sputum) or biopsy (lymph node, bone marrow) in the appropriate setting. Microscopic examination may reveal yeast forms extracellularly and within phagocytes. Histology may demonstrate either a granulomatous (in the immunocompetent), suppurative, or necrotizing (in the immunocompromised) response.
- Culture—treatment may need to be initiated, while culture is ongoing. Typically takes 4–7 days, but occasionally weeks. At 25°C, grows as a mould with sporulating structures. May convert to yeast form at 37°C. This dimorphism is not seen in other members of the genus *Penicillium*.
- Serological assays are not widely used due to limited data on their accuracy.

Treatment

May need to be initiated prior to culture completion. Beware of interactions between azoles and antiretrovirals. Consider therapeutic drug level monitoring.[7]

- Severe or CNS involvement—2 weeks IV amphotericin, followed by 10 weeks PO itraconazole. Voriconazole may also be effective.
- Mild—PO itraconazole 400mg/day for 8 weeks.
- HIV-infected patients—should be started on ART within 2–4 weeks of antifungal treatment commencing. Secondary prophylaxis with PO itraconazole 200mg/day should continue until CD4 >100 cells/mm^3 for at least 6 months.

Reference

7 Panel on Opportunistic Infections in HIV-Infected Adults and Adolescents. *Guidelines for the prevention and treatment of opportunistic infections in HIV-infected adults and adolescents: recommendations from the Centers for Disease Control and Prevention, the National Institutes of Health, and the HIV Medicine Association of the Infectious Diseases Society of America*. Available at: https://aidsinfo.nih.gov.

Chapter 10

Protozoa

Plasmodium species (malaria) 512
Babesia 515
Toxoplasma gondii 517
Cryptosporidium 520
Cystoisospora 522
Cyclospora 523
Trypanosoma 523
Trypanosoma cruzi 523
Trypanosoma brucei complex 525
Leishmania 527
Giardia lamblia 530
Trichomonas vaginalis 532
Entamoeba histolytica 533
Free-living amoebae 535
Microsporidia 537

Plasmodium species (malaria)

Malaria, an infection caused by *Plasmodium* spp., has affected mankind for millennia. The word malaria means 'bad air', and refers to the association between the illness and the marshes where *Anopheles* mosquitoes breed. Although malaria has virtually disappeared from Europe and the USA (apart from imported cases), it remains a major problem in tropical countries where it causes an estimated 216 million cases and 655 000 deaths per year.

Plasmodium species

Five *Plasmodium* spp. cause human infection:

- *P. falciparum* can invade RBCs of all ages, may be drug-resistant, and is responsible for most severe, life-threatening infections. It does not produce dormant liver stages (hypnozoites) or cause relapse.
- *P. vivax* and *P. ovale* cause clinically similar, milder infections. They produce hypnozoites and may cause relapse months after the initial infection.
- *P. malariae* rarely causes acute illness in normal hosts, does not produce hypnozoites, but may persist in the bloodstream for years.
- *Plasmodium knowlesi* causes malaria in macaques and has recently been recognized as a cause of human malaria in South East Asia. Microscopically, it resembles *P. malariae* but can cause fatal disease (like *P. falciparum*).

Mixed infections may occur in 5–7% of patients.

Life cycle

Humans acquire malaria from sporozoites transmitted by the bite of the female *Anopheles* mosquito. Sporozoites travel through the bloodstream and enter hepatocytes. Here they mature into tissue schizonts which rupture and release merozoites into the bloodstream. These invade RBCs and mature into ring forms, then trophozoites, and finally schizonts, before rupturing to release merozoites. Alternatively, some erythrocytic parasites develop into gametocytes (sexual forms), which are ingested by the mosquito and complete the sexual life cycle. In *P. vivax* and *P. ovale* infections, some parasites remain dormant in the liver as hypnozoites for months, before they mature into tissue schizonts.

Epidemiology

The epidemiology of malaria varies and depends on a number of factors: climate, *Plasmodium* spp. and life cycle, efficiency of transmission by vectors, and drug resistance. Thus, in sub-Saharan Africa, *P. falciparum* can survive as a result of the year-round presence and efficient transmission by its mosquito vectors (*Anopheles gambiae* and *Anopheles funestus*). In contrast, *P. vivax*, which is found in more temperate zones, requires hypnozoites to sustain its transmission.

Pathogenesis

The following mechanisms contribute to the pathogenesis of severe falciparum malaria:

- *cytoadherence*—adherence of parasitized RBCs to the vascular endothelium is mediated by *P. falciparum*-infected erythrocyte membrane protein 1 (PfEMP1), which binds to specific endothelial receptors, e.g. thrombospondin, CD36, ICAM-1, VCAM1, and ELAM1. This results in peripheral sequestration of parasites, which protects them from removal from the circulation as they pass through the spleen, and oxidant damage as they pass through the lungs;
- *rosetting*—PfEMP1 also binds to complement receptor-1, resulting in clustering of unparasitized red cells around parasitized red cells;
- *hyperparasitaemia* (>5%)—is associated with a greater risk of death, particularly in non-immune patients. Reasons for this include more severe metabolic effects, e.g. hypoglycaemia and lactic acidosis.

Clinical features

- Fevers (cyclical or continuous with intermittent spikes).
- Malarial paroxysm—chills, high fever, sweats.
- Complications—cerebral malaria, pulmonary oedema, severe anaemia, hypoglycaemia, jaundice, acute kidney injury, acidosis.

Laboratory diagnosis

- Thick and thin blood smears, stained with Field's stain or Giemsa stain, examined under light microscopy. Giemsa is better for species identification.
- Malaria dipstick tests, e.g. OptiMAL-IT® and Paracheck-Pf®. These detect plasmodial lactate dehydrogenase (LDH) and offer a rapid diagnostic near-patient test. Some tests enable distinction of species.
- Laboratory findings—haemolytic anaemia, thrombocytopenia (common), uraemia, hyperbilirubinaemia, abnormal LFTs, coagulopathy.

Treatment

See Box 10.1.

- Antimalarials (➔ see Antimalarials, pp. 112–3)—remain the mainstay of therapy, but successful treatment is threatened by increasing drug resistance. The main classes of drugs are:
  - quinoline derivatives (chloroquine, quinine, mefloquine, halofantrine);
  - antifolates (pyrimethamine, sulfonamides);
  - ribosomal inhibitors (tetracycline, doxycycline, clindamycin);
  - artemisinin derivates (artemisinin, artemether, artemotil, artesunate);
  - artemisinin derivatives are the treatment of choice and show rapid parasite clearance, and have low toxicity and limited resistance (in South East Asia). Despite superior efficacy to quinine, IV artesunate is not licensed in the UK.
- *Supportive therapy*—good supportive therapy, with careful management of seizures, pulmonary oedema, acute renal failure, and lactic acidosis, is essential in severe malaria. Exchange transfusion may be helpful in hyperparasitaemia.

Box 10.1 Malaria treatment and prevention guidelines

Treatment

- UK guidelines:
  - Lalloo D, Shingadia D, Pasvol G, *et al*. UK malaria treatment guidelines. *J Infect* 2016;72(6):635–64
  - Public Health England. Guideline for malaria prevention in travellers from the UK 2015
  - Both available at 🖱 www.britishinfection.org/guidelines-resources/published-guidelines/
  - See also sections on treatment and prophylaxis of malaria in the *BNF* (🖱 www.bnf.org)
- US guidelines:
  - Treatment of malaria (guidelines for clinicians) 2013. Available at 🖱 http://www.cdc.gov/malaria/resources/pdf/clinicalguidance.pdf
  - *The Yellow Book*. CDC health information for international travel 2016, Chapter 3, Malaria. Available at 🖱 wwwnc.cdc.gov/travel/yellowbook/2016/infectious-diseases-related-to-travel/malaria
- World Health Organization:
  - 2015 *Guidelines for the treatment of malaria*, third edition. Available at 🖱 www.who.int/malaria/publications/atoz/9789241549127/en/

- *Adjunctive therapies*—adjunctive therapies for severe malaria have proved disappointing. Monoclonal antibodies directed against TNF-α reduced fever but showed no effect on mortality and may have increased morbidity. Dexamethasone has been shown to increase the duration of coma and was associated with poorer outcome in cerebral malaria.

Prevention

(See Box 10.1.)

- *Insecticide-treated bed nets* have been shown to reduce intradomiciliary vector populations and protect against infection.
- *Insect repellents*, such as diethyltoluamide (DEET), reduce the risk of transmission in areas where mosquitoes are active before bedtime.
- *Chemoprophylaxis*, taken rigorously, is efficacious in reducing the incidence of malaria in travellers.
- *Vaccines*—a number of candidate vaccines using various antigens have been developed. Of these, the RTS,S/AS01E vaccine looks to be the most promising.

Babesia

Babesiosis is a zoonotic infection caused by *Babesia* spp., a malaria-like parasite that parasitizes erythrocytes of animals and causes fever, haemolysis, and haemoglobinuria. It typically causes mild illness in humans, but fulminant disease may occur in asplenic or immunosuppressed patients.

The parasite

There are >70 *Babesia* spp. worldwide that infect a wide range of mammals and birds. *Babesia* spp. have traditionally been classified into four clades:

- clade 1 contains *Babesia microti* spp. that cause disease in the USA and Japan;
- clade 2 contains *Babesia duncani* and *B. duncani*-like organisms that cause disease in the western USA;
- clade 3 contains *Babesia divergens* that causes disease in cattle in Europe, *B. divergens*-like organisms that cause disease in humans in Europe and the USA, and *Babesia venatorum* that causes human disease in Europe;
- clade 4 contains *Babesia bovis* and *Babesia bigemina* that rarely cause disease in humans.

Babesia spp. vary in length from 1 to 5 micrometres, and are pear-shaped, oval, or round; their ring conformation and peripheral location in erythrocytes may lead to their misidentification as *P. falciparum*. *Babesia* spp. are transmitted from their animal reservoir to humans via a tick vector *Ixodes scapularis* (USA) or *Ixodes ricinus* (Europe). The tick has three developmental stages (larva, nymph, and adult) and requires a blood meal, often from different mammalian species (e.g. deer, rodent) to mature to the next stage.

Epidemiology

The first fatal human case of babesiosis was reported in 1996. Since then, >2700 cases have been reported worldwide, most from the north-eastern coastal regions of the USA. Based on seroprevalence data, most infections appear to be subclinical. Transfusion-associated, transplacental, and perinatal transmission may occur. The clinical features of babesiosis vary markedly between regions. Virtually all of the European cases have been caused by *B. bovis* or *B. divergens*, have occurred in splenectomized patients, and have had a fulminant and usually fatal course. In contrast, epidemiological data from the USA suggest that most infections are caused by *B. microti* and are mild or subclinical; clinical infections are more likely in the asplenic, immunosuppressed, elderly, or patients with concomitant Lyme disease. Risk factors for severe disease include age >50 years, splenectomy, HIV infection, immunosuppression, and therapy with anti-TNF agents (infliximab, etanercept) or anti-CD20 antibody (rituximab).

Clinical features

- Clinical features include fever, chills, malaise, fatigue, anorexia, headache, myalgia, arthralgia, nausea, vomiting, abdominal pain, dark urine, depression, and emotional lability. Photophobia, conjunctival injection, retinal infarcts, sore throat, and cough have also been described.
- Clinical features of severe disease include ARDS, CCF, acute kidney injury, liver failure, and DIC.

- Laboratory abnormalities include haemolytic anaemia, reticulocytosis, normal or low WCC, thrombocytopenia, raised erythrocyte sedimentation rate (ESR), positive direct Coombs' test, abnormal LFTs, renal impairment, and reduced serum haptoglobin levels.
- Urinalysis reveals haemoglobinuria and proteinuria.

Laboratory diagnosis

- Microscopy—examination of thick and thin blood smears stained with Giemsa or Wright stains show parasitized erythrocytes, sometimes with diagnostic tetrads ('Maltese cross') of merozoites. *Babesia* spp. can be distinguished from *P. falciparum* by its lack of haemozoin and the absence of schizonts and gametocytes.
- Serology—indirect immunofluorescent antibody titre for *B. microti* is available from CDC Atlanta. A titre of ≥1:256 is considered diagnostic for acute *B. microti* infection.
- Molecular methods—a PCR-based assay may be used for the detection of low levels of parasitaemia.

Treatment

- Treatment is indicated for: (i) symptomatic patients with babesial parasites detected on microscopy or babesial DNA detected by PCR; (ii) asymptomatic patients with babesial parasites detected on microscopy or babesial DNA detected by PCR for ≥3 months; and (iii) patients with babesial parasites detected on microscopy or babesial DNA detected by PCR for ≥3 months after initiation of therapy.
- For patients with mild *B. microti* infection, atovaquone plus azithromycin for 7–10 days is the preferred regimen, as it is better tolerated than quinine plus clindamycin (also given for 7–10 days).
- For patients with severe disease, quinine plus clindamycin is recommended, as there is more experience with this regimen. Longer durations of therapy may be required for severe disease—up to 6 weeks in immunosuppressed patients.
- Exchange transfusion is used in critically ill patients with high-grade parasitaemia (≥10%).

Prevention

- Avoid exposure to ticks in endemic areas between May and September.
- Wear light-coloured, long-sleeved clothing, and tuck trousers into socks or boots.
- Use insect repellent (e.g. DEET) on skin and clothes.
- Carefully remove any ticks.
- Discourage blood donations from donors in endemic areas between May and September, from donors with fevers 2 months prior to donation, and from donors with a history of tick bite.

Toxoplasma gondii

Toxoplasmosis is a zoonotic infection caused by *T. gondii*, a coccidian parasite of cats that affects humans and other mammals as intermediate hosts. Although infection with *T. gondii* is common, it rarely causes disease, apart from in congenitally acquired infection and in patients with cell-mediated immunodeficiency, especially AIDS.

Classification

T. gondii belongs to subphylum *Apicomplexa*, class *Sporozoa* and exists in three forms: the oocyst (which releases sporozoites), the tissue cyst (which contains bradyzoites), and the tachyzoite.

Life cycle

Oocysts are produced in the cat's intestine and shed in its faeces. Once outside the cat, the oocysts sporulate and develop sporozoites. Oocysts are ingested by other animals and release sporozoites, which develop into tachyzoites. These infect a wide variety of cells, multiply rapidly to form rosettes, lyse the cells, and spread to other cells or parts of the body. In the tissues, formation of tissue cysts may occur, with slowly replicating bradyzoites inside them.

Epidemiology

Toxoplasmosis is a worldwide zoonosis infecting a wide variety of mammals. Human infection occurs through the ingestion of:

- tissue cysts in raw or undercooked meat;
- food or water contaminated with oocysts;
- transplacental transmission from mother to fetus;
- rarely, through organ transplantation from a seropositive donor, contaminated blood transfusion, or needlestick injury.

In HIV-infected patients, cerebral toxoplasmosis is usually due to reactivation of latent infection due to advanced immunosuppression (CD4 count <100 cells/mm^3). The incidence of toxoplasmosis amongst HIV-infected individuals is directly related to the seroprevalence of *T. gondii* antibodies in the general population. Thus, rates are higher in Western Europe and Africa than in the USA. However, the introduction of HAART and use of co-trimoxazole prophylaxis for PCP have resulted in a dramatic fall in the incidence of toxoplasmosis in the developed world.

Pathogenesis

T. gondii penetrates intestinal epithelial cells and multiplies intracellularly. Organisms spread to the regional lymph nodes before being carried to distant organs in the lymphatics and blood. Infection with *T. gondii* induces both humoral and cellular immune responses, which are important for the early clearance of organisms from the blood and limit the parasite burden in other organs. Cyst formation is responsible for persistent or latent infection; the main sites are the brain, skeletal and cardiac muscle, and the eye. In immunocompetent individuals, initial infection is often asymptomatic; chronic/latent infection is not clinically significant, and immunity is lifelong. In immunosuppressed patients, toxoplasmosis may be caused by primary infection but is usually due to reactivation of latent infection. The histological features of cerebral toxoplasmosis include: focal (or diffuse) necrotizing encephalitis, microglial nodules, multiple brain abscesses, hydrocephalus.

Clinical features

- *Immunocompetent patients*—10–20% of infections are symptomatic. Clinical features include lymphadenopathy and/or an infectious mononucleosis-like syndrome. Rarely, severe disseminated disease (myocarditis, pericarditis, pneumonitis, ARDS, polymyositis, hepatitis, encephalitis) may occur.
- *Immunodeficient patients*—toxoplasmosis in HIV-negative patients is associated with organ transplants and lymphoma, and presents with CNS, myocardial, or pulmonary involvement. In AIDS patients, cerebral toxoplasmosis is the commonest diagnosis and presents subacutely with focal neurological symptoms. Other manifestations include spinal cord involvement, pneumonitis, chorioretinitis, pituitary abnormalities, orchitis, and GI involvement.
- *Ocular toxoplasmosis*—*T. gondii* is an important cause of chorioretinitis. Congenitally acquired infection usually presents in the second or third decade of life, with bilateral disease, macular involvement, and old retinal scars. Post-natal infection usually presents in the fourth to sixth decade of life, with unilateral involvement and macular sparing. Ocular toxoplasmosis has also been reported in HIV-infected patients, especially from Brazil.
- *Congenital toxoplasmosis*—the incidence of fetal infection varies with trimester: 10–25% in the first trimester, 30–54% in the second trimester, 60–65% in the third trimester. The risk of severe congenital infection is highest in the first and second trimesters (weeks 10–24). Clinical features include: chorioretinitis, strabismus, blindness, seizures, microcephaly, intracranial calcification, hydrocephalus, anaemia, jaundice, rash, encephalitis, pneumonitis, diarrhoea, hypothermia. In contrast, infants who acquire infection in the third trimester may be born with subclinical infection but, if untreated, may go on to develop disease, e.g. chorioretinitis or developmental delay.

Laboratory diagnosis

- Serology—this remains the mainstay of diagnosis. The main problem with serological tests is that antibodies are present in many healthy individuals and persist at high levels for years. Different tests measure different antibodies, and there is no single test that can be used to differentiate acute from chronic infection. A combination of tests is often used:
  - IgG antibodies usually appear within 1–2 weeks, peak at 1–2 months, and persist for life. The most widely used tests are: ELISA, indirect fluorescent antibody (IFA) test, modified direct agglutination test (DAT), IgG avidity test, and Sabin–Feldman dye test (gold standard);

  - IgM antibodies may appear and decline more rapidly than IgG antibodies. However, high IgM levels may persist for years, limiting its use as the sole marker of acute infection. Various tests exist: ELISA (false positives with antinuclear antibody (ANA) and rheumatoid factor), IFA, and IgM immunosorbent agglutination assay (ISAGA);
  - IgA antibodies have higher sensitivity than the IgM assays for the diagnosis of congenital toxoplasmosis;
  - IgE antibodies are present for a shorter duration than IgM or IgA and may be useful for diagnosing recently acquired infection.
- PCR—the detection of *T. gondii* DNA in body fluids and tissues has been used to diagnose all forms of *Toxoplasma* infection, including intrauterine infection and disseminated disease. Sensitivity is 15–85% in blood/buffy coat, and 11–77% in CSF.
- Isolation—isolation of *T. gondii* from blood, body fluids, placenta, or fetal tissues is diagnostic of acute infection. Isolation may be performed by tissue culture (3–6 days) or mouse inoculation.
- Histology—demonstration of tachyzoites in tissues or body fluids is diagnostic of acute infection. Various staining methods may be used, e.g. fluorescent antibody staining, immunoperoxidase, ELISA, fluorescein-labelled monoclonal antibodies, EM, Wright–Giemsa staining of centrifuged deposit/smear.
- Antigen-specific lymphocyte transformation and typing—lymphocyte proliferation in response to *T. gondii* antigens is a sensitive and specific indicator of previous infection in adults and has been used to diagnose congenital infection. An increase in CD8+ T cells may occur with acute infection in immunocompetent adults.

Radiological features

Radiological imaging is helpful in patients with CNS disease. In neonates with congenital toxoplasmosis, ultrasound or CT may demonstrate intracranial calcification and ventricular dilatation. In immunodeficient adults with cerebral toxoplasmosis, CT typically shows multiple ring-enhancing lesions. However, scans may be normal or show solitary lesions or cortical atrophy. MRI appears to be more sensitive than CT and is the imaging modality of choice.

Treatment

(See references 1,2.)

Currently recommended drugs act primarily against the tachyzoite form and do not eradicate the encysted form. Pyrimethamine is the most effective agent and should be given with folinic acid to prevent bone marrow suppression. A second drug, sulfadiazine or clindamycin, is also given. Alternative agents include co-trimoxazole or pyrimethamine plus one of azithromycin, clarithromycin, atovaquone, or dapsone.

- *Immunocompetent adults*—do not usually require treatment, unless symptoms are severe and persistent, visceral disease is overt, or infection is parenterally acquired.

- *Immunodeficient patients*—acute/primary therapy is recommended for 3–6 weeks, followed by lifelong maintenance therapy/secondary prophylaxis. AIDS patients with cerebral toxoplasmosis usually respond clinically within 2 weeks; those who do not should be investigated for other alternative diagnoses, e.g. CNS lymphoma.
- *Ocular toxoplasmosis*—treatment may not be required for small peripheral retinal lesions in immunocompetent adults but is generally indicated for lesions that threaten or cause visual loss.
- *Toxoplasmosis in pregnancy*—patients with suspected acute toxoplasmosis in pregnancy should be referred to a specialist unit for further investigation and management. Treatment with spiramycin reduces the risk of transmission to the fetus. As spiramycin does not cross the placenta, if fetal infection occurs, treatment should be changed to pyrimethamine (not in the first trimester) and sulfadiazine.
- *Congenital toxoplasmosis*—infants with congenital toxoplasmosis should be referred to a specialist unit. Treatment is with pyrimethamine and sulfadiazine for up to 12 months.

Prevention

- Prevention of primary infection in susceptible individuals, e.g. pregnant women and immunosuppressed patients is by education:
  - avoid contact with cat faeces in gardens and cat litters;
  - avoid ingestion of undercooked meat.
- For HIV-infected patients with CD4 count <200 cells/mm^3, primary prophylaxis with co-trimoxazole has been shown to reduce the incidence of cerebral toxoplasmosis. Prophylaxis may be discontinued when CD4 count remains persistently >200 cells/mm^3.
- Some countries, e.g. France and Austria, advocate monthly screening of seronegative pregnant women during pregnancy.

References

1 Panel on Opportunistic Infections in HIV-Infected Adults and Adolescents. *Guidelines for prevention and treatment of opportunistic infections in HIV-infected adults and adolescents: recommendations from the Centers for Disease Control and Prevention, the National Institutes of Health, and the HIV Medicine Association of the Infectious Diseases Society of America*. Available at: http://aidsinfo.nih.gov/contentfiles/lvguidelines/adult_oi.pdf.

2 Nelson M, Dockrell DH, Edwards S; BHIVA Guidelines Subcommittee. *British HIV Association and British Infection Association guidelines for the treatment of opportunistic infection in HIV-seropositive individuals 2011*. Available at: http://www.bhiva.org/documents/Guidelines/OI/hiv_v12_is2_Iss2Press_Text.pdf.

Cryptosporidium

Cryptosporidium is an intracellular protozoan, first described in 1907 in mice and thought to be rare and clinically insignificant for 50 years. It has since been recognized as a common enteric pathogen and is associated with waterborne outbreaks and diarrhoea in children and adults. It infects and replicates in epithelial cells of the digestive and respiratory tracts of most vertebrates. Twenty species are recognized; *Cryptosporidium parvum* is the most important species.

Life cycle

Ingestion of oocysts is followed by encystation, usually following exposure to digestive enzymes or bile acids, then release of four sporozoites which attach to the epithelial cell wall. Sporozoites mature asexually into meronts and release merozoites intraluminally. Some of these re-invade the host cells (autoinfection), while others mature sexually into oocysts which are excreted in the faeces.

Epidemiology

Cryptosporidium is a ubiquitous enteric pathogen of all age groups. Transmission occurs by person-to-person, animal-to-person, waterborne, or, less commonly, food-borne spread. The prevalence of faecal oocyst excretion varies from 1–3% in industrialized countries to 5–10% in Asia and Africa. Seroprevalence data indicate that cryptosporidiosis is commoner than surveys of faecal oocyst excretion demonstrate, e.g. 25–35% seroprevalence in Europe and North America. Crytosporidiosis has been recognized as an important cause of diarrhoea in HIV/AIDS patients. Other risk factors: malnutrition, immunoglobulin deficiencies, intercurrent viral infections, diabetes mellitus, organ transplantation, haematological malignancies.

Clinical features

- Symptoms usually develop 7–10 days after ingestion of oocysts:
    - GI symptoms—diarrhoea (may be copious), cramping abdominal pains, anorexia, nausea, vomiting, toxic megacolon (rare);
    - other symptoms—low-grade fever, weakness, malaise, fatigue, cholecystitis (especially HIV patients), hepatitis, pancreatitis, reactive arthritis, respiratory symptoms, disseminated disease. Recovery depends on the immune status of the patient—immunocompetent have self-limiting disease.

Diagnosis

- Stool microscopy—examination of several specimens may be required (intermittent shedding). Most laboratories use a faecal concentration method, followed by microscopy using a modified acid-fast stain—oocysts stain red/pink (carbol fuchsin) against a blue (methylene blue) or green (malachite green) counterstain. Other stains include safranin–methylene blue, methenamine silver–nigrosin acridine orange, auramine–rhodamine, and auramine–carbol fuchsin.
- Antigen detection—immunofluorescent monoclonal antibody or ELISA tests may be used to detect cryptosporidial antigens in clinical or water specimens.
- Serology is primarily used as an epidemiological tool, rather than for acute diagnosis.
- PCR-based assays have been developed and can distinguish between genotypes. They may be helpful in the investigation of outbreaks.
- Histology has low sensitivity and is now rarely used.

Treatment

- Disease is usually self-limiting in immunocompetent patients, and supportive therapy (hydration, parenteral nutrition) is key.
- When specific treatment is required, nitazoxanide is the preferred agent.
- In HIV-infected patients, ART is the key intervention. For patients with severe symptoms, antidiarrhoeal agents and enteral/parenteral nutrition may be considered. The benefit of nitazoxanide or paromomycin in HIV-infected patients has not been established.

Prevention

- Prevention of exposure in 'at-risk' individuals, e.g. water filters, avoiding exposure to human and animal faeces, boiling water during outbreaks.
- Prophylaxis against *Cryptosporidium* in HIV-infected patients is not recommended; one report suggested that clarithromycin or rifabutin given as MAC prophylaxis may be beneficial.

Cystoisospora

Cystoisospora belli (formerly known as *Isospora belli*) is a coccidian GI parasite, first described in 1915.

Epidemiology

C. belli is found worldwide but predominantly causes infections in tropical and subtropical climates. Infection may occur in immunosuppressed patients (HIV infection, HTLV-1 infection, lymphoblastic lymphoma, T-cell leukaemia, non-Hodgkin's lymphoma) and immunocompetent patients. Transmission is by the faeco-oral route with ingestion of sporulated oocysts in contaminated food and water.

Clinical features

It causes a self-limiting diarrhoeal illness in immunocompetent patients but may cause chronic or severe diarrhoea in immunocompromised individuals, especially HIV-infected patients. Rare presentations include disseminated disease, cholecystitis, and reactive arthritis.

Laboratory diagnosis

In cases of heavy infection, oocysts may be seen in a wet mount of the stool. However, shedding may be intermittent, requiring the examination of several stools and the use of acid-fast stains or immunofluorescent techniques. A real-time PCR assay has been developed but is not widely available.

Treatment

- Supportive therapy with fluid resuscitation and nutritional support may be required for patients with severe diarrhoea.
- Treatment is with co-trimoxazole 960mg bd for 7–10 days for immunocompetent patients.
- In immunosuppressed patients, treatment with co-trimoxazole 960mg qds for 10 days, followed by 960mg three times a week, has been shown to be beneficial. Alternative agents include ciprofloxacin (inferior efficacy), pyrimethamine, and nitazoxanide.

Cyclospora

Epidemiology

Cyclospora cayetanensis was first described in humans in Papua New Guinea in 1977. Since then, it has emerged as a worldwide cause of diarrhoea in travellers, children, and HIV-infected patients. Transmission is by contaminated food and water. Most of the early cases were described in Nepal, Peru, and Haiti. More recently, outbreaks have been associated with the importation of fruits and vegetables from endemic areas.

Clinical features

The clinical features of the disease vary according to the type of patient. In endemic areas, infection may be asymptomatic or mild and self-limiting. In non-endemic areas, clinical features include anorexia, fatigue, nausea, abdominal pain, diarrhoea, fever, and weight loss. In immunocompromised/ HIV-infected patients, symptoms may be severe and last longer.

Laboratory diagnosis

Diagnosis is by microscopic detection of oocysts in stool, using modified acid-fast or safranin stains. UV autofluorescence of oocysts is both rapid and sensitive, but not specific.

Treatment

Treatment is with co-trimoxazole (960mg bd for 7 days for immunocompetent patients, 960mg qds for 10 days followed by lifelong suppressive therapy in HIV patients, until CD4 count consistently >200 cells/mm^3).

Trypanosoma

The genus *Trypanosoma* consists of ~20 species of protozoa. They are common animal pathogens causing severe disease in domestic animals. Three species infect humans:

- *T. cruzi* which causes Chagas' disease;
- *T. brucei gambiense* causes West African sleeping sickness;
- *T. brucei rhodesiense* causes East African sleeping sickness.

Trypanosoma cruzi

Chagas' disease is a zoonosis caused by the protozoan parasite *T. cruzi*. The disease is endemic in wild and domestic animals in Central and South America and is estimated to infect 8–10 million people. It is transmitted by triatome or 'kissing' bugs. Humans are considered accidental hosts. Transmission of *T. cruzi* may also occur through vertical transmission, blood transfusion, organ transplantation, oral transmission (contaminated food), and laboratory exposure.

Life cycle

The parasites multiply in the midgut of the insects as promastigotes. In the hindgut, they transform into trypomastigotes which pass out in the faeces during blood meals. Transmission to a second mammalian host occurs when breaks in the skin, mucous membranes, or conjunctivae are contaminated with bug faeces. The parasites enter host cells, transform into amastigotes, and multiply and differentiate into trypomastigotes. The cell ruptures, releasing the parasites which invade local tissue and spread haematogenously.

Pathogenesis

In acute Chagas' disease, the inflammatory lesion that develops at the site of entry is called the chagoma. Trypomastigotes released by cell rupture may be detected by microscopic examination of the blood. Muscles are the most heavily parasitized tissues and result in chronic complications, e.g. cardiac and GI disease.

Clinical features

There are five main clinical presentations.

- *Acute Chagas' disease* is usually an illness of children. An inflammatory lesion called a chagoma develops at the site of entry. Romaña's sign (painless periorbital oedema) may be seen if the site of entry is the conjunctivae. Localized signs may be followed by fever, malaise, anorexia, oedema, lymphadenopathy, and hepatosplenomegaly. CNS involvement is rare but carries a poor prognosis. Severe myocarditis with CCF may also occur. The acute illness usually resolves, and the patient enters the asymptomatic phase.
- *Indeterminate form (latent disease)* is characterized by the absence of symptoms and signs of infection, a normal ECG, and normal radiological investigations (e.g. CXR and barium studies), with serological/ parasitological evidence of chronic *T. cruzi* infection. No formal guidelines exist for monitoring patients with asymptomatic infection.
- *Chronic cardiac cardiomyopathy*—cardiac disease may become symptomatic many years after the primary infection. The heart is the commonest site, and clinical features are dizziness, syncope, chest pain, arrhythmias, CCF, pulmonary and systemic emboli, and stroke. Cardiac examination may reveal apical heave, prominent mitral or tricuspid regurgitation, and wide splitting of the second heart sound. CXR shows cardiomegaly, and ECG typically shows right bundle branch block. Death occurs within months of developing cardiac failure.
- *GI disease*—this usually affects 10–15% of patients with chronic Chagas' disease and presents between the ages of 20 and 40 years. Patients present with symptoms of achalasia and megaoesophagus, e.g. dysphagia, odynophagia, cough, chest pain, and regurgitation. Aspiration pneumonitis is common and may be fatal. An increased incidence of oesophageal cancer has been reported. Patients with megacolon present with constipation, abdominal pain, intestinal obstruction, or bowel perforation.
- *Disease in immunosuppressed patients*—reactivation of *T. cruzi* may occur in immunosuppressed patients, e.g. solid organ transplantation, HIV infection. The clinical presentation is similar to acute Chagas' disease but may be more severe, with CNS involvement.

Diagnosis

Diagnosis of Chagas' disease is based on:

- history of exposure to *T. cruzi*, e.g. residence or travel to an endemic area, blood transfusion in an endemic area;
- acute Chagas' disease—wet prep or Giemsa smear for detection of circulating parasites. In immunocompromised patients, other specimens may need to be examined, e.g. lymph node, bone marrow aspirates, pericardial fluid, CSF. If the smear is negative, culture of blood or specimens in liquid media or xenodiagnosis may be attempted;
- chronic Chagas' disease is diagnosed by detection of IgG antibodies to the parasite. Many serological assays are available, but their performance is variable;
- PCR assays have been developed over the past 20 years. Sensitivity is usually >90% (range 47–100%).

Treatment

The current treatment of Chagas' disease is far from ideal.

- Indications for treatment—acute infection, early congenital infection, children with chronic *T. cruzi* infection, reactivated infection in immunosuppressed patients.
- Benznidazole, a nitroimidazole derivative, is the preferred agent, as it is better tolerated than nifurtimox. Side effects include rash, peripheral neuropathy, and bone marrow suppression. Concurrent alcohol use can result in disulfiram effects and should be avoided.
- Nifurtimox, a nitrofuran derivative, is the alternative agent and is better tolerated in children. Side effects include nausea, vomiting, abdominal pain, weight loss, and neurological symptoms.
- Both agents are contraindicated in pregnancy, and in patients with severe renal and hepatic dysfunction.
- Chronic infection—treatment is supportive. Pacemakers are helpful in patients with bradyarrhythmias. Megaoesophagus may be treated with balloon dilatation/myomectomy of the lower oesophageal sphincter. Megacolon is managed with high-fibre diet and laxatives/enemas. Surgery may be required for complications.

Trypanosoma brucei complex

Human African trypanosomiasis (HAT) or sleeping sickness is caused by protozoan parasites that belong to the *T. brucei* complex:

- *T. brucei rhodesiense* that causes East African trypanosomiasis;
- *T. brucei gambiense* that causes West African trypanosomiasis.

They are morphologically indistinguishable and transmitted by tsetse flies (*Glossina* spp.), but the clinical features of infection differ in presentation and prognosis. A third species *T. brucei brucei* is an animal pathogen.

Life cycle

Tsetse flies ingest trypomastigotes during a blood meal from an infected mammalian host. Once in the midgut, the short, stumpy trypomastigotes transform into long, slender, procyclic trypomastigotes. After several cycles of replication, they migrate to the salivary glands where they differentiate into epimastigotes and continue to multiply. The epimastigotes transform into infective trypomastigotes which are inoculated into a second mammalian host at the next blood meal. African trypanosomes differ from *T. cruzi* in that they exhibit antigenic variation and are thus able to evade the host immune response.

Pathogenesis

The pathogenesis of African sleeping sickness is complex and incompletely understood. An acute inflammatory lesion (trypanosomal chancre) develops at the site of the tsetse fly bite. Multiplication of the parasite occurs in this lesion, resulting in inflammation, oedema, and local tissue destruction. The parasites spread to the local lymph nodes and then disseminate in the bloodstream. In stage 1 disease (haemolymphatic), there is widespread lymphadenopathy and histiocytic infiltration, followed by fibrosis. The heart may be involved. Stage 2 disease (meningoencephalitic) is characterized by CNS invasion.

Clinical features

- West African trypanosomiasis is caused by *T. brucei gambiense*. Infected humans are the main reservoir of infection. A trypanosomal chancre develops 1–2 weeks after the tsetse fly bite and resolves within several weeks. Early infection (stage 1) is marked by the onset of intermittent high fevers, posterior cervical lymphadenopathy (Winterbottom's sign), hepatosplenomegaly, transient oedema, pruritus, and rash. Late infection (stage 2) is characterized by the insidious onset of neurological symptoms (headache, somnolence, listless gaze, extrapyramidal signs) and CSF abnormalities.
- East African trypanosomiasis is caused by *T. brucei rhodesiense*. Infected wild animals are the main reservoir of infection. The illness is more acute than the West African disease, with onset of symptoms a few days after the insect bite. Intermittent fever and rash are common features—lymphadenopathy is less prominent than in West African disease. Cardiac manifestations, such as arrhythmias and CCF, may result in death prior to the onset of CNS disease. Untreated, this condition is fatal in weeks to months.

Diagnosis

The diagnosis of HAT is based on:

- history of exposure, e.g. residence in, or travel to, an endemic area;
- compatible clinical features;
- blood smear examination for trypanosomes (wet prep and Giemsa stain) is more likely to be positive in the haemolymphatic stage and in East African trypanosomiasis (higher parasitaemia). Serial specimens should be examined. Blood concentration techniques or buffy coat examination may increase sensitivity;

Table 10.1 Treatment of African trypanosomiasis

	Stage 1 disease	Stage 2 disease
T. brucei gambiense	Pentamidine OR suramin	Eflornithine plus nifurtimox OR eflornithine OR melarsoprol
T. brucei rhodesiense	Suramin	Melarsoprol

- tissue aspirate examination of chancre fluid or lymph nodes for trypanosomes (wet prep and Giemsa stain);
- CSF examination which shows increased cell count, increased CSF pressure, and elevated IgM and total protein concentrations. A patient with any CSF abnormalities should be regarded as having CNS disease;
- bone marrow aspiration may be helpful in patients whose other tests are negative;
- serology—antibody tests for *T. brucei gambiense* are available but have variable sensitivity and specificity. The test that is most frequently used in the field is the card agglutination tests for *T. gambiense* trypanosomes (CATT). Antigen detection ELISA tests have been developed but are not commercially available;
- molecular tests—have been used for subspeciation in research settings.

Treatment

A number of drugs are available to treat African trypanosmiasis (see Table 10.1):

- melarsoprol (➔ see Antiprotozoal drugs, p. 121);
- pentamidine (➔ see Antiprotozoal drugs, pp. 122–3);
- suramin (➔ see Antiprotozoal drugs, p. 123);
- eflornithine (➔ see Antiprotozoal drugs, pp. 120–1).

The treatment of African trypanosomiasis depends on the infecting species, drug resistance patterns, and stage of disease.

Prevention

The prevention of HAT relies on two strategies—vector control (aerial insecticide spraying, tetse fly traps, reduction of wild animal populations) and surveillance (with early treatment of identified cases). Travellers to endemic areas are advised to avoid areas where tsetse flies are endemic, wear protective clothing, and use insect repellents. There is no vaccine.

Leishmania

Leishmaniasis is caused by various *Leishmania* spp. that vary in their geographical distribution and clinical features. There are three clinical syndromes, each of which may be caused by several species:

- visceral leishmaniasis (kala-azar);
- cutaneous leishmaniasis;
- mucosal leishmaniasis (espundia);
- post-kala-azar dermal leishmaniasis.

The parasite

Leishmania spp. have a dimorphic life cycle and live in macrophages as intracellular amastigotes in mammalian hosts and extracellular promastigotes in the gut of their sandfly vectors. *Leishmania* spp. cannot be differentiated on the basis of morphology. Speciation was initially based on epidemiological and clinical features; several molecular assays are now used.

Epidemiology

- Visceral leishmaniasis has a wide geographical distribution. It is caused by *Leishmania donovani* spp. (India, Pakistan, Nepal, East Africa, Eastern China), *Leishmania infantum* (Middle East, Mediterranean, Balkans, central and South West Asia, North and West China, North and sub-Saharan Africa), or *Leishmania chagasi* (Latin America). Rarely, *Leishmania amazonensis* or *Leishmania tropica* may cause visceral leishmaniasis.
- Cutaneous leishmaniasis is also widely distributed. The classic form of Old World cutaneous leshmaniasis, the oriental sore, is found in the Middle East, the Mediterranean, Africa, India, and Asia. It is usually caused by *L. major, L. tropica, Leishmania aethiopica*, and occasionally by *L. donovani* and *L. infantum*. New World cutaneous leishmaniasis is endemic in Latin America. It is caused by *Leishmania brazilensis, Leishmania mexicana, Leishmania panamensis*, and occasionally by *L. chagasi*.
- Mucosal leishmaniasis (espundia) mainly occurs in Latin America and is usually caused by *L. braziliensis*.

Clinical features

- *Visceral leishmaniasis*—incubation period 3–8 months. Onset may be acute or gradual. Symptoms include abdominal enlargement, fever, weakness, anorexia, and weight loss. Examination shows pallor, hepatosplenomegaly ± lymphadenopathy. The skin becomes dry, thin, scaly, and discoloured (kala-azar = black fever). Haemorrhage may occur at various sites. Secondary infections are common in advanced disease and may lead to death. Laboratory findings include renal impairment, anaemia, leucopenia, and hypergammaglobulinaemia. Visceral leishmaniasis may be the presenting feature of HIV infection.
- *Cutaneous leishmaniasis*—incubation period 2 weeks to several months. A wide variety of skin lesions may occur, from small, dry, crusted lesions (usually *L. tropica*) to large, deep ulcers with a granulating base and overlying exudate (usually *L. braziliensis*). Lesions may be single or multiple and tend to occur on exposed areas. Secondary bacterial infections and lymphadenopathy may occur.
- *Mucosal leishmaniasis*—a small proportion of patients with cutaneous leishmaniasis develop mucous membrane involvement of the nose, oral cavity, pharynx, and larynx months to years after their skin lesions have healed. Symptoms include nasal stuffiness, discharge, or epistaxis. The nasal septum may be destroyed, resulting in nasal collapse. Perforation may occur through the nose or soft palate. Occasionally, patients may be unable to eat or may develop aspiration pneumonia.

Diagnosis

- *Visceral leishmaniasis*—tissue biopsy of the spleen, bone marrow, lymph node, or liver may confirm the diagnosis. Amastigotes may be seen in Wright- or Giemsa-stained smears. Specimens should be inoculated into special media (e.g. Novy, McNeal and Nicoll medium, Schneider insect medium) and cultured at 22–26°C. Motile promastigotes develop after days to weeks. Anti-leishmanial antibodies may be present at high titre in immunocompetent patients but may be absent or at low titre in HIV-infected patients. False-positive reactions occur with leprosy, Chagas' disease, malaria, schistosomiasis, toxoplasmosis, or cutaneous leishmaniasis. A urinary antigen test has been developed.
- *Cutaneous leishmaniasis*—skin biopsies taken from the edge of a lesion may show amastigotes on Wright or Giemsa staining. Lesions may also be injected and aspirated with saline, and examined for amastigotes. Samples may be cultured using special media (➔ see bullet point above). Anti-leishmanial antibodies may be present in some patients. The leishmanin (Montenegro) skin test becomes positive during the course of the disease but is no longer used. PCR-based assays are highly sensitive for the diagnosis of cutaneous leishmaniasis.
- *Mucosal leishmaniasis*—a definitive diagnosis is made by the identification of amastigotes in tissue biopsies or isolation of promastigotes in culture. However, the diagnosis is often presumptive and based on the presence of a characteristic scar and positive leishmanin skin test or anti-leishmanial antibodies.
- *Serology*—serum antibody tests, e.g. ELISA, IFA, and the DAT, have high sensitivity, but low specificity because of cross-reaction with other infections. A urine antigen test (KAtex) has high specificity, but low sensitivity.
- *Molecular tests*—PCR-based assays are available for the diagnosis of visceral and cutaneous leishmaniasis.

Treatment

- *Visceral leishmaniasis*—liposomal amphotericin B has the highest therapeutic efficacy and lowest toxicity profile. Conventional amphotericin B is used but carries a risk of renal toxicity. Pentavalent antimonial compounds (e.g. sodium stibogluconate and meglumine antimoniate) have been used for decades. The standard dose is 20mg/kg/day for 28–30 days. Side effects include cardiotoxicity, pancreatitis, myalgia and arthralgia, nausea, vomiting, abdominal pain, headache, fatigue, rash, elevated LFTs, and decreased Hb, WCC, and platelet counts. Alternative agents include PO miltefosine (2.5mg/kg/day for 28 days) or IV or IM paromomycin (12–20mg/kg/day for 21–28 days). Observational studies and small trials suggest that combination therapy is the way forward, but published data are sparse.
- *Cutaneous leishmaniasis*—many lesions will resolve without treatment. Uncomplicated disease is treated with local therapy, e.g. cryotherapy, thermotherapy, intralesional pentavalent antimony compounds, TOP paromomycin, photodynamic therapy. Complicated disease is treated with systemic therapy, e.g. PO fluconazole, ketoconazole, or miltefosine. Parenteral systemic therapy is sometimes indicated—options include pentavalent antimony compounds, amphotericin, and pentamidine.

Prevention

Prevention strategies include:

- control of sandfly vectors (insecticides, bed nets);
- control of animal reservoirs (difficult);
- treatment of infected humans.

Although there is no effective form of immunoprophylaxis, there are ongoing efforts to produce a vaccine.

Giardia lamblia

G. lamblia, a flagellated intestinal protozoan, is a common cause of diarrhoea throughout the world.

The pathogen

The differentiation of *Giardia* spp. has traditionally relied on the morphological features and the identity of the host. However, they may now be classified on the basis of antigen, isoenzyme, and genetic analysis. *G. lamblia* is the only species that infects humans. The life cycle consists of two stages: trophozoite and cyst.

Epidemiology

G. lamblia has a worldwide distribution and is the most commonly identified intestinal parasite. It is usually acquired by ingestion of contaminated water or food but may also be spread by person to person (children in day-care centres, institutionalized people, sexual). Natural or experimental infections with *Giardia* spp. have been documented for many mammalian species; whether these act as reservoirs for transmission to humans is less clear.

Pathogenesis

Infection occurs after ingestion of as few as 10–25 cysts. After encystation, trophozoites colonize and multiply in the small bowel. The production of GI secretory IgA antibodies appears to be key in preventing and clearing infection. The cellular immune response is also important in clearing infection, by coordinating IgA secretion and cellular cytotoxicity. Susceptibility to giardiasis has been seen in patients with common variable immune deficiency, X-linked agammaglobulinaemia, previous gastric surgery, or reduced gastric acidity.

Clinical features

- Incubation period—symptoms develop 1–2 weeks after ingestion of cysts; detection of cysts in the stool may take longer.
- Clinical features include asymptomatic cyst passers (5–15%), diarrhoeal syndrome (25–50%), and subclinical infection (35–70%).
- Symptomatic giardiasis is characterized by diarrhoea, abdominal cramps, bloating, flatulence, malaise, nausea, anorexia, and weight loss. Initially, stools may be profuse and watery, but later may become greasy and foul-smelling and may float (steatorrhoea). Vomiting, fever, and tenesmus are less common.

- Unusual features include urticaria, reactive arthritis, biliary disease, and gastric infection (if achlorhydria).
- Severe volume depletion may occur in young children and pregnant women, necessitating hospital admission.

Diagnosis

The diagnosis should be considered in all patients with chronic diarrhoea, particularly if associated with malabsorption or weight loss.

- Stool examination—a wet mount of fresh liquid stool may show motile trophozoites; iodine staining may reveal cysts. Formol-ether concentration techniques may increase the yield.
- Antigen detection assays detect *G. lamblia* by immunofluorescence or ELISA. They are most useful in investigating outbreaks and testing patients after treatment.
- Duodenal string test (Entero-Test) may be helpful in difficult cases.
- Duodenal aspirate and biopsy are more invasive but may help to exclude other diagnoses.
- Antibody tests are not widely available but are useful in distinguishing acute from past infection, and in epidemiological surveys.
- *In vitro* culture and molecular assays are available in research settings.

Treatment

- Treatment is recommended for symptomatic individuals. Acquired lactose intolerance occurs in 20–40% of cases, so patients should be advised to avoid lactose-containing foods for a month after treatment.
- Metronidazole is the drug of choice and has an efficacy of 75–100%. Drug resistance can be induced *in vitro* and may occur *in vivo*. Side effects: metallic taste, nausea, dizziness, headache, disulfiram reaction (with alcohol), neutropenia (rare). Concerns about teratogenicity mean that it is contraindicated in pregnancy (first trimester) and not recommended in children.
- Tinidazole (➲ see Antiprotozoal drugs, p. 124), another nitroimidazole, can be given as a single dose, and has fewer side effects and an efficacy of >90%.
- Nitazoxanide has been found to be at least as effective as metronidazole, with an efficacy of 81–85%.
- Albendazole and mebendazole (➲ see Antihelminthic drugs, p. 124) have been shown to have similar efficacy to metronidazole, and fewer side effects than metronidazole and tinidazole.
- Paromomycin has been shown to have an efficacy of 55–90%. It has poor intestinal absorption and is used for patients in whom other agents are contraindicated. Side effects include nausea, diarrhoea, and abdominal pain.
- Furazolidone (➲ see Nitrofurans, pp. 66–7), a nitrofuran, has a lower efficacy rate (80%) but is available as a liquid suspension. Side effects: GI symptoms, brown discoloration of urine, mild haemolysis (in G6PD deficiency).
- Quinacrine is an alternative and has an efficacy of 90%. Side effects: nausea, vomiting, abdominal cramps, yellow discoloration of skin, urine, and sclera (rare), exfoliative dermatitis (rare).

Prevention

- Good sanitation with proper treatment of public water supplies.
- Boiling or purification of water with chlorine- or iodine-based preparations in endemic areas.
- Prevention of person-to-person spread by good personal hygiene/ handwashing/avoidance of orogenital or oro-anal sex.
- Breastfeeding reduces the risk of *Giardia* infection in infants in developing countries.

Trichomonas vaginalis

T. vaginalis, a flagellated protozoan, is the commonest non-viral STI.

The pathogen

On microscopic examination of genital specimens, *T. vaginalis* is a pear-shaped organism (10 × 7 micrometres) with twitching motility. There are four anterior flagellae that arise from a single stalk and a fifth flagellum which is embedded in the undulating membrane.

Epidemiology

The incidence appears to be declining in Western Europe and the USA. Trichomoniasis is usually sexually transmitted, and its incidence is highest in women with multiple partners, in patients with other STIs, and in HIV-infected patients. Trichomoniasis is occasionally acquired non-venereally (e.g. in institutionalized patients) or by vertical transmission during delivery.

Pathogenesis

All areas of the cell surface are capable of phagocytosis and can ingest bacteria, leucocytes, erythrocytes, and epithelial cells. Trichomonads appear to damage the genital epithelium by direct contact, which is mediated by surface proteins, and cause micro-ulceration. Specific virulence factors have not been defined, and the immune response is incompletely understood. *T. vaginalis* activates the alternative complement pathway and attracts neutrophils which may kill the protozoan.

Clinical features

- The incubation period is 5–28 days.
- Symptoms often begin or worsen during periods and include vaginal discharge (may be smelly or itchy), dyspareunia, dysuria, and lower abdominal discomfort.
- Signs include vulvar erythema, yellow/green or frothy vaginal discharge, vaginal inflammation, and punctate haemorrhages on the cervix ('strawberry cervix').
- Most infected men are asymptomatic, but those who are symptomatic may have urethritis that is clinically indistinguishable from other causes of non-gonococcal urethritis.
- Complications of vaginal trichomoniasis include vaginitis emphysematosa (gas-filled blebs in the vaginal wall), vaginal cuff cellulitis after hysterectomy, premature labour, and low-birthweight infants.

Diagnosis

- Diagnosis relies on identification of the organism in genital specimens.
- The wet mount will identify organisms in 48–80% of infected women and 50–90% of infected men.
- Various staining methods (e.g. Gram, Giemsa, Pappenheim, and acridine orange) are less sensitive than the wet mount.
- Other methods (e.g. direct fluorescent antibody staining, latex agglutination, ELISA, DNA probe, and PCR-based assays) are more sensitive than wet prep, but less sensitive than culture.
- Culture remains the most sensitive technique, and trichomonads can be cultured on a variety of media; modified Diamond's media is the best.
- Serological diagnosis is hampered by low sensitivity and poor specificity, particularly in high-risk populations.

Treatment

- Metronidazole (➲ Nitroimidazoles, p. 64) is the treatment of choice and can be given as a single 2g dose or in divided doses for 7 days. The main disadvantage of a single dose is the risk of reinfection if the partner is not treated simultaneously.
- Alternative drugs include tinidazole which can be given as a single dose.
- Patients should be advised to avoid alcohol because of the risk of a disulfiram reaction with metronidazole and tinidazole.

Prevention

- General advice about prevention of STIs.
- Use of barrier contraceptive methods, e.g. condoms and spermicides.

Entamoeba histolytica

E. histolytica is a common cause of diarrhoea worldwide, particularly in the tropics. It can also cause extraintestinal disease, e.g. abscesses in the liver, lung, heart, and brain. *Entamoeba coli, E. hartmanni, E. polecki, Endolimax nana*, and *iodamoeba buetschlii* are generally considered nonpathogenic and reside in the large intestine of the human host.

The parasite

E. histolytica is one of three intestinal amoebae that infect man. The others (*Entamoeba dispar* and *Entamoeba moshkovskii*) are morphologically identical and non-pathogenic. The organism exists in two forms: the trophozoite (10–60 micrometres with a single nucleus ± ingested erythrocytes) and the cyst (5–20 micrometres with four nuclei). Ingestion of the cyst results in excystation in the small bowel and trophozoite infection of the colon, resulting in symptoms. When conditions are no longer favourable, the trophozoite encysts and is passed out in the faeces. Cysts remain viable for weeks or months in moist environments.

Epidemiology

Ten per cent of the world's population is estimated to be infected with *E. histolytica*. There is a wide geographical variation in prevalence, ranging from ≤5% in developed countries to 20–30% in the tropics. Risk factors for amoebiasis in endemic areas include low socio-economic status, poor sanitation, and overcrowding. In low-prevalence countries, certain groups are at higher risk: immigrants or travellers from endemic regions, institutionalized individuals, and promiscuous male homosexuals. Factors associated with severe disease: neonates, pregnancy, corticosteroid therapy, and malnutrition.

Clinical features

The clinical features of amoebiasis can be divided into intestinal and extraintestinal syndromes.

- Intestinal manifestations include asymptomatic infection, symptomatic non-invasive infection, amoebic dysentery (gradual onset, abdominal pain/tenderness, bloody diarrhoea), fulminant colitis (rare but carries a high mortality), toxic megacolon and chronic colitis, amoeboma (annular lesion of the colon), and perianal ulceration.
- Amoebic liver abscess—this is the commonest extraintestinal manifestation and typically presents 8–20 weeks after return from an endemic area. Clinical features include fever, right upper quadrant pain, anorexia, malaise, weight loss, cough, and hiccough. Rupture of the abscess can cause pleural infection or peritonitis.
- Pleuro-pulmonary infection—risk factors include malnutrition, alcoholism, and atrial septal defect. Clinical features include a serous pleural effusion, amoebic empyema, consolidation, lung abscess, or hepato-bronchial fistula.
- Cardiac infection—this is very rare and occurs after rupture of a liver abscess into the pericardium. It presents with chest pain, cardiac failure, and pericardial tamponade.
- Brain abscess—results from haematogenous spread.

Diagnosis

- Stool microscopy remains the cornerstone of diagnosis, but sensitivity is poor, and multiple specimens may need to be examined. A fresh liquid stool should be examined by wet mount for motile trophozoites. A formol-ether concentrate with examination of iodine-stained deposit increases the likelihood of seeing cysts.
- Stool culture is more sensitive than microscopy, but not routinely available.
- Colonoscopy and biopsy may be helpful in confirming the diagnosis in patients with colitis. Endoscopic features include punctate haemorrhages and ulcers, but may appear normal in early disease.
- Antigen testing—stool and serum antigen tests are rapid, sensitive, and specific, and can distinguish between *E. histolytica* and other species.
- Serological tests, e.g. indirect haemagglutination assays are helpful in the diagnosis of invasive intestinal amoebiasis, but titres may be negative in early disease and remain high for years. Other less sensitive assays (e.g. counterimmunoelectrophoresis or gel diffusion precipitation) wane more rapidly and may be helpful in diagnosing acute disease.
- Molecular methods—detection of parasite DNA or RNA in faeces can differentiate between species but is mainly a research tool.

- Imaging studies, e.g. ultrasound, CT, or MRI scans, are useful in assessing patients with suspected amoebic liver abscess. Aspiration of the abscess yields a brown, odourless, sterile liquid, which may show trophozoites. The main risk of aspiration is peritoneal spillage/peritonitis. Many cases may be diagnosed and treated with aspiration.

Treatment

The treatment of amoebiasis is complicated by a number of factors, including a variety of clinical syndromes, varying sites of action of different drugs, and the availability of different drugs in different countries.

- Intraluminal carriage (e.g. asymptomatic cyst passers) should be treated because of the risk of invasive disease. Possible regimens include: paromomycin, diloxanide furoate, or diiodohydroxyquin.
- Invasive intestinal disease (e.g. dysentery, colitis) should be treated with metronidazole or tinidazole, followed by a luminal agent (➔ see bullet point above). Surgery is required for peritonitis or toxic megacolon.
- Extraintestinal amoebiasis (e.g. liver abscess) should be treated by metronidazole, followed by an intraluminal agent (➔ see bullet point above). In severely ill patients, emetine or dehydroemetine (less toxic) may be added for the first few days. Aspiration or percutaneous drainage is usually only required for large cysts or to confirm the diagnosis. Surgical attempts to correct amoebic bowel perforation or peritonitis should be avoided.

Prevention

- Avoid ingestion of contaminated water and food.
- In endemic areas, vegetables should be treated with a detergent and soaked in acetic acid or vinegar. Water should be boiled, as purification with chlorine or iodine may not be sufficient to kill cysts.
- Avoid sexual practices that involve faeco-oral contact.
- Development of oral and parenteral vaccines is in progress.

Free-living amoebae

Human infection with free-living amoebae is infrequent but may be severe and life-threatening. Three clinical syndromes occur:

- primary amoebic meningoencephalitis, caused by *Naegleria fowleri*;
- granulomatous amoebic encephalitis (GAM), caused by *Acanthamoeba* spp. and *Ballamuthia mandrillaris*;
- amoebic keratitis, caused by *Acanthamoeba* spp.

Naegleria fowleri

- *Epidemiology*—found throughout the world in soil, rivers, lakes, and thermally polluted water; grows well in temperatures up to 45°C. Causes primary amoebic encephalitis in children and young adults who have recently swum in warm freshwater lakes or ponds.
- *Pathogenesis*—amoebae penetrate the olfactory mucosa and enter the CNS through the cribriform plate, resulting in a diffuse meningoencephalitis, purulent leptomeningitis, and cortical haemorrhages.

- *Clinical features*—symptoms occur 1–7 days after exposure. Patients may initially report changes in smell or taste, followed by an abrupt onset of fever, anorexia, nausea, vomiting, headache, meningism, and altered mental status. Patients rapidly progress to coma and death within a week. Myocarditis is found in 7–16% of patients at autopsy, but patients do not appear to develop arrhythmias or heart failure.
- *Diagnosis* is based on clinical suspicion and confirmed by the demonstration of trophozoites in the CSF. A variety of molecular assays have been developed. Serological tests are not helpful, as the majority of adults tested in endemic areas, e.g. Florida, have antibody.
- *Treatment*—the optimal treatment is unknown. Only 11 survivors are reported in the literature, the majority of whom were macrolide-treated with amphotericin and rifampicin. Other agents that may be active are fluconazole, miltefosine, and azithromycin.

Acanthamoeba species

- *Epidemiology*—*Acanthamoeba* spp. have been isolated from soil, water, and air. Serological surveys indicate that exposure is common, and the organism may be isolated in pharyngeal swabs from healthy people. Encephalitis tends to occur in debilitated or immunosuppressed patients, e.g. HIV infection, liver disease, diabetes mellitus, chronic renal failure, SLE, malignancy, chemotherapy, organ transplantation, and corticosteroid therapy. In contrast, keratitis occurs in healthy patients.
- *GAM* has an insidious onset and presents with focal neurological deficits. Clinical features include altered mental status, seizures, fever, headache, hemiparesis, meningism, visual disturbance, and ataxia. The duration of CNS illness until death is 7–120 days. Other clinical syndromes include skin lesions, pneumonitis, adrenalitis, leucocytoclastic vasculitis, and osteomyelitis.
- *Amoebic keratitis* is associated with minor corneal trauma or the use of soft contact lenses. Clinical features include a foreign body sensation, followed by severe pain, photophobia, tearing, blepharospasm, conjunctivitis, and blurred vision. The diagnosis is often delayed because of initial misdiagnosis or periods of temporary remission.
- *Diagnosis*—GAM is usually diagnosed post-mortem but may be diagnosed ante mortem by brain biopsy. CT brain scans have shown multiple lucent, non-enhancing lesions. LP is contraindicated because of the risk of herniation. When performed, CSF examination has been non-diagnostic with elevated WCCs and protein and decreased glucose levels. The diagnosis of amoebic keratitis depends on the demonstration of *Acanthamoeba* in corneal scrapings, contact lenses, or contact lens fluid by histology or culture. Corneal scrapings may be examined by wet mount for motile trophozoites, or fixed and stained using a variety of stains. A non-nutrient agar overlaid with *E. coli* is most commonly used for culture. Molecular techniques include PCR and DNA probes.
- *Treatment*—the optimal treatment for GAM is unknown. Drugs that are active *in vitro* include propamidine, pentamidine, ketoconazole, miconazole, paromomycin, neomycin, 5-flucytosine, and, to a lesser extent, amphotericin. Combination therapy with miltefosine, fluconazole, and pentamidine isethionate has been recommended.

Co-trimoxazole, metronidazole, and a macrolide may be added. The treatment of amoebic keratitis involves aggressive surgical debridement and topical therapy with miconazole, propamidine isethionate, and neosporin for 4–6 weeks.

Ballamuthia mandrillaris

- *Epidemiology*—*B. mandrillaris* is a soil inhabitant which contaminates fresh water. It causes GAM in both immunocompetent and immunocompromised hosts.
- *Clinical features*—some patients present with a skin lesion (non-ulcerated plaque), followed by neurological symptoms, whereas others present with meningoencephalitis. Clinical features include fever, malaise, headache, nausea, vomiting, seizures, and focal neurological signs. Death occurs 1 week to several months after onset of symptoms.
- *Diagnosis*—CT brain scan shows multiple hypodense lesions with mass effect. CSF abnormalities include mononuclear pleocytosis (10–500 cells), raised protein, and low glucose. Brain biopsy specimens may demonstrate the cyst and trophozoite. Previously, *B. mandrillaris* was difficult to distinguish from *Acanthamoeba* spp., but an IFA and a cell-free growth medium have been developed.
- *Treatment*—the optimal treatment is unknown. Survivors have been treated with a combination of pentamidine, 5-flucytosine, fluconazole, and a macrolide.

Microsporidia

The microsporidia are a diverse group of obligate intracellular, spore-forming protozoa that belong to the phylum *Microspora*, order *Microsporida*. Comparative molecular phylogenetic studies support a relationship between microsporidia and fungi. Over 1300 species exist, and 14 species have been implicated in human disease, with *Enterocytozoon bieneusi* and *Encephalitozoon* spp. being the commonest pathogens.

Epidemiology

Human infection has been reported worldwide (except in Antarctica). Most severe infections are associated with immunocompromise, e.g. HIV infection, organ transplantation, corticosteroid therapy. However, infections are becoming increasingly recognized in immunocompetent patients, e.g. residents of, or travellers from, tropical countries. Routes of transmission include food-borne, waterborne, person-to person spread, inhalation/aerosol, or zoonotic spread.

Pathology

Microsporidia can infect many different organs:

- eye—punctate epithelial keratopathy;
- respiratory tract—rhinitis, sinusitis, nasal polyposis, tracheitis, bronchitis, bronchiolitis ± pneumonia;
- GU tract—chronic and granulomatous interstitial nephritis, acute tubular necrosis, microabscesses, granulomas, necrotizing ureteritis and cystitis, prostatic abscess;

- GI and hepatobiliary tract—enteritis, ulceration, mucosal invasion, granulomatous hepatitis, and cholecystitis;
- CNS—ring-enhancing lesion with central areas of necrosis filled with spores/macrophages, surrounded by microsporidia-filled astrocytes;
- musculoskeletal system—myositis, muscle fibrosis.

Clinical features

The clinical manifestations of microsporidiosis can be divided into two groups, according to the host's immune status.

Immunocompetent patients

- Intestinal infections caused by *E. bieneusi* or *Encephalitozoon intestinalis* are commonest. Presents with watery diarrhoea, nausea, abdominal pain, and fever, and is usually self-limiting.
- Ocular infections are rare and may present with corneal stromal infection or keratoconjunctivitis.
- Cerebral infections, endocarditis, and myositis have also been reported.

HIV-infected patients

- *E. bieneusi* typically causes intestinal infections with chronic diarrhoea, anorexia, weight loss, and malabsorption. CD4 counts are typically <100 cells/mm^3. Patients may also develop cholecystitis or cholangitis with fever, nausea, vomiting, and abdominal pain.
- *E. intestinalis* causes intestinal and systemic infections that appear similar to those caused by *E. bieneusi*. Disseminated disease, particularly to the kidneys, may occur.
- *Encephalitozoon hellem* and *Encephalitozoon cuniculi* can both cause keratoconjunctivitis sicca. Patients often have laboratory evidence of disseminated infection and may present with bronchiolitis, sinusitis, nephritis, cystitis, urethritis, prostatitis, hepatitis, peritonitis, cerebral infection, or nodular skin infections.
- Myositis may be caused by various microsporidial species, e.g. *Pleistophora* spp., *Trachipleistophora hominis, Brachiola vesicularum*.
- Systemic infections due to other microsporidial species have been described in case reports.

Diagnosis

- Stool microscopy is the commonest test but requires special stains, e.g. modified trichrome stain, calcofluor white stain, indirect immunofluorescent stains.
- Cytology is used for diagnosis of microsporidiosis in other organs. Various stains may be used, e.g. Weber, Gram, Giemsa, Steiner silver, trichrome blue, chemifluorescent stains.
- Histology remains important in the diagnosis of microsporidiosis. Various stains may be used, e.g. modified Gram, Giemsa, PAS, and Steiner silver stains.
- EM may be useful to identify microsporidia to genus or species level.
- Nucleic acid amplification assays—several PCR-based assays have been developed for species-specific diagnosis. They are usually restricted to a few research laboratories.

- Immunofluorescent detection methods using polyclonal antisera can detect microsporidia (except *E. bieneusi*) in most clinical specimens. Sensitivity is poor in stool specimens.
- Serology is unhelpful in the diagnosis of microsporidiosis.
- Tissue culture is only available in a few specialist laboratories.

Treatment

- GI infection—albendazole is effective against most microsporidia species, particularly *Encephalitozoon* infections, but has minimal activity against *E. bieneusi*. Fumagillin is used for *E. bieneusi* infection (side effects: nausea, vomiting, bone marrow toxicity). Nitazoxanide may also be effective for *E. bieneusi* infections in HIV-infected patients.
- Ocular infections—TOP fumagillin is used, and concomitant albendazole is warranted, particularly if there is evidence of systemic infection. TOP voriconazole has been used in keratitis.

Prevention

Meticulous handwashing and adherence to existing guidelines for the general prevention of opportunistic infections in HIV-infected patients are pertinent. As yet, there are no clinical trial data to support antimicrobial prophylaxis. HAART may be important in preventing microsporidiosis.

Chapter 11

Helminths

Nematodes 542
Ascaris lumbricoides 543
Trichuris trichiura 544
Ancylostoma duodenale and *Necator americanus* 545
Strongyloides stercoralis 546
Enterobius vermicularis 548
Cutaneous larva migrans 550
Toxocariasis 550
Trichinella species 552
Dracunculus medinensis 553
Filariasis 554
Loa loa 556
Onchocerca volvulus 557
Cestodes 559
Trematodes (flukes) 563
Abdominal angiostrongyliasis 568
Anisakiasis 569
Capillariasis 569

Nematodes

There are >60 species of nematodes or roundworms that infect humans, some of which are shown in Table 11.1. They are the commonest human parasites and are estimated to infect 3–4 billion people worldwide. Helminth infections are a major public health burden in the developing world. All nematodes are elongated, cylindrical, non-segmented organisms, with a smooth cuticle and body cavity containing a digestive tract and reproductive organs.

Intestinal nematodes

Intestinal nematodes are the largest group of human helminths. The commonest intestinal nematodes (*A. lumbricoides, A. duodenale, N. americanus,* and *T. trichiura*) cannot reproduce in humans and are referred to as geohelminths, as their eggs have to develop in the soil. The exceptions are *S. stercoralis* and *E. vermicularis*, which can be transmitted from person to person.

Tissue nematodes

The tissue-dwelling roundworms are also a major public health problem, particularly in the tropics. Some affect humans only, while others have an animal reservoir. All of the parasites have a complex life cycle involving intermediate hosts, except *Trichinella* spp. Adult worms do not multiply in humans, so the worm load and severity of disease depend on intensity of exposure.

Table 11.1 Medically important nematodes

Type	Disease	Species
Intestinal	Ascariasis	*Ascaris lumbricoides*
	Trichuriasis	*Trichuris trichiura*
	Hookworm	*Ancylostoma duodenale* *Necator americanus*
	Strongyloidiasis	*Strongyloides stercoralis*
	Pin worm	*Enterobius vermicularis*
Tissue	Trichinosis	*Trichinella spiralis*
	Dracunculiasis	*Dracunculus medinensis*
	Filariasis	*Wuchereria bancrofti* *Brugia malayi* *Brugia timori*
	Onchocerciasis	*Onchocerca volvulus*

Ascaris lumbricoides

Ascariasis is the commonest helminthic infection of humans, with an estimated prevalence of >1 billion. It is caused by *A. lumbricoides* (roundworm) and is found worldwide, most commonly in the tropics.

The parasite

The adult worms (white or reddish yellow, 15–35cm in length) live in the small intestine and have a lifespan of 10–24 months. Each female produces up to 200 000 ova/day, which pass out in the faeces. When ingested, the eggs hatch in the small intestine, penetrate the intestinal wall, migrate through the venous system to the lungs where they break into the alveoli, migrate up the bronchial tree, before they are swallowed and develop into mature worms in the intestine.

Epidemiology

Ascaris infection is commonest in young children but can occur at any age. Transmission is by the faeco-oral route and is enhanced by the high output of ova and their ability to survive unfavourable environmental conditions. In endemic areas, most people have light to moderate worm burdens.

Clinical features

Most infected patients are asymptomatic. Clinical features depend on the site and intensity of infection.

- Pulmonary manifestations occur during larval migration through the lungs. Patients may present with Löeffler's syndrome (respiratory symptoms, pulmonary infiltration, and peripheral eosinophilia).
- GI manifestations include malnutrition, malabsorption, steatorrhoea, and intestinal obstruction.
- Biliary obstruction may cause abdominal pain, cholangitis, pancreatitis, and obstructive jaundice.
- Ectopic infections occur rarely, e.g. umbilical or hernial fistulae, Fallopian tubes, bladder, lungs, and heart.

Diagnosis

- Stool microscopy—may be negative until 40 days after infection. The eggs are oval-shaped with a thick, mamillated shell and measure 45–70 micrometres (length) by 35–50 micrometres (breadth) (see Fig. 11.1). Sometimes an adult worm is passed.
- Eosinophilia—may be seen in early infection, infection when the larvae migrate through the lungs. Serum IgE and IgG may also be raised.
- Serology—usually used for epidemiological studies, rather than diagnosis.

Treatment

- Albendazole (400mg stat) or mebendazole (100mg bd for 3 days or 500mg stat) are the treatments of choice.
- Alternative agents include ivermectin, nitazoxanide, piperazine citrate, and levamisole.
- Endoscopic or surgical intervention may be required for biliary/intestinal obstruction.

Trichuris trichiura

Trichuriasis is one of the most prevalent helminthic infections—it is estimated that one-quarter of the world's population carries the parasite. Infection is mainly asymptomatic, but heavy infection may cause anaemia, bloody diarrhoea, growth retardation, or rectal prolapse.

The parasite

T. trichiura principally infects humans, residing in the caecum and ascending colon. The mean lifespan of adult worms is 1 year, and each female worm produces 5–20 000 eggs per day. After excretion, embryonic development occurs over 2–4 weeks. The embryonated egg is ingested, and the larva escapes its shell, penetrating the small intestinal mucosa, before migrating down into the caecum or colon. The anterior whip-like portion remains embedded in the mucosa, while the shorter posterior end is free in the lumen.

Epidemiology

T. trichiura has a worldwide distribution but is commoner in most tropical environments. Infection results from ingestion of embryonated eggs by direct contamination of hands, food, or drink, or indirectly through flies or other insects. The intensity of infections is usually light; heavy infection is commoner in children.

Clinical features

Infection is mainly asymptomatic, but heavy infection may present with a variety of symptoms:

- iron deficiency anaemia;
- acute GI symptoms—diarrhoea (often containing mucus and/or blood), nocturnal soiling, dysentery;
- chronic colitis with growth retardation;
- rectal prolapse.

Diagnosis

- Stool microscopy reveals the characteristic lemon-shaped ova (52 × 22 micrometres) (see Fig. 11.1). The Kato-Katz technique can be used to quantify egg numbers which tend to correlate with worm burden.
- Proctoscopy or colonoscopy may demonstrate adult worms (shaped like a whip) protruding from the bowel mucosa.

Treatment

Albendazole (400mg od for 3 days) or mebendazole (100mg bd for 3 days) are the treatments of choice. Ivermectin has some activity but is not as effective as albendazole or mebendazole. For mass community therapy in developing countries, a combination of ivermectin plus albendazole or mebendazole is used.

Prevention

Improved sanitation and meticulous handwashing may help to prevent infection.

Ancylostoma duodenale and *Necator americanus*

Human hookworm infection is estimated to affect 740 million people worldwide. It is caused by two species *A. duodenale* and *N. americanus*.

The parasite

Adult hookworms are small, cylindrical (1cm long), and greyish-white in colour. They live in the upper small intestine, attached to the mucosa. Adult worms produce about 7000 eggs per day. They pass out in the stool and hatch into larvae. Skin penetration requires contact with contaminated soil. The larvae are carried in the venous circulation to the lungs where they migrate up the respiratory tree to be swallowed and carried to the small intestine.

Epidemiology

The prevalence of hookworm infection is highest in sub-Saharan Africa, Asia, Latin America, and the Caribbean. Transmission requires human faecal contamination of the soil, favourable conditions for larvae (warmth, moisture, and shade), and contact of human skin with contaminated soil. Transmission may also occur from mother to child, either transplacentally or during breastfeeding.

Clinical features

- *Skin rash*—patients may present early in the disease with 'ground itch', intense pruritus, erythema, and a papular/vesicular rash at the site of larval penetration.
- *Pulmonary manifestations*—Löeffler's syndrome (respiratory symptoms, pulmonary infiltration, and eosinophilia) is caused by migration of larvae through the lungs.
- *Acute GI symptoms*—these include nausea, vomiting, diarrhoea, and abdominal pain.
- *Iron deficiency anaemia* is the commonest manifestation. The average daily blood loss is 0.2mL for *A. duodenale*, and 0.03mL for *N. americanus*. Protein energy malnutrition is a common complication.

Diagnosis

- Stool microscopy for ova is diagnostic, but not very sensitive, so serial tests may be required. The ova are ovoid and thin-shelled, and measure 58 × 36 micrometres. See Fig. 11.1.
- Eosinophilia is usually mild and varies during the course of the disease.

Treatment

- Albendazole (400mg stat) or mebendazole (100mg bd for 3 days) are the treatments of choice.
- Iron replacement therapy for iron deficiency anaemia.

Prevention

- Hygiene measures, including safe drinking water, properly cleaning and cooking food, handwashing, and wearing shoes.
- Regular antihelminthic therapy for populations at risk, e.g. children, pregnant women, and women of childbearing age in endemic countries.
- Development of a human vaccine is under way.

Strongyloides stercoralis

Strongyloidiasis, caused by the helminth *S. stercoralis*, may cause asymptomatic eosinophilia or disseminated infection in immunocompromised individuals.

The parasite

S. stercoralis worms can survive as parasitic forms in humans or free-living forms in the soil. Adult worms inhabit the small intestine where the females deposit ova. Eggs hatch in the mucosa, releasing larvae, and enter the intestinal lumen where they pass out in the faeces. The usual route of infection is through skin contact with contaminated soil. Humans can also be infected via the faeco-oral route. The larvae migrate through the bloodstream to the lungs where they migrate up the respiratory tree to be swallowed to the small intestine.

Epidemiology

S. stercoralis infection is endemic in tropical and subtropical regions and occurs sporadically in temperate climates, often in immigrants, travellers, military personnel, and institutions. The risk of developing hyperinfection syndrome is increased if CMI is impaired, e.g. congenital immunodeficiency, alcoholism, malignancy, BMT, corticosteroid or cytotoxic therapy. Patients with HTLV-1 infection are also at increased risk of disseminated disease, which is greater than in patients with HIV infection. Other risk factors include hypogammaglobulinaemia and anti-TNF receptor therapy.

Clinical features

- Asymptomatic infection occurs in about one-third of infected people.
- *Skin rash*—patients may present with a pruritic papulo-vesicular rash at the site of larval penetration (ground itch); 5–22% of patients develop an urticarial rash which starts perianally and extends to the buttocks, thighs, and abdomen. Also present with larva currens.
- *Pulmonary manifestations*—patients may present with Löeffler's syndrome (respiratory symptoms, pulmonary infiltration, and eosinophilia) caused by migration of larvae through the lungs.
- *Abdominal symptoms* are common and include colicky abdominal pain, diarrhoea, passage of mucus, nausea, vomiting, weight loss, malabsorption, and protein-losing enteropathy. Eosinophilia is common.

- *Hyperinfection syndrome*—massive larval invasion may occur with autoinfection, particularly in immunocompromised hosts, e.g. patients with leukaemia, lymphoma, or lepromatous leprosy, those receiving corticosteroids or with HIV infection. Clinical features include shock, severe abdominal pain, ileus, pulmonary infiltrates, and Gram-negative bacillary meningitis or septicaemia. Mortality is high.

Diagnosis

- *Stool microscopy*—this is notoriously insensitive (<50%) for the detection of larvae which are excreted intermittently.
- *Duodenal aspirates* or the string test (Enterotest)—sometimes used in patients with negative stool samples.
- *Molecular tests*—PCR tests to detect *Strongyloides* in stool samples are not widely available.
- *Serology*—ELISA tests are useful for diagnosing strongyloidiasis in immunocompetent individuals but may be negative in immunocompromised patients.
- *Endoscopy*—this is rarely required to diagnose strongyloidiasis but may be performed in the investigation of patients with GI symptoms. Larvae may be seen on mucosal biopsies.

Treatment

- Ivermectin is the treatment of choice for uncomplicated infections. It is usually administered as two single 200 micrograms/kg doses, either on consecutive days or 2 weeks apart. Immigrants from areas of Africa that are endemic for loiasis should be screened for this prior to treatment, as ivermectin may precipitate encephalopathy in patients with high levels of microfilaraemia.
- Albendazole (400mg bd for 3–7 days) is also effective against strongyloidiasis.
- Disseminated disease/hyperinfection syndrome—the optimal treatment is uncertain. Treatment is with ivermectin, alone or in combination with albendazole, until symptoms resolve and stool tests have been negative for 2 weeks. For patients who cannot tolerate oral therapy, alternative (unlicensed) regimens include s/c ivermectin or a parenteral veterinary formulation. In immunocompromised patients, reduction of immunosuppressive therapy is an important adjunct to antihelminthic therapy.

Prognosis

The prognosis of strongyloidiasis is good, apart from in patients with disseminated infection/hyperinfection syndrome which has a high case fatality rate.

Prevention

Prevention of disease is by wearing shoes and avoiding contact with infected soil in endemic areas.

Enterobius vermicularis

Infection with *E. vermicularis* (pinworm) is highly prevalent in both temperate and tropical climates. Pinworm infection is commonest in children and institutionalized populations.

The parasite

E. vermicularis is a small, white, thread-like worm which inhabits the caecum and ascending colon of humans. Female worms contain about 11 000 ova and live for 11–35 days. The gravid females migrate at night to the perianal region where they deposit their eggs. The eggs embryonate within hours and are transferred from the perianal region to clothing, bedding, dust, and air. The commonest route of transmission, however, is via the patient's hands.

Epidemiology

The prevalence of pinworm is highest in children aged 5–10 years. Pinworm is primarily a family or institutional infection, with no particular socioeconomic associations. As the lifespan of the worm is relatively brief, and eggs can only survive out of the body for 20 days, long-standing infections must be due to continuous reinfection.

Clinical features

- Most infected patients are asymptomatic.
- Perianal/perineal pruritus and disturbed sleep are the commonest symptoms.
- Occasionally, migration of the worms may cause ectopic disease, e.g. appendicitis, salpingitis, oophoritis, vulvovaginitis, ulcerative bowel lesions, peritoneal inflammation.

Diagnosis

- A 'sellotape slide' is used to collect worms from the perianal region.
- The ova are oval-shaped, but flattened on one side, and measure 56 × 27 micrometres. See Fig. 11.1.
- The number of examinations is correlated with the rate of detection, e.g. 50% for a single examination, 90% for three examinations.
- All family members of an affected individual should be screened for infection.

Treatment

- Albendazole (400mg stat, repeated at 2 weeks) or mebendazole (100mg stat, repeated at 2 weeks) are the treatments of choice.
- Pyrantel pamoate (11mg/kg, maximum dose 1g) is an alternative but has GI, hepatic, and neurological side effects.
- Ivermectin (200 micrograms/kg, two doses 10 days apart) has also been used.

Prevention

Although good personal hygiene is a useful general principle, its role in the management of enterobiasis is debatable.

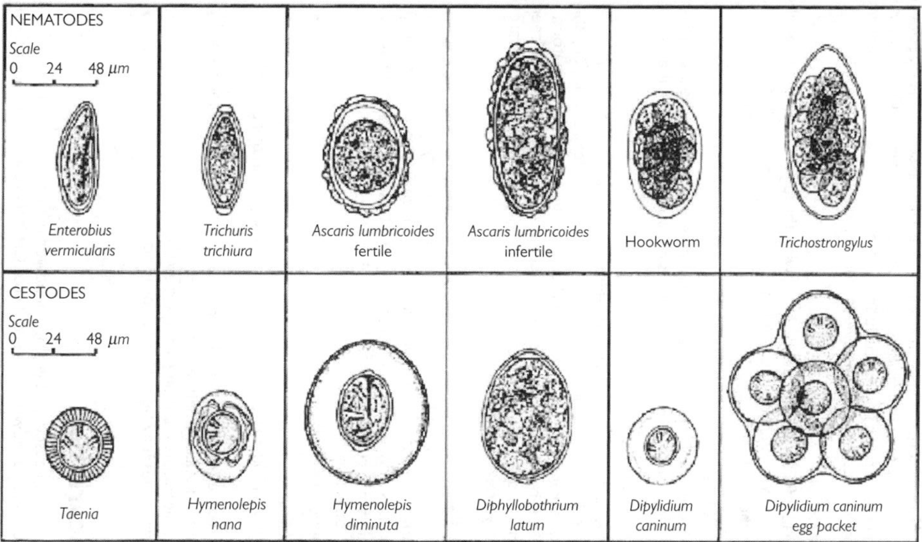

Fig. 11.1 Identification of helminth ova (nematodes and cestodes).

Cutaneous larva migrans

Cutaneous larva migrans (creeping eruption) is characterized by an erythematous, pruritic, serpiginous skin lesion. It is usually caused by the dog or cat hookworm *Ancylostoma braziliense* or *Ancylostoma caninum*. Other worms that can cause similar findings include *Unicinaria stenocephala, Bunostomum phlebotomum, S. stercoralis*, and *Gnathostoma spinigerum*.

The parasite

The larvae infect dogs or cats by burrowing through the skin. The adults live in the host's intestine and shed eggs in the faeces, which develop into larvae in the sandy soil.

Epidemiology

Infections are commonest in warmer climates, especially in holidaymakers who visit tropical sandy beaches. Infection is commoner in children than adults.

Clinical features

- Cutaneous disease—the larvae penetrate the skin of humans (an accidental host), causing tingling, itching, and vesicle formation. They then migrate through the skin, causing a characteristic raised, erythematous, pruritic, serpiginous track. In severe infections, many tracks may be seen.
- Pulmonary disease—haematogenous dissemination to the lungs is rare and may present with chronic cough.

Diagnosis

- The diagnosis is usually made based on clinical history (walking or lying on sand) and characteristic serpiginous rash. The main differential diagnosis is larva currens (strongyloidiasis) which migrates more quickly (1cm in 5min, compared with 1cm per hour).
- Skin biopsy may show an eosinophilic inflammatory infiltrate, but the migrating parasite is rarely found.

Treatment

- Ivermectin (200 micrograms stat for 1–2 days) is the treatment of choice.
- Albendazole (400mg od for 3 days) is an alternative. For patients with extensive disease, treatment may be extended to 7 days.
- Topical agents, e.g. tiabendazole, are available.
- Antihistamines may be helpful for pruritus.

Toxocariasis

Toxocariasis is caused by the dog roundworm *Toxocara canis* or, less commonly, the cat roundworm *Toxocara cati*. Clinical presentations include visceral larva migrans (VLM) and ocular toxocariasis.

The parasite

The lifecycle of *T. canis* and *T. cati* occur in dogs and cats, respectively. Eggs are shed in the stool of the definitive host, and humans are infected accidentally by ingestion of eggs in faecally contaminated soil or encysted larvae in the tissues of infected hosts. Following ingestion, the eggs hatch and penetrate the intestinal wall before being carried to other tissues, e.g. liver, heart, lungs, brain, eyes, and muscles.

Epidemiology

Toxocariasis has a worldwide distribution and is commonest in tropical rural populations. The prevalence of infection is unknown, but seroepidemiological surveys show prevalence rates ranging from 3% to 54%. Most seropositive people are asymptomatic. VLM is commoner in children, whereas ocular larva migrans (OLM) may occur in children or adults.

Clinical features

- Most infections are asymptomatic.
- VLM—presents with hepatitis and pneumonitis, as the larvae migrate through the organs. May also result in fever, anorexia, malaise, irritability, and pruritic urticarial rash. CNS manifestations include eosinophilic meningoencephalitis, space-occupying lesion, myelitis, and cerebral vasculitis.
- OLM—presents with visual impairment and a whitish, elevated granuloma on eye examination. May present with uveitis, papillitis, or endophthalmitis.

Diagnosis

- The diagnosis is usually made clinically in a young child with typical clinical features and a history of exposure to puppies.
- A definitive diagnosis is made by finding larvae in the tissues by histological examination.
- Laboratory abnormalities include eosinophilia, leucocytosis, and hypergammaglobulinaemia.
- Serological tests, e.g. ELISA, may help to confirm the diagnosis (but may also be positive in asymptomatic patients). The sensitivity is lower in OLM than VLM.
- Molecular methods—PCR assays for *Toxocara* detection have been described but are not commercially available.
- Eosinophils may be detected in BAL fluid and CSF in patients with pulmonary and CNS involvement, respectively.
- Imaging studies—hepatic, pulmonary, and cerebral lesions may be detected by ultrasound (liver lesions), CT, and MRI scans.

Treatment

- The optimal treatment is unknown, and patients with mild symptoms may recover without antihelminthic therapy.
- VLM—for patients with moderate/severe symptoms, treatment with albendazole (800mg bd for 2 weeks (adults) and 400mg bd for 2 weeks (children)) may be warranted. In cases with pulmonary, cardiac, or CNS involvement, concomitant corticosteroids should be given.
- OLM—there are some reports of response to treatment with albendazole which should be given with concomitant corticosteroids.

Prevention

Prevention measures include good hygiene practices, routine deworming of pets, timely disposal of pet faeces, and handwashing after contact with pets.

Trichinella species

Trichinellosis (trichinosis) is a parasitic infection caused by nematodes of the genus *Trichinella*. Most infections are asymptomatic, but heavy exposure may cause fever, diarrhoea, periorbital oedema, and myositis.

The parasite

The genus *Trichinella* comprises eight species, seven of which cause human disease: *Trichinella spiralis* (commonest), *Trichinella nativa, Trichinella nelsoni, Trichinella britovi, Trichinella pseudospiralis, Trichinella murrelli*, and *Trichinella papuae*. The cysts are ingested in undercooked meat, and the larvae liberated by acid–pepsin digestion of the cysts in the stomach. The larvae invade enterocytes where they develop into adult worms. The adult worms may disseminate in the bloodstream and seed the skeletal muscles where they encyst.

Epidemiology

Trichinella spp. have a worldwide distribution and infect a wide range of animals, e.g. pigs, rats, horses, bears, foxes, wild boar, and big cats. The prevalence of human infection is highest in China, Thailand, Argentina, Bolivia, Mexico, the former USSR, and Romania. Humans are infected by consumption of raw or undercooked meat.

Clinical features

- The severity of infection correlates with the number of ingested larvae—the incubation period is 7–30 days.
- Mild infections may be subclinical.
- In heavy infections, two clinical stages occur. The intestinal stage occurs 2–7 days after ingestion and may be asymptomatic or present with abdominal pain, nausea, vomiting, and diarrhoea. This is followed by the muscle stage when larvae disseminate and become encysted in the host muscle.
- Cardiac disease—myocarditis and arrhythmias may occur and are associated with high mortality.
- Neurological disease—meningitis or encephalitis may occur.
- Pulmonary disease—may occur early due to larval migration and present with a dry cough. Respiratory myositis (intercostal, diaphragmatic, upper airways) may develop in response to encysted larvae. Secondary bacterial pneumonia may also occur.
- Renal involvement is rare and only occurs in severe disease.

Diagnosis

- The diagnosis should be suspected in any patient who presents with fever, periorbital oedema, and myositis, particularly if there is a history of ingestion of undercooked meat.
- Routine laboratory tests show eosinophilia, raised ESR, elevated creatine phosphokinase (CPK), and LDH levels.
- Serology—antibodies are detectable 3 weeks after infection. Various assays may be used, e.g. ELISA, immunofluorescence, indirect haemagglutination, precipitin, and bentonite flocculation assays.

- Molecular tests—DNA detection assays have been developed.
- Muscle biopsy—is diagnostic but is not usually required, unless there is diagnostic uncertainty.

Treatment

- Most *Trichinella* infections are mild and self-limiting and do not require antihelminthic treatment. Most patients are treated symptomatically with bed rest and analgesics.
- Management of severe disease (CNS, cardiac, or pulmonary involvement) consists of antihelminthic therapy and corticosteroids. Albendazole (400mg bd for 10–14 days) or mebendazole (200–400mg tds for 3 days, then 400–500mg tds for 10 days) are the treatments of choice. Prednisolone should be administered concomitantly (30–60mg/day for 10–15 days).

Prevention

The most effective way to prevent trichinosis is to cook meat properly. Freezing at −15°C for 3 weeks or irradiation of packed meat will also kill larvae.

Dracunculus medinensis

Dracunculiasis (guinea worm infection) occurs after drinking water containing crustaceans infected with the larvae of *D. medinensis*.

The parasite

After ingestion of crustaceans containing *D. medinensis*, the larvae are released in the stomach, pass into the small intestine, penetrate the mucosa, and reach the retroperitoneum where they mature and mate. About a year later, the female worm migrates to the subcutaneous tissues of the legs. The overlying skin ulcerates, and a portion of the worm protrudes. On contact with water, large numbers of larvae are released where they are ingested by crustaceans, and the lifecycle continues.

Epidemiology

D. medinensis is found predominantly in Africa where water supplies are used both for drinking and for bathing.

Clinical features

- There are often no clinical signs, until the worm reaches the skin surface.
- Initially, a stinging papule develops on the lower leg.
- Some patients may develop generalized symptoms such as urticaria, nausea, vomiting, diarrhoea, and dyspnoea.
- Over the next few days, the lesion vesiculates and ruptures and forms a painful ulcer. If the area is rinsed with water, a milky fluid containing larvae wells up.
- Discharge continues intermittently over weeks, and the worm is slowly absorbed or extruded, after which the ulcer heals.
- Multiple ulcers may occur, and secondary infection is common.

Diagnosis

The diagnosis is mainly clinical, but larvae may be seen on examination of the discharge fluid.

Treatment

- Treatment consists of removal of the worm by gradually rolling it around a small stick. Unerupted worms may be removed by minor surgery under local anaesthesia.
- Secondary bacterial infections should be treated with antibiotics.

Prevention

Boiling, chlorinating, or sieving drinking water prevents guinea worm infection. In West Africa, major advances in prevention have dramatically reduced infection rates.

Filariasis

Filariasis is caused by three species of nematodes (roundworms) that inhabit the lymphatics and subcutaneous tissues: *Wuchereria bancrofti*, *Brugia malayi*, and *Brugia timori*.

The parasites

After the bite of an infected mosquito, larvae enter the lymphatics and lymph nodes where they mature into white, thread-like adult worms. The adults live for 5 years, and females discharge microfilariae into the bloodstream, usually around midnight. In the South Pacific, the peak is less pronounced and occurs during the day.

Epidemiology

It is estimated that 120 million people are infected with these parasites.

- *W. bancrofti* occurs throughout the tropics and subtropics.
- *B. malayi* occurs mainly in South East Asia.
- *B. timori* is restricted to Timor in Indonesia.

Humans are the only host for *W. bancrofti*, but *B. malayi* has been found in felines and primates. Only a small proportion of people who are bitten by infected mosquitoes develop clinical disease.

Clinical features

- Most patients are asymptomatic, despite microfilaraemia.
- Acute infection may present with acute adenolymphangitis (ADL), acute dermatolymphangioadenitis (DLA), filiarial fever, and tropical pulmonary eosinophilia.
- Chronic manifestations include lymphoedema (which may progress to elephantiasis) and hydrocele (which may be unilateral or bilateral).
- Renal involvement with discharge of lymph into the renal pelvis causes chyluria, which can result in anaemia and hypoproteinaemia.

Diagnosis

- Blood smear—a blood sample should be taken between 10 p.m. and 2 a.m. (apart from if the patient is from the South Pacific when they may be taken in the daytime) and stained with Giemsa or Wright's stain. Microfilariae are occasionally seen in hydrocele fluid, chylous urine, or lymph node aspirates.
- Circulating filarial antigen (CFA) assays are available for *W. bancrofti* infections and can be performed at any time of day.
- Serological tests may be positive but do not distinguish the different species, or current from past infection. Immunoassays and PCR-based assays have been developed.
- Molecular tests—species-specific PCR tests are only available in the research setting.
- Ultrasonography of the lymphatic vessels in the spermatic cord may show motile adult worms.
- Evaluation for co-infection with onchocerciasis and loiasis—in areas where these diseases are endemic, they should be excluded prior to administering treatment for filariasis, as severe inflammatory reactions may occur.

Treatment

- Diethylcarbamazine (DEC; see ➔ p. 125) (6mg/kg/day for 12 days) is the treatment of choice for lymphatic filariasis. Side effects: fever, headache, nausea, arthralgia.
- Doxycycline (200mg/day for 4–6 weeks) has macrofilaricidal activity and reduces pathology in mild to moderate disease.
- Patients with concomitant infection with onchocerciasis (➔ see *Onchocerca volvulus*, pp. 557–8) should be treated with ivermectin (150 micrograms/kg stat), followed by standard treatment for filariasis.
- Patients with concomitant loiasis (➔ see *Loa loa*, pp. 556–7) and <2500 *Loa loa* microfilariae/mL of blood can be treated with DEC (8–10mg/kg/day for 21 days). Patients with higher levels of *Loa loa* microfilaraemia should be treated with doxycycline (200mg/day for 4–6 weeks) or albendazole (200–400mg daily for 21 days).
- Mass drug treatment of populations in endemic areas use yearly single dose of DEC alone or in combination with albendazole or ivermectin.

Prevention

Mass drug administration to reduce the reservoir of microfilariae has been the cornerstone of prevention. Vector control using insecticide-treated bed nets has been useful in areas where anopheline mosquitoes transmit *W. bancrofti*. Travellers to endemic areas should be advised to avoid mosquito bites (protective clothing, insect repellent).

Loa loa

Loiasis is caused by *Loa loa* and characterized by transient subcutaneous swellings (Calabar swellings). Occasionally, worms can migrate through the subconjunctiva, causing conjunctivitis.

The parasite

The white, thread-like worms measure 30–70 × 0.3mm and migrate through the connective tissues. The microfilariae measure 300 × 8 micrometres and appear in the blood during the day.

Epidemiology

Loa loa is endemic in West and Central Africa. It is transmitted to humans by the bite of the *Chrysops* fly (tabanid fly, horse or deer fly).

Clinical features

- Many patients are asymptomatic but often have eosinophilia.
- The characteristic feature is transient oedematous swellings (Calabar swellings), which are caused by worms migrating through the subcutaneous tissues. They are usually preceded by localized pain and itching, are solitary and commonly found around joints, and may last for days to weeks.
- Occasionally, a worm may migrate across the subconjunctiva, causing conjunctivitis.
- Complications include worms in the penis or breast tissue, endomyocardial fibrosis, cardiomyopathy, retinopathy, encephalopathy, peripheral neuropathy, arthritis, lymphadenitis, and pleural effusion.

Diagnosis

- The diagnosis is often clinical, based on finding typical clinical features in a patient from West or Central Africa.
- Detection of organisms—the diagnosis is confirmed by demonstrating microfilariae in the subcutaneous tissues, the eye, or a peripheral blood smear taken between 10 a.m. and 2 p.m.
- Serology—these are helpful in travellers and expatriates, but not in residents of endemic areas.
- Other tests—a quantitative real-time PCR-based assay has been developed but is not widely available. Tests that detect circulating *Loa loa* antigens are under development.

Treatment

- DEC (➔ see Antihelminthic drugs, p. 125) eliminates microfilariae from the blood but does not kill adult worms. Treatment may precipitate encephalopathy in patients with high microfilarial loads. Treatment for patients without detectable microfilaraemia is with DEC 9mg/kg/day for 21 days. Treatment for patients with microfilaraemia is with a graded dosing schedule, increasing from 1mg/kg/day to 9mg/kg/day over a total of 21 days.
- Albendazole is an alternative agent with macrofilaricidal activity, causing sterilization or death of adult worms; it has no significant effect on microfilariae.

- Ivermectin is no longer a preferred treatment. It has rapid microfilaricidal activity and can precipitate encephalitis and/or shock, particularly in patients with high levels of microfilaraemia. It should be given as pre-treatment in patients who are co-infected with *Loa loa* and onchocerciasis.

Prevention

- Avoid insect bites (protective clothing, insect repellent) in endemic areas.
- Mass treatment with DEC or ivermectin interrupts transmission in endemic areas.
- Temporary visitors to endemic areas may take prophylactic DEC (300mg weekly).

Onchocerca volvulus

Onchocerciasis (river blindness) is caused by the nematode *O. volvulus* and characterized by blindness and skin disease.

The parasite

O. volvulus is transmitted to humans by the *Simulium* blackfly. After a bite, the larvae penetrate the skin and migrate into the connective tissues where they develop into filiform adults. The worms are often found tangled in nodules of subcutaneous tissue. Each female produces large numbers of microfilariae that migrate through the skin and connective tissues.

Epidemiology

Onchocerciasis is the second leading cause of blindness worldwide. One hundred and twenty million people are at risk, and 37 million people are estimated to be infected. It occurs in West, Central, and East Africa, with scattered foci in Central and South America.

Clinical features

- Ocular onchocerciasis—the first sign is the presence of microfilariae in the eye on slit lamp examination. Additional manifestations include punctate keratitis, sclerosing keratitis, uveitis, optic atrophy, and chorioretinitis.
- Onchocercal skin disease—generalized itching is often the first symptom. Early signs include pruritic inflammatory papules, nodules, and plaques. The skin may become lichenified, atrophied, and depigmented. Lymphadenopathy may develop, particularly in the inguinal region. Fibrosis of lymph nodes may result in lymphatic obstruction and elephantiasis.
- Subcutaneous nodules—fibrous nodules (onchocercomata) containing adult worms may develop over bony prominences.
- Systemic features include fever, weight loss, backache, and musculoskeletal pains.

Diagnosis

- Skin snips—detection of microfilariae is diagnostic, but skin snips may be negative in early disease. A minimum of two, and ideally six, snips should be taken and incubated in saline for 24h prior to examination.
- Slit lamp examination—this may demonstrate microfilariae in the anterior chamber of the eye.
- Mazotti test—this consists of a 50mg PO dose of DEC (➔ see Antihelminthic drugs, p. 125), which results in microfilarial death and exacerbation of symptoms. It should only be used in patients with suspected onchocerciasis, and negative skin snips and slit lamp examination. It is contraindicated in heavily infected individuals because of the risk of severe reactions.
- Patch test—a topical preparation of DEC can be administered to the skin to assess for a local skin reaction. It is a useful alternative to skin snips in low-prevalence areas, as it is cheap, non-invasive, and more sensitive than skin snips.
- Serology—serological tests are not very reliable, as the prevalence of positive serology is high in the absence of active infection in adults returning from endemic areas and can remain positive for years. There is also significant cross-reactivity in ELISAs between different filarial parasites.
- Antigen tests—these may be more reliable than serology, as they are only positive in patients with active infection.
- Molecular tests—highly sensitive PCR assays have been developed but are not routinely available.
- Ultrasound—this may identify adult worms within subcutaneous nodules.

Treatment

- Ivermectin (➔ see Antihelminthic drugs, p. 125) is the treatment of choice—it kills microfilariae and has some effect on adult worms (macrofilariae). Side effects include fever, pruritus, headache, and arthralgia.
- Doxycycline (➔ see Tetracyclines, pp. 56–8) is active against *Wolbachia*, the endosymbiotic bacteria within *O. volvulus*, and thus is macrofilaricidal. Doxycycline (100mg/day for 6 weeks), followed by a single dose of ivermectin (150 micrograms/kg stat), has been shown to be effective. Rifampicin and azithromycin also have activity against *Wolbachia*.
- Other agents—moxidectin is a veterinary deworming agent that has macro- and microfilaricidal activity. Closantel, another veterinary drug, is also a potential therapy.

Prevention

- Avoid insect bites (protective clothing, insect repellents).
- Vector control with larvicides is being used in West Africa.
- There is no vaccine.

Cestodes

Human cestode (tapeworm) infections occur in one of two forms: mature tapeworms residing in the gut, or larval cysts in the tissues. The form that the infection takes depends on the species. The medically important cestodes are summarized in Table 11.2.

Parasite structure

The parasitic cestodes are flatworms (platyhelminths). The worms consist of several parts: a head (scolex, which has suckers and sometimes hooks), a short neck, and a strobila (a segmented tail made of proglottids). The proglottid has both male and female sexual organs and is responsible for egg production. They become gravid and eventually break free of the tapeworm, releasing eggs in the stool or outside the body.

Parasite life cycle

Cestodes divide their life cycle between two animal hosts: the definitive carnivorous host and the intermediate herbivorous/omnivorous host. Mature tapeworms reside in the intestinal tract of the definitive host and shed eggs into the stool. The eggs may be embryonated (can immediately infect the intermediate host) or non-embryonated (require development outside the body). The intermediate host is infected by the ingestion of eggs that hatch in the intestine, releasing an oncosphere. This penetrates the gut mucosa and spreads through the circulation to the tissues where it forms a larval cyst. The life cycle is completed when the carnivorous host ingests the cyst-infected tissues of the intermediate host.

Taenia saginata (beef tapeworm)

- The parasite—adult worms are long (up to 10m in length) and contain >1000 proglottids, each capable of producing thousands of eggs.
- Epidemiology—transmitted to humans by ingestion of larval cysts in rare or undercooked meat from infected cattle. Common in cattle-breeding areas of the world such as Central Asia, the near East, and Central and

Table 11.2 Medically important cestodes

Type of cestode	Disease	Species
Intestinal	Tapeworm	*Taenia saginata*
		Taenia solium
		Diphyllobothrium latum
		Hymenolepis nana
Invasive	Cysticercosis, echinococcosis	*Taenia solium*
		Echinococcus granulosus
		Echinococcus vogeli
		Echinococcus multilocularis

Eastern Africa where prevalence of infection may be >10%. Areas of lower prevalence (<1%) include Europe, South East Asia, and Central America,
- Clinical features—patients are usually asymptomatic, but a minority complain of nausea, anorexia, and abdominal pain. The proglottids are motile and may be seen on the perineum or clothing.
- Diagnosis is confirmed by examination of proglottids (with 15–20 lateral uterine branches). The eggs are morphologically indistinguishable from those of *T. solium*. See Fig. 11.1.
- Treatment is with praziquantel (5–10mg/kg) or niclosamide (2g) PO stat.

Taenia solium (pork tapeworm)

- The parasite—*T. solium* tapeworms may live for 10–20 years and grow up to 8m in length.
- Epidemiology—humans can be definitive or intermediate hosts for *T. solium*. Individuals who ingest larval cysts in raw or undercooked pork acquire pork tapeworm; those who ingest eggs develop tissue infection with cysts (cysticercosis; ➔ see Neurocysticercosis, pp. 731–2). *T. solium* infection is endemic in Mexico, Central and South America, South East Asia, India, the Philippines, and southern Europe.
- Clinical features—most patients are asymptomatic, unless autoinfection with parasite eggs occurs.
- Diagnosis—infection is readily diagnosed by detection of eggs in the stool (morphologically indistinguishable from those of *T. saginata*). Definitive diagnosis is by examination of the proglottids (with 7–13 lateral uterine branches). See Fig. 11.1.
- Treatment is with praziquantel (5–10mg/kg) or niclosamide (2g) PO stat.

Diphyllobothrium latum (fish tapeworm)

- The parasite—*D. latum* tapeworms may grow up to 25m in length. The tapeworm takes 3–6 weeks to mature and may survive for >30 years.
- Epidemiology—human infection is acquired by ingesting uncooked freshwater fish containing cysts. Areas of endemic infection (>2% prevalence) include Siberia, Scandinavia and other Baltic countries, North America, Japan, and Chile where there is stable zoonotic transmission through other animal hosts, e.g. seals, cats, bears, foxes, and wolves.
- Clinical features—infection is usually asymptomatic, but patients may report weakness, dizziness, salt cravings, diarrhoea, or intermittent abdominal discomfort. Prolonged/heavy infection may lead to megaloblastic anaemia caused by vitamin B_{12} deficiency ± folate deficiency.
- Diagnosis—stool examination shows operculated eggs (45–65 micrometres). Recovery of proglottids (with a characteristic central uterus) also confirms the diagnosis. See Fig. 11.1.
- Treatment is with praziquantel (5–10mg/kg) or niclosamide (2g) PO stat. Mild vitamin B_{12} deficiency resolves with eradication of the tapeworm; severe deficiency requires parenteral treatment.

Hymenolepis nana (dwarf tapeworm)

- The parasite—*H. nana* is the only tapeworm that can be transmitted directly from human to human. Adult tapeworms measure 15–50mm.
- Epidemiology—areas of endemic infection (up to 26%) include Asia, southern and eastern Europe, Central and South America, and Africa. Infection is commoner in children and institutionalized patients.
- Clinical features—heavy infection may be associated with abdominal cramps, nausea, diarrhoea, and dizziness. See Fig. 11.1.
- Diagnosis is made by identification of eggs (30–47 micrometres, with a characteristic double membrane) in the stool.
- Treatment is with praziquantel (25mg/kg PO stat, repeated after 1 week) or niclosamide (2g PO daily for 1 week).

Cysticercosis

- The parasite—cysticercosis is an infection with larval cysts of the cestode *T. solium* (➔ see *Taenia solium* (pork tapeworm), p. 560).
- Epidemiology—infection is acquired by consumption of *T. solium* eggs and occurs wherever *T. solium* infection is prevalent. The cumulative risk of infection increases with age, the frequency of pork consumption, and poor household hygiene.
- Clinical features—infected individuals may harbour multiple cysts throughout the body but are often asymptomatic. Symptoms may develop because of local inflammation at the site of infection. Serious disease is rare but occurs with cardiac or CNS involvement (neurocysticercosis; see ➔ p. 731–2). The latter may present with focal symptoms, seizures, chronic meningitis, or spinal cord compression. Neurocysticercosis is the commonest cause of seizures in Central America. Racemose cysticercosis is an aggressive form of basilar neurocysticercosis, resulting in coma and death.
- Diagnosis—asymptomatic patients may be diagnosed incidentally by detection of calcified cysts on plain radiographs. Neurocysticercosis may be diagnosed by CT or MRI scan, which show multiple enhancing and non-enhancing unilocular cysts. Diagnosis may be supported by a positive ELISA, indicating prior exposure to *T. solium* antigens, but patients infected with other helminths may have cross-reactive antibodies. Immunoblotting techniques using purified glycoprotein from cyst fluid may be more sensitive/specific.
- Treatment—seizures should be treated with anti-epileptic medication, and hydrocephalus with shunting. Surgical resection is the treatment of choice for symptomatic cysts outside the CNS. Albendazole (15mg/kg/day, usually 800mg/day in two divided doses) is the treatment of choice. Duration of therapy ranges from 3–7 days for single lesions to 10–14 days for parenchymal disease and 4 weeks for subarachnoid disease. Praziquantel (50–100mg/kg/day in three divided doses) is an alternative. Combination therapy with albendazole and praziquantel is generally safe and may be more effective than albendazole alone. Corticosteroids should be administered to patients with parenchymal neurocysticercosis receiving treatment with antiparasitic therapy, to

reduce inflammation associated with the dying organisms. Doses are typically 1mg/kg/day of prednisone or prednisolone or 0.1mg/kg/day of dexamethasone for 5–10 days, followed by a rapid taper.

Echinococcosis

- The parasite—the canine tapeworms *Echinococcus* spp. inadvertently infect humans, causing visceral cysts. *Echinococcus granulosus* causes cystic echinococcosis, and *Echinococcus multilocularis* causes alveolar echinococcosis. Two other species *Echinococcus vogeli* and *Echinococcus oligarthrus* rarely cause polycystic echinococcosis.
- Epidemiology—infection is acquired by ingestion of parasite eggs excreted by tapeworm-infected animals. *E. granulosus* is prevalent in South America, the Middle East and Eastern Mediterranean, some sub-Saharan African countries, China, and the former Soviet Union, and is transmitted by sheep, goats, horses, camels, and domestic dogs. *E. multilocularis* is found in Central Europe, much of Russia, the Central Asian republics, north-eastern, north-western, and western China, the north-western portion of Canada, and Western Alaska, and is transmitted by dogs and foxes.
- Clinical features—the hydatid cysts of *E. granulosus* usually affect the liver (50–70%) or lungs (20–30%) but may affect any organ of the body, e.g. heart, kidneys, bones, CNS, and eyes. They are often asymptomatic and found incidentally on radiological imaging. Symptoms may occur as a result of expansion or rupture into adjacent organs. Cyst rupture may cause a severe allergic reaction or seeding to distant organs. Alveolar cyst disease caused by *E. multilocularis* may be asymptomatic or present with malaise, weight loss, and right upper quadrant pain. Complications include biliary disease, portal hypertension, and Budd–Chiari syndrome. Extrahepatic disease is rare; multiorgan involvement.
- Diagnosis—infection is detected by radiological imaging (ultrasound, CT or MRI scan); may be confirmed serologically by ELISA or Western blot assay. This confirms exposure to the parasite and is more sensitive for *E. multilocularis* than *E. granulosus* infections.
- Treatment—asymptomatic cysts may be monitored, whereas symptomatic cysts should be treated. The optimal treatment is by surgical resection of the whole cyst 30min after instillation of a cysticidal agent, e.g. 30% saline, iodophor, or 95% ethanol. Perioperative antihelminthic agents (e.g. albendazole 400mg bd or mebendazole 40–50mg/kg/day in three divided doses) may be given, and care must be taken to prevent cyst rupture or spillage during surgery. For inoperable cysts, medical therapy improves symptoms (55–79%), although cure rates are low (29%). In patients treated surgically, an antiparasitic agent, preferably albendazole, is continued for at least 2 years. In inoperable patients, treatment is considered for years, and possibly for life. The PAIR procedure (puncture, aspiration, injection, and re-aspiration) is more popular, as it is less invasive than surgery.

Trematodes (flukes)

Flukes are parasitic worms of the class *Trematoda*. They are usually oval-shaped and vary in length (1mm to several cm). Structurally, they have an oral sucker, a ventral sucker (usually), a blind bifurcate intestinal tract, and prominent reproductive organs. The human flukes belong to the digenetic group in which sexual reproduction is followed by asexual multiplication. Most human parasites are hermaphrodites, except *Schistosoma* spp.

Schistosoma species

- Humans are the principal host of the five *Schistosoma* spp. (see Table 11.3). Adult worms live in the venous plexus of the urinary bladder (*S. haematobium*) or the portal venous system (*S. mansoni, S. japonicum*) where they mate and shed their eggs. Eggs are passed out in the urine or faeces and hatch in fresh water, releasing miracidia that enter the snail (intermediate host). The miracidia multiply asexually in the snail and eventually release cercariae. These infective forms penetrate human skin and migrate through the lungs and the liver, before passing to their final habitat.
- *Epidemiology*—200 million people worldwide are estimated to be infected with *Schistosoma* spp. Each species has a specific geographical location: *S. haematobium* (Africa, the Middle East), *S. mansoni* (Arabia, Africa, South America, the Caribbean), *S. japonicum* (the Far East), *S. mekongi* (South East Asia), *S. intercalatum* (West and Central Africa). Two factors are responsible for endemicity—the presence of the snail vector and contamination of fresh water by human waste.
- *Pathogenesis*—the disease syndromes that characterize schistosomiasis coincide with the three stages of parasite development:
  - cercariae penetrate the skin to cause a rash;

Table 11.3 Medically important trematodes

Type of fluke	Disease	Species
Blood	Schistosomiasis	*Schistosoma haematobium*
		Schistosoma japonicum
		Schistosoma mansoni
		Schistosoma mekongi
		Schistosoma intercalatum
Liver	Clonorchiasis	*Clonorchis sinensis*
	Opisthorchiasis	*Opisthorcis felineus*
		Opisthorcis viverrini
	Fascioliasis	*Fasciola hepatica*
Intestinal	Fasciolopsiasis	*Fasciolopsis buski*
	Heterophyiasis	*Heterophyes heterophyes*
Lung	Paragonimiasis	*Paragonimus westermani*

  - some weeks after infection, the mature worms deposit their eggs; this may be accompanied by acute schistosomiasis (Katayama fever);
  - production of large numbers of eggs results in chronic granulomatous inflammation and fibrosis of the urinary tract or portal venous system.
- Clinical features of schistosomiasis include:
  - swimmer's itch—a papular, pruritic dermatitis that occasionally occurs 24h after penetration of the skin by cercariae. It appears to be a sensitization phenomenon, as it rarely occurs on primary exposure;
  - acute schistosomiasis or Katayama fever—occurs 4–8 weeks after infection and is characterized by fever, chills, sweating, headache, cough, hepatosplenomegaly, and lymphadenopathy. Peripheral eosinophilia is common. Symptoms usually resolve within a few weeks, but rarely death may occur;
  - chronic schistosomiasis—occurs in patients with heavy infestation;
  - intestinal schistosomiasis, caused by *S. mansoni, S. japonicum*, or *S. mekongi*, may present with fatigue, colicky abdominal pain, diarrhoea, dysentery, chronic granulomatous bowel lesions, mucosal ulceration, or anaemia. *S. intercalatum* infection may also present with symptoms;
  - hepatic schistosomiasis—also caused by *S. mansoni, S. japonicum*, or *S. mekongi*; may present with hepatomegaly, portal hypertension, splenomegaly, oesophageal varices, or decompensated liver disease. *S. mekongi* infection may also present with hepatomegaly;
  - urinary schistosomiasis—caused by *S. haematobium*, causes granulomatous inflammation in the bladder and ureters. Patients may complain of dysuria and terminal haematuria. Haematospermia is common. Progression of disease may cause urinary obstruction with hydronephrosis and hydroureter;
  - CNS schistosomiasis—rare, but complicates 3% of *S. japonicum* infections. It may present with a space-occupying lesion, encephalopathy, or seizures. *S. haematobium* and *S. mansoni* may cause spinal cord lesions and present with a transverse myelitis.
- *Diagnosis*—the diagnosis should be suspected in any patient with compatible symptoms and an appropriate travel history. The diagnosis is confirmed by detection of eggs in a terminal urine specimen collected between 12 and 2 p.m. (*S. haematobium*), or in faeces examined by the Kato thick smear procedure (other species; see Fig. 11.2). Schistosomiasis may also be diagnosed by finding eggs in tissue biopsy specimens of rectal, intestinal, liver, or bladder biopsies. Serodiagnostic tests do not distinguish between recent and past infection—they are most useful in returning travellers (➔ see Imported fever, pp. 584–6).
- *Management*—praziquantel is the treatment of choice. The dose is 40mg/kg (in one or two doses) for *S. haematobium, S. mansoni*, and *S. intercalatum*, or 60mg/kg (in two or three doses) for *S. japonicum* and *S. mekongi*. Side effects are mild: abdominal discomfort, fever, and headache. Drug resistance may become a problem in endemic areas with mass treatment. Adjunctive treatment with corticosteroids is given in Katayama fever and CNS disease.

Clonorchiasis

- *Clonorchis sinensis* (Chinese or oriental liver fluke) is a parasite of fish-eating mammals in the Far East. The adult flukes are flat, elongated worms (15 × 3mm) that inhabit the distal biliary capillaries where they deposit small, yellow, operculated eggs (30 × 14 micrometres). The eggs pass out in the stool and are ingested by snails, inside which they hatch into miracidia. Miracidia multiply into cercariae that pass into the water and penetrate fresh water where they encyst as metacercariae. Humans are infected by ingestion of raw or undercooked fish. Once ingested, the metacercariae excyst in the duodenum and migrate to the bile ducts.
- *Epidemiology*—millions of humans are estimated to be infected, mainly in China, Hong Kong, Korea, and Vietnam.
- *Clinical features*—most infected people are asymptomatic. Heavy infection may result in cholangitis and cholangiohepatitis. Infection has been associated with an increased risk of cholangiocarcinoma.
- *Diagnosis*—infection is confirmed by demonstration of characteristic operculated, embryonated eggs in the stool (see Fig. 11.2).
- *Management*—praziquantel 25mg/kg tds for 2 days, or albendazole 10mg/kg/day for 7 days. Surgery is needed rarely to relieve biliary obstruction.

Opisthorciasis

- *Opisthorcis felineus* and *Opisthorcis viverrini* are common liver flukes of cats and dogs that are occasionally transmitted to humans. The life cycle is similar to *C. sinensis*.
- *Epidemiology*—*O. felineus* is endemic in South East Asia and eastern Europe, whereas *O. viverrini* is found in Thailand.
- *Clinical features*—mild or moderate infection is usually asymptomatic. Biliary tract symptoms and ultrasonographic signs are commoner in patients aged 20–40 years with heavy infection. An association between *O. viverrini* infection and cholangiocarcinoma has been reported in Thailand.
- *Diagnosis*—this is confirmed by the detection of eggs in the stool (see Fig. 11.2).
- *Management*—praziquantel is the drug of choice.

Fascioliasis

- *Fasciola hepatica* is a liver fluke of sheep and cattle that can infect humans. The adult worms are large, flat, brown, and leaf-shaped, (2.5 × 1cm) and live in the biliary tract of their mammalian host. The large, oval, yellow-brown, operculated eggs (140 × 75 micrometres) pass out in the faeces and complete their development in water.

  The miracidia hatch and enter the snail intermediate host where they multiply into unforked-tail cercariae. These emerge and undergo encystment into metacercariae on aquatic plants, grasses, and sometimes soil. After ingestion, the metacercariae excyst, releasing larvae that penetrate the intestinal wall, peritoneum, and liver capsule to migrate to the biliary tract.
- *Epidemiology*—infection is commoner in sheep- and cattle-rearing areas, e.g. South America, Europe, Africa, China, and Australia.

- *Clinical features*—*F. hepatica* infection has two distinct clinical phases:
  - acute hepatic migratory phase, characterized by fever, right upper quadrant pain, hepatomegaly, and peripheral eosinophilia. Nodules or linear tracks may be seen on ultrasound, CT, or MRI scan;
  - chronic biliary phase which may be asymptomatic or present with biliary obstruction or cirrhosis.
- *Diagnosis*—this is confirmed by detection of characteristic ova in the stool or bile (see Fig. 11.2). Serological tests may also be helpful.
- *Management*—triclabendazole 10mg/kg PO one dose is the treatment of choice. Alternatives: nitazoxanide (500mg bd for 7 days) or bithionol.

Fasciolopsiasis

- *Fasciolopsis buski* is a large intestinal fluke (2–7.5cm in length) which is endemic in South East Asia and the Far East. It inhabits the duodenum and jejunum, producing large, operculated eggs (135 × 80 micrometres), which are excreted and hatch into miracidia in fresh water. These enter the snail intermediate host where they multiply and develop into cercariae which encyst into metacercariae on aquatic plants. Humans are infected by ingestion of contaminated plants. The metacercariae excyst in the intestine and develop into adult worms.
- *Clinical features*—fasciolopsiasis is usually asymptomatic, but heavy infection may present with diarrhoea, abdominal pain, or malabsorption.
- *Diagnosis*—this is confirmed by detection of eggs in the stool (see Fig. 11.2).
- *Management*—praziquantel 25mg/kg tds for 1 day.

Heterophyiasis

- *Heterophyes heterophyes* is a tiny intestinal fluke (<2mm in length) which is endemic in the Nile Delta, South East Asia, and the Far East. The life cycle is similar to *F. buski* (➔ see Fasciolopsiasis above), except that the metacerceriae encyst in fish. Humans are infected by consumption of undercooked fish.
- *Clinical features*—infection may present with abdominal pain and diarrhoea.
- *Diagnosis*—adult worms produce small, operculated eggs (30 × 15 micrometres), which may be detected in the stool (see Fig. 11.2).
- *Management*—praziquantel 25mg/kg tds for 2 days.

Paragonimiasis

- *Paragonimus westermani* is a lung fluke that is widely distributed (West Africa, the Indian subcontinent, the Far East, Central and South America).
- *Life cycle*—adult worms inhabit the lungs and produce golden brown, operculated eggs that pass into the bronchioles and are coughed up or are swallowed and pass out into the faeces. In fresh water, the eggs mature and release miracidia that infect the snail intermediate host. After 3–5 months, cerceriae are released and infect freshwater crustaceans (crayfish and crabs) where they encyst in the muscles. Humans are infected by ingestion of raw or pickled crustaceans.

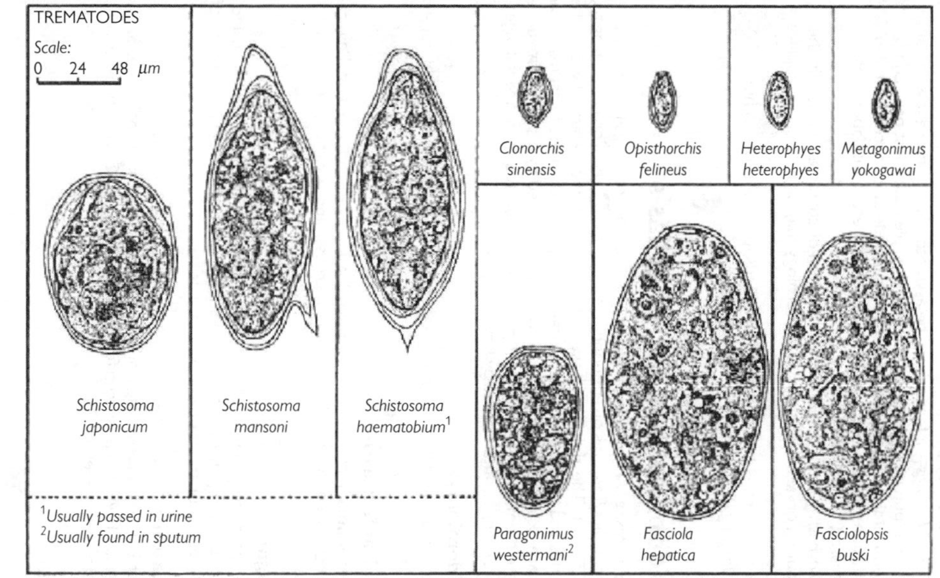

Fig. 11.2 Identification of trematode eggs.

The metacercariae excyst in the intestine, penetrate the intestinal wall, enter the peritoneal cavity, and migrate through the diaphragm and pleural cavities to the lungs. Worms may also lodge in the peritoneal cavity or the brain.

- *Clinical features*—infection may be asymptomatic or present with cough, brown sputum, intermittent haemoptysis, pleuritic chest pain, and peripheral eosinophilia. Complications include lung abscess and pleural effusion. Ectopic infection is rare and may present with abdominal masses, epilepsy, or focal neurological signs.
- *Diagnosis*—this is confirmed by detection of characteristic eggs in the sputum or faeces (see Fig. 11.2). Serology may be helpful in ectopic infections.
- *Management*—praziquantel 25mg/kg tds for 2 days, or biothionol 30–50mg/kg PO every other day for 10 days.

Abdominal angiostrongyliasis

The parasite *Angiostrongylus cantonensis*, a rodent parasite, may cause abdominal symptoms or eosinophilic meningitis (➔ see Chronic meningitis, pp. 724–6). The definitive host is the rat where the parasite lives in the arteries and arterioles of the ileocaecum. Eggs hatch in the intestinal tissue and are excreted in the faeces, before being ingested by a slug intermediate where a similar cycle occurs. Humans may be infected by accidental ingestion of foods contaminated by larvae or slugs.

Epidemiology

Infection usually affects children in Central and South America and, rarely, Africa.

Clinical features

Patients usually complain of abdominal pain, fever, and vomiting. Physical findings include fever, abdominal tenderness, and a right lower quadrant mass (50%).

Diagnosis

The syndrome resembles appendicitis, apart from the presence of eosinophilia. Radiological features are non-specific. Serology and PCR detection of DNA exist but are not routinely available.

Treatment

Most patients undergo laparotomy and removal of infected tissue. Some patients have been successfully treated with DEC and tiabendazole. Alternative: mebendazole.

Anisakiasis

Anisakis and *Phocanema* are parasites of marine mammals, e.g. dolphins, seals, and whales. The eggs are excreted in the faeces and hatch as free-swimming larvae that are ingested by crustaceans and then by fish and squid. Humans are accidentally infected, following ingestion of raw or poorly cooked seafood.

Epidemiology

Infection occurs most frequently in countries where raw fish is consumed, e.g. Japan and the Netherlands.

Clinical features

Symptoms usually occur 48h after ingestion and are caused by penetration of the worms into the GI tract. Gastric anisakiasis is usually caused by *Phocanema* and characterized by abdominal pain, nausea, and vomiting. Small intestinal involvement is usually caused by *Anisakis* and characterized by lower abdominal pain and signs of obstruction. Symptoms may become chronic with development of abdominal masses. Occasionally, acute allergic symptoms, e.g. urticaria and anaphylaxis, may also occur with *Anisakis*.

Diagnosis

The diagnosis should be suspected in any patient with a history of ingestion of raw fish and abdominal symptoms. Leucocytosis commonly occurs with intestinal involvement; eosinophilia is rare. Gastric anisakiasis is confirmed by upper GI endoscopy and histological examination of biopsy specimens. Intestinal anisakiasis is confirmed by radiological features of obstruction and detection of eosinophils in aspirated ascites. Serological tests are not routinely available.

Treatment

Symptoms usually improve without specific therapy but may resolve more quickly if gastric worms are removed by endoscopy. Occasionally, removal of an intestinal mass may be required.

Prevention

Anisakiasis may be prevented by cooking or freezing fish for 24h prior to ingestion.

Capillariasis

Although the life cycle of *Capillaria philippinensis* is incompletely understood, its larvae have been found in freshwater fish and are known to be infectious for human and birds. After ingestion of raw fish, the larvae invade the jejunum and ileum and produce both eggs and larvae. The parasite multiplies in the gut and may cause autoinfection and overwhelming infection (similar to *S. stercoralis*; ➲ see *Strongyloides stercoralis*, pp. 546–7).

Epidemiology

Infections usually occur in the Philippines and Thailand, but two cases have been reported in the Middle East.

Clinical features

These are consistent with malabsorption and protein-losing enteropathy, and include abdominal pain, vomiting, diarrhoea, abdominal distension, borborygmi, malaise, weight loss, and peripheral oedema.

Diagnosis

This is confirmed by detecting ova or larvae in the stool. There are no serological tests.

Treatment

Treatment is with mebendazole or albendazole. Mortality rates of up to 30% have been reported in untreated patients.

Chapter 12

Ectoparasites

Introduction *572*
Hexapoda 572
Arachnida 575

Introduction

An ectoparasite is an organism that survives through interaction with the cutaneous surface of the host (e.g. obtaining a blood meal or living in the skin). Most ectoparasites belong to the phylum *Arthropoda*. Two classes are important in human disease: *Hexapoda* (six-legged insects, e.g. lice, bugs, flies, mosquitoes) and *Arachnida* (eight-legged mites, spiders, and ticks). Ectoparasitic diseases are a common health problem in non-industrialized tropical countries.

Hexapoda

Lice (pediculosis)

Aetiology

Three species of sucking lice affect humans: *Pediculus humanus capitis* (head louse), *Pediculus humanus humanus* (body louse), and *Phthirus pubis* (pubic or crab louse). The first two species are morphologically similar with small, flat, elongated bodies and pointed heads. The pubic louse is shorter and wider, and resembles a crab. Small ovoid eggs (nits) are laid by the adult female and adhere to hair and clothing; 7–10 days later, the nymphs emerge, and, after three successive moults, the adult lice develop and mate. The females produce up to 300 eggs per day for 3–4 weeks until they die. Lice pierce the skin, inject saliva, and defecate while feeding.

Epidemiology

Lice infestations occur worldwide, are transmitted by direct contact, and are associated with poor hygiene and overcrowding. Lice cause skin disease and can also act as vectors for other infectious diseases, e.g. epidemic typhus (*R. prowazekii*), trench fever (*B. quintana*), and relapsing fever (*Borrelia recurrentis*).

Clinical features

- *P.h. capitis* affects the scalp and causes pruritus. Complications include secondary bacterial infection and regional adenopathy.
- *P.h. corporis* is usually found in the seams of clothing. Symptoms include pruritus, erythematous macules, papules, and excoriations, usually on the trunk. Complications include impetigo, hyperpigmentation, and hyperkeratosis.
- *P. pubis* resides in the pubic hair but may also be found in eyebrows, eyelashes, and axillary and chest hair. Symptoms include pruritus, erythematous macules, papules and excoriations, but are usually less severe than with other species. Small greyish-blue macules (maculae ceruleae), caused by injection of an anticoagulant, may be seen. Eyelash infestation may be associated with nits at the base of the eyelashes and crusting of the eyelids.

Diagnosis

Diagnosis is usually clinical but may be confirmed by microscopic examination of the organism.

Management

- *P.h. capitis*—nits can be removed by combing wet hair with a fine-toothed comb. Topical treatments include pyrethroids (e.g. permethrin 1%), malathion 0.5% (requires prolonged application, malodorous, may be irritant to the eyes), benzyl alcohol 5% lotion, lindane shampoo/lotion (neurotoxicity, poor efficacy), spinosad, and TOP ivermectin. Systemic treatment, e.g. ivermectin or co-trimoxazole, is reserved for those who fail topical therapy.
- *P.h. corporis*—body lice can be eradicated by discarding the clothing, washing clothes in a hot cycle, and ironing the seams or dusting clothing with 1% malathion powder or 10% DDT (dichlorodiphenyltrichloroethane) powder. Occasionally, a topical pediculicide, e.g. permethrin 5% cream, may be required.
- *P. pubis* may be treated with the same agents as head lice (see above). Eyelid infestation may be treated by applying a thick layer of petrolatum bd for 8 days, or 1% yellow oxide of mercury qds for 2 weeks.
- Pruritus is treated symptomatically with antihistamines and topical corticosteroids. Secondary bacterial infection should be treated with an oral antistaphylococcal agent, e.g. flucloxacillin.

Scabies

Aetiology

S. scabiei var. *hominis* is an eight-legged mite that resides in human skin. The adult female lays 2–3 eggs per day, which burrow into the skin. After 72–84h, the larvae emerge and, after several moults, develop into adults and mate. The males die shortly afterwards, but the gravid female lives for 4–6 weeks.

Epidemiology

Scabies occurs worldwide, and epidemics are associated with poverty, malnutrition, overcrowding, and poor hygiene. Scabies is transmitted by direct contact or by fomites.

Clinical features

- Human scabies—symptoms include intense pruritus (more severe at night). Signs include linear burrows, erythematous papules, excoriations, and occasionally vesicles. Complications include secondary bacterial infection and hypersensitivity reactions, e.g. eczematous eruption, nodular scabies.
- Norwegian scabies is a severe variant which may occur in institutionalized, debilitated, or immunosuppressed patients. Cutaneous lesions are hyperkeratotic, crusted nodules or plaques, and nail involvement may occur. Complications include secondary bacterial infection, septicaemia, and even death.
- Animal scabies—humans may occasionally be infected by *S. scabiei* var. *canis* from their pet dog. Skin lesions are pruritic, papular, or urticarial.

Diagnosis

Diagnosis is usually clinical but may be confirmed by microscopic examination of skin scrapings for the organism, egg, or faeces.

Management

- Permethrin 5% cream applied for 8–10h is the most effective treatment.
- PO ivermectin 200 micrograms/kg is an alternative—two doses are as effective as permethrin. Its use is favoured in institutional outbreak settings. It should not be used in pregnant women or children.
- Other agents include lindane (neurotoxic), benzyl benzoate, crotamiton, malathion, and sulphur in petrolatum.
- Pregnant women and children may be treated with sulphur in petrolatum daily for 3 days.
- Secondary bacterial infection should be treated with an antistaphylococcal agent, e.g. PO flucloxacillin.
- Household members and close contacts should be treated simultaneously. Infected clothing and bed linen should be washed and dried on a hot cycle.

Myiasis

Epidemiology

Myiasis is an infestation caused by the larvae (maggots) of dipterous (two-winged) flies. It occurs more commonly in tropical climates and is an important veterinary problem. Human disease occurs as a result of travel to an endemic area or exposure to infected animals.

Aetiology

A number of species may cause myiasis:

- *Dermatobia hominis* (human or tropical botfly);
- *Cordylobia anthropophaga* (tumbu fly);
- *Cordylobia rodhaini*;
- *Oestrus ovis* (sheep botfly);
- *Gasterophilus* spp. (horse botfly);
- *Hypoderma bovis* (cattle botfly);
- *Cuterebra* spp. (North American botfly);
- *Cochliomyia hominivorax* (New World screwworm);
- *Chrysomya bezziana* (Old World screwworm).

Clinical features

- Furunculoid myiasis is usually caused by *D. hominis, C. anthropophaga*, or *C. rodhaini*, and occurs in travellers returning from Latin America or Africa. It is characterized by single or multiple cutaneous nodules, each containing a larva. A central punctum develops and may exude serosanguineous or purulent fluid. *D. hominis* infestations occur in the scalp, face, and extremities, and may be associated with local pain. *C. anthropophaga* usually affects the trunk, buttocks, and thighs. *C. rodhaini* is similar, but lesions are larger and more painful.
- Subcutaneous infestation is caused by *Gastrophilus* spp. and characterized by migratory integumomiasis (creeping eruption), which is due to migration of larvae through the skin. *H. bovis* may cause similar lesions, which become furunculoid as the larvae mature.
- Wound myiasis may be caused by *C. hominivorax* or *C. bezziana*, and is characterized by local tissue destruction and secondary bacterial infection.

- Ophthalmomyiasis is caused by *O. ovis* and may be superficial (ophthalmomyiasis externa), with conjunctivitis, lid oedema, and punctate keratopathy, or deep (ophthalmomyiasis interna) with invasion of the globe.

Management

- Cutaneous myiasis—removal of the larvae from the affected tissue may be achieved by occlusion of the punctum, e.g. with white soft paraffin or cling film, which encourages the larva to partially emerge from the punctum to avoid asphyxiation. It can then be removed with forceps. Surgical excision may be required.
- Wound myiasis—treatment requires removal of larvae and wound debridement.
- Ophthalmomyiasis—external infection is managed by removal of larvae under local anaesthetic, using forceps and slit lamp examination. With internal infection, dead larvae (without associated inflammation) may be left *in situ*. Inflammation requires topical corticosteroids and mydriatics. Surgical intervention is indicated for live larvae or involvement of critical structures.

Arachnida

Mites

Aetiology

Mites belong to the class *Arachnida*. They occur worldwide and may be free-living or parasitize plants, insects, animals, and humans. The mites that infect humans include:

- chiggers (harvest mite, red bug, trombiculid mite);
- animal mites, e.g. *S. scabiei* var. *canis, Cheyletiella* spp., *Liponyssoides sanguineus, Ornithonyssus bacoti*;
- bird mites, e.g. *Dermanyssus gallinae*;
- food, grain, and straw mites;
- follicle mites, e.g. *Demodex folliculorum, Demodex brevis*;
- house dust mites, e.g. *Dermatophagoides pteronyssinus, Dermatophagoides farinae*;
- scabies (➔ see Scabies, pp. 573–4).

Clinical features

Mites may cause cutaneous disease in humans or act as vectors for infectious diseases, e.g. rickettsial diseases (➔ see Rickettsial diseases, pp. 344–6), Q fever (➔ see *Coxiella burnetii*—ACDP 3, pp. 346–8), tularaemia (➔ see *Francisella*, pp. 317–8), and plague (➔ see *Yersinia pestis*, pp. 314–5).

Management

Treatment of mite bites is symptomatic, with oral antihistamines or topical corticosteroids. Most lesions resolve within a week. Secondary bacterial infection should be treated with an antistaphylococcal antibiotic.

Ticks

Ticks are bloodsucking arthropods of the class *Arachnida*. There are three classes: *Ixodidae* (hard ticks), *Argasidae* (soft ticks), and *Nuttalliellidae* (with characteristics of both).

Epidemiology

Ticks occur worldwide and are important vectors of infectious diseases, e.g. Lyme disease (➔ see Lyme disease, pp. 338–40), babesiosis (➔ see Babesia, pp. 515–6), erlichiosis, rickettsial diseases (➔ see Rickettsial diseases, pp. 344–6), Q fever (➔ see *Coxiella burnetii*—ACDP 3, pp. 346–8), tularaemia (➔ see *Francisella*, pp. 317–8), and relapsing fever (➔ see *Borrelia* species, pp. 337–8).

Clinical features and management

- Tick bites—most bites are asymptomatic. Attached ticks should be removed with forceps to prevent disease transmission. After removal, a pruritic, erythematous papule or plaque may persist for 1–2 weeks. Sometimes a tick bite granuloma may develop.
- Tick paralysis is a rare complication of prolonged attachment of certain tick species. Clinical features are of an ascending paralysis caused by a neurotoxin in the tick salivary gland. Symptoms usually resolve with removal of the tick. A hyperimmune globulin against *Ixodes holocyclus* is effective against tick paralysis caused by this species.

Part 4

Clinical syndromes

13 Fever 579

14 Respiratory, head, and neck infections 589

15 Cardiovascular infections 629

16 Gastrointestinal infections 643

17 Urinary tract infections 677

18 Sexually transmitted infections 693

19 Neurological infections 717

20 Ophthalmological infections 745

21 Skin and soft tissue infections 757

22 Bone and joint infections 773

23 Pregnancy and childhood 785

24 Immunodeficiency and HIV 809

25 Health protection 843

Chapter 13

Fever

Fever: introduction *580*
Sepsis *580*
Pyrexia of unknown origin *582*
Imported fever *584*
Eosinophilia in travellers *586*

Fever: introduction

Fever has been recognized as a clinical syndrome since the sixth century BC. Several centuries later, Hippocratic physicians proposed that body temperature was a balance between the four corporal humours—blood, phlegm, black bile, and yellow bile. Devices to measure body temperature have been around since the first century BC. Thermometry became a part of clinical practice in 1868, when Wunderlich declared 37.4°C (98.6°F) to be the normal body temperature and described the diurnal variation of body temperature.

Definitions

The definitions of sepsis are constantly evolving. 'Sepsis-3'[1], published in February 2016, moved away from the use of SIRS in the identification of sepsis focussing instead on life-threatening organ dysfunction.

- *Fever*—defined as 'a state of elevated core temperature which is often, but not necessarily, part of the defensive responses of a multicellular organism (the host) to the invasion of live (microorganisms) or inanimate matter recognized as pathogenic or alien to the host'.
- *Infection*—the presence of organisms in a normally sterile site, usually accompanied by a host inflammatory response.
- *Bacteraemia*—the presence of bacteria in the blood; may be transient.
- *Systemic inflammatory response syndrome (SIRS)*—response to a wide variety of clinical insults which include infectious and non-infectious causes.
- *Sepsis*—a clinical syndrome defined as life-threatening organ dysfunction caused by a dysregulated immune response to infection.
- *Septic shock*—that subset of sepsis in which underlying circulatory and cellular/metabolic abnormalities are profound enough to increase mortality.

Sepsis

Sepsis is a clinical syndrome characterized by systemic inflammation caused by infection. There is a continuum of severity, ranging from sepsis to septic shock. In the USA, over 1.6 million cases of sepsis occur every year, with a mortality rate of 20–50%. Mortality of septic shock is 40–50%.

Clinical features

'Sepsis-3' proposes using the Sequential (sepsis-related) Organ Failure Assessment (SOFA) score to assess organ dysfunction in the presence of infection. Full details are available at the reference below. These changes will take time to become fully operationalized in health-care institutions. At present most hospitals will use these clinical definitions:

- *Sepsis* is defined as the presence of infection with systemic manifestations, including: (i) physiological variables, e.g. temperature >38.3°C or <36°C, pulse >90 beats/min, systolic blood pressure <90mmHg, respiratory rate >20/min, altered mental state, significant oedema or positive fluid balance, hyperglycaemia; (ii) inflammatory variables, e.g. leucocytosis >12 000 cells/microlitre, leucopenia <4000 cells/microlitre, C-reactive protein (CRP) >2 standard deviations above normal, plasma procalcitonin > 2 standard deviations above normal value; (iii) organ dysfunction, e.g. arterial hypoxaemia, acute oliguria, creatinine increase >44.2 micromoles/L, coagulation abnormalities, ileus, thrombocytopenia, hyperbilirubinaemia; (iv) tissue perfusion variables, e.g. decreased capillary refill, hyperlactataemia.

- *Severe sepsis* refers to sepsis-induced tissue hypoperfusion or organ dysfunction with any of the following thought to be due to the infection: (i) sepsis-induced hypotension; (ii) lactate above ULN; (iii) urine output <0.5mL/kg/h for 2h, despite adequate fluid resuscitation; (iv) acute lung injury with PaO_2/FiO_2 ratio <250 in the absence of pneumonia as infection source; (v) acute lung injury with PaO_2/FiO_2 ratio <200 in the presence of pneumonia as infection source; (vi) serum creatinine >176.8 micromoles/L; (vii) serum bilirubin >34.2 micromoles/L; (viii) platelet count <100 000/microlitre; (ix) coagulopathy INR >1.5.

Laboratory diagnosis

- Routine investigations may show a number of abnormalities, as described in ➔ Clinical features above.
- BCs and samples from suspected sites of infection (e.g. sputum, urine, stool, pus) should be taken for culture, ideally prior to administration of antimicrobial therapy.

Management

(See reference 2.)

- *Therapeutic priorities*—these include early initiation of supportive care to correct physiological abnormalities and institution of appropriate therapy for sepsis.
- *Stabilize respiration*—supplemental oxygen should be given to all patients with sepsis, and oxygen saturations monitored. Intubation and mechanical ventilation may be required. A CXR and arterial blood gas (ABG) should be obtained.
- *Assess perfusion*—blood pressure should be assessed early and often. An arterial line may be required in patients who are shut down or have labile blood pressures.
- *Establish central venous access*—a CVC is inserted in most patients with severe sepsis, in order to infuse fluids and medications and to collect blood samples.
- *Initial resuscitation*—goals during the first 6h, as suggested by the Surviving Sepsis Campaign Guidelines, include: (i) central venous pressure 8–12mmHg; (ii) central venous (superior vena cava) or mixed venous oxygen saturation 70% or 65%, respectively; (iii) mean arterial pressure ≥65mmHg; (iv) urine output ≥0.5mL/kg/h.
- *Restoration of perfusion*—rapid infusion of large volumes of IV fluid are administered, often in 500mL boluses. Careful monitoring is required, as patients may develop non-cardiogenic pulmonary oedema.

Vasopressors, e.g. noradrenaline, may be required in patients who remain hypotensive, despite adequate fluid resuscitation. Additional therapies, such as inotropic therapy (e.g. dobutamine) or red cell transfusions, are sometimes given.

- *Identification of septic focus*—prompt identification and treatment of the focus of infection are essential. Biomarkers of sepsis, e.g. procalcitonin, TREM-1 (triggering receptor expressed on myeloid cells-1), and CD64 expression on neutrophils, may be useful to suggest bacterial infection.
- *Antimicrobial therapy*—this should be instigated promptly; the empirical regimen will depend on the likely source of infection, local antibiotic policies, and antibiotic resistance profiles. Poor outcome is associated with delayed or inappropriate therapy.
- *Additional therapies*—glucocorticoid therapy may be of benefit in patients with severe septic shock. Nutritional support improves nutritional outcomes in critically ill patients, but its impact on clinical outcomes from sepsis is uncertain. Intensive insulin therapy is helpful in diabetic patients with hyperglycaemia and insulin resistance. One study has suggested that external cooling may be helpful in patients with severe sepsis. Sepsis treatment protocols also appear to improve outcome.

Reference

1 Singer M, *et al.*; The Third International Consensus Definitions for Sepsis and Septic shock (Sepsis-3). *JAMA* 2016; **315**(8): 801–10.

2 Dellinger RP, Levy MM, Rhodes A, *et al.*; the Surviving Sepsis Campaign Guidelines Committee including the Pediatric Subgroup (2013). *Surviving Sepsis Campaign. International guidelines for management of severe sepsis and septic shock: 2012*. Available at: http://www.survivingsepsis.org/Guidelines/Pages/default.aspx.

Pyrexia of unknown origin

Definition

The first definition of pyrexia of unknown origin (PUO) was proposed by Petersdorf and Beeson in 1961: 'fever of >38.3°C (101°F) on several occasions persisting without diagnosis for at least 3 weeks despite at least 1 week's investigation in hospital'.

Since then, the definition has been modified to reflect changes in medical practice, and there are now four different subtypes:

- classic PUO (>38°C for >3 weeks, >2 visits, or 3 days in hospital);
- nosocomial PUO (>38°C for 3 days, not present or incubating on admission);
- immune-deficient PUO (>38°C for >3 days, negative cultures after 48h);
- HIV-related PUO (>38°C for >3 weeks for outpatients or >3 days for inpatients).

Causes of pyrexia of unknown origin

(See reference 3.)

- *Classic PUO*—although a wide variety of conditions can cause classic PUO, most fall into five categories:
  - infections (27–50%), e.g. abscesses, endocarditis, TB, complicated UTIs. Some causes show distinct geographical variation, e.g. visceral leishmaniasis (Spain), melioidosis (South East Asia);
  - neoplasms (13–25%), e.g. lymphoma;
  - connective tissue disorders (9–17%), e.g. Still's disease, SLE, rheumatoid arthritis, temporal arteritis, polymyalgia rheumatica;
  - miscellaneous disorders (15–21%);
  - undiagnosed conditions (5–23%).

The relative frequency of disorders within these five categories varies according to the era in which the study was conducted, geographical region, age of the patient, and type of hospital.

- *Nosocomial PUO* presents as fever after hospitalization for at least 24h. Risk factors include intravascular devices, urinary or respiratory tract instrumentation, surgical procedures, immobility, and drug therapy. However, knowledge is limited due to lack of published data.
- *Immune-deficient PUO* occurs in patients receiving cytotoxic therapy or with haematological malignancies. Because of impaired immune function, signs of inflammation may be modest, leading to atypical presentations. During episodes of neutropenia, infections caused by pyogenic bacteria are commonest. In patients with impaired CMI, viral infections are commoner.
- *HIV-related PUO* may occur with primary infection or in advanced disease where it is due to opportunistic infections (e.g. mycobacteria, visceral leishmaniasis, *P. jirovecii*, bacterial infections, CMV, toxoplasmosis, cryptococcosis) or malignancies.

Evaluation of pyrexia of unknown origin

- *History and examination*—a comprehensive history should include details of recent travel, contact with persons who have a similar illness, exposure to animals, work environment, past medical history, drug history, and family history for hereditary causes of fever. A careful physical examination may reveal clues as to the aetiology, e.g. stigmata of endocarditis. The presence of fever should be verified, although fever patterns are neither sensitive nor specific enough to be diagnostically reliable.
- *Laboratory investigations* include simple blood tests (e.g. FBC, CRP, ESR, biochemical profile including LFTs, CPK) and urinalysis. BCs (at least three sets drawn from different sites at different times) should be taken prior to initiation of antimicrobial therapy. Serology may be helpful for viral infections (e.g. hepatitis A, B, and C, EBV, CMV, and HIV) and autoimmune disorders (e.g. ANA, antineutrophil cytoplasmic antibody (ANCA), and rheumatoid factor). Serum protein electrophoresis may be helpful.
- *Imaging studies*—all patients should have a chest radiograph. Further radiological imaging should be guided by the clinical presentation, e.g. abdominal ultrasound, CT chest/abdomen, fluorodeoxyglucose

positron emission tomography (FDG-PET) scans. Venous duplex scans of the lower extremities may reveal deep vein thromboses.

- *Invasive procedures*—directed diagnostic biopsies may be helpful, e.g. liver, lymph node, temporal artery, pleural, pericardial, or bone marrow biopsies.
- *Therapeutic trials*—these may confound or delay the diagnosis of PUO. Thus, therapeutic trials should be reserved for those few patients in whom all other approaches have failed or for the occasional patient who is too ill for therapy to be withheld.

Management

A fundamental principle of management of classic PUO is that therapy should be delayed, until the cause has been identified, so that it can be targeted appropriately. However, this ideal is frequently ignored in clinical practice and may confound or delay the diagnosis of PUO. In contrast, for neutropenic sepsis, which carries a high risk of serious bacterial infections, empiric broad-spectrum antibiotic therapy should be started immediately after appropriate cultures are taken.

Prognosis

Nine to 51% of cases of PUO defy diagnosis. Prognosis depends on the cause of the fever and the underlying disease. Elderly patients and those with malignant disease have the poorest prognosis. Diagnostic delay adversely affects outcome in intra-abdominal infections, disseminated TB and fungal infections, and recurrent PEs. Patients who have undiagnosed PUO after extensive evaluation generally have a favourable outcome (5-year mortality rate of 3.2%).

Reference

3 Durack DT. Fever of unknown origin. In: Mackowiak PA (ed). *Fever. Basic mechanisms and management*, second edition. Philadelphia: Lippincott-Raven, 1997: pp. 237–49.

Imported fever

Fever in returning travellers is estimated to affect 22–64% of the 50 million people who travel from industrialized countries to the developing world each year. Although most illnesses are mild, up to 8% of people are ill enough to seek medical attention; 0.1% require medical evacuation, and 1 in 100 000 dies. An increased risk of travel-associated infections is seen in people who visit family and friends abroad and in adventure travellers.

Clinical features

A 2006 report from 30 GeoSentinel sites in developed countries provided clinical-based surveillance information on 17 353 ill travellers who returned from travel in developing countries and were seen between June 1996 and August 2004.[4] The primary manifestations for approximately two-thirds of the returned travellers fell into five major syndrome categories: systemic febrile illness without localizing findings, acute diarrhoea, dermatological disorders, chronic diarrhoea, and non-diarrhoeal GI disorders.

Patients may present with a wide spectrum of disease,[5] ranging from asymptomatic carriage to fulminant disease (see Table 13.1).

Table 13.1 Causes of imported fever

Incubation	Syndrome	Causes
<14 days	Undifferentiated fever	Malaria, dengue, rickettsial spotted fevers, scrub typhus, leptospirosis, bacterial gastroenteritis, typhoid, acute HIV
	Fever with respiratory symptoms	Influenza, legionellosis, Q fever, acute histoplasmosis, acute coccidioidomycosis
	Fever with CNS symptoms	Bacterial meningitis, viral meningitis, encephalitis, cerebral malaria, typhoid, typhus, rabies, arboviral encephalitis, *A. cantonensis* eosinophilic meningitis, polio, East African trypanosomiasis
	Fever with haemorrhage	Meningococcaemia, leptospirosis, *Streptococcus suis*, malaria, VHFs
14 days to 6 weeks		Malaria, typhoid, hepatitis A, hepatitis E, acute schistosomiasis, amoebic liver abscess, leptospirosis, acute HIV infection, East African trypanosomiasis, VHFs, Q fever, brucellosis, ascariasis, Chagas' disease
>6 weeks		Malaria, TB, hepatitis B, hepatitis E, visceral leishmaniasis, lymphatic filariasis, schistosomiasis, amoebic liver abscess, chronic mycosis, rabies, African trypanosomiasis, HIV, brucellosis

History and examination

The following are essential in the assessment of a returning traveller:

- geography—countries visited or passed through, urban or rural, dates of travel and duration of stay in each place, means of transportation, accommodation;
- activities and exposures—sexual or other intimate contact, animal contact, insect bites, exposure to blood or needles, food and beverages, soil and water contact;
- host factors—age, gender, past medical history, past surgery, past infections and vaccines, current medications including immunosuppressive/immunomodulatory drugs, pre-travel immunizations, antimalarial chemoprophylaxis;
- symptoms—nature and duration of symptoms;
- physical findings—fever, rash, lymphadenopathy, splenomegaly, genital lesions, retinal or conjunctival haemorrhages, neurological signs. Findings that require urgent intervention are confusion, lethargy, meningism, hypotension, respiratory distress, and haemorrhagic manifestations.

Laboratory investigations

- FBC, WCC, and differential, thick and thin films for malaria.
- Urea, creatinine, electrolytes, LFTs, CRP.
- Urinalysis, microscopy and culture.
- Stool for microscopy (ova, cyst, parasites) and culture.

- Skin scrapings or biopsy of lesions.
- Sputum microscopy and culture.
- BCs.
- Serology.
- Imaging, e.g. CXR, abdominal ultrasound.
- Bone marrow examination may be helpful in certain conditions.

Treatment

- Supportive treatment (mild infections or those with no treatment).
- Specific treatment according to the causative organism.

Prevention

- Pre-travel vaccination and antimalarial prophylaxis, if indicated.
- Advice regarding risk avoidance, e.g. water purification, avoiding uncooked food, barrier contraception.

References

4 Freedman DO, Weld LH, Kozarsky PE, *et al.*; GeoSentinel Surveillance Network. Spectrum of disease and relation to place of exposure among ill returned travelers. *N Engl J Med*. 2006;**354**:119–30.

5 Ryan ET, Wilson ME, Kain KC. Illness after international travel. *N Engl J Med*. 2002;**347**:505–16.

Eosinophilia in travellers

Eosinophilia in returning travellers and migrants is common. Helminth infection accounts for most in which a cause is identified, and many patients experience little in the way of significant symptoms. However, some helminths have the potential for causing significant health problems. The pattern of disease tends to differ between migrants from, and travellers making short trips to, the regions in which infection is acquired. The former are more likely to experience a larger burden of infection or present with the complications of chronic infection (e.g. bladder cancer or portal hypertension due to chronic schistosomiasis); the latter are more likely to present with features of acute infection (e.g. Löeffler's syndrome) and higher eosinophil counts.

General points when assessing a patient

- History—a detailed travel history is important. Some organisms can be acquired worldwide (e.g. *Strongyloides*), others in specific regions (e.g. *T. solium*), and still others are more geographically restricted (e.g. schistosomiasis). Establish dates of symptom onset, timings of water exposure, foods eaten, specific regions visited within a country, and any activities undertaken.
- The asymptomatic patient with eosinophilia—it is worthwhile performing stool microscopy and *Strongyloides* serology on such patients. Other screening tests may be appropriate, depending on the region visited (e.g. terminal urine microscopy and filarial serology in those returning from Africa). Some authorities recommend empirical albendazole as treatment for undiagnosed ascariasis/hookworm infection in patients with a suitable travel history and transient eosinophilia. Those with the necessary expertise should make such decisions.

- Timing of investigations—eosinophilia can occur briefly in association with the tissue migration phase of infection, and eggs/larvae may not yet be detectable. Stool microscopy then becomes positive after eosinophilia resolves. Serological tests are likely to become positive only 4–12 weeks after infection, and many of these tests cross-react between helminth species.
- Those with sustained eosinophilia in whom no diagnosis is reached or with symptoms that are not in keeping with a parasitic infection should be investigated for other infectious causes (e.g. fungi, HIV) and non-infectious causes such as allergy, malignancy (especially leukaemia and lymphoma), and connective tissue disease.

Eosinophilia with specific symptoms

- Fever with or without respiratory symptoms—Katayama fever (➔ see *Schistosoma* species, pp. 563–4), Löeffler's syndrome (➔ see *Strongyloides stercoralis*, pp. 546–7), acute toxocariasis (➔ see Toxocariasis, pp. 550–1), tropical pulmonary eosinophilia due to filarial infection (➔ see Filariasis, pp. 554–5), pulmonary hydatid disease (➔ see Echinococcosis, p. 562), paragonimiasis (➔ see Paragonimiasis, pp. 566–8). Also consider endemic fungi (e.g. coccidiomycosis; ➔ see *Coccidioides immitis*—ACDP 3, pp. 505–8) and non-infectious causes (drugs, connective tissue diseases).
- GI symptoms—*Strongyloides* (➔ see *Strongyloides stercoralis*, pp. 546–7), schistosomiasis (➔ see Trematodes (flukes), pp. 563–8), ascariasis (➔ see *Ascaris lumbricoides*, p. 543), tapeworm (➔ see Cestodes, pp. 559–62), hookworm (➔ see *Ancylostoma duodenale* and *Necator americanus*, pp. 545–6), whipworm (➔ see *Trichuris trichiura*, p. 544), *Enterobius vermicularis* (➔ see heading title, p. 548), trichinellosis (➔ see *Trichinella* species, pp. 552–3).
- Right upper quadrant pain, with or without jaundice—hydatid disease of the liver (➔ see Echinococcosis, p. 562), fasciola hepatica (➔ see Fascioliasis, pp. 565–6), schistosomiasis (➔ see Trematodes (flukes), pp. 563–4).
- Neurological symptoms—ask the laboratory to specifically examine the CSF for eosinophils. Causes include gnathostomiasis, neurocysticercosis meningitis (➔ see Cysticercosis, pp. 561–2), neurological schistosomiasis (➔ see *Schistosoma* species, pp. 563–4), toxocariasis (➔ see Toxocariasis, pp. 550–1), and endemic fungi (➔ see *Histoplasma capsulatum*, pp. 498–503). Also consider non-infectious causes such as lymphoma and vasculitis.
- Rash, itch, urticaria—onchocerciasis (➔ see *Onchocerca volvulus*, pp. 557–8), larva currens due to *Strongyloides* (➔ see *Strongyloides stercoralis*, pp. 546–7), lymphatic filariasis (➔ see Filariasis, pp. 554–5), loiasis (calabar swellings; ➔ see *Loa loa*, pp. 556–7), gnathostomiasis, trichinellosis (➔ see *Trichinella* species, pp. 552–3), swimmer's itch due to exposure to avian schistosomiasis.
- Urinary symptoms—schistosomiasis.

Further reading

Checkley AM, Chiodini PL, Dockrell DH, *et al.*; British Infection Society and Hospital for Tropical Diseases. Eosinophilia in returning travellers and migrants from the tropics: UK recommendations for investigation and initial management. *J Infect.* 2010;**60**:1–20.

Chapter 14

Respiratory, head, and neck infections

Common cold 590
Pharyngitis 591
Retropharyngeal abscess 593
Quinsy (peritonsillar abscess) 594
Lemierre's syndrome 595
Croup 596
Epiglottitis 597
Bacterial tracheitis 598
Laryngitis 598
Sinusitis 599
Mastoiditis 601
Otitis externa 602
Otitis media 603
Dental infections 605
Lateral pharyngeal abscess 606
Acute bronchitis 606
Chronic bronchitis 607
Bronchiolitis 609
Community-acquired pneumonia 611
Atypical pneumonias 615
Aspiration pneumonia 617
Hospital-acquired pneumonia 617
Ventilator-associated pneumonia 618
Pulmonary infiltrates with eosinophilia 619
Empyema 619
Lung abscess 621
Cystic fibrosis 623
Bronchiectasis 625
Pulmonary tuberculosis 627

Common cold

The term applied to the acute minor coryzal illness caused by viruses belonging to a number of different families.

Aetiology

- Over 200 subtypes of virus have been associated with the common cold.
- Rhinoviruses (of which there are >100 subtypes) account for 30–50% of cases.
- Other causes include coronaviruses (10–15%), influenza, parainfluenza, RSV, adenoviruses, enteroviruses, bocaviruses, and human metapneumovirus.
- Twenty-five per cent of cases are attributed to agents as yet unidentified.
- Re-exposure may result in reinfection, but symptoms tend to be milder.

Epidemiology

- Rhinoviruses and parainfluenza viruses tend to occur in autumn and late spring. RSV and coronaviruses tend to cause epidemics in winter and spring. Enteroviruses tend to cause illness in summer. Adenoviruses are usually not seasonal but cause outbreaks in institutions.
- In developed countries, adults experience on average 2–3, and preschool children 5–7, colds a year. Smokers tend to experience more significant symptoms.
- The prime reservoir for cold viruses is the upper airway of young children, and spread occurs in schools and the home. Mothers have higher secondary attack rates than fathers.
- Spread is by hand contact (either directly or via fomites) or by droplet transmission.

Pathogenesis

- The pathological mechanisms of different viruses differ. All invade the mucosa of the upper respiratory tract, and sloughed nasal columnar epithelial cells may be identified in the nasal secretions.
- Chemical mediators (cytokines, histamine, prostaglandin) and activation of parasympathetic nervous pathways cause inflammation and engorging of blood vessels of the nasal turbinates, with congestion and discharge.
- Peak of rhinovirus cold symptoms coincides with maximal viral shedding.
- Cold viruses may affect the bacterial flora of the respiratory tract and facilitate secondary bacterial infections.

Clinical features

- Incubation 12 h to 3 days. Symptoms: nasal discharge, congestion, sneezing, cough, sore throat. Fever is mild and commoner in children.
- Symptoms reach peak severity by day 3. Most resolve by 1 week; some last up to 2 weeks. Conjunctivitis may be seen in adenovirus and enterovirus infection.
- Complications include acute rhinosinusitis, LRTIs, acute otitis media.

Diagnosis

- Identification of the causative agent is unhelpful in uncomplicated cold.
- Important to recognize secondary bacterial sinusitis (0.5–2% of cases) and otitis media (2% of cases). Marked pharyngeal inflammation or exudates raise the possibility of streptococcal, adenovirus, HSV, or EBV infection.
- Rapid antigen detection tests for GAS may be useful in those with prominent pharyngeal symptoms.

Treatment

- Patients should be encouraged to wash their hands and take measures to avoid contamination of others at the peak of symptoms.
- Sedating antihistamines provide relief from sneezing, discharge, and cough.
- NSAIDs, such as naproxen, reduce cough.
- Decongestants may be given topically or orally. Rebound nasal congestion may follow withdrawal of topical agents after prolonged use.
- Topical anaesthetic-containing lozenges may relieve sore throat.
- Large doses of vitamin C may have a modest therapeutic effect but have no demonstrable preventative effect in controlled trials.
- There is no role for antibiotics in uncomplicated cold.

Pharyngitis

Pharyngitis is an infection/irritation of the pharynx and/or tonsils.

Aetiology

- Forty to 60% viral. The commonest causes are influenza, parainfluenza, coronavirus, rhinovirus, adenovirus, enterovirus, RSV, metapneumovirus, HSV, EBV, CMV, and HIV.
- Five to 40% bacterial—GAS commonest.
- Other causes—allergy, trauma, toxins, malignancy.
- It is important to distinguish pharyngitis from more serious conditions such as epiglottitis and para-/retropharyngeal abscess.

Pathogenesis

- Bacteria or viruses invade the pharyngeal mucosa, causing a local inflammatory response. Certain viruses (rhinovirus) promote nasal secretions which cause secondary pharyngeal irritation.
- Streptococcal protein/toxins facilitate local invasion and may lead to complications such as rheumatic fever and post-streptococcal glomerulonephritis.

Epidemiology

- Commonest in children. Cases of both viral and bacterial aetiology peak amongst school-aged children (4–7 years).
- GAS account for 30% of childhood pharyngitis and 15% of adult cases. *M. pneumoniae* and *Chlamydophila pneumoniae* are common causes amongst teenagers and young adults.
- Consider gonococcal pharyngitis if there is a history of orogenital contact.

Clinical features

- Viral and bacterial causes are not easily distinguished clinically.
- General features—fever, malaise, sore throat, myalgia. On examination, erythema and oedema of the tonsils and pharyngeal mucosa.
- Purulent tonsillar exudate suggests streptococcal infection or EBV.
- Conjunctivitis suggests adenovirus.
- Vesicles suggest HSV or Coxsackie A infection.
- Chest signs may indicate LRTIs by *M. pneumoniae* or *C. pneumoniae*. Hepatosplenomegaly may be seen in EBV infection.
- GAS infection—5–15% of cases. Occur in winter to early spring. Consider if: abrupt onset, recent contact with others diagnosed with GAS, headache, vomiting, no cough, swollen and tender cervical lymphadenopathy, high WCC. *Complications: rheumatic fever (1 in 400 untreated GAS infections), glomerulonephritis, abscess, TSS, airway obstruction.* Pharyngitis caused by group C, G, and F streptococci resemble GAS, but without the immunological sequelae.
- Other bacteria—*Arcanobacterium haemolyticus* (5%—common in young adults, causing outbreaks of a scarlet fever-like rash), *M. pneumoniae* (young adults with headache, pharyngitis, chest symptoms, cough), *C. pneumoniae* (similar to *M. pneumoniae*—pharyngitis may precede pulmonary infection), *N. gonorrhoeae* (rare—usually follows orogenital contact), *C. diphtheriae* (rare in the developed world—risk of airway obstruction), *Borrelia* spp.
- *Candida* spp. (particularly in immunocompromised), irritation (dry air, post-nasal drip, allergy, oesophageal reflux, smoking).
- Differential diagnosis—diphtheria, mycoplasmal pneumonia, parapharyngeal abscess, malignancy.

Investigations

- Throat swab—antigen tests and culture are highly sensitive and widely used in the USA. High rates of asymptomatic carriage. Antigen tests do not detect group C or G streptococci or other bacterial pathogens. Culture for *N. gonorrhoeae*, if indicated.
- Consider specific tests for other causes—EBV, *C. pneumoniae, M. pneumoniae*.
- Serology—a rise in ASOT confirms GAS infection retrospectively. Viral serology may be useful in retrospect.

Management

- General—assess airway, sepsis, hydration; exclude abscess.
- Most cases are viral, do not need antibiotic treatment, and resolve spontaneously within 10 days. Early treatment of GAS infection reduces the incidence of immunological sequelae. Antibiotic therapy may prevent suppurative complications.
- Although their value might be questioned, most people would treat suspected GAS infection and all patients who appear unwell, e.g. phenoxymethylpenicillin for 10 days. Avoid ampicillin or amoxicillin in those in whom EBV infection has not been excluded. Rates of recurrence are higher in those who do not complete the 10-day course.
- Recurrent tonsillitis—treat with β-lactamase-stable agents such as clindamycin. Consider ENT referral—tonsillectomy may be appropriate.

Complications

LRTI, suppurative complications (abscess, sinusitis, otitis media, epiglottitis, mastoiditis), non-suppurative sequelae of GAS infection. Scarlet fever (➲ see Bacterial causes of childhood illness, pp. 804–8) may be seen in association with a streptococcal infection at any site.

Retropharyngeal abscess

Infection causing abscess in one of the deep spaces of the neck. Potentially life-threatening due to risk of airway compromise, but rare in developed countries where antibiotic usage in the treatment of URTI is widespread. Commonest in 2–4 year olds but can affect any age. Other pharyngeal abscesses (lateral pharyngeal, peritonsillar) are commoner in older children/adults.

Pathogenesis

- The retropharyngeal space is located posterior to the pharynx, anterior to the cervical vertebrae, and extends from the base of the skull to the level of the tracheal bifurcation.
- It may become infected by contiguous spread (e.g. an URTI that has spread to the retropharyngeal lymph nodes) or through direct inoculation by penetrating trauma or instrumentation (feeding tube insertion, endoscopy, intubation, head and neck surgery, fish bone).

Clinical features

- Patients may have experienced previous URTI (perhaps weeks previously) and may not recall specific trauma (e.g. running and falling with a lollipop in the mouth).
- Symptoms—fever, chills, malaise, voice change (classically a duck quack—'*cri du canard*'), sore throat, dysphagia, neck stiffness, sensation of a lump in the throat, pain in back and shoulders on swallowing. Difficulty breathing is a serious sign that may herald airway obstruction.
- On examination—fever, sepsis, unilateral lymphadenopathy, neck mass, mass in posterior pharyngeal wall on oral examination (30% of cases), signs of vascular complications (jugular vein thrombophlebitis, carotid rupture—bleeding from the ear, nose, or mouth and ecchymosis in the neck).
- Consider the diagnosis in those with fever, neck stiffness, and normal LP.
- Complications—mass effect (e.g. expansion against the trachea causing airway compression), abscess rupture (pus aspiration may lead to pneumonia), spread of infection (inflammation and destruction of adjacent tissues—mediastinitis, pericarditis, empyema, jugular vein thrombosis, carotid artery rupture, osteomyelitis of the cervical vertebrae leading to subluxation and spinal cord damage). The infection itself may rarely develop into necrotizing fasciitis and sepsis.

Diagnosis

- Laboratory tests—FBC (raised WCC), throat swab, and BCs.
- Radiology—lateral soft tissue X-ray of the neck (inspiration with the neck in normal extension) may show widening of the prevertebral

tissue and gas. Contrast CT is more useful. MRI produces more detailed images, but these are usually unnecessary, and children often require sedation.
- Microbiology—usually polymicrobial members of the oropharyngeal flora: Gram-positive bacteria (GAS, *S. aureus*) and anaerobes (*Fusobacteria, Prevotella, Veillonella* spp.) predominate. *Haemophilus* spp, occasionally found.
- Consider TB and coccidiosis in patients with risk factors who fail to respond to standard antibiotic therapy.
- Differential diagnosis—other infections (e.g epiglottitis, peritonsillar abscess, croup, tracheitis, diphtheria), trauma, foreign body, angio-oedema, anaphylaxis, cystic hygroma, tumour.

Management

- Supportive care—secure airway, maintain hydration, adequate analgesia.
- Urgent ENT referral for incision and drainage; 30% require a surgical airway.
- Antibiotic therapy—IV benzylpenicillin and clindamycin, or cephalosporin and metronidazole empirically. Antibiotics may be tailored to the causative organism once identified. Oral step-down therapy is usually with co-amoxiclav or clindamycin.

Complications

- Airway obstruction.
- Septicaemia.
- Aspiration pneumonia if the abscess ruptures into the airway.
- Internal jugular vein thrombosis.
- Jugular vein suppurative thrombophlebitis (Lemierre's syndrome).
- Carotid artery rupture.
- Mediastinitis.
- Atlantoaxial dislocation.

Quinsy (peritonsillar abscess)

- Relatively common infection of the peritonsillar space (between the capsule of the palatine tonsil and the pharyngeal muscles), which usually follows bacterial pharyngitis but may arise *de novo*.
- One-third of cases occur in children. Peak incidence age 20–30 years.
- Usually polymicrobial—predominant organisms are GAS, *S. aureus*, and respiratory anaerobes (*Fusobacterium, Prevotella*, and *Veillonella* spp.). Can sometimes be caused by *Haemophilus* spp.
- Symptoms—sore throat, fever, muffled voice, drooling, and dysphagia.
- Examination—asymmetrical tonsillar enlargement and neck swelling, maybe a palpable fluctuant mass, and bad breath. Cervical lymphadenopathy may be present. Trismus may render examination impossible. USS or CT may be useful in such patients.

- Diagnosis—laboratory tests include FBC, biochemistry, and a throat swab. Imaging is not usually necessary. A lateral neck X-ray may be taken to exclude epiglottitis and retropharyngeal abscess. A CT scan is the imaging modality of choice and distinguishes quinsy from peritonsillar cellulitis.
- Differential diagnosis—severe tonsillopharyngitis, epiglottitis, retropharyngeal or parapharyngeal abscess.
- Management—ENT referral for consideration of surgical drainage and IV benzylpenicillin or co-amoxiclav. Perimucosal needle aspiration may be appropriate in patients who can tolerate it, with no evidence of deep neck tissue extension, sepsis, or toxicity. Material can also be obtained for culture. Complication: airway obstruction.
- Complications—airway obstruction, aspiration pneumonia, septicaemia, internal jugular vein thrombosis, Lemierre's syndrome, carotid artery rupture, pseudoaneurysm of the carotid artery, mediastinitis, necrotizing fasciitis, sequelae of GAS infection.
- Prognosis—treatment success is 90–95% for appropriately treated uncomplicated abscesses, with a 10–15% recurrence rate (the majority very shortly after the initial episode, suggesting ongoing infection). Such patients may benefit from interval tonsillectomy.

Lemierre's syndrome

- Definition—an infection of the posterior compartment of the lateral pharyngeal space, complicated by jugular vein suppurative thrombophlebitis.
- Epidemiology—usually occurs in young, healthy adults; mean age 20 years. Often preceded by pharyngitis.
- Microbiology—usually caused by *Fusobacterium necrophorum*. Other pathogens include other *Fusobacterium* spp. (e.g. *F. nucleatum*), *E. corrodens*, *Porphyromonas asaccharolytica*, streptococci including GAS, and *Bacteroides* spp.
- Clinical features—presents with fever, rigors, respiratory distress, and neck/throat pain. Examination of the oropharynx may reveal erythema, ulceration, or a pseudomembrane. There may be tenderness, swelling, or induration over the internal jugular vein or along the sternocleidomastoid muscle. Septic emboli to the lungs are common, resulting in lung abscesses and empyema. Metastatic infection may occur.
- Diagnosis—USS, CT, and MRI confirm the diagnosis. The organism may be grown from blood or pus.
- Treatment—prolonged antibiotic therapy with a β-lactam/β-lactamase inhibitor combination (e.g. piperacillin–tazobactam or co-amoxiclav). Surgery may be required for ongoing sepsis which fails to respond to antimicrobial therapy, e.g. lung abscess, empyema. The role of anticoagulation is controversial.

Croup

Croup is an acute respiratory illness of the larynx and trachea (laryngotracheitis) characterized by cough, hoarseness and stridor. It is usually caused by viruses.

Epidemiology

- A common illness in young children (around 10% of LRTIs). Usually affects children aged 6–36 months, rare after the age of 6.
- Viral causes include parainfluenza viruses, RSV, human coronavirus NL63 (HCoV-NL63), measles (where it is endemic), influenza viruses, rhinovirus, enteroviruses (especially Coxsackie types A9, B4, and B5, and echovirus types 4, 11, and 21), and human metapneumovirus.
- *M. pneumoniae* has been associated with mild cases of croup. Secondary bacterial infections may occur, e.g. *S. aureus*, GAS, *S. pneumoniae*.

Clinical features

- It is vital to distinguish croup from epiglottitis (➔ see Epiglottitis, pp. 597–8).
- Children usually have a short history of URTI with sore throat, mild cough, and fever. The onset of croup often occurs at night with barking, 'seal-like' cough, and hoarseness. Stridor and dyspnoea may develop. The child may sit forward to aid breathing. Auscultation can reveal rhonchi and wheeze in severely affected children. Some develop pneumonia. Respiratory rates of 40/min are not unusual. Symptoms fluctuate, improving or worsening within an hour, tending to be more severe in the evening.
- In severe cases, exhaustion or severe obstruction may necessitate respiratory support or intubation.
- *Indicators of impending respiratory failure*—stridor at rest (may be quiet), sternal wall retractions, lethargy or decreased level of consciousness, paradoxical breathing, quiet breath sounds.
- Some children experience repeated episodes of croup (spasmodic croup), perhaps related to airway hyper-reactivity and allergic disease.

Diagnosis

- Diagnosis is clinical, and croup must be differentiated from other causes of stridor (e.g. foreign body) and bacterial epiglottitis. Epiglottitis has a more rapid course, and children tend to be more toxic with dysphagia and drooling. Croup's distinctive cough is also absent.
- General laboratory features—WCC may be normal or raised; hypoxia is seen in most hospitalized children, and hypercapnia in half.
- Viral identification—immunofluorescence and RT-PCR may allow rapid identification of a causative agent.
- Serology is not useful in the diagnosis of croup.

Management

- Patients unwell enough to require hospitalization require close observation to identify signs of airway obstruction, exhaustion, and respiratory failure requiring intubation and ventilation. Interventions,

such as blood sampling, should be kept to the minimum necessary to avoid exacerbating anxiety and breathlessness.
- Humidified air or humidified oxygen, as indicated for hypoxaemia (oxygen saturations <92%) or respiratory distress.
- Corticosteroid therapy—a single dose of dexamethasone (0.6mg/kg PO, IV, or IM) reduces the proportion of those with mild disease requiring further medical attention. It is beneficial in cases of moderate and severe croup, equal to, or more efficacious than, nebulized steroids. Although it is not routinely indicated in the treatment of croup, a single dose of nebulized budesonide (2mg [2mL solution] via nebulizer) may provide an alternative to IM or IV dexamethasone for children with vomiting or severe respiratory distress.
- Nebulized racemic adrenaline (0.05mL/kg per dose (maximum of 0.5mL) of a 2.25% solution diluted to 3mL total volume with normal saline) is given via a nebulizer over 15min—diminishes subglottic swelling and produces clinical improvement in those children with severe stridor. Fast-acting, but improvement is transitory—around 2h. It does not improve oxygenation but results in less frequent need for intubation due to exhaustion.
- There is no role for antibiotics in the management of croup in the absence of concomitant bacterial infection.

Epiglottitis

A potentially life-threatening condition of inflammation, oedema, and obstruction of the epiglottis and surrounding structures. Classically, a disease of children (aged 3–7 years) traditionally caused by *H. influenzae* type B. Since the introduction of Hib vaccination, it may be caused by a variety of organisms, e.g. *H. influenzae* (types A and F, and non-typeable), streptococci, *S. aureus* including MRSA. In adults, it may be caused by a wide range of bacteria, viruses, and fungi. In immunocompromised patients, *P. aeruginosa* and *Candida* spp. have been reported.

Clinical features

- Abrupt onset of severe sore throat and fever, with stridor, drooling, anxiety, and refusal to eat. Children may adopt the typical posture—sitting up, leaning forward, and looking seriously unwell.
- Attempting to examine the throat (e.g. use of a tongue depressor) may result in total airway obstruction, as may IV cannulation. These should be deferred, until anaesthetic support is present.
- Complications—epiglottic abscess, bacteraemia, pneumonia, meningitis, arthritis, cellulitis.

Management

- Securing the airway is the absolute priority. Once the airway is secured, mortality is <1%. Outcome is significantly better with elective intubation than emergency intubation. Patients should be monitored in an intensive care setting.

- Antibiotics—IV ceftriaxone or cefotaxime usually for 7–10 days. In the USA, anti-MRSA therapy (e.g. vancomycin or clindamycin) is also recommended.
- Glucocorticoids—the role of glucocorticoids in airway management is controversial.
- Prophylaxis—rifampicin should be given to the patient and all household/day-care contacts, including adults, if there are other susceptible (unvaccinated or immunocompromised) children in the family.
- Mortality—around 0% with a quick diagnosis in specialist centres, 9–18% where diagnosis is delayed, 6% where patients are managed without intubation.

Investigations

- All investigations should follow securing the airway.
- WCC and inflammatory markers are raised.
- Cultures—blood and throat swabs.
- Radiology—lateral neck X-ray may show an enlarged epiglottis protruding from the anterior wall of the hypopharynx ('thumb sign').
- Differential—croup, diphtheria, inhaled foreign body.

Bacterial tracheitis

An atypical form of croup, its clinical picture having more in common with epiglottitis. It is uncommon, tending to affect older children. Those with a history of either recent intubation or viral illness are at greater risk. Presentation is with an abrupt onset of fever, stridor, and breathlessness with large amounts of purulent sputum. Progression can be rapid, necessitating intubation. Obstruction is subglottic, the epiglottis itself being only minimally inflamed. Organisms that may be recovered include *S. aureus*, group A, β-haemolytic streptococci, and (prior to vaccination) *H. influenzae* type B. Antibiotics should be given promptly, and direct laryngoscopy can confirm the diagnosis and provide local secretions for culture.

Laryngitis

Aetiology

An inflammation of the larynx that may be caused by any of the major respiratory viruses, including rhinovirus, influenza, parainfluenza, adenovirus, and coronavirus. It can be a feature of streptococcal sore throat. Other common bacterial agents associated with laryngitis include *M. catarrhalis*, *H. influenzae*, *M. pneumoniae*, and *C. pneumoniae*. Worldwide, diphtheria continues to be an important cause. Uncommon causes include *Candida*, *C. immitis*, *C. neoformans*, TB, and blastomycosis.

Clinical features

Most cases occur in adults between 18 and 40 years of age. It is a feature in 38% of cases of pneumonia, 24% of cases of children with sore throat, and 75% of toddlers with croup. It presents as a hoarse or harsh voice, with lowered pitch, episodes of aphonia, and sore throat. Duration: 3–8 days.

Treatment

Management is symptomatic (analgesia and voice rest). Routine antibiotics are not recommended. Treatment should be directed at the underlying cause.

Sinusitis

Inflammation of the paranasal sinuses usually due to viral, bacterial, or fungal infection, or non-infectious causes. Acute sinusitis lasts <4 weeks, and chronic sinusitis lasts >4 weeks.

Aetiology

- Bacterial sinusitis:
  - community-acquired—*S. pneumoniae, H. influenzae*, α-haemolytic streptococci, *M. catarrhalis*;
  - nosocomial—*P. aeruginosa, K. pneumoniae, Enterobacter* spp., *P. mirabilis, S. marcescens, S. aureus*.
- Viral sinusitis—rhinovirus, influenza, parainfluenza, adenovirus.
- Fungal sinusitis—usually occurs in patients with diabetes mellitus or immunocompromise: *Mucor, Rhizopus, Aspergillus, Absidia*, and *Basidiobolus* spp.
- Non-infectious causes—chemical irritants, tumours, foreign bodies, Wegener's granulomatosis (now called 'granulomatosis with polyongitis' (GPA)).

Epidemiology

- One to 5% of European adults are diagnosed with acute sinusitis each year.
- Viral sinusitis is seen as part of the common cold from autumn to spring. Cases of acute community-acquired bacterial sinusitis peak in association with these (occur in around 0.5% of colds).
- Non-viral cases occur throughout the year in association with allergy, swimming, nasal polyps, foreign bodies, tumour, immunodeficiency, CF.
- Nosocomial cases (often polymicrobial) may occur secondary to head trauma, prolonged nasotracheal/NG intubation, neutropenia, diabetic ketoacidosis, corticosteroids, or broad-spectrum antibiotic use.

Pathogenesis

- Viral—90% of patients with a cold develop viscous discharge and reduced clearance of secretions from sinuses, which may be due to local viral infection or the effect of inflammatory mediators.
- Bacterial—the majority of cases probably occur by spread of nasopharyngeal organisms to the usually sterile sinuses. Sinus

obstruction prevents effective clearance, and bacterial growth leads to destruction of epithelial cells, inflammatory infiltration, and the formation of mucus/pus.
- Fungal sinusitis may be non-invasive (two forms: allergic fungal sinusitis or sinus mycetoma) or invasive (occurs in hospitalized or immunocompromised patients). There are three forms of invasive sinusitis—acute fulminant (high mortality rate), chronic, and granulomatous.

Clinical features

- Viral infections—cough, sneeze, nasal discharge (clear or purulent) and obstruction, headache, and facial pressure may occur in viral infections.
- Bacterial infections—high fever and facial pain are characteristic. Sphenoid sinus infection may cause severe headache and sensory changes. Advanced frontal sinusitis may cause swelling and oedema of the forehead, as pus collects under the periosteum.
- Nosocomial cases—infection may not be apparent if the patient is unwell or unconscious (on ICU).
- Allergic fungal sinusitis—consider in patients with intractable sinusitis, and a history of allergic rhinitis and nasal polyposis.
- Sinus mycetoma—symptoms of sinusitis plus gravel-like material from the nose. Often found incidentally on CT scan.
- Acute invasive fungal sinusitis—fever, cough, nasal discharge, headache, confusion, dark ulcers on the septum/turbinates/palate.
- Chronic invasive fungal sinusitis—long history; may have reduced vision or ocular mobility (mass in the superior orbit).
- Granulomatous invasive fungal sinusitis—chronic sinusitis and proptosis, bone erosion. Often rapidly progressive.

Complications

Meningitis, brain abscess, subdural empyema, cavernous sinus and cortical vein thrombosis, orbital cellulitis and abscess, Pott's puffy tumour (osteomyelitis, usually staphylococcal, of the frontal bone).

Diagnosis

- Most cases are diagnosed clinically. Consider a bacterial aetiology in those whose symptoms fail to improve or worsen after 1 week.
- Nosocomial cases present during the second week of hospitalization.
- Radiology—an air–fluid level on skull X-ray correlates well with a positive bacterial aspirate culture, but sensitivity is low.
- Microbiology—sinus cavity specimens must be collected by sinus puncture and aspiration via the antrum below the inferior turbinate; 60% of aspirates are positive in suspected bacterial sinusitis.

Treatment

- Two-thirds of cases resolve spontaneously, reflecting the fact that many of these have a viral aetiology.
- Decongestants may relieve symptoms of obstruction but have no effect on sinus drainage.

- Patients who do not respond to antimicrobial therapy should be considered for sinus puncture and lavage to avoid progression.
- Bacterial disease—treatment is usually given empirically. Co-amoxiclav, cefuroxime, and quinolones, such as levofloxacin, have been shown to be effective, and treatment should be continued for 10 days. Those with severe infection or complications, such as intracranial extension, should receive IV therapy with broad-spectrum agents, until culture results are available. These groups require CT or MRI imaging and may need diagnostic LP or surgical interventions. Nosocomial cases may require broader therapy than community-acquired disease.
- Fungal infection (community-acquired) is effectively treated by surgical debridement. Complicated cases/immunocompromised patients are likely to need a combination of surgical and antifungal therapy.

Mastoiditis

A suppurative infection of the mastoid air cells, and the commonest complication of acute otitic media.

Pathogenesis

The mastoid bone is penetrated by air spaces that are lined with modified respiratory mucosa and are connected via the antrum to the middle ear. It is adjacent to many important structures: the posterior and middle cranial fossae, the sigmoid and lateral sinuses, the facial nerve canal, and the semicircular canals. Infection of the mastoid leads to the collection of purulent exudates within the air cells. The thin bony septae necrose, and pus coalesces into cavities.

Epidemiology

The epidemiology is similar to acute otitis media, with the highest incidence seen in children <2 years old. Recurrent acute otitis media is a risk factor.

Microbiology

The commonest causes are *S. pneumoniae* (particularly serotype 19A), GAS, *S. aureus*, and rarely *P. aeruginosa*.

Clinical features

Acute mastoiditis is accompanied by acute middle ear infection. Shortly after the onset of the signs of acute otitis media, pain, swelling, and erythema develop over the mastoid. The pinna may be displaced downwards, and tympanic perforation is followed by a purulent discharge. Chronic disease may lead to erosion through the roof of the antrum (causing a temporal lobe abscess) or extend posteriorly (where it may cause thrombosis of the lateral sinus).

Diagnosis

Plain X-ray may show something of the destruction of bony septa and inflammation of the air cells. CT scan demonstrates the extent of the disease. It is useful to obtain fresh pus, as it exudes from the tympanic membrane, to enable culture of material from the middle ear.

Treatment

- Treatment is with systemic antibiotics providing cover for *S. pneumoniae* and *H. influenzae*, as well as *S. aureus* and Gram-negative organisms in cases that have had a prolonged course. Therapy can be modified, once culture results are available.
- Mastoidectomy is indicated in those cases where a mastoid abscess has formed, and should be performed once sepsis has been adequately controlled.

Otitis externa

Inflammation of the external auditory canal—may be caused by bacteria, viruses, fungi, or non-infectious causes (e.g. allergic or dermatological conditions).

Pathogenesis

The external auditory canal is around 2.5cm long. The lateral half is cartilaginous, and the medial half runs through the temporal bone, with a narrowing at the junction between the two. The bacterial flora is that of skin elsewhere: *S. epidermidis*, *S. aureus*, and some anaerobes. In situations in which the skin becomes damaged, these organisms may proliferate, resulting in infection and inflammation of the skin itself. In addition to native organisms, invasive disease may be caused by Gram-negative species such as *P. aeruginosa*. Fungal species, such as *Aspergillus* and *C. albicans*, may also cause otitis externa.

Clinical features and therapy

- Acute localized otitis externa—may be due to a pustule (*S. aureus*) or erysipelas (GAS) involving the canal. There may be regional lymphadenopathy. Systemic antibiotics are usually curative—surgical drainage is rarely necessary.
- Acute diffuse otitis externa—a large portion of the canal skin becomes oedematous, red, itchy, and painful. Gram-negative bacteria (e.g. *P. aeruginosa*) are important. Cases occur in humid weather and may be associated with swimming. Irrigation with saline and alcohol/acetic acid mixes may help. Neomycin/hydrocortisone ear drops or oral antibiotics with topical hydrocortisone reduce inflammation and speed resolution.
- Chronic otitis externa—due to discharge through a perforated tympanic membrane secondary to chronic suppurative otitis media which results in irritation of the external canal. Rare causes: TB, leprosy, sarcoid.
- Invasive otitis externa—a severe necrotizing infection usually caused by *P. aeruginosa*. It is seen in the elderly, diabetic, and immunocompromised, and characterized by infection spreading from the skin of the external auditory canal to the tissue, vessels, and bone beneath. Symptoms: pain and tenderness of the tissue around the ear, pus discharging from the canal. Disease may be life-threatening in those cases where the sigmoid sinus, skull base, and meninges become involved. Cranial nerves VII, IX, X, and XI may be affected (sometimes

permanently). Diagnosis can be confirmed, and the extent of tissue damage ascertained, on CT or MRI. Necrotic tissue may need removing, and topical steroids and antipseudomonal antibiotics combined with systemic therapy for 4–6 weeks. Any underlying disease should be identified and treated.

Otitis media

An acute inflammatory condition characterized by fluid in the middle ear. It is a common cause of fever, pain, and hearing impairment in children and may cause sequelae in adults.

Epidemiology

- The most frequent diagnosis made by GPs in those <15 years old. By the age of 3 years, two-thirds of children have had at least one episode. Complicates one-third of respiratory infections and occurs at higher rates in children attending day-care centres.
- Most children with recurrent or severe disease have no obvious predisposition. Increased risk in those with anatomical abnormalities (e.g. cleft uvula) and immune deficiency (e.g. HIV infection).
- Commoner in males and tends to be more severe in Native Americans and Australian aborigines.

Pathogenesis

- Dysfunction of the Eustachian tube, e.g. due to mucosal congestion, leads to accumulation of middle ear secretions which provide a hospitable environment for bacteria.
- *S. pneumoniae* is the most frequent bacterial cause of otitis media. *H. influenzae* is the second commonest cause, of which only 10% are caused by type B. Other bacterial causes include GAS and *M. catarrhalis*. Causes of chronic suppurative otitis media: *P. aeruginosa, S. aureus, Corynebacterium* spp., and *K. pneumoniae*. Uncommon causes: *C. trachomatis* (in infants <6 months of age), diphtheria, TB.
- Respiratory viruses (e.g. rhinovirus, RSV, influenza) cause up to 25% of clinical cases and may co-infect with bacteria.

Clinical features

- Acute otitis media—fluid in the middle ear, with features of acute illness such as ear pain, discharge, hearing loss, fever, and lethargy. Vertigo, nystagmus, and tinnitus may occur. Tympanic erythema is an early feature but is not specific to middle ear infection. Otitis media with effusion ('glue ear') is seen in 10% of children (90% of those with cleft palates). The presence of fluid is associated with hearing impairment, and children with a history of recurrent episodes of acute otitis media show delay in speech and language abilities.
- Chronic suppurative otitis media—inflammation of the middle ear lasting ≥6 weeks and associated with discharge. Some authorities consider a single infection that resolves leaving a persistent effusion as 'chronic otitis media'.

Diagnosis

- Detecting fluid—use techniques that assess the mobility of the tympanic membrane (e.g. pneumatic otoscopy, tympanometry) or the difference in acoustic reflectivity between a fluid-filled or air-filled middle ear.
- Culture—not usually attempted. Causative organisms are well defined and routinely covered in antibiotic therapy. Take BCs and local samples if patients are severely unwell or have infection elsewhere.
- Even after therapy and the resolution of acute features, fluid persists for some weeks (10% of children still have fluid at 3 months after infection). Tympanocentesis may be warranted in those with immune impairment, those unresponsive to antibiotic therapy, or the critically ill.

Management

- Acute otitis media—uncomplicated cases with no systemic features usually resolve without antibiotic therapy (~25% are viral). Consider antibiotics after 72h if no improvement or if symptoms worsen. Agents must achieve good middle ear penetration, e.g. PO amoxicillin (erythromycin if allergic). Co-amoxiclav or ceftriaxone should be considered if there is no improvement after 24–48h. Ensure Gram-negative coverage in newborn infants, the immunosuppressed, or suppurative chronic otitis media. If the tympanic membrane has perforated, culture and sensitivity testing of discharge may guide antibiotic choice.
- Recurrent episodes of acute infection:
  - antibiotic prophylaxis (e.g. PO amoxicillin) may benefit those experiencing well-documented recurrent episodes. Consider it in those experiencing two episodes in the first 6 months of life or three episodes in 6 months for older children. It reduces the number of febrile episodes attributable to otitis media. Risk of side effects and selection of resistant organisms. Patients should be reviewed monthly and assessed for the presence of an asymptomatic effusion;
  - xylitol is a polyol sugar alcohol which inhibits bacterial colonization and, used by children in chewing gum form (five times a day!), has been shown to reduce the number of episodes of acute otitis media;
  - pneumococcal vaccination prevents otitis media caused by *S. pneumoniae* and is not very effective in children under 2 years of age due to poor immunological response. Hib vaccination only prevents 10% of cases caused by *H. influenzae* (90% are non-type B).
- Persistent effusion—systemic antibiotics are not usually indicated. Refer to ENT if 'glue ear' persists for >1–2 months. Interventions include:
  - myringotomy—once commonplace, now used only in cases of intractable pain, for drainage of a persistent effusion unresponsive to medical therapy, or to speed the resolution of mastoid infection;
  - adenoidectomy—may improve Eustachian tube function in selected children and reduce the time spent with effusion;
  - tympanostomy tubes—placed in the tympanic membrane to allow ventilation and drainage in cases of persistent effusions unresponsive to medical therapy over 3 months.

- Chronic suppurative otitis media—thorough cleaning with microsuction may resolve long-standing infection. Acute exacerbations of chronic infection will require systemic therapy with broad cover (e.g. amoxicillin and metronidazole) and may need to be given parenterally.

Dental infections

Pathogenesis

- Fermentation of dietary carbohydrates by bacteria (e.g. *S. mutans* and lactobacilli) leads to acid production and dental caries.
- Dental caries erode the protective enamel, allowing bacteria access to the dentine and pulp. In the pulp, infection may track through the root, reaching the medullary cavity of the maxilla or mandible.
- Advanced infection perforates the bony cortex, draining into tissues of the oral cavity or deep fascial planes. Neutropenic patients are at particular risk of sepsis and airway compromise.

Clinical features

- Local infections—local pain, oedema, and sensitivity to percussion and temperature. Severe local infections may be associated with abscess formation.
- Mandibular infection—pain and local swelling (e.g. infection of the mandibular incisors causing submental space infection may produce midline swelling beneath the chin; sublingual space infection may cause swelling of the floor of the mouth and tongue elevation). Retropharyngeal infection may follow molar infection (➔ see Retropharyngeal abscess, pp. 593–4). Horner's syndrome or cranial nerve palsies may follow involvement of deep areas of the neck.
- Buccal space infection due to infection of posterior teeth may cause facial oedema. Masticator space infection causes trismus, is typically indicated by cheek oedema, and is due to infection of posterior teeth, usually premolar or molar.
- Ludwig's angina—a severe cellulitis of the floor of the mouth; 75% of odontogenic cases follow infection of the second or third mandibular molars. Features: elevation/swelling of the tongue, drooling, airway obstruction, sensation of choking/suffocating (from which it gets its name). It is polymicrobial in nature and can cause widespread infection.
- Vincent's angina—an acute necrotizing ulcerative gingivitis, which presents with oral pain, bleeding gums, fetid breath, fever, anorexia, and lymphadenopathy. Caused by invasive fusiform bacteria and spirochaetes. On examination, patients have ulcerated interdental papillae, with necrosis and pseudomembrane formation over the tonsils and gums. Differential includes candidiasis, HSV stomatitis, and diphtheria. Material swabbed from the affected area should be cultured. Treatment: phenoxymethylpenicillin and metronidazole or co-amoxiclav. Risk factors: poor dental hygiene, smoking, severe intercurrent illness. A rare complication in the immunocompromised is progression to noma, a gangrenous stomatitis.

Management

- Airway protection is paramount.
- Dental X-ray, facial series, or soft tissue X-ray of the neck may help localize the region involved. A CT scan is necessary in more advanced infections.
- Localized infections may respond to oral antibiotics. Patients who appear unwell should be given IV antibiotics initially. More extensive infection and abscesses may require surgical intervention.

Lateral pharyngeal abscess

- Infection of lateral pharyngeal space may complicate pharyngitis, tonsillitis, mastoiditis, and dental abscesses.
- Caused by mixed organisms.
- Anterior infection may present with fever, pain, trismus, swelling below the mandible, dysphagia, and displacement of the tonsil towards the midline. Posterior infection may present with sepsis and little pain.
- Complications—systemic sepsis, respiratory obstruction (laryngeal oedema), thrombosis of internal jugular, erosion of the internal carotid.
- Management—airway protection, parenteral antibiotic, and surgical drainage.

Acute bronchitis

A syndrome of tracheal and bronchial inflammation associated with respiratory infection. Diagnoses peak in the winter months and are made most frequently in children <5 years of age.

Aetiology

- Viral causes commonest—influenza A and B, parainfluenza, coronavirus (types 1–3), rhinovirus, RSV, and human metapneumovirus.
- Other less common pathogens—*M. pneumoniae*, *C. pneumoniae*, and *B. pertussis*.

Pathogenesis

- The exact nature of pathogenesis varies between viruses. Some (e.g. influenza) invade the lower respiratory tract. Others (e.g. rhinovirus) do not, and symptoms may be secondary to inflammatory mediators. Either way, the outcome is an inflamed, oedematous tracheobronchial tree with increased secretions. The extent of epithelial damage varies with the aetiological agent.
- Attack severity may be increased by exposure to irritants, such as cigarette smoke, and may lead to long-term airway damage. Patients with acute bronchitis are more likely to have a history of atopic disease, which may be associated with airway hyper-reactivity. Some progress to develop adult-onset asthma.

Clinical features

- Severe, prolonged cough distinguishes acute bronchitis from other respiratory syndromes such as the common cold. It lasts over 4 weeks in over 40% of patients. May be productive early on, but typically dry.
- Cough and respiration may be associated with retrosternal pain in those cases with severe tracheal inflammation. Dyspnoea and more severe respiratory symptoms are seen only in those with underlying chest disease. Fever is seen in some cases—most frequently with agents such as influenza or *M. pneumoniae*.

Diagnosis

- Bronchitis is a diagnosis of exclusion, and a complete history and examination should be performed, seeking any more serious cause of cough.
- Respiratory virus PCR may aid in the identification of viral causes of acute bronchitis. Rapid tests for influenza are sometimes used.
- Cultures of respiratory secretions may be useful in looking for specific agents such as *B. pertussis*, but routine bacteriological culture is unhelpful in defining a cause of bronchitis. Serological tests may be used to confirm infection with *M. pneumoniae* and *C. pneumoniae*, but are not helpful in the acute setting.
- Those in whom cough persists beyond a reasonable duration of illness should be investigated for other causes (e.g. foreign body, TB, malignancy).

Treatment

- Treatment is mainly symptomatic, e.g. NSAIDs, aspirin, paracetamol, and/or ipratropium bromide.
- There is no good evidence for the use of cough suppressants.
- Short courses of inhaled steroids are widely used, but their efficacy remains unproven.[1]
- Guidelines from NICE advise not treating uncomplicated acute bronchitis with antibiotics. For patients at risk of significant complications (e.g. due to heart, lung, renal, liver, neuromuscular disease, immunosuppression, or frailty), further investigation, management, and possible initiation of antimicrobial therapy may be warranted.
- Smoking should be discouraged.

Reference

1 Schroeder K, Fahey T. Over-the-counter medications for acute cough in children and adults in ambulatory settings. *Cochrane Database Syst Rev*. 2004;4:CD001831.

Chronic bronchitis

Defined as a cough productive of sputum on most days during at least 3 months of 2 successive years, which cannot be attributed to other specific diseases (e.g. TB, bronchiectasis). Where airflow obstruction exists, the patient is considered to have COPD, which may coexist with emphysema.

Epidemiology

- Common, affecting 10–25% of the adult population. Men are affected more than women, and it is commoner in those >40 years of age.
- Associations—cigarette smoking (although only 15% of smokers develop chronic bronchitis), pollution, and exposure to allergens.

Pathogenesis

- Even modest smoking is associated with increased alveolar macrophages, inflammation of the respiratory bronchioles, epithelial hyperplasia, and fibrosis of the bronchiolar and alveolar walls.
- The inflammation and oedema seen in patients with chronic bronchitis result from the interaction between exogenous irritants and the pathological response, including: an increase in bronchial mucus-secreting cells, granulocytic infiltration in response to chemokines produced by epithelial cells, increased airway secretions, and the production of neuropeptides promoting bronchospasm.
- Acute exacerbations of disease may be related to bacterial infections. Pathogenic bacteria can be cultured from the bronchi of most chronic bronchitics (as well as those with other lung pathologies such as TB), and the development of purulent sputum is not associated with the appearance of specific organisms but does correlate with an increase in number. *H. influenzae* and *S. pneumoniae* are found in half of chronic bronchitics. Organisms such as *M. pneumoniae, S. aureus*, and Gram-negative organisms are identified infrequently. One-third of acute exacerbations are thought to be due to viral infections.

Clinical features

- Frequent productive cough, most severe in the morning when patients may produce large amounts of sputum, which may be mucoid and white or obviously purulent in appearance.
- Patients may be incapacitated only when they develop acute infections; however, most patients have some degree of airflow limitation. COPD exists as a spectrum of clinical disease, with emphysema predominant at one end (breathless, less sputum, fewer infections, barrel chest with hyperexpanded, clear lungs) and bronchitis predominant at the other (productive coughing, frequent infections, wheeze, widespread crepitations, and right heart failure in severe cases).

Diagnosis

- Acute exacerbations of chronic bronchitis can be difficult to identify. Most patients do not develop fever or leucocytosis. Diagnosis is made on symptoms such as an increase in sputum production or a change in colour with increasing cough and breathlessness.
- CXR is useful only in the exclusion of other illnesses.

Treatment

General measures

- Exclude other causes of recurrent chest infections and have a high index of suspicion for lung malignancy.

- Smoking cessation, weight control, avoidance of environmental irritants, and assessment for allergic disease.
- Record of baseline spirometry, ABG, and oxygen saturations.
- Pneumococcal and influenza vaccinations.
- Pulmonary rehabilitation programmes and postural drainage where appropriate.

Maintenance therapy to improve airflow obstruction symptoms

- For example, regular inhaled steroids, β2-agonists, anticholinergic agents. Oral steroids as required.
- Prophylactic antibiotics may be useful in selected patients with very frequent exacerbations (four or more per year)—most specialists believe they do not have a role in routine treatment due to concerns over the development of resistance. RCTs prior to 1970 demonstrated that chronic bronchitis patients using prophylactic antibiotics had a small, but significant, reduction in exacerbations, compared to placebo, and antibiotics significantly reduced the number of days of disability per person per month treated. There are no contemporary studies.

Intensive therapy for acute exacerbations

- Intensification of normal therapy (e.g. course of oral steroids).
- Antibiotic therapy—infection can cause respiratory decompensation (a common cause of death in these patients), and, despite difficulties in assessing their efficacy, antibiotic therapy does improve clinical outcome. They are usually given PO for 7–10 days. Specific agents are best determined locally and with reference to previous microbial sensitivities.

Bronchiolitis

An acute infection of the lower respiratory tract, characterized by the acute onset of wheeze and associated with cough, nasal discharge, breathlessness, and respiratory distress.

Aetiology

- RSV is the commonest cause, followed by rhinovirus. Less common causes include parainfluenza virus, human metapneumovirus, influenza virus, adenovirus, coronavirus, and human bocavirus. With molecular diagnostics, two or more viruses are detected in approximately one-third of young children hospitalized with bronchiolitis.
- *M. pneumoniae* is an uncommon cause.

Epidemiology

- In temperate regions, cases peak in winter and early spring (RSV), with small peaks in autumn (parainfluenza). Most cases occur in children aged between 2 and 10 months.
- Estimated incidence varies widely; 80% of children have evidence of previous RSV infection by their second birthday. A UK study estimated the total mean annual incidence of hospital admissions of children aged <1 year attributable to RSV at 28.3 per 1000.

- Factors associated with high rates of hospitalization with bronchiolitis—young age, young maternal age, living in crowded/polluted areas, large number of siblings, airway hyper-reactivity, RSV identified as cause.

Pathogenesis

- Virus infects the upper respiratory mucosa and spreads to the lower airways. Bronchial and bronchiolar inflammation and necrosis follow, with oedema and peribronchiolar mononuclear cell infiltration. In severe cases, interstitial pneumonitis may develop.
- Inflammation and oedema reduce the airway calibre. Necrotic material may block small airways. Distally trapped air is later absorbed, resulting in multiple areas of atelectasis and a low ventilation/perfusion ratio. Children become breathless and tachypnoeic, developing respiratory distress and respiratory failure in severe cases.
- Infants who develop wheeze with respiratory virus infection in early life are more likely to have some form of recurrent lower respiratory tract disease. Whether this is related to a propensity to atopy or pre-existing lung dysfunction or having a viral aetiology is not clear.

Clinical features

- Mild fever and signs of URTI. Progresses after 2–3 days to lower respiratory tract features, with cough, raised respiratory rate, anorexia, lethargy, and wheeze. Fever may resolve.
- Severe cases develop tachypnoea, tachycardia, and signs of increased breathing work (nasal flaring, chest wall retraction, grunting). Cyanosis is rare, even in the presence of hypoxia. Apnoea is relatively common in young infants hospitalized with RSV infection.
- Auscultatory findings are variable—wheeze, crepitations, decreased breath sounds in severe cases. Other findings: dehydration, otitis media, diarrhoea. Symptoms begin to settle after 2–3 days, with recovery taking 2 weeks or more.

Diagnosis

- General features—the WCC may be elevated in severe cases. CXR findings include hyperinflation, hyperlucent parenchyma, and multiple areas of atelectasis, and pneumonia may be present. Findings do not correlate with clinical severity.
- Diagnosis is usually clinical in the setting of a seasonal outbreak. Other causes of wheeze and dyspnoea must be considered (e.g. a first episode of asthma, gastric reflux and aspiration, CCF, or airway obstruction by a foreign body).
- The specific agent may be identified from respiratory secretions (preferably an NPA) by respiratory virus PCR. Positive predictive value diminishes outside the setting of an epidemic. Serology is rarely helpful.

Treatment

- General measures—oxygen to maintain the saturation above 92%, and ventilation if indicated. Bronchodilators are often given but are of limited benefit. Corticosteroids are often used and have been reported to bring about a modest improvement in symptoms, but with no effect

on the duration of hospitalization. Saline drops or nasal bulb suction may relieve nasal congestion.
- Ribavirin may be given to hospitalized infants at risk of severe disease by aerosol for 8–12h a day for 2–5 days. Such children include those with underlying cardiac or respiratory disease, or the premature. Although it has been shown to speed the improvement in oxygenation, its use does not result in shorter hospital stays.

Prevention

Immunoprophylaxis with palivizumab, a humanized monoclonal antibody against the RSV F glycoprotein, decreases the risk of hospitalization due to RSV illness amongst infants with bronchopulmonary dysplasia, premature birth, and congenital heart disease.

Complications

- Infants with underlying cardiac or pulmonary disease or immunodeficiency are at greatest risk of severe disease.
- Although up to 75% of infants requiring hospital admission have recurrent episodes of bronchospasm within the first 2 years after recovery, the number continuing to experience such episodes drops year by year. The majority with long-term problems tend to either have a predisposition to atopy or have reduced lung function at birth.

Community-acquired pneumonia

Epidemiology

- Incidence >1 per 100 people per year; 20–40% of cases require hospital admission. Mortality varies with the patient group (overall 5–10%, 50% in those requiring ICU admission).
- Peak age 50–70 years, and onset in mid winter and early spring; 58–89% have an underlying disease (e.g. COPD, diabetes, cardiovascular disease, immunosuppression, etc.).
- Some organisms are acquired by person-to-person spread or are existing commensals (*S. pneumoniae, H. influenzae*). Others are acquired from the environment (*L. pneumophila*) or animals (*C. psittaci*).
- ~80% of CAP is managed in primary care—viruses, *S. pneumoniae*, and *M. pneumoniae* are the commonest causes.
- Risk factors—extremes of age, smoking, COPD, diabetes, cardiovascular disease, severe intercurrent illness, recent anaesthetic/intubation, immunosuppression.

Aetiology

- Organisms vary with country, study, age, and patient group (e.g. *Moraxella* and *H. influenzae* are commoner in COPD).
- Pneumonia in childhood is usually viral.
- Common bacterial isolates vary with age:
  - 0–1 month—*E. coli*, GBS, *L. monocytogenes*;
  - 1–6 months—*C. trachomatis, S. aureus*, RSV;
  - 6 months to 5 years—RSV, parainfluenza viruses;

- 5–15 years—*M. pneumoniae*, influenza;
- 16–30 years—*M. pneumoniae, S. pneumoniae*;
- older adults—*S. pneumoniae, H. influenzae*.

- Some infections, e.g. *M. pneumoniae*, are associated with epidemics.
- *S. pneumoniae* infection is associated with viral illness, e.g. influenza.
- Mixed infections are commoner in the elderly—*S. aureus* and Gram-negatives are seen more frequently amongst those in residential care.
- Severe disease occurs with *S. pneumoniae*, MRSA, *L. pneumophila*, and Gram-negative organisms. Mortality is 20–53%.
- Rare causes of pneumonia include anthrax, plague, and melioidosis.
- *P. jirovecii* (➔ see *Pneumocystis jirovecii*, p. 482) is an important cause in HIV-infected patients, who are also at increased risk of infection with mycobacteria, *C. neoformans*, and viruses (e.g. CMV).

Clinical features

- History—most patients present with sudden-onset chills, fever, cough, mucopurulent sputum, pleuritic chest pain, fatigue, anorexia, sweats, and nausea; 20% do not have cough. Ask about predisposing conditions, travel, and exposure to animals.
- Symptoms and signs—fever, tachypnoea, tachycardia, postural blood pressure drop (may indicate dehydration), and consolidation (absent in ~70%). Signs of respiratory distress in severe cases. All findings are less pronounced in the elderly in whom presentation may be insidious (confusion, abdominal pain). Other findings: herpes labialis (40% of pneumococcal pneumonia patients), bullous myringitis (*Mycoplasma* pneumonia).

Investigations

- Blood tests—FBC shows neutrophilia, or neutropenia if very unwell. Biochemical abnormalities include raised urea, hyponatraemia (especially elderly due to SIADH), abnormal LFTs (especially *Legionella*), raised CRP.
- CXR changes are non-specific:
  - lobar consolidation, cavitation, and effusions suggest a bacterial cause;
  - CXR worse than examination findings suggest mycoplasmal or viral pneumonia;
  - diffuse bilateral involvement may suggest PCP, *Legionella* infection, or primary viral pneumonia;
  - pneumatoceles may be seen in pneumonia caused by *S. aureus, K. pneumoniae, H. influenzae*, and *S. pneumoniae*.
- CT is helpful in recurrent pneumonias or those unresponsive to therapy (e.g. to identify a tumour). In immunocompromised patients, some pathogens (e.g. *Aspergillus*) have typical CT appearances, which may aid diagnosis.

Microbiological investigations

- Microbiological tests are not routinely recommended for patients managed in the community—consider in those who do not respond to empirical antibiotic therapy or in whom unusual pathogens are suspected.

- BC—positive in only 1–16% of hospitalized patients with CAP (≤25% of cases of pneumococcal pneumonia).
- Sputum examination has low sensitivity; >50% of sputum cultures are negative, even in proven bacterial cases. Sputum examination is, however, useful in the identification of organisms such as *Legionella* spp., *Pseudomonas* spp., *Burkholderia* spp., and MTB.
- Serology—severely ill patients who have had symptoms for 5–7 days should have serum tested for antibodies to atypical pathogens (*Legionella, Mycoplasma*, and *Chlamydia* spp.) A second specimen is taken 7–10 days later.
- Antigen testing—urinary *Legionella* antigen testing should be performed on all patients with severe disease and at least 5 days of symptoms. Some authorities also recommend pneumococcal antigen testing.
- BAL—a bronchoscope is used to instil sterile fluid into a segment of the lung, and the fluid examined microscopically and cultured. A threshold of 10^4 cfu/mL is used to define significant isolates. It is particularly useful in the diagnosis of MTB, *P. jiroveci*, CMV, and VAP.
- Pleural fluid sampling—where positive, pleural fluid cultures are specific for the organism causing the underlying pneumonia. Fluid analysis helps differentiate other causes of lung disease (e.g. TB, tumour).
- Other tests—immunofluorescence or PCR for respiratory viruses; immunofluorescence for *Chlamydia* spp.; cold agglutinins for *M. pneumoniae* (<25% positive); lung biopsy (e.g. immunosuppressed patients with no diagnosis).

Severity assessment

- The CURB-65 score (*C*onfusion, *U*rea, *R*espiratory rate, *B*lood pressure, age *65* or over) enables rapid assessment of severity and guides initial management (see Fig. 14.1).
- Additional adverse features—hypoxia regardless of oxygen therapy (arterial oxygen saturation (SaO_2) <92% or partial pressure of arterial oxygen (PaO_2) <8kPa), bilateral or multilobe involvement on CXR, positive BCs, WCC <4 × 10^9/L or >20 × 10^9/L.
- Severity should be reassessed regularly during the course of the illness.

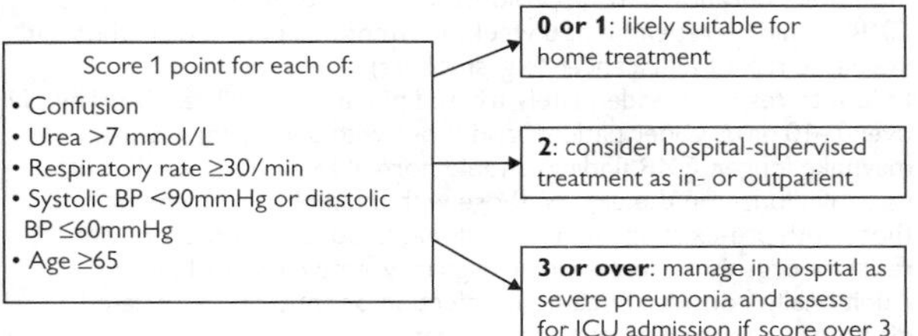

Fig. 14.1 The CURB-65 severity assessment tool. BP, blood pressure.

Management

- See BTS guidelines for CAP, 2009 update.[2]
- General—IV fluids, appropriate oxygen therapy (with repeated ABG in those with COPD), fluids, frequent reassessment of progress and severity, particularly aimed at the early identification of those who may require ICU support.
- Antibiotics—empirical therapy should be started as soon as possible:
  - CURB-65 score 0 or 1—amoxicillin 500mg to 1g tds PO. Alternatives: erythromycin 500mg qds PO, or clarithromycin 500mg bd PO;
  - CURB-65 score 2—amoxicillin 500mg tds PO and erythromycin 500mg qds PO (or clarithromycin 500mg bd PO);
  - CURB-65 score ≥3—co-amoxiclav 1.2g tds IV plus erythromycin 500mg qds PO;
  - older fluoroquinolones (e.g. ciprofloxacin) are not recommended for empirical treatment due to poor activity against *S. pneumoniae*. Newer agents (e.g. levofloxacin and moxifloxacin) may be used.
- Antibiotic therapy should be tailored to the causative organism in the light of microbiological data:
  - *S. pneumoniae*—amoxicillin or benzylpenicillin;
  - *M. pneumoniae*—erythromycin or clarithromycin;
  - *C. pneumoniae*—erythromycin or clarithromycin;
  - *C. psittaci*—doxycycline;
  - *C. burnetii*—doxycycline;
  - *Legionella* spp.—clarithromycin ± rifampicin;
  - *H. influenzae*—amoxicillin (non-β-lactamase producer) or co-amoxiclav (β-lactamase producer);
  - Gram-negative enteric bacilli—cefuroxime, cefotaxime, or ceftriaxone;
  - *P. aeruginosa*—ceftazidime and gentamicin or tobramycin;
  - *S. aureus* (methicillin-sensitive)—flucloxacillin ± rifampicin;
  - MRSA—vancomycin.
- IV antibiotics should be switched to oral therapy as soon as there is evidence of clinical improvement (preferably within 48h). However, IV treatment may be continued in patients with severe infections caused by *Legionella, S. aureus*, or aerobic Gram-negatives.
- Three to 5 days' therapy is usually sufficient in uncomplicated cases. Treatment duration may be prolonged to 7–21 days in severe disease.
- CXR should be repeated at 6 weeks if symptoms persist or in those at increased risk of lung cancer (e.g. smokers).
- Failure to respond—adequately treated pneumonia will resolve clinically over 7–10 days. Older patients and those with underlying disease may take longer. CXR findings should normalize within 4 weeks but may take longer in the elderly, those with multilobe involvement, and those with pre-existing pulmonary disease. Consider infection with resistant organisms, underlying malignancy, empyema, or lung abscess. Additionally, consider IV catheter infection or antibiotic-associated diarrhoea in those with prolonged fever.

Complications

- Parapneumonic effusion.
- Empyema (➔ see Empyema, pp. 619–21).
- ARDS.
- Sepsis syndrome.
- Metastatic infection (meningitis, arthritis, endocarditis).
- Rare neurological sequelae may follow *M. pneumoniae* infection, e.g. meningoencephalitis, cranial nerve palsies, and GBS.

Prevention

Two vaccines are available: PPSV23, a polysaccharide vaccine, made from the 23 capsular serotypes that cause over 90% of invasive infections, and PCV13, a protein conjugate vaccine.

Reference

2 British Thoracic Society; Community Acquired Pneumonia in Adults Guideline Group (2009). *Guidelines for the management of community acquired pneumonia in adults: update 2009*. Available at: https://www.brit-thoracic.org.uk/document-library/clinical-information/pneumonia/adult-pneumonia/bts-guidelines-for-the-management-of-community-acquired-pneumonia-in-adults-2009-update/.

Atypical pneumonias

These account for 7–28% of CAP. The term was originally used to describe cases that failed to respond to penicillin or sulfa drugs and those in which no organism was identified. More recently, it has meant those cases that start with an apparently mild respiratory tract illness (which may last up to 10 days), followed by pneumonia with dyspnoea and cough, with or without sputum. Clinical signs tend to be milder than the CXR would suggest. It usually involves the lower lobes and may be unilateral or bilateral. The clinical course is usually benign, although certain organisms may cause extrapulmonary symptoms (e.g. mycoplasmal infection and neurological sequelae) or severe disease (e.g. *Legionella*). CXR tends to improve faster than typical pneumonia. It is good practice to avoid the term 'atypical pneumonia', although it is still useful to refer to 'atypical organisms', as they have certain features in common—they tend not to be respiratory tract colonizers; they affect healthy individuals of all age groups; they occur in epidemics, and they do not respond to penicillin.

Mycoplasma pneumoniae

(➔ See *Mycoplasma*, pp. 350–2.)

- Causes autumn epidemics every 4–8 years (more frequently within closed populations such as prisons). Commonest in children >4 years and young adults.
- Certain respiratory viruses cause a similar clinical picture (e.g. influenza, parainfluenza, adenovirus, RSV).
- Resolves without complications in the majority of cases, although the illness may last a few weeks, with a protracted cough.
- Difficult to culture—diagnosis is usually retrospective by serology.
- Serum cold agglutination is a non-specific test (positive in 50–70% of patients after 7–10 days of infection).

- CXR appearance is of basal atelectasis or involvement of a single lower lobe, sometimes a nodular infiltration resembling that associated with other diseases with granulomatous pathology such as TB, mycoses, and sarcoidosis.
- Treatment is with erythromycin or clarithromycin.
- Rare complications—pericarditis, arthritis, Stevens–Johnson syndrome, haemolytic anaemia, thrombocytopenia, CNS infections, GBS, peripheral neuropathy, other neurological manifestations, and ocular complications.

Legionella pneumophila

(➲ See *Legionella*, pp. 318–20.)

- Accounts for 1–20% of CAP cases. Commoner in summer.
- The organism colonizes water piping systems, and outbreaks are associated with acquisition from contaminated water sources, including cooling systems, showers, decorative fountains, humidifiers, respiratory therapy equipment, and whirlpool spas.
- Risk factors—smoking, diabetes, malignancy, AIDS, end-stage renal disease, alcohol abuse.
- Clinical features—1- to 2-day prodrome (mild headache and myalgias) is followed by high fever, chills and rigors, cough (non-productive, becoming productive as the disease progresses), dyspnoea, pleuritic chest pain, haemoptysis, nausea, vomiting, diarrhoea, abdominal pain, altered mental status, arthralgias, and myalgias. Consider it in those with a high fever, multilobar involvement, a need for ICU, and rapidly evolving GI, neurological, and radiographic abnormalities. Laboratory abnormalities include DIC, SIADH, abnormal LFTs, and renal impairment.
- Treatment—clarithromycin ± rifampicin.
- Mortality rate of 25% (may be related to co-morbidities).

Chlamydophila pneumoniae

(➲ See *Chlamydophila pneumoniae*, p. 355.)

- Accounts for 3–10% of CAP cases in adults.
- Causes mild pneumonia or bronchitis in adolescents and young adults.
- Incidence is highest in the elderly who may experience more severe disease and repeated infections.
- Mortality rate ~9%.

Chlamydophila psittaci

(➲ see *Chlamydophila psittaci*, pp. 354–5.)

- Usually associated with exposure to birds—pet shop employees and poultry industry workers are at risk.
- Clinical spectrum ranges from an asymptomatic infection to fulminant toxicity.
- Consider in those patients with pneumonia, splenomegaly, and a history of bird exposure (especially sick birds).
- May develop rash, hepatitis, haemolytic anaemia, DIC, meningoencephalitis, or reactive arthritis.
- Treatment—tetracycline.
- Mortality rate <1%.

Coxiella burnetii

(➔ see *Coxiella burnetii*—ACDP 3, pp. 346–8.)

- An intracellular pathogen found worldwide, with the exception of New Zealand. Highly prevalent in parts of Spain and France (second commonest cause of CAP in some regions).
- Reservoir primarily farm animals (e.g. cattle, goats, sheep). Excreted in urine, milk, and faeces, and attains high concentration in birth products.
- Rare human-to-human transmission from exposure to the placenta of an infected woman and from blood transfusions.
- Acute Q fever may cause a febrile illness, pneumonia, or hepatitis.
- Most cases of acute Q fever resolve spontaneously within 2 weeks, but 14–21 days of treatment with doxycycline reduces symptom duration.

Aspiration pneumonia

Elderly patients, those with neurological impairment (e.g. acute phase of stroke), and others with altered consciousness (e.g. alcoholics) and abnormal swallow/gag reflexes are at risk of aspiration. Acid aspiration results in the release of proinflammatory cytokines that recruit neutrophils into the lung. These are thought to be the key mediators of acute lung injury, with bacterial pneumonia developing several days later, perhaps facilitated by bronchial obstruction by inhaled debris (e.g. peanut). Abscess and empyema are not uncommon. Anaerobes on their own or mixed with aerobes are the commonest bacteriological findings (e.g. *Bacteroides, Fusobacterium*). Bronchoscopy may be indicated to provide material for culture and exclude foreign bodies.

Hospital-acquired pneumonia

- HAP is the leading cause of infection-related deaths in hospital. Defined as pneumonia developing >48h after admission.
- Sixty per cent of cases are caused by aerobic Gram-negatives, the majority being enterobacteria and *Pseudomonas* spp. Other causes include *S. aureus, S. pneumoniae*, and anaerobes. Nosocomial outbreaks of viral pneumonia are not uncommon.
- Risk factors:
  - patient-related—age >70 years, severe underlying disease, malnutrition, coma, metabolic acidosis, and possibly sinusitis;
  - infection control-related—poor HCW hand hygiene, contaminated respiratory equipment;
  - intervention-related—sedatives, corticosteroids and cytotoxic drugs, prolonged antibiotic use, ventilation (risk of acquiring pneumonia 20 times that of unventilated patients).
- Treatment—antimicrobial therapy should be based upon risk factors for MDR pathogens, including recent antibiotic therapy (if any), the

resident flora in the hospital or ICU, the presence of underlying diseases, and available culture data. Empiric broad-spectrum therapy is recommended, e.g. piperacillin–tazobactam. Once the results of pre-therapy cultures are available, therapy should be narrowed, based upon the susceptibility pattern of the pathogens identified.

Ventilator-associated pneumonia

VAP complicates the course of 8–28% of patients receiving mechanical ventilation.[3]

- Causes—the predominant organisms responsible for infection are *P. aeruginosa*, *S. aureus*, enterobacteria, *Haemophilus* spp., and *Acinetobacter* spp., but aetiological agents vary according to the ICU, duration of inpatient stay, and prior antibiotic use. Polymicrobial infections are common.
- Pathogenesis—intubation compromises the natural barrier between the oropharynx and trachea, and also facilitates entry of bacteria into the lung by pooling and leakage of contaminated secretions around the endotracheal tube cuff.
- Risk factors—hypoalbuminaemia, age ≥60 years, ARDS, COPD, coma, burns, trauma, organ failure, gastric aspiration, gastric colonization and pH, upper respiratory tract colonization, sinusitis, H2 receptor antagonists, paralytic agents, prior antibiotics, continuous sedation, mechanical ventilation >2 days, re-intubation, tracheostomy, NG tube, supine position.
- Clinical features—the diagnosis of VAP is based on three features: systemic signs of infection, new or worsening pulmonary infiltrates, bacteriological evidence of parenchymal infection. Presents with purulent secretions, CXR changes, neutrophilia, fever, and increased ventilatory requirements. Differential includes: PE, ARDS, aspiration (chemical pneumonitis).
- Diagnosis—can be difficult. Quantitative cultures of endotracheal aspirates may be misleading, as they may only reflect upper respiratory tract colonizers. Bronchoscopic sampling provides lower respiratory tract samples for microbiological analysis. This may be directed (i.e. in an area of maximal pulmonary infiltrate) or non-directed. Quantitative BAL cultures indicate the likelihood of infection, with $>10^4$ organisms/mL being diagnostic of infection. Some authorities recommend surveillance BALs in patients on the ICU.
- Treatment[4]—this should be targeted against the likely organism and antimicrobial susceptibility pattern. In early-onset VAP (≤4 days after hospital admission), the organisms are community-acquired and unlikely to be MDR. Treatment should be with ceftriaxone or a fluoroquinolone or ertapenem. In late-onset VAP (>4 days after hospital admission), organisms are likely to be hospital flora and MDR. Treatment is with an antipseudomonal cephalosporin or piperacillin-tazobactam or carbapenem plus a fluoroquinolone or an aminoglycoside. Vancomycin should be added if there is a possibility of MRSA.
- Prognosis—mortality ranges from 24% to 76%.

References

3 Chastre J, Fagon JY. Ventilator-associated pneumonia. *Am J Respir Crit Care Med*. 2002;**165**:867–903.
4 American Thoracic Society; Infectious Diseases Society of America. Guidelines for the management of adults with hospital-acquired, ventilator-associated, and healthcare-associated pneumonia. *Am J Respir Crit Care Med*. 2005;**171**:388–416.

Pulmonary infiltrates with eosinophilia

The differential diagnosis is broad and includes:
- tropical eosinophilia;
- parasitic infections, e.g. *Ascaris* or *Strongyloides*;
- TB;
- brucellosis;
- psittacosis;
- coccidioidomycosis;
- histoplasmosis;
- bronchopulmonary *Aspergillus*;
- drug allergy;
- sarcoidosis;
- Churg–Strauss syndrome;
- eosinophilic leukaemia;
- hypersensitivity pneumonitis.

Empyema

Microbial infection of the pleural space—prognosis can be poor in those cases where diagnosis is missed or therapy inadequate.

Aetiology

- Usually secondary to pneumonia. Cases may occur with no evidence of pneumonia (primary empyema). Other precipitants: surgery, trauma, oesophageal perforation, chest drains.
- Common organisms in cases secondary to pneumonia: *S. aureus*, *S. pneumoniae*, and *S. pyogenes*. *H. influenzae* has declined since the introduction of the Hib vaccine.
- Cases associated with aspiration or arising from GI sites are more likely to be due to anaerobic organisms. Those associated with subdiaphragmatic disease are often polymicrobial. Aerobic Gram-negative organisms are common in cases complicating trauma or surgery and those associated with serous effusions.
- The immunocompromised have higher rates of Gram-negative and fungal empyema generally in the context of disseminated disease.

Clinical features

- Chest pain, breathlessness, weight loss, night sweats, fever. Examination reveals only the signs of the effusion in most cases.
- Consider in patients with persistent fever already receiving antibiotics for pneumonia.

- Consider oesophageal rupture in those who develop a pleural effusion soon after significant retching or vomiting.

Diagnosis

See BTS guidelines for the management of pleural infection.[5]

- Radiology—CXR shows pleural effusion. Ultrasound permits diagnostic aspiration and the identification of loculated effusions. Contrast CT distinguishes empyema from most lung abscesses and is used to monitor treatment.
- Diagnostic sampling—should be performed in all patients with a pleural effusion in the context of pneumonia or sepsis. Samples should be kept tightly sealed on ice to prevent changes in pH and glucose. The presence of pus cells or high numbers of microorganisms on Gram stain confirms diagnosis. Cultures may be negative in patients receiving antibiotics.
- Biochemical tests—empyema is confirmed by measurement of pH (<7.2), glucose (<2.2mmol/L), and LDH (>1000IU/L). Low pH values (pH 6–6.7) should raise the suspicion of oesophageal rupture or chronic empyema (see Table 14.1). Remember low pH/glucose may occur in TB, malignancy etc.
- Culture-negative cases—consider BC, urine antigen testing for *Legionella* or histoplasmosis, pleural biopsy in suspected TB (95% positive on histology, compared to 23% by pleural fluid culture/microscopy), serology for *E. histolytica* (positive in 98% of patients with pleural amoebiasis), microscopy/culture of empyema pus for AFB in those at risk of nocardiosis, examination of stool/sputum for eggs in cases with pleural or blood eosinophilia suggestive of paragonimiasis.

Management

Empyema requires prompt treatment to prevent complications and the need for surgical drainage. Involve a respiratory specialist.

- Drainage—indications for chest tube insertion are: (1) purulent pleural fluid; (2) pleural fluid pH <7. 2; (3) positive pleural fluid Gram stain or culture; (4) loculated pleural collections; (5) large non-purulent pleural effusions; and (6) poor response to antimicrobial therapy alone.

Table 14.1 Pleural fluid characteristics in empyema

Stage	Pleural fluid findings	Comments
Simple parapneumonic effusion	Clear fluid; pH >7.2; LDH <1000IU/L, glucose >2.2mmol/L; no organisms on culture or Gram stain	Will usually resolve with antibiotics alone. Perform chest tube drainage for symptom relief, if required
Complicated parapneumonic effusion	Clear or cloudy fluid; pH <7.2, LDH >1000IU/L, glucose <2.2mmol/L; may be Gram stain- or culture-positive	Requires chest tube drainage
Empyema	Purulent fluid; may be Gram stain- or culture-positive	Requires chest tube drainage

- Antibiotics—the regimen should be guided by culture results. Culture-negative cases should receive antibiotics covering community-acquired and anaerobic organisms (e.g. ceftriaxone and metronidazole). Broader-spectrum cover should be initiated in cases of hospital-acquired empyema. Consider adding a macrolide in cases of suspected *Legionella* infections. Once the fever has settled, convert to oral antibiotics, and continue treatment for at least 3 weeks.
- Intrapleural administration of fibrinolytic agents (e.g. streptokinase, urokinase, and tissue plasminogen activator) has been assessed as a way to improve drainage of loculated parapneumonic effusions and empyemas. Data regarding the benefit of intrapleural fibrinolysis have been conflicting, but a recent review concluded that it was potentially beneficial.[6]
- Consider bronchoscopy if there is a high index of suspicion of bronchial obstruction.
- In patients with persistent sepsis and/or residual pleural effusion, review the diagnosis, and perform a CT chest to confirm chest tube position and effusion anatomy, and look for obstructing lesions, etc.
- Surgery—patients should be considered for surgery if they have ongoing sepsis with a persistent pleural collection by day 7, despite chest tube drainage and antibiotics. Modalities include video-assisted thoracoscopic surgery (VATS), open thoracic drainage, or thoracotomy and decortication.

References

5 British Thoracic Society; Pleural Disease Guideline Group (2010). *BTS pleural disease guideline 2010*. Available at: https://www.brit-thoracic.org.uk/document-library/clinical-information/pleural-disease/pleural-disease-guidelines-2010/pleural-disease-guideline/.

6 Janda S, Swiston J. Intrapleural fibrinolytic therapy for treatment of adult parapneumonic effusions and empyemas: a systematic review and meta-analysis. *Chest*. 2012;**142**:401–11.

Lung abscess

Lung abscess is defined as necrosis of the pulmonary parenchyma caused by microbial infection, resulting in a pus-filled fluid cavity.

Pathogenesis

- Bacteria are usually endogenously acquired from the flora of the upper respiratory tract. Most follow aspiration in the context of states of altered consciousness (e.g. alcoholism, stroke) or dysphagia (e.g. neurological disease).
- Other associations—intestinal obstruction, periodontal disease or gingivitis, septic embolization, bronchiectasis, immunosuppression, and pharyngeal instrumentation (e.g. endotracheal intubation). Up to 5% of PEs may become secondarily infected.
- Lung regions that are dependent when lying flat are commonly affected—the posterior segment of the right upper lobe and apical segments of the lower lobes. Bases may be affected in cases of subdiaphragmatic extension (e.g. amoebic liver abscess).
- Multiple abscesses follow septic embolization (e.g. *S. aureus* right heart endocarditis) or bacteraemia (enteric Gram-negatives and anaerobes).

Microbiology

- Most frequently caused by oral anaerobes, e.g. *Peptostreptococcus, Prevotella, Bacteroides* (usually not *B. fragilis*), and *Fusobacterium* spp.
- The commonest non-anaerobes are *S. milleri* and other microaerophilic streptococci.
- Other bacterial causes include *S. aureus, K. pneumoniae*, other Gram-negative bacilli, GAS, *B. pseudomallei, H. influenzae* type B, *Legionella, Nocardia*, and *Actinomyces* spp.

Clinical features

- Cases diagnosed late may present with several weeks or months of cough, low-grade fever, weight loss, anaemia, and clubbing. Sputum is copious and may be foul-smelling. Findings are those of a severe pneumonia, with or without effusion.
- In cases of secondary lung abscess, the primary lesion may also be apparent (endocarditis, subphrenic infection, etc.) and lung lesions multiple (e.g. *S. aureus* in IDUs).
- Necrotizing pneumonia—seen in severe cases of anaerobic infection and may affect a single segment or extend to involve one or both lungs, with associated empyema. Disease rapidly spreads, destroying large volumes of parenchyma. Patients appear ill with a pronounced leucocytosis. Pulmonary actinomycosis may present similarly.
- Amoebic lung abscesses—features of coexistent liver abscess and presents with cough productive of brown-red (anchovy sauce) sputum.
- Complications—empyema (one-third of cases), brain abscess, localized bronchiectasis. TB should be considered in the differential diagnosis.

Diagnosis

- Radiology—CXR may reveal a cavity with an air–fluid level. CT scan facilitates the detection of smaller lesions.
- Microbiology—sputum culture is helpful only in the diagnosis of amoebic infection. Culture of empyema fluid or percutaneous transtracheal aspiration (CT-guided) is useful where possible. Quantitative culture of bronchoscopic sampling can provide good results. It is essential samples are placed in anaerobic conditions for transport to the laboratory. BCs may be positive but may not reveal the entire infecting flora.

Treatment

- Empirical therapy while awaiting culture—community-acquired cases, e.g. ceftriaxone and metronidazole; nosocomially acquired infection (cover for *S. aureus*), e.g. piperacillin/tazobactam. Vancomycin should be considered if local rates of MRSA warrant it.
- Antibiotics should be given for 2–4 months. Patients should be monitored carefully for relapse.
- Bronchoscopy and postural physiotherapy may facilitate drainage.
- Surgical resection is rarely required outside the context of malignancy.

Prognosis

- Overall mortality is <15% for anaerobic lung abscesses, and ~25% for anaerobic necrotizing pneumonia.
- Mortality is higher in acute pneumonias caused by organisms such as *S. aureus*.

Cystic fibrosis

CF is the commonest autosomal recessive disease amongst Caucasian populations (affecting 1 in 2000–3000 live births). CF usually presents with respiratory infections and pancreatic insufficiency.

Pathogenesis

CF is caused by mutations in the CF transmembrane conductance regulator (CFTR) protein, which is found in all exocrine tissues. Defective transport of chloride and other ions leads to thick, viscous secretions in the lungs, pancreas, liver, intestine, and reproductive tract, and to increased sweat chloride levels.

Microbiology

- *S. aureus*—most prevalent organism in childhood, persists in adulthood.
- *H. influenzae*—affects 20–30% of children, less prevalent in adults.
- *P. aeruginosa*—colonizes in childhood or early adolescence; >80% are infected by adulthood. Early non-mucoid isolates can be eradicated. Later isolates produce large amounts of mucoid polysaccharide (alginate), are difficult to eradicate, and are associated with greater mortality than non-mucoid strains. Chronic infection is associated with rapid decline in lung function and increased mortality.
- *B. cepacia* complex—an important and highly transmissible group of pathogens, intrinsically resistant to aminoglycosides and polymyxins. May be difficult to identify, requiring specific isolation media ± referral to reference laboratory. Colonized patients should be separated from the non-colonized. Infection with *B. cenocepacia* can lead to a rapid deterioration in pulmonary function, bacteraemia, and even death amongst adolescents and young adults (cepacia syndrome).
- Other pathogens—non-typeable *H. influenzae, S. maltophilia, Achromobacter* (formerly *Alcaligenes*) *xylosoxidans*, NTM (e.g. *M. abscessus* complex, MAC), *Aspergillus* spp.

Clinical features

- Reflect obstruction of organs by viscous secretions and the presence of chronic bacterial lung infection.
- General features—chronic cough, wheeze, recurrent pneumonia, sinusitis, clubbing, haemoptysis, pneumothorax, signs of respiratory impairment. Hypoxia and CO_2 retention are uncommon. The CXR may show airway thickening, retained secretions, and bronchiectasis.
- Acute respiratory infections—patients often produce a large amount of purulent sputum, even when well. Episodes of deterioration are associated with increased volume and purulence of sputum, dyspnoea,

wheeze, chest ache, anorexia, and malaise. High fever or sepsis is unusual, despite the large number of organisms in the secretions (10^8 organisms/mL of sputum). CXR may be unchanged from the patient's normal film. Forced expiratory volume in 1s (FEV_1) falls, returning to pre-infection levels with successful antibiotic therapy.
- Other clinical features include meconium ileus, distal ileal obstruction, rectal prolapse, biliary disease, infertility, musculoskeletal disorders, recurrent venous thrombosis, nephrolithiasis, and nephrocalcinosis.

Management

The aims are to slow lung damage by removing viscous airway secretions, control bacterial infection, and monitor the appearance of highly transmissible or antibiotic-resistant organisms. Antibiotics need to be given to CF patients for longer and at frequent, higher doses than non-CF patients. Outpatient IV antibiotic therapy may be given via a long line. Those requiring very frequent antibiotics may require insertion of a Port-a-cath.

- *General measures*—postural drainage, deep breathing, coughing, exercise, aerosolized DNase I (reduces mucus viscosity, clears airway secretions), inhaled steroids, bronchodilators (helpful in some patients). Pneumococcal and annual influenza vaccinations are recommended. Lung transplantation should be considered if life expectancy is <2 years and quality of life is severely impaired despite medical therapy.
- Antimicrobial prophylaxis—controversial. A Cochrane review[7] found that antibiotic prophylaxis against *S. aureus* infection reduced isolation of *S. aureus* from the sputum but had no impact on lung function. Whereas the US guidelines do not recommend it, the UK Cystic Fibrosis Trust recommends PO flucloxacillin from diagnosis until the age of 2 years, and some UK clinics promote lifelong prophylaxis.[8]
- Eradication of *Pseudomonas* colonization—the first isolation of a non-mucoid *Pseudomonas* strain should be treated with the aim of eradication (e.g. 6 weeks of PO ciprofloxacin 750mg bd with nebulized colistimethate sodium 1 mega unit bd).
- Long-term management of *Pseudomonas* colonization—patients with established colonization may benefit from long-term nebulized antibiotics (e.g. colistimethate sodium or tobramycin) to reduce the bacterial burden; studies have shown improved lung function and reduced episodes of respiratory illness in such patients. Some centres advocate elective courses of IV antipseudomonal therapy every 3 months to reduce the frequency of exacerbations and consequent lung damage. There is no evidence to support this.
- Treatment of acute exacerbations—the patient's most recent sputum culture result should be used to guide therapy. Broad-spectrum oral agents are beneficial, despite the presence of resistant *P. aeruginosa*. High doses and prolonged therapy (3–4 weeks) are recommended. Aggressive IV therapy is indicated in those patients who do not respond to oral treatment. Such therapy is usually directed at *P. aeruginosa*, e.g. ceftazidime and an aminoglycoside. Once-daily aminoglycoside dosing is as effective as three times a day and is associated with reduced toxicity in children. *H. influenzae* and *S. aureus* should be treated if isolated, even if the patient is asymptomatic. *B. cepacia* is very resistant and

should be treated with a combination of two or three agents such as ceftazidime and an aminoglycoside. Nebulized vancomycin can be used to treat MRSA colonization of sputum, but IV therapy is required for exacerbations. Parenteral therapy may be given on an outpatient basis and should continue for 10–14 days or longer. *Aspergillus* is frequently cultured from sputum. Treatment (steroids ± antifungals) is indicated only for ABPA, if present.

References

7 Smyth AR, Walters S. Prophylactic anti-staphylococcal antibiotics for cystic fibrosis. *Cochrane Database Syst Rev*. 2012;**12**:CD001912.
8 Antibiotic treatment for cystic fibrosis, Third edition, May 2009. Available at https://www.cysticfibrosis.org.uk/the-work-we-do/clinical-care/consensus-documents.

Bronchiectasis

Bronchiectasis is a respiratory condition characterized by chronic daily cough, mucopurulent sputum production, and bronchial wall thickening and luminal dilatation on CT chest.

Epidemiology

- The prevalence of bronchiectasis is unknown but probably varies between countries.
- Prevalence increases with age, and the condition is commoner in women.

Aetiology and pathogenesis

- Induction of bronchiectasis requires an infectious insult and impaired drainage, airway obstruction (e.g. foreign body, tumour, anatomical abnormality), or a defect in host defence (e.g. ciliary dyskinesia, α1-antitrypsin deficiency, hypogammaglobulinaemia, immunosuppression).
- Conditions associated with bronchiectasis include CF, Young's syndrome, rheumatoid arthritis, Sjögren's syndrome, and rarely SLE and Marfan's syndrome.
- A number of pulmonary infections have been associated with the development of bronchiectasis, e.g. pertussis, MTB, NTM infections, ABPA.
- Organisms isolated during acute exacerbations include *H. influenzae, M. catarrhalis, S. aureus, P. aeruginosa*, and less commonly *S. pneumoniae*.

Clinical features

- The classic feature is chronic cough, productive of mucopurulent sputum for months to years. Other symptoms include dyspnoea, wheezing, rhinosinusitis, fatigue, haemoptysis, and pleuritic chest pain.
- Physical findings include crackles, wheezing, and finger clubbing.

Diagnosis

- Initial assessment should include FBC, immunoglobulins, IgG subclass levels, pneumococcal antibody titres before, and 4 weeks after, pneumococcal vaccination, and *CFTR* gene mutation analysis.

- A sputum sample should be sent for smear and culture for pyogenic bacteria, mycobacteria, and fungi.
- Total serum IgE, *Aspergillus* IgE and IgG antibodies, α1-antitrypsin levels, and rheumatoid factor should be checked, if clinically indicated.
- Lung function tests show an obstructive defect.
- Other tests include examination of the ciliary epithelium (suspected ciliary dysfunction) or IGRA (in patients at risk of TB).

Imaging

- CXR findings include linear atelectasis, dilated and thickened airways ('tramline' thickening or ring shadows), and irregular peripheral opacities (mucus plugs).
- CT scan is the imaging modality of choice—characteristic features include airway dilatation, lack of tapering, bronchial wall thickening, mucopurulent plugs/debris with distal airway trapping, and cysts of the bronchial wall.

Management

- Treatment of the underlying disease—in most cases, it is not possible to treat the underlying disease, as bronchiectasis is a result of previous infection or problems with clearing secretions. Some conditions may be treated to prevent disease progression, e.g. NTM infections, primary immunodeficiencies, ABPA.
- Acute exacerbations—most afebrile, clinically stable patients can be treated as outpatients. The initial selection of an oral antibiotic is usually based on previous sputum microbiology results and tailored in light of new culture results. Treatment is usually given for 10 days or 14 days if *P. aeruginosa* is isolated. Inpatient treatment is required for patients with fever, tachypnoea, hypoxia, hypotension, or failure to improve with oral antibiotics.
- Inhaled glucocorticoids are not routinely used, unless there is concomitant asthma.
- Other medications that are used in selected patients include bronchodilators, medications to reduce gastro-oesophageal reflux, and immunizations.
- Prevention of exacerbations—for patients with recurrent exacerbations, preventative therapy with macrolides may be indicated. Chest physiotherapy may help to clear the airways and prevent exacerbations. There are insufficient data to support the use of nebulized saline, inhaled mannitol, or acetylcysteine.
- Patients with severe haemoptysis may require interventions to control bleeding, e.g. bronchial artery embolization or surgery.
- Surgical resection of bronchiectatic lung or lung transplantation may be required in some cases.

Further reading

Pasteur MC, Bilton D, Hill AT; British Thoracic Society Bronchiectasis non-CF Guideline Group. British Thoracic Society guideline for non-CF bronchiectasis. *Thorax*. 2010;**65** Suppl 1:i1–58.

Pulmonary tuberculosis

TB is caused by the MTB complex which comprises seven closely related species—*M. tuberculosis* (➔ see *Mycobacterium tuberculosis*—ACDP 3, pp. 355–9), *M. bovis, M. africanum, M. microti, M. canetti, M. caprae*, and *M. pinnipedii*.

Epidemiology

TB is estimated to infect >2 billion people (one-third of the world's population). In 2014, there were 9.6 million new cases of TB and 1.5 million deaths worldwide[9]. An estimated 1.2 million cases were HIV-infected, and 0.4 million deaths occurred in this group. Over 50% of cases were in South East Asia and the Western Pacific, and a further quarter were in Africa, which had the highest death rates. In 2014, an estimated 480 000 people developed MDR-TB, and an estimated 190 000 died. XDR-TB is estimated to affect 9.7% of patients with MDR-TB.

Pathogenesis

- Primary disease—TB is transmitted by inhalation of infected droplet nuclei which results in primary infection in the lungs. If the innate immune system of the host fails to eliminate the infection, the bacilli proliferate inside alveolar macrophages, resulting in the formation of a granulomatous tubercle. If bacterial replication is not controlled, the tubercle enlarges, and the bacilli enter local draining lymph nodes, causing lymphadenopathy (Ghon focus). Bacteraemia may accompany initial infection. Failure by the host to mount an effective cell-mediated response and tissue repair leads to progressive destruction of the lung. Unchecked bacterial growth may lead to haematogenous spread of bacilli to produce disseminated TB.
- Latent disease—in most individuals (90%), MTB infection is contained initially by host defences, and infection remains latent. However, latent infection has the potential to develop into active disease at any time.
- Reactivation disease—this results from proliferation of previously dormant bacteria seeded at the time of the primary infection. Reactivation disease occurs in ~10% of cases. Risk factors include increased age, HIV infection, corticosteroid use, inhibitors of TNF-α and its receptor, end-stage renal disease, diabetes mellitus, and lymphoma.

Clinical features

The clinical presentations of pulmonary TB include:

- primary TB—symptoms include fever, pleuritic chest pain, and less commonly retrosternal pain, fatigue, cough, arthralgia, and pharyngitis. The CXR may be normal or show hilar adenopathy, pleural effusions, and upper or lower lobe pulmonary infiltrates.
- Reactivation TB—symptoms include fever, night sweats, cough, weight loss, fatigue, chest pain, and haemoptysis. The CXR typically shows upper lobe pulmonary infiltrates, but other findings include hilar adenopathy, infiltrates or cavities in the middle or lower lung zones, pleural effusions, and solitary nodules.

- Endobronchial TB—occurs in 10–40% of patients with pulmonary TB and presents acutely with cough, sputum production, wheezing, haemoptysis, and chest pain. The CXR may be normal or show upper lobe infiltrates and cavitation.
- Other presentations—these include laryngeal TB, lower lung field TB, and tuberculoma.
- Complications—these include haemoptysis, pneumothorax, bronchiectasis, extensive tissue destruction, septic shock, malignancy, venous thromboembolism, and chronic pulmonary aspergillosis.

Diagnosis

(See references 10, 11.)

- Sputum smear microscopy—this remains the commonest diagnostic method. Special stains, e.g. ZN or auramine phenol, show AFB. Fluorescence microscopy increases sensitivity.
- Mycobacterial culture—this is the diagnostic gold standard but may not be available in resource-limited settings. Automated liquid culture systems, e.g. the MGIT, are increasingly being used.
- NAATs—these detect MTB complex DNA; are more sensitive in smear-positive than smear-negative cases. Automated NAAT systems, e.g. the Xpert® Rif/TB assay, which simultaneously detect MTB DNA and rifampicin resistance, are increasingly being used.
- Drug susceptibility testing (DST)—this is performed at reference laboratory level.
- IGRAs—these are used for the diagnosis of latent TB infection.

Management

- For drug-susceptible pulmonary TB, the standard short-course regimen is 2-month initiation phase with four drugs (rifampicin, isoniazid, pyrazinamide, ethambutol), followed by a 4-month continuation phase with two drugs (rifampicin and isoniazid).
- For suspected MDR- and XDR-TB, the regimen should be modified to include several drugs to which the isolates are likely to be susceptible—seek expert advice. These treatment regimens are more toxic and much longer than regimens for drug-susceptible TB. Patients must be monitored closely for toxicity and response to treatment.

References

9 World Health Organization (2015). *Global tuberculosis report 2015*. Available at: http://www.who.int/tb/publications/global_report/en/.

10 Public Health England (2014). *Tuberculosis in the UK 2014 report*. Available at: https://www.gov.uk/government/uploads/system/uploads/attachment_data/file/360335/TB_Annual_report__4_0_300914.pdf.

11 National Institute for Health and Care Excellence (2016). *Tuberculosis*. NICE guideline 33. Available at: https://www.nice.org.uk/guidance/ng33.

Chapter 15

Cardiovascular infections

Infective endocarditis *630*
Intravascular catheter-related infections *632*
Endovascular infections *634*
Myocarditis *636*
Pericarditis *638*
Mediastinitis *640*

Infective endocarditis

IE is characterized by infection of the endocardial surface of the heart. It may be classified as acute, subacute, or chronic, depending on the time course of the infection. It is now more commonly classified according to the type of valve (native or prosthetic) and the aetiological agent (e.g. staphylococcal, streptococcal, enterococcal, fungal, culture negative, etc.).

Epidemiology

The incidence of IE is estimated to be 0.16–5.4 cases per 1000 hospital admissions. Most patients are aged 30–60 years; male > female. The disease is uncommon in children in the absence of a predisposing condition. Risk factors include congenital heart disease, rheumatic heart disease, degenerative heart disease, prosthetic valves, IVCs, IDU, and mitral valve prolapse.

Pathogenesis

The development of IE requires the simultaneous occurrence of a number of events: alteration of the valvular surface, deposition of platelets and fibrin, colonization by bacteria, bacterial multiplication, and development of a vegetation.

Aetiology

- Eighty per cent of cases of native valve endocarditis are due to streptococci (viridans group, *S. gallolyticus*) or staphylococci.
- *S. aureus* is the commonest isolate in IDUs and tricuspid valve IE.
- *S. epidermidis* is the commonest isolate in early (<2 months) prosthetic valve endocarditis (PVE).
- Enterococcal endocarditis is usually associated with malignancy or manipulation of the GU or GI tracts.
- Other organisms, e.g. *Corynebacteria, Listeria, Bacillus, Salmonella, E. coli, Enterobacter, Citrobacter*, and *Pseudomonas* spp., are uncommon.
- HACEK organisms or fungi are associated with large vegetations.
- Culture-negative endocarditis (~5%) may be caused by *C. burnetii, Chlamydia* spp., *Legionella* spp., *M. pneumoniae, Bartonella* spp., and *Brucella* spp.
- Polymicrobial infections occur in 1–2%.

Clinical features

- The incubation period may vary from days to weeks.
- Symptoms are protean and include fever, chills, weakness, dyspnoea, sweats, anorexia, weight loss, malaise, cough, skin lesions, stroke, nausea, vomiting, headache, myalgia, arthralgia, oedema, chest pain, abdominal pain, delirium, coma, haemoptysis, and back pain.
- Physical findings include fever, cardiac murmur, Roth spots, clubbing, splinter haemorrhages, Osler's nodes, Janeway lesions, petechiae, peripheral emboli, splenomegaly, and septic complications (pneumonia, meningitis, mycotic aneurysms; ➔ see Endovascular infections, pp. 634–6).

Laboratory diagnosis

- BCs are positive in approximately two-thirds of cases. Three BC sets should be obtained in the first 24h and incubated for 3 weeks.
- Blood tests may show elevated ESR (90–100%), anaemia (70–90%), leucocytosis (20–30%), leucopenia (5–15%), and thrombocytopenia (5–15%). Hypergammaglobulinaemia (20–30%) may result in false-positive results for rheumatoid factor and VDRL. Renal impairment and hypocomplementaemia occur in 5–15%.
- Urinalysis is frequently abnormal with proteinuria (50–60%), microscopic haematuria (30–60%), gross haematuria, pyuria, bacteriuria, red cell casts, and white cell casts.
- Serology is useful for diagnosis of culture-negative endocarditis.
- Echocardiography—transthoracic echocardiography (TTE) allows visualization of vegetations in 60–75% of cases, compared with >95% with transoesophageal echocardiography (TOE).
- ECG—lengthening of the PR interval in aortic valve endocarditis indicates aortic root involvement.

Duke criteria

This schema stratifies patients with suspected IE into three categories:

- definite—identified histopathologically or by clinical criteria. Clinical diagnosis requires the presence of two major criteria, one major and two minor criteria, or five minor criteria:
  - major criteria—≥2 positive BCs (or a single positive culture for *C. burnetii*), echocardiographic evidence for endocardial involvement;
  - minor criteria—predisposing condition (heart condition, IDU), temp >38°C, vascular phenomena, immunological phenomena, microbiological evidence (not satisfying major criteria).
- possible—one major and one minor criteria, or three minor criteria;
- rejected—firm alternative diagnosis, rapid resolution with no or short-course antibiotics, no pathological evidence of IE.

Management

- Antimicrobial therapy is targeted at the causative organism:
  - UK endocarditis guidelines;[1]
  - US endocarditis guidelines.[2]
- Surgery is indicated in patients with life-threatening CCF or cardiogenic shock due to surgically treatable valvular disease, if the patient has a reasonable prospect of recovery. Surgery is recommended for annular or aortic abscesses, heart block, recurrent emboli on therapy, antibiotic-resistant infections, and fungal endocarditis.

Prevention

There are few data to support antimicrobial prophylaxis for the prevention of IE. For detailed recommendations, see NICE guidelines for prevention of endocarditis,[3] and American Heart Association guidelines for prevention of endocarditis.[4]

References

1 Gould FK, Denning DW, Elliot TS, *et al.*; Working Party of the British Society for Antimicrobial Chemotherapy. Guidelines for the diagnosis and antibiotic treatment of endocarditis in adults: a report of the Working Party of the British Society for Antimicrobial Chemotherapy. *J Antimicrob Chemother*. 2012;**67**:269–89.

2 Baddour LM, Wilson WR, Bayer AS, *et al.* Infective endocarditis: diagnosis, antimicrobial therapy, and management of complications: a statement for healthcare professionals from the Committee on Rheumatic Fever, Endocarditis, and Kawasaki Disease, Council on Cardiovascular Disease in the Young, and the Councils on Clinical Cardiology, Stroke, and Cardiovascular Surgery and Anesthesia, American Heart Association: endorsed by the Infectious Diseases Society of America. *Circulation*. 2005;**111**:e394–434.

3 National Institute for Health and Care Excellence (2008). *Prophylaxis against infective endocarditis: antimicrobial prophylaxis against infective endocarditis in adults and children undergoing interventional procedures*. NICE clinical guideline 64. Available at: http://www.nice.org.uk/guidance/CG64.

4 Wilson W, Taubert KA, Gemitz M, *et al.* Prevention of infective endocarditis: guidelines from the American Heart Association: a guideline from the American Heart Association Rheumatic Fever, Endocarditis, and Kawasaki Disease Committee, Council on Cardiovascular Disease in the Young, and the Council on Clinical Cardiology, Council on Cardiovascular Surgery and Anesthesia, and the Quality of Care and Outcomes Research Interdisciplinary Working Group. *Circulation*. 2007;**116**:1736–94.

Intravascular catheter-related infections

Definitions

- *Catheter colonization*—significant growth of organism in quantitative or semi-quantitative culture from catheter tip, subcutaneous segment, or catheter hub.
- *Phlebitis*—induration, erythema, pain, or tenderness around the exit site.
- *Exit site infection*—exudate at exit site yielding microorganism or phlebitis <2cm from the exit site plus signs of infection (fever, pus) ± BSI.
- *Tunnel infection*—phlebitis ≥2cm from the exit site, along the subcutaneous tract of the catheter ± BSI.
- *Pocket infection*—infected fluid in subcutaneous pocket of implanted intravascular device, often associated with local erythema, induration, tenderness, rupture and drainage, and necrosis of skin ± BSI.
- *BSI*—bacteraemia or fungaemia in a patient who has an intravascular device and ≥1 positive BC obtained from a peripheral vein and no obvious source (apart from the device).

Epidemiology

In the USA, >200 000 nosocomial BSIs occur per year; most of these are related to intravascular devices. Risk factors for IVC-related infections include type of catheter, site of catheter, duration of placement, and hospital demographics.

Aetiology

- Staphylococci, e.g. CoNS, *S. aureus*.
- Aerobic Gram-negative bacilli, e.g. *E. coli, Klebsiella* spp., *Pseudomonas* spp., *Enterobacter* spp., *Serratia* spp., *Acinetobacter* spp.
- Fungi, e.g. *C. albicans, Candida* spp., *M. furfur*.

Clinical features

The clinical features are unreliable. The most sensitive clinical features, e.g. fever and chills, lack specificity, whereas inflammation and purulence at the catheter site are specific but not sensitive.

Diagnosis

- Rapid diagnostic techniques, e.g. Gram stain or acridine orange stain, may be used for diagnosis of exit site infections but have poor sensitivity.
- Cultures of IVC tips—semi-quantitative (roll plate) or quantitative (flush, vortex, or sonication) methods have greater specificity than qualitative methods.
- Paired BCs drawn through IVC and percutaneously—all patients with suspected IVC-related infections should have two sets of BCs drawn, at least one peripherally. A positive culture from a line requires clinical interpretation, whereas a negative culture virtually excludes catheter-related BSI.
- Quantitative cultures of CVC and peripheral blood samples—a 5- to 10-fold difference in colony count between the central and peripheral cultures, or an absolute colony count of >100 cfu/mL from a central culture supports the diagnosis of catheter-related BSI.
- Differential time to positivity for CVC and peripheral cultures—this method takes advantage of continuous blood culture monitoring, e.g. by radiometric methods to compare differential times to positivity between central and peripheral cultures. It correlates well with quantitative methods and is suitable for use in routine laboratories.

Management

- See IDSA guidelines for management of IVC-related infections.[5]
- PVCs—remove IVC; swab the exit site if pus present, and take two sets of BCs before starting antimicrobial therapy.
- Non-tunnelled CVCs—if there are local or systemic signs or positive BCs, the CVC should be removed, antimicrobial therapy started, and the CVC replaced at a new site:
  - complicated infections (septic thrombosis, endocarditis, osteomyelitis): remove the CVC, and treat with systemic antimicrobials for 4–6 weeks;
  - uncomplicated CoNS infection: remove the CVC, and treat with 5–7 days of systemic antibiotics;
  - uncomplicated *S. aureus* bacteraemia: remove the CVC, and treat with 14 days of systemic antibiotics (if negative TOE) or 4–6 weeks of antibiotics (if positive TOE);
  - uncomplicated Gram-negative bacteraemia: remove the CVC, and treat with 10–14 days of systemic antibiotics;
  - uncomplicated candidaemia: remove the CVC, and treat with antifungals for 14 days after the last positive BC.
- Tunnelled CVCs and implanted devices (IDs)—investigations should be performed to establish the CVC or ID as the source of infection:
  - tunnel infection or port abscess: remove the CVC/ID, and treat with systemic antibiotics for 10–14 days;

- complicated infections (septic thrombosis, endocarditis, osteomyelitis): remove the CVC/ID, and treat with systemic antibiotics for 4–6 weeks;
- uncomplicated CoNS infection: retain the CVC/ID, and treat with 7 days of systemic antibiotics plus antibiotic lock therapy for 10–14 days. Remove the CVC/ID if persistent bacteraemia or clinical deterioration;
- uncomplicated *S. aureus* bacteraemia: remove the CVC/ID, and treat with 14 days of systemic antibiotics (if negative TOE) or 4–6 weeks of antibiotics (if positive TOE). For salvage therapy, see IDSA guidelines;[5]
- uncomplicated Gram-negative bacteraemia: remove the CVC/ID, and treat with 10–14 days of systemic antibiotics.

Prevention

See IDSA guidelines for the prevention of intravascular catheter-related infections.[6]

References

5 Mermel LA, Allon M, Bouza E, *et al*. Clinical practice guidelines for the diagnosis and management of intravascular catheter-related infection: 2009 Update by the Infectious Diseases Society of America. *Clin Infect Dis*. 2009;**49**:1–45.

6 O'Grady NP, Alexander M, Burns LA, *et al*.; Healthcare Infection Control Practices Advisory Committee (HICPAC). Guidelines for the prevention of intravascular catheter-related infections. *Clin Infect Dis*. 2011;**52**:e162–93.

Endovascular infections

Persistent bacteraemia (i.e. multiple BCs taken on different occasions which are positive for the same isolate) suggests endovascular infection. These include endocarditis, IVC-related infections, mycotic aneurysms, pacemaker infections, and vascular graft infections.

Mycotic aneurysm

- *Definition*—a mycotic aneurysm may be any extra- or intracardiac aneurysm of infectious origin, except syphilitic aortitis.
- *Aetiology*—in the pre-antibiotic era, mycotic aneurysms were usually associated with IE and caused by streptococci and staphylococci. Today mycotic aneurysms are usually due to haematogenous seeding of atherosclerotic vessels or trauma. Pathogens include *S. aureus*, *Salmonella* spp., aerobic Gram-negative bacilli, *L. monocytogenes*, *B. fragilis*, group A and C streptococci, *C. septicum*, enterococci, and pneumococci.
- *Clinical features*—symptoms and signs of IE (➔ see Infective endocarditis, pp. 630–2) may be present. Intracranial mycotic aneurysms are usually silent but may present with headache, homonymous hemianopia, or focal neurological symptoms and signs. Symptomatic intracranial haemorrhages carry a high mortality. Visceral mycotic aneurysms are uncommon. The commonest location is the superior mesenteric artery, but other sites include the hepatic artery, coeliac

artery, external iliac artery, and femoral, peripheral, and carotid arteries. Aortic aneurysms are usually associated with infected atherosclerotic lesions and present with fever, back or abdominal pain ± draining cutaneous sinus.

- *Diagnosis*—BCs may identify the causative organism in 50–85%. Echocardiography is useful to visualize aortic valve mycotic aneurysms. CT brain scan may show intracerebral haemorrhages, although cerebral angiography is the investigation of choice for intracranial mycotic aneurysms. Magnetic resonance (MR) angiography is less invasive but less sensitive. Abdominal X-ray may show calcified abdominal aorta. CT or MRI abdomen are less sensitive than angiography for intra-abdominal aneurysms.
- *Management*—intracranial mycotic aneurysms should be treated with antimicrobial therapy, monitored by angiography, and excised if they enlarge or bleed. Infected atherosclerotic aneurysms should be operated on before rupture occurs, and systemic antibiotics continued for 6–8 weeks post-operatively. Peripheral vessel mycotic aneurysms are managed by surgical resection/reconstruction and antibiotic therapy.

Pacemaker infections

- Pacemaker infections affect 1–7% of procedures. Superficial infections involve the generator pocket and/or subcutaneous electrode. Deep infections involve the transvenous intravascular electrode ± generator.
- *Aetiology*—CoNS and *S. aureus* are the commonest isolates. Other organisms include *Enterobacteriaceae* spp., *P. aeruginosa, C. albicans*, streptococci, enterococci, *Corynebacteria* spp., *Listeria* spp., and *Aspergillus* spp.
- *Clinical features*—infections confined to the generator pocket usually present with local swelling, erythema, tenderness ± discharge through the incision site or fistula ± systemic symptoms. Infection of the epicardial electrodes may be associated with pericarditis (➔ see Pericarditis, pp. 638–9), mediastinitis (➔ see Mediastinitis, pp. 640–1), bacteraemia, and systemic symptoms. Infection of the intravascular portion presents with clinical features of endocarditis (➔ see Infective endocarditis, pp. 630–2).
- *Management*—superficial infection confined to the subcutaneous elements may be treated by a one-stage exchange under antimicrobial cover. For pacemaker endocarditis, the generator and electrodes should be removed transcutaneously, if possible, but surgical extraction may be required. A temporary pacing system is inserted, and at least 2 weeks' systemic antimicrobial therapy is given before insertion of a permanent system. A full course of endocarditis therapy should be given; this may need to be extended if there is evidence of metastatic infection.

Vascular graft infections

- *Epidemiology and pathogenesis*—the incidence of vascular graft infection is 1–5%. Three mechanisms are thought to be responsible for infection: intraoperative contamination (commonest), extension from adjacent infected tissue, haematogenous seeding.

- *Aetiology*—*S. aureus* is the commonest cause. However, a wide range of organisms may cause infection, e.g. *Enterobacteriaceae* spp., CoNS, enterococci, streptococci, *P. aeruginosa, Bacteroides* spp., and corynebacteria.
- *Clinical features*—these depend on the site of the graft infection:
  - inguinal graft infections present with an inguinal mass ± pain, erythema, fever, and sinus formation;
  - abdominal graft infections present with fever, abdominal pain or mass, retroperitoneal bleeding, lower extremity emboli, and GI bleeding due to erosion into the GI tract.
- *Diagnosis*—superficial graft infections may be readily diagnosed clinically. Deep grafts may require radiological imaging (e.g. CT or MRI abdomen) to confirm the infection. BCs are often negative, unless infection involves the graft lumen.
- *Management*—surgical resection of the infected graft and revascularization (preferably through an extra-anatomic, uninfected route) is the treatment of choice. Systemic antimicrobial therapy is given for 4–6 weeks post-operatively. If the arterial stump is found to be infected at the time of surgery, culture-specific antimicrobial therapy is given for 6 months post-operatively. Salvage therapy with long-term suppressive antibiotic therapy is sometimes given for vascular graft infections that are not surgically resectable.

Myocarditis

An inflammatory disease of the myocardium, which may be caused by a variety of infectious and non-infectious causes. May be acute, subacute, or chronic, and focal or diffuse.

Aetiology

- Myocardial injury may be a consequence of direct cell damage by an infectious agent, by a circulating toxin, or by immune reactions following infection. The cause is not identified in most cases.
- Viruses are the commonest agents in the developed world, e.g. measles, influenza, polio, mumps, adenovirus, and the group B Coxsackie viruses.
- Bacterial infection may cause myocarditis through immunological mechanisms (e.g. Lyme disease, acute rheumatic fever) or through direct myocardial infection with associated inflammation (e.g. brucellosis, meningococcal, streptococcal, and staphylococcal sepsis, *Legionella* spp., *M. pneumoniae*, and *C. psittaci* infection). Toxin-mediated damage is seen in infection by *C. diphtheriae* and *C. perfringens*.
- Parasitic causes include trypanosomal disease, e.g. *T. cruzi* is a common cause in South America.
- Disseminated infection in the immunocompromised may lead to myocarditis (e.g. *Toxoplasma, Aspergillus*, and *Cryptococcus* spp.). Cardiac dysfunction may be clinically apparent in up to 20% of AIDS patients, with echocardiographic abnormalities in up to 65% of AIDS patients.

Pathogenesis

The pathological process varies according to the mechanism of the injury and whether it is acute or chronic. All lead to an inflammatory infiltrate and damage to adjacent myocardial cells. In addition, some agents damage vascular endothelial cells. Routine histology rarely allows a definitive aetiological diagnosis. Where normal cardiac function is regained, histological abnormalities may lag behind clinical improvement. Cases that leave permanent damage are marked by interstitial fibrosis and a loss of muscle fibres.

Clinical presentation

- Myocarditis may be asymptomatic or result in severe heart failure or sudden death.
- Myocarditis should be considered in a young person developing cardiac abnormalities in the context of a recognized systemic illness or in an otherwise well individual developing unexpected heart failure or arrhythmias (e.g. supraventricular tachycardia (SVT) or extrasystoles).
- Fever, malaise, upper respiratory tract symptoms, tachycardia, dyspnoea, and chest pain may precede Coxsackie virus myocarditis.
- On examination, there may be cardiomegaly, murmurs, and signs of cardiac failure.
- Pericarditis may coexist.

Diagnosis

- Diagnosis can be difficult in those cases occurring in the context of fulminant systemic infection.
- ECG changes are non-specific (e.g. sequential ST elevation and T wave inversion).
- Around one-third of patients with biopsy-proven myocarditis have raised troponin levels.
- Echocardiography may demonstrate systolic dysfunction and can be used to track the progression of disease.
- MRI scanning is a sensitive means of detecting myocardial inflammation.
- Endomyocardial biopsy is considered the gold standard for diagnosis but can miss cases in which disease is focally distributed, and timing is critical—most experts believe it is not warranted in most cases.
- Demonstrating a viral cause requires isolation of the virus or viral material from the myocardium. Generally, diagnosis is inferred by serology (e.g. Lyme disease) or detection of the organism in other specimens (e.g. stool or blood).

Treatment

- Therapy should be directed at the causative agent where possible.
- General measures include bed rest (exercise is associated with increased death in mouse models) and management of heart failure and arrhythmias. Most patients recover completely.
- Severe cases may require cardiac assist devices.
- Steroids are of no benefit and are probably deleterious overall. Immunoglobulin administration may help certain subgroups (e.g. CMV myocarditis). Antivirals may be of benefit in the future.

Differential diagnosis

Pericarditis, idiopathic congestive cardiomyopathy, acute rheumatic fever, non-infectious myocarditis (collagen vascular disease, thyrotoxicosis, drug- or radiation-induced).

Pericarditis

An inflammation of the pericardium which may be acute or chronic.

Aetiology

- 'Idiopathic' cases account for up to 86% of cases and are probably viral.
- Viruses—Coxsackie B virus, adenovirus, hepatitis C, CMV, echovirus, influenza virus (including H1N1), EBV, parvovirus B19, and HHV-6.
- Bacteria—before antibiotics became widely available, bacterial pericarditis (e.g. *S. aureus* and *S. pneumoniae*) was a recognized complication of pneumonia. Bacterial pericarditis is now uncommon and tends to occur following Gram-negative infection in older people with predisposing conditions, e.g. oesophageal perforation, head/neck infections (usually anaerobes), and in cases of meningococcal septicaemia. Other bacterial causes include *M. pneumoniae*, *L. pneumophila*, and *H. influenzae*. Tuberculous pericarditis is a major cause of heart failure in sub-Saharan Africa—chronic disease is associated with constrictive pericarditis.
- Fungi—these include *H. capsulatum*, *C. immitis*, *Aspergillus* spp., *C. neoformans*, and *Candida* spp.
- Parasites—these include *T. gondii*, *E. histolytica*, and *T. canis*.

Pathogenesis

- Viruses reach the pericardium haematogenously, and infection results in inflammation of both the visceral and parietal pericardium, with or without a pericardial effusion. Most patients recover—some may experience episodes of relapse, a phenomenon that is probably related to immune mechanisms, rather than persistent viral infection. It is rare that viral pericarditis leads to constriction.
- Bacterial infection may occur as a result of direct inoculation (trauma or surgery), contiguous spread (e.g. endocarditis or untreated pneumonia), or bacteraemia. Fluid is usually grossly purulent, and subsequent organization with adhesions may lead to constriction.
- TB pericarditis may arise from haematogenous spread (during primary infection), lymphatic spread (from the regional lymph nodes), or contiguous spread (from infected lung or pleura). Initial fibrin deposition, granuloma formation, and polymorphonuclear cell infiltration are followed by the development of a serous/serosanguinous effusion with lymphocytes and plasma cells. Later, the pericardium is thickened by fibrin deposition and granulomas. In late disease, the pericardial space is taken up with adhesions and fibrous tissue, leading to constriction.

Clinical presentation

- Idiopathic or viral pericarditis—retrosternal chest pain, radiating to the shoulder/neck and aggravated by breathing or lying flat. Fever may be present, along with flu-like features.
- Bacterial pericarditis is usually seen in the context of severe systemic infection with an acutely ill patient. Chest pain and pericardial rubs may be reported in less than one-third of patients. Bacterial pericarditis may be recognized late, after the onset of haemodynamic complications.
- TB pericarditis has an insidious onset with chest pain, weight loss, night sweats, cough, and breathlessness. The classic clinical finding is a pericardial rub. Where the effusion is significant, there may be jugular venous distension and pulsus paradoxus.

Diagnosis

- Diagnosis is often made clinically and depends on the history.
- The ECG is abnormal in 90% of cases (due to diffuse subepicardial inflammation), with 50% showing the classic findings of early ST elevation in multiple leads, resolving over a few days to be replaced with T wave flattening/inversion.
- Echocardiography is useful in diagnosing and assessing effusions and the extent of any compromise.
- Virus isolation from throat swabs or stool, or acute and convalescent viral serology, may lead to a diagnosis but rarely affect management.
- Diagnostic sampling may be indicated if the effusion persists for >3 weeks, when TB, fungal infection, malignancy, or connective tissue disorders should be considered.
- Pericardiotomy with biopsy is preferable to pericardiocentesis, as it has a higher diagnostic yield and fewer complications.

Treatment

- Viral/idiopathic—bed rest, analgesia, and monitoring for haemodynamic complications. Steroids should be avoided in the acute phase, due to frequent concomitant myocarditis in which steroids are contraindicated. They may, however, have a role in preventing recurrent pericarditis, once a patient has recovered. Colchicine may also be useful.
- Purulent bacterial—surgical drainage and appropriate antibiotic therapy are essential. Early pericardiocentesis may be lifesaving, but fluid often reaccumulates. Overall mortality, however, remains at around 30%—particularly in those cases associated with endocarditis or following surgery.
- TB—antituberculous therapy should be initiated. Constrictive pericarditis may develop in up to half of patients, despite this. Steroids (prednisolone 60mg for 4 weeks, then reducing over 7 weeks), in addition to antituberculous therapy, reduce the need for repeat drainage, as well as result in a modest reduction in those developing constriction. Those developing haemodynamic compromise secondary to effusion reaccumulation or progressive pericardial thickening benefit from early surgery (pericardectomy).

Mediastinitis

Acute mediastinitis is an uncommon, but potentially devastating, infection involving the mediastinal structures.

Epidemiology and pathogenesis

- Primary infection is rare. Almost all cases are secondary to:
  - cardiothoracic surgery, now the commonest cause;
  - oesophageal perforation, e.g. iatrogenic, trauma, spontaneous;
  - head and neck infections, e.g. odontogenic, Ludwig's angina, pharyngitis, tonsillitis, epiglottitis, parotitis;
  - spread from other infections, e.g. pneumonia, empyema, subphrenic abscess, pancreatitis, skin or soft tissue infections of the chest wall, osteomyelitis of the sternum, clavicle, ribs, or vertebrae, haematogenous seeding.

Aetiology

- The spectrum of organisms causing infection varies strikingly according to the underlying cause.
- Post-surgical infections are usually monomicrobial and caused by MSSA (45%), MRSA (16%), Gram-negative bacilli (17%), CoNS (13%), and streptococci (5%).
- Oesophageal perforation or head and neck infections are usually polymicrobial and caused by oral streptococci (e.g. viridans streptococci, peptococci, peptostreptococci) and anaerobic Gram-negative bacilli (e.g. *Bacteroides* spp., *Fusobacterium* spp., *Prevotella* spp., *Porphyromonas* spp.)

Clinical features

- The clinical manifestations also depend on the underlying cause.
- Head and neck infections usually present with fever, pain, and swelling of the affected site.
- Oesophageal perforation may be obvious or clinically inapparent.
- Symptoms include chest pain (site depends on the location of infection), respiratory distress, and dysphagia.
- Physical signs include fever, tachycardia, crepitus, and oedema of the head and neck. Hamman's sign (a crunching sound heard over the precordium synchronous with the cardiac rhythm) is due to emphysema of the mediastinum.
- Post-cardiothoracic mediastinitis usually presents within 2 weeks of surgery, with fever, wound erythema/discharge, and chest pain (often pleuritic). Sternal instability, wound dehiscence, and chest wall emphysema may occur.

Diagnosis

- Blood tests show leucocytosis and raised inflammatory markers. BCs may yield the causative organism(s).
- CXR may show mediastinal widening, air–fluid levels, and subcutaneous or mediastinal emphysema.
- CT thorax is particularly useful in post-operative mediastinitis to distinguish superficial wound infections from deep retrosternal infections.

Management

- Prompt surgical intervention is required with drainage, debridement, and repair (in cases due to oesophageal perforation). Post-operative mediastinitis may be managed by the open technique (wound debrided and left open to heal by secondary intention) or the closed technique (debridement, primary closure, and irrigation through drains).
- Appropriate parenteral antibiotic therapy should be initiated as soon as the diagnosis is made. Empiric therapy should cover the most likely organisms (e.g. penicillin and metronidazole or clindamycin for head and neck/oesophageal infections, and vancomycin and meropenem for post-operative mediastinitis).

Complications

- Pericardial effusion/cardiac tamponade.
- Pleural effusions/empyema.
- Peritonitis.
- Sternal osteomyelitis (post-operative mediastinitis).

Chapter 16

Gastrointestinal infections

Oesophagitis *644*
Peptic ulcer disease *645*
Infectious diarrhoea *647*
Enteric fever *649*
Cholera *652*
Clostridium difficile diarrhoea *654*
Cholecystitis *656*
Acute cholangitis *658*
Pancreatitis *659*
Primary peritonitis *661*
Secondary peritonitis *662*
Peritoneal dialysis peritonitis *664*
Diverticulitis *666*
Intra-abdominal abscess *667*
Liver abscess *670*
Acute hepatitis *671*
Chronic hepatitis *673*
Other gastrointestinal infections *674*

Oesophagitis

Inflammation of the oesophagus, generally non-infectious (e.g. gastro-oesophageal reflux), but may also be caused by a variety of infectious agents, usually in the context of impaired immunity (HIV, transplant recipients, or those receiving cancer chemotherapy).

Aetiology

- *Candida*—*C. albicans* is the commonest cause of oesophagitis. Other *Candida* spp. are less commonly isolated. Colonization is seen in 20% of the population (particularly those receiving antacid therapy). Infection follows when breakdown of local and systemic defences permit invasion to the deeper epithelial layers. Endoscopy reveals yellow-white plaques adhering to a hyperaemic oesophagus (usually the distal third). Removing these reveals an inflamed, friable surface. Perforation occurs rarely. Predisposing factors: acute or advanced HIV infection, diabetes mellitus, haematological malignancy, broad-spectrum antibiotic therapy, corticosteroid therapy, conditions that impair oesophageal motility (systemic sclerosis, achalasia), reflux oesophagitis.
- *CMV*—seen usually in AIDS patients (the cause in around 30% of such patients reporting oesophageal symptoms) or the severely immunosuppressed. Endoscopy may demonstrate large ($10cm^2$), shallow 'punched-out' ulcers. Diagnosis is best made by histopathological examination of biopsies obtained from the ulcer edge and base, which show enlarged endothelial cells with large intranuclear inclusions. Isolation of CMV in culture is not reliable due to contamination from blood or saliva. Co-infection with HSV or *Candida* spp. is common.
- *HSV*—usually seen in those with significant immunosuppression; rare in healthy adults. HSV-1 is commoner than HSV-2. Accounts for up to 16% of HIV patients with oesophageal symptoms. Presentation may be with odynophagia, chest pain, fever, nausea, and vomiting; <25% may develop clinically significant GI bleeding. Oral/labial or cutaneous HSV infection may be apparent (<38% of cases). Endoscopy reveals multiple small, superficial ulcers in the distal third of the oesophagus. Large confluent ulcers and denuded epithelium may be seen as infection progresses. Viral PCR of brushing or biopsies is the most sensitive means of diagnosis.
- *Idiopathic ulceration*—extensive ulceration may occur in those with acute or advanced HIV, or in mild form in the otherwise healthy. These may be attributed to unrecognized infectious agents. A course of prednisolone (40mg a day for 14 days, then tapered to stop) improves symptoms in the majority of HIV-related aphthous ulceration.

Clinical features

Patients present with difficulty in, or pain on, swallowing. Liquids may be better tolerated than solids. Pain may be worse with acidic substances. Severe ulcerative oesophagitis can cause such severe pain that oral intake is limited to the point of weight loss and dehydration. GI bleeding can occur. Oesophagitis can exist in the absence of symptoms (<41%). Fever may be seen in those with CMV or mycobacterial infection. Vomiting is commoner with CMV than other causes. The presence of oral lesions may be indicative of the cause of oesophagitis (e.g. oral thrush, or herpetic ulceration).

Diagnosis and treatment

Accurate diagnosis of oesophageal candidiasis requires endoscopic brushing (with a sheathed cytology brush) and biopsy. The gross appearance can mislead—white lesions may be seen with HSV, CMV, and candidal infection. Histopathological examination and viral PCR may identify viral causes. Fungal culture is useful only in the management of refractory cases, e.g. to identify the species and sensitivities.

Management

- Diagnostic endoscopy may not always be feasible (bleeding, severe pain, critical illness), particularly in those patients developing oesophagitis secondary to cancer chemotherapy. Empirical treatment for *Candida* and HSV infection may be appropriate (e.g. IV amphotericin and aciclovir), particularly if symptoms are very severe or oral thrush/HSV stomatitis are apparent.
- Patients receiving immunosuppressant therapy may need drug level monitoring if treated with antifungals such as fluconazole.
- *Candida* spp.—fluconazole PO or IV for 14–21 days.
- HSV—aciclovir IV for 7–14 days or PO for 14–21 days.
- CMV—ganciclovir IV for 14–21 days.

Oesophagitis in AIDS patients

- Oesophageal symptoms are seen in 40–50% of patients with AIDS at some point in their illness and affect nutritional status and morbidity.
- *Candida* oesophagitis is commonest and can be treated empirically with fluconazole in mild cases if oral thrush is observed in a symptomatic patient (70% will have oesophageal involvement). Alternative agents include itraconazole solution, voriconazole, posaconazole or IV echinocandins (caspofungin, micafungin, or anidulafungin). Amphotericin is now rarely used, as it is more toxic than other agents.
- Viruses cause one-third of cases (often in association with candidiasis). Three-quarters will have a partial or complete response to induction therapy with antiviral drugs, but relapses are common without maintenance treatment; 70% of HSV oesophagitis responds to aciclovir, but relapse is seen in 15% within 4 months.
- Other rare causes of oesophagitis in HIV: EBV, MAC, *C. neoformans, Cryptosporidium, Actinomyces.*

Peptic ulcer disease

H. pylori is a motile, curved GNR that lives within the mucus layer overlying the gastric (and occasionally duodenal or oesophageal) mucosa. It is present in most people with peptic ulcer disease, increasing the risk of several inflammatory and neoplastic processes. All clinical isolates of *H. pylori* produce urease. It has been isolated from people in all parts of the world—humans appear to be the major reservoir, with transmission likely to be via faeco-oral, and possibly oral–oral, routes. Rates of colonization are equal between men and women. Carriage is near universal by age 20 years in developing countries. Prevalence is over 50% by age 50 years in the UK. One to 3% of those who remain free of the organism by adulthood acquire the bacteria each year.

Clinical features

- Acute acquisition—may cause an acute upper GI illness with nausea and abdominal discomfort, with vomiting, burping, and fever lasting 3–14 days. However, infection is clinically silent in most individuals. There have been some documented cases of acute self-limiting infection.
- Persistent colonization—*H. pylori* persists for decades in the majority of people. Acute symptoms do not recur in most, although the incidence of non-ulcer dyspepsia is slightly higher in colonized individuals.
- Duodenal ulceration—90% have *H. pylori* infection. The organism is found only in areas of metaplastic gastric-type epithelium, and its presence is associated with an over 50 times greater risk of duodenal ulceration.
- Gastric ulceration—50–80% are colonized with *H. pylori*. A greater proportion of gastric ulcers are associated with NSAID or aspirin use.
- Gastric carcinoma—the presence of *H. pylori* has been identified as a risk factor for gastric carcinoma. It induces a chronic gastritis which is thought to lead to atrophic and metaplastic changes over decades. However, *H. pylori* is neither necessary nor sufficient for oncogenesis.
- Gastric lymphoma—colonization is strongly associated with mucosa-associated lymphoid tissue (MALT) tumours (lymphomas arising from B lymphocytes). There is evidence to suggest that eradication may lead to improvement in tumour histology.
- Oesophageal disease—as the incidence of *H. pylori* colonization falls, it appears the incidence of gastro-oesophageal reflux disease (GORD), Barrett's oesophagus, and oesophageal adenocarcinoma are on the rise. Certain *H. pylori* strains may have an inverse association with Barrett's oesophagus. It has been shown that eradication of *H. pylori* in those with duodenal ulceration doubles the rate of GORD development, and patients with GORD are less likely to be colonized with *H. pylori* than controls.

Diagnosis

- Endoscopy with biopsy—*H. pylori* infection is diagnosed by one of three methods: biopsy urease test, histology, or less commonly bacterial culture. Antral biopsies can be tested for urease activity using commercial tests (e.g. CLO test), which detect the production of ammonia from urea which results in a colour change. Gastric biopsy histology may demonstrate *H. pylori* and also provides information about the presence of gastritis, intestinal metaplasia, or MALT. Bacterial culture and sensitivity testing of *H. pylori* are difficult and rarely performed.
- Serology—ELISA tests detect IgG, which is positive in nearly all colonized patients (sensitivity 90–100%, specificity 76–96%). Local prevalence of *H. pylori* infection affects the positive predictive value of antibody tests. Inaccurate tests are commoner in the elderly and in those with cirrhosis.

Treatment

- Various treatment regimens for the treatment of *H. pylori* have been evaluated in clinical trials, but the optimal therapy has not been defined.
- The incidence of metronidazole resistance varies with geography—80–90% in the tropics and up to 50% in some European countries. The incidence of macrolide resistance is 4–12%.
- Triple therapy—this is used in areas with low levels of clarithromycin resistance (<15%). The commonest regimen is a PPI plus amoxicillin (1g bd) and clarithromycin (500mg bd) for 7–14 days. Metronidazole (250mg qds) may be used, instead of amoxicillin, in penicillin-allergic patients.
- Quadruple therapy—this is indicated in areas with high levels of resistance to clarithromycin or metronidazole, or in patients who have recent or repeated exposure to either drug. It consists of a PPI combined with bismuth (525mg qds) and two antibiotics, e.g. metronidazole (250mg qds) and tetracycline (500mg qds) for 10–14 days. Doxycycline (100mg bd) may be used as an alternative to tetracyline.
- Other regimens—one study has shown that a combination of levofloxacin, omeprazole, nitazoxanide, and doxycycline for 7–10 days had a higher cure rate than triple therapy.
- Sequential therapy—this 10-day regimen consists of a PPI plus amoxicillin for 5 days, followed by PPI plus clarithromycin and metronidazole for 5 days. Levofloxacin may be used as an alternative to amoxicillin (if penicillin allergy) or clarithromycin (if resistance is high).
- Multiple trials have shown that sequential therapy and quadruple therapy are equally effective in treatment-naïve patients.

Infectious diarrhoea

Definitions

- Gastroenteritis is inflammation of the stomach and intestinal epithelium.
- Diarrhoea is the passage of ≥3 loose/liquid stools within 24h.
- Food poisoning is vomiting and/or diarrhoea caused by eating food contaminated with microorganisms or toxins (bacterial or otherwise, e.g. poisonous mushrooms).
- Dysentery is bloody diarrhoea with mucus, tenesmus, pain, and fever usually caused by bacterial, parasitic, or protozoan infection.

Aetiology

- Some individuals are at higher risk (e.g. previous gastric surgery, immunodeficiency), and recent antibiotic use predisposes to antibiotic-associated diarrhoea. Bacterial infections are commoner in the tropics. In the UK, causes of gastroenteritis include:
  - general patients—viruses (50–70% of cases, e.g. rotavirus, norovirus), *Campylobacter, Shigella, Salmonella, C. perfringens, S. aureus, B. cereus, E. coli, C. difficile*, parasites (10–15%, e.g. *Giardia, Cryptosporidium*);

- immunosuppressed patients—general causes plus increased *E. coli*, *Cryptosporidium*, mycobacteria, microsporidia, CMV, and HSV (especially HIV patients with CD4 count <200/mm^3);
- returning travellers—enterotoxigenic *E. coli* (30–70%), *Shigella* spp. (5–20%), *Salmonella* spp. (5%), *Campylobacter* (5–20%), *V. parahaemolyticus* (shellfish), viral (10–20%), protozoal (5–10%).

Clinical features

- History:
  - nature of the diarrhoea—blood, mucus, or pus? Is it painful? Watery diarrhoea with blood or mucus implies large bowel pathology; fatty or smelly diarrhoea suggests small bowel involvement;
  - timing (acute or chronic)—an abrupt onset suggests bacterial and viral infections. Chronic diarrhoea is more characteristic of parasites and may also occur with non-infectious causes, e.g. IBD or malignancy;
  - food history—specific restaurant, reheated food, unusual diets, fish;
  - are other people affected—is it an outbreak, and, if so, what was the source?
  - recent antibiotic use (in community or hospital);
  - foreign travel—country, city, or rural, with reference to timing of possible exposures, e.g. food from a street vendor;
  - risk factors for immunosuppression.
- Examination:
  - is the patient febrile, systemically unwell, and shocked? Consider infection, as well as surgical causes, e.g. diverticulitis;
  - wasting implies a longer-standing problem, e.g. small bowel malabsorption, immunosuppression, malignancy;
  - rectal examination—blood, mucus, faecal occult blood, impacted faeces causing overflow diarrhoea, rectal carcinoma.
- When GI symptoms are followed by neurological signs, think of *Clostridium botulinum* (nausea, dry mouth, cranial nerve palsies, and descending weakness with respiratory and autonomic dysfunction), or *C. jejuni* infection-associated GBS (occurs 1–3 weeks after GI symptoms).
- Differential diagnosis—non-infectious causes of food poisoning include mushrooms and metal poisoning. Non-infectious causes of diarrhoea include perforation, appendicitis, diverticulosis, IBD, colonic malignancy, ischaemic colitis, malabsorption, irritable bowel syndrome, constipation with overflow, thyrotoxicosis, drugs, and autonomic neuropathy.

Investigations

- Blood tests—anaemia or macrocytosis may be due to malabsorption. Renal failure may occur with dehydration or HUS. Blood film shows red cell fragmentation in HUS.
- Sigmoidoscopy may show inflamed colonic mucosa ± pseudomembranes (*C. difficile* colitis). Biopsies may be taken to exclude IBD.
- Abdominal X-ray or CT abdomen may be necessary to exclude surgical causes.

- Stool samples should be sent to the laboratory for:
  - microscopy—blood and pus cells indicate infectious diarrhoea (e.g. *Salmonella, Shigella*, or *Campylobacter* spp.) or IBD. Ova, cysts, and parasites may be diagnostic in patients with a history of foreign travel. Modified ZN stain for *Cryptosporidium* (preschool children and the immunocompromised);
  - culture—detects specific pathogens such as *Salmonella* spp., *Shigella* spp., *C. jejuni, E.coli* O157, *Yersinia* spp., and *Vibrio* spp.; special media are required;
  - toxin detection—either the toxin itself within stool (e.g. *C. difficile*) or the toxin gene in isolated organisms (e.g. *E. coli* O157).

Management

- Oral rehydration is sufficient in mild cases. Oral rehydration salts are commercially available. Patients with moderate or severe dehydration require IV replacement or fluid and electrolytes.
- Antibiotics are not generally indicated in immunocompetent patients. The exceptions are: early *C. jejuni* enteritis, *Y. enterocolitica* infections (children and the immunocompromised), *S. dysenteriae*, severe *S. enteritidis* and *S. typhimurium* infections (e.g. bacteraemia), *G. lamblia*, and *E. histolytica*.
- Antispasmodic agents—useful in mild diarrhoea without blood. Do not use if there is a suggestion of dysentery.

Public health aspects

All cases of suspected food poisoning or dysentery should be notified to public health. PHE has issued guidelines for the prevention of person-to-person spread following GI infections.[1]

Reference

1 Working Group of the former PHLS Advisory Committee on Gastrointestinal Infections. Preventing person-to-person spread following gastrointestinal infections: guidelines for public health physicians and environmental health officers. *Commun Dis Public Health*. 2004;7:362–84. Available at: http://www.hpa.org.uk/cdph/issues/CDPHvol7/No4/guidelines2_4_04.pdf.

Enteric fever

The clinical and pathological features of typhoid fever were first described in the nineteenth century by Louis (1829) and then by Jenner (1850). The term enteric fever was proposed by Wilson in 1869. Typhoid Mary (Mary Mallon) worked as a cook in New York in the early 1900s and infected 49 people with typhoid, three of whom died. She was forcibly quarantined and died after almost 30 years in isolation. The species that cause enteric fever are *S. enterica* serotype Typhi and *S. enterica* serotype paratyphi A, B, or C.

Epidemiology

Enteric fever is a global health problem, affecting an estimated 12–33 million people per year. The disease is endemic in many developing countries, e.g. Indian subcontinent, Asia, Africa, and Central and South America. The organisms are spread by ingestion of faecally contaminated food or water.

Direct person-to-person spread is rare, and laboratory transmission has been reported. Outbreaks in developing countries may result in high morbidity and mortality. In developed countries, infection is usually associated with international travel, although food-borne outbreaks do occur.

Pathogenesis

Inoculum size and decreased gastric acidity are important determinants of disease severity. The ability of the organisms to survive within macrophages is essential to disease pathogenesis and spread. Organisms multiply in Peyer's patches, then enter the bloodstream and re-invade the small bowel, causing bleeding and peritonitis. The Vi antigen of S. typhi prevents antibody-mediated opsonization, increases resistance to peroxide, and confers resistance to complement-mediated lysis.

Clinical features

- The incubation period ranges from 5 to 21 days, depending on the inoculum size, age, gastric acidity, and host immune status.
- Abdominal symptoms (e.g. diarrhoea, constipation, or abdominal pain) may initially develop, then resolve. This is followed by non-specific symptoms (e.g. chills, diaphoresis, headache, anorexia, cough, weakness, sore throat, muscle pains, dizziness, delirium, or psychosis), prior to the onset of fever.
- On examination, patients are acutely ill with fever, rose spots, abdominal tenderness, and hepatosplenomegaly. Cervical lymphadenopathy, respiratory crepitations, cholecystitis, pancreatitis, seizures, or coma may also occur.
- Complications occur in the third or fourth week of illness and include intestinal perforation or haemorrhage, endocarditis, pericarditis, hepatic or splenic abscesses, and orchitis.
- Mortality rates are <1% in developed countries but may be as high as 10–30% in developing countries, as a result of delayed treatment or MDR strains.
- Long-term carriage (presence of salmonellae in stool or urine for >1 year) occurs in 1–4% of patients with S. typhi. It is associated with biliary abnormalities, concurrent infection with *S. haematobium*, and an increased risk of developing cholangiocarcinoma.

Diagnosis

- Culture—definitive diagnosis requires isolation of the organism from cultures of blood (40–80% positive,), stool (30–40% positive), or bone marrow (50–90% positive). Other diagnostic samples include urine, rose spots, or duodenal contents. A combination of specimens increases the likelihood of diagnosis. Cultures should be tested for sensitivity to nalidixic acid, as resistant organisms have reduced susceptibility to fluoroquinolones.
- Serology—tests like the Widal test detect antibodies to S. typhi. They are of limited clinical utility in endemic areas, because they do not distinguish recent from past infection. Newer ELISA and dipstick tests are better, but their sensitivity and specificity are not adequate for routine diagnostic use.

Management

- The emergence and spread of MDR strains (resistant to ampicillin, co-trimoxazole, and chloramphenicol) and increasing resistance to fluoroquinolones have made treatment challenging.
- Antibiotic selection depends on local resistance patterns, patient age, whether oral medications are feasible, and the clinical setting.
- Fluoroquinolones—are the first-line treatment for uncomplicated enteric fever, apart from in areas with high rates of resistance. Regimens include ciprofloxacin (500mg bd) or ofloxacin (400mg bd) for 7–10 days. They are bactericidal, concentrate intracellularly and in the bile, and result in faster resolution of fever.
- Ceftriaxone (2–3g daily IV) for 7–14 days is indicated in severe systemic disease and in patients with suspected fluoroquinolone resistance.
- Alternative agents include: (i) cefixime (20mg/kg/day PO in two divided doses) for 7–14 days, (ii) azithromycin (1g PO stat, followed by 500mg daily for 5–7 days or 1g daily for 5 days), or (iii) chloramphenicol (2–3g PO in four divided doses) for 14 days.
- Corticosteroids—early studies in the 1980s suggested that dexamethasone was associated with reduced mortality in critically ill patients treated with chloramphenicol. It is not certain whether these findings would be confirmed in the post-chloramphenicol era.
- Surgery—this is indicated in patients with ileal perforation.

Relapse

This may occur 2–3 weeks after treatment in 1–6% of patients. These are treated with an additional course of therapy to which the organism is susceptible.

Chronic carriage

Chronic carriage with excretion of organisms in the stool occurs in 1–6% of patients—rates are higher in patients with biliary tract abnormalities. Carriers do not develop recurrent disease but pose a risk to others, particularly if they are food handlers. Eradication therapy with fluoroquinolones for 4 weeks is indicated. Cholecystectomy may be required.

Prevention

- There are two vaccines available for protection against S. typhi—neither is completely effective nor do they provide protection against S. paratyphi.
- The live oral vaccine Ty21a has an efficacy of 35% and 58% at year 1 and year 2, respectively.
- The parenteral Vi polysaccharide vaccine has an efficacy of 69% and 59% at year 1 and year 2, respectively.
- Immunization is recommended for travellers to high-risk areas such as the Indian subcontinent.

Cholera

Cholera is an acute diarrhoeal disease caused by *V. cholerae*, a highly motile, halophilic, curved GNR. The disease is caused by toxigenic strains. *V. cholerae* is classified on the basis of the O-antigen. Over 200 serotypes exist, but only *V. cholerae* O1 and O139 cause epidemics. *V. cholerae* O1 is the predominant cause of cholera worldwide. *V. cholerae* O1 has two major serotypes (Inaba and Ogawa) and two biotypes (El Tor and classical).

Epidemiology

- Cholera has the ability to cause both epidemics with pandemic potential and to remain endemic in affected areas.
- Epidemic cholera affects non-immune individuals of all ages, occurs after a single introduction, spreads by the faeco-oral route, and has high secondary spread.
- Endemic cholera affects children aged 2–15 years, has an aquatic or asymptomatic human reservoir, and is spread by water or food or faeco-orally. Immunity increases with age, and secondary spread is variable. Cases show seasonal variation.
- Six pandemics occurred between 1817 and 1923 caused by *V. cholerae* O1 classic biotype originating from the Indian subcontinent. The seventh originated in Indonesia in 1961 caused by *V. cholerae* O1 El Tor biotype. Following the 2010 Haiti earthquake there was a huge O1 outbreak—the worst in recent history.
- In 1992, a new epidemic caused by *V. cholerae* O139 occurred in India and Bangladesh. This has subsequently subsided.

Pathogenesis

The infectious dose varies from 10^2 to 10^8 organisms. Reduced gastric acidity is associated with an increased severity of disease. Pathogenic strains have two virulence factors—cholera toxin and toxin co-regulated pilus. The latter is pilus that aggregates organisms on the surface of the small intestine. The toxin has a B subunit that binds to gangliosides on the epithelial surface and allows the A subunit to enter the cell. Once inside the cell, the A subunit increases cAMP activity, resulting in chloride secretion at the apical surface and concurrent losses of sodium and water.

Clinical features

- Infection with *V. cholerae* results in a spectrum of disease, from asymptomatic to severe diarrhoea.
- Abdominal pain, vomiting, and borborygmi are common early symptoms.
- Fever is uncommon, occurring in <5% of cases.
- Severe disease is characterized by profuse watery diarrhoea ('rice water stool') and can result in hypovolaemia and electrolyte loss. Patients may be anxious, restless, or obtunded, with sunken eyes, dry mucous membranes, and loss of skin elasticity. Severe disease is commoner in pregnancy and associated with fetal loss in up to 50%.

- Complications—hypoglycaemia, coma, acute kidney injury, pneumonia, bacteraemia (rare), 'cholera sicca' (fluid accumulation in the intestinal lumen without diarrhoea).

Laboratory diagnosis

- Dark-field microscopy—of fresh rice water stools shows large numbers of motile vibrios whose movement can be blocked by specific antisera.
- Stool culture—on selective media (thiosulfate citrate bile salts sucrose agar or tellurite taurocholate gelatin agar), followed by identification using biochemical tests. Serogroup and serotype are determined by specific antibodies.
- Rapid tests—these include commercial immunochromatographic lateral flow devices, e.g. Crystal VC™ dipstick.

Management

(See references 2, 3, and 4.)

- The goal of therapy is to restore fluid losses rapidly and safely.
- Evaluate the patient for the degree of dehydration: mild (<5% fluid loss), moderate (5–10% fluid loss), or severe (>10% fluid loss).
- Rehydrate the patient in two phases: intensive phase (2–4h); maintenance phase (until diarrhoea resolves).
- Use IV fluids only for: severely dehydrated patients in rehydration phase (50–100mL/kg/h); moderately dehydrated patients who cannot tolerate oral fluids; high stool volumes (>10mL/kg/h) in maintenance phase.
- Use oral hydration salts (OHS) for patients in maintenance phase (800–1000mL/h), matching input with output.
- Discharge patients when all the following criteria are fulfilled: oral intake ≥1000mL/h; urine volume ≥400mL/h; stool volume ≤400mL/h.
- Antimicrobial agents play a secondary role in treatment and have been shown to reduce duration and volume of diarrhoea. Oral tetracycline (500mg qds PO for 3 days) or doxycycline (300mg stat PO) are the agents of choice in adults with sensitive strains. Alternative agents include: furazolidone (100mg qds PO for 3 days), co-trimoxazole (960mg bd PO for 3 days), ciprofloxacin (20mg/kg stat), or azithromycin (20mg/kg stat).

Prevention

- A clean water supply and good sanitation are the cornerstones of prevention.
- Vaccines—two oral cholera vaccines are available: (i) WC-rBS, a killed whole-cell vaccine of *V. cholerae* O1 and recombinant cholera toxin B subunit, and (ii) bivalent killed whole-cell vaccine containing *V. cholerae* O1 and O139.

References

2 Seas C, DuPont HL, Valdez LM, Gotuzzo E (1995). Practical guidelines for the treatment of cholera. *Drugs*. **51**:966–73.

3 Morris JGJr (2003). Cholera and other types of vibriosis: a story of human pandemics and oysters on the half shell. *Clin Infect Dis*. **37**:272–80.

4 Sack DA, Sack RB, Nair GB, Siddique AK (2004). Cholera. *Lancet*. **363**:223–33.

Clostridium difficile diarrhoea

Diarrhoea is the commonest complication of antibiotic therapy, occuring in up to 15% of those receiving β-lactam antibiotics and 25% of those receiving clindamycin. *C. difficile* is the frequent cause (20–30% of antibiotic-associated diarrhoea, 50–75% of antibiotic-associated colitis).

Epidemiology

- Antibiotic-associated diarrhoea and colitis were reported soon after the widespread use of antibiotics. In 1978, *C. difficile* was identified as the main causative agent and largely attributed to clindamycin. Since then, it has been associated with a range of antibiotics, including penicillins, cephalosporins, and fluoroquinolones.
- Between 1989 and 1992, a strain of *C. difficile* resistant to clindamycin, the 'J strain', was implicated in large outbreaks in the USA.
- From 2003 to 2006, *C. difficile* infections became more frequent, severe, and resistant to treatment in North America and Europe. These were attributed to a new strain designated B1, NAP1, or ribotype 027. This strain occurred in older hospitalized patients, and was associated with fluoroquinolone use and high rates of colectomy and death.
- Since 2005, *C. difficile* ribotype 078 has emerged in the Netherlands. It also caused severe disease but was community-acquired, occurred in a younger population, and is genetically similar to porcine isolates.
- Transmission—patients with *C. difficile* carriage, whether symptomatic or not, are a reservoir for environmental contamination. *C. difficile* is highly transmissible via fomites, as well as the hands, clothing, and stethoscopes of HCWs.
- Risk factors for CDAD—antibiotic use, hospitalization, advanced age, severe illness, gastric acid suppression, enteral feeding, GI surgery, obesity, cancer chemotherapy, haematopoietic stem cell transplantation.

Microbiology

- *C. difficile* is an anaerobic, Gram-positive, spore-forming, toxin-producing bacillus, which is difficult to culture on conventional media. It exists in spore form in the environment and converts to its vegetative form in the colon where it produces toxins.
- *C. difficile* produces two potent exotoxins—toxin A (enterotoxin) and toxin B (cytotoxin). Toxin A activates neutrophils and causes mucosal injury, fluid secretion, and inflammation. Toxin B is essential for virulence and ten times more potent than toxin A.

Clinical features

- Infection with toxigenic *C. difficile* may be asymptomatic (particularly in neonates) or symptomatic, or cause fulminant colitis. Markers of severe disease include high WCC, raised blood creatinine, fever, low albumin, as well as clinical features.
- Carrier state—about 20% of hospitalized adults carry *C. difficile* and shed it in their stools but do not have diarrhoea.

- *C. difficile* diarrhoea—symptoms commonly start 5–10 days after antibiotic therapy (<10 weeks after therapy has finished). Features include fever, abdominal pain, and leucocytosis.
- Pseudomembranous colitis—patients present with symptoms of colitis and have yellow/white pseudomembranes visible on sigmoidoscopy/colonoscopy.
- Fulminant colitis—presents with severe abdominal pain and distension, fever, hypovolaemia, marked leucocytosis, and lactic acidosis. Toxic megacolon is a clinical diagnosis based on systemic symptoms plus colonic dilatation >7cm on abdominal X-ray. Bowel perforation leads to peritonitis.
- Other presentations—protein-losing enteropathy with ascites, CDAD in IBD, appendicitis, skin and soft tissue infection, splenic abscess, osteomyelitis, Reiter's syndrome (all rare).
- Differential diagnosis—other infectious causes of diarrhoea, adverse drug reaction, ischaemic colitis, IBD.

Diagnosis

- Requires the presence of diarrhoea and either a stool test positive for *C. difficile* toxins or toxigenic *C. difficile* or endoscopic/histological evidence of pseudomembranous colitis.
- EIA for *C. difficile* GDH—useful as a screening test, as glutamate dehydrogenase (GDH) is produced by all *C. difficile* isolates, but its detection does not distinguish between toxigenic and non-toxigenic strains.
- EIA for *C. difficile* toxins A and B—sensitivity is about 75%, and specificity is up to 99%.
- PCR tests—real-time PCR tests that detect toxin A and B genes are highly sensitive (potential for false-positive results). Often used in combination with EIA tests.
- Cell culture cytotoxicity assay—the gold standard test that detects the cytopathic effects of *C. difficile* toxins on fibroblast monolayers. Highly sensitive, but labour-intensive and slow (2 days).
- Cepheid Xpert® *C. difficile* PCR assay—97% sensitivity and 93% specificity, compared with cytotoxicity assay.
- Culture—culture on selective anaerobic plates is also highly sensitive but is slow and does not distinguish toxigenic from non-toxigenic strains.
- Endoscopy—colonoscopy or sigmoidoscopy and biopsy are a useful adjunct in the following situations: (i) high clinical suspicion of CDAD with negative laboratory tests, (ii) prompt diagnosis before laboratory tests available, (iii) failure to respond to therapy, and (iv) atypical presentation with ileus or minimal diarrhoea.

Management

(See reference 5.)

- General measures—isolate the patient; implement infection control measures; discontinue the precipitating drug; replace fluid/electrolyte losses, and avoid antimotility agents.
- Non-severe disease—PO metronidazole (500mg tds). Vancomycin is an option, but there is concern that overuse may lead to the selection of VRE.

- Severe disease—PO vancomycin (125mg qds) for 10–14 days (lower failure rates and faster response than metronidazole). Consider fidaxomicin in those with severe disease at high risk of relapse. Consider IV metronidazole (400mg tds) and PR vancomycin (500mg in 100mL of normal saline qds) in those unable to take oral therapy.
- Recurrent disease—occurs in ~25% of patients, usually 1–3 weeks after completing therapy. Options for treatment of the initial recurrence include metronidazole (non-severe), vancomycin (severe), or fidaxomicin (200mg bd for 10 days). Second relapses are treated with tapering doses of vancomycin (125mg qds for 7–14 days, then slowly reducing over 5 weeks). Alternatives: fidaxomicin (200mg bd for 10 days) or vancomycin (125mg qds for 14 days), followed by rifaximin (400mg bd for 14 days).
- Surgery is rarely necessary but is lifesaving in cases of toxic megacolon or perforation. Mortality in such cases is around 35%.
- Alternative therapies—these include: (i) probiotics, (ii) faecal bacteriotherapy, (iii) anion-binding resins, (iv) IVIG. Of these, there is only good evidence for faecal bacteriotherapy, with reported response rates of <90%.[6]

Prevention

Limit the use of inciting agents, e.g. antibiotics and PPIs. Infection control measures, such as handwashing, universal precautions, and phenolic disinfectants for environmental cleaning, are of proven benefit in reducing *C. difficile* transmission in health-care settings.

References

5 Public Health England (2013). *Updated guidance on the management and treatment of Clostrdium difficile infection*. Available at: https://www.gov.uk/government/publications/clostridium-difficile-infection-guidance-on-management-and-treatment.

6 van Nood E, Vrieze A, Nieuwdorp M, *et al* (2013). Duodenal infusion of donor feces for recurrent *Clostridium difficile*. *N Engl J Med*. **368**:407–15.

Cholecystitis

Inflammation of the gall bladder which may develop acutely or gradually over time. Acute cholecystitis presents with fever and right upper quadrant pain and is usually related to gallstone disease. Acalculous cholecystitis (without gallstones) presents in a similar fashion usually in critically ill patients. Chronic cholecystitis is characterized by chronic inflammation of the gall bladder and is usually asymptomatic or minimally symptomatic.

Pathogenesis

Ninety per cent of patients have gallstones impacted in the cystic duct. The consequent increase in intraductal pressure impairs blood supply and lymphatic drainage. Tissue necrosis and bacterial proliferation follow within the gall bladder. Complications occur in 10–15% of cases: gall bladder empyema, emphysematous cholecystitis (elderly diabetic men), gall bladder perforation and peritonitis, pericholecystic abscess, intraperitoneal abscess, cholangitis, liver abscess, pancreatitis, bacteraemia. The differential diagnosis includes: MI, ulcer perforation, intestinal obstruction, right lower lobe pneumonia.

Clinical features

Early obstruction may cause only mild epigastric pain and nausea. Transient cases may settle in 1–2h. Persistent obstruction sees the symptoms localize to the right upper quadrant and increase in severity with signs of peritoneal irritation (shoulder tip pain). The gall bladder may be palpable in 30–40% of cases. Patients with acute cholecystitis often have a positive 'Murphy's sign'—pain on inspiration, as the gall bladder descends towards, and presses against, the examining fingers. Fever may occur. Most patients settle within 4 days, with 25% requiring surgery or developing complications. Complications include: (i) gall bladder gangrene, (ii) gall bladder perforation, (iii) cholecystoenteric fistula, (iv) gallstone ileus, and (v) emphysematous cholecystitis.

Diagnosis

- Blood tests—WCC is usually raised; 50% of patients have mild elevations of bilirubin; 40% have raised AST, 25% raised ALP.
- Microbiology—bacteria may be isolated from bile, even in asymptomatic cases of cholecystitis. Rates of bile infection rise with the duration of symptoms and the age of the patient, and in jaundiced patients (particularly with common bile duct (CBD) obstruction). The organisms isolated are those of the intestinal flora: enteric Gram-negative bacilli (*E. coli, Klebsiella, Enterobacter, Proteus* spp.), enterococci, and anaerobes (*Bacteroides*, clostridia, *Fusobacterium* spp.). Anaerobic organisms may be found in polymicrobial infection and are often isolated following biliary tract procedures.
- Radiology—CXR is of limited use. Gas in the gall bladder wall or lumen is diagnostic of emphysematous cholecystitis. USS is the diagnostic study of choice, showing a sensitivity of around 90% (presence of stones, thickened gall bladder wall, dilated gall bladder lumen, pericholecystic collection). Cholescintigraphy (hepatobiliary iminodiacetic acid (HIDA) scan) may be indicated if the diagnosis remains unclear after ultrasonography. Magnetic resonance cholangiopancreatography (MRCP) is used to examine the intra- and extrahepatic bile ducts—its role in the diagnosis of acute cholecystitis is limited. Abdominal CT is usually unnecessary but may show gall bladder wall oedema, pericholecystic stranding, and high attenuation bile.

Treatment

- Supportive therapy—IV fluids, analgesia, fasting, NG tube if vomiting.
- Antibiotic therapy—acute cholecystitis is primarily an inflammatory process, and the role of antibiotics is not clear, apart from in patients with sepsis (fever and raised WCC). Nevertheless, antibiotics are often given because of the risk of gall bladder empyema and pericholecystic abscesses. The empiric choice should be active against the most likely organisms, e.g. *E. coli*, enterococci, *Klebsiella* spp. *Enterobacter* spp.

Commonly used regimens include amoxicillin/metronidazole/gentamicin, ceftriaxone and metronidazole, or ciprofloxacin and metronidazole. Therapy should be tailored in the light of any positive cultures.

- Surgery—immediate cholecystectomy may be preferred amongst patients who are hospitalized with acute cholecystitis and good candidates for surgery, as it has been associated with reduced perioperative morbidity and mortality and shorter lengths of hospital stay. Some surgeons prefer to treat with antibiotics and delay surgery (>7 days after admission). Laparoscopic cholecystectomy is the preferred option.

Acute cholangitis

Clinical syndrome characterized by fever, jaundice, and abdominal pain. Usually caused by bacterial infection in patients with biliary obstruction, e.g. gallstones, benign stenosis, malignancy.

- *Aetiology*—similar to acute cholecystitis, i.e. *E.coli, Klebsiella, Enterobacter* spp., enterococci, anaerobes.
- *Clinical features*—onset is acute with fever, jaundice, and abdominal pain (Charcot's triad—seen in 50–75% of cases). The presence of confusion and hypotension (Reynold's pentad) suggests suppurative cholangitis and is associated with significant morbidity and mortality. Septic shock may lead to multiorgan failure.
- *Diagnosis*—the 2013 Tokyo guidelines propose the diagnosis should be suspected if the patient has fever/shaking or has evidence of inflammation (abnormal WCC, raised CRP etc.), and either jaundice or abnormal liver enzymes (ACP, GGT, ALT, AST). The diagnosis can be considered definite if, in addition, the patient has biliary dilatation on imaging or evidence of a cause (stone etc.).
- *Differential diagnosis*—acute cholecystitis, liver abscess, infected choledochal cyst, Mirizzi syndrome, biliary leak, acute pancreatitis, appendicitis, acute diverticulitis, intestinal perforation, right lower lobe pneumonia.
- *Treatment*—management of sepsis, e.g. oxygen, fluid resuscitation, monitoring. Antibiotic therapy—initial broad-spectrum therapy based on likely organisms and local resistance patterns. Biliary drainage—usually endoscopic sphincterotomy with stone removal ± stent insertion. If endoscopic drainage is not feasible/successful, either percutaneous transhepatic cholangiography (PTC) or open surgical drainage may be required.
- *Prognosis*—reported mortality rates range from 2% to 65%.

Pancreatitis

Pancreatitis is an inflammation of the pancreas, which may be acute or chronic (>4 weeks' symptoms) in nature.

Causes of acute pancreatitis

- Gallstones, biliary sludge.
- Alcohol.
- Smoking.
- Hypertriglyceridaemia.
- Post-ERCP.
- Hypercalcaemia.
- Genetic mutations, e.g. *PRSSI, CFTR, SPINK1*, and *CTRC* genes.
- Drugs, e.g. diuretics, sulfonamides, aminosalicylic acid, 6-mercaptopurine, valproic acid, didanosine, pentamidine, tetracycline, azathioprine, oestrogens.
- Viruses, e.g. mumps, Coxsackie virus, hepatitis B, CMV, VZV, HSV, HIV.
- Bacteria, e.g. *Mycoplasma, Legionella, Leptospira, Salmonella*.
- Fungi, e.g. *Aspergillus*.
- Parasites, e.g. *Toxoplasma, Cryptosporidium, Ascaris*.
- Toxins, e.g. the venom of the brown recluse spider, some scorpions, the Gila monster lizard.
- Trauma.
- Pancreas divisum.
- Vascular disease, e.g. vasculitis, atheroembolism, hypotension.
- Pregnancy.
- Idiopathic.

Clinical features

- Symptoms—patients usually present with acute-onset, severe abdominal pain, which is usually epigastric (or in the right upper quadrant) and radiates through to the back. It may be associated with nausea and vomiting (>90%), dyspnoea (ARDS, pleural effusions), or hypotension.
- Examination findings—epigastric tenderness, generalized abdominal tenderness, abdominal distension, hypoactive bowel sounds, jaundice (if biliary obstruction). Patients with severe pancreatitis may have fever, tachypnoea, hypoxia, and hypotension. Three per cent of patients may have discoloration around the umbilicus (Cullen sign) or in the flanks (Grey Turner sign), indicating retroperitoneal haemorrhage. Rarely, patients may have panniculitis (subcutaneous fat necrosis). There may also be signs related to the cause, e.g. alcoholic liver disease, hyperlipidaemia, or mumps parotitis.

Laboratory diagnosis

- Serum amylase rises within 6–12h of onset and returns to normal after 3–5 days. It is usually >3 times the ULN but may not rise to this level in patients with alcoholic pancreatitis or hypertriglyceridaemia-related pancreatitis. It has a sensitivity of 67–83% for the diagnosis of acute pancreatitis.

- Serum lipase rises within 4–8h of onset, peaks at 24h, and returns to normal within 8–14 days. It has a sensitivity of 82–100% for the diagnosis of acute pancreatitis.
- Blood tests—FBC, electrolytes, ALT, AST, bilirubin, calcium, and albumin should be obtained to rule out other causes of acute abdominal pain.
- A pregnancy test should be performed in all women of childbearing age.

Imaging

- Plain radiographs—abdominal X-ray may be unremarkable or show a sentinel loop (localized ileus of the small bowel) or a colon cut-off sign (lack of air in the distal colon, caused by colonic spasm secondary to pancreatic inflammation) in severe disease. CXR may show a raised hemidiaphragm, pleural effusions, basal atelectasis, pulmonary infiltrates, or ARDS.
- Ultrasound—the pancreas is diffusely enlarged and hypoechoic, and there may be gallstones, peripancreatic fluid, or evidence of pancreatic necrosis. However, in 25–35% of cases, the pancreas may not be visible because of small bowel ileus.
- CT scan—this may show focal or diffuse enlargement of the pancreas with heterogeneous enhancement with IV contrast, necrotizing pancreatitis, or gallstones.
- MRI scan—has a higher sensitivity for the diagnosis of early acute pancreatitis, compared with CT scan, and can better characterize the pancreatic and bile ducts and complications of acute pancreatitis.

Management

- The severity of acute pancreatitis should be assessed for fluid losses, organ failure, and using SIRS and APACHE scores.
- Patients with severe acute pancreatitis adverse features should be admitted to ICU for management.
- Fluid replacement—aggressive fluid resuscitation (5–10mL/kg/h) may be required initially, and fluid requirements should be reassessed at frequent intervals during the first 24–48h.
- Pain control—opiates are safe and effective at providing pain control in acute pancreatitis.
- Nutrition—patients with mild pancreatitis can be managed with fluids, until they are able to tolerate oral nutrition. Those with moderate to severe pancreatitis may require enteral nutrition.
- Antibiotics—prophylactic antibiotics are not recommended, but antibiotics should be commenced if the patient develops an extrapancreatic infection (25% of cases), which is associated with increased mortality.
- Monitoring—patients should be closely monitored with respect to vital signs, fluid balance, electrolytes, and serum glucose for the first 24–48h.

Primary peritonitis

Infection of the peritoneal cavity that is not related to an intra-abdominal surgical treatable source. It can occur in any age group and is most commonly associated with cirrhosis of the liver.

Aetiology

- Children—associated with post-necrotic cirrhosis, nephrotic syndrome, and UTI but can occur in those with no predisposing condition. Its incidence has fallen in children with the use of antibiotics.
- Adults—at-risk groups: hepatic cirrhosis with ascites, chronic active hepatitis, CCF, metastatic malignancy, SLE, HIV. A cause of decompensation in those with previously stable chronic liver disease.

Pathogenesis

- Infection is acquired via the lymph and blood (particularly in those with portosystemic shunting in association with cirrhosis which may increase the rates and duration of bacteraemia), by bacterial transmural migration from the gut lumen, or via the Fallopian tubes in women (e.g. gonococcal or chlamydial perihepatitis).
- Enteric organisms account for nearly 70% of infections in cirrhotic patients (*E. coli*, *K. pneumoniae*, enterococci, and other streptococci). *S. aureus* and anaerobes are less commonly isolated. Bacteraemia may occur in up to 75% of those with aerobic organisms. Unusual causes of peritonitis include MTB and *C. immitis*—such organisms are usually found in disseminated infection. *S. pneumoniae* is the commonest cause in HIV-infected patients.

Clinical features

- An acute febrile illness with fever, diffuse abdominal pain, nausea/vomiting, diarrhoea, and rebound tenderness on examination. Resembles acute appendicitis. The onset may be insidious, and patients can present with signs of infection/sepsis and no localizing features.
- Cirrhotic patients may have other features of chronic liver disease and develop hepatic encephalopathy.
- Paralytic ileus, hypotension, and hypothermia are signs of severe disease and associated with poor survival.
- Tuberculous peritonitis is gradual in onset, with fever, weight loss, night sweats, and abdominal distension.
- Gonococcal or chlamydial perihepatitis is usually seen in women. Presents with pain, guarding, and tenderness in the right upper quadrant.

Diagnosis

- Abdominal paracentesis is indicated in all cirrhotic patients with ascites. Ascitic fluid should be sent for cell count, Gram stain, culture, and protein concentration. Culture yield is improved by the direct inoculation of 10mL of fluid into BC bottles at the bedside. A positive Gram stain is diagnostic but is negative in 60% of cirrhotics with infection. Ascitic fluid neutrophil count of >500/microlitre is the best single predictor of peritonitis (86% sensitive, 98% specific)—generally

a threshold of 250/microlitre is used (93% sensitive, 94% specific). Improved diagnostic accuracy is achieved by combining cell counts and the ascitic fluid pH (neutrophil count >500/microlitre and an ascitic fluid pH <7.35 gives 100% sensitivity and 96% specificity).
- BCs may be positive in approximately one-third of patients. The diagnosis of primary peritonitis can be made only after other potential primary sources of infection have been excluded.
- Contrast-enhanced CT can help identify intra-abdominal sources of infection.
- Some surgeons will exclude appendicitis in children only at operation. Tuberculous peritonitis may be confirmed at operation or histology/culture of peritoneal biopsies.

Treatment

- Treat those patients with positive cultures or Gram stain, regardless of the cell count (nearly 40% of those with positive cultures and normal cell counts go on to develop peritonitis), and all culture-negative patients with raised cell counts.
- Initial treatment is empirical, while culture results are awaited—ampicillin in combination with an aminoglycoside, or a third-generation cephalosporin (avoids the risks of nephrotoxicity). Patients with primary peritonitis respond within 48h to appropriate antibiotic therapy. Antibiotics are usually given for 10–14 days.
- Follow-up peritoneal fluid cell counts are useful but not essential.
- In those who do not respond, another primary source of infection should be considered (e.g. perforation, intra-abdominal abscess).

Prevention

- Antimicrobial prophylaxis (e.g. ciprofloxacin) decreases the frequency of primary peritonitis in certain high-risk groups (patients with ascites admitted with GI bleeds, those awaiting liver transplantation, those with ascitic protein levels <1g/dL) but does not confer a survival advantage.

Secondary peritonitis

Secondary peritonitis occurs as a result of a breach in the mucosal barrier, resulting in spillage of organisms from the GI or GU tracts into the peritoneal cavity. This normally occurs in the context of intra-abdominal infections (e.g. appendicitis, diverticulitis) or surgery (abdominal, gynaecological, or obstetric).

Aetiology

- Most cases are due to infection by the commensal flora of the mucous membranes within the abdominal cavity. Peritonitis also complicates an exogenously acquired visceral infection (e.g. *S. aureus*, MTB).
- Infection is usually polymicrobial. The commonest isolates are *E. coli, B. fragilis*, enterococci, other *Bacteroides* spp., *Fusobacterium, C. perfringens, Peptococcus*, and *Peptostreptococcus*. Antibiotic-resistant organisms are more likely to be found amongst those patients who

acquire peritonitis while receiving antibiotics in hospital (e.g. *Candida*, enterococci, *Enterobacter, Serratia, Acinetobacter* spp.). Vaginal flora, e.g. GBS, may be present after vaginal surgery or labour.

Pathogenesis

- Many anaerobic infections are synergistic, e.g. facultative anaerobes providing a sufficiently reduced environment for the establishment of obligate anaerobic organisms.
- Leaking bile or acid may cause a chemical peritonitis that leads to inflammation, necrosis, and further intra-abdominal damage, facilitating the establishment of bacterial infection.
- Local response—local inflammatory response of peritoneum leads to fluid production and granulocyte entry to the peritoneal cavity. The exudate contains fibrinogen which forms plaques around inflamed surfaces aimed at localizing infection and may later lead to adhesions. Some instances of infection may be contained and resolve. Others may lead to local abscess formation. If localization fails completely, diffuse peritonitis may result.

Clinical features

- Symptoms—initial features are those of the primary disease process (e.g. appendicitis). Moderate abdominal pain, aggravated by movement, becomes more severe and diffuse, as infection spreads throughout the abdomen. Pain may reduce in intensity and become more focal if localization strategies are effective. Other: vomiting, fever, distension, anorexia, inability to pass flatus, thirst.
- Signs—patient lying still, alert, and restless at first, later becoming listless. Fever is usually present. Hypothermia may be noted in early chemical peritonitis and is a severe sign late in the course of patients presenting with sepsis. Tachycardia, hypotension, tachypnoea, abdominal tenderness (maximal over primarily affected organ) with rebound and guarding, and bowel sounds present initially later disappear. Some of these features may be masked in patients receiving glucocorticoids or whose abscess has been localized away from the anterior abdominal wall (e.g. subphrenic).

Diagnosis

- Laboratory tests—peripheral WCC 17 000–25 000 cells/mL with a left shift (in some situations, massive peritoneal inflammation may lead to low peripheral WCC with an extreme shift to immature forms), haemoconcentration, elevated amylase, acidosis in late disease, features of underlying condition (diabetic ketoacidosis (DKA), haematuria, pyuria, pancreatitis).
- Radiology—contrast CT is the preferred initial study; plain erect chest and abdominal X-ray: signs of inflammation, free air, distended loops of adynamic bowel, signs of the underlying condition (obstruction, volvulus, intussusception, gall bladder calcification); USS may be limited by the presence of air-filled loops of bowel.
- BCs.

- Peritoneal lavage or aspiration may be appropriate in some situations.
- Differential diagnosis—pneumonia, sickle-cell anaemia, herpes zoster, DKA, porphyria, familial Mediterranean fever, SLE, uraemia.

Treatment

- General measures—fluid resuscitation, circulatory and respiratory support, appropriate surgical interventions. Exclude pregnancy.
- Antimicrobial therapy—broad-spectrum antimicrobial therapy should be started immediately after taking BCs. Combinations of two or three antibiotics are used to provide good activity against aerobes and anaerobes, e.g. IV cephalosporin, metronidazole ± gentamicin, or IV co-amoxiclav ± gentamicin. Detailed culture and sensitivity results may take several days, as cultures are often mixed and some organisms are slow-growing. Antibiotics may not need to be active against every organism isolated—the elimination of the majority may allow host defences to eliminate the remainder. Antifungal therapy (e.g. amphotericin) should be used if *Candida* spp. are isolated; 5–7 days of treatment should be sufficient after adequate surgical intervention, depending on the severity of infection and clinical response. Conversion to oral therapy may be indicated in those patients with a good response.

Prognosis

- Survival depends on age, co-morbid conditions, duration of peritoneal contamination, the primary process, and microorganisms involved.
- Mortality ranges from 3.5% in those with early infection caused by penetrating trauma to 60% in those with established infection and secondary organ failure. Death is thought to follow uncontrolled cytokine release.

Prevention

Pre/perioperative antibiotics reduce infections in clean, contaminated surgery (e.g. appendectomy for appendicitis without rupture, penetrating wounds of the abdomen, vaginal hysterectomy in premenopausal women). Post-operative infection rates fall from 20–30% to 4–8% with prophylactic antibiotic use in such infections.

Peritoneal dialysis peritonitis

Peritonitis was a common complication of PD, until Tenckhoff introduced his improved catheter in 1968. Rates fell further, as techniques and bag adapters, etc. improved. However, it still occurs at around one episode per patient year, with up to 70% of patients experiencing an episode of infection in their first year of dialysis. Recurrent infection is one of the commonest reasons for discontinuing CAPD (20–30% of patients). Prognosis is good—mortality is <1%.

Pathogenesis

Infection is commonly acquired by contamination of the catheter by skin organisms. Enteric organisms may be cultured from the skin of some CAPD patients. Organisms can also enter via the catheter exit site and through contamination of the dialysate delivery system, as well as transmurally in the manner seen in some cases of primary peritonitis.

Microbiology

Gram-positive organisms account for 50% of isolates (CoNS, *S. aureus*, streptococci, enterococci, and diphtheroids). Gram-negative infections account for 15% (*E. coli, Klebsiella, Enterobacter*, and *Pseudomonas*) and polymicrobial infections for 4%. Anaerobes and yeasts are uncommon isolates. ~20% of cases are culture-negative. *Pseudomonas* and fungal peritonitis are difficult to eradicate and require catheter removal. TB peritonitis should be suspected in patients from TB-endemic areas with lymphocytic peritoneal fluid and culture-negative peritonitis. NTM may also cause PD peritonitis.

Clinical features

Patients are often unaware of an antecedent event, e.g. possible contamination or breaks in sterile technique. There may be a history of recent exit site or tunnel infection. The commonest symptoms are abdominal pain and cloudy peritoneal fluid. Other symptoms include fever, abdominal tenderness, nausea, diarrhoea, and hypotension.

Diagnosis

Peritoneal fluid should be taken from the catheter under sterile technique. It is usually cloudy in appearance. A WCC >100 cells/mm^3 (>50% neutrophils) is indicative of infection. Eosinophilia may be seen after tube placement (an allergic reaction to the tubing) and in some cases of fungal infection. A predominance of lymphocytes may be seen in mycobacterial infection. Gram stain is positive in less than half of the cases. BCs are rarely positive. Fluid should be inoculated into BC bottles. Yield can be improved by culturing the sediment of 50mL of the centrifuged fluid.

Differential diagnosis

Other causes of cloudy peritoneal fluid include chemical peritonitis, eosinophilia of the effluent, haemoperitoneum, malignancy, chylous effluent, and specimen taken from a 'dry' abdomen.

Treatment

- General measures—heparin (500 units/L of dialysate) may be used to help lyse or prevent fibrin clots. Analgesia for abdominal pain.
- Bacterial—intraperitoneal antibiotics are preferred and can be given with each exchange (continuous dosing) or od (intermittent dosing). Empirical therapy should cover both Gram-positive and Gram-negative organisms, according to local antibiotic policies and then guided by the Gram stain and culture results. Treatment should continue for between 10 and 21 days, or for 1 week after catheter removal. Most patients improve within 2–4 days. Those who do not should be re-evaluated, and unusual (e.g. fungi) or resistant organisms considered, as well as alternative diagnoses.
- Fungal—most cases can be treated with amphotericin which can be given intraperitoneally but may cause abdominal pain. Most patients

with fungal infections will require catheter removal and IV therapy. Flucytosine may be used, but levels must be carefully monitored. Some *Fusarium* spp. are resistant to amphotericin.
- Catheter removal—up to 20% of patients require catheter removal. Indications for catheter removal include: refractory peritonitis, relapsing peritonitis, refractory exit site/tunnel infection, fungal peritonitis, mycobacterial peritonitis, and multiple enteric organisms.

Prevention

Good technique helps reduce infection rates, e.g. exit site care, connection methods, patient training. Antibiotic prophylaxis may be of some benefit in those patients undergoing extensive dental procedures or lower GI endoscopy. Further details are available in the guidelines produced by the International Society for Peritoneal Dialysis.[7]

Reference

7 Li PK, Szeto CC, Piraino B, *et al.*; International Society for Peritoneal Dialysis (2010). Peritoneal dialysis-related infections recommendations: 2010 update. *Perit Dial Int.* **30**:393–423. Available at: www.pdiconnect.com/content/30/4/393.full.pdf+html.

Diverticulitis

Pathogenesis

Diverticulae are sac-like protrusions of the colonic wall. They are associated with a low-fibre diet, constipation, and obesity. Diverticulosis is the presence of diverticulae and affects >10% of those over 45 years of age, and 80% of those over 85 years. Acute (uncomplicated) diverticulitis is defined as inflammation of the diverticulae—it occurs in 20% of patients with diverticulae and is commoner in the elderly and those with extensive disease. Complicated diverticulitis is defined as acute diverticulitis with one of the following complications: abscess, colovesical or colovaginal fistula, perforation, or obstruction.

Presentation

Abdominal pain is the commonest symptom and usually affects the left lower quadrant (sigmoid colon). However, it may occur in the right lower quadrant (mimicking appendicitis) or suprapubically. The pain is usually constant and lasts for several days. Fifty per cent of patients report previous episodes. Other symptoms include nausea, vomiting, fever, a palpable mass, localized peritoneal signs, altered bowel habit (constipation or diarrhoea), or urinary symptoms (bladder irritation).

Diagnosis

Acute diverticulitis should be suspected in a patient with lower abdominal pain/tenderness. The diagnosis is usually confirmed by abdominal CT scan or ultrasound. Blood WCC is often elevated, but this is neither sensitive nor specific. Differential diagnosis includes acute appendicitis, IBD, ischaemic colitis, infectious colitis, and colorectal cancer.

Management

- Uncomplicated diverticulitis—this can usually be treated conservatively with bowel rest and oral antibiotics (e.g. co-amoxiclav) for 10–14 days. Success rates range from 70% to 100%.
- Complicated disease—broad-spectrum IV antibiotic therapy (e.g. piperacillin–tazobactam) is required until symptoms start to settle, followed by oral antibiotics for a total period of 10–14 days.
- Drainage of diverticular abscesses—this can be performed percutaneously under radiological guidance. Surgical drainage is indicated if symptoms are not controlled after 3–5 days.
- Surgery—this is indicated in patients who present with sepsis or diffuse peritonitis, or who fail medical therapy or percutaneous drainage of abscesses.
- After recovery—~6 weeks after recovery from acute diverticulitis, patients should undergo colonoscopy to exclude other pathologies (e.g. colonic carcinoma) and evaluate the extent of the diseases.

Intra-abdominal abscess

Intra-abdominal abscesses may complicate peritonitis of any cause. Primary abscesses develop following primary peritonitis. Secondary abscesses may follow appendicitis, diverticulitis, biliary tract lesions, pancreatitis, IBD, perforated peptic ulcers, trauma, and surgery.

Pathogenesis

Infections are usually polymicrobial, with anaerobes isolated in up to 70% of cases. Other organisms include *Enterobacteriaceae*, *S. milleri*, enterococci, *P. aeruginosa*, and *S. aureus*. Abscess location is related to that of the primary disease and the direction of peritoneal drainage (e.g. most appendicitis-related abscesses occur in the right lower quadrant or pelvis).

Clinical features

These include high/fluctuating fever, rigors, abdominal pain, and tenderness over the affected area. Specific features will vary with the location, e.g. subphrenic abscesses may cause costal tenderness and chest signs on examination. Presentation can be acute or chronic (particularly subphrenic abscesses where the patient has been receiving antibiotics), and may follow primary abdominal disease (e.g. pancreatitis) or abdominal surgery with a prolonged recuperation.

Diagnosis

Ultrasound, CT, or MRI scans are the most effective means of identifying abscesses. A pleural effusion on CXR may indicate a subphrenic abscess. The diagnosis is confirmed by radiologically guided diagnostic aspiration. Samples should be sent to the laboratory for microscopy and culture.

Treatment

- Drainage is key—percutaneous drainage (radiologically guided) is suitable for unilocular collections that are readily accessible, are not vascular, and are likely to drain easily by simple dependent drainage. Repeat scanning should be used to confirm resolution, following adequate drainage. Surgical drainage is usually required for multiple or loculated abscesses, or those with very viscous pus.
- Antibiotics—agents should be directed against the most likely organisms, e.g. *Enterobacteriaceae* and anaerobes. Therapy should be started immediately after BCs have been taken. The antimicrobial regimen should be tailored to culture results. Repeat samples may be required in patients with prolonged antimicrobial therapy.

Retroperitoneal abscess

- Abscesses may form in the retroperitoneal space, following direct extension of infection from a retroperitoneal structure (e.g. pyelonephritis, spinal osteomyelitis), intra-abdominal sepsis, traumatic haemorrhage, or bacteraemia.
- Common organisms include *S. aureus* and coliforms. Anaerobes and polymicrobial infections are less common. MTB may be seen in endemic areas.
- Clinical features—patients present with fever, abdominal/flank/lumbar pain, and a palpable mass. If the psoas sheath is involved, there may be pain on hip flexion.
- Diagnosis is made by CT or MRI scan. BCs and aspirated pus should be sent to the laboratory for culture.
- Management is by surgical drainage and empirical broad-spectrum IV antibiotic therapy, while awaiting results of cultures. Treatment should be tailored to culture results.

Pancreatic abscess

- Up to 9% of patients with acute pancreatitis develop a pancreatic abscess. Abscesses may also develop, following penetration by a peptic ulcer or secondary infection of a pancreatic pseudocyst. Up to 50% of abscesses are polymicrobial. Haematogenous seeding of bacteria may explain those abscesses caused by single organisms.
- Clinical features—presents with failure to improve or abrupt deterioration following initial recovery from acute pancreatitis. Most patients experience abdominal pain radiating to the back, with fever and vomiting. Rarer manifestations include jaundice, distension, peritonitis, abdominal mass. Serum amylase may be elevated.
- Diagnosis—USS and CT demonstrate the abscess in the majority of cases, but distinguishing the abscess from a pseudocyst may require guided diagnostic needle aspiration.
- Treatment—surgical drainage/debridement is essential (53–86% survival). Percutaneous drainage may be helpful in some patients requiring stabilization prior to surgery but is rarely sufficient. Initial antibiotic therapy needs to be broad and can later be adjusted according to sensitivity testing.

- Complications—retroperitoneal extension of infection; fistula formation between the abscess and the stomach, duodenum, or colon; erosion of major blood vessels causing intra-abdominal haemorrhage.

Splenic abscess

- Uncommon and may be due to bacteraemic seeding of infection (e.g. bacterial endocarditis, IDU), splenic infarction (e.g. blunt trauma, sickle-cell disease), or direct extension of intra-abdominal infection. They are usually multiple.
- Aetiology—causes include *S. aureus*, streptococci, *Enterobactericeae*, anaerobes, and *Candida* spp. Around a quarter are polymicrobial.
- Clinical features—left upper quadrant pain with shoulder tip discomfort and fever. Multiple small abscesses may not cause spleen enlargement.
- Diagnosis—CXR may demonstrate an elevated hemidiaphragm, basal pulmonary infiltrates, or pleural effusion. Ultrasound, CT, or MRI scanning confirm the diagnosis.
- Treatment—initial antibiotic therapy must be broad-spectrum (e.g. cephalosporin and metronidazole) and modified, following culture results. Multiple or large single abscesses may necessitate splenectomy. Incision and drainage may be preferred in cases where the spleen is held by extensive adhesions.

Psoas abscess

- A psoas (or iliopsoas) abscess is a collection of pus in the iliopsoas muscle compartment. It may arise by haematogenous or lymphatic spread from a distant site (primary abscess) or from contiguous spread from adjacent structures (secondary abscess), e.g. vertebrae, hip arthroplasty, GI tract, GU tract, aorta.
- Aetiology—primary psoas abscesses are usually monomicrobial, e.g. *S. aureus*, streptococci, *E. coli*, and MTB (in endemic areas). Secondary psoas abscesses may be monomicrobial or polymicrobial (21–55%, often enteric organisms).
- Clinical features—fever, back or flank pain, inguinal mass, limp, anorexia, weight loss. On examination, patients may have a lumbar lordosis and a flexed hip—pain is exacerbated by extending the hip (psoas sign).
- Diagnosis—this may be suspected clinically and confirmed by CT scan. Identification of the causative organism requires aspiration/drainage and culture of pus. BCs are positive in 41–68% of cases.
- Treatment—drainage may be performed percutaneously (under ultrasound or CT guidance) or by an open surgical procedure. Empiric antibiotic therapy should cover the most likely organisms (*S. aureus* and enteric organisms) and be tailored in light of culture results. The optimal duration of therapy is uncertain—usually 3–6 weeks after drainage.
- Outcome—mortality rates vary from 2.4% (primary abscesses) to 19% (secondary abscesses). Risk factors include advanced aged, delayed or inadequate treatment, bacteraemia, and *E. coli* infections. Relapse may occur in 15–36% of cases.

Liver abscess

Liver abscesses account for 48% of visceral abscesses and 13% of intra-abdominal abscesses. The estimated incidence is 2.3 cases per 100 000 population, and they occur more frequently in women than men. Risk factors include diabetes mellitus, underlying hepatobiliary or pancreatic disease, and liver transplantation.

Aetiology

- Most pyogenic liver abscesses are polymicrobial with mixed enteric organisms and anaerobes.
- *S. milleri* (*S. anginosus*) group are important causes.
- *S. aureus*, *S. pyogenes*, and other Gram-positive cocci are recognized pathogens in certain circumstances.
- *K. pneumoniae* is an important emerging pathogen, especially in East Asia where it has been associated with underlying colorectal cancer.
- *Candida* spp. have also been implicated in up to 22% of cases.
- Tuberculous abscesses should be considered in endemic areas and in cases with sterile cultures.
- *B. pseudomallei* (melioidosis) is an important pathogen in South East Asia.
- *E. histolytica* (amoebic liver abscess) should be considered in those who come from/have travelled to an endemic area.

Presentation

- Pyogenic liver abscess—presents with fever and abdominal pain, over days or weeks. Other symptoms include nausea, vomiting, anorexia, and weight loss. About 50% of patients have hepatomegaly, right upper quadrant tenderness, or jaundice.
- Amoebic liver abscess—usually presents with 1–2 weeks of right upper quadrant pain and fever 8–20 weeks after returning from an endemic area. Other symptoms include sweating, anorexia, malaise, weight loss, cough, and hiccough. There may be a history of previous dysentery, although diarrhoea is present in <30% of cases. Examination may reveal tender hepatomegaly (50%) and jaundice (10%).

Diagnosis

- Radiology—plain CXR may reveal elevation of the right hemidiaphragm, with a right pleural effusion or gas in the abscess cavity. USS or CT scan are most useful and may be used to guide diagnostic aspiration.
- Blood tests—WCC, CRP, and LFTs may be raised.
- BCs—positive in 50% of patients with pyogenic liver abscesses.
- Aspirates—should be examined by microscopy for *E. histolytica* trophozoites and cultured aerobically and anaerobically. Pus from amoebic liver abscesses is brown, foul-smelling (anchovy pus), and culture-negative.
- Serology and antigen detection—99% of patients with amoebic liver abscess develop antibodies, which are detectable after 7 days, but do not distinguish recent from past infection. More recent tests based on *E. histolytica* antigens, which wane over time, may be more useful in endemic areas.

Treatment

- Pyogenic liver abscesses—the mainstay of treatment is drainage and antibiotic therapy. For single abscesses, percutaneous aspiration or catheter drainage is appropriate. Repeat aspiration may be required in up to 50% of cases. The drain should be kept in, until drainage is minimal. Indications for surgical drainage include: (i) large (>5cm), multiple, loculated, or viscous abscesses; (ii) failure to respond to percutaneous drainage within 7 days; and (iii) underlying disease requiring surgical management. Empiric broad-spectrum IV antibiotic therapy should be started as soon as the diagnosis is suspected and tailored in light of culture results. The optimal duration of treatment is unknown, but antibiotics are usually continued for 4–6 weeks.
- Amoebic liver abscesses—metronidazole (➡ see *Entamoeba histolytica*, pp. 533–5) is the treatment of choice and has a >90% cure rate. Alternatives include tinidazole and nitazoxanide. Following this treatment, a luminal agent (e.g. paromomycin) is required to eliminate intraluminal cysts. Aspiration is probably not necessary, unless the lesion is very large, threatens to rupture, or fails to respond to medical therapy. The mortality rate of uncomplicated amoebic abscesses is under 1%. Higher mortalities are associated with those abscesses that rupture into the peritoneum (18%), pericardium (30%), or pleura/ bronchi (6%).

Acute hepatitis

An acute inflammation of the liver characterized by hepatocyte damage and elevations in serum AST and AST. May be caused by a variety of infectious and non-infectious agents.

Aetiology

- Hepatitis viruses—HAV (➡ see Hepatitis A virus, pp. 411–2), HBV (➡ see Hepatitis B virus, pp. 413–7), HCV (➡ see Hepatitis C virus, pp. 418–21), HDV (➡ see Hepatitis D virus, pp. 417–8), HEV (➡ see Hepatitis E virus, pp. 421–3).
- Other viruses—EBV (➡ see Epstein–Barr virus, pp. 402–5), CMV (➡ Cytomegalovirus, pp. 405–8), HSV (➡ see Herpes simplex, pp. 396–9), VZV (➡ see Varicella-zoster virus, pp. 399–402), measles (➡ see Measles, pp. 384–6), rubella (➡ see Rubella, pp. 389–90), adenovirus (➡ Adenovirus, pp. 436–8), Coxsackie B, Enterovirus, and yellow fever virus (➡ see Yellow fever, pp. 455–6).
- Non-viral infectious diseases—syphilis (➡ see Syphilis, pp. 714–6), leptospirosis (➡ see *Leptospira* species, pp. 340–2), Q fever (➡ see *Coxiella burnetii*—ACDP 3, pp. 346–8), sepsis, legionellosis (➡ see *Legionella*, pp. 318–20), tuberculosis (➡ see *Mycobacterium tuberculosis*—ACDP 3, pp. 355–9), brucellosis (➡ see *Brucella*—ACDP 3, pp. 311–3), tularaemia (➡ see *Francisella*—ACDP 3, pp. 317–8), plague (➡ see *Yersinia pestis*—ACDP 3, pp. 314–5).
- Drug-induced hepatitis, e.g. paracetamol, isoniazid, rifampicin, pyrazinamide, phenytoin, and halothane.

- Toxins, e.g. mushrooms, herbal medicines.
- Alcoholic hepatitis.
- Sepsis.
- Ischaemic hepatitis.
- Heat stroke.
- Muscle disorders (e.g. polymyositis), seizures, heavy exercise.
- Autoimmune hepatitis.
- Wilson's disease.
- Budd–Chiari syndrome.
- Sinusoidal obstruction syndrome (veno-occlusive disease).
- HELLP (haemolysis, elevated liver enzymes, low platelets) syndrome.

Clinical features

- There are no clinical features that distinguish the various causes.
- Acute viral hepatitis can be divided into four clinical stages: incubation period, pre-icteric phase, icteric phase, and convalescence.
- Clinical features may range from asymptomatic disease to anorexia, malaise, abdominal pain, and jaundice to fulminant hepatic failure.
- Hepatitis B and C may cause immune complex-mediated diseases, e.g. serum sickness, polyarteritis nodosa (HBV), glomerulonephritis, mixed cryoglobulinaemia.
- Fulminant viral hepatitis, characterized by liver failure and hepatic encephalopathy, occurs within 8 weeks after onset of symptoms.

Diagnosis

- Routine blood tests—AST and ALT are usually dramatically elevated, and bilirubin may be variably elevated. A prolonged PT is rare and suggests severe hepatic necrosis.
- Serology—anti-HAV IgM, HBsAg and anti-HBc IgM, and anti-HCV should be performed initially. If these are negative, other diagnoses should be considered.
- Liver ultrasound is usually normal in acute viral hepatitis. Abnormalities, e.g. hepatic lesions, cirrhosis, portal hypertension, or ascites suggest alternative diagnoses.
- Liver biopsy may be performed to establish the diagnosis in acute hepatitis with negative serology.

Management

- Supportive care—most patients with acute viral hepatitis do not require hospitalization, unless they are at risk of dehydration, have clinical evidence of liver failure, or have a rising bilirubin or PT. Bed rest and alcohol avoidance are recommended, while patients are symptomatic. Most medications should be avoided, but symptomatic therapy for nausea or pain may be required. Vitamin K may be given if the PT is prolonged.
- Treatment—there is no specific treatment for acute viral hepatitis. Corticosteroids have been recommended for cholestatic hepatitis and fulminant hepatic failure, although clinical trials have failed to show benefit. IFN-α has also been used in fulminant HBV, but the evidence is poor. There is some evidence that treatment of acute HCV infection with IFN-β may prevent chronic infection.

- Monitoring—inpatients should be monitored regularly for signs of liver failure and with blood tests (bilirubin, AST, ALT, and PT). Hepatitis serology should be rechecked after 6 months to determine chronicity.
- Liver biopsy may be performed for various reasons, e.g. diagnostic uncertainty, if >1 cause is a possibility, or if specific treatment is being considered.
- Liver transplantation is the only available treatment for fulminant hepatic failure, and patients should be promptly referred for consideration of transplantation.

Chronic hepatitis

This is used to describe chronic inflammation of the liver (lasting >6 months) and may be caused by a variety of infectious and non-infectious agents.

Causes

- Chronic viral hepatitis: HBV (➔ see Hepatitis B virus, pp. 413–7), HCV (➔ see Hepatitis C virus, pp. 418–21), HDV (➔ see Hepatitis D virus, pp. 417–8), HEV (➔ see Hepatitis E virus, pp. 421–3).
- Autoimmune hepatitis.
- Hereditary haemochromatosis.
- Wilson's disease.
- α1-antitrypsin deficiency.
- Fatty liver and non-alcoholic steatohepatitis (NASH).
- Alcoholic liver disease.
- Drug-induced liver disease.
- Hepatic granulomas—infectious, drug-induced, neoplastic, idiopathic.

Clinical features

There are no specific clinical features, and many patients remain asymptomatic, until they develop end-stage liver disease. Non-specific features (e.g. fatigue and right upper quadrant discomfort) are common. Symptoms, such as jaundice, weight loss, abdominal distension, or confusion, suggest decompensation. Examination may show signs of chronic liver disease (e.g. palmar erythema, Dupuytren's contractures, jaundice, spider naevi, hepatosplenomegaly, caput medusae, ascites). Clinical features of hepatic encephalopathy include confusion, drowsiness, asterixis, ophthalmoplegia, and ataxia.

Diagnosis

- Routine blood tests—AST and ALT are usually elevated, and bilirubin may be variably elevated. A prolonged PT suggests hepatic failure. A low albumin occurs in cirrhosis.
- Serology—HBsAg and anti-HCV should be performed for patients with suspected chronic viral hepatitis. If these are negative, other diagnoses should be considered.
- Liver ultrasound may show hepatomegaly or cirrhosis, portal hypertension, or ascites. Hepatic lesions may be due to hepatocellular carcinoma.

- Liver biopsy may be performed to establish the diagnosis in chronic hepatitis with negative serology or to determine the degree of fibrosis in patients with suspected cirrhosis. In patients with deranged clotting, this may be performed by the transjugular route.

Management

- Chronic HBV infection is usually treated with antiviral agents (➔ see Antivirals for hepatitis B, pp. 97–9), e.g. IFN-α, lamivudine, adefovir dipivoxil, and entecavir. Tenofovir (TDF) also has anti-HBV activity and should be used to treat HIV/HBV co-infected patients. Liver transplantation may be performed for patients with end-stage liver disease. However, the risk of reinfection is 20%, even with prophylaxis (lamivudine and polyclonal anti-hepatitis B immunoglobulin, HBIG). ➔ See Treatment, pp. 416–7 for full details.
- Chronic HCV infection can also be treated with antiviral therapy.[8,9] Sofosbuvir-based regimes appear as effective in HCV/HIV co-infected patients as HCV monoinfected patients. ➔ See Treatment, pp. 420–1 for more details.
- HCV genotype 3 infection—patients should be treated with sofosbuvir and weight-based ribavirin for 24 weeks.
- HCV and HIV co-infection—studies with PEG-IFN and ribavirin have shown lower response rates in HIV/HCV co-infected patients, compared with HCV monoinfected patients. As of 2013, sofosbuvir had been studied in 223 HIV/HCV co-infected patients and had similar response rates as HCV monoinfected patients.
- Patients with compensated cirrhosis—sofosbuvir and ribavirin appear to be safe in this patient population.
- Liver transplantation—end-stage liver disease secondary to chronic HCV is the leading indication for hepatic transplantation. The use of sofosbuvir and ribavirin in patients with compensated cirrhosis awaiting transplantation seems to be a safe and effective strategy when the timing of transplantation can be predicted. HCV recurrence occurs in >95% of patients after liver transplantation. The best strategy to prevent or treat reinfection has not yet been established.

References

8 American Association for the Study of Liver Diseases; Infectious Diseases Society of America (2014). *Recommendations for testing, managing, and treating hepatitis C*. Available at: http://www.hcvguidelines.org/sites/default/files/full_report.pdf.

9 European Association for the Study of the Liver (2014). *EASL recommendations on treatment of hepatitis C 2014*. Available at: http://files.easl.eu/easl-recommendations-on-treatment-of-hepatitis-C.pdf.

Other gastrointestinal infections

Mesenteric adenitis

- Inflammation of the mesenteric lymph nodes—may be acute or chronic, depending on the infecting agent. Organisms are thought to pass through intestinal lymphatics to the lymph nodes where they produce inflammation and sometimes suppuration. Commonest in children <15 years of age.

- Causes—these include *Yersinia* spp., *Staphylococcus* spp., *E. coli*, *Streptococcus* spp., MTB, *G. lamblia*, non-typhoidal salmonellae, and viruses (e.g. Coxsackie and adenovirus).
- Clinical features—fever, abdominal pain, and tenderness. It may be difficult to distinguish clinically from appendicitis.
- Diagnosis—ultrasound or CT scan may demonstrate enlarged mesenteric lymph nodes. The key feature in diagnosis is to recognize appendicitis and other problems requiring surgical intervention; <20% of appendectomies may reveal evidence of non-specific mesenteric adenitis. BCs may be positive in those bacterial cases that progress to sepsis. Serological tests may demonstrate evidence of *Y. enterocolitica* infection.
- Treatment—patients with mild symptoms need only supportive care. Ill patients with more obvious evidence of infection require antibiotic treatment.
- Complications—abscess formation, sepsis, peritonitis.

Typhlitis

- Inflammation of the caecum. May occur in patients with HIV or severe neutropenia. It is thought that bacteria from the lumen invade ulcerations in the bowel wall during periods of neutropenia, proliferate, and produce exotoxins, causing damage to the gut wall.
- Clinical features—resembles acute appendicitis, with fever, pain, and rebound tenderness in the right iliac fossa. Rapid progression to an acute abdomen may occur.
- Treatment—broad-spectrum IV antibiotic therapy (aerobic and anaerobic cover) with surgical resection of necrotic bowel is recommended, as the mortality rate of severe cases of neutropenic enterocolitis is >50%.

Tropical sprue/enteropathy

- A syndrome of acute or chronic diarrhoea, weight loss, and malabsorption of at least two nutrients, which is believed to follow an intestinal microbial infection that causes enterocyte injury and bacterial overgrowth. Villous destruction and demonstrable nutrient malabsorption occur in varying degrees. It has been described in tropical climates throughout the world, but primarily in South East Asia and the Caribbean.
- Clinical features—symptoms develop over months, after several years resident in an affected area. It presents with weight loss, fatigue, and the features of the loss of specific nutrients—commonly folate, vitamin B_{12}, and iron.
- Diagnosis—there are no specific tests. Laboratory studies reveal the features of the specific nutritional deficiencies (e.g. megaloblastic anaemia). Stool studies may demonstrate fat malabsorption, and small bowel biopsy may show villous atrophy. The diagnosis is one of exclusion.
- Treatment—management is by nutritional support and antibiotic therapy (e.g. tetracycline or metronidazole for 6–12 months).

Whipple's disease

- A rare chronic and systemic infectious disorder, caused by a Gram-positive bacterium *T. whipplei*. Clinical manifestations probably follow a disordered host response to the organism's infiltration of various body tissues. The organism is taken up into tissue macrophages, which may be seen with PAS staining.
- Predominantly affects middle-aged Caucasian men. Patients with HIV infection do not develop the disease, and one small study found *T. whipplei* DNA in 35% of healthy volunteers.
- Clinical features—presents with arthritis, fever, diarrhoea, abdominal pain, and weight loss (90%). Malabsorption follows disruption of the villous architecture. Cardiovascular (endocarditis), respiratory, and CNS (supranuclear ophthalmoplegia, cerebellar ataxia, disinhibition, meningoencephalitis) involvement may occur.
- Diagnosis—biopsy of affected organs (small bowel, synovium, brain, endocardium) to demonstrate the typical histopathology (not pathognomonic and may be seen with *Mycobacterium avium intracellulare* (MAI), cryptococcosis, or other parasitic infections usually observed in patients who are immunosuppressed with HIV disease) and DNA testing for *T. whipplei*. Some experts recommend PCR testing of skin biopsy regardless of involvement, reporting high diagnostic yield.
- Treatment—prolonged course of antibiotics, e.g. 2 weeks of IV ceftriaxone, followed by 1 year of co-trimoxazole. PCR may be the best way to demonstrate remission—therapy should be continued if patients remain positive, perhaps with an alternative regime. Malnourished patients will need nutritional support and vitamin supplementation.
- Prognosis—almost universally fatal within 12 months, if untreated. Most treated patients do well, apart from those who have CNS disease or those who relapse (17–35%).

Chapter 17

Urinary tract infections

Introduction *678*
Cystitis *679*
Acute pyelonephritis *681*
Chronic pyelonephritis *683*
Renal abscess *685*
Catheter-associated urinary tract infections *686*
Prostatitis *688*
Epididymitis *689*
Orchitis *691*

Introduction

Definitions

- The term 'urinary tract infection' (UTI) covers the whole spectrum of infection, from asymptomatic bacteriuria to severe pyelonephritis.
- Uncomplicated UTI is considered to be infection of a structurally and functionally normal urinary tract, e.g. acute cystitis in women.
- A complicated UTI is associated with an underlying factor that increases the risk of failing therapy, e.g. diabetes mellitus, pregnancy, symptoms >7 days, HAI, urinary tract obstruction, renal failure, presence of urinary catheter/stent/nephrostomy tube, recent urinary tract instrumentation, anatomic or functional abnormality of the urinary tract, history of childhood UTI, renal transplantation, immunosuppression.
- All UTIs in men, pregnant women, and children are considered complicated. Any patient with a complicated UTI should be referred to a specialist for assessment and follow-up.

Epidemiology

- Asymptomatic bacteriuria occurs in all age groups and does not necessarily result in clinical infection.
- Infants—incidence of UTI 1–2%, commoner in males.
- Children—asymptomatic bacteriuria and UTI commoner in girls. UTI is rare in boys and suggests a structural abnormality.
- Women—asymptomatic bacteriuria occurs in 1–3% of non-pregnant women and 2–9.5% of pregnant women. Ten to 20% of women experience symptomatic UTI during their life. Risk factors: frequent sexual intercourse, diaphragm use, spermicide use, lack of urination after intercourse, and history of recurrent infections. Twenty to 30% of pregnant women with untreated asymptomatic bacteriuria go on to develop acute pyelonephritis.
- Men—asymptomatic bacteriuria <0.1%. Circumcision is associated with a decreased risk of UTI.
- Elderly—10% of men and 20% of women aged >65 years have bacteriuria. Risk factors: prostatic disease, poor bladder emptying, perineal soiling, and urinary tract instrumentation.
- Hospitalized patients—high rates of bacteriuria; 10% of catheterized patients develop UTI. Other risk factors: female diabetics, pregnant black women with sickle-cell trait, those with interstitial renal disease, renal transplant recipients.
- Renal transplant patients—asymptomatic bacteriuria is associated with a high incidence of pyelonephritis and the risk of graft loss.

Aetiology

- Seventy-five to 95% of acute community infections are due to *E. coli*. Other organisms include *P. mirabilis*, *K. pneumoniae*, and *S. saprophyticus*.
- The microbial spectrum for complicated UTIs is broader and includes the above, as well as *Serratia, Pseudomonas, Enterobacter, Providencia*, enterococci, staphylococci, and fungi.

- Polymicrobial infections are common in those with structural abnormalities, as are antibiotic-resistant organisms (secondary to antibiotic exposure and instrumentation).
- Fungi (particularly *Candida*) occur in patients with indwelling catheters receiving antimicrobial therapy.
- *S. aureus* infection is usually haematogenous and associated with renal/perinephric abscesses.
- Adenoviruses (especially type 11) are implicated in acute haemorrhagic cystitis in children and allogenic BMT recipients.

Diagnosis

- Specimen collection—urine may be collected by midstream clean-catch (to reduce the number of urethral organisms collected), by catheterization, or by suprapubic aspiration of the bladder.
- Urine dipstick analysis—pyuria (10–50 white cells/mm^3 of urine) is non-specific and does not necessarily indicate infection, but most patients with UTI have pyuria. The leucocyte esterase test is sensitive (75–96%) and specific (94–98%) for detecting >10 white cells/mm^3 of urine. Haematuria may be seen in certain infections, but calculi, tumour, vasculitis, glomerulonephritis, and renal TB should be considered. Proteinuria is common in UTI and should be <2g/24h. The dipstick nitrite test detects the products of bacterial nitrate reduction. It may be falsely negative in the presence of diuretic use, low dietary nitrate, or organisms that do not produce nitrate reductase (e.g. *Enterococcus, Pseudomonas*, and *Staphylococcus*). The combined sensitivity/specificity of dipstick leucocyte/nitrite testing is 79.2% and 81%, respectively.
- Urine culture—patients with UTI usually have $\geq 10^5$ organisms/mL of urine in properly collected specimens. Patients without infection will have counts of $<10^4$ organisms/mL of urine. However, symptomatic infections can result with counts of 10^4–10^5 organisms/mL of urine. These criteria apply to Gram-negative organisms. Infection caused by Gram-positive organisms, fastidious bacteria, and fungi rarely reach over 10^4 bacteria/mL.
- BCs—should be taken if systemic infection is a possibility.
- Urological assessment—exclude anatomical abnormalities, stones, tumours in patients with recurrent UTIs, complicated UTIs, or UTIs in men, pregnant women, infants, and children.

Cystitis

An infection of the bladder characterized by dysuria, frequency, and urgency. These symptoms may also be related to urethritis or inflammation without infection. Non-bacterial causes of cystitis include infectious agents (viral, mycobacterial, chlamydial, and fungal species) and non-infectious precipitants (radiation, chemical, autoimmune, hypersensitivity, and interstitial cystitis). Consider these non-bacterial causes in cases of cystitis that are culture-negative and fail to respond to antibiotic therapy.

Clinical features

- These include dysuria, urgency, hesitancy, polyuria, incomplete voiding, urinary incontinence, haematuria, and suprapubic or low back pain.
- Elderly patients may present with confusion and no localizing features.
- Constitutional symptoms, such as fever, are mild or absent.

Management

(See reference 1.)

- General measures—these include hydration, management of diabetes, and investigation and management of obstruction or structural abnormalities.
- Antibiotic therapy—all symptomatic infections should be treated, and empirical regimes based on local resistance data. The resolution of bacteriuria is related to the concentration of the antimicrobial agent achieved in the urine—dosage modifications are necessary in patients with renal insufficiency for agents excreted primarily by the kidney:
  - cystitis in women—appropriate empiric agents include nitrofurantoin (100mg bd for 5 days), co-trimoxazole (960mg bd for 3 days), fosfomycin (3g stat), or pivmecillinam (400mg bd for 5 days). Alternative agents include fluoroquinolones or co-amoxiclav;
  - cystitis in pregnant women—appropriate regimens include nitrofurantoin (5 days), co-amoxiclav (3–7 days), cefpodoxime (3–7 days), or fosfomycin (3g stat dose);
  - cystitis in men—appropriate agents include ciprofloxacin, levofloxacin, or co-trimoxazole for 7–14 days. Nitrofurantoin and β-lactams should be avoided, as they do not achieve adequate tissue concentrations and would be less effective for occult prostatitis;
  - cystitis in children—antibiotic treatment will depend on the age of the child, the likely pathogens, and local resistance patterns. Seek expert advice.

Recurrent infection

May follow relapse (bacteriuria with the same organism that was present when treatment was started) or reinfection (bacteriuria with a different organism from that before treatment). Reinfection with the same organism may occur if it has persisted in nearby areas, e.g. vagina.

- Relapse—consider renal involvement (necessitating a longer course of therapy 2–6 weeks), a structural abnormality (e.g. calculi, obstruction—consider urological investigation), or chronic prostatitis (➔ see Prostatitis, pp. 688–9). Certain patients experiencing repeated relapses in whom surgical correction is not indicated or is not feasible may be appropriate for long-term antibiotic therapy. Such patients should have regular urine cultures (looking for antibiotic resistance), assessment of renal function, and renal imaging. There is no consensus on how long prophylaxis should last. Rates of infection return to pre-treatment levels once therapy is stopped. Cranberry juice *does* reduce the frequency of episodes, compared to placebo.
- Reinfection—certain patients experience repeated reinfections (with successful clearance following appropriate therapy between each

episode). Those cases related to sexual intercourse may benefit from post-coital voiding. One RCT demonstrated reduced recurrence rates on taking a single dose of antibiotic (co-trimoxazole) up to 2h after intercourse.[2] Where no associated precipitating event can be identified, long-term chemoprophylaxis may be appropriate, particularly in children who may be at risk of renal damage.

Prognosis

- Children—those without obstruction (e.g. urethral valves) or vesico-ureteric reflux (VUR) have a good prognosis. Obstruction can lead to severe destruction of the renal parenchyma. VUR is seen in 30–50% of children with bacteriuria and can lead to renal scarring. Infants and preschool children are at greatest risk. Severe reflux may lead to repeated infection and renal impairment. Reflux alone, particularly intrarenal reflux, may be capable of causing renal scarring, even in the absence of infection. Infection exacerbates reflux, which reduces with the elimination of bacteriuria.
- Adults—once a woman has had a UTI, she is more likely to go on to have further episodes. There may be a role for prophylactic antibiotic therapy in women with recurrent uncomplicated UTIs.

Urethral syndrome

Seen in women with acute onset of urinary symptoms (dysuria, etc.), but with $<10^5$ bacteria/mL. Studies have shown that the majority of these patients have genuine infection, with a low number of organisms confined to the lower urinary tract. Others may represent patients with sterile pyuria and urethritis secondary to infection with *C. trachomatis* or *N. gonorrhoeae*. However, some patients with the syndrome have no pyuria and persistently sterile cultures—vaginitis and genital herpes should be excluded.

References

1 International Clinical Practice Guidelines for the Treatment of Acute Uncomplicated Cystitis and Pyelonephritis in Women: A 2010 Update by the Infectious Diseases Society of America and the European Society of Microbiology and Infectious Diseases. *Clin Infect Dis*. 2011;**52**:e103–20.

2 BMJ Clinical Evidence. Available at: http://www.clinicalevidence.com/x/index.html.

Acute pyelonephritis

Infection of the kidney, which may be caused by ascending infection from the bladder or by seeding of the kidneys during bacteraemia. Uncomplicated pyelonephritis occurs in non-pregnant women, and the annual incidence of pyelonephritis is 1.2–1.3 cases per 100 000 women. Complicated pyelonephritis is progression of disease to emphysematous pyelonephritis, real corticomedullary abscess, perinephric abscess, or papillary necrosis.

Clinical features

Clinical symptoms of pyelonephritis include symptoms of cystitis, plus fever, chills, nausea, vomiting, flank pain, and tenderness. May rarely present with sepsis, shock, acute renal failure (ARF), and multiorgan failure.

Microbiology

- *E.coli* is the commonest isolate in uncomplicated pyelonephritis. Other species include *P. mirabilis, K. pneumoniae*, and *S. saprophyticus*.
- Complicated pyelonephritis is caused by the above organisms, as well as *Pseudomonas, Serratia, Providencia*, enterococci, staphylococci, and fungi.

Diagnosis

- Usually easily diagnosed in women, but may be less obvious in men, the elderly, and the hospitalized in whom infection may develop insidiously. For general points on the diagnosis of UTI, ➲ see Introduction, pp. 678–9).
- Urinalysis—pyuria is present in most cases; haematuria is unusual and suggests another pathology.
- Urine culture—all patients with presumed pyelonephritis should be tested because of the possibility of antibiotic resistance.
- BCs—up to 20% are positive.
- Imaging—is indicated for patients who fail to respond to 48–72h therapy or are severely ill with pyelonephritis. Other indications include history of renal stones, symptoms of renal colic, diabetes mellitus, previous urological surgery, immunosuppression, and repeated episodes of urosepsis. Ultrasound or CT scan are useful to demonstrate renal tract abnormalities—the latter may be contraindicated in those with renal impairment if IV contrast is required.

Management

(See reference 3.)

- General—rehydration, antipyretics, analgesics.
- Antibiotic therapy—start empirically, as guided by local resistance patterns, while awaiting culture and sensitivity testing.
- Uncomplicated pyelonephritis in non-hospitalized patients—ciprofloxacin 500mg bd for 7 days is appropriate (where the incidence of fluoroquinolone resistance in community uropathogens is <10%). If the rate of fluoroquinolone resistance is >10%, then a single dose of ceftriaxone or gentamicin may be given, pending culture results.
- Hospitalized patients would be treated with IV antibiotics, based on local antibiotic susceptibility data. Possible regimens include: (i) a fluoroquinolone, (ii) gentamicin ± ampicillin, (iii) extended-spectrum cephalosporin or β-lactam ± gentamicin, and (iv) a carbapenem.
- Surgery may be required in some patients with predisposing conditions who fail to respond to therapy and in those developing certain complications, e.g. renal cortical abscess, corticomedullary abscess, emphysematous pyelonephritis.

Prevention

- Cases with an obvious precipitant—practice changes (e.g. different means of contraception, administration of prophylactic antibiotics, early identification and treatment of lower UTIs) may prevent them.
- Long-term catheter-related infections—ensure a closed system; consider intermittent or suprapubic catheterization.
- Renal transplant recipients—antibiotic prophylaxis may be given to some groups of patients in the first 6–12 months after transplantation.

Prognosis

- ARF is rare outside the context of hypovolaemia, obstruction, or sepsis. It may follow papillary necrosis, which may be seen in those with diabetes mellitus, sickle-cell disease, or urinary tract obstruction.
- Renal scarring:
  - children—seen in 6–15% of children after a febrile UTI. This is often associated with a degree of VUR (thought to be congenital), and patients with scarring are at risk of hypertension and renal impairment in later life. This risk increases with delayed treatment in those experiencing recurrent infection;
  - adults—a single episode of acute pyelonephritis in an adult woman leads to renal scarring in 46%, as demonstrated by Tc99m-labelled DMSA (dimercaptosuccinic acid) scanning 10 years later. Acute pyelonephritis in pregnancy may lead to acute renal impairment, ARF, ARDS, low-birthweight children, preterm delivery, and sepsis. Renal scarring is four times more likely after pyelonephritis in pregnant women than in non-pregnant women. Renal impairment is seen particularly in infections causing severe papillary necrosis.
- Pyelonephritis becomes potentially fatal when secondary conditions develop such as emphysematous pyelonephritis (20–80% mortality rate), perinephric abscess (20–50% mortality rate), or sepsis.
- Acute renal transplant pyelonephritis occurring in the first 3 months after transplant has a significant association with graft loss (>40%) by 96 months, compared to all renal transplant cases, with or without the occurrence of pyelonephritis at any time after the transplant up to 96 months (25–30%).

Reference

3 Gupta K, Hooton TM, Naber KG, *et al.*; Infectious Diseases Society of America; European Society for Microbiology and Infectious Diseases (2011). International clinical practice guidelines for the treatment of acute uncomplicated cystitis and pyelonephritis in women: A 2010 update by the Infectious Diseases Society of America and the European Society of Microbiology and Infectious Diseases. *Clin Infect Dis*. **52**:e103–20.

Chronic pyelonephritis

Chronic diffuse interstitial inflammation which may be caused by several conditions, including obstruction, calculi, analgesic nephropathy, hypokalaemic nephropathy, renal TB, and following acute pyelonephritis in childhood in the context of VUR.

Chronic pyelonephritis secondary to vesico-ureteric reflux

VUR is congenital incompetence of the ureterovesical valve due to an abnormally short intramural segment of the ureter. The condition is present in 30–40% of young children with symptomatic UTIs and in almost all children with renal scars. VUR may also be acquired by patients with a flaccid bladder due to spinal cord injury. This may lead to reflux nephropathy. Sometimes this diagnosis is established, based on radiological evidence obtained during an evaluation for recurrent UTI in young children. Infection without reflux is less likely to produce injury.

- *Symptoms*—patients with chronic pyelonephritis present with fever, lethargy, nausea and vomiting, flank pain, and dysuria, and children may fail to thrive. Hypertension may be noted.
- *Investigations*—pyuria, proteinuria (poor prognostic feature), urine cultures (negative cultures do not exclude the diagnosis), demonstration of renal stones/dilatation (IV urogram, renal USS), reflux (voiding cystourethrogram, cystoscopy), and renal scarring (radioisotopic scanning with technetium DMSA).
- *Management*—infection should be treated, and underlying structural abnormalities corrected (e.g. ureteric reimplantation).
- *Complications*—proteinuria, focal glomerulosclerosis, renal impairment secondary to scarring (rate of progress of scars can be slowed by speedy institution of appropriate antibiotic therapy), pyonephrosis (if obstructed), nephrosis (may occur in cases of obstruction), hypertension (increases rate of decline in renal function), xanthogranulomatous pyelonephritis.

Emphysematous pyelonephritis

- A severe, necrotizing, acute, multifocal bacterial nephritis, with extension of the infection through the renal capsule. Gas is found in the renal substance and perinephric space.
- Eighty-five to 100% of cases are seen in patients with diabetes mellitus.
- Most cases due to *Enterobacteriaceae*.
- Patients present with fever, chills, pain, flank mass (50%), crepitation (over thigh or flank), and urinary symptoms.
- Diagnosis is confirmed by CT scan.
- Treatment—antibiotics, drainage, nephrectomy.
- Mortality—60% in those with gas within the kidney alone and managed with antibiotics and drainage, 80% in those with gas extending to the perinephric space and managed by antibiotic therapy alone, 20% in those managed by nephrectomy.

Xanthogranulomatous pyelonephritis

- A rare, serious, debilitating illness characterized by a chronic inflammatory mass originating in the renal parenchyma. Gross appearance: mass of yellow tissue composed of lipid-laden macrophages and inflammatory cells (perhaps with an abscess cavity), regional necrosis, and haemorrhage.
- Causes—often associated with infection by *Proteus, E. coli*, or *Pseudomonas* spp. in the context of chronic obstruction (stones are seen in 75% of patients, e.g. staghorn calculus).
- Patients are often immunocompromised or diabetic, and it is four times commoner in women than men.
- Clinical features—patients appear chronically ill, with dull persistent flank pain, fever, weight loss, and fistulae (pyelocutaneous and ureterocutaneous fistulae have been described). Can present acutely with fever and flank pain. Renal function is reduced in almost all cases.
- Diagnosis—CT scan helps diagnosis. Resembles a neoplastic lesion in its radiographic appearance and tendency to involve adjacent structures, including the psoas muscle and perirenal space. Renal pelvis is dilated.

Many are confirmed only at operation. Bacteria are not typically cultured from the urine, but, if culture is positive, the commonest organisms are *P. mirabilis*, *E. coli*, and *Pseudomonas* spp.
- Treatment—appropriate antibiotic therapy may be important in initial stabilization, but definitive therapy is always surgical, usually nephrectomy. Other factors complicating response to therapy: obstructing calculus, renal papillary necrosis.

Renal abscess

Perinephric abscess

- Follows chronic or recurrent pyelonephritis, rupture or extension of suppuration within the kidney, or haematogenous dissemination from another site. Located between the renal capsule and surrounding fascia and may extend to involve the GI tract, groin, lung (pleuritic pain, raised hemidiaphragm, pleural effusion), and psoas (may be signs of psoas irritation, e.g. scoliosis, pain on hip flexion).
- Clinical features—presentation is insidious, with fever, chills, unilateral flank pain (70%), dysuria (40%), nausea, vomiting, weight loss (25%), flank tenderness, abdominal tenderness (60%), referred pain (i.e. hip, thigh, or knee), flank or abdominal mass (<50%), pyuria (70%), sterile urine (40%), and bacteraemia (40%).
- Diagnosis is often not apparent—one-third of patients are diagnosed at autopsy. CT scan confirms the diagnosis. USS may be falsely negative. MRI defines the extension.
- Treatment—drainage is always required. Specific agents providing pseudomonal or enterococcal coverage may be indicated. Other organisms that have been reported include TB and fungi. Nephrectomy may be necessary.
- Mortality <50%, less if recognized early and managed appropriately (e.g. surgery and aminoglycoside with antistaphylococcal agent).

Renal corticomedullary abscess

- Usually associated with urinary tract abnormalities and commonly caused by *Enterobacteriaceae*. Disease is part of a spectrum that ranges from acute focal bacterial nephritis affecting a single lobe to severe emphysematous pyelonephritis. Males and females are equally affected in most cases.
- Clinical features—fever, chills, flank pain, nausea, vomiting (usually absent in cortical abscesses), flank mass, hepatomegaly. Urinary symptoms may be absent (but seen more frequently than with cortical abscesses), and urinalysis is normal in 30%.
- Diagnosis is best confirmed by CT. Microbiology: MSU, BCs, culture of pus obtained by CT/USS-guided aspiration or drainage.
- Treatment is by antibiotic therapy (e.g. ciprofloxacin and gentamicin) and drainage or surgical intervention. Structural abnormalities should be corrected, e.g. obstruction relieved.

Renal cortical abscess

- Uncommon and usually due to the haematogenous spread of *S. aureus*, most commonly from a skin infection. Risk factors include IDU, diabetes mellitus, and haemodialysis. Microabscesses forming in the cortex coalesce to form a circumscribed abscess over days to months. Commoner in men than women.
- Clinical features—the onset is often insidious. Symptoms include fever, chills, back pain, abdominal pain, flank mass, and rarely urinary symptoms (if the abscess communicates with, and involves, the collecting system).
- Diagnosis best confirmed by CT, and this or USS may be used to guide aspiration or drainage.
- Microbiology—MSU (culture is usually normal), BCs (often negative), culture of aspirated pus.
- Treatment—IV antibiotics (e.g. high-dose flucloxacillin for 4 weeks) and drainage (for all but the smallest abscesses) which may be successfully achieved percutaneously. Nephrectomy rarely required.

Catheter-associated urinary tract infections

UTIs associated with urinary catheters are the leading cause of secondary health care-associated bacteraemia. ~20% of hospital-acquired bacteraemias arise from the urinary tract, and the associated mortality is about 10%.

Pathogenesis of urinary tract infections

- Catheterization thwarts a number of the defence mechanisms that reduce the incidence of UTI in healthy individuals.
- Organisms may be introduced from the perineum or the urethra at the time of catheter insertion, contaminate the collecting device, or enter via the space between the catheter and the urethral mucosa.
- Once in the urinary tract, organisms are not eliminated as efficiently as is usual and can reach large numbers within a couple of days. Some are capable of producing biofilms which facilitate their growth. An inflammatory response may result in cystitis and pyuria. Organisms may ascend and cause upper UTI.
- Risk factors associated with catheter-associated bacteriuria include the duration of catheterization, female sex, older age, diabetes mellitus, bacterial colonization of the drainage bag, and errors in catheter care.

Short-term catheterization

Up to 25% of patients have a catheter in at some point during a hospital stay. The rate of bacteriuria is 3–10% per day of catheterization. Common organisms: *E. coli* (24%), *Candida* spp. (26%), *P. aeruginosa*, *K. pneumoniae*, *P. mirabilis*, enterococci, and CoNS. Most bacteriuric episodes in this group are caused by a single organism. Organisms isolated from the catheter itself may not be found in the urine. Most episodes of bacteriuria are asymptomatic, but 10–25% develop symptoms of UTI. Bacteraemia is uncommon but occurs at higher rates in bacteriuric patients undergoing instrumentation (e.g. prostatectomy).

Long-term catheterization

The two most frequent indications are urinary incontinence (women) and outflow obstruction (men). Such patients may be catheterized for months to years. All develop bacteriuria at some point, and certain species possess adhesins that enable them to persist in the catheterized urinary tract. Polymicrobial bacteriuria is seen in 95% of long-term catheterized patients. Mildly symptomatic UTIs occur fairly regularly, most lasting only a day and resolving without treatment. Bacteraemia occurs in 4–10% of institutionalized patients undergoing catheter removals or replacements, often following the development of acute pyelonephritis. Other complications of long-term catheterization: symptomatic UTI, catheter obstruction (by bacteria, crystals, protein, glycocalyx), urinary stones, chronic renal inflammation, peri-urinary infection, bladder metaplasia, malignancy (in very long-term patients). Some of the complications of long-term catheterization once seen in spinal injury patients are now seen much less frequently, as such individuals manage themselves with intermittent catheterization.

Prevention

- Patients should be catheterized for clear indications only. Incontinence, in particular, may be more appropriately managed by other means.
- When urethral catheterization cannot be avoided, carers should be meticulous in maintaining a closed collection system, and the catheter should be used for as short a period as possible.
- Alternatives to indwelling urethral catheterization: conveens (lower incidence of bacteriuria, but have infection risks and other complications of their own), intermittent catheterization, suprapubic catheterization (cleaner skin region is associated with lower rate of infection).
- A single dose of gentamicin at insertion may reduce infection.

Treatment

- Asymptomatic bacteriuria—no evidence that treating catheterized patients with bacteriuria in the absence of symptoms significantly reduces the number of people who go on to develop symptoms. Long-term catheterized patients treated with antibiotics for bacteriuria, regardless of symptoms, showed no difference in the number of febrile episodes. Certain situations do warrant treatment: identification of organisms with a high incidence of bacteraemia (e.g. *S. marcescens*), control of organisms associated with an outbreak of UTI in an institution, and bacteriuria in those patients at high risk of serious complications (e.g. pregnant women, immunosuppressed patients), or patients undergoing urological surgery.
- Symptomatic catheter-associated UTI—cultures of blood and urine should be taken. Patients are treated with empirical IV antibiotics, based on local antibiotic susceptibility patterns and previous infections. Therapy can be modified in light of culture results and given orally once the patient is afebrile. Treatment duration is usually 7–14 days. Bacteria may persist in the catheter biofilm, and it is sensible to remove or replace the catheter, if possible.
- Candiduria—seen in many catheterized patients and particularly related to hospitalization and previous antibiotic exposure. It is usually

asymptomatic. Catheter removal resolves it in 40%; changing the catheter resolves it in 20%. Patients who must remain catheterized and continue to have candiduria may benefit from a course of fluconazole if they have a non-krusei candidal cystitis. Systemic therapy with IV amphotericin or fluconazole and possibly surgery may be indicated. Complications: fever, renal/perirenal abscess, fungus balls in the bladder and renal pelvis, dissemination.

Prostatitis

Up to 50% of men will experience symptoms of prostatitis at some time in their lives.

Acute bacterial prostatitis

- Clinical features—symptoms are those of a lower UTI (dysuria, frequency) and possibly obstruction (due to prostatic oedema), and fever. On examination: lower abdominal/suprapubic discomfort, extreme tenderness, firm prostate on PR examination.
- Investigations—urinalysis shows pyuria, and cultures are positive. The usual pathogens are *E. coli, Proteus* spp., other *Enterobacteriaceae (Klebsiella, Enterobacter, Serratia* spp.), and *P. aeruginosa*. BCs may be positive either spontaneously or following vigorous PR.
- Management—response to antimicrobial therapy is usually rapid; agents should provide good coverage of *Pseudomonas*, enterococci, and *Enterobacteriaceae*. Urinary retention is best managed by suprapubic catheterization to avoid obstructing the drainage of prostatic secretions.
- Complications—prostatic abscess, prostatic infarction, chronic prostatitis.

Chronic bacterial prostatitis

- Chronic/recurrent bacterial infections of the prostate which occurs in young and middle-aged men. Risk factors include previous acute prostatitis, history of prior manipulation of the urinary tract, voiding symptoms, diabetes, smoking, and higher prostate volumes.
- Patients often experience repeated infections with the same organism and are asymptomatic between episodes, with a normal prostate on examination.
- GNRs are the commonest cause, with *E. coli* causing ~75–80% of episodes. *E. faecalis, K. pneumoniae, P. mirabilis, P. aeruginosa*, and other Gram-negative bacilli are the next most commonly reported organisms. *S. aureus* and streptococcal species are occasional pathogens.
- Diagnosis is usually clinical, as obtaining prostatic fluid or urine sample post-prostatic massage requires specialist input.
- Treatment is usually with a fluoroquinolone for 6 weeks. Co-trimoxazole is an alternative, but longer courses may be required to achieve cure. Long treatment courses fail in one-third, cure one-third, and bring about resolution, while on treatment, with subsequent relapse in one-third. These poor results may be a consequence of poor drug penetration into the prostatic parenchyma or perhaps infected calculi

serving as persistent foci for infection. Those not cured may remain asymptomatic on long-term low-dose suppressive antibiotic therapy, despite the persistence of prostatic bacteria.

Chronic prostatitis/chronic pelvic pain syndrome

- The largest subset of patients with symptoms of prostatitis. There is no history of bacteriuria or evidence of infection.
- Symptoms—difficulty voiding, erectile dysfunction, and a dull aching pain which may be pelvic, perineal, suprapubic, scrotal, or inguinal and is exacerbated by ejaculation. Examination is unremarkable.
- Some patients may have leucocytes in semen or prostatic secretions (expressed by digital massage), whereas others have no evidence of inflammation. Although the reason for this is not known, patients with leucocytes are more likely to have bacteria in their prostatic parenchyma, and it is suggested that those without are experiencing a non-infectious disease.

Asymptomatic inflammatory prostatitis

Prostate inflammation with no symptoms. Such patients may be identified in working up the cause of a raised prostate-specific antigen (PSA), with prostate biopsy showing a simple inflammatory process.

Granulomatous prostatitis

A histological reaction that may follow acute bacterial prostatitis, tuberculous prostatitis (and that following BCG therapy for transitional cell carcinoma of the bladder), and systemic mycoses. It may cause an indurated, firm, or nodular prostate, clinically indistinguishable from that caused by malignancy.

Prostatic abscess

- A rare complication of acute bacterial prostatitis. Patients most commonly affected: those with urinary tract obstruction or foreign bodies, those with diabetes, the immunocompromised, and those not adequately treated for their acute episode.
- Most cases are caused by the common uropathogens acquired by the ascending route and, rarely, organisms such as *S. aureus*.
- Symptoms resemble those of acute bacterial prostatitis: fever, dysuria, and signs of urinary sepsis. A fluctuant area of the prostate may be apparent on PR.
- Definitive diagnosis can be made by USS, CT scan, or MRI scan of the pelvis.
- Treatment—drainage and appropriate antibiotics.

Epididymitis

An inflammatory reaction of the epididymis caused by infection or trauma. There are two distinct patterns of infective epididymitis: sexually transmitted and non-specific (non-sexually transmitted) bacterial epididymitis. Underlying GU tract abnormalities are common only in the latter group.

General features

- Symptoms—painful swelling of the scrotum which may be acute (over 1–2 days) or more gradual in onset, dysuria with or without urethral discharge. Fever may be present, particularly in hospitalized patients who develop the condition following urinary tract manipulation.
- Examination—tender swelling and erythema of the scrotum, usually unilateral. Early in disease, swelling may be localized to one portion of the epididymis. Consequent involvement of the associated testis is common, producing epididymo-orchitis. Secretion of inflammatory fluid can lead to the development of a hydrocele.

Non-specific bacterial epididymitis

- The commonest pathogens in men >35 years are *Enterobacteriaceae* and *Pseudomonas* spp. Other infectious agents: MTB (tuberculous epididymitis is the commonest form of male genital TB), systemic mycoses (e.g. *Blastomycetes*).
- Patients often have an underlying urinary tract pathology or a history of recent GU tract manipulation (cases may occur weeks or months after the intervention), particularly if bacteriuric at the time. Bacterial prostatitis or long-term urethral catheters are other important predisposing factors.
- Complications—testicular infarction, scrotal abscess, pyocele, scrotal sinus, infertility, chronic epididymitis.
- Management—empirical antibiotics aimed at covering GNRs and Gram-positive cocci, while awaiting urinary cultures. Bed rest, scrotal elevation, analgesics. Some complications may require surgical intervention.

Sexually transmitted epididymitis

- The commonest form in young men.
- Major pathogens—*C. trachomatis, N. gonorrhoeae*.
- Many patients do not complain of discharge. *Chlamydia* spp. may be carried for prolonged periods (≥1 month) before developing symptoms.
- Diagnosis requires a high index of suspicion and appropriate cultures. The patient should be evaluated for the presence of other STIs, and sexual partners followed up. Underlying GU abnormalities are uncommon in this group.
- Treatment—specific therapy covering both chlamydial and gonococcal infections. If symptoms do not subside within 3 days of therapy or tenderness/swelling persists on completion, the diagnosis should be reviewed. Consider abscess, infarction, malignancy, and tuberculous/fungal epididymitis.
- Complications—abscess, testicular infarction, infertility, chronic epididymitis.

Orchitis

Less common than epididymitis or prostatitis. Blood-borne dissemination is the major route of infection.

Viral orchitis

Viruses are by far the commonest cause, e.g. mumps, Coxsackie B virus. Mumps rarely causes orchitis in pre-pubescent males but is seen in 20% of post-pubertal patients. Testicular pain and swelling follow 4–6 days after parotitis and may be seen even in the absence of parotitis; 70% of cases are unilateral. Contralateral involvement may occur a few days after the first testicle. Symptoms range from mild discomfort to severe pain, with nausea, vomiting, prostration, fever, and constitutional symptoms. Mild cases resolve within 4–5 days; severe ones may take 3–4 weeks; 50% of patients experience some degree of testicular atrophy. Testicular atrophy has been documented in 30–50% after mumps orchitis—impaired fertility occurs in 13%, but sterility is rare.

Bacterial orchitis

Isolated bacterial orchitis is extremely rare. It usually follows from contiguous spread from an infected epididymis. Most cases of pyogenic orchitis are caused by *E. coli, K. pneumoniae, P. aeruginosa*, staphylococci, and streptococci. Patients are acutely ill with a high fever, marked discomfort, testicular swelling, and nausea and vomiting. Pain radiates to the inguinal canal. There is usually an acute hydrocele, and the testis is swollen and tender. Overlying skin may be erythematous and oedematous. Treatment is as for bacterial epididymitis. Complications (e.g. infarction, abscess) may require surgery.

Chapter 18

Sexually transmitted infections

Introduction *694*
Bacterial vaginosis *695*
Vulvovaginal candidiasis *697*
Genital warts *699*
Tropical genital ulceration *701*
Genital herpes *703*
Pelvic inflammatory disease *705*
Toxic shock syndrome *707*
Gonorrhoea *709*
Chlamydia *711*
Trichomoniasis *713*
Syphilis *714*

Introduction

STIs have been on the rise in the UK and many other Western countries in recent years, fuelled by a decline in the practice of 'safer sex'. The most severely affected groups are younger females and homosexual men. The number of new STI diagnoses made in UK GUM clinics continues to rise, with an increase of 2–3% each year since 2003.

Risk factors

The risk factors that influence an individual's chance of acquiring a particular STI are broadly the same for all STIs. This means that patients with one STI should be assessed for the presence of others, including syphilis and HIV. Risk factors include: the number of sexual partners an individual has, failure to use barrier contraception, frequency of partner change, lower socio-economic status, age <25 years, residence in an inner city, symptomatic partner, sexual orientation (syphilis, gonorrhoea, HIV, and hepatitis B are more prevalent amongst MSM in the UK), and sexual practices (orogenital and anogenital contact).

Contact tracing

During the Second World War, fears of a UK STI epidemic led to laws enabling the compulsory treatment of a sexual contact named by >1 person with a diagnosed STI. These laws were repealed after the war and led to the concept of partner notification. Partner notification aims to prevent reinfection of treated persons and break any chain of onward STI transmission. Patients are encouraged to notify their sexual partners of any infection risk, with the help and advice of trained health advisers. This process should be carried out by a GUM clinic, and it is essential that individuals experiencing such infections are referred. It may be appropriate to treat asymptomatic contacts presumptively. Partner notification is voluntary in the UK, but a legal requirement in some states of the USA and Sweden.

Patient assessment

- History—last intercourse, contraceptive method, nature of sexual contacts and number, frequency of partner change, sexual orientation, sexual practices, previous history of STI, previous treatments received, menstrual history, drug use, foreign travel.
- Examination—skin (rashes, lesions), lymphadenopathy, hair loss, jaundice, mucosal lesions, conjunctivitis, urethritis, arthritis, detailed examination of the genitalia, including a speculum examination of women and the subpreputial space and male urethra in men. A rectal examination and proctoscopy may be indicated.
- Tests—samples of genital secretions should be taken; in practice, this will usually be done by an experienced individual in the GUM clinic. In men: urethral swab (*Chlamydia*) and smear for Gram stain and culture (*N. gonorrhoeae*); in women: high vaginal swab in Stuart's media for microscopy and culture (*Candida, G. vaginalis*, anaerobes, *Trichomonas*), endocervical swab (*C. trachomatis*). Other tests: swab ulcers for HSV culture and dark microscopy for syphilis, blood serology for syphilis, hepatitis, and HIV.

Differential diagnoses

- Men with urethritis—*N. gonorrhoeae*, non-gonococcal urethritis (*Chlamydia*, trichomoniasis, UTI).
- Balanitis—if associated with ulcers or blisters, consider causes of genital ulceration. If associated with erythema or excoriation, consider *Chlamydia*, causes of urethritis, trichomoniasis, *Candida*, and bacterial infection. Non-STI causes—consider dermatological causes such as dermatitis, lichen simplex, lichen planus, etc.
- Vulval irritation/pain—if associated with ulcers/blisters, consider causes of genital ulceration. Otherwise, consider candidiasis (especially if pregnant, diabetic, discharge, or recent antibiotics), trichomoniasis, and BV. Non-STI causes: dermatological conditions, especially atopic vulvitis, and consider vulval intraepithelial neoplasia.
- Abnormal vaginal discharge—watery white/grey with fishy smell, consider BV; white curdy discharge with vulval rash, consider candidiasis; malodorous green/yellow discharge, consider trichomoniasis. Other: gonorrhoea, *Chlamydia*, cervical herpes simplex. Non-STI causes: retained foreign body (e.g. tampon).
- Anogenital ulceration—herpes (preceded by vesicles), syphilis, tropical. Non-STI causes: neoplasia, drug reactions, Behçet's disease, trauma.
- Genital lumps—genital warts, molluscum contagiosum, condylomata lata. Non-STI causes: folliculitis, lichen planus, keratoacanthoma, carcinoma.
- Infestations that may be transmitted sexually include pubic lice and scabies.

Bacterial vaginosis

BV causes vaginal discharge in ≤50% of symptomatic women (the other causes are vulvovaginal candidiasis and trichomoniasis). Rather than being due to a single organism, BV is caused by complex changes in the balance of the microbiological flora.

Epidemiology

- Worldwide prevalence ranges from 11% to 48% in women of childbearing age.
- Risk factors for acquisition—new or multiple sexual partners, vaginal douching, smoking. It can occur in women who have never had vaginal intercourse.

Pathology

- Lactobacilli produce H_2O_2 which lowers the pH—the loss of these organisms permits an increase in pH and overgrowth of vaginal anaerobes. These produce proteolytic enzymes which degrade vaginal peptides into offensive-smelling products and promote discharge and exfoliation of the epithelial layers.
- A reduction in the normally dominant lactobacilli and increase in other organisms, such as *G. vaginalis, Prevotella* spp., *Porphyromonas* spp., *Bacteroides* spp., *Peptostreptococcus* spp., *M. hominis, U. urealyticum*, and *Mobiluncus* spp.

Clinical features

- Fifty to 75% of cases are asymptomatic.
- Thin, white, fishy smelling discharge, most noticeable after intercourse.
- May be associated with cervicitis which may or may not occur in the presence of simultaneous chlamydial or gonococcal infection.
- Vaginal pain or vulval irritation is uncommon.
- Complications—pregnant women with BV have a higher rate of preterm delivery; BV is associated with endometritis, post-partum fever, and infections following gynaecological surgery; it is a risk factor for HIV acquisition and transmission, and acquisition of HSV-2, *Chlamydia*, and gonorrhoea.

Diagnosis

- The Amsel criteria—sensitivity is 90%, specificity 77% if three of the four criteria are present. Remember that trichomonal infection may cause the first three findings:
    - homogeneous, watery, white-grey discharge coating the vaginal walls;
    - vaginal pH > 4.5;
    - positive amine test—add 10% KOH to a sample of discharge—positive if produces a fishy odour;
    - the presence of 'clue cells' (epithelial cells studded with adherent coccobacilli) on a saline wet mount—the single best predictor of BV. At least 20% of epithelial cells should be clue cells in those women with BV. Gram staining is the most sensitive, but impractical in standard clinical practice.
- No bacteria are specific for BV, and bacterial culture is not useful.
- Diagnostic card tests for pH indicate the presence of amines.

Differential diagnosis

Trichomoniasis, atrophic vaginitis (dyspareunia and inflammation are present in these cases).

Management

(See reference 1.)

- Infection resolves spontaneously in one-third of cases.
- Treatment may reduce the risk of acquiring other STDs.
- Who to treat:
    - all women presenting with symptoms—oral treatment is safe in pregnancy and not associated with adverse fetal effects;
    - asymptomatic women proceeding to abortion or hysterectomy—reduces the risk of post-operative infection;
    - asymptomatic pregnant women with previous preterm delivery may also benefit from treatment. BV is associated with a higher rate of preterm birth (perhaps due to chorioamnionitis), but studies have not demonstrated that treating it brings about a significant reduction. However, treating BV in those women with a history of preterm delivery is associated with reduced rates of preterm pre-labour rupture of membranes and low-birthweight babies. Consider screening those women with a history of preterm labour for BV.

- Regimes:
    - metronidazole—500mg bd PO for 7 days (single 2g dose has lower efficacy and is no longer recommended) or 5g od PV of 0.75% metronidazole gel for 5 days. Early cure rates >90%, 80% at 4 weeks;
    - clindamycin—300mg bd PO for 7 days or 100mg ovules od PV for 3 days. The use of clindamycin may be associated with the acquisition of clindamycin-resistant anaerobes. No resistance to metronidazole has been demonstrated;
    - other agents—tinidazole, secnidazole, and probiotics have been used.
- Thirty per cent of patients experience recurrence within 3 months. A prolonged (e.g. 14 days) or alternative treatment course should be used in such patients. Those who experience multiple relapses may benefit from a long-term maintenance regime of twice-weekly PV metronidazole gel. Clindamycin should not be used for this purpose.
- Treating partners does not appear to reduce recurrence. Sexual intercourse appears to play a role in disease activity. Some studies have reported reduced rates of recurrence when male sexual partners used condoms routinely during coitus or when women remained abstinent.

Reference

1 Clinical Effectiveness Group, British Association for Sexual Health and HIV (2012). *UK national guideline for the management of bacterial vaginosis 2012*. Available at: http://www.bashh.org/documents/4413.pdf.

Vulvovaginal candidiasis

Vulvovaginal candidiasis accounts for one-third of cases of vaginitis.

Epidemiology

- *Candida* spp. may be found in the lower genital tract of 10–20% of asymptomatic women.
- It is common, with 29–49% of premenopausal women reporting at least one episode. It is less common in post-menopausal women.
- Candidal infection is uncommon in prepubertal women but does occur in children who have had recent antibiotic therapy, wear nappies, or are immunosuppressed.
- There is an increase in incidence at the time at which most women begin regular sexual activity.

Pathology

- *C. albicans* is the cause of 80–92% of cases, but the incidence of other *Candida* spp., such as *C. glabrata*, may be increasing as a result of increasing use of over-the-counter drugs.
- Sporadic episodes usually occur with no identifiable predisposing factor. Risk factors include: diabetes mellitus, immunosuppression, recent antibiotic use, oral contraceptive use, or oestrogen therapy.

Clinical features

- Pruritus, dysuria, dyspareunia, soreness.
- There may be discharge which might be white and clumpy, or thin and watery, but it is often absent, with only vulvar and vaginal erythema on examination.
- Recurrent infection—defined as ≥4 episodes a year and seen in 5–8% of women. Predisposing factors, such as diabetes, are seen in a minority, and susceptibility seems to be largely determined genetically. Behavioural factors seem to play a part—a 2-fold increase in risk has been associated with the consumption of cranberry juice, the use of sanitary towels, and sexual lubricants.

Diagnosis

- Self-diagnosis unreliable—one study demonstrated that only 34% of those women self-diagnosing candidal infection actually had it.
- A wet mount of the discharge with 10% KOH may allow recognition of yeast and hyphae, but microscopy is negative in around 50%.
- Vaginal pH is around 4–4.5 (unlike trichomonal infection or BV).
- Perform culture in patients with persistent discharge or recurrent symptoms unresponsive to azole treatment—they may have non-albicans *Candida* infection. Routine culture is unhelpful.
- As well as other infective causes, consider allergic reactions and contact dermatitis in the differential.

Management

(See reference 2.)

- Treatment is indicated for symptoms. Asymptomatic carriage does not require therapy.
- Ninety per cent of cases represent uncomplicated infections (healthy, non-pregnant women with mild/moderate symptoms, infrequent episodes and infection with *C. albicans*). Oral and topical treatments are similarly effective, with topical therapy relieving symptoms more rapidly, but oral being preferred by women, e.g. PO fluconazole.
- Ten per cent of cases are complicated (infection with non-albicans spp., severe symptoms, four or more episodes per year, and those cases occurring in the pregnant, uncontrolled diabetics, or the immunosuppressed).
- The immunosuppressed and those with severe symptoms are unlikely to respond to short treatment courses—7–14 days of topical therapy, or two doses of PO fluconazole (150mg) 72h apart, is indicated.
- *C. glabrata* infection—50% of women infected with this species fail treatment with azoles. Moderate success may be seen with intravaginal boric acid, and >90% cure may be seen with TOP flucytosine cream.
- Pregnancy—treat only for symptoms using a topical imidazole for 7–14 days (e.g. clotrimazole). Oral azoles are contraindicated in pregnancy. Vaginal candidiasis is not associated with adverse outcomes in pregnancy.
- Recurrent infection (four or more episodes per year)—aim to eliminate risk factors (e.g. better glucose control, lower oestrogen-containing contraceptives, behavioural changes where appropriate).

After the initial treatment course, long-term suppressive therapy (e.g. fluconazole 150mg PO weekly for 6 months) is effective at preventing relapses. However, more than half are likely to experience further infections in the months following cessation of suppressive therapy. These patients should be treated acutely once again, and then given a year of suppressive treatment after culture confirmation of relapse. Development of azole resistance has not yet been associated with long-term therapy in this setting.
- Most experts do not recommend treatment of asymptomatic sexual partners.

Reference

2 Clinical Effectiveness Group, British Association for Sexual Health and HIV (2007). *United Kingdom national guideline on the management of vulvovaginal candidiasis (2007)*. Available at: http://www.bashh.org/documents/1798.pdf.

Genital warts

Anogenital warts are one of the commonest sexually transmitted viral infections. They are caused by HPV, a highly infectious dsDNA virus, of which there are over 70 distinct subtypes. Ninety per cent of cases are related to subtypes 6 and 11. Subtypes 16 and 18 are associated with squamous cell carcinoma.

Epidemiology

- Exposure is usually sexual, and incubation is from a few weeks to several months. The risk of disease increases with the number of sexual partners. Women tend to be affected more than men in most settings.
- Anal disease can occur in women as a result of extension of perineal infection or receptive anal intercourse. Men usually experience lesions on the shaft of the penis or the preputial cavity. Anal lesions are commoner among MSM but also occur among heterosexual men.
- The prevalence of anogenital warts is higher amongst those who are HIV-positive or have other STD. The risk increases with lower CD4 counts and decreases with ART.
- Most infections are cleared within 2 years, but persistent infections can occur and are associated with the development of squamous cell carcinoma.

Clinical features

- Those with a small number of lesions may experience no symptoms.
- A larger number of lesions may be associated with pruritus, bleeding, dysuria, PV discharge, pain, and tenderness.
- Rarely, warts may form larger exophytic masses that can interfere mechanically with intercourse, defecation, and even childbirth.
- Anal disease may cause strictures.

Diagnosis

- Usually made visually. Lesions are pink and can take the form of flattened papules or the more classic verrucous papilliform warts.

Application of 5% acetic acid causes lesions to turn white. This is not specific for anogenital warts, however.

- Anoscopy, colposcopy, etc. allows the extent of disease to be assessed.
- Biopsy should be performed where the diagnosis is in doubt, in immunocompromised patients (higher risk of malignancy), and in cases that do not respond to therapy.
- The differential includes: condyloma lata (flat, velvety lesions of secondary syphilis), anogenital squamous cell carcinoma (may coexist with genital warts), vulvar intraepithelial neoplasia, skin tags, and molluscum contagiosum.

Management

Spontaneous regression is seen in up to 30% of immunocompetent cases by 3 months. The choice of therapy, where indicated, is governed by the number and extent of the lesions. All modalities have high rates of recurrence. Women should have a Pap smear. Small external lesions can be managed by the application of a topical treatment, either in clinic or by the patient where appropriate. Large, multiple, or internal lesions should be referred to a surgeon or gynaecologist, and pathological studies undertaken where indicated.[3]

- Chemical agents:
  - podophyllin contains an anti-mitotic agent which stops the cell cycle in metaphase, causing cell death; a 25% solution is administered 1–2 times per week—usually at a clinic—and achieves clearance rates of 20–50% at 3 months. It should be applied to small areas of skin, allowed to dry, and washed off 6h later. It should not be used on the cervix or vaginal epithelium (burns). It is contraindicated in pregnancy (teratogenic);
  - podophyllotoxin is a related agent that can be self-administered to external warts, with similar rates of success;
  - trichloroacetic acid acts by protein coagulation and has similar rates of success and similar side effects to podophyllin. It can be used on internal lesions and during pregnancy. Neighbouring skin can be protected from its caustic effects by the application of petroleum jelly prior to use;
  - fluorouracil/adrenaline gel injected intralesionally can achieve an initial cure rate of up to 60%, but half relapse by 3 months.
- Immuno-modulation:
  - imiquimod is applied topically as a cream to external lesions only and acts by cytokine induction. It achieves high rates of clearance (over 80%) and low rates of recurrence (under 20%);
  - IFN-α given systemically achieves similar rates of clearance as thermocoagulation but has higher rates of recurrence.
- Surgery—ablation or excision should be performed where medical therapies have failed or are not indicated (e.g. due to size). Cryotherapy with liquid nitrogen or a cryoprobe is safe in pregnancy and achieves clearance rates of over 90% at 3 months—repeated applications are required. Laser therapy is expensive, requires anaesthesia, and places the operator at risk of developing warts. It achieves cure rates of almost 100% at 1 year. Surgical excision has clearance rates of 36% at 3 months.

As well as the standard risks associated with anaesthesia and surgery, patients may develop strictures. Excised lesions should be examined pathologically for signs of malignancy.
- Newer therapies include TOP cidofovir, TOP BCG, and infrared coagulation.

Reference

3 Clinical Effectiveness Group, British Association for Sexual Health and HIV (2015). *UK national guidelines on the management of anogenital warts 2015*. Available at: http://www.bashh.org/documents/UK%20national%20guideline%20on%20Warts%202015%20FINAL.pdf.

Tropical genital ulceration

Genital ulceration is much commoner in patients presenting with STI in the developing world and an important factor in the spread of HIV. The common causes of genital ulcers in the developed world (HSV and syphilis) remain common in developing regions (e.g. HSV remains the top cause in Jamaica and South Africa) but may be pushed out of the top place by certain other infections (e.g. chancroid in Rwanda). Diagnosing lesions clinically can be difficult—syphilis classically causes a single painless ulcer, but so may HSV and LGV. Where facilities allow, investigations should include: serologic testing for syphilis, a diagnostic evaluation for herpes, and, where appropriate, Gram stain and culture on selective media (for *H. ducreyi*).

Chancroid

- Caused by *H. ducreyi*, a fastidious GNR.
- It produces a potent 'cytolethal distending toxin' which is likely to contribute to both the formation of ulcers and their slow healing.
- Incubation after infection is around 1 week, following which painful, erythematous papules develop on the external genitalia (prepuce, corona, or glans in men; the labia, vagina, and perianal areas in women), develop into pustules, and then erode into sloughy, non-indurated haemorrhagic ulcers. Lesions are usually multiple, often developing on adjacent skin surfaces (thigh, scrotum), and suppurative inguinal lymphadenopathy is common (sometimes forming fluctuant buboes). Co-infection with HIV may result in atypical presentations with multiple lesions, extragenital involvement, and delayed response to treatment.
- Diagnosis is by clinical appearance and culture and Gram stain (organisms clump in parallel strands—'school of fish' appearance) of material from the ulcer or aspirated lymph nodes. Enriched culture media are required. PCR-based tests are in development.
- Treatment is with azithromycin 1g PO stat or ceftriaxone 1g IM stat or ciprofloxacin 500mg PO stat or ciprofloxacin 500mg bd PO for 3 days or erythromycin 500mg qds PO for 7 days (recommended for HIV-infected patients).[4]

Lymphogranuloma venereum

- Genital ulcer disease caused by the L1, L2, and L3 serovars of *C. trachomatis*. Endemic in areas of East and West Africa, India, South East Asia, and the Caribbean. Since 2003, a series of outbreaks of LGV have been reported in MSM. In 2004, PHE (formerly the HPA) launched an enhanced surveillance programme.

- Asymptomatic infection in women is common and may serve as a reservoir. Incubation is 3–12 days. Primary infection is characterized by a transient, painless genital ulcer. Direct local extension leads to a secondary lesion 2–6 weeks later—an inflammatory reaction in the inguinal lymph nodes, with fever, headache, weight loss ± pneumonia, meningoencephalitis, and arthritis. Lymphadenopathy may be so severe as to bulge on each side of the inguinal ligament ('groove sign'). An inflammatory mass may form in the rectum, leading to pain, constipation, tenesmus, and rectal discharge. LGV proctitis may be confused with IBD. Late disease may lead to fibrosis and strictures in the anogenital tract, genital elephantiasis, anal fistulae, frozen pelvis, and infertility.
- Diagnosis is based on clinical features. Culture of pus from lesions and nodes is possible but rarely practical in regions where the disease occurs. Chlamydial serology is useful but not specific for serovars. PCR-based tests are available.
- Treatment is with doxycycline 100mg bd PO or erythromycin 500mg qds PO for 21 days.[5]

Granuloma inguinale (donovanosis)

- Caused by *Klebsiella granulomatis*.
- Endemic in Western New Guinea, the Caribbean, Southern India, South Africa, South East Asia, Australia, and Brazil; granuloma inguinale (or donovanosis) is primarily an STI causing indolent, painless, non-purulent ulceration. Infection may also be acquired faecally and by passage through an infected birth canal.
- After an incubation of 1–3 months, the 'beefy red' ulcers appear on the prepuce or labia and enlarge over months to 5cm in diameter or more. Auto-inoculation may see ulcers forming on adjacent skin. Local extension and fibrosis occur, and late lesions may cause elephantiasis-like swelling of the external genitalia. Regional lymphadenopathy is rare, but metastatic spread to the bones, joints, and liver has been reported.
- Diagnosis is clinical and by microscopy of Giemsa-stained material from ulcers which may demonstrate bipolar intracellular bacteria ('Donovan bodies'—a characteristic safety-pin appearance). Culture is extremely difficult and rarely performed.
- Treatment—donovanosis may be treated with a variety of antibiotics which should be given for a minimum of 3 weeks or until the lesions have healed. Azithromycin 1g weekly or 500mg daily is recommended by the Australian antibiotic guidelines. The US CDC recommends the following regimens: (i) co-trimoxazole 960mg bd, (ii) doxycycline 100mg bd, (iii) erythromycin 500mg qds, or (iv) ciprofloxacin 500mg bd. An aminoglycoside (e.g. gentamicin 1mg/kg tds IV) may be added if there is no initial response (which may be seen in HIV-positive patients).[6]

References

4 Clinical Effectiveness Group, British Association for Sexual Health and HIV (2014). *UK national guideline on the management of chancroid 2014*. Available at: http://www.bashh.org/documents/Chancroid%202014%20.pdf.

5 Clinical Effectiveness Group, British Association for Sexual Health and HIV (2013). *2013 UK national guideline on the management of lymphogranuloma venereum*. Available at: http://www.bashh.org/documents/2013%20LGV%20guideline.pdf.

6 Clinical Effectiveness Group, British Association for Sexual Health and HIV (2011). *United Kingdom national guideline for the management of donovanosis (granuloma inguinale) 2011*. Available at: http://www.bashh.org/documents/3194.pdf.

Genital herpes

Genital herpes simplex infections are a major public health problem across the world. Like all herpesviruses, herpes simplex establishes a latent state, following primary infection, and may reactivate, causing episodic local disease.

Epidemiology

- HSV-2 is the commonest cause of genital herpes, but an increasing number of cases are due to HSV-1 infection.
- Asymptomatic HSV-2 infection is more likely in those previously infected with HSV-1, and vice versa.
- The incidence of genital herpes has been increasing in the UK, and the presence of HSV-related ulcers is associated with an increased risk of HIV transmission.

Clinical features

- Incubation is usually 3–7 days. Primary infection is characterized by local burning, followed by a painful genital vesicular eruption. These vesicles then rupture, forming ulcers. Other symptoms: fever, dysuria, tender inguinal lymphadenopathy, headache, herpetic proctitis. New lesions appear for around a week. Resolution over 1–3 weeks. Up to 60% of primary cases are asymptomatic; thus, the first clinical attack may actually represent the first reactivation.
- Recurrent attacks tend to be less severe with a shorter duration of symptoms and infrequent systemic features. Up to half of patients with reactivation experience prodromal symptoms (local tingling, shooting pains). The majority of patients developing primary infection will experience a recurrence within the first year. Prolonged first episodes are associated with earlier and more frequent relapses. Recurrence rates are much higher with HSV-2 infection and in immunosuppressed patients.
- Rare extragenital features of primary infection include: meningitis, urinary retention due to autonomic dysfunction, and distant skin lesions.
- Subclinical viral shedding can occur in the absence of lesions. This is of importance, as it leads to unrecognized transmission to neonates and sexual partners. It is commoner with HSV-2.

Diagnosis

- Type-specific antibodies to HSV develop in the first few weeks of infection and are maintained indefinitely. Commercial tests are available, but a positive test does not allow one to distinguish present from previous infection.
- Viral culture from lesions allows definitive diagnosis—it is more likely to be positive if the fluid is taken from vesicles that have not yet ruptured.
- Viral antigen detection tests are available and allow rapid, type-specific diagnosis.
- PCR-based viral detection is rapid and specific, and allows recognition of asymptomatic viral shedding.

Management

- Symptomatic treatment—saline bathing, analgesia, and topical local anaesthetic agents (e.g. 5% lidocaine) ointment for painful micturition. Hospitalization may be required for urinary retention, meningism, or severe constitutional symptoms. If catheterization is required (e.g. autonomic disturbance or pain), the suprapubic route may be better to reduce pain, aid recognition of return of normal micturition, and reduce the risk of ascending infection.
- Antiviral treatment—this is indicated within 5 days of onset or while new lesions are forming. Recommended regimens include: (i) aciclovir 300mg 5 times a day for 5 days, (ii) aciclovir 400mg tds for 5 days, (iii) valaciclovir 500mg bd for 5 days, and (iv) famciclovir 250mg tds for 5 days. Antivirals reduce the severity and duration of episodes but do not alter the natural history of the disease. Topical agents are less effective. IV aciclovir is indicated if patients are unable to take oral therapy.
- Recurrent disease—episodic antiviral therapy reduces the duration and severity of recurrent episodes. Recommended regimens include: (i) aciclovir 300mg 5 times a day for 5 days, (ii) aciclovir 400mg tds for 5 days, (iii) valaciclovir 500mg bd for 5 days, and (iv) famciclovir 125mg bd for 5 days. Alternative short-course regimens include: (i) aciclovir 800mg tds for 2 days, (ii) famciclovir 1g bd for 1 day, and (iii) valaciclovir 500mg bd for 3 days.
- Suppressive antiviral therapy—patients with frequent recurrences (>4 per year) may benefit from suppressive antiviral therapy. Recommended regimens include: (i) aciclovir 400mg bd, (ii) aciclovir 200mg qds, (iii) famciclovir 250mg bd, and (iv) valaciclovir 500mg od for up to 1 year.
- HIV-infected patients who develop severe genital herpes should be given secondary prophylaxis with antivirals if their CD4 count is under 100 cells/mm^3.[7]

Reference

7 Clinical Effectiveness Group, British Association for Sexual Health and HIV (2014). *UK national guideline on the management of anogenital herpes 2014*. Available at http://www.bashh.org/documents/HSV_2014%20IJSTDA.pdf.

Pelvic inflammatory disease

An acute infection of the female upper genital tract which may involve the uterus, Fallopian tubes, ovaries, and even adjacent pelvic structures.

Epidemiology

- The majority of cases present within 1 week of menses, which is thought to enhance the ascent of vaginal organisms.
- Those at greatest risk of PID are those with multiple sexual partners. It is rarely seen in celibate women and those in long-standing monogamous relationships.
- Other risk factors include: age (highest incidence in those aged 15–25 years), the presence of symptomatic STI in the partner, previous PID, and possibly vaginal douching.

Microbiology

- *N. gonorrhoeae* accounts for approximately one-third of cases.
- *C. trachomatis* serovars D–K account for 30–50% of cases. The introduction of screening for *C. trachomatis* infection has reduced the incidence of PID.
- Other organisms—older studies isolated GAS and GBS (rarely enterococci), *E. coli, Klebsiella* spp., *P. mirabilis, Haemophilus* spp., *Bacteroides/Prevotella* spp., *Peptococcus*, and *Peptostreptococcus* spp. A more recent study found an association between GAS and *H. influenzae* and severe disease.

Clinical features

- Infection of the upper genital structures may precipitate any or all of endometritis, salpingitis, oophoritis, peritonitis, and perihepatitis.
- Symptoms—lower abdominal pain which may start during or shortly after menses, vaginal discharge, abnormal uterine bleeding. Rebound tenderness is common in the lower quadrants, and fever is seen in half of patients. Those with perihepatitis may also develop upper abdominal pain. The uterus and adnexae will be tender on pelvic examination.
- PID can be a subclinical disease and cause of infertility—one-third of women with no history of PID were found to have *C. trachomatis* in the upper genital tract, with no clinical findings except infertility.

Diagnosis

- Consider the diagnosis in patients with abdominal pain *and* one of: cervical or uterine/adnexal tenderness, fever >38°C, raised WCC, abnormal cervical or vaginal discharge, or raised inflammatory markers.
- Investigations include:
  - microscopy of vaginal discharge—if this demonstrates Gram-negative intracellular diplococci, the probability of PID is high;
  - laparoscopy—although specificity approaches 100%, laparoscopy has been found to be only around 50% sensitive in the diagnosis of PID. It should be considered in patients who do not respond to empirical therapy within 72h (less if acutely ill) and those in whom there is a high suspicion of an alternative diagnosis (e.g. appendicitis);

- endometrial biopsy—the demonstration of plasma cell endometritis is a common finding in cases of clinical PID, but it is also found in asymptomatic women with no other evidence of PID;
- other tests—transvaginal ultrasound has a low specificity and sensitivity for PID but is useful in the identification of pelvic abscesses; positive DNA testing for gonococcus and *Chlamydia* increases clinical probability.

- Confirmed cases are considered to be those with pelvic pain/tenderness *and* one of: endometritis/salpingitis on biopsy, *N. gonorrhoeae* or *C. trachomatis* in the genital tract, salpingitis seen on laparoscopy or laparotomy, isolation of pathogenic bacteria from the upper genital tract, or inflammatory pelvic peritoneal fluid with no other cause.
- All patients should have a pregnancy test and urinalysis.
- Differential diagnosis—appendicitis, cholecystitis, IBD, UTI, dysmenorrhoea, ectopic pregnancy, ovarian cyst/torsion/tumour.

Treatment

- Most people can be treated as outpatients. Consider admitting pregnant women, those failing to respond to oral medications, those with severe clinical features (high fever, vomiting, severe pain), and those with tubo-ovarian abscesses or likely to require surgical intervention.
- Selected antibiotics should cover *N. gonorrhoeae, C. trachomatis*, GAS and GBS, anaerobes, and the common Gram-negative enterics. Avoid fluoroquinolones (increase *N. gonorrhoeae* resistance). Suitable regimes include:
  - outpatient therapy—ceftriaxone 500mg IM stat, followed by doxycycline 100mg PO bd for 14 days *and* metronidazole 400mg tds PO for 14 days. Alternative regimens: (i) ofloxacin 400mg bd PO plus metronidazole 400mg tds PO for 14 days, (ii) ceftriaxone 500mg IM stat, followed by azithromycin 1g PO weekly for 2 weeks, and (iii) moxifloxacin 400mg od PO for 14 days;
  - inpatient therapy—IV therapy should be given until 24h after clinical improvement and then changed to an oral regimen to complete a 14-day course. Regimens include: (i) ceftriaxone 2g od IV plus doxycycline 100mg PO or IV bd, followed by doxycycline 100mg bd PO plus metronidazole 400mg tds PO and (ii) clindamycin 900mg tds IV *and* gentamicin 5–7mg/kg od IV, followed by clindamycin 450mg tds PO (or metronidazole 400mg tds PO) plus metronidazole 400mg tds PO.
- As with all STIs, contacts should be traced, and patients should be counselled and screened for HIV, hepatitis, etc., where indicated.[8]

Reference

8 Clinical Effectiveness Group, British Association for Sexual Health and HIV (2011). *UK national guideline for the management of pelvic inflammatory disease 2011*. Available at: http://www.bashh.org/documents/3572.pdf.

Toxic shock syndrome

A syndrome of fever, skin rash, and shock due to toxins produced by certain organisms, e.g. *S. aureus* (➔ see *Staphylococcus aureus*, pp. 234–6), GAS (➔ see Group A *Streptococcus*, pp. 249–51), and *C. sordellii* (➔ see Other clostridia, pp. 270–1).

Epidemiology

- Staphylococcal TSS—classically associated with tampon use. Around half of cases are now non-menstrual (e.g. surgical and post-partum wound infections, mastitis, septorhinoplasty, sinusitis, osteomyelitis, arthritis, burns, skin and soft tissue infections, respiratory infections following influenza, and enterocolitis.
- Streptococcal TSS—associated with severe invasive GAS infections, e.g. necrotizing skin and soft tissue infections, bacteraemia, and pneumonia. Risk factors for development of severe GAS include minor trauma, NSAIDs, recent surgery, viral infections (e.g. influenza, varicella), post-partum state.
- *C. sordellii* TSS—this is associated with gynaecological procedures, childbirth, abortion, and injecting drug users.

Pathogenesis

- Staphylococcal TSS—TSST-1 was the initial exotoxin isolated from cases reported in 1981. It is found in 90–100% of *S. aureus* strains associated with menstrual TSS and 40–60% of non-menstrual cases. The staphylococcal enterotoxins A, B, C, D, E, and H have also been implicated in TSS. They act as superantigens, activating large numbers of T cells and massive cytokine production.
- Streptococcal TSS—streptococcal pyogenic exotoxins A, B, and C (SPEA, SPEB, SPEC) acts as superantigens, resulting in T-cell proliferation and production of cytokines that mediate shock and tissue injury.
- *C. sordellii* TSS—the production of two cytotoxins, lethal toxin (LT) and haemorrhagic toxin (HT), causes diffuse capillary leak, oedema, and shock. Another toxin *C. sordellii* neuraminidase modifies vascular adhesion molecules and stimulates promyelocytic proliferation.

Clinical features

- Staphylococcal TSS—symptoms develop rapidly, 2–3 days after the onset of menstruation or surgery, in otherwise healthy individuals. Clinical features include fever, hypotension, and skin lesions (erythroderma, diffuse macular rash, mucosal hyperaemia, ulceration, desquamation of the palms and soles 1–2 weeks after illness onset). Myalgia, weakness, and raised CK are common. Diarrhoea is common, and renal failure and CNS symptoms (confusion, seizures) may occur. Recurrent TSS may occur days to months after the initial episode, usually in patients who have not been treated adequately or who fail to develop an appropriate antibody response.
- Streptococcal TSS—typically presents with pain prior to developing symptoms of infection. Clinical features include localized swelling and erythema, followed by bruising, sloughing of the skin, and progression

to necrotizing fasciitis or myositis. Twenty per cent develop an influenza-like illness with fever, chills, myalgia, nausea, vomiting, and diarrhoea. Fever is common, but hypothermia may occur. Patients may be normotensive at presentation but rapidly become hypotensive. Altered mental status occurs in 50% of patients. Complications include bacteraemia, renal failure, ARDS, DIC, and rarely Waterhouse–Friderichsen syndrome.

- *C. sordellii* TSS—characterized by rapid onset of severe illness/septic shock in previously healthy individuals. Early symptoms include nausea, vomiting, lethargy, 'flu-like' symptoms, and abdominal pain/tenderness. This is followed by development of massive generalized tissue oedema, pleural, pericardial, and peritoneal effusions, refractory hypotension, and absence of fever. Laboratory tests show profound leucocytosis and haemoconcentration.

Diagnosis

- Staphylococcal TSS—the US CDC clinical criteria for staphylococcal TSS[9] include: (i) fever, (ii) hypotension, (iii) rash, (iv) desquamation, (v) involvement of three or more systems (e.g. GI, muscular, mucous membranes, renal, hepatic, haematological, CNS), and (vi) negative tests (e.g. blood, throat, and CSF cultures for other pathogens; negative serology for measles, leptospirosis, RMSF).
- Streptococcal TSS—the Working Group on Severe Streptococcal Infections clinical diagnostic guidelines[10] include: (i) isolation of GAS from a normally sterile site AND (ii) hypotension (systolic blood pressure ≤90mmHg in adults or <5th percentile for age in children) PLUS (iii) two or more of the following: renal dysfunction, coagulopathy, liver dysfunction, ARDS, erythematous macular rash, soft tissue necrosis (e.g. necrotizing fasciitis, myositis, gangrene).
- *C. sordellii* TSS—the diagnosis should be suspected in young women with rapid clinical deterioration following a gynaecological procedure, abortion, or delivery, and in IDUs. BCs are positive in 20% of cases. Vaginal and/or wound specimens should be cultured.

Management

- Supportive therapy—patients may require extensive fluid replacement (10–20L/day) to maintain tissue perfusion. Vasopressors, e.g. (dopamine and noradrenaline) may be required.
- Surgery—for menstrual TSS, foreign bodies should be removed, and surgical drainage/debridement may be required for post-surgical cases. Extensive surgical debridement is required for necrotizing fasciitis cases.
- Staphylococcal TSS—while it is not clear whether antibiotics are required in the acute management of staphylococcal TSS, they are important in preventing recurrent disease. Clindamycin *may* be more effective than antibiotics acting solely on the bacterial cell wall, as it suppresses protein synthesis (and therefore potentially toxin production). Empirical treatment is with clindamycin 600mg IV tds and vancomycin 30mg/kg/day IV in two divided doses. Treatment should be for 14 days.

- Streptococcal TSS—empirical treatment for streptococcal TSS is clindamycin 900mg tds IV plus piperacillin–tazobactam 4.5g tds IV (or meropenem 1g tds IV if penicillin-allergic). Once the diagnosis is confirmed, treatment should be changed to benzylpenicillin 4 million units every 4h plus clindamycin 900mg tds IV. The duration of therapy is 14 days after the last surgical debridement.
- *C. sordellii* TSS—empirical treatment is with clindamycin 900mg tds IV plus piperacillin–tazobactam 4.5g tds IV. Once the diagnosis is confirmed, treatment should be changed to benzylpenicillin 4 million units every 4h plus clindamycin 900mg tds IV.
- Adjunctive therapies—these include: (i) IVIG—there are no trials to demonstrate the effectiveness of IVIG in the management of staphylococcal or streptococcal TSS. Case reports suggest it may be of benefit in severe cases that fail to respond to fluids and vasopressors; (ii) corticosteroids—there is no evidence to suggest the use of steroids affects outcome in staphylococcal TSS; (iii) hyperbaric oxygen—this has been reported in a few cases of streptococcal TSS; and (iv) *C. sordellii* anti-toxin—there is evidence of benefit in a mouse model of *C. sordellii* TSS, but no clinical data.

Prognosis

- Staphylococcal TSS—death usually occurs within a few of days of presentation but can occur up to 2 weeks later. Causes of death include cardiac arrhythmias, respiratory failure, and bleeding. Mortality in menstrual cases is around 1.8%, non-menstrual cases 6%.
- Streptococcal TSS—the mortality rate is 30–70% in adults, and 18% in children.
- *C. sordellii* TSS—mortality is high and ranges from 50% to 100%.

References

9 Centers for Disease Control and Prevention (1997). Case definitions for infectious conditions under public health surveillance. *MMWR Recomm Rep.* **46**(RR-10):1–55.

10 The Working Group on Severe Streptococcal Infections (1993). Defining the group A streptococcal toxic shock syndrome. Rationale and consensus definition. *JAMA*. **269**:390–1.

Gonorrhoea

A purulent infection of mucous membranes (e.g. urethra, rectum, cervix, conjunctiva, pharynx) caused by *N. gonorrhoeae*.

Epidemiology

- Infection is common across the world. In the developing world, perinatal transmission and neonatal eye infections remain a significant problem.
- It is the second commonest STI in the UK, affecting predominantly young people (peaking in males aged 20–24 years and females aged 16–19 years), with the highest rates in deprived urban areas. Infection is concentrated amongst MSM and black ethnic minority populations.
- The recent increase in incidence and growing prevalence of antimicrobial resistance have made it a major public health concern.

- Resistance to first-line antibiotic treatment is related to an increased risk of treatment failure (with consequent disease complications) and onward transmission within a community. In 2005, 21% of isolates were resistant to ciprofloxacin overall (42.4% amongst homosexual men and 11.3% amongst heterosexual men), and 17.9% of isolates were resistant to penicillin. Therefore, first-line therapy should be ceftriaxone or cefixime.

Clinical features

- Incubation is 2–5 days. Lower genital tract infection may be asymptomatic or cause urethritis, with purulent discharge and dysuria in men and endocervicitis with PV discharge, itch, and dysuria in women. Although infection of the female urethra, pharynx, and rectum (common in homosexual men, uncommon otherwise and causing discharge and tenesmus) are probably common, they are usually asymptomatic.
- Retrograde spread may occur, causing salpingitis/endometritis, PID, and tubo-ovarian abscesses in up to 20% of women with cervicitis. In rare cases, frank peritonitis or perihepatitis (Fitz-Hugh–Curtis syndrome) are seen. Men with gonococcal urethritis can develop epididymitis or epididymo-orchitis.
- Disseminated gonococcal infection may follow around 1% of genital infection; 75% of such cases occur in women who are at increased risk if mucosal infection occurs during menstruation or pregnancy. Features include: rash, fever, arthralgias, migratory polyarthritis, septic arthritis, endocarditis, and meningitis.
- Neonates acquiring infection intrapartum present with ophthalmia neonatorum and disseminated infection. Conjunctivitis can also occur in adults, following direct inoculation of organisms, and may lead to blindness.

Diagnosis

- NAATs—these have become the screening test of choice for asymptomatic individuals with urethral and endocervical infection, and for rectal and pharyngeal infection in MSMs. They are highly sensitive (>96%) and positive tests from extragenital sites and, in low prevalence populations (<1% prevalence), require confirmatory testing.
- Microscopy—provides rapid, near-patient diagnosis in symptomatic patients and shows Gram-negative diplococci within polymorphonuclear cells. Sensitivity is high in men with urethral discharge (>95% sensitive) and lower in asymptomatic males (50–75%) and in women with endocervical discharge (30–50% sensitive). It should not be performed on pharyngeal or rectal specimens.
- Culture—all infected areas should be swabbed and plated onto selective media, both to confirm diagnosis and to provide antibiotic susceptibility data. Culture has a sensitivity of 85–95% for urethral and endocervical infection.
- Disseminated infection—joint effusions, blood, and CSF should be sent for culture and Gram stain, where appropriate. Negative cultures do not rule out disseminated infection.

- Test of cure (TOC)—this is recommended following treatment of gonococcal infections, because of treatment failures and increasing antimicrobial resistance. Where universal TOC is not feasible, it is recommended for the following populations: persisting symptoms/signs, pharyngeal infection, treatment with a second-line regimen, pregnant women.[11]

Management

- Indications for treatment—these include: (i) identification of Gram-negative intracellular diplococci on microscopy of a genital tract smear, (ii) a positive culture of *N. gonorrhoeae* from any site, (iii) a positive NAAT from any site, (iv) a recent sexual partner of confirmed case of gonococcal infection, and (v) consider on epidemiological grounds in sexual assault cases.
- Antibiotics—first-line therapy is ceftriaxone 500mg IM single dose plus azithromycin 1g PO single dose. Alternative regimens include: (i) cefixime 400mg PO single dose (treatment failures reported), (ii) spectinomycin 2g IM single dose, (iii) cefotaxime 500mg IM single dose, (iv) cefoxitin 2g IM single dose (with probenecid 1g PO), (v) cefpodoxime 200mg PO single dose, and (vi) quinolones (e.g. ciprofloxacin 500mg PO single dose) not recommended apart from for infections that are confirmed to be sensitive.[12]

References

11 Clinical Effectiveness Group, British Association for Sexual Health and HIV (2012). *United Kingdom national guideline for gonorrhoea testing 2012*. Available at: http://www.bashh.org/documents/4490.pdf.

12 Bignell C, Fitzgerald M; Guideline Development Group; British Association for Sexual Health and HIV UK (2011). UK national guideline for the management of gonorrhoea in adults, 2011. *Int J STD AIDS*. **22**:541–7. Available at: http://www.bashh.org/documents/3920.pdf.

Chlamydia

Epidemiology

The commonest STI in the UK, with rates highest in the under 25s. A significant number of cases are asymptomatic, and 10–40% of untreated infected women develop PID, making it an important reproductive health issue. The number of cases in the UK has been rising steadily since the mid 1990s, prompting the initiation of a national screening programme. The responsible organisms are *C. trachomatis* serovars D–K (see *Chlamydia*, p. 352).

Clinical features

- Incubation period is 1–3 weeks.
- Around 50% of infected males and 80% of infected females are asymptomatic—such infection may persist for many years, if untreated.
- Symptoms—mucopurulent cervicitis in females and urethritis with dysuria and discharge in males. Ascending genital tract infection may lead to PID in women and is the commonest cause of epididymitis in men under 35 years. Proctitis and pharyngitis occur in men and women.

- Other presentations—LGV (the cause of 10% of genital ulcers in tropical countries; ➲ see Tropical genital ulceration, pp. 701–3), neonatal conjunctivitis, and neonatal pneumonia may occur in children born to infected mothers.
- Complications—PID (➲ see Pelvic inflammatory disease, pp. 705–6), Reiter's disease (urethritis, conjunctivitis, reactive arthritis), perihepatitis, conjunctivitis.
- Co-infection of *Chlamydia* and gonorrhoea is common (40% of women and 20% of men with *Chlamydia* also have gonorrhoea).

Diagnosis

- NAATs—these have become the diagnostic test of choice, as they are highly sensitive (90–95%). Appropriate samples in women include self-taken vaginal swab, first-catch urine sample (65–100% sensitive), or endocervical swab (in those undergoing speculum examination). Appropriate samples in men include first-catch urine sample or urethral swab. Pharyngeal and rectal swabs recommended in MSMs.
- EIAs—these are no longer recommended because of low sensitivity (40–60%).
- Direct fluorescent antibody tests (DFAs)—routine use not recommended, as labour-intensive, although sensitivity may be >80%.
- Cell culture—not routinely recommended, as low sensitivity (60–80%), requires expertise, and is expensive.[13]

Management

- General measures—patients should be advised to avoid sexual intercourse until treatment has finished (or for 7 days after azithromycin treatment). Patients should be offered screening for other STIs, including HIV and HBV screening, and vaccination. All contacts should be offered the same tests.
- Antibiotics—doxycycline 100mg bd PO for 7 days or azithromycin 1g single dose (the drug of choice for reasons of compliance). Alternative regimens are erythromycin 500 mg bd for 10–14 days or ofloxacin 200 mg bd or 400 mg od for 7 days. First-time cure rates of over 95%.
- Pregnancy—doxycycline is contraindicated. Patients should be treated with erythromycin 500mg qds PO for 7–14 days or amoxicillin 500mg tds PO for 7 days or azithromycin 1g PO single dose (*BNF* caution).
- Recurrent infection is usually due to reinfection by untreated partners. Female partners of men with urethritis should be treated, whether or not there is evidence of infection, given the high risk of asymptomatic disease.[14]

References

13 Clinical Effectiveness Group, British Association for Sexual Health and HIV (2010). *Chlamydia trachomatis UK testing guidelines*. Available at: http://www.bashh.org/documents/3352.pdf.

14 British Association for Sexual Health and HIV (2006). *2006 UK national guideline for the management of genital tract infection with Chlamydia trachomatis*. Available at: http://www.bashh.org/documents/65.pdf.

Trichomoniasis

An infection caused by the flagellated protozoan *T. vaginalis* (➔ see *Trichomonas vaginalis*, pp. 532–3), which may be asymptomatic (particularly in men) or lead to vaginal discharge, dysuria, and lower abdominal pain in women or urethritis in men.

Epidemiology

- Transmission is by sexual contact, and its incidence is highest in women with multiple sexual partners and those with other STIs, including HIV. Vertical transmission may take place during delivery.
- Non-sexual transmission (e.g. by contact with contaminated linen in institutions) occurs but is very rare.

Clinical features

- Incubation is 5–28 days.
- Infection is asymptomatic in 10–50% of women and 15–50% of men.
- Symptoms tend to develop during menstruation or pregnancy (higher vaginal pH provides a favourable environment for parasite replication) and include: frothy, yellow vaginal discharge (may be itchy and smelly), dyspareunia, dysuria, and lower abdominal pain.
- On examination, the vulva may be erythematous, with obvious discharge, vaginal inflammation, and punctate haemorrhages on the cervix ('strawberry cervix'). Symptomatic men experience a urethritis indistinguishable from other causes of non-gonococcal urethritis.
- Complications—vaginitis emphysematosa (gas-filled blebs in the vaginal wall), vaginal cuff cellulitis after hysterectomy, premature labour, low-birthweight infants.

Diagnosis

- Microscopy—phase-contrast or dark-ground microscopy of wet preparation of genital specimens will demonstrate the motile flagellated protozoans in 48–80% of infected women and 50–90% of infected men.
- Culture is more sensitive than microscopy but requires specialist media, e.g. InPouch™ TV media or Diamond's media.
- Point-of-care tests, e.g. OSOM® *Trichomonas* rapid test has a sensitivity of 80–94% and a specificity of >95%.
- NAATs offer the highest sensitivity and are becoming the gold standard.

Management

Metronidazole 2g stat dose or tinidazole 2g stat dose. Partners and asymptomatic individuals should be treated.[15]

Reference

15 Clinical Effectiveness Group, British Association for Sexual Health and HIV (2014). *United Kingdom national guideline on the management of Trichomonas vaginalis 2014*. Available at: http://www.bashh.org/documents/UK%20national%20guideline%20on%20the%20management%20of%20TV%20%202014.pdf.

Syphilis

Caused by *T. pallidum* subspecies *pallidum* (➔ see *Treponema* species, pp. 335–6).

Epidemiology

- Generally transmitted by sexual contact; can also be transmitted vertically and via blood transfusions. Highest rates are seen in adults.
- Cases of syphilis have risen dramatically in the UK since the late 1990s, driven by outbreaks in London and Manchester.
- HIV infection is associated with treatment failures and more frequent, earlier neurological disease.

Clinical features

- *Primary syphilis*—after an incubation period of 14 days to 3 months, a painless, erythematous papule develops. This ulcerates, forming a painless, 'punched-out' chancre on the genitalia (rarely on the mouth, hands, and anus). Associated with regional lymphadenopathy. Multiple chancres can occur, particularly in HIV-infected patients. They are highly infectious and heal spontaneously after 1–2 months.
- *Secondary syphilis*—organisms disseminate from the chancre, causing symptoms 1–6 months later:
  - rash—localized or diffuse mucocutaneous rash may be macular, papular, pustular, or mixed. Involves the trunk, limbs, palms, and soles. Mucosal ulcers may occur. Condylomata lata occur in warm, moist areas (e.g. skinfolds) and are highly infectious;
  - early neurosyphilis (commoner in HIV)—may be asymptomatic (CSF findings: pleocytosis, raised protein, decreased glucose, reactive CSF VDRL test), presents with syphilitic meningitis (chronic basal meningitis with headache and cranial nerve palsies—fever is usually absent) or causes meningovascular syphilis (headache, fits, limb paralysis). May also present with stroke, cervical myelopathy, and hemiplegia;
  - other features—fever, sore throat, 'snail-track ulcers' in the mouth, lymphadenopathy, malaise, hepatitis, periostitis, iritis, arthritis, glomerulonephritis.
- *Latent syphilis*—spontaneous resolution of secondary syphilis occurs at 3–12 weeks. During the latent period, patients are asymptomatic, and infectivity is low, but up to one-quarter of patients experience recrudescence of disease. Early latent syphilis is the period up to 2 years after primary infection, and late latent syphilis occurs after 2 years.
- *Late/tertiary syphilis*—rare, follows a latent period of 2–20 years; characterized by chronic inflammation:
  - gummatous syphilis—granulomatous lesions usually affecting the skin, mucous membranes, and bone or organs, causing local destruction (e.g. saddle nose). Gummata may be indurated, nodular, or ulcerated and can be painful;
  - cardiovascular syphilis—endarteritis of the aorta leads to aortic regurgitation (may present with angina and left ventricular failure

(LVF)) and aneurysm formation (ascending aorta). Other large arteries may be affected. VDRL can be negative;
  - late neurosyphilis—two forms: (i) general paresis of the insane (presents with gradual confusion, hallucinations, delusions, fits, cognitive impairment, tremor of the lips and tongue, brisk reflexes, extensor plantars, Argyll Robertson pupils), and (ii) tabes dorsalis (atrophy of the dorsal columns of the spinal cord with autonomic neuropathy and cranial nerve lesions). Presents with ataxia, sensory loss, sphincter disturbance, shooting pains, sensory loss, and arreflexia.
- *Congenital syphilis*—there are two forms:
  - early congenital syphilis occurs within 2 years of birth and presents with rash, condylomata lata, vesiculobullous lesions, snuffles, haemorrhagic rhinitis, osteochondritis, periostitis, pseudoparalysis, mucous patches, perioral fissures, hepatosplenomegaly, generalized lymphadenopathy, non-immune hydrops, glomerulonephritis, neurological or ocular involvement, haemolysis and thrombocytopenia;
  - late congenital syphilis presents after 2 years with interstitial keratitis, Clutton's joints, Hutchinson's incisors, mulberry molars, high palatal arch, rhagades, deafness, frontal bossing, short maxilla, protuberance of the mandible, saddle nose deformity, sternoclavicular thickening, paroxysmal cold haemoglobinuria, and neurological or gummatous involvement.

Diagnosis

- Microscopy—detection of organisms on dark-field microscopy or immunofluorescence of samples taken from chancre exudates.
- PCR-based tests can be used to confirm the diagnosis or to test samples taken from oral lesions, which may be contaminated by commensal spirochaetes, e.g. *Treponema macrodentium* and *Treponema microdentium*.
- Serology[16]—here are two types of serological tests; may be negative in HIV-infected persons (➔ see *Treponema* species, pp. 335–6).
  - specific treponemal tests, e.g. treponemal EIAs to detect IgM and IgG, TPHA, *T. pallidum* particle assay (TPPA), and FTA-ABS. IgM is detectable towards the end of week 2, and IgG by week 4–5. Specific tests are invariably positive in secondary and early latent syphilis;
  - non-treponemal/cardiolipin tests, e.g. VDRL/RPR. A quantitative test should be done to stage the disease and monitor treatment. A positive IgM and a VDRL titre >16 indicate the need for treatment. A false-negative VDRL/RPR test can occur in secondary or early latent syphilis due to the prozone effect.
- CSF findings—in asymptomatic neurosyphilis, include pleocytosis, low glucose, raised protein, and a positive VDRL test (may be negative in HIV). Symptomatic patients have more severe CSF changes, and the CSF VDRL is almost always positive. CSF changes occur in general paresis (elevated lymphocytes, raised protein, and positive CSF VDRL) but are variable in tabes (may be normal; 25% of CSF VDRL tests non-reactive).

- Primary syphilis—dark-field or immunofluorescence microscopy of samples taken from chancre exudates. PCR-based tests for oral lesions or to confirm microscopy findings. VDRL may be positive in around 75%, TPHA in around 90%.
- Secondary syphilis—VDRL present at high titre in almost 100%, TPHA positive in 100%. CSF-VDRL is usually positive in early neurosyphilis.
- Latent infection—VDRL falls with time and following treatment, so a negative test does not rule out infection. TPHA remains positive.
- Tertiary syphilis—in gummatous syphilis, both VDRL and TPHA are positive. In contrast, in syphilitic aortitis and late neurosyphilis, VDRL may be only weakly positive or even negative. TPHA is positive.
- A CXR should be performed in late latent syphilis or if there are signs of aortic disease. Neurological imaging should be performed in those with neurological symptoms/signs.

Management

- All patients should be tested for other STIs and HIV infection.
- Early syphilis—benzathine benzylpenicillin 2.4 million IU IM stat as two injections into separate sites, or doxycycline 100mg bd for 14 days, or erythromycin 500mg qds for 14 days. Penicillin treatment may be complicated by the Jarisch–Herxheimer reaction (➔ see *Borrelia* species, Treatment, p. 338).
- Late syphilis—benzathine benzylpenicillin 2.4 million IU IM as two injections into separate sites weekly for 3 weeks, or doxycycline 100mg bd PO for 28 days.
- Neurosyphilis—benzylpenicillin 3–4 million IU IV 4-hourly for 14 days, or procaine benzylpenicillin G 2.4 million IU IM daily with probenecid 500mg PO qds for 14 days, or ceftriaxone 2g IV od for 14 days, or doxycycline 200mg PO bd for 28 days.
- Treatment success is assessed by symptoms and repeat VDRL. Repeat LP in neurosyphilis at 3–6 months and 3-monthly thereafter until CSF normal and CSF VDRL non-reactive. Failure to achieve resolution by 2 years should prompt retreatment.[17]

References

16 Egglestone SI, Turner AJ (2003). Serological diagnosis of syphilis. PHLS Syphilis Serology Working Group. *Commun Dis Public Health*. 3:158–62.

17 Kingston M, French P, Goh B, *et al.*; Syphilis Guidelines Revision Group 2008, Clinical Effectiveness Group (2008). UK National Guidelines on the Management of Syphilis 2008. *Int J STD AIDS*. 19:729–40. Available at: http://www.bashh.org/documents/1879.pdf.

Chapter 19

Neurological infections

Acute meningitis 718
Bacterial meningitis 718
Viral meningitis 722
Chronic meningitis 724
Tuberculous meningitis 726
Cryptococcal meningitis 727
Coccidioidal meningitis 728
Histoplasma meningitis 729
Neuroborreliosis 730
Neurocysticercosis 731
Encephalitis 732
Brain abscess 737
Subdural empyema 739
Epidural abscess 740
CSF shunt infections 741

Acute meningitis

Definition

Acute meningitis is defined as a syndrome characterized by the onset of meningeal symptoms (headache, neck stiffness, vomiting, photophobia), and cerebral dysfunction (confusion, coma) over hours to days. It is identified by an abnormal number of white blood cells in the CSF. Table 19.1 summarizes the causes.

Table 19.1 Causes of acute meningitis

Category	Causes
Bacteria	GBS, *E. coli*, *L. monocytogenes*, *K. pneumoniae*, *H. influenzae*, *S. pneumoniae*, *N. meningitidis*, *Klebsiella* spp., *Salmonella* spp., *S. marcescens*, *P. aeruginosa*, *Enterobacter* spp., *S. aureus*, *S. epidermidis*, *Propionibacterium acnes*
Viruses	Enteroviruses, mumps virus, measles virus, herpesviruses, influenza and parainfluenza viruses, HIV, arboviruses, lymphocytic choriomeningitis virus
Rickettsia	*R. rickettsii*, *R. conorii*, *R. prowazekii*, *R. typhi*, *R. tsutsugamushi*, *Erlichia* spp.
Protozoa	*N. fowleri*, *Acanthamoeba* spp., *A. cantonensis*
Helminths	*S. stercoralis*
Other infectious diseases	IE, parameningeal foci of infection, viral post-infectious syndromes, post-vaccination
Medications	Antimicrobials, non-steroidals, azathioprine, OKT-3, cytosine arabinoside, carbamazepine, immune globulin, ranitidine
Systemic diseases	SLE
Procedure-related	Post-neurosurgery, spinal anaesthesia, intrathecal injections
Miscellaneous	Seizures, migraine, Mollaret's meningitis

Bacterial meningitis

The cause of acute bacterial meningitis depends on the age, immune status, and whether there has been recent head trauma or neurosurgery (see Table 19.2). The initiation of infection usually begins with nasopharyngeal colonization by a new organism, followed by systemic invasion. Important bacterial virulence factors include fimbriae, bacterial capsule, and production of IgA proteases. Host factors that predispose to meningitis include splenectomy and complement deficiencies.

Table 19.2 Causes of bacterial meningitis

Age/condition	Common organisms
0–4 weeks	GBS, *E. coli*, *L. monocytogenes*, *K. pneumoniae*, *Enterococcus* spp., *Salmonella* spp.
4–12 weeks	GBS, *E. coli*, *L. monocytogenes*, *K. pneumoniae*, *H. influenzae*, *S. pneumoniae*, *N. meningitidis*
3 months to 18 years	*H. influenzae*, *N. meningitidis*, *S. pneumoniae*
18–50 years	*N. meningitidis*, *S. pneumoniae*, *S. suis*
>50 years	*S. pneumoniae*, *N. meningitidis*, *L. monocytogenes*, *aerobic Gram-negative bacilli*, *S. suis*
Immunocompromised	*S. pneumoniae*, *N. meningitidis*, *L. monocytogenes*, aerobic Gram-negative bacilli (e.g. *E. coli*, *Klebsiella* spp., *Salmonella* spp., *S. marcescens*, *P. aeruginosa*)
Basal skull fracture	*S. pneumoniae*, *H. influenzae*, GAS
Head trauma, post-neurosurgery	*S. aureus*, *S. epidermidis*, aerobic Gram-negative bacilli
CSF shunt	*S. aureus*, *S. epidermidis*, *P. acnes*, aerobic Gram-negative bacilli

Clinical features

- Classical features include fever, headache, meningism (neck stiffness, photophobia, positive Kernig's sign and Brudzinski's sign), and cerebral dysfunction (confusion and/or reduced conscious level).
- Seizures occur in 30% of patients. Cranial nerve palsies (especially III, IV, VI, and VII) and focal signs are seen in 10–20% of cases. Hemiparesis may be due to a subdural effusion.
- Papilloedema is rare (<1%).
- Skin rash (initially macular, then petechial) occurs in patients with meningococcal septicaemia but can occur in pneumococcal, *H. influenzae*, or *S. suis* septicaemia.
- Rhinorrhoea or otorrhoea suggests basal skull fracture.
- Patients with *L. monocytogenes* have an increased risk of seizures and focal signs; some patients present with ataxia, cranial nerve palsies, and nystagmus caused by rhomboencephalitis.
- Neonates may present with non-specific symptoms, e.g. temperature instability, listlessness, poor feeding, irritability, vomiting, diarrhoea, jaundice, respiratory distress. Seizures occur in 40%, and a bulging fontanelle is a late sign.
- Elderly patients may present insidiously with confusion, lethargy, obtundation, no fever, and variable signs of meningeal inflammation.

Diagnosis

The diagnosis is confirmed by examination and culture of the CSF. In bacterial meningitis, the following are typically seen:

- opening pressure >18mm of CSF;
- CSF WCC 1000–5000 cells/mm^3 (range 100–10 000);
- CSF neutrophils ≥80%;
- CSF protein 0.1–0.5g/dL;
- CSF glucose ≤40mg/dL or ≤2.2mmol/L;
- CSF lactate ≥35mg/dL or ≥1.9mmol/L;
- Gram stain positive in 60–90%;
- culture positive in 70–85%;
- bacterial antigen detection positive in 50–100%;
- bacterial PCR positive in 90%.

Management

- For acute management, ➔ see flow chart in back cover.
- Empirical antimicrobial therapy should be commenced immediately, pending investigations (see Table 19.3).

If the CSF Gram stain or culture is positive, treatment should be tailored to the infecting organism (see Table 19.4).

- Adjunctive corticosteroids have been recommended for the treatment of acute bacterial meningitis.[1] The recommended regimen was dexamethasone 10mg qds for 4 days, administered before or with the first dose of antibiotic. However, data from the developing world[2,3] and a recent systematic review only recommend their use in high income-countries.[4]
- Reduction of raised ICP may be achieved by various methods—elevating the head of the bed to 30° to maximize venous drainage, hyperventilation to cause cerebral vasoconstriction, and use of hyperosmolar agents, e.g. mannitol.
- Neurosurgery may be required in certain circumstances—persistent CSF leak after basal skull fracture, congenital defects leading to recurrent meningitis, subdural empyema.

Prevention

- Vaccination—Hib and meningitis C conjugate vaccine are part of the routine childhood immunization schedule in the UK. The quadrivalent meningitis vaccine (ACYW135) is recommended for patients with complement or properdin deficiency, asplenic patients, travellers to endemic areas, and medical or laboratory personnel routinely exposed to *N. meningitidis*. *S. pneumoniae* vaccination is recommended in certain high-risk groups, e.g. age >65 years, chronic cardiovascular, pulmonary, renal, or liver disease, diabetes mellitus, alcoholism, CSF leak, asplenia, HIV, haematological and other malignancies, BMT patients, immunosuppressive therapy.
- Chemoprophylaxis should be given within 24h to household contacts, kissing contacts, and medical personnel involved in resuscitation of the index case. Rifampicin is the agent of choice for *H. influenzae* type B meningitis. For *N. meningitidis*, the agents used are rifampicin (600mg bd for 2 days), ciprofloxacin (500mg stat), or ceftriaxone (250mg IM). NB. Rifampicin interacts with the OCP and may reduce its efficacy. Penicillin is not recommended to prevent secondary cases of *S. pneumoniae*

Table 19.3 Empirical antibiotic therapy

Age/condition	Empiric therapy
Age 0–4 weeks	Ampicillin + cefotaxime or aminoglycoside
Age 4–12 weeks	Ampicillin + cefotaxime or ceftriaxone
Age 3 months to 18 years	Cefotaxime or ceftriaxone
Age 18–50 years	Ceftriaxone or cefotaxime ± vancomycin
Age >50 years	Ceftriaxone or cefotaxime + ampicillin
Immunocompromised	Vancomycin + ampicillin + ceftazidime or meropenem
Health care-associated meningitis	Vancomycin + ceftazidime or meropenem
Basal skull fracture	Cefotaxime or ceftriaxone
Head trauma/ neurosurgery	Vancomycin + ceftazidime
CSF shunt	Vancomycin + ceftazidime
β-lactam allergy	Vancomycin + moxifloxacin ± co-trimoxazole (if *Listeria* suspected)

Table 19.4 Specific antibiotic therapy

Organism	Antimicrobial therapy
S. pneumoniae	Penicillin MIC <0.06 micrograms/mL: benzylpenicillin Penicillin MIC ≥0.12 and <1 microgram/mL: ceftriaxone Penicillin MIC ≥1 microgram/mL: ceftriaxone plus vancomycin
N. meningitidis	Penicillin MIC <0.1 microgram/mL: benzylpenicillin or ampicillin Penicillin MIC 0.1–1 microgram/mL: ceftriaxone
L. monocytogenes	Ampicillin or benzylpenicillin
GBS	Ampicillin or benzylpenicillin
E. coli	Ceftriaxone or cefotaxime
P. aeruginosa	Ceftazidime or meropenem
H. influenzae	β-lactamase-negative: ampicillin β-lactamase-positive: ceftriaxone
S. aureus	Meticillin-susceptible: flucloxacillin Meticillin-resistant: vancomycin
Enterococcus spp.	Ampicillin-susceptible: ampicillin + gentamicin Ampicillin-resistant: vancomycin + gentamicin Ampicillin- and vancomycin-resistant: linezolid

meningitis but is recommended for children with sickle-cell disease, although the optimum duration is unknown. IV ampicillin, penicillin, clindamycin, or erythromycin are recommended for pregnant women colonized with GBS or with obstetric risk factors for invasive disease. Meningitis C vaccination should be given for unvaccinated close contacts of meningitis C cases.

References

1 de Gans J, van de Beek D (2002). Dexamethasone in adults with bacterial meningitis. *N Engl J Med*. **347**:1549–56.
2 Nguyen TH, Tran TH, Thwaites G, *et al* (2007). Dexamethasone in Vietnamese adolescents and adults with bacterial meningitis. *N Engl J Med*. **357**:2431–40.
3 Scarborough M, Gordan SB, Whitty CJ, *et al* (2007). Corticosteroids for bacterial meningitis in adults in sub-Saharan Africa. *N Engl J Med*. **357**:2441–50.
4 Brouwer MC, McIntyre P, Prasad K, *et al* (2013). Corticosteroids for acute bacterial meningitis. *Cochrane Database Syst Rev*. **6**:CD004405.

Viral meningitis

Viruses are the major cause of the aseptic meningitis syndrome. This is usually characterized by lymphocytic pleocytosis in the CSF and sterile bacterial cultures.

Causes

- Enteroviruses are the leading cause of viral meningitis, e.g. echoviruses, Coxsackie viruses, enteroviruses 70 and 71.
- Arboviruses that cause meningitis include St Louis encephalitis virus, California, Eastern equine, Western equine, Venezuelan equine, and Colorado tick fever.
- Mumps virus is a common cause in unimmunized populations. CNS disease may occur in the absence of parotitis and is usually a benign self-limited disease.
- Herpesviruses include HSV-1 and HSV-2, VZV, CMV, EBV, and HHV. Although all of these can cause meningitis, HSV are the commonest cause and are often associated with primary genital HSV-2 infection.
- HIV may cause meningitis as part of primary infection.
- Lymphocytic choriomeningitis virus (LCMV) is a rare cause of aseptic meningitis. It usually occurs in laboratory personnel, pet owners, or persons living in unsanitary conditions.

Pathogenesis

After colonization of mucosal surfaces, the virus invades and replicates prior to haematogenous dissemination. CNS invasion may occur by several mechanisms: via the cerebral microvascular endothelial cells, via the choroid plexus epithelium, or by spread along the olfactory nerve. Once CNS invasion occurs, inflammatory cells accumulate, leading to the release of inflammatory cytokines, e.g. IL-6, IFN-γ, IL-1β, and synthesis of immunoglobulins, e.g. oligoclonal IgG.

Clinical features

- Enterovirus—in neonates, fever is accompanied by vomiting, anorexia, rash, and upper respiratory tract symptoms. Meningeal signs (nuchal rigidity, bulging anterior fontanelle) may be present or absent, and focal signs are uncommon. A severe form may occur in the early neonatal period with hepatic necrosis, myocarditis, necrotizing enterocolitis, and encephalitis. In older children and adults, symptoms are milder with fever, headache, neck stiffness, and photophobia. There may be non-specific symptoms, e.g. anorexia, vomiting, rash, diarrhoea, cough, pharyngitis, and myalgia. Other clues include community enteroviral epidemics, maculopapular or pustular rashes, conjunctivitis, pleurodynia, pericarditis, and herpangina.
- Mumps virus—CNS symptoms usually occur 5 days after the onset of parotitis. Other findings include salivary gland enlargement (50%), neck stiffness, lethargy, and abdominal pain.
- Herpesviruses—HSV-2 meningitis presents with classical symptoms. Complications include urinary retention, dysaesthesia, paraesthesiae, neuralgia, motor weakness, paraparesis, difficulties in concentration, and impaired hearing; these usually resolve within 3–6 months. EBV meningitis is associated with pharyngitis, lymphadenopathy, and splenomegaly. VZV meningitis is associated with a characteristic, diffuse vesicular rash.
- HIV—HIV-infected patients may present with a typical aseptic meningitis syndrome, associated with acute primary HIV infection.
- LCMV—this is usually a biphasic illness that starts with non-specific viral symptoms, followed by improvement; 15% of patients develop severe headache, photophobia, lightheadedness, myalgia, and pharyngitis. Occasionally, arthritis, orchitis, myopericarditis, and alopecia may occur.

Diagnosis

- CSF examination—CSF pleocytosis (100–1000 cells/mm^3) usually occurs. This may show a neutrophil predominance initially but becomes lymphocytic over 6–48h. CSF protein level may be normal or mildly elevated. CSF glucose level is normal or mildly reduced.
- Viral culture—enteroviral meningitis may be identified by tissue culture, although sensitivity is only 65–75%. Prolonged or asymptomatic viral shedding may occur. LCMV is diagnosed by viral culture of blood or CSF (early infection) or urine (later infection). HSV-2 has been cultured from the CSF and buffy coat of some patients. HIV has been isolated from the CSF of some patients with neurological disease. Arboviruses may be cultured from blood and CSF.
- Serology—rapid diagnosis of enteroviral infections is possible by detection of enteroviral IgM antibodies; the specificity of some tests is unsatisfactory. A 4-fold rise in mumps antibody titres confirms the diagnosis of mumps meningitis. A salivary antibody test has been developed that looks promising. LCMV and arboviral infections are usually diagnosed serologically.

- Molecular methods—cDNA nucleic acid probes for enteroviruses have been developed but have poor specificity (≤33%). PCR-based assays for enteroviruses are more promising, with higher sensitivity and specificity than tissue culture. PCR-based assays are the diagnostic test of choice for herpesvirus infections, e.g. HSV-2, CMV, VZV. HIV RNA has been isolated from the CSF of some patients with meningitis.

Differential diagnosis

The following may mimic viral meningitis:

- syphilitic meningitis (➲ see Syphilis, pp. 714–6);
- Lyme disease (➲ see Lyme disease, pp. 338–40);
- RMSF;
- erlichiosis;
- cryptococcal meningitis (➲ see *Cryptococcus*, pp. 480–1);
- coccidioidomycosis (➲ see *Coccidioides immitis*—ACDP 3, pp. 505–8);
- tuberculous meningitis (➲ see *Mycobacterium tuberculosis*—ACDP 3, pp. 355–9);
- parameningeal bacterial infections, e.g. epidural/subdural abscess, otitis media, sinusitis;
- *A. cantonensis* meningitis;
- leptomeningeal neoplasmas;
- drug-induced meningitis, e.g. NSAIDs, co-trimoxazole, IVIG, rofecoxib, cetuximab, antiepileptics, OKT-3.

Management

- Treatment of viral meningitis is mainly supportive, e.g. analgesics, antipyretics.
- Pleconaril has been used for enteroviral meningitis.
- IV aciclovir is used for meningitis associated with HSV infection.
- No specific antiviral therapy exists for arboviruses, mumps virus, or LCMV meningitis
- ART may be indicated for HIV infection but is not usually given in primary infection.

Chronic meningitis

Chronic meningitis is a syndrome characterized by the subacute onset of meningoencephalitic symptoms (fever, headache, nausea, vomiting, neck stiffness, lethargy, and confusion) and CSF abnormalities which persist for at least 4 weeks There are a large number of infectious and non-infectious causes (see Table 19.5).

Clinical features

- History—an exposure history may suggest certain infections, e.g. TB, brucellosis, cysticercosis, coccidioidomycosis, histoplasmosis, Lyme disease, syphilis, or HIV infection. In non-infectious cases, there may be a history of pre-existing systemic disease.
- Examination—diagnostic physical findings are rare. Skin lesions may be found in cryptococcosis, sarcoidosis, *Acanthamoeba* infection, coccidioidomycosis, blastomycosis, and secondary syphilis.

Table 19.5 Causes of chronic meningitis/meningoencephalitis

	Syndrome	Causes
Infectious	Meningitis	*Acanthamoeba* spp., *A. cantonensis*, brucellosis, candidiasis, coccidioidomycosis, cryptococcosis, *Ehrlichia chaffeensis, F. tularensis*, histoplasmosis, *Leptospira* spp., *Listeria* spp., Lyme disease, sporotrichosis, syphilis, TB, Whipple's disease
	Focal lesions	Actinomycosis, blastomycosis, cysticercosis, aspergillosis, nocardiosis, schistosomiasis, toxoplasmosis, TB
	Encephalitis	African trypanosomiasis, CMV, enterovirus (hypogammaglobulinaemia), EBV, HIV, HTLV, HSV, measles, SSPE, rabies, VZV
Non-infectious	Meningitis	Drugs (NSAIDs, IVIG, intrathecal agents), Behçet's disease, benign lymphocytic meningitis, CNS vasculitis, Fabry's disease, granulomatous angiitis, malignancy, sarcoidosis, SLE, Wegener's granulomatosis, Vogt–Koyanagi–Harada disease

Subcutaneous nodules may be found in cysticercosis and metastatic carcinoma. Lymphadenopathy and hepatomegaly suggest systemic disease. Eye examination may show choroidal tubercles, sarcoid granulomas, papilloedema, iritis, or uveitis. Neurological examination is non-discriminatory—focal signs indicate a cerebral mass lesion; hydrocephalus and cranial nerve palsies indicate basal meningitis; peripheral neuropathy suggests sarcoidosis or Lyme disease.

Laboratory diagnosis

- Blood tests—in addition to routine blood tests (FBC, ESR, CRP, creatinine, LFTs), the following may be indicated: Mantoux test, BC for fungi and mycobacteria, serology for HIV and syphilis, serum cryptococcal antigen, ANA, and ANCA. Depending on the patient's exposure history, the following tests may be indicated: serology for *Brucella, B. burgdorferi, Histoplasma, Coccidioides*.
- Radiology—a CXR and CT or MRI brain scan should be performed in all cases. Meningeal enhancement and hydrocephalus are common findings.
- CSF examination should be performed in all cases (unless contraindicated by scan findings). The CSF should be analysed for cell count and differential, protein, glucose, and lactate (see Table 19.6). Diagnostic tests include Gram stain and culture, ZN stain for mycobacteria, India ink and cryptococcal antigen, and syphilis serology. Depending on the patient's exposure history, the following tests may be indicated: CSF antibodies to *Histoplasma, Coccidioides, Blastomycosis, T. solium, Brucella*, and measles virus.

Table 19.6 CSF findings in chronic meningitis

CSF characteristic	Causes
Lymphocytic pleocytosis	Viral causes, TB meningitis
Neutrophilic pleocytosis	Actinomycosis, nocardiosis, HIV-associated CMV, early MTB infection, aspergillosis, candidiasis
Eosinophilic pleocytosis	*Angiostrongylus, Coccidioides*, cysticercosis, schistosomiasis, lymphoma, chemical
Pleocytosis <50 cells/microlitre	Behçet's disease, benign lymphocytic meningitis, carcinoma, HIV-associated cryptococcosis, sarcoidosis, vasculitis
Low CSF glucose	Actinomycosis, nocardiosis, carcinoma, cysticercosis, fungi, TB, syphilis, toxoplasmosis, chronic enterovirus, HIV-associated CMV, sarcoidosis, subarachnoid haemorrhage

In cases where the diagnosis remains obscure, the following tests may be helpful: repeat Mantoux test or TB IGRA; immunoglobulins, serum angiotensin-converting enzyme (ACE); CSF antibody for *S. schenkii*; and enteroviral culture and PCR. Biopsy of the brain or other tissues may also be indicated.

Management

- Specific therapy is tailored according to the cause of chronic meningitis (for further details, see section on the causative organism).
- Therapeutic trials may be indicated when a specific cause is not found, despite comprehensive evaluation. Response to treatment may be slow, making interpretation difficult. Attempts to establish a diagnosis should be continued during therapeutic trial. In areas where TB is endemic, tuberculous meningitis (see next section) is the commonest cause of chronic meningitis, and empirical therapy is often initiated if the clinical presentation and CSF indices are compatible. Positive cultures or a clinical response to treatment are indications for continuing therapy. In areas where TB is not endemic, chronic meningitis is usually not infectious.

Tuberculous meningitis

- Caused by *M. tuberculosis* (➔ see *Mycobacterium tuberculosis*—ACDP 3, pp. 355–9). There are three forms of CNS TB—tuberculous meningitis, intracranial tuberculoma, and spinal tuberculous arachnoiditis.
- Pathogenesis—primary infection or reactivation of latent infection results in bacillaemia and seeding of the brain and meninges. Rupture of these foci into the subarachnoid space results in a proliferative basal arachnoiditis, vasculitis, and communicating hydrocephalus.

- Clinical features of TB meningitis—non-specific, with gradual onset of meningeal symptoms, cranial nerve palsies (III, IV, and VI), hemiplegia or paraplegia, and urinary retention. CXR is abnormal in 50% of cases and may show pulmonary or miliary TB. CT or MRI brain scan may show hydrocephalus, basal meningeal enhancement, infarcts, or tuberculomas. There are three clinical stages which are prognostically useful: (i) stage 1—Glasgow coma scale (GCS) 15/15 with no focal neurological signs, (ii) stage 2—GCS 15 with focal signs or GCS 11–14, and (iii) stage 3—GCS ≤10. In areas with high HIV prevalence, TB meningitis may be a primary presentation of HIV infection or present as IRIS after initiation of ART.
- Laboratory diagnosis—CSF findings include lymphocytic pleocytosis (100–500 cells/mm^3), increased CSF protein, and decreased CSF glucose levels. Neutrophils may predominate in early disease and in HIV-infected patients. Diagnosis confirmed by detection of *M. tuberculosis* by CSF ZN smear or culture. Smear positivity rates are generally low (10–22%) but may be increased to >50% if the spun deposit of a large volume of CSF (5–10mL) is examined meticulously. PCR detection of mycobacterial DNA shows a sensitivity of 27–85% and a specificity of 95–100%. CSF cultures are positive in 38–88% of cases.
- Management—the optimum drug choice and duration of treatment have not been established in clinical trials. The UK and US TB treatment guidelines both recommend a four-drug initiation phase (rifampicin, isoniazid, pyrazinamide, and ethambutol) for 2 months, followed by a two-drug continuation phase (rifampicin and isoniazid) for 10 months. As isoniazid and pyrazinamide are the only two drugs that have good CSF penetration, some experts recommend continuing pyrazinamide during the continuation phase. Studies from India and South Africa suggest that 6 months of therapy may be adequate. Adjunctive dexamethasone has been shown to reduce short-term mortality. Treatment with higher doses of rifampicin and fluoroquinolones may reduce mortality and are being assessed in RCTs. A clinical trial of early versus deferred ART in HIV-associated TB meningitis showed no survival benefit, and an increased frequency of severe adverse effects in the early ART arm.

Cryptococcal meningitis

- There are estimated to be ~960 000 cases of cryptococcal meningitis globally each year, with 600 000 deaths. The highest incidence is in sub-Saharan Africa, followed by South and South East Asia. Most patients are immunocompromised. Advanced HIV infection (CD4 count <100 cells/mm^3) is a major risk factor, but others include glucocorticoid therapy, solid organ transplantation, malignancy (especially haematological), sarcoidosis, and liver failure.
- *C. neoformans* var. *neoformans* occurs worldwide and tends to cause disease in immunocompromised patients. *C. neoformans* var. *gatii* occurs in tropical and subtropical climates, and tends to affect non-immunocompromised patients.

- Clinical features—subacute presentation with fever, meningoencephalitis, visual loss, and focal signs (<30%).
- Laboratory diagnosis—CSF findings include raised CSF pressure, lymphocytic pleocytosis (40–400 cells/mm^3), low CSF glucose (55%), and positive India ink stain (≤50%). CSF findings may be normal in HIV patients. Serum and CSF cryptococcal antigen tests can increase the diagnostic rate to ≥90%. CSF cultures are positive in 75% of patients. Cultures of blood, urine, and sputum may increase the diagnostic rate.
- Management:
  - HIV-infected patients—induction therapy with amphotericin deoxycholate (0.7mg/kg/day IV) plus flucytosine (100mg/kg/day in four divided doses) for 2 weeks. If there is clinical improvement after 2 weeks, change to consolidation therapy with fluconazole (400mg/day PO) for 8 weeks, followed by maintenance therapy with fluconazole (200mg/day PO) for a minimum of 1 year. This may be discontinued in asymptomatic patients with CD4 counts >100 cells/mm^3, who have an undetectable HIV viral load on ART for >3 months, and who have received a minimum of 1 year of azole maintenance therapy.
  - HIV-negative transplant patients—induction therapy with liposomal amphotericin (3–4mg/kg/day IV) or amphotericin lipid complex (5mg/kg/day IV) plus flucytosine (100mg/kg/day in four divided doses) for at least 2 weeks. This is followed by a consolidation therapy with fluconazole (400–800mg/day PO) for 8 weeks, followed by maintenance therapy with fluconazole (200–400mg/day PO) for 6–12 months.
  - HIV-negative non-transplant patients—induction therapy with amphotericin deoxycholate (0.7–1mg/kg/day IV) plus flucytosine (100mg/kg/day in four divided doses) for at least 4 weeks. This is followed by consolidation therapy with fluconazole (400mg/day PO) for 8 weeks, then maintenance therapy of fluconazole (200mg/day PO) for 6–12 months.

Further reading

Perfect JR, Dismukes WR, Dromer F, *et al* (2010). Clinical practice guidelines for the management of cryptococcal disease: 2010 update by the Infectious Diseases Society of America. *Clin Infect Dis*. **50**:291–322.

Coccidioidal meningitis

- Coccidioidomycosis is caused by *Coccidioides* spp. (➔ see *Coccidioides immitis*—ACDP 3, pp. 505–8), a dimorphic fungus that is endemic in the desert areas of south-western USA, and Central and South America. Two species cause disease—*C. immitis* (California) and *Coccidioides posadasii* (Arizona, Texas, Central and South America). The exact incidence of coccidioidal meningitis is unknown, but disseminated coccidioidomycosis occurs in 8% of reported cases, of which 17% involve the CNS. In contrast to non-CNS infections, mortality is high—95% if untreated.

- Clinical features—CNS involvement may be part of generalized coccidioidomycosis or may be the only site of extrapulmonary disease. Meningitis usually occurs within weeks or months of primary infection, although it can present years afterwards. Persistent headache is the main symptom (75% of cases), but the clinical syndrome is indistinguishable from other causes of chronic meningitis. Rarer clinical features include tremor, papilloedema, cranial nerve palsies, cerebral infarction, focal neurological deficits, and gait abnormalities.
- Laboratory diagnosis—the CSF usually has raised WCC, which is predominantly lymphocytic, although CSF neutrophilia or eosinophilia may occur. The CSF glucose is low, and the CSF protein is elevated. Rarely, the organisms may be seen on CSF microscopy. CSF cultures are positive in 15–30% of cases. CSF antibodies are positive in 55–95% of patients; ELISA to spherule is more sensitive than complement fixation tests (CFTs). A serum CFT titre of 1:16 is supportive of the diagnosis. Skin tests with spherulin are positive in 33–55% of patients. Occasionally, meningeal biopsy may be required to establish the diagnosis.
- Imaging—CT or MRI scanning may identify abnormalities such as hydrocephalus, basal meningitis, and cerebral infarction; these are not specific to coccidioidal meningitis.
- Management—fluconazole (400mg/day) is associated with a 70% response rate. Higher fluconazole doses (800–1000mg/day) may be used in patients who do not initially respond. Itraconazole (200mg bd or tds) has been reported to have similar efficacy. Intrathecal amphotericin deoxycholate (0.01–1.5mg daily to weekly) has been used in patients who do not respond to oral azole therapy. Treatment is usually started at low dose and escalated, as tolerated. This is usually given by direct cisternal injection or via an Ommaya reservoir. Voriconazole and posaconazole have been used as salvage therapy in patients who develop disease progression on fluconazole. Hydrocephalus may require a ventriculoperitoneal (VP) shunt.

Further reading

Galgiani JN, Ampel NM, Blair JE, *et al.*; Infectious Diseases Society of America (2005). Coccidioidomycosis. *Clin Infect Dis.* **41**:1217–23.

Histoplasma meningitis

- Caused by *H. capsulatum* (➔ see *Histoplasma capsulatum*—ACDP 3, pp. 498–503), which is found worldwide but particularly in North America (especially the mid-Western states) and Central America. The commonest presentation is pulmonary disease, but disseminated infection may occur in 1 in 2000 patients with acute infection. Risk factors for disseminated infection include HIV infection, solid organ transplantation, treatment with TNF-α inhibitors, and extremes of age.
- Clinical features—these are non-specific with fever and gradual onset of meningitic symptoms over weeks or months. Oral mucosal lesions occur in 16% of patients and are commoner than skin lesions. Other

manifestations of disseminated infection may be seen including weight loss, lymphadenopathy, hepatomegaly, and splenomegaly.

- Laboratory diagnosis—CSF examination shows lymphocytic pleocytosis, with low glucose and raised protein levels. CSF microscopy is rarely positive. CSF cultures are positive in 27–65% of cases. Large volumes of CSF (10–20mL) should be cultured, on at least two occasions to improve diagnostic yield. Detection of serum and CSF antibodies is the most sensitive test, but problems occur with cross-reactivity to other fungi. *Histoplasma* polysaccharide antigen may be detected in blood, urine, or CSF in 61% of patients. Three sets of BCs should also be taken. Bone marrow culture should be considered in patients with suspected disseminated disease.
- Management—treatment is with amphotericin (0.7–1.0mg/kg/day). Liposomal formulations of amphotericin achieve higher concentrations in blood and brain, and may be useful in CNS disease (e.g. AmBisome® 5mg/kg/day IV for 4–6 weeks). Following induction therapy, itraconazole (400–600mg/day) should be given for at least 1 year to prevent relapse. LPs should be performed weekly for 6 weeks, then every 2 weeks to assess response. Treatment should be monitored with serum and/or urine *Histoplasma* antigen tests every 4–6 months during therapy. Initial response rates are good (60–80%), but relapse rates are high, resulting in an overall cure rate of 50%.

Further reading

Wheat LJ, Freifeld AG, Kleiman MB, *et al.*; Infectious Diseases Society of America (2007). Clinical practice guidelines for the management of patients with histoplasmosis: 2007 update by the Infectious Diseases Society of America. *Clin Infect Dis*. **45**:807–25.

Neuroborreliosis

- Neuroborreliosis is a manifestation of Lyme disease, a tick-borne illness caused by *Borrelia* spp. (➔ see *Borrelia* species, pp. 337–40). There are three pathogenic species—*B. burgdorferi*, *B. afzelii*, and *B. garinii*. All three species cause disease in Europe; *B. burgdorferi* causes disease in the USA, and *B. afzelii* and *B. garinii* cause disease in Asia.
- Clinical features—early infection is characterized by flu-like symptoms and a characteristic rash (erythema chronicum migrans) which is seen in 80% of patients. Joint involvement occurs more frequently in the USA than in Europe. The nervous system is the third commonest site and is involved in 10–15% of patients. Many patients develop non-specific symptoms (e.g. headache, fatigue, cognitive slowing, memory difficulty), but these do not constitute CNS infection. Neuroborreliosis is characterized by chronic meningitis, cranial nerve palsies, Lyme encephalomyelitis, and benign intracranial hypertension. CNS involvement may occur weeks or months after the tick bite. Peripheral nerve involvement may also occur, e.g. radiculoneuritis, mononeuritis multiplex.
- Laboratory diagnosis—CSF examination shows lymphocytic pleocytosis. CSF protein concentration is raised, but CSF glucose is usually normal.

Diagnosis is confirmed by positive serology in the context of an appropriate exposure history. Serology is insensitive in early disease, and false-positive and false-negative results are a considerable problem. The most specific test is detection of *B. burgdorferi* antibodies in the CSF, and comparison of CSF and serum antibody levels by an immunocapture assay. PCR detection of *B. burgdorferi* has poor sensitivity (25–38%), but high specificity. Elevated levels of the chemokine CXCL13 have been reported in CNS Lyme disease. Imaging—MRI scan may show evidence of encephalomyelitis. Electrophysiological studies—electromyography (EMG) and nerve conduction studies may be useful in patients with peripheral neuropathy.

- Management—IV ceftriaxone 2g/day for 14–28 days.
  Alternatives: cefotaxime 2g IV tds or benzylpenicillin 18–24 million units IV per day in six divided doses. Adults with penicillin allergy may be treated with doxycycline 200–400mg/day in two divided doses.

Further reading

Wormser GP, Dattwyler RJ, Shapiro ED, *et al* (2006). The clinical assessment, treatment, and prevention of lyme disease, human granulocytic anaplasmosis, and babesiosis: clinical practice guidelines by the Infectious Diseases Society of America. *Clin Infect Dis*. **43**:1089–134.

Neurocysticercosis

- Caused by *T. solium* (➲ see Cestodes, pp. 559–62), the commonest parasitic disease of the CNS. Infection is endemic in Mexico, Central and South America, the Caribbean, sub-Saharan Africa, India, and China.
- Clinical features—these depend on whether the cysts are localized to the parenchyma or extra-parenchymal tissues. Parenchymal cysts are associated with focal or generalized seizures; if there are large numbers of cysts associated with oedema, there may also be headache, nausea, vomiting, impaired consciousness, reduced visual acuity, and fever. Extra-parenchymal cysts are associated with symptoms of hydrocephalus, e.g. headache, nausea, vomiting, altered mental status, reduced visual acuity. Spinal cysticercosis may present with radicular pain, paraesthesiae, and sphincter disturbance. Ocular cysticercosis may present with impaired vision, diplopia, and eye pain.
- Imaging—CT scan may show calcified lesions. MRI is better for smaller lesions, as well as intraventricular and subarachnoid lesions. Spinal imaging should be performed in patients with basal subarachnoid neurocysticercosis. Plain X-rays may show skeletal muscle calcification.
- Laboratory diagnosis—CSF examination shows lymphocytic or eosinophilic pleocytosis, normal or low CSF glucose (25%), and normal or elevated CSF protein. A number of serological tests exist for serum and CSF. Antibody tests include ELISAs, CFTs, radioimmunoassays, haemagglutination assays, and immunoblots. Antigen tests may detect specific antigens or unfractionated antigens (poor sensitivity and specificity). The test of choice is the enzyme-linked immunoelectrotransfer blot (EITB) assay which has a higher sensitivity (83–100%) and specificity (~100%) than older assays. Brain biopsy is only warranted in cases where non-invasive testing is non-diagnostic.

- Management—the initial approach is to control or prevent seizures with antiepileptic medications. The role of antihelminthic therapy remains controversial, but potential benefits include resolution of active cysts, decreased risk of seizures, and decreased recurrence of hydrocephalus. Potential risks include exacerbation of symptoms caused by increased inflammation around degenerating cysts. Albendazole (800mg/day in two divided doses) is the treatment of choice of 3–14 days, depending on the number of cysts. Longer courses (≥28 days) may be required for extra-parenchymal disease. Praziquantel (50–100mg/kg/day in three divided doses) is an alternative. Corticosteroids should be given to reduce CNS inflammation but can reduce praziquantel levels. Surgical intervention (e.g. ventriculostomy or VP shunt) is required for patients with symptomatic hydrocephalus.

Encephalitis

- Encephalitis is an inflammatory process in the brain accompanied by cerebral dysfunction.
- It may be caused by infectious agents (mainly viruses) or non-infectious conditions (e.g. vasculitis, autoimmune diseases, or paraneoplastic syndromes). In some cases, there may be features of meningitis, and it is referred to as meningoencephalitis.
- The incidence of encephalitis varies according to geography and population; the estimated incidence in industrialized countries is 0.7–13.8 cases per 100 000 population.
- The diagnostic evaluation of a patient with encephalitis should be individualized and guided by epidemiological clues (see Table 19.7), clinical presentation (see Table 19.8), and laboratory tests (see Table 19.9).

Clinical features

- Viral encephalitis is characterized by alterations in consciousness, progressing from mild lethargy to confusion, to stupor and coma.
- Some patients may present with features of meningitis.
- Focal neurological signs frequently develop, and seizures are common.
- Motor weakness, attenuation of reflexes, and extensor plantar responses may be seen.
- Some viruses may cause CNS symptoms as part of a post-infectious encephalomyelitis, e.g. mumps, measles, rubella, influenza.
- Certain diseases are associated with characteristic symptoms or signs (see Table 19.8).

Diagnosis

- CSF examination is essential. In viral encephalitis, the CSF pleocytosis is variable (10–2000 cells/mm^3), and lymphocytes usually predominate. In early disease, however, there may be no cells or neutrophils in the CSF. Red cells may be found in HSV encephalitis. CSF protein is usually increased. CSF glucose is usually normal or slightly low. All patients should have CSF PCR for HSV, VZV, and enteroviruses performed. Additional CSF diagnostic studies should be performed, guided by epidemiological risk factors and clinical findings (see Table 19.9).

Table 19.7 Epidemiological factors and causes of encephalitis[5,6]

Risk factor	Potential causes
Agammaglobulinaemia	Enterovirus, *Mycoplasma pneumoniae*
Age	
- Neonates	HSV-2, CMV, rubella, *L. monocytogenes*, syphilis, *T. gondii*
- Infants and children	Eastern equine encephalitis, Japanese encephalitis, Murray Valley encephalitis, influenza, La Crosse virus
- Elderly	Eastern equine encephalitis, St Louis encephalitis, West Nile virus, sporadic CJD, *L. monocytogenes*
Animal contact	
- Bats	Rabies, Nipah virus
- Birds	West Nile virus, Eastern and Western equine encephalitis, St Louis encephalitis, Murray Valley encephalitis, Japanese encephalitis, *C. neoformans*
- Cats	Rabies, *C. burnetii, B. henselae, T. gondii*
- Dogs	Rabies
- Horses	Eastern, Western, and Venezuelan equine encephalitis, Hendra virus
- Old world primates	B virus
- Raccoons	Rabies, *Baylisascaris procyonis*
- Rodents	Eastern and Venezuelan equine encephalitis, tick-borne encephalitis, Powassan virus, La Crosse virus, *B. quintana*
- Sheep and goats	*C. burnetii*
- Skunks	Rabies
- Swine	Japanese encephalitis, Nipah virus
- White tailed deer	*B. burgdorferi*
Immunocompromised persons	CMV, EBV, HHV-6, HIV, JC virus, VZV, West Nile virus, *L. monocytogenes*, MTB, *C. neoformans*, *Coccidioides* spp., *Histoplasma* spp., *T. gondii*
Ingestion of food/drink	
- Raw/partially cooked meat	*T. gondii*
- Raw meat/fish/reptiles	*Gnathostoma* spp.
- Unpasteurized milk	Tick-borne encephalitis, *L. monocytogenes, C. burnetii*
Insect bites	
- Mosquitoes	Dengue, Chikungunya, Eastern, Western, and Venezuelan equine encephalitis, St Louis encephalitis, Murray Valley encephalitis, Japanese encephalitis, West Nile virus, La Crosse virus, *P. falciparum*
- Sandflies	*B. bacilliformis*
- Ticks	Tick-borne encephalitis, Powassan virus, *R. ricketsii, Erlichia chaffeensis, Anaplasma phagocytophilum, C. burnetii, B. burgdorferi*
- Tsetse flies	*T.b gambiense, T.b rhodesiense*

(Continued)

Table 19.7 (*Contd.*)

Risk factor	Potential causes
Occupation	
- Exposure to animals	See above for specific animals
- Laboratory workers	West Nile virus, HIV, *C. burnetii*, *Coccidioides* spp.
- Health-care workers	VZV, HIV, influenza, measles, MTB
- Veterinarians	Rabies, *Bartonella* spp., *C. burnetii*
Person-to-person transmissions	Influenza, VZV, HSV (neonatal), mumps, measles, rubella, polio, enteroviruses, EBV, HHV-6, HIV, Venezuelan equine encephalitis virus (rare), Nipah virus, B virus, West Nile virus (transfusion, breastfeeding), rabies virus (transplantation), *M. pneumoniae*, MTB, syphilis
Recreational activities	
- Camping/hunting	See mosquitoes/ticks above
- Caving	Rabies, *Histoplasma* spp
- Sexual contact	HIV, syphilis
- Swimming	Enteroviruses, *N. fowleri*
Season	
- Late summer/ early autumn	Enteroviruses, agents transmitted by mosquitoes and ticks
- Winter	Influenza virus
Transfusion and transplantation	CMV, EBV, HIV, West Nile virus, tick-borne encephalitis, rabies, iatrogenic CJD, syphilis, *A. phagocytophilum, R. rickettsii, C. neoformans, Coccidioides* spp., *H. capsulatum, T. gondii*
Travel	
- Africa	Rabies, West Nile virus, *P. falciparum*, *Trypanosoma* spp.
- Central America	Rabies, Eastern, Western and Venezuelan equine encephalitis, St Louis encephalitis, *R. rickettsii*, *P. falciparum, T. solium*
- North America	Eastern and Western equine encephalitis, West Nile virus, *B. burgdorferi, E. chaffeensis, A. phagocytophilum*, *Coccidioides* spp.
- South America	Rabies, Eastern, Western and Venezuelan equine encephalitis, St Louis encephalitis, *R. rickettsii*, *B. bacilliformis* (Andes), *P. falciparum, T. solium*
- Australia	Murray Valley encephalitis, Japanese encephalitis, Hendra virus
- Europe	West Nile virus, tick-borne encephalitis, *A. phagocytophilum, B. burgdorferi*
- India, Nepal	Rabies, Japanese encephalitis,
- Middle East	West Nile virus, *P. falciparum*
- Russia	Tick-borne encephalitis
- South East Asia/China/ Pacific Rim	Japanese encephalitis, tick-borne encephalitis, Nipah virus, *P. falciparum, Gnathastoma* spp., *T. solium*

Table 19.7 (*Contd.*)

Risk factor	Potential causes
Vaccination status	
- Unvaccinated	VZV, mumps, measles, rubella, polio, Japanese encephalitis
- Recent vaccination	Acute disseminated encephalomyelitis

Table 19.8 Clinical features and causes of encephalitis[5,6]

Clinical presentation	Potential causes
Hepatitis	*C. burnetii*
Lymphadenopathy	HIV, EBV, CMV, measles, rubella, West Nile virus, syphilis, *Bartonella* spp., MTB, *T. gondii*, *T. brucei gambiense*
Parotitis	Mumps
Rash	VZV, rubella, some enteroviruses, HIV, HHV-6, B virus, West Nile virus, *R. rickettsii*, *M. pneumoniae*, *B. burgdorferi*, syphilis, *E. chaffeensis*, *A. phagocytophilum*
Respiratory	Influenza, adenovirus, Venezuelan equine encephalitis, Nipah virus, Hendra virus, *C. burnetii*, *M. pneumoniae*, MTB, *H. capsulatum*
Retinitis	CMV, West Nile virus, *B. henselae*, syphilis
Urinary symptoms	St Louis encephalitis (early)
Cerebellar ataxia	VZV (children), EBV, mumps, St Louis encephalitis, *T. whipplei*, *T. brucei gambiense*
Cranial nerve abnormalities	HSV, EBV, *L. monocytogenes*, MTB, syphilis, *B. burgdorferi*, *T. whipplei*, *C. neoformans*, *Coccidioides* spp., *H. capsulatum*
Dementia	HIV, sporadic and variant CJD, measles (SSPE), syphilis, *T. whipplei*
Myorhythmia	*T. whipplei* (oculomasticatory)
Parkinsonism	Japanese encephalitis, St Louis encephalitis, West Nile virus, Nipah virus, *T. gondii*, *T brucei gambiense*
Flaccid paralysis	Japanese encephalitis, West Nile virus, tick-borne encephalitis, enterovirus-71, Coxsackie viruses, polio
Rhomboencephalitis	HSV, West Nile virus, enterovirus-71, *L. monocytogenes*

Table 19.9 Laboratory diagnosis of encephalitis[5,6]

Class of organism	Diagnostic tests
Viruses	CSF PCR for HSV-1, HSV-2, VZV, enteroviruses, EBV, CMV Throat swab/respiratory specimens for respiratory virus PCR Blister fluid for HSV, VZV PCR Serology for HIV, EBV, mumps, measles, rubella, West Nile virus, Eastern, Western, and Venezuelan equine encephalitis, La Crosse virus
Bacteria	CSF and blood cultures Serology for *B. henselae, C. burnetii, M. pneumoniae, T. whipplei*
Rickettsiae and Erlichiae	Serology for *R. rickettsii, E. chaffeensis, A. phagocytophilum* Blood smears for *E. chaffeensis, A. phagocytophilum*
Spirochaetes	CSF and serology for syphilis and *B. burgdorferi*
Mycobacteria	Sputum and CSF for microscopy (acid-fast stain), mycobacterial culture and TB PCR CSF and blood cultures
Fungi	Serum and CSF cryptococcal antigen Urine and CSF *Histoplasma* antigen Serum and CSF for *Coccidioides*
Protozoa	Blood film for malaria Blood, CSF, bone marrow films and serology for *T. brucei gambienese* and *T. brucei rhodesiense* Serology for *T. gondii*
Helminths	CSF eosinophilia, identification of worm in tissues and serology for *Gnathostoma* spp. Serology of cyst fluid or CSF for *T. solium*

- Serology—all patients should have an HIV test performed. Other tests should be guided by epidemiological and clinical features (see Table 19.9).
- Imaging—MRI is more sensitive than CT scan.
- EEG—is not helpful, apart from to identify patients with non-convulsive seizures.
- Brain biopsy—this is occasionally performed for diagnostic reasons.

Treatment

- The treatment of encephalitis is mainly supportive.
- Empirical therapy—all patients should be treated with IV aciclovir to cover HSV (the most frequent cause of encephalitis). Other empirical antimicrobial agents should be initiated on the basis of epidemiological and clinical features (e.g. ceftriaxone for presumed bacterial meningitis, doxycycline for rickettsial infections, etc.).
- Specific therapy—this should be tailored to the causative organism. For detailed guidance, see IDSA guidelines.

Prevention

Some diseases may be prevented by vaccination, e.g. mumps, measles, rubella, polio, rabies, Japanese B encephalitis.

References

5 Tunkel AR, Glaser CA, Bloch KC, et al.; Infectious Diseases Society of America (2008). The management of encephalitis: clinical practice guidelines by the Infectious Diseases Society of America. *Clin Infect Dis*. **47**:303–27.
6 Solomon T, Michael BD, Smith PE, et al.; National Encephalitis Guidelines Development and Stakeholder Groups (2012). Management of suspected viral encephalitis in adults—Association of British Neurologists and British Infection Association National Guidelines. *J Infect*. **64**:347–73.

Brain abscess

A focal intracerebral infection that begins as a local area of cerebritis and develops into a collection of pus surrounded by a well-vascularized capsule. Bacteria may enter the brain by direct spread from contiguous areas (e.g. ear, sinus, dental infections, or post-neurosurgery) or by haematogenous spread from elsewhere (e.g. endocarditis, or pulmonary, intra-abdominal, or skin infections).

Epidemiology

Brain abscesses are an uncommon, but severe, disease. They tend to occur more frequently in males, with a median age of presentation of 30–40 years. Case fatality rates range from 0% to 24%.

Aetiology

Brain abscesses may be caused by a broad range of organisms, some of which are associated with predisposing conditions (see Table 19.10).

Clinical features

The clinical features of brain abscess are initially non-specific, often resulting in delayed diagnosis. Headache is the commonest symptom (69%) and may be localized to the side of the abscess. Other symptoms/signs include fever (45–53%), focal neurological deficits (50%), seizures (25%), and neck stiffness (15%). Nausea, vomiting, cranial nerve palsies, and papilloedema indicate raised ICP. Changes in mental status (lethargy, coma) and associated with poor outcome.

Diagnosis

- Imaging—a CT scan with contrast should be performed urgently to confirm the diagnosis. Early cerebritis appears as an area of low density, which does not enhance with contrast. As the lesion enlarges, it develops an inflammatory capsule that enhances with contrast. MRI is more sensitive than CT and also visualizes the brainstem better.
- An LP is contraindicated if there are focal symptoms or signs, because of the risk of brainstem herniation. If bacterial meningitis is suspected, BCs should be taken and an LP deferred until a mass lesion is excluded by CT/MRI scan.

Table 19.10 Factors predisposing to cerebral abscess

Predisposing condition	Microorganisms
Otitis media/mastoiditis	Streptococci, *Enterobacteriaceae, Bacteroides* spp., *P. aeruginosa*
Sinusitis	Streptococci, *Haemophilus* spp., *Bacteroides* spp., *Fusobacterium* spp.
Dental sepsis	Streptococci, *Haemophilus* spp., *Bacteroides* spp., *Fusobacterium, Prevotella*
Pulmonary/pleural sepsis	Streptococci, *Fusobacterium, Actinomyces, Bacteroides, Prevotella* spp., *Nocardia* spp.
Endocarditis	*S. aureus*, streptococci
Congenital heart disease	Streptococci, *Haemophilus* spp.
Urinary tract	*Enterobacteriaceae, P. aeruginosa*
Head trauma	*S. aureus, Enterobacter* spp., *Clostridium* spp.
Neurosurgery	*Staphylococcus* spp., *Streptococcus* spp., *P. aeruginosa, Enterobacter* spp.
Immunocompromised hosts	*T. gondii, L. monocytogenes, N. asteroides, Aspergillus, C. neoformans, C. immitis, Candida* spp., mucormycosis, zygomycosis
HIV infection	*T. gondii, Nocardia* spp., *Mycobacterium* spp., *L. monocytogenes, C. neoformans*

- Culture—if single or multiple ring-enhancing lesions are seen, then the patient should be referred for CT-guided or surgical aspiration. Samples should be sent for microscopy and culture, including TB and fungal cultures. 16S rRNA PCR may be helpful in culture-negative cases. BCs should also be taken.
- Serology—this is helpful in cases of cerebral toxoplasmosis (➔ see *Toxoplasma gondii*, pp. 517–20) and neurocysticercosis (➔ see Neurocysticercosis, pp. 731–2).

Treatment

- For a brain abscess arising from dental/sinus/ear infections, empirical therapy with ceftriaxone 2g bd IV and metronidazole 500mg tds IV is appropriate.
- For brain abscesses arising from haematogenous spread (e.g. endocarditis), vancomycin 15–20mg/kg/dose every 8–12h (maximum 2g per dose) can be added to the above regimen.
- For brain abscesses occurring post-neurosurgery, empirical therapy with vancomycin 15–20mg/kg/dose every 8–12h (maximum 2g per dose) and ceftazidime 2g tds IV or meropenem 2g tds IV is appropriate.

- Once culture results are available, treatment can be rationalized according to antimicrobial sensitivities. Antimicrobial therapy is given for 2–4 weeks IV, followed by 2–4 weeks PO. The usual duration of therapy is 6–8 weeks, but patients with multiple lesions or multiloculated lesions or those who are immunocompromised may require longer courses.
- Adjunctive corticosteroids should be given to patients with significant oedema and mass effect.[7]

Reference

7 Infection in Neurosurgery Working Party of the British Society for Antimicrobial Chemotherapy. The rational use of antibiotics in the treatment of brain abscess. *Br J Neurosurg*. 2000;**14**:525–30.

Subdural empyema

A collection of pus in the space between the dura and the arachnoid.

Epidemiology

Accounts for 15–20% of localized intracranial infections. Risk factors: sinusitis, otitis media, mastoiditis, skull trauma, neurosurgery, infection of pre-existing subdural haematoma, cranial traction devices, nasal surgery, ethmoidectomy, or polypectomy. Metastatic infection accounts for ~5%. A complication of meningitis in infants.

Aetiology

Causative organisms include streptococci, staphylococci, aerobic Gram-negative bacilli, and anaerobes. Polymicrobial infections are common. Post-operative/traumatic empyemas are usually caused by staphylococci or aerobic Gram-negative bacilli. Unusual causes include *Salmonella* spp., *P. acnes*, MTB, and *Candida* spp.

Clinical features

Acute onset of fever, headache (may be localized), vomiting, altered mental state (disorientation, drowsiness, coma), and focal neurological signs (hemiparesis, cranial nerve palsies, dysphasia, homonymous hemianopia, cerebellar signs). About 80% of patients have meningeal symptoms/signs. Seizures occur in ≤50% of cases. There may be rapid neurological deterioration with signs of raised ICP and cerebral herniation. Complications: septic venous thrombosis, cerebritis, cerebral abscess. In infants with subdural empyema, persistent fever, decline in neurological status, and seizures are seen. Spinal epidural abscess presents with radicular pain and signs of spinal cord compression.

Diagnosis

Consider the diagnosis in any patient with meningism and focal neurological signs. LP is contraindicated. CT or MRI brain scan shows a crescentic or elliptical area of hypodensity with contrast enhancement. MRI is more sensitive than CT.

Management

Subdural empyema is an emergency and requires immediate surgical management. Samples should be sent for urgent microscopy and culture. Commence IV antibiotics immediately after aspiration, based on the likely infecting organisms, e.g. ceftriaxone and metronidazole. Vancomycin should be added for suspected staphylococcal infection. Tailor treatment to culture results, once available. Outcome is related to the conscious level at presentation (>90% for patients who are awake/alert and <50% in patients who are unresponsive to pain); 10–44% of survivors experience permanent neurological sequelae.

Epidural abscess

A localized collection of pus between the dura mater and the overlying skull or vertebral column. May be complicated by subdural empyema.

Epidemiology

The epidemiology of cranial epidural abscess is similar to that of subdural empyema. Spinal epidural abscess usually occurs following haematogenous spread from another site of infection or by extension of vertebral osteomyelitis. Risk factors: bacteraemia, diabetes mellitus, skin infections, spinal trauma/surgery, decubitus ulcers, LP, epidural anaesthesia/analgesia.

Aetiology

The causes of cranial epidural abscess are similar to those of subdural empyema. *S. aureus* is the commonest cause of spinal epidural abscess. Others include aerobic and anaerobic streptococci, aerobic Gram-negative bacilli (e.g. *E. coli* and *P. aeruginosa*); 5–10% are polymicrobial. Unusual causes include *Nocardia*, MTB, and fungi.

Clinical features

- The presentation of cranial epidural abscess may be insidious, masked by the primary focus of infection, e.g. sinusitis, otitis media. Headache is common, and focal neurological signs and seizures eventually develop, followed by signs of raised ICP.
- Gradenigo's syndrome, characterized by unilateral facial pain and cranial nerve V and VI palsies, may occur if the abscess is close to the petrous bone.
- Spinal epidural abscess may present acutely (hours to days with haematogenous seeding) or chronically (weeks to months with vertebral osteomyelitis). Pain is the commonest symptom (70–90%), followed by fever (60–70%). There are four clinical stages: (i) back pain and tenderness; (ii) nerve root pain; (iii) spinal cord symptoms, e.g. motor or sensory deficits, sphincter dysfunction; and (iv) paralysis.

Diagnosis

Gadolinium-enhanced MRI is the diagnostic investigation of choice; abscesses appear as low-density lesions with linear enhancement.

Management

Cranial epidural—surgical drainage and antibiotics (3–6 weeks after drainage). Spinal epidural abscess—surgical decompression (laminectomy) and antibiotics. Empirical therapy should cover staphylococci (e.g. vancomyin) and aerobic Gram-negative bacilli (e.g. ceftriaxone, ceftazidime, or meropenem). The outcome of spinal epidural abscess depends on the level of neurological deficit before decompression. Complete recovery is possible if neurological signs have been present for <24h.

CSF shunt infections

Infection is a frequent complication of neurosurgical procedures used to treat hydrocephalus, occurring in ~5–15% of cases. The types of device that may become infected are:

- ventriculo-atrial (VA), VP, or ventriculopleural shunt;
- Ommaya drains;
- external ventricular drains (EVDs);
- lumbar–peritoneal or lumbar–pleural shunt.

Shunt infections may be classified as internal (associated with CSF abnormalities) or external (associated with soft tissue abnormalities).

Aetiology

- *S. epidermidis* is the commonest isolate.
- *S. aureus*, including MRSA.
- Streptococci, enterococci.
- *P. acnes, C. jeikeium.*
- Gram-negative organisms, including *P. aeruginosa*.
- Mycobacteria.
- Fungi.

Pathogenesis

The mechanisms of infection are: (i) contamination (at implantation of the device), (ii) externalization (erosion of shunt through the skin), (iii) retrograde (perforation of VP shunt through the bowel), and (iv) haematogenous (rare).

Clinical features

- These depend on age of the patient, site of infection, and whether there is raised ICP.
- Symptoms include fever, headache, nausea, vomiting, neck stiffness, and impaired conscious level.
- VA shunts may present with fever, bacteraemia, and endocarditis.
- VP shunts may present with fever, nausea, and abdominal pain.
- External shunt infections present with soft tissue infection.

Laboratory diagnosis

- CSF examination—direct aspiration of the shunt is preferred over ventricular tap or LP, if possible. CSF samples should be taken for urgent microscopy, culture, protein, and glucose. All abnormal results should be confirmed by a second sample within 24h, unless the clinical condition mandates immediate treatment.
- Blood tests—FBC, differential WCC, urea and electrolytes (U&Es), glucose, LFTs, ESR, CRP. NB. A normal WCC, ESR, and CRP do not exclude shunt infection.
- BCs—90% positive with VA shunt infections.
- CT/MRI brain scan to look for raised ICP.
- Urine dipstick for haematuria and proteinuria—VA shunts may be associated with shunt nephritis.
- CXR if VA or ventriculopleural shunt.
- Abdominal ultrasound/CT scan if abdominal symptoms/signs and VP or lumbar peritoneal shunt.
- Consider echocardiogram if VA shunt.

Management

- CSF shunt infections should be managed by neurosurgeons, with ID/microbiology input. Management should include device removal, external drainage, and subsequent shunt replacement once the CSF is sterile.
- External shunt infections—drainage of pus, removal of infected device and bone flap if present, soft tissue closure if possible, insertion of a temporary device at a new site, interval antibiotics for 7–14 days, followed by replacement with a new permanent device.
- Internal shunt infections—shunt removal, EVD placement or ventricular taps, interval antibiotics for 7–14 days, followed by insertion of a new device when CSF sterility is achieved.
- Empiric antibiotic therapy should be with vancomycin IV (1g bd IV; monitor levels) and intrathecally (10mg od intrathecal). IV meropenem (2g tds) should be added if there are abdominal symptoms or Gram-negative organisms seen in the CSF. Consider gentamicin IV (5mg/kg od IV) and intrathecally (1–5mg od; monitor levels) if there is evidence of endocarditis.
- Specific antibiotic therapy should be tailored in light of culture results and clinical response.
- Salvage therapy—in some cases, e.g. CoNS infections where shunt removal is not possible, salvage therapy may be attempted with vancomycin and rifampicin (but there are insufficient data to support this strategy).[8,9]

Prognosis

- The prognosis of internal shunt infections varies:
    - IV plus intrathecal antibiotic therapy with two-stage exchange—90% cure;
    - IV antibiotic therapy with one-stage exchange—70% cure;
    - IV plus intrathecal antibiotic therapy—40% cure;
    - IV antibiotic therapy alone—20% cure;
    - salvage therapy (for CoNS infection only) without shunt exchange (but with an Ommaya reservoir), using intrathecal vancomycin and PO rifampicin—40–99% cure.

References

8 Working Party on the Use of Antibiotics in Neurosurgery of the British Society for Antimicrobial Chemotherapy (1995). Treatment of infections associated with shunting for hydrocephalus. *Br J Hosp Med*. **53**:368–73.

9 Infection in Neurosurgery Working Party of the British Society for Antimicrobial Chemotherapy (2000). Management of neurosurgical patients with postoperative bacterial or aseptic meningitis or external ventricular drain-associated ventriculitis. *Br J Neurosurg*. **14**:7–12.

Chapter 20

Ophthalmological infections

Periorbital infections 746
Orbital infections 747
Conjunctivitis 749
Keratitis 751
Uveitis 753
Endophthalmitis 754

Periorbital infections

Blepharitis

Inflammation of the eyelids. Bacterial infection is usually secondary to minor trauma and often occurs in association with seborrhoeic dermatitis, acne rosacea, and pubic lice infestations.

Anterior blepharitis

Affects the lid where eyelashes attach and is usually caused by bacteria colonizing the base of the eyelashes (e.g. *S. aureus*). Infection of the pilosebaceous glands of Zeiss and Moll may result in an abscess (a 'stye'). Anaerobic infection may follow certain injuries, e.g. bites. Symptoms: erythema, pruritus, and crusting of lid margins. Chronic infections are caused by infection with *S. aureus*, CoNS, and more rarely *Pseudomonas* spp., *P. mirabilis*, or *C. ochracea*. Clinical features: hyperaemia, crusted exudates around the base of the lashes, lash loss. Exclude the presence of lice and their eggs. CMI mechanisms have been implicated in the pathogenesis of chronic blepharitis.

Posterior blepharitis

Affects the inner portion of the eyelid where it contacts the eye and due to meibomian gland dysfunction and infection. May present acutely as an 'internal stye' or hordeolum (pain and swelling are usually apparent on the conjunctival surface of the lid), or chronically as a painless cyst (chalazion). Symptoms: eye-watering, foreign body, or burning sensation. An internal stye may rarely progress to cause preseptal cellulitis.

Treatment

Eyelid hygiene may be sufficient in most cases. Blepharitis thought to be infectious in nature should be treated with a topical antibiotic, the frequency and duration of treatment determined by the severity (chloramphenicol bd for up to 2 weeks). Chalazion may require incision and drainage. Cases following trauma may require oral therapy with anaerobic cover, e.g. animal bites. Predisposing conditions should be treated, e.g. lice (malathion), acne rosacea (PO tetracycline), seborrhoeic dermatitis (topical antifungal/steroid combinations).

Other causes of lid inflammation: cosmetic contact allergy, molluscum contagiosum, louse infestation (e.g. *P. pubis*), dermatoblepharitis secondary to HSV infection or spread of adjacent impetigo.

Infections of the lacrimal apparatus

The lacrimal gland is found at the lateral upper lid margin. It produces around 10mL of tears a day, the act of blinking serving to smear the tear film from the lateral to the medial edge of the eye surface. Drainage is via the puncta at the inner canthus into the canaliculi, and from here to the lacrimal sac, the nasolacrimal duct, and out into the nose.

Canaliculitis

Low-grade inflammation of the canaliculi usually chronic and due to infection by *Propionibacterium* spp. or *Actinomyces*. Forms gritty casts that obstruct the lacrimal duct, leading to eye-watering, chronic conjunctivitis, and nasal lid swelling. Treatment: antibiotic irrigation with canaliculotomy and curettage where necessary.

Dacryocystitis

Inflammation of the lacrimal sac usually in the setting of obstruction of the sac or duct (congenital, secondary to infection, tumour, or trauma). Common in infants, resolving spontaneously by 12 months of age. Organisms include *S. pneumoniae*, *S. aureus*, and *P. aeruginosa*. Recurrent cases may be seen with sarcoidosis or *C. trachomatis*. The only symptom may be eye-watering. Acute cases follow obstruction of both the proximal and distal ends of the drainage system, e.g. sarcoidosis, trauma. The main symptom is pain in the region of the tear sac. It may be possible to express purulent material through the lacrimal puncta. Cases may require dacryocystorhinostomy. Orbital cellulitis is a serious complication of acute dacryocystitis. Treatment: in the newborn, lacrimal sac massage may be sufficient to resolve the blockage, and most cases will resolve with time; if not, probing may resolve the problem. Adults: systemic antibiotics.

Dacryoadenitis

Inflammation of the lacrimal gland. Symptoms: localized tenderness/swelling of the outer upper eyelid, with conjunctivitis and periorbital oedema. Pyogenic bacteria are the usual causes. Viral infections may be seen in children, e.g. mumps. Ocular motility defects may occur. Chronic infections may be caused by TB, syphilis, leprosy, and fungi. Treatment: systemic antibiotics; drainage if a collection develops.

Mikulicz syndrome: dacryoadenitis associated with inflammation and swelling of the salivary glands (of any aetiology).

Orbital infections

The orbital septum is a fibrous sheet lying beneath the orbicularis oculi. It extends from the periosteum of the orbit and fuses to the levator aponeurosis in the upper lids and orbital retractor in the lower lids. It acts as a physical barrier to infection. Orbital cellulitis (infection within the septum) is an ophthalmic emergency and must be differentiated from the less devastating preseptal cellulitis (see Table 20.1). Early involvement of an ophthalmologist is essential. Children with preseptal infection are at high risk of progressing to orbital cellulitis, due to the undeveloped nature of the orbital septum, and should be managed as orbital cellulitis.

Preseptal (periorbital) cellulitis

An infection of the superficial skin around the eyes, anterior to the orbital septum. It may follow infection of adjacent structures (e.g. dacryocystitis) or trauma.

- *Aetiology*—*S. aureus, S. pneumoniae*, other streptococci, *H. influenzae* (if unvaccinated), anaerobes. Rare causes include *Acinetobacter* spp., *Nocardia* spp., *B. anthracis, P. aeruginosa, N. gonorrhoeae, Proteus* spp., *P. multocida*, MTB, and *Trichophyton* spp.
- *Clinical features*—ocular pain, eyelid swelling and erythema, low-grade fever. Proptosis and impairment of eye movements are not seen—their presence suggests orbital cellulitis (➔ see Orbital (post-septal)

cellulitis below). Optic nerve function is normal. Complications include progression to orbital cellulitis and CNS infections.

- *Investigations*—Gram stain and culture of any discharge, CT/MRI scan if any question of orbital involvement.
- *Management*—oral antibiotics are sufficient in simple cases (e.g. flucloxacillin 500mg qds with metronidazole 400mg tds, both for 7 days). Alternative regimens include clindamycin monotherapy or co-trimoxazole plus amoxicillin or co-amoxiclav or cefpodoxime or cefdinir. IV antibiotics may be required, particularly if *H. influenzae* is suspected. Ensure anaerobic cover if infection developed following trauma (e.g. bite).

Orbital (post-septal) cellulitis

An acute infection involving the contents of the orbit (fat and ocular muscles). This is an ophthalmic emergency because of the risk of visual loss and posterior extension to the cavernous sinus (with possible thrombosis and death). Most cases result from contiguous spread from infected sinuses but can occur as a result of trauma, otitis media, and dental infection.

- *Aetiology*—*S. aureus, S. anginosus* (*milleri*) group, *S. pneumoniae*, GAS, anaerobes, and Gram-negatives (particularly in those cases following chronic sinus infection). Rare causes: *H. influenzae*, anaerobes, *A. hydrophila, P. aeruginosa, E. corrodens*, MTB, *Aspergillus* spp., mucormycosis.
- *Clinical features*—ocular pain, swelling, eyelid erythema (may be absent), painful eye movements, proptosis, ophthalmoplegia, diplopia. Fever is commoner in orbital cellulitis than preseptal cellulitis. Late signs: increased orbital pressure, reduced corneal sensation, and congestion of retinal veins. Complications include subperiosteal abscess, orbital abscess, loss of vision (3–11%), central retinal artery occlusion, cavernous sinus thrombosis, brain abscess, and death (1–3%).
- *Investigations*—CT scan of the orbits/sinuses is indicated if there are any of the following features: proptosis, pain on eye movement, limitation of eye movements, double vision, loss of vision, oedema extending beyond the eyelid margin, signs/symptoms of CNS involvement, inability to examine the patient fully, failure to improve within 24–48h of starting antibiotic therapy. Gram stain and culture of material, if possible. BCs

Table 20.1 Orbital versus preseptal cellulitis

	Preseptal	Orbital
Proptosis	Absent	Present
Ocular motility	Normal	Painful and restricted
Visual acuity	Normal	Reduced in severe cases
Colour vision	Normal	Reduced in severe cases
Relative afferent pupillary defect	Normal	Present in severe cases

Reproduced from Denniston A and Murray P, *Oxford Handbook of Ophthalmology*. Oxford: Oxford University Press, 2005, with permission from Oxford University Press.

should be taken prior to antibiotics but are rarely positive. If surgical intervention is performed, the organism may be recovered from material, despite empirical antibiotic therapy.

- *Treatment*—empiric antibiotics should be started as soon as possible, e.g. ceftriaxone and metronidazole ± vancomycin if MRSA is suspected/ possible. Urgent ophthalmology opinion and ENT review (if sinus surgery may be required). Continuing deterioration on therapy suggests the development of an abscess, and a repeat CT should be performed, with a view to surgical drainage if necessary. The management of fungal orbital cellulitis is a complex mix of surgical debridement and antifungal therapy.

Conjunctivitis

Conjunctivitis is the commonest ocular inflammation and may be a primary/ local infection or part of a systemic infection (e.g. leptospirosis, measles). Some organisms (e.g. *C. trachomatis*) cause very specific syndromes, but most cannot be distinguished clinically. Viruses are the commonest cause. Acute conjunctivitis resolves within 4 weeks; chronic conjunctivitis persists for ≥4 weeks. Conjunctivitis is typically self-limiting but can progress to potentially sight-threatening infections.

Aetiology

- Viruses—the commonest cause, e.g. adenovirus, Coxsackie A24, enterovirus 70, HSV, VZV, smallpox, vaccinia, rubella, rubeola, mumps, influenza, EBV.
- Chlamydia—*C. trachomatis, C. pneumoniae*.
- Bacterial—*S. aureus, S. pneumoniae, H. influenzae, Moraxella* spp., *C. diphtheriae, Neisseria* spp., and enteric GNRs.
- Parasitic—*Leishmania* spp., *Trypanosoma* spp., microsporidia, cryptosporidia, fly larvae, *Loa loa, P. pubis* (pubic lice), *Demodex* (mites).
- Fungal—*Candida* spp., *Blastomyces* spp., *S. schenkii*.
- Allergic or toxic—allergens, cosmetics, soaps, detergents, medications.

Clinical features

- Irritation and itching are the commonest symptoms. Ocular pain is unusual, unless there is ulceration, e.g. HSV or corneal involvement.
- Visual acuity is normal or slightly reduced (unless the cornea is involved).
- Skin lesions are seen with HSV, VZV, poxviruses, immune-mediated diseases, e.g. Stevens–Johnson syndrome.
- Conjunctival hyperaemia is worse in the periphery than in the limbal region.
- Ocular secretion may be due to increased lacrimal flow or impaired drainage.
- Conjunctival oedema (chemosis) may be marked, resulting in an inability to close the eyelids.
- Conjunctival papillae—conjunctival inflammation may result in dilated subepithelial blood vessels that become surrounded by an inflammatory

infiltrate to form mounds called papillae. Commoner in bacterial and allergic conjunctivitis.

- Conjunctival follicles—small, elevated clusters of lymphocytes, similar to papillae, but with no central vascular core. Most commonly associated with viral, chlamydial, or toxic conjunctivitis.
- Membrane and pseudomembranes—inflammatory exudate may coalesce, forming a yellow-white membrane overlying the palpebral conjunctiva. Commoner in viral and bacterial conjunctivitis.
- Conjunctival phlyctenules—a phlyctenule is a whitish, nodular collection located at or near the limbus, often in the centre of a hyperaemic area. It is a delayed-type hypersensitivity reaction and is associated with *S. aureus* and MTB.
- Conjunctival granuloma—a granulomatous nodule of inflammatory cells. Seen in Parinaud's oculoglandular conjunctivitis, foreign body, TB, and sarcoidosis, and sometimes in chlamydial or fungal conjunctivitis.
- Corneal involvement—may be mild (superficial epithelial erosions) or severe (ulceration or perforation). Corneal dendritic ulceration is a feature of HSV conjunctivitis. Symptoms include foreign body sensation, pain, decreased visual acuity, and photophobia.
- Lymphadenopathy—preauricular adenopathy is a non-specific finding associated with viral, chlamydial, and gonococcal causes of conjunctivitis. Submandibular and submental adenopathy are uncommon but may be present in Parinaud's oculoglandular conjunctivitis.

Diagnosis

- Laboratory investigations are not usually performed for most cases of conjunctivitis, especially if a viral aetiology is suspected.
- All cases of ophthalmia neonatorum (conjunctivitis occurring within the first month of life) should be investigated with smears and cultures for bacteria and viruses. The commonest causes are *C. trachomatis* and *N. gonorrhoeae*. Others causes include *S. aureus, S. pneumoniae, Pseudomonas* spp., *S. flexneri, M. catarrhalis*, and HSV.
- Swabs and conjunctival scrapings should be taken for Gram stain, culture (on blood, chocolate, and Sabouraud agar), and *Chlamydia* and viral diagnostics (e.g. immunofluorescent staining, PCR, etc.).

Management

- Treatment should be directed at the likely cause.
- Acute bacterial conjunctivitis—topical antibiotic eye drops (e.g. chloramphenicol, trimethoprim and polymyxin B, fluoroquinolone, or azithromycin drops) or ointment (e.g. erythromycin, bacitracin, or bacitracin and polymyxin B).
- Viral conjunctivitis usually resolves spontaneously and is usually treated supportively, e.g. artificial tears and cold compresses. There is no role for antivirals or corticosteroids.
- Chlamydial conjunctivitis—trachoma is treated with azithromycin 20mg/kg stat or doxycycline for 21 days, or erythromycin for 14 days. Adult inclusion conjunctivitis is treated with doxycycline or erythromycin for 3 weeks; sexual partners should be treated simultaneously.

- *N. gonorrhoeae* or *N. meningitidis*—IV ceftriaxone for 1–3 days. Patients with gonococcal conjunctivitis should be screened and treated for other STIs.
- Chronic bacterial conjunctivitis—treat with appropriate antibiotic therapy (e.g. against *S. aureus*) and aggressive lid hygiene.
- Microsporidia—PO albendazole or TOP fumagillin.

Keratitis

Keratitis is an inflammation of the cornea that may be caused by infectious or non-infectious agents. Any corneal inflammation is potentially sight-threatening and requires prompt investigation/management, as corneal perforation can occur within 24h. Subsequent endophthalmitis may lead to loss of vision or even loss of the eye.

Aetiology

- Microbial agents do not usually cause keratitis in immunocompetent patients with an intact corneal epithelium. Exceptions include *N. gonorrhoeae, L. monocytogenes, Shigella* spp., and *Corynebacterium* spp.
- Risk factors—trauma, contact lens use, contaminated cleaning fluids, immunological impairment secondary to malnutrition, alcoholism or diabetes, recent or pre-existing eye disease (e.g. sicca syndrome, recent topical steroid use).
- Bacteria—the commonest cause of keratitis. Causes include *Staphylococcus* spp., *Streptococcus* spp., *Corynebacterium* spp., *Bacillus* spp., *Propionibacterium* spp., *Pseudomonas* spp., *Haemophilus* spp., *Moraxella* spp., *N. gonorrhoeae*, and *Enterobacteriaceae*.
- Mycobacteria—MTB, *M. chelonae, M. gordonae*, MAI.
- *C. trachomatis*.
- Spirochaetes—*T. pallidum, B. burgdorferi*.
- Viruses—HSV, VZV, vaccinia, adenovirus, enterovirus, molluscum contagiosum, EBV, Coxsackie virus, measles.
- Fungi—*Fusarium* (commonest), *Aspergillus, Curvularia, Paecilomyces, Phialophora, Blastomyces, Sporothrix, Exophiala, Pseudallescheria, Scedosporium*, and *Alternaria* spp.
- Parasites—*Acanthamoeba, O. volvulus, Leishmania*, microsporidia, and *Trypanosoma* spp.

Clinical features

- Rapid onset of eye pain is characteristic and may hinder physical examination. Topical anaesthesia may facilitate eye examination but can result in further epithelial damage.
- Eye pain is accompanied by conjunctival injection, tearing, photophobia, blepharospasm, and decreased visual acuity.
- Other features include corneal infiltrate, epithelial defects (visualized by fluorescein stain under cobalt blue light), stromal suppuration, corneal oedema, corneal neovascularization, intraocular inflammation (white cells or protein flare in the anterior chamber, hypopyon, synechiae, glaucoma), and loss of corneal tissue (keratolysis).

Diagnosis

- Because of the limited amount of tissue available, extreme care must be taken in the collection, transport, and processing of specimens.
- Corneal scrapings (or biopsies) should be taken using sterile technique and transferred to glass slides and appropriate culture media. It may also be helpful to culture material from the conjunctiva, eyelids, contact lenses/solutions/storage cases.
- For viruses, samples should be collected into viral transport media. PCR assays enable rapid diagnosis of HSV and VZV.

Management

Patients may need to be admitted to hospital for management, particularly if there is evidence of corneal thinning.

- Bacterial keratitis—broad-spectrum topical therapy, e.g. cephalosporin (or vancomycin) and an aminoglycoside (gentamicin or tobramycin), is given for severe keratitis. Topical fluoroquinolones are increasingly being used. The use of topical corticosteroids is controversial. Supportive measures: topical cycloplegics, temporary soft contact lens for corneal ulceration.
- Chlamydial keratitis—systemic antimicrobials, e.g. PO tetracycline, erythromycin, or azithromycin. Sexual partners should be treated simultaneously.
- Interstitial keratitis—an immune phenomenon associated with syphilis and Lyme disease. Specific therapy may be indicated for the primary disease but has little impact on the cornea. Topical corticosteroids may be helpful.
- HSV keratitis—acute infection requires topical (1% trifluridine eye drops for ≥7 days) or systemic therapy (aciclovir, famciclovir, or valaciclovir for 14–21 days).
- VZV keratitis—acute herpes zoster ophthalmicus requires antiviral therapy (aciclovir, famciclovir, or valaciclovir), pain management (e.g. amitriptyline). Exposure keratopathy—topical antibiotic ointment (to prevent secondary bacterial infection). Dendritiform keratopathy—3% vidarabine ointment or 1% trifluridine drops or oral antivirals. Immune keratopathy—topical corticosteroids. General measures—non-steroidal analgesia and cycloplegics.
- Ocular vaccinia—TOP 1% trifluridine drops or 3% vidarabine ointment. IVIG not indicated, unless required for other reasons, e.g. eczema vaccinatum, progressive vaccinia.
- Viral keratoconjunctivitis—no specific treatment required; supportive treatment only, e.g. artificial tears ± cycloplegics. If severe symptoms, topical steroids and cycloplegics may be helpful.
- Fungal keratitis—topical agents (e.g. amphotericin, flucytosine, fluconazole, and itraconazole) have poor corneal penetration. May require combined topical and systemic therapy for months.
- Parasitic keratitis—the optimal treatment for *Acanthamoeba* keratitis is unknown, and various agents have been used, e.g. diamidines, biguanides, aminoglycosides, and azoles. Onchocerciasis is treated with ivermectin. Microsporidia may be treated with albendazole.

Uveitis

Uveitis is an inflammation of the uveal tract (iris, ciliary body, choroid) or adjacent ocular structures such as the retina. Inflammation may occur in different anatomical regions of the eye, e.g. anterior (commonest), intermediate, posterior, or panuveitis. Uveitis may be caused by infections, autoimmune conditions, or rarely trauma; 50% are idiopathic. Some infectious causes may affect particular locations. Aspiration of aqueous or vitreous material may allow identification of the causative organism. Involve an ophthalmologist early in management.

Classification

- *Anterior uveitis*—inflammation affects the iris (iritis), anterior ciliary body (cyclitis), or both (iridocyclitis). It presents with a unilateral red eye, deep ocular pain, a tender eyeball, irregular/constricted pupil, photophobia, and eye-watering. Most cases are associated with autoimmune conditions (45%) or are idiopathic (40%). Infectious causes include HSV, syphilis, TB, Lyme disease, and leprosy.
- *Intermediate uveitis*—inflammation involving the anterior vitreous and adjacent portion of the retina. Most cases have an unknown aetiology (69%) or are due to sarcoidosis or multiple sclerosis. Lyme disease causes <1%.
- *Posterior uveitis*—inflammation involving the choroid (choroiditis), retina (retinitis), or both (choroidoretinitis). More likely to be painless and present with floaters. Over 40% of cases are due to infection, e.g. *Toxoplasma*, CMV, acute retinal necrosis (HSV), *Toxocara*, syphilis, and *Candida*.
- *Panuveitis*—inflammation involving all parts of the uvea. Causes: mostly autoimmune, idiopathic (25%), and infections (10%), e.g. syphilis, TB, and *Candida*.

Aetiology

- *Infectious*—these include bacteria, spirochaetes, viruses, fungi, and parasites (see Table 20.2). These affect different populations and have distinctive clinical presentations.
- *Systemic inflammatory conditions associated with uveitis*—these include spondyloarthritides (e.g. ankylosing spondylitis, reactive arthritis, psoriatic arthritis, IBD, sarcoidosis, Behçet's disease, tubulointerstitial nephritis and uveitis (TINU) syndromes, juvenile idiopathic arthritis, Kawasaki disease, relapsing polychondritis, Sjögren's syndrome, SLE, Wegener's granulomatosis, Vogt–Koyanagi–Harada (VGK) syndrome, Blau syndrome).
- *Syndromes confined to the eye*—pars planitis is a relatively common form of uveitis restricted to the pars plan a (between the retina and ciliary body); may be associated with multiple sclerosis or sarcoidosis. Sympathetic ophthalmia is inflammation of the contralateral eye that occurs weeks to a year after trauma to one eye. Birdshot choroidopathy.
- *Masquerade syndromes*—these include ocular lymphoma, melanoma or retinoblastoma, leukaemia, giant retinal tears, retinal ischaemia, retinitis pigmentosa.

Diagnosis

- The diagnosis of uveitis is almost always presumptive, as the uvea cannot be biopsied without risking sight. The aqueous and vitreous humours may be sampled, but these samples rarely yield a diagnosis.
- Molecular diagnostic techniques may be helpful, e.g. PCR for HSV, VZV, and CMV. Serology is unhelpful, apart from in the diagnosis of syphilis, Lyme disease, and SLE.
- A CXR may be useful to look for TB or sarcoidosis.

Treatment

The treatment of the infectious causes of uveitis is the same as the treatment for CNS infection caused by the same pathogen. Systemic corticosteroids may be given in some conditions, e.g. ocular syphilis.

Endophthalmitis

Inflammation of the ocular cavity (aqueous and vitreous humours). Usually caused by bacteria or fungi, which may be introduced into the eye from an external (exogenous) source (e.g. trauma, surgery, keratitis, bleb-related) or enter the eye haematogenously from a distant (endogenous) site of infection, e.g. endocarditis. Panophthalmitis refers to inflammation of all ocular tissue.

General features

- Symptoms—eye pain, redness, lid swelling, decreased visual acuity, headache, photophobia, discharge. Fungal endophthalmitis may have a more indolent course, with symptoms developing over days to weeks. Consider in anyone with a history of penetrating injury with a plant substance or soil-contaminated foreign body. Symptoms of the primary source of infection may be seen in endogenous cases (e.g. fever, meningism).
- Signs—lid swelling/erythema, inflamed conjunctiva, hypopyon, chemosis, corneal oedema, discharge, reduced/absent red reflex, papillitis, cotton-wool spots, vitritis, fluffy yellow-white retinal or vitreoretinal lesions of growing fungi, fever, and, late in panophthalmitis, proptosis.

Aetiology

- Bacterial—the commonest infectious cause. Onset is abrupt, and progression rapid. Most cases are seen after intraocular surgery. Slit-lamp examination is necessary to confirm the diagnosis and detect early signs of infection. Two types:
    - exogenous—symptoms develop 24–48h after eye trauma, later in patients undergoing extracapsular cataract extraction (<5 days post-operatively). Ocular surface flora are responsible for the majority of infections, and preoperative conjunctival sterilization may reduce the incidence. Common post-operative causes: CoNS, coryneforms, *S. aureus*. Common post-traumatic causes: *S. aureus, B. cereus*, GAS, coliforms, anaerobes, *Pseudomonas* spp. Delayed endophthalmitis

Table 20.2 Infectious causes of uveitis

Bacteria	Viruses	Fungi	Parasites
TB	CMV	Aspergillosis	Toxocariasis
Syphilis	EBV	Blastomycosis	Toxoplasmosis
Cat scratch disease	HSV	Candidiasis	*Acanthamoeba*
NTM	VZV	Coccidioidomycosis	Cysticercosis
Leprosy	HIV	Cryptococcosis	Onchocerciasis
Leptospirosis	HTLV-1	Histoplasmosis	
Lyme disease	Mumps	*P. jiroveci*	
Propionibacteria	Parechovirus	Sporotrichosis	
RMSF	Rubella		
Whipple's disease	Rubeola		
	Vaccinia		
	West Nile virus		
	Chikungunya virus		

after cataract extraction in patients with an intraocular lens may run a chronic course—associated organisms include *P. acnes*, *Corynebacterium* spp., CoNS, and NTM. Visual outcome after recovery is poor.
- Endogenous—tends to affect the posterior segment of the eye. Patients are usually very unwell and often immunocompromised. Foci of primary infection include meningitis, endocarditis, pneumonia, abdominal infection, and dental procedures. Causes: *S. aureus*, *S. pneumoniae*, and GAS.

- Fungal—increasing in incidence with the use of immunosuppressive agents and antibiotics. Haematogenous cases are most commonly caused by *Candida* spp. Cases have occurred in healthy patients, following injections of contaminated anaesthetic. Ocular features may arise many days after *Candida* being recovered from the blood. Patients are often sick (e.g. ventilated on the ICU) and may not report early visual symptoms. Have a low threshold for ocular examination of such patients. *Aspergillus* enophthalmitis may occur in seriously immunosuppressed patients and IDUs. Other causes: *C. neoformans, B. dermatitidis, H. capsulatum, Nocardia* spp.
- Viral—HSV, VZV, and CMV cause a spectrum of eye disease from acute retinal necrosis (usually healthy patients) to progressive outer retinal necrosis (severely immunocompromised patients). CMV retinitis is seen in AIDS patients and those receiving chemotherapy for acute leukaemia and malignant lymphomas. Measles retinopathy may be seen 6–12 days after skin rash, and chorioretinitis can be a complication of SSPE.
- Parasitic—causes include *T. gondii* and *T. canis*.

Diagnosis

Early recognition and prompt microbiological investigations are essential if functional vision is to be salvaged in bacterial endophthalmitis. Samples from the vitreous humour have the greatest yield. It may also be appropriate to obtain material from the anterior chamber and any wound. Surgical specimens should be examined. Gram, Giemsa, and PAS stains should be performed, and samples cultured for aerobic and anaerobic bacteria, mycobacteria, and fungi. ELISA or PCR testing of samples may also be appropriate. BCs should be taken if the patient is systemically unwell. Viral retinitis may have a characteristic appearance on fundoscopy, and urgent specialist examination is indicated.

Treatment

Successful outcome is dependent upon a low threshold of clinical suspicion for diagnosing infectious endophthalmitis. Urgent specialist referral is indicated.

- Bacterial—broad-spectrum intravitreal antibiotics (vancomycin, amikacin, ceftazidime) should be started immediately after urgent diagnostic aspirates and modified in the light of culture results. Those with visual acuity of light perception or worse benefit from immediate vitrectomy; those with better vision than this do no better with vitrectomy and intravitreal antibiotics than with biopsy and intravitreal antibiotics (unless perhaps they are diabetic). Outcome is influenced by the time to diagnosis and appropriate treatment and the virulence of the organism—*P. aeruginosa* and *S. aureus* can destroy the eye within 24h of presentation. There may be a role for early corticosteroids.
- Fungal—*Candida*: systemic and intravitreal amphotericin with vitrectomy in those cases with intravitreal abscess. *Aspergillus*: vitrectomy and high-dose IV amphotericin. 5-flucytosine may be used in combination. Prognosis is poor. Steroids are contraindicated.
- Viral—a combination of systemic and, in some cases, intraocular antiviral agents is indicated.

Chapter 21

Skin and soft tissue infections

Skin and soft tissue infections: introduction *758*
Bite infections *760*
Surgical site infections *760*
Clostridial gas gangrene (myonecrosis) *762*
Necrotizing fasciitis *763*
Pyomyositis *764*
Fungal skin infections *766*
Viral skin infections *768*
Miscellaneous skin infections *770*

Skin and soft tissue infections: introduction

Impetigo

- Caused by *S. aureus* and/or GAS. Commonly affects children in tropical/subtropical regions; also prevalent in temperate regions in summer months.
- Clinical features—occurs on the face and extremities. Lesions start as small vesicles that develop into flaccid bullae that rupture, releasing a yellow discharge that forms thick crusts.
- Treatment—mupirocin is the best topical agent. Patients who have numerous lesions or who do not respond to topical treatment should receive oral antibiotics, e.g. flucloxacillin or cefalexin. If MRSA is suspected/isolated, then treatment with doxycycline, clindamycin, or co-trimoxazole are appropriate.

Folliculitis

- A superficial infection of the hair follicles and apocrine structures.
- Aetiology—*S. aureus* (commonest), *P. aeruginosa* ('hot tub' folliculitis), *Enterobacteriaceae* (complication of acne), *Candida* spp., and *M. furfur* (in patients taking corticosteroids). Eosinophilic pustular folliculitis occurs in AIDS patients.
- Clinical features—lesions consist of small, erythematous, pruritic papules, often with a central pustule.
- Treatment—empiric treatment is with PO flucloxacillin. If the clinical response is slow, consider other pathogens.

Cutaneous abscesses

- Collections of pus within the dermis and deeper skin structures.
- Usually polymicrobial containing skin/mucous membrane flora; *S. aureus* is the sole pathogen in ~25% of cases.
- Clinical features—painful, tender, fluctuant nodules, usually with an overlying pustule and surrounded by a rim of erythematous swelling.
- Treatment is with incision and drainage. Antibiotics are rarely necessary, unless there is extensive infection or systemic toxicity, or the patient is immunocompromised.

Furuncles and carbuncles

- A furuncle (boil) is a deep inflammatory nodule that usually develops from preceding folliculitis. Furuncles usually occur in areas of the hairy skin, e.g. face, neck, axillae, and buttocks.
- A carbuncle is a larger, deeper lesion made of multiple abscesses extending into the subcutaneous fat. Usually occur at the nape of the neck, on the back, or on the thighs. Patients may be systemically unwell.
- Outbreaks of furunculosis caused by MSSA and MRSA have been described in groups of individuals with close contact, e.g. families, prisons, and sports teams.

- Most furuncles may be treated with application of moist heat which promotes localization and spontaneous drainage. Large lesions require surgical drainage. Systemic antibiotics are indicated if fever, cellulitis, or lesions are located near the nose or lip. Control of outbreaks may require washing with chlorhexidine soaps, no sharing of cloths or towels, laundering of clothing, towels, and bedclothes, and eradication of staphylococcal carriage in colonized persons.

Ecthyma

- Punched-out ulcers surrounded by raised violaceous margins.
- Caused by *S. aureus* or GAS. Similar lesions (ecthyma gangrenosum) may occur with *P. aeruginosa* in neutropenic patients.
- Empiric treatment is with flucloxacillin or cephalexin (unless cultures yield streptococci alone, in which case penicillin is appropriate). Antipseudomonal agents, e.g. piperacillin-tazobactam, should be given for *P. aeruginosa* infections.

Erysipelas

- An acute spreading skin infection with prominent lymphatic involvement. Usually affects children, infants, and the elderly. Predisposing factors include skin lesions, venous stasis, paraparesis, diabetes mellitus, and alcohol abuse.
- Causes—GAS (commonest), group C and G streptococci, *S. aureus*, or GBS.
- Clinical features—painful, erythematous, oedematous lesion with an elevated, sharply demarcated border. Usually occurs on the face or legs. Systemic symptoms are common; 5% are bacteraemic.
- Treatment is with flucloxacillin or clindamycin. If cultures yield streptococci, treatment with penicillin is appropriate.

Cellulitis

- An acute spreading infection of the skin that extends into the subcutaneous tissues. *S. aureus* and streptococci are the main causes. Clues to other causes include physical activities, trauma, water contact, and animal, insect, or human bites and immunosuppression. Examples include *Enterobacteriaceae, L. pneumophila, A. hydrophila, V. vulnificus, E. rhusiopathiae*, and *C. neoformans*.
- Clinical features—spreading erythematous, hot, tender lesion, usually accompanied by systemic symptoms.
- The diagnosis is usually clinical, as cultures are rarely positive.
- Treatment—empiric treatment is with IV flucloxacillin or clindamycin. Vancomycin, teicoplanin, linezolid, or daptomycin are indicated for MRSA cellulitis. Gram-negative and anaerobic cover may be required for cellulitis in the context of diabetic ulcers. The affected limb should be immobilized and elevated.

Further reading

Stevens DL, Bisno AL, Chambers HF, *et al* (2014). Practice guidelines for the diagnosis and management of skin and soft tissue infections: 2014 update by the Infectious Diseases Society of America. *Clin Infect Dis*. **59**:147–59.

Bite infections

Animal bites

- Aetiology—these are usually caused by domestic pets (e.g. dogs or cats) but may be caused by exotic pets or wild animals. Most infections are polymicrobial. The predominant pathogens are the oral flora of the biting animal, e.g. *P. multocida, C. canimorsus, Bacteroides* spp., *Fusobacterium* spp., *Prevotella* spp., *Porphyromonas* spp., *Propionibacterium* spp., and peptostreptococci. Secondary bacterial infection with *S. aureus* or GAS may occur.
- Clinical features—patients who present >8h after injury usually have established infection, which may be purulent or non-purulent.
- Diagnosis—this is clinical, but samples may be taken to identify the causative organisms. Complications include septic arthritis, osteomyelitis, subcutaneous abscesses, tendonitis, and bacteraemia.
- Management—wounds *should* be irrigated copiously with sterile saline, and any debris removed; debridement is rarely necessary. Wounds should be steri-stripped, but not sutured (except facial wounds by a plastic surgeon). Empiric antibiotic therapy is with PO amoxicillin/clavulanic acid. Alternatives include PO doxycycline or IV piperacillin–tazobactam or carbapenems. A tetanus booster should be given to those whose vaccination status is unknown. Rabies vaccination should be considered for animal bites in endemic regions. Prophylactic valaciclovir should be considered for monkey bites (simian herpesvirus).

Human bites

- Aetiology—human bites result from aggressive behaviour and are often more serious than animal bites. The causative organisms are usually the oral flora of the biter, e.g. oral streptococci, staphylococci, *Haemophilus* spp., *E. corrodens, Fusobacterium* spp., *Prevotella* spp., *Porphyromonas* spp., and rarely *Bacteroides* spp. Human bites may also potentially transmit viral infections, e.g. HBV, HCV, and HIV.
- Clinical features—bite wounds may be occlusive injuries (where teeth bite the body part) or clenched-fist injuries (where one person's fist hits the other person's teeth). Complications of closed-fist injuries include tendon or nerve damage, fractures, septic arthritis, or osteomyelitis.
- Management—the principles are the same as for animal bites, e.g. wound irrigation and prophylactic antimicrobial therapy (➔ see Animal bites above). Hand injuries should be evaluated for complications by a hand surgeon. PEP (➔ see Prevention, p. 417) of hepatitis B and HIV (➔ see Table 6.5) should be considered if the source is potentially infected.

Surgical site infections

- Infections of surgical wounds are common adverse events following surgery. The frequency of SSIs is related to the category of operation and is highest with contaminated or high-risk surgical procedures. There are three categories of SSI:

- superficial incisional SSI—involves subcutaneous tissue, occurs within 30 days of operation;
- deep incisional SSI—involves muscle and fascia, occurs within 30 days of operation (or 1 year if prosthesis inserted);
- organ/space SSI—involves any part of the anatomy (organs or spaces) other than the incisional site.

Aetiology and pathogenesis

The commonest organisms are *S. aureus* and MRSA. Others include CoNS, aerobic Gram-negative bacilli, *Bacillus* spp., and corynebacteria. SSIs that occur after an operation on the GI tract or female genitalia have a high probability of having mixed flora. The presence of prosthetic material greatly reduces the number of organisms that are required to initiate infection.

Clinical features

- Most SSIs have no clinical manifestations for at least 5 days after the operation, and many may not become apparent for up to 2 weeks.
- Local signs of pain, swelling, erythema, and purulent drainage are usually present. Fever may not be present until a few days later.
- In morbidly obese patients or in patients with deep, multilayer wounds, e.g. thoracotomy, the external signs of SSIs may appear late.

Diagnosis

(See reference 1.) The diagnosis is usually clinical, but samples of fluid or tissue should be sent to the laboratory for Gram stain and culture.

Management

- The primary therapy for SSIs is to open the incision, debride the infected material, and continue dressing changes until the wound heals by secondary intention.
- Although patients commonly receive antibiotics for SSIs, there is little or no evidence supporting this practice.
- A common practice, endorsed by expert opinion, is to open all infected wounds. If there is minimal evidence of invasive infection (<5cm of erythema) and if the patient has minimal systemic signs of infection (temperature <38°C, WCC <12), antibiotics are unnecessary. For patients with a temperature of >38°C or WCC >12, a short course of antibiotics (24–48h) may be indicated.
- In Enigma, PHE performs surveillance of SSIs.[2]

References

1 Stevens DL, Bisno AL, Chambers HF, *et al* (2014). Practice guidelines for the diagnosis and management of skin and soft tissue infections: 2014 update by the Infectious Diseases Society of America. *Clin Infect Dis*. **59**:147–59.

2 Public Health England (2014). *Surveillance of surgical site infections in NHS hospitals in England 2013/14*. Available at: https://www.gov.uk/government/uploads/system/uploads/attachment_data/file/386927/SSI_report_2013_14_final__3_.pdf.

Clostridial gas gangrene (myonecrosis)

This is a rapidly progressive, life-threatening skeletal muscle infection caused by *Clostridium* spp. (clostridial myonecrosis).

Aetiology and pathogenesis

- Gas gangrene usually occurs following muscle injury and contamination of the wound by soil or foreign material containing clostridial spores. *C. perfringens* is the predominant cause (80–95%), and its pathological effects are mediated by α and λ toxins.
- Spontaneous or non-traumatic gas gangrene may occur in the absence of an obvious wound. This form is usually caused by *C. septicum* and associated with intestinal abnormalities, e.g. colonic cancer, diverticulitis, bowel infarction, necrotizing enterocolitis.
- Other organisms include *C. novyi, C. bifermentans, C. histolyticum*, and *C. fallux*. Organisms, such as *E. coli, Enterobacter* spp., or enterococci, may be isolated, reflecting contamination of the wound.

Clinical features

- The incubation period is usually 2–3 days but may be shorter.
- Patients present with acute onset of excruciating pain and signs of shock (fever, tachycardia, hypotension, jaundice, renal failure).
- Local oedema and tenderness may be the only early signs, or there may be an open wound, herniation of muscle, a serosanguinous and foul-smelling discharge, crepitus, skin discoloration, and necrosis.
- Progression is rapid, and death may occur within hours.

Diagnosis

- The diagnosis is usually clinical but may be confirmed by Gram stain of the wound or aspirate.
- Liquid anaerobic cultures may be positive within 6h.
- Plain radiographs may show gas in the affected tissues.

Management

- Emergency surgical exploration and debridement of the affected area should be performed.
- Empirical antibiotic therapy with piperacillin–tazobactam plus vancomycin (if risk of MRSA) is appropriate, pending cultures.
- Definitive treatment for clostridial myonecrosis is with penicillin and clindamycin.
- Hyperbaric oxygen therapy is not recommended, as its benefit is unproven and it may delay resuscitation/surgery.

Further reading

Stevens DL, Bisno AL, Chambers HF, *et al* (2014). Practice guidelines for the diagnosis and management of skin and soft tissue infections: 2014 update by the Infectious Diseases Society of America. *Clin Infect Dis*. **59**:147–59.

Necrotizing fasciitis

A severe acute infection involving the superficial and deep fascia.

Aetiology

- Type I necrotizing fasciitis involves at least one anaerobic species (e.g. *Bacteroides* or *Peptostreptococcus* spp.), as well as one or more facultative anaerobic species (e.g. non-GAS, *E. coli, Enterobacter, Klebsiella, Proteus* spp.).
- Type II necrotizing fasciitis is usually caused by GAS alone or in combination with other species (e.g. *S. aureus*). Infections caused by *A. hydrophila* (associated with freshwater injury) and *V. vulnificus* (associated with seawater injury or oyster ingestion in patients with cirrhosis) have been reported.

Epidemiology

In the USA, the estimated incidence of invasive GAS infection is 3.5 cases per 100 000 persons—necrotizing infections account for 6% of these. Risk factors include diabetes mellitus, IDU, obesity, immunosuppression, surgery, and traumatic wounds. The incidence of invasive GAS infections appears to be increasing.

Clinical features

- Necrotizing fasciitis most commonly affects the lower limbs but may affect any part of the body. The affected area is usually red, hot, swollen, and exquisitely tender/painful. There is rapid progression with skin discoloration, crepitus, bulla formation, and cutaneous gangrene. The affected area becomes anaesthetic as a result of small vessel thrombosis and destruction of superficial nerves. Systemic toxicity is common.
- In the newborn, necrotizing fasciitis may complicate omphalitis and spread to involve the abdominal wall, flanks, and chest wall.
- Fournier's gangrene is a form of necrotizing fasciitis that affects the male genitals and is usually polymicrobial.
- Craniofacial necrotizing fasciitis is usually associated with trauma and caused by GAS.
- Cervical necrotizing fasciitis is usually associated with dental or pharyngeal infections and is polymicrobial.

Diagnosis

- Surgery—the diagnosis of necrotizing fasciitis is a clinical one that is confirmed by surgical exploration and debridement. The tissues appear swollen, with dull, grey fascial appearances, a thin exudate, and easy separation of tissue planes by blunt dissection.
- Microbiology—surgical samples should be sent for urgent Gram stain and culture. BCs are positive in about 60% of cases. Skin aspirates are not as reliable as deep tissue samples.
- Histopathology—characteristic features include extensive tissue destruction, blood vessel thrombosis, and abundant bacteria spreading along fascial planes.

- Imaging—plain X-rays and CT or MRI scans may demonstrate subcutaneous and fascial oedema and gas in the tissues but should never delay surgical exploration.

Management

(See reference 3.)

- Emergency surgical exploration and debridement confirm the diagnosis and are the mainstay of therapy.
- Empirical therapy—this should be broad, e.g. piperacillin–tazobactam plus clindamycin, pending culture results. Add vancomycin if MRSA is a possible cause. Clindamycin has anti-toxin effects against toxin-producing strains of streptococci and staphylococci.
- Specific therapy for proven GAS necrotizing fasciitis is with penicillin and clindamycin.
- Adjunctive therapies—high-dose IVIG has been shown to improve 30-day survival in a small study of 21 adults with streptococcal TSS,[4] with or without necrotizing fasciitis. The role of hyperbaric oxygen therapy is unproven.

Outcome

Necrotizing fasciitis is associated with considerable mortality, even with optimal therapy—21% in type I and 14–34% in type II necrotizing fasciitis.

References

3 Stevens DL, Bisno AL, Chambers HF, *et al* (2014). Practice guidelines for the diagnosis and management of skin and soft tissue infections: 2014 update by the Infectious Diseases Society of America. *Clin Infect Dis*. **59**:147–59.

4 Kaul R, McGeer A, Norrby-Teglund A, *et al* (1999). Intravenous immunoglobulin therapy for streptococcal toxic shock syndrome—a comparative observational study. The Canadian Streptococcal Study Group. *Clin Infect Dis*. **28**:800–7.

Pyomyositis

Pyomyositis is a purulent infection of skeletal muscle, usually with abscess formation, that arises from haematogenous spread.

Epidemiology

Most cases occur in the tropics where it affects two age groups: children (aged 2–5 years) and adults (aged 20–45 years). In temperate climes, pyomyositis usually affects adults or the elderly. Males are more commonly affected than females. Patients in temperate regions often have a predisposing condition, e.g. HIV infection, diabetes mellitus, malignancy, cirrhosis, renal insufficiency, organ transplantation, immunosuppressive therapy. Other risk factors include trauma, IDU, and concurrent infections (e.g. toxocariasis, VZV).

Aetiology

S. aureus accounts for 90% of tropical cases and 75% of temperate cases. GAS account for 1–5% of cases. *E. coli* ST131 is an emerging cause in patients with haematological malignancy. Uncommon causes include groups B, C, and G streptococci, *S. pneumoniae*, and *S. anginosus*. Rare causes include *Enterobacteriaceae*, *Y. enterocolitica*, *N. gonorrhoeae*, *H. influenzae*,

A. hydrophila, anaerobes, *B. mallei*, *B. pseudomallei*, *A. fumigatus*, *Candida* spp., MTB, and MAC.

Clinical features

Between 20% and 50% of cases have had recent blunt trauma or vigorous exercise of the affected area. The disease usually affects the lower extremity (thigh, calf, gluteal muscles), but any muscle group may be affected. Multifocal infection occurs in up to 20% of cases. Patients should be evaluated for complications of bacteraemia, e.g. endocarditis. There are three clinical stages:

- stage 1 (invasive stage)—crampy local muscle pain, swelling, and low-grade fever. Induration of the affected muscle and leucocytosis may be present;
- stage 2 (suppurative stage)—this occurs 10–21 days after onset of symptoms, and most patients present at this stage. Clinical features include fever, exquisite muscle tenderness, and oedema. An abscess may be clinically apparent, aspiration of which yields pus. There is marked leucocytosis;
- stage 3 (systemic stage)—the affected muscle is fluctuant. Patients may present with complications of *S. aureus* bacteraemia, e.g. septic shock, endocarditis, septic emboli, pneumonia, pericarditis, septic arthritis, brain abscess, and ARF. Rhabdomyolysis may occur.

Diagnosis

- Early pyomyositis may be difficult to differentiate from a number of other conditions, e.g. thrombophlebitis, muscle haematoma, muscle rupture, PUO, osteomyelitis. Iliacus pyomyositis may mimic septic arthritis of the hip, and iliopsoas pyomyositis may mimic appendicitis.
- Imaging—MRI is the optimal imaging technique and may show muscle enhancement and intramuscular abscesses. CT may detect muscle swelling and well-delineated abscesses. Ultrasound may be helpful, both diagnostically and therapeutically.
- Microbiology—diagnostic aspirates prior to antibiotic therapy are helpful to define the microbiology of the infection. BCs are positive in 10% of tropical cases and 35% of temperate cases.

Management

- Antibiotics—although stage 1 disease can be treated with antibiotics alone, most patients present with stage 2/3 disease and require antibiotics and drainage. Empiric therapy should be directed against *S. aureus* and streptococci, e.g. flucloxacillin or vancomycin (if there is a risk of MRSA). For immunocompromised patients, broader-spectrum therapy is indicated, e.g. piperacillin–tazobactam ± vancomycin. Antibiotic therapy should be tailored in the light of culture results and continued for 3–4 weeks.
- Drainage—percutaneous drainage can be useful both to secure a microbiological diagnosis and as a therapeutic measure. This may be CT-guided or ultrasound-guided. If there is deep infection or extensive muscle involvement, open surgical intervention, including fasciotomies, may be required.

Further reading

Stevens DL, Bisno AL, Chambers HF, *et al* (2014). Practice guidelines for the diagnosis and management of skin and soft tissue infections: 2014 update by the Infectious Diseases Society of America. *Clin Infect Dis*. **59**:147–59.

Fungal skin infections

Fungi may cause primary infection of the skin or present with cutaneous manifestations of systemic disease.

Candida

(➲ see *Candida* species, pp. 472–3.)

- Localized skin infections—'erosio interdigitalis blastomycetica' (between fingers and toes), folliculitis, mastitis, intertrigo, nappy rash, paronychia, onychomycosis, balanitis.
- Generalized cutaneous candidiasis—in which lesions spread and become confluent, affecting widespread areas of the trunk, thorax, and extremities (uncommon).
- Chronic mucocutaneous candidiasis—a group of candidal infections that fail to respond to normally adequate therapy, resulting in complications such as oesophageal stenosis, alopecia, and disfigurement of the face, scalp, and hands. These failures seem to be associated with immunological abnormalities. Most cases present in infancy or by the age of 20 years. There is a wide spectrum of severity. Up to half of patients subsequently develop certain endocrinopathies (e.g. hypoparathyroidism). Most patients have good life expectancies. The commonest cause of death is bacterial sepsis, rather than disseminated candidiasis. Chronic mucocutaneous disease is very difficult to treat. IV amphotericin is initially effective, but most patients relapse on its cessation. Months or years of treatment with azoles may be necessary.

Malessezia furfur

Causes pityriasis versicolor (a superficial skin infection characterized by hypopigmented lesions, usually confined to the trunk and proximal limbs), folliculitis, as well as IV line infections. *Malessezia* spp. have been implicated in the pathogenesis of seborrhoeic dermatitis. (➲ see *Malessezia* infections, pp. 478–9).

Aspergillus

Cutaneous infection is rare, usually occurring in burn wounds or neutropenic patients at the site of IVC insertion. Commoner is otomycosis, caused by *A. niger* in those with chronic otitis externa. Cleaning and topical therapy with an agent such as 3% amphotericin or clotrimazole is curative. (➲ see *Aspergillus*, pp. 484–8).

Mucormycosis

Infection by fungi belonging to the order *Mucorales*. Risk factors: immunosuppression, transplantation, diabetes mellitus, trauma. Presents with chronic ulcer or cellulitis—if unrecognized, the organism penetrates deeper into the skin, with vascular invasion, necrosis, and possible dissemination (➲ see Mucormycosis, pp. 489–90).

Eumycetoma

Chronic, slow-growing, destructive fungal infection of the hands or feet. Found worldwide in tropical regions, but rare in temperate areas (➲ see Eumycetoma, pp. 491–2).

Pseudallescheria boydii

May cause eumycetoma, skin and soft tissue infection, abscesses (➲ see *Pseudallescheria boydii*, pp. 494–5).

Scedosporium prolificans

Extremely rare. Focal (e.g. osteoarticular) disease in the immunocompetent, disseminated infection (including skin) in the immunocompromised (e.g. those undergoing BMT) (➲ see *Scedosporium prolificans*, p. 495).

Fusarium species

Rare in immunocompetent people. Skin lesions start as macules and progress to necrotic papules. Systemic infection is seen in patients with acute leukaemia with prolonged neutropenia and those undergoing BMT (➲ see *Fusarium* species, p. 495).

Sporothrix schenckii

Inoculated into skin at sites of minor trauma. May cause either a fixed plaque, or painless smooth or verrucous erythematous nodular papules, with secondary lesions that follow the routes of lymphatic vessels (➲ see *Sporothrix schenckii*, pp. 495–7).

Chromomycosis

An itchy, small, pink papule is followed by crops of either warty, violaceous nodules or firm tumours, which may enlarge, forming groups with ulceration and dark, haemopurulent material on the surface. Satellite lesions may occur. Some people develop annular, papular lesions, with active edges and healing in the centre which can become scarred or form keloid. Fibrosis and oedema of the affected limb may occur in severe cases (➲ see Chromomycosis, pp. 497–8).

Dermatophytes

A group of fungi capable of invading the dead keratin of skin, hair, and nails. Clinical classification is by the body area involved: tinea capitis (scalp hair and the commonest in children), tinea corporis (trunk and limbs), tinea manuum and pedis (palms and soles, and the commonest overall worldwide), tinea cruris (groin), tinea barbae (beard area and neck), tinea faciale (face), tinea unguium (nail—also known as onychomycosis) (➲ see Dermatophytes, pp. 492–4).

Cutaneous manifestations of systemic fungal infection

- Systemic fungal infections that present with cutaneous disease include:
  - disseminated candidiasis;
  - cryptococcosis (➲ see *Cryptococcus*, pp. 480–1);

- *P. marneffei* (➔ see *Penicillium marneffei*—ACDP 3, pp. 509–10);
- *B. dermatitidis* (➔ see *Blastomyces dermatitidis*—ACDP 3, pp. 503–5);
- *C. immitis* (➔ see *Coccidioides immitis*—ACDP 3, pp. 505–8);
- *P. brasiliensis* (➔ see *Paracoccidioides brasiliensis*—ACDP 3, pp. 508–9);
- *Fusarium* spp. (➔ see *Fusarium* species, p. 495);
- *S. prolificans* (➔ see *Scedosporium prolificans*, p. 495);
- mucormycosis (➔ see Mucormycosis, pp. 489–90).

Viral skin infections

Herpes simplex virus

Cutaneous manifestations of HSV infection (➔ see Herpes simplex, pp. 396–9) include:

- pharyngitis/gingivostomatitis—the commonest presentation of primary HSV-1, generally seen in children and young adults. General features: fever, malaise, difficulty chewing, cervical lymphadenopathy. Ulcers and exudative lesions are found on the posterior pharynx and sometimes the tongue, buccal mucosa, and gums. Patients with eczema may develop severe disease (eczema herpeticum), which may disseminate, requiring systemic therapy. HSV has been associated with up to 75% of cases of erythema multiforme;
- recurrent herpes labialis—the most frequent manifestation of HSV-2 reactivation. May be asymptomatic or present with symptoms that are milder and of shorter duration than primary infection. Mild prodromal tingling is followed by the development of lesions within 48h and usually resolve within 5 days. Immunosuppressed patients may experience severe mucositis, with spread to skin surrounding the mouth;
- herpetic whitlow—HSV infection of the finger which may result from auto-inoculation (existing oral or genital infection) or by direct inoculation from some other environmental source. Presents with vesicles ± regional lymphadenopathy;
- *Herpes gladiatorum*—mucocutaneous infection of surfaces such as chest, ears, face, and hands seen in rugby players and wrestlers.

Varicella-zoster virus

(➔ See Varicella-zoster virus, pp. 399–402.)

- Chickenpox—90% of cases occur in children under 13 years of age. Incubation is 10–14 days and may be followed by a 1- to 2-day febrile prodrome before the onset of constitutional symptoms (malaise, itch, anorexia) and rash. Lesions start as maculopapules (<5mm across), progressing to vesicles which quickly pustulate and form scabs which fall off 1–2 weeks after infection. They appear in successive crops over 2–4 days, starting on the trunk and face and spreading centripetally. May rarely involve the mucosa of the oropharynx and vagina. Complications include secondary bacterial infection, pneumonitis, and encephalitis. Disease may be severe in pregnancy and the immunocompromised.
- Shingles (herpes zoster—localized recurrence of varicella virus)—causes a unilateral vesicular eruption in a dermatomal distribution (most

commonly thoracic and lumbar), often preceded by 2–3 days of pain in the affected area. Maculopapular lesions evolve into vesicles, with new crops forming over 3–5 days. Resolution may take 2–4 weeks. Complications include keratitis (herpes zoster ophthalmicus), Ramsay–Hunt syndrome (cranial nerve VIII palsy), encephalitis, and paralysis (anterior horn cell involvement).

Smallpox

(➔ See Poxviruses, pp. 444–5.)

- Smallpox is caused by variola virus, an orthopoxvirus. There are two strains: variola major (mortality 20–50%) and variola minor (mortality <1%).
- The last reported case was in Somalia in 1977, and the virus was declared eradicated by the WHO in 1980. Virus stocks exist in two laboratories, and there are concerns about its potential use as a bioterrorism agent (➔ see Bioterrorism, pp. 846–8).
- The incubation period is 10–12 days and is followed by a prodromal period of 1–2 days. The centrifugal rash is initially maculopapular and progresses to vesicles, pustules, and scabs over 1–2 weeks. Death may occur with fulminant disease.
- Diagnosis may be confirmed by EM or PCR (to differentiate it from other poxviruses).
- There is no specific treatment. Management is by isolation of cases to prevent transmission.

Monkeypox

(➔ See Poxviruses, pp. 444–5.)

- Monkeypox caused by an orthopoxvirus.
- It causes a vesicular illness in monkeys and rodents in West and Central Africa. Infection may sporadically be transmitted to humans. A large outbreak in humans in the USA was traced to importation and sale of exotic pets. The disease is similar to, but less severe than, smallpox.
- Diagnosis is by EM or PCR (to differentiate it from other poxviruses).
- Management is symptomatic, as there is no specific treatment.

Orf

(➔ See Poxviruses, pp. 444–5.)

- Orf is caused by a parapoxvirus and primarily affects sheep and cattle. Humans are infected, following direct exposure to infected animals.
- It presents with vesicular rash on sites of contact, e.g. hands and arms. This progresses to pustules which coalesce, scab, and gradually resolve over weeks.
- Diagnosis is by virus culture and identification of the virus by EM.
- Management is symptomatic, as there is no specific treatment.

Molluscum contagiosum

(➔ See Molluscum contagiosum, p. 445.)

- Molluscum contagiosum is caused by a poxvirus.
- It is spread by close human contact and may cause severe, generalized disease in HIV-infected patients.

- The lesions are small, firm, umbilicated papules, which occur on exposed epithelial surfaces or the genitalia. Lesions may resolve spontaneously or persist for months or years.
- Diagnosis is confirmed by histology or EM.
- Management is with local therapy, e.g. laser, cryotherapy, or incision and curettage. One small, uncontrolled study of three patients has shown benefit with cidofovir.

Miscellaneous skin infections

Cutaneous anthrax

- Cutaneous anthrax is caused by *B. anthracis* (➔ see *Bacillus anthracis*—ADCP 3, pp. 258–60). It usually affects humans who are in direct contact with infected animals (e.g. cattle and sheep) or animal products.
- The lesion begins with a pruritic papule that enlarges to form an ulcer surrounded by vesicles and then develops into an eschar surrounded by oedema. There may be regional lymphangitis, lymphadenopathy, and systemic symptoms.
- Diagnosis is confirmed by microscopy and culture of the vesicle fluid. If the patient has received antibiotics or cultures are negative, a punch biopsy may be taken for immunohistochemistry or PCR.
- Antimicrobial therapy does not accelerate healing of the skin lesion but may reduce oedema and systemic symptoms. Empiric therapy is with PO ciprofloxacin for 5–9 days; the duration of treatment should be increased to 60 days if inhalational anthrax is a possibility.

Erysipeloid

- Erysipeloid is caused by *E. rhusiopathiae* (➔ see *Erysipelothrix rhusiopathiae*, pp. 265–6). It usually affects people who handle fish, marine mammals, poultry, or swine.
- After exposure, a red maculopapular lesion develops, usually on the fingers or hands. Erythema spreads centrifugally, with central clearing. A blue ring with a peripheral red halo may appear. Regional lymphangitis/lymphadenopathy occurs in approximately one-third of cases. A severe, generalized cutaneous infection may also occur.
- Diagnosis is confirmed by culture of a lesion aspirate and/or biopsy specimen; BCs are rarely positive.
- Untreated erysipeloid resolves during a period of 3–4 weeks, but treatment probably hastens healing and perhaps reduces systemic complications. Treatment is with PO penicillin or amoxicillin for 7–10 days.

Cat scratch disease

- Cat scratch disease is mainly caused by *B. henselae* (➔ see *Bartonella* species, pp. 348–50).
- A papule or pustule develops 3–30 days after a scratch or a bite. Regional adenopathy occurs ~3 weeks after inoculation, and ~10% of nodes suppurate. Extranodal disease (e.g. CNS, liver, spleen, bone, and lung) occurs in 2% of cases.

- Diagnosis is by serology (poor specificity), PCR, or histology (Warthin–Starry silver stain).
- Treatment is with PO azithromycin for 5 days. Clinical response is rarely dramatic, but lymphadenopathy usually resolves by 6 months.

Bacillary angiomatosis

Bacillary angiomatosis may be caused by *B. henselae* or *B. quintana*. It usually occurs in immunosuppressed patients, especially AIDS.

Further reading

Stevens DL, Bisno AL, Chambers HF, *et al* (2014). Practice guidelines for the diagnosis and management of skin and soft tissue infections: 2014 update by the Infectious Diseases Society of America. *Clin Infect Dis*. **59**:147–59.

Chapter 22

Bone and joint infections

Septic arthritis 774
Septic bursitis 775
Reactive arthritis 776
Osteomyelitis 778
Prosthetic joint infections 780
Diabetic foot infections 783

Septic arthritis

An inflammatory reaction of the joint space caused by an infectious agent. It is usually caused by bacteria but may be caused by mycobacteria or fungi.

Aetiology

- *S. aureus* (commonest cause).
- Streptococci, e.g. groups A, B, C, and G streptococci, *S. pneumoniae*.
- CoNS.
- *E. coli*.
- *H. influenzae*.
- *N. gonorrhoeae*.
- *N. meningitidis*.
- *P. aeruginosa*.
- *Salmonella* spp.
- Others, e.g. *P. multocida, C. canimorsis, E. corrodens, S. moniliformis, Brucella* spp., *B. pseudomallei, Clostridium* spp.
- Polymicrobial infections.

Epidemiology

The reported incidence of septic arthritis varies from two to five cases per 100 000 population or 8–27% of adults presenting with painful joints. Risk factors for septic arthritis include age >80 years, diabetes mellitus, rheumatoid arthritis, prosthetic joint, recent joint surgery, skin infection/ulcers, intra-articular corticosteroid infection, injection drug use, and alcoholism.

Pathogenesis

Septic arthritis usually occurs after haematogenous seeding of pathogenic microorganisms but may occur via direct inoculation, e.g. injection, surgery, or trauma.

Clinical features

- Children and adults with acute septic arthritis usually present with fever (60–80%) and monoarticular involvement (90%).
- The knee is the most commonly affected joint, followed by the hip. Clinical features include pain, swelling, and reduced mobility in the joint.
- Polyarticular infections occur in 10–20% of patients, especially those with rheumatoid arthritis and viral causes.
- Infections with mycobacteria or fungi usually have an insidious onset.

Differential diagnosis

- Inflammatory arthritides.
- Post-infectious arthritis.
- Chronic bacterial arthritis, e.g. *B. burgdorferi, Brucella* spp., *T. whipplei, N. asteroides*.
- Viruses, e.g. parvovirus B19, hepatitis B, mumps, rubella, HTLV-1, HIV, lymphocytic choriomeningitis virus, Chikungunya virus, and Ross River virus.
- Mycobacteria, e.g. MTB (commonest), *M. kansasii, M. marinum*, MAI, *M. fortuitum, M. haemophilum, M. leprae*.

- Fungi, e.g. *S. schenkii, B. dermatitidis, C. immitis, P. braziliensis, C. albicans, P. boydii.*
- Parasites, e.g. filarial infections, schistosomiasis.

Diagnosis

- *Laboratory investigations* frequently show a raised WCC and inflammatory markers. Aspiration of the joint reveals a purulent synovial fluid, with an elevated WCC (50 000–100 000 cells/mm^3), mostly neutrophils. Gram stain is positive in 29–50%, and culture is positive in 80–90% of cases. False-positive Gram stains may occur with artefacts from stain, mucin, and cellular debris. Direct inoculation of the synovial fluid into BC bottles may improve recovery of pathogens. Samples should also be sent for microscopy for crystals. BCs are positive in ~50% of cases.
- *Imaging*—radiographs of the affected joint may be normal at presentation. Typical changes are periarticular soft tissue swelling, fat pad oedema, periarticular osteoporosis, loss of joint space, periosteal reactions, erosions, and loss of subchondral bone. Ultrasound can be used to confirm an effusion and guide aspiration. CT and MRI are highly sensitive for imaging early septic arthritis. CT is better for imaging bone lesions. MRI may not distinguish septic arthritis from inflammatory arthropathies.

Management

- *Drainage* of the joint, either by closed aspiration or arthroscopic washout, should be performed urgently. Open drainage may be required either when repeated drainage has failed to control the infection or for drainage of hip joints. Prosthetic joint infections often require removal of the prosthesis.
- *Antimicrobial therapy*—should be guided by the initial Gram stain findings. If the Gram stain is negative, then IV piperacillin–tazobactam ± vancomycin is a reasonable choice. Definitive therapy should be tailored to the organism isolated and its antimicrobial susceptibility pattern. Treatment is usually for 3 weeks.
- *Adjunctive therapy*—short-course systemic corticosteroid treatment has been shown to be of benefit in children with haematogenous bacterial arthritis.

Septic bursitis

- Septic bursitis is an inflammation of the bursa that is due to infection.
- It occurs as a result of bacterial inoculation, which may be direct (e.g. trauma, corticosteroid injection) or spread from nearby soft tissues (e.g. cellulitis) or haematogenously (e.g. endocarditis).
- Aetiology—*S. aureus* is the commonest cause (>80%), followed by streptococci (usually β-haemolytic streptococci). Other organisms include CoNS, enterococci, *E. coli, P. aeruginosa*, and anaerobes. Polymicrobial infections occur in 10–36% of cases. Subacute/chronic bursitis may occur with *B. abortus*, MTB, NTM, fungi, and algae.

- Clinical features—patients typically present with fever, pain, erythema, and warmth around the affected bursa. The most commonly affected sites are the olecranon, and pre-patellar and infra-patellar bursae. The blood WCC, ESR, and CRP are usually raised. Bacteraemia is rare in the absence of deep bursitis.
- Diagnosis—aspiration of the affected bursa is indicated, and the fluid should be examined microscopically for cells, organisms, and crystals and cultured. A WCC of >2000 cells/mm^3 was reported to have 94% sensitivity and 79% specificity for the diagnosis of septic bursitis. The Gram stain is reported to be 15–100% sensitive in septic bursitis.
- Imaging—not usually required, unless there is a history of trauma or concern about foreign body penetration. If septic bursitis of a deep bursa (e.g. ischiogluteal bursa) is suspected, then a CT or MRI scan may be indicated.
- Differential diagnosis—this includes cellulitis, crystal-induced bursitis, acute monoarthritis, haemobursa, non-septic bursitis, and patellar osteomyelitis.
- Treatment—includes aspiration, which is useful both diagnostically and therapeutically, and antibiotics. Empiric antibiotic therapy should cover *S. aureus*, e.g. flucloxacillin or vancomycin (if there is a risk of MRSA). Immunosuppressed patients should receive broad-spectrum therapy, e.g. piperacillin–tazobactam ± vancomycin, while awaiting culture results. Antibiotic therapy should be tailored in the light of culture results. The duration of therapy is determined by clinical response but is typically 2–3 weeks.

Reactive arthritis

Reactive arthritis is defined as an arthritis that arises during or soon after an infection elsewhere, but in which microorganisms cannot be recovered from the joint. Patients with Reiter's syndrome—a clinical triad of arthritis, urethritis, and conjunctivitis—comprise a subset of patients with reactive arthritis.

Aetiology

Reactive arthritis is associated with a number of GI and urogenital pathogens:

- *C. trachomatis*;
- *Yersinia* spp.;
- *Salmonella* spp.;
- *Shigella* spp.;
- *Campylobacter*;
- *E. coli*;
- *C. difficile*;
- *C. pneumoniae*.

Epidemiology

Reactive arthritis is a relatively uncommon disease, affecting young adults. It has an estimated annual incidence of 0.5–27 per 100 000 adults. Most cases occur sporadically, but clusters may follow point source infection outbreaks.

Pathogenesis

- The pathogenesis of the condition is not fully understood; it probably represents an abnormal host response to infectious agents.
- Associated with the presence of HLA-B27 which is found in >90% of patients with Reiter's syndrome.

Clinical features

- Patients may report previous GI or GU symptoms, and typically present 1–4 weeks after the precipitating infection.
- Musculoskeletal symptoms—acute-onset asymmetric oligoarthritis, often affecting the lower extremities; 50% have upper extremity involvement, and some have small joint polyarthritis. Axial arthritis involving the spine or sacroiliac joints is uncommon. Enthesitis (inflammation of the ligaments) can occur and most often affect the Achilles tendon and plantar fascia. Some patients develop dactylitis (sausage digits).
- Extra-articular symptoms—these include conjunctivitis, anterior uveitis, episcleritis, corneal ulcers, GU symptoms (dysuria, pelvic pain, urethritis, cystitis, cervicitis, salpingo-oophoritis, prostatitis, balanitis), mouth ulcers, constitutional symptoms (fever, malaise, headache, weight loss), rashes (keratoderma blenorrhagica, erythema nodosum), nail changes, and pericarditis (rare).

Diagnosis

- There is no diagnostic test for reactive arthritis.
- Inflammatory markers—ESR and CRP may be elevated.
- Stool samples are rarely positive for bacterial pathogens, as the diarrhoea has usually resolved at the time of clinical presentation.
- Urine and genital swabs may be positive for *Chlamydia* by NAATs, even in the absence of symptoms.
- Serological testing (for *Yersinia, Salmonella, Campylobacter*, and *Chlamydia* spp.) is not diagnostically helpful but may be epidemiologically useful.
- Patients may be HLA-B27-positive.
- Imaging—X-rays may show evidence of arthritis and enthesitis.
- Synovial fluid examination shows a raised WCC (2000-64 000 white cells/mm^3), with a neutrophil predominance. Histology shows non-specific changes.

Management

- Treatment is controversial.
- Antibiotics—these may be indicated if there is evidence of ongoing GU infection or carriage of bacterial pathogens. A systematic review and meta-analysis of antibiotics versus placebo for the treatment of reactive arthritis found no difference in remission of arthritis.
- Anti-inflammatory drugs—NSAIDs (e.g. naproxen, diclofenac, or indometacin) are given for symptomatic relief of acute arthritis.
- Glucocorticoids—intra-articular or systemic glucocorticoids may be used in patients who do not respond adequately to NSAIDs.
- Disease-modifying drugs—sulfasalazine, methotrexate, etanercept, or infliximab may be used in refractory cases.

Prognosis

- The clinical course of reactive arthritis is highly variable and probably depends on the triggering pathogen and the genetic background of the host.
- The disease usually lasts 3–5 months, and most patients remit within 6–12 months.
- Fifteen to 20% may experience chronic arthritis.

Osteomyelitis

Osteomyelitis is an infection of the bone characterized by progressive bone destruction and formation of sequestra.[1]

Pathogenesis

Osteomyelitis can occur as a result of haematogenous seeding, contiguous spread from adjacent infected tissues, or traumatic or surgical inoculation of microorganisms. Inflammatory exudate in the bone marrow leads to increased medullary pressure, with extension of the exudate to the bony cortex where it can rupture through the periosteum. If this occurs, the periosteal blood supply is interrupted, leading to necrosis and separation of dead bone (sequestrum). This is followed by bone formation (involucrum) at the site of periosteal damage.

Classification

Two classification systems exist.[2]

- *The Cierny–Mader system*—is a functional classification, based on the affected portion of bone and physiological status of the host, and is useful in guiding therapy. There are four anatomical types: stage 1 = medullary osteomyelitis, stage 2 = superficial osteomyelitis, stage 3 = localized osteomyelitis, stage 4 = diffuse osteomyelitis. There are three physiological classes: A = normal host, B = host with local (BL) or systemic (Bs) compromise, C = treatment worse than disease.
- *Lee and Waldvogel system*—is essentially an aetiological classification, based on duration of illness (acute or chronic), mechanism of illness (contiguous or haematogenous), and presence or absence of vascular insufficiency. It is less helpful in terms of treatment.

Aetiology

- Haematogenous osteomyelitis is usually monomicrobial, while contiguous osteomyelitis may be monomicrobial or polymicrobial. In patients with sinuses, the superficial flora may not represent the true pathogen.
- *S. aureus* and CoNS are the commonest cause of osteomyelitis, accounting for >50% of cases.
- Less common causes (>25%) include streptococci, enterococci, *Pseudomonas* spp., *Enterobacter* spp., *Proteus* spp., *E. coli, Serratia* spp., and anaerobes.
- Rare causes (<5%) include MTB, MAC, rapidly growing mycobacteria, dimorphic fungi, *Candida* spp., *Aspergillus* spp., *Mycoplasma* spp., *T. whipplei, Brucella* spp., *Salmonella* spp., and *Actinomyces* spp.

Clinical features

- Acute osteomyelitis usually presents with subacute to chronic onset of pain around the affected site. Systemic symptoms and local findings (e.g. swelling, tenderness, warmth, and erythema) may be present or absent, particularly in osteomyelitis affecting the vertebrae, hip, and pelvis.
- Chronic osteomyelitis may present with pain, swelling, erythema, and the presence of a sinus tract. Deep or extensive ulcers that fail to heal with prolonged antibiotic therapy may also indicate underlying osteomyelitis. If bone is felt when probing an ulcer, this is sufficient to diagnose osteomyelitis.

Diagnosis

Diagnosis is often suspected clinically and may be confirmed by a combination of radiological, microbiological, and histopathological investigations.

- *Blood tests*—the blood WCC may be normal or raised; inflammatory markers (ESR and CRP) are often elevated. BCs are more likely to be positive in vertebral disease and in haematogenous osteomyelitis affecting the clavicle and pubis.
- *Radiology*—although insensitive, a plain radiograph is readily available and inexpensive, and may show changes after 10–14 days. Bone scans are sensitive but non-specific. CT or MRI scans are expensive but highly sensitive and specific, and have become the investigations of choice. MRI may be contraindicated in patients with metalware; these may also cause artefacts on CT.
- *Biopsy*—an open or percutaneous bone biopsy should be taken, preferably prior to commencing antibiotic therapy. Cessation of antibiotics 48–72h prior to biopsy may increase the microbiological yield. Samples should be sent for both microbiology and histology. Sinus tract swabs are of dubious value, as they may represent colonizing flora.

Management

- *General principles*—owing to the lack of good clinical trial data, most of the recommendations for the management of osteomyelitis come from animal models, retrospective cohort studies, and expert opinion. The goal of therapy is to eradicate infection and restore/preserve function. Osteomyelitis in adults is usually treated with a combination of surgical debridement and antibiotic therapy.
- *Surgery*—the principles of surgical therapy are debridement of infected tissue, removal of metalware, management of dead space (using a flap), wound closure, and stabilization of infected fractures.
- *Antimicrobial therapy*—choice of antimicrobial therapy depends on the organism isolated and its drug susceptibility results. The optimal duration of treatment is not known, but most experts advocate 4–6 weeks of IV therapy. The addition of rifampicin to β-lactams has been shown to be effective in animal models of staphylococcal osteomyelitis and is often used in infections, particularly those involving prosthetic material. Once patients are clinically stable, they may be discharged from hospital and treated with outpatient antimicrobial therapy via a long-term IV catheter, if appropriate.

- *Adjunctive therapy*—hyperbaric oxygen has been shown to be effective in animal studies, but there are inadequate data to support this approach in humans. Negative pressure wound therapy (vacuum-assisted closure) is being increasingly used and may accelerate wound healing in complex wounds and in diabetic patients.

Complications

- Sinus tract formation.
- Pathological fractures.
- Haematogenous spread and sepsis.
- Tumours in patients with long-standing (4–5 years) osteomyelitis, e.g. squamous cell carcinoma (commonest), fibrosarcoma, myeloma, lymphoma, plasmacytoma, angiosarcoma, rhabdomyosarcoma, and malignant fibrous histiocytoma.

References

1 Lew DP, Waldvogel FA (2004). Osteomyelitis. *Lancet*. **364**:369–79.
2 Mader JT, Shirtliff M, Calhoun JH (1997). Staging and staging application in osteomyelitis. *Clin Infect Dis*. **25**:1303–9.

Prosthetic joint infections

Epidemiology

- PJIs complicate 0.5–1% of hip replacements and 0.5–2% of knee replacements, resulting in considerable morbidity and expense.
- For knee replacements, the risk of PJI is highest (1.5%) in the first 2 years after implantation, falling to 0.5% in years 2–10 after joint replacement.
- Risk factors for PJI include: advanced aged, diabetes mellitus, rheumatoid arthritis, high body mass index, nasal colonization with *S. aureus*, prior infection of the joint or adjacent bone, prior surgery to the joint, bacteraemia during the previous year, non-surgical trauma to the joint, prolonged surgery, peri- or post-operative infections, post-operative bleeding/haematoma, and early-onset SSI.
- The risk of relapse depends on the type of surgical procedure, co-morbidities, and the organism causing PJI, and can be 10–20%.

Classification and aetiology

- *Early-onset PJI* (<3 months after surgery)—these are usually acquired during implantation or as a result of post-operative wound infection. They are often caused by virulent organisms such as *S. aureus*, Gram-negative bacilli, anaerobes, and polymicrobial infections.
- *Delayed-onset PJI* (3–12 months after surgery)—these are also usually acquired during implantation. They are often caused by less virulent pathogens such as CoNS, *Propionibacterium* spp., and enterococci.
- *Late-onset PJI* (>12 months after surgery)—these usually occur as a result of haematogenous spread from another site (e.g. STI, UTI, vascular catheter). These are usually caused by *S. aureus*, β-haemolytic streptococci, and Gram-negative bacilli.

- Rarer causes include corynebacteria, fungi, and mycobacteria.
- The development of PJI is enhanced in the presence of a foreign body (the prosthesis), which reduces the number of bacteria required to induce infection and promotes biofilm formation.

Clinical features

- *Early-onset PJI*—these present acutely with fever, joint pain, swelling and erythema, and wound discharge. Often associated with haematoma formation or superficial necrosis of the skin.
- *Delayed-onset PJI*—these present subacutely with persistent joint pain, with or without implant loosening. Fever occurs in <50%. Sinus tract formation and intermittent discharge may be seen.
- *Late-onset PJI*—these present with acute onset of symptoms in a previously well-functioning joint.

Differential diagnosis

The differential diagnosis of PJI includes aseptic loosening, dislocation, gout, haemarthrosis, and osteolysis.

Diagnosis

- *Blood tests*—ESR and CRP are usually elevated in PJI but may also be elevated post-surgery and in coexisting rheumatoid disease. Procalcitonin has low sensitivity for the diagnosis of PJI. IL-6 levels may be more helpful than CRP.
- *Plain X-rays*—may show abnormal lucency (>2mm) at the bone cement surface, periosteal reaction, cement fractures, changes in position of the prosthetic components, and movement of components on stress views. However, these changes are evident in 50% of cases and may also occur with prosthetic loosening.
- *Imaging*—radioisotope scans are generally unhelpful, as they may be abnormal for up to 12 months following surgery. The use of CT scans is limited by metal implant artefacts. Likewise, MRI scans are contraindicated with metal implants (unless made of titanium or tantalum).
- *Arthrocentesis*—synovial fluid should be aspirated using aseptic technique, and sent for cell count, microscopy, and culture. The synovial fluid cell count may be elevated, and a neutrophil percentage of >65% has a high sensitivity and specificity for the diagnosis of PJI. The Gram stain is only positive in 32%. Culture is more sensitive (86–92%) and specific (82–97%). Antibiotics should ideally be withheld for 2 weeks prior to sampling to increase sensitivity of culture.
- *Operative samples* (arthroscopic or open surgical)—are used to make a definitive diagnosis. Several (3–6) operative samples of tissue and fluid should be taken, ideally prior to antibiotic therapy, and sent for microbiology and histology. Three positive cultures for the same organism give a 94.8% probability of PJI. Histopathological examination may show an acute inflammatory infiltrate; the optimum number of neutrophils per high-power field is not known, but thresholds of 5–10 have been used.

- *Blood cultures*—these should be taken in patients with fever and acute onset of symptoms.
- *Explant sonication*—sonication of an explanted prosthesis can improve the yield of microbiological diagnosis, compared to culture, particularly in patients who have received antibiotics.

Management

- *General principles*—the management of PJI usually involves both surgery and antibiotic therapy. The type of surgery and choice/duration of antibiotics depends on the time frame of the infection, the organism, and the individual patient circumstances. Surgical options include revision arthroplasty (one- or two-stage), debridement and implant retention, or resection arthroplasty without reimplantation.
- *Two-stage revision*—this involves prosthesis resection, debridement of soft tissue, and placement of joint spacer. IV antibiotics are administered for 4–6 weeks, after which a new prosthesis is implanted. Success rates of 90% have been reported. The use of antibiotic-impregnated spacers (prior to reimplantation) and antibiotic-impregnated cement (at reimplantation) is common, although clinical trial data are lacking.
- *One-stage revision*—this involves prosthesis resection, debridement of soft tissue and bone, and reimplantation of a new prosthesis during the same operation. This approach may be used in patients with easily treatable organisms and a good soft tissue envelope. Success rates of up to 80% have been reported. IV antibiotics ideally in combination with oral rifampicin if treating a susceptible staphylococcal infection are given for 4–6 weeks. After this, oral suppressive antibiotic therapy may be required.
- *Debridement and implant retention (DAIR)*—this involves debridement, polyethylene liner exchange, and retention of the prosthesis. It is appropriate in certain situations: (i) early-onset PJI (within 30 days of implantation, <3 weeks of symptoms) with a well-fixed prosthesis and no sinus tract and (ii) patients for whom other surgical strategies are too high risk. Initial therapy for *S. aureus* infections is pathogen-specific IV therapy, in combination with PO rifampicin for 4–6 weeks. This is followed by oral suppressive therapy for 3–6 months. For non-staphylococcal infections, pathogen-specific IV or oral therapy (with high bioavailability) for 4–6 weeks followed by oral suppressive therapy.
- *Permanent resection arthroplasty*—this is reserved for patients who are not suitable for any of the previous surgical options. Patients with hip PJI undergo resection arthroplasty (Girdlestone procedure), and those with knee PJI undergo resection arthroplasty and arthrodesis.
- *Long-term suppressive antibiotic therapy*—this is given in special circumstances, e.g. prosthesis removal impossible, prosthesis not loose, pathogen relatively avirulent, pathogen highly sensitive to oral antibiotic, patient able to tolerate long-term oral antibiotics.

Prevention

PJIs may be prevented by perioperative antimicrobial prophylaxis, meticulous surgical technique, filtered laminar airflow systems in operating theatres, early recognition, and prompt treatment of wound infections.

Further reading

Osmon DR, Berberi EF, Berendt AR, *et al.*; Infectious Diseases Society of America (2013). Diagnosis and Management of Prosthetic Joint Infection: Clinical Practice Guidelines by the Infectious Diseases Society of America. *Clin Infect Dis*. **56**:1–25.

Diabetic foot infections

A diabetic foot infection may be defined as any inframalleolar infection in a patient with diabetes mellitus. The commonest lesion is an infected diabetic ulcer, but the spectrum of infections is broad and may include paronychia, cellulitis, myositis, abscesses, necrotizing fasciitis, septic arthritis, tendonitis, and osteomyelitis.

Epidemiology

Foot infections in diabetic patients are common, debilitating, and difficult to manage. Risk factors include: peripheral sensory, motor, and/or autonomic neuropathy, neuro-osteopathic deformity (e.g. Charcot joint), vascular insufficiency, hyperglycaemia leading to poor immune function and wound healing, patient disabilities (e.g. poor vision, limited mobility, previous amputations), maladaptive patient behaviours (inadequate foot care or footwear), and health system failure (inadequate education and management of diabetes and foot care).

Aetiology

A number of organisms may be associated with various syndromes (see Table 22.1).

Table 22.1 Aetiology of diabetic foot infections

Foot infection syndrome	Pathogens
Cellulitis	β-haemolytic streptococci (groups A, B, C, and G), *S. aureus*
Infected ulcer, antibiotic-naïve	Often monomicrobial: *S. aureus* or β-haemolytic streptococci (groups A, B, C, and G)
Infected ulcer, chronic, previous antibiotic therapy	Usually polymicrobial: *S. aureus*, β-haemolytic streptococci (groups A, B, C, and G), *Enterobacteriaceae*
Macerated ulcer	*P. aeruginosa* ± other organisms as above
Long-standing, non-healing wound, prolonged antibiotic therapy	Usually polymicrobial with antibiotic-resistant organisms: aerobic Gram-positive cocci (*S. aureus*, CoNS, enterococci), diphtheroids, *Enterobacteriaceae, Pseudomonas* spp., non-fermentative GNRs, fungi
'Fetid foot': extensive necrosis or gangrene	Mixed aerobic Gram-positive cocci (*S. aureus*, CoNS, enterococci), *Enterobacteriaceae*, non-fermentative GNRs, obligate anaerobes

Clinical features

These can range from mild to severe and life-threatening:

- foot ulcer with no signs of infection;
- foot ulcer with surrounding inflammation or cellulitis <2cm from the edge of the wound;
- local complications—cellulitis >2cm from the edge of the wound, lymphangitis, spread beneath the superficial fascia, deep tissue abscess, gas gangrene, involvement of muscle, tendon, or bone;
- systemic toxicity or metabolic instability—fever, chills, tachycardia, hypotension, confusion, vomiting, leucocytosis, acidosis, hyperglycaemia, uraemia.

Diagnosis

- Diagnosis is based on clinical features. It is important to assess perfusion (peripheral pulses), as well as sensation (using a monofilament). Use a Doppler ultrasound to determine ankle–brachial pressure indices (ABPIs).
- Imaging, e.g. MRI scan, may be helpful to determine the extent of infection, e.g. deep collections, osteomyelitis.
- Deep tissue specimens (not superficial swabs) should be taken and sent to the laboratory for microscopy and culture prior to commencing antimicrobial therapy.

Management

See NICE and IDSA guidelines below.[3,4]

- Determine the need for hospitalization.
- Stabilize the patient if systemically unwell, and correct any metabolic abnormalities.
- Antibiotics—do not give antibiotics for uninfected ulcers. Initial empiric therapy should be based on the severity of infection and available microbiological data, e.g. Gram stain. Oral antibiotics may be sufficient for mild infections. For more severe infections, broad-spectrum IV therapy may be required.
- Assess the need for surgery—patients with severe infections, e.g. necrotizing fasciitis, gas gangrene, extensive tissue loss, critical limb ischaemia, should be referred for urgent surgical review.
- Wound care plan—the wound should be dressed in a way that permits daily inspection. Special aids may be available to offload pressure on the wound.
- Adjunctive therapies—vacuum-assisted wound closure has been beneficial in one study. The use of G-CSF shows no clear benefits.

References

3 National Institute for Health and Care Excellence (2011). *Diabetic foot problems. Inpatient management of diabetic foot problems*. NICE clinical guideline 119. Available at: https://www.nice.org.uk/guidance/cg119.

4 Lipsky BA, Berendt AR, Cornia PB, *et al.*; Infectious Diseases Society of America (2012). 2012 Infectious Diseases Society of America clinical practice guideline for the diagnosis and treatment of diabetic foot infections. *Clin Infect Dis*. **54**:132–73

Chapter 23

Pregnancy and childhood

Congenital infections *786*
Maternal infections associated with neonatal morbidity *789*
Management of rash contact in pregnancy *790*
Rash illnesses in pregnancy *792*
Prevention of congenital/perinatal infection *794*
Chorioamnionitis *796*
Puerperal sepsis *797*
Neonatal sepsis *799*
Viral causes of childhood illness *801*
Enteroviral infections *803*
Bacterial causes of childhood illness *804*

Congenital infections

Congenital infections may be acquired *in utero* or perinatally. The acronym TORCH has been used to describe a group of infections which generally cause mild or inapparent infections in the mother, yet may cause severe disease in neonates:

- *T*oxoplasmosis;
- *O*thers (e.g. syphilis, parvovirus B19, enterovirus, and VZV);
- *R*ubella;
- *C*ytomegalovirus;
- *HSV*.

Long-term consequences include growth retardation, microcephaly, congenital defects with long-term sequelae, and progressive disease in childhood. They may also present with unusual exanthemata, organomegaly, or thrombocytopenia in the neonatal period. Any infant with features of congenital infection should be tested for these possible causes. The practice of screening mothers in pregnancy varies geographically, e.g. the UK screens for syphilis and rubella, but not for toxoplasmosis.

Toxoplasmosis

- Caused by *T. gondii* (➲ see *Toxoplasma gondii*, pp. 517–20)
- Maternal infection—may be subclinical or present with an infectious mononucleosis-like illness with lymphadenopathy.
- Fetal infection—risk of transmission is lowest in the first trimester (but associated with more severe abnormalities) and highest in the last trimester. Most infants are asymptomatic at birth but may present with fever, rash, jaundice, hepatosplenomegaly, microcephaly, seizures, thrombocytopenia, and lymphadenopathy (rare). The classic triad of congenital toxoplasmosis is chorioretinitis, hydrocephalus, and intracranial calcifications. Sequelae include intellectual disability, deafness, and spasticity.
- Diagnosis—IgM typically becomes positive in the first few days of life. If the infant's IgM titres are negative or equivocal, then IgA and IgE titres should be performed. Repeat testing at 10 days of age can help, as can serial testing during the first year of life. Maternal IgG wanes between 6 and 12 months of age, so high IgG levels at 1 year confirms the diagnosis.
- Treatment—maternal infection is treated with spiramycin which reduces fetal infection rate. Refer to a specialist centre for treatment and ultrasound monitoring of the fetus. Congenital infection—treat with pyrimethamine, sulfadiazine, and folinic acid for 1 year, under specialist guidance.

Syphilis

- Caused by *T. pallidum* (➲ see *Treponema* species, pp. 335–6).
- Maternal infection—risk of congenital infection is 50% in primary and secondary syphilis, 40% in latent infection, and 10% in tertiary syphilis. Maternal infection should be detected by routine antenatal screening.

- Fetal infection—clinical features include stillbirth, intrauterine growth restriction (IUGR), non-immune hydrops, rhinitis, skin rash, hepatosplenomegaly, 'mulberry molars', 'saber shins', saddle nose deformity, interstitial keratitis, cranial nerve VIII deafness, and peg-shaped incisors.
- Diagnosis—based on serology or positive dark-field microscopy or staining for treponemes in samples from the placenta or umbilical cord.
- Treatment—maternal infection treated with penicillin. Neonates should be treated for neurosyphilis (cannot be excluded).

Parvovirus B19

- Maternal infection—presents with fever, malaise, polyarthralgia, coryza, and rash. May be mistaken for rubella. (➔ See Management of rash contact in pregnancy, pp. 790–1.)
- Fetal infection—anaemia leading to non-immune hydrops. Fetal loss 9–13%.
- Diagnosis—IgM and IgG serology in the mother. Fetal infection can be diagnosed by amniotic fluid sampling for parvovirus DNA PCR or fetal blood sampling for serology (1% risk of fetal loss).
- Treatment—mild to moderate anaemia is well tolerated and resolves without sequelae. Severe anaemia requires intrauterine blood transfusion.

Enterovirus

- Maternal infection—usually mild or asymptomatic. Enteroviruses do not readily cross the placenta or cause fetal disease, miscarriage, or preterm birth. Vertical transmission more likely to occur in the perinatal period.
- Fetal infection—this can range from rashes and aseptic meningitis to fulminant disease (e.g. myocarditis, hepatitis, encephalitis). The latter are associated with group B Coxsackie virus serotypes 2 and 5 and echovirus 11. Nosocomial transmission between infants can occur via the hands of HCWs.
- Diagnosis—enterovirus PCR of clinical specimens or serology (limited utility in acute infection as serotype-specific).
- Treatment—IVIG has been given to neonates with myocarditis.

Varicella-zoster

- Maternal infection—primary VZV infection presents with a vesicular rash and is associated with increased morbidity in the mother, e.g. pneumonitis. (➔ See Rash illnesses in pregnancy, pp. 792–4.)
- Fetal infection—primary VZV infection during the first half of pregnancy has been associated with a 1–2% risk of congenital varicella syndrome—limb hypoplasia, cicatricial lesions, psychomotor retardation, cutaneous scars, chorioretinitis, cataracts, cortical atrophy, microcephaly, microphthalmus, and IUGR. Primary VZV immediately before or after delivery may cause neonatal varicella which can present with a rash or disseminated infection.
- Diagnosis—usually clinical. May be confirmed by VZV PCR of skin lesions in the mother or infant.
- Treatment—aciclovir PO or IV for the mother. VZIG for the neonate if the mother develops chickenpox within 5 days of delivery.

Rubella (German measles)

- Congenital rubella syndrome has become rare in developed countries since the introduction of routine childhood vaccination.
- Maternal infection—may be asymptomatic or present with a rash illness. Prodromal symptoms include fever, conjunctivitis, coryza, sore throat, cough, headache, and malaise. Polyarthritis/polyarthralgia are potential sequelae. (➔ See Rash illnesses in pregnancy, pp. 792–4.)
- Fetal infection—the risk of infection varies with trimester—81% in the first trimester, 25% in the second trimester, and 35–100% in the third trimester. The risk of congenital detects is limited to the first trimester. Clinical features include 'blueberry muffin skin', cloudy cornea, cataracts, glaucoma, microphthalmia, sensorineural deafness, PDA, AV septal defects, pulmonary artery stenosis, microcephaly, meningoencephalitis, IUGR, hepatosplenomegaly, interstitial pneumonitis, radiolucent bone lesions, haemolytic anaemia, and thrombocytopenia.
- Diagnosis—IgM in neonatal serum or cord blood in infants at birth and 1 month. Monitoring of IgG at 3, 6, and 12 months may also confirm congenital or early post-natal infection. Rubella virus PCR of clinical specimens (may not be available).
- Treatment—none available.

Cytomegalovirus

- Maternal infection—infection is usually asymptomatic (90%) but may present with an infectious mononucleosis-like syndrome. Occurs in 1–2% of seronegative women during pregnancy; a small number of cases are due to viral reactivation.
- Fetal infection—infection of the neonate may occur *in utero* or perinatally. The rate of transmission increases with gestational age—36.5% in the first trimester, 40.1% in the second trimester, and 65% in the third trimester. Five to 15% of newborns of mothers with primary CMV infection are symptomatic at birth. Clinical features include IUGR, microcephaly, periventricular calcifications, sensorineural deafness, blindness with chorioretinitis, mental retardation, hepatosplenomegaly, thrombocytopenic purpura, and haemolytic anemia. Symptomatic newborns have a mortality rate of about 5%, and 50–60% develop neurological sequelae, e.g. progressive hearing loss, visual loss, cognitive impairment.
- Diagnosis—serological testing of symptomatic mothers. Amniocentesis for CMV DNA PCR. Detection of CMV in the urine or saliva within the first 3 weeks of life.
- Treatment of mother is rarely indicated. Antiviral treatment of symptomatic neonates may decrease morbidity/mortality.

Herpes simplex

- Maternal infection—primary infection presents with a vesicular genital rash. ~15% of all pregnant women with a history of genital HSV infection experience recurrent lesions at delivery. Around 2% of pregnant women with a history of recurrent HSV infection are asymptomatically shedding at the time of delivery.

- Fetal infection—usually acquired intrapartum but may be acquired *in utero*. Seventy-five to 90% of infants with neonatal HSV are born to infected asymptomatic mothers who have no known history of genital HSV. Oral–labial herpes presents a greater risk of post-natal HSV acquisition than genital HSV. Clinical features include skin lesions, chorioretinitis, microcephaly, hydranencephaly, and microphthalmia. While primary HSV infections in the first trimester are associated with higher rates of spontaneous abortion and stillbirth, infection later in pregnancy appears more likely to be associated with preterm labour or growth restriction. Of greatest concern is the risk of primary infection acquired at birth, which could lead to herpetic meningitis.
- Diagnosis—usually clinical in the mother. May be confirmed by HSV PCR of blister fluid or serology.
- Treatment—first and second trimesters: treat the mother with PO or IV aciclovir. Third trimester or genital lesions at time of delivery—deliver by Caesarean section. For women with a history of genital HSV, some recommend suppressive antiviral therapy from 36 weeks' gestation. Infants born to women with active lesions should be isolated, and the infant closely observed during the first month of life for features of neonatal HSV infection.

Maternal infections associated with neonatal morbidity

Pelvic inflammatory disease

PID is associated with chlamydial infection in over 50% of cases, and gonorrhoea in around 14%. Many cases are asymptomatic. Pregnant women with PID should be treated with IV antibiotics, as it is associated with an increase in preterm delivery, and maternal and fetal morbidity (e.g. ophthalmia neonatorum).

Listeria monocytogenes

Pregnant women are 20 times more likely to contract listeriosis than other adults; ~33% of all cases of listeriosis occur during pregnancy. Acquisition is mainly by the ingestion of contaminated food. Pregnant patients are often asymptomatic or present with a flu-like febrile illness. These mild symptoms notwithstanding, listeriosis can still lead to premature delivery, neonatal sepsis, and stillbirth. Placental transfer of the organism can cause amnionitis, with spontaneous septic abortion or premature labour with delivery of an infected baby. Fetal infection may cause sepsis, meningoencephalitis, or disseminated infection with microabscesses. Neonatal infection has a mortality of around 50%, particularly in early-onset sepsis (➔ see Neonatal sepsis, pp. 799–801). Late-onset infection typically presents as meningitis at 3–4 weeks of age.

Management

Prevention is by avoidance of potentially contaminated foods. Treatment is with ampicillin (or co-trimoxazole in those with serious penicillin allergies; it has not been approved for use in pregnancy).

Other

- Malaria (➡ see *Plasmodium* species (malaria), pp. 512–4).
- Varicella-zoster and herpes simplex (➡ see Herpes simplex, pp. 396–9 and Varicella-zoster virus, pp. 399–402).
- Hepatitis B (➡ see Hepatitis B virus, pp. 413–7).
- GBS (➡ see Group B *Streptococcus*, pp. 252–3).
- Chorioamnionitis (➡ see Chorioamnionitis, pp. 796–7).
- Leptospirosis (➡ see *Leptospira* species, pp. 340–2).
- *U. urealyticum* (➡ see *Mycoplasma*, pp. 350–2).
- *M. hominis* (➡ see *Mycoplasma*, pp. 350–2).

Management of rash contact in pregnancy

See also the PHE guidance on rashes in pregnancy and the DH *Green Book*.[1,2]

Contact with a non-vesicular rash

The important infective causes are measles, rubella, and parvovirus B19. Intervention is indicated for other possible causes in the absence of the development of symptoms in the pregnant woman. *All* pregnant women with contact with a non-vesicular rash illness should be investigated for asymptomatic parvovirus B19 infection, and for asymptomatic rubella infection, unless there is satisfactory evidence of past rubella infection (vaccine or natural infection). A significant contact is defined as being in the same room for a significant period of time (>15min) or face-to-face contact.

- *Rubella*—a mother is extremely unlikely to be susceptible to rubella if she has had at least two previous positive rubella antibody tests or at least two doses of rubella vaccine documented, or one vaccine dose followed by one positive rubella antibody test. She should be reassured but told to re-attend if a rash develops. If rubella susceptibility is possible, a serum sample should be taken and tested for rubella-specific IgG and IgM.
- If IgG-positive and IgM-negative, the mother can be considered immune with no evidence of recent primary infection. If IgG levels are low, it is worth repeating the test—there are rare occasions when IgG may precede IgM positivity in primary infection.
- If IgM and IgG are negative, the patient is susceptible.
- If IgM is detected, further advice should be sought—the control of rubella in the UK means that *most* rubella-specific IgM-positive results do not reflect recent rubella. Unless seroconversion has been demonstrated, further specialist testing is required.
- *Parvovirus B19*—all women should be investigated for asymptomatic infection. This should not be delayed, pending the development of symptoms, as asymptomatic infection is just as likely as symptomatic to infect and damage the fetus, and active management of the infected fetus reduces the risk of poor outcome. Maternal serum should be taken as soon after rash contact as possible and tested for parvovirus B19-specific IgG and IgM.

- If IgM, but not IgG, is detected, tests should be repeated on another fresh serum sample.
- If IgG is detected and IgM is not present, the mother can be reassured.
- If both IgG and IgM are negative, another sample should be taken 1 month after the last contact. If these remain negative, the mother can be reassured she has not been infected but informed that she is susceptible. If the mother is found to have developed asymptomatic infection, she should be managed, as detailed in ➲ Rash illnesses in pregnancy, p. 792–4.
- *Measles*—if epidemiological and clinical features suggest the source patient has measles, passive prophylaxis with IM HNIG should be considered. This should be given as soon as possible after exposure and certainly within 6 days—it attenuates maternal illness but does not confer any benefit on the fetus. If the mother has received two doses of the measles vaccine, the probability of becoming infected is very low. If vaccination history is negative or uncertain, serum should be taken for an urgent measles IgG and results awaited, before giving HNIG. If IgG-positive within 10 days of contact, no further action is required. If measles IgG is not present, HNIG should be given, and serological tests repeated at 3 weeks. There is no point in giving HNIG if the contact was >10 days prior to presentation.

Contact with a vesicular rash

- Pregnant women who are exposed to varicella or herpes zoster in pregnancy should seek medical attention as soon as possible. Contact is considered significant if the mother was in the same room for 15min or more or had face-to-face contact of any duration.
- They can be reassured that they are protected if they themselves have a history of varicella or herpes zoster.
- If there is an uncertain or absent history of infection, the mother's susceptibility should be determined urgently by VZV IgG testing. VZIG should be offered to VZV IgG-negative women within 10 days of exposure (or within 10 days of rash onset in cases of continuous household exposure, e.g. an infected child in the house). The 10-day administration window allows ample time for antibody testing before proceeding with administration of VZIG. Around 50% of women who receive VZIG following household exposure will develop chickenpox; another 25% are infected subclinically. However, disease is attenuated (the risk of fatal varicella is estimated to be about five times higher in pregnant than non-pregnant adults, with fatal cases concentrated late in the second or early third trimester), and the risk of fetal infection reduced. NB. If contact was before the infectious period (i.e. >48h before chickenpox rash onset or before the appearance of shingles vesicles), VZIG is not indicated.

References

1 Public Health England (2011). *Guidance on viral rash in pregnancy*. Available at: https://www.gov.uk/government/publications/viral-rash-in-pregnancy.

2 Public Health England (2013). *The Green Book: immunisation against infectious disease*. Available at: https://www.gov.uk/government/collections/immunisation-against-infectious-disease-the-green-book.

Rash illnesses in pregnancy

(See also the PHE guidance on rashes in pregnancy and the DH *Green Book*.)[3,4]

Rubella, parvovirus B19, and VZV are the infections of most relevance because of their potential impact on the fetus and neonate. With the exception of varicella, these infections do not have a specific impact on the fetus beyond 20 weeks' gestation. Investigation is recommended at any gestational age; age calculation may not be accurate, and achieving an accurate diagnosis is helpful in guiding the advice given to the mother regarding contact with other pregnant women and neonates (e.g. antenatal clinics). Other infections (enterovirus, infectious mononucleosis, syphilis, *Streptococcus*, meningococcus) are managed as normal in the mother, and the neonate should be followed up. *NB. If investigation is commenced some weeks after rash or contact, it may not be possible to confirm or refute a possible diagnosis.*

Patients presenting with a non-vesicular rash

All pregnant women with a non-vesicular rash illness compatible with rubella or parvovirus B19 should be investigated simultaneously for both infections, *regardless* of previous history, immunization, or prior testing.

- Rubella infection—around 1–2% of young pregnant women in the UK are susceptible, and the rates of infection following contact are high. Maternal infection is extremely rare in the UK today.
    - Risk of adverse fetal outcome—90% at a gestational age <11 weeks, 20% at 11–16 weeks, falling to a minimal risk of deafness at 16–20 weeks, and no increased risk after this time.
    - Management of pregnant women with proven primary or symptomatic reinfection with rubella varies with the gestation at which infection took place and the individual circumstances of the woman. The only available intervention is termination of pregnancy.
    - There is a low, but significant, risk to the fetus in maternal asymptomatic reinfection within the first 16 weeks of gestation. It may be that further fetal investigation by virus detection (to ascertain whether infection has occurred) is warranted. Such investigations are, however, invasive and risk adverse outcome.
- Parvovirus B19—40–50% of young pregnant mothers are susceptible, and the UK rates of infection are around 1 in 400 infections at present.
    - Fetal infection at <20 weeks' gestation is associated with a 9% excess fetal loss and 3% rate of hydrops fetalis (of which ~50% die).
    - Maternal parvovirus B19 infection diagnosed during pregnancy—the fetus should be scanned by USS 4 weeks after the onset of illness or date of seroconversion, and then at 1- to 2-weekly intervals until 30 weeks' gestation. If findings suggest the development of hydrops fetalis, the patient should be referred to a fetal medicine unit for consideration of fetal blood sampling and intrauterine transfusion (improves outcome). Termination is not recommended.

Patients presenting with a vesicular rash

~10% of young pregnant women are susceptible to VZV infection and are at risk of severe disease, particularly in the late second and early third trimester. The case fatality rate for women developing varicella in pregnancy is 1 in 1000. They must be advised to consult their GP at the first sign of chickenpox, and those with suspected chickenpox should avoid contact with others who might be at risk (other pregnant women and neonates).

- *Diagnosis*—if clinical diagnosis cannot be made with some certainty, confirm varicella infection by virus antigen or virus detection in the vesicle fluid and urgent serological testing for VZV IgM.
- *Management*—women presenting within 24h of onset of the first observable lesion should be offered 7 days' aciclovir or valaciclovir. Antivirals are not recommended in those presenting over 24h after rash onset (no evidence that they alter the clinical course in uncomplicated cases).
  - Uncomplicated cases can be managed at home with daily review, but those in whom fever persists and fresh vesicles are appearing 6 or more days after initial presentation should be referred to hospital. Also consider hospitalization in those patients who are approaching term, have a bad obstetric history, are smokers, have chronic lung disease, or have poor social circumstances, or if the GP is unable to monitor the patient closely.
  - Severe disease—pneumonitis, neurological symptoms other than headache, haemorrhagic rash/bleeding, severe extensive rash or numerous mucosal lesions, significant immunosuppression. Urgent hospital review is indicated. Those with severe disease should be referred to specialist isolation facilities under the joint care of an obstetrician, ID specialist, and paediatrician. Treatment is with IV aciclovir for at least 5 days.
- The fetus—consequences of primary maternal varicella in the first 20 weeks include spontaneous miscarriage in the first trimester and the risk of congenital varicella syndrome (~1% in the first 12 weeks, and 2% between weeks 13 and 20 of pregnancy). Features: dermatomal skin scarring, eye defects (chorioretinitis, cataract, micro-ophthalmia), limb hypoplasia, and neurological abnormalities (microcephaly, cortical atrophy, mental retardation, bladder and bowel dysfunction).
  - Infection before 20 weeks' gestation—perform a specialist ultrasound at 5 weeks post-infection (or 16–20 weeks' gestation), looking for polyhydramnios, microcephaly, hyperechogenic liver foci, and hydrops fetalis. A neonatal eye examination should be performed at birth.
  - Infection after 20 weeks' gestation—congenital varicella syndrome does not occur, but maternal infection up to 1 week from delivery may lead to herpes zoster in an otherwise healthy infant. Occasional reports of mild fetal damage up to 28 weeks' gestation.
  - Infection from 1 week before to 1 week after delivery—may lead to severe neonatal varicella. Such infants should be given prophylactic VZIG, with aciclovir if maternal disease onset was 4 days before to 2 days after delivery. For management of disease exposure in neonates, ➲ see p. 795.

References

3 Public Health England (2011). *Guidance on viral rash in pregnancy*. Available at: https://www.gov.uk/government/publications/viral-rash-in-pregnancy.

4 Public Health England (2013). *The Green Book: immunisation against infectious disease*. Available at: https://www.gov.uk/government/collections/immunisation-against-infectious-disease-the-green-book.

Prevention of congenital/perinatal infection

General points

- Any strategy aimed at preventing congenital/perinatal infection should start well before conception with education and general public health measures, e.g. vaccination against diseases, such as rubella which are associated with congenital/perinatal disease, and, in some countries, screening for GBS carriage.
- Infection history and rash contact advice—midwives should ask all pregnant women at booking whether they have previously had chickenpox or shingles, and, if they have not, advise that they make urgent contact if they develop a rash in pregnancy or have contact in pregnancy with someone with a rash.
- In the UK, all maternal booking bloods are screened as a matter of course for evidence of immunity to:
  - rubella—<2% of pregnant women are non-immune and should be vaccinated post-partum. Vaccination in pregnancy is not recommended;
  - syphilis—to prevent congenital syphilis in the neonate;
  - hepatitis B—identification of maternal infection allows a course of active and passive immunization to be undertaken in at-risk neonates after birth, in an attempt to prevent infection.
- Routine maternal HIV screening is recommended in the UK, so measures can be taken to prevent vertical transmission.
- Pregnancies complicated by congenital infection should be referred to regional fetomaternal medicine centres. Amniocentesis is the method of choice for fetal sampling in those cases of possible congenital infection in which such invasive investigations may be warranted. Maternal investigations for possible infective causes in cases of fetal hydrops, fetal brain lesions, unexplained severe growth restriction, or *in utero* demise are recommended.
- Certain interventions may prevent or reduce neonatal acquisition, or treat infections in neonates exposed *in utero*. These are detailed in further sections below.
- Infants in whom congenital infection is suspected and those born preterm, where infection may have played a role, need follow-up with a paediatric neurologist.

Preventing neonatal varicella

- Give VZIG to:
  - those whose mothers develop varicella from 7 days before to 7 days after delivery, as they will not be protected by maternal antibody;
  - those who are VZV antibody-negative (i.e. born to susceptible uninfected mothers) and are exposed to varicella or herpes zoster in the first 7 days of life;
  - those born before 28 weeks' gestation or weighing <1kg exposed to varicella or herpes zoster, as transfer of maternal IgG antibodies may be inadequate. Some infants beyond 28 weeks' gestation at birth may become VZV antibody-negative if they are >60 days old or have had repeated blood samples, despite a maternal history of varicella or zoster—serological testing is recommended.
- IV aciclovir should be:
  - given urgently to those infants developing varicella despite VZIG;
  - considered as prophylactic treatment in those infants whose mothers develop varicella from 4 days before to 2 days after delivery (high risk of fatal outcome despite VZIG prophylaxis).
- Mothers with varicella can breastfeed, but, if they have lesions close to the nipple, they should express milk from the affected breast until the lesions have crusted. This milk can be fed to the baby if they are covered by VZIG and/or aciclovir.
- If other children in the family have varicella, and the mother has had varicella (or is VZV antibody-positive), there is no reason to prevent a new baby from going home. If the mother is susceptible, contact with siblings with varicella should be delayed, until the new baby has reached 7 days of age.

Preventing neonatal HIV

Neonatal HIV transmission is a significant problem, particularly in resource-poor countries with a high prevalence of maternal HIV. Maternal transmission can occur *in utero* by passage of the virus across the placenta, during delivery from blood and placental fluids, and through breast milk. Transmission can be reduced by delivering through Caesarean section, avoidance of breastfeeding (advice that may be impractical in certain developing countries), and maternal ART. Untreated, most maternally infected children die by 10 years of age. For more details, ➔ see HIV prevention, pp. 840–2.

Preventing neonatal hepatitis B

In contrast to adult infection, most (90%) neonates infected with hepatitis B perinatally go on to become chronic carriers. All infants born to HBsAg-positive mothers should receive IM hepatitis B immune globulin within 12h of birth, along with their first dose of hepatitis B vaccine (into the *other* thigh). This strategy is effective in 90% of cases; a Cochrane review reported the relative risk of developing hepatitis B infection as 0.08, compared to no intervention.[5] The second and third vaccine doses are given at 1 and 6 months, respectively, with testing to confirm immunity at 1 year.

Prevention and treatment of other neonatal infections

Preventing other infections requires a combination of good maternal health (aiming to reduce the chance of uterine or intrapartum transmission) and a low threshold for investigating and treating at-risk neonates when infection develops if severe disease is to be avoided. Specific interventions are indicated in certain cases of GBS infection (➔ see Group B *Streptococcus*, pp. 252–3), neonatal HSV infection (➔ see Herpes simplex, pp. 396–9), toxoplasmosis (➔ see *Toxoplasma gondii*, pp. 517–20), and neonatal CMV infection (➔ see Cytomegalovirus, pp. 405–8).

Reference

5 Lee C, Gong Y, Brok J, Boxall EH, Gluud C (2006). Hepatitis B immunisation for newborn infants of hepatitis B surface antigen-positive mothers. *Cochrane Database Syst Rev.* 2:CD004790.

Chorioamnionitis

Inflammation of the chorion and amnion, the membranes surrounding the fetus. The early recognition of maternal chorioamnionitis is important, as it is associated with early-onset bacterial infections of the neonate, with consequent neonatal morbidity and mortality.

Aetiology

Usually chorioamnionitis is associated with a bacterial infection. Organisms residing in the vagina and cervix ascend into the uterus, initiating infection of the fetal membranes and amniotic fluid. Ascending infection may be facilitated by poor urogenital hygiene and certain sexual practices. Villitis is seen in around 6% of placentas after delivery (not necessarily due to infection). Conservative estimates place the incidence of infective chorioamnionitis at around 1% of all deliveries. Chorioamnionitis (which may be clinically silent) greatly increases the risk of preterm labour. The risk of developing chorioamnionitis is highest following PROM or prolonged labour. Maternal mortality is rare. More significant is the impact on the neonate. The risk of neonatal infection increases with the time from membrane rupture.

Although bacterial vaginosis is an important cause of premature labour, overt neonatal infection is uncommon.

Clinical features

Fever (>37.8°C), maternal tachycardia, less commonly fetal tachycardia (>160 beats/min), purulent amniotic fluid or vaginal discharge, uterine tenderness, raised maternal WCC. The presence of at least two of these features is associated with an increased risk of neonatal sepsis. Remember that mothers with genuine chorioamnionitis may be asymptomatic. Epidural anaesthesia during labour may be associated with a low-grade fever that can prompt suspicion of maternal chorioamnionitis. The reasons for this are not clear.

Diagnosis

Usually made clinically in the intrapartum period. Antenatal screening examinations may have detected GBS carriage, itself associated with an increased risk of chorioamnionitis. Asymptomatic mothers presenting with premature labour or PROM should have silent chorioamnionitis excluded (e.g. amniotic fluid examination).

- Amniotic fluid examination—amniotic fluid may be obtained by amniocentesis, if appropriate (risk of rupturing fetal membranes if intact). It can be examined for white cells, pH, glucose, cytokine levels, and microscopy and microbiological culture performed. Certain centres perform PCR to detect common causes of infection.
- Blood tests—WCC (may be raised in mothers who have been given steroids), CRP, BCs if febrile.
- Histology—diagnosis may be confirmed or refuted only on histological examination of the placenta, fetal membranes, and umbilical cord for evidence of inflammation and infection.
- Neonates born to mothers with suspected chorioamnionitis should be assessed for evidence of sepsis.

Management

- Mothers presenting with PROM and no obvious infection—a balance needs to be struck between avoiding the complications of prematurity and those of chorioamnionitis. Subclinical infection may be a precipitant of PROM. Mothers are usually given steroids to promote fetal maturation prior to delivery. In the absence of clinical infection, there is no evidence that prophylactic antibiotics improves outcome, but they are normally given, along with steroids. The mother and fetus must be assessed regularly for signs of distress or the onset of chorioamnionitis.
- Mother presenting with acute chorioamnionitis—delivery must be expedited. If signs of fetal distress develop, emergency delivery may be necessary. Antibiotics should *not* be withheld with the intention of obtaining neonatal cultures.
- Mothers in preterm labour or with PROM at <36 weeks' gestation should receive prophylactic antibiotics, as should mothers in labour at term with risk factors for fetal GBS infection (➲ see Group B *Streptococcus*, pp. 252–3).
- The standard drug treatment of the mother with chorioamnionitis includes clindamycin and an aminoglycoside. Ampicillin or penicillin may have already been given to some mothers as prophylaxis against GBS infection of the neonate. Ampicillin covers GBS, *Haemophilus* spp., most enterococci strains, and *Listeria* spp.
- The infant should be assessed and treated for any evidence of infection.

Puerperal sepsis

Any infection following delivery is classified as post-partum or puerperal infection. Puerperal pyrexia is defined as a maternal temperature of >38°C on >1 occasion on the first 14 days after delivery; 90% of infections are genital or urinary in origin.

Aetiology

- Sources of infection include endometritis (commonest), wound infections, perineal cellulitis (usually seen around day 2 after delivery), mastitis, pneumonia (a complication of anaesthesia), retained products of conception, UTIs, and septic pelvic phlebitis (pregnant women are at increased risk of thrombosis).

- Risk factors include: Caesarean delivery, PROM, frequent cervical examination, internal fetal monitoring, pre-existing pelvic infection, diabetes, and obesity.
- The uterine cavity is normally sterile until rupture of the amniotic sac, and the organisms isolated in endometritis are those normally present in the bowel, vagina, perineum, and cervix. Uterine infections are most likely following prolonged rupture of the membranes and after instrumental delivery. Genital tract infections may be polymicrobial and include *E. coli*, GAS, GBS, *Bacteroides*, and *Clostridium* spp.

Clinical features

- The source of infection may be indicated by the history. Was the delivery vaginal (with or without instruments?) or Caesarean? Did PROM occur? Was there intrapartum fever?
- Patients may be febrile and shocked, and may have symptoms and signs indicative of the causative infection. Look for signs of UTI, DVT, wound infection, respiratory symptoms (pneumonia or septic PE), abdominal pain and tenderness on bimanual examination with foul-smelling vaginal discharge (suggestive of endometritis—although GAS infections are associated with odourless lochia), and evidence of mastitis.

Diagnosis and management

- *Investigations*—FBC, U&E, BCs, urine cultures; swab and culture any wounds or discharges; swab for *Chlamydia* from the cervix and lochia. Pelvic USS may help detect pelvic abscesses or infected haematomas. Contrast abdominal CT may be required if non-pregnancy-related abdominal sources of infection are suspected.
- *Management*—fluid resuscitation and respiratory support, if required. Antibiotic therapy should be guided by the likely source of infection. Avoid tetracyclines if breastfeeding. Mild cases of endometritis may be managed by broad-spectrum PO antibiotics (e.g. co-amoxiclav); moderate to severe cases require IV therapy. Mastitis should respond to PO flucloxacillin—mothers should continue to express milk to prevent blockage and breast engorgement. Check for abscess development. Treat UTI/pyelonephritis, as indicated. Septic pelvic thrombosis requires anticoagulation and broad-spectrum antibiotics. Infected wounds may need surgical debridement or drainage, in combination with antibiotic therapy.
- If the patient fails to respond, check the culture results and appropriateness of antibiotic therapy; exclude pelvic/abdominal collections and abscesses (wound, breast). If sensitivities are not available, consider adding gentamicin and changing to a third-generation cephalosporin. Early surgical referral is essential if there is evidence of spreading skin infection despite antibiotic therapy—consider synergistic gangrene. Urgent surgical debridement may be required.
- If GBS, *Chlamydia*, or *N. gonorrhoeae* are cultured, inform the paediatrician or family GP, so infection can be excluded in the child.

Neonatal sepsis

This is defined as sepsis occurring within 4 weeks of birth:

- early onset—within 7 days, associated with microbes acquired from the mother, either transplacentally or intrapartum; 85% of early-onset cases present within 24h of delivery;
- late onset—after 7 days, associated with organisms acquired from the environment (e.g. caregivers, or urinary or vascular devices);
- premature infants experience the most rapid onset;
- certain viral infections may cause an indistinguishable clinical picture.

Epidemiology

- Incidence of culture-proven sepsis is 2/1000 live births in the USA, but up to 7–13% of neonates may be evaluated for sepsis due to the non-specific nature of the early signs.
- Neonatal sepsis contributes up to 15% of all neonatal deaths from meningitis and 4% of all neonatal deaths.
- Risk factors:
    - early-onset sepsis—maternal colonization with GBS, PROM, prolonged rupture of membranes, prematurity, maternal UTI, chorioamnionitis, maternal fever >38°C at delivery, poor maternal nutrition, recurrent abortion, meconium staining, congenital abnormalities;
    - late-onset sepsis—prematurity, central venous catheterization (duration >10 days), continuous positive-pressure nasal cannula, H_2 antagonist/PPI use, GI tract pathology.

Aetiology

- Early onset—GBS, *E. coli, H. influenzae, L. monocytogenes*.
- Late onset—CoNS, *S. aureus, Klebsiella* spp., *E. coli, Pseudomonas* spp., *Candida* spp., *Enterobacter* spp., *Serratia* spp., *Acinetobacter* spp., GBS, anaerobes.

Clinical features

- Pneumonia—neonates may aspirate organisms during delivery or have developed intrauterine pneumonia following aspiration of amniotic fluid. Signs: tachypnoea, cyanosis, grunting, apnoea, costal/sternal retractions, nasal flaring. CXR may show bilateral consolidation and pleural effusions. *Klebsiella* spp. and *S. aureus* may generate severe lung damage with abscesses and empyema. Early-onset GBS pneumonia may be fulminant, with significant mortality.
- Cardiac features—overwhelming sepsis may be associated with pulmonary hypertension, decreased cardiac output, and hypoxia. Late features: overt shock, pallor, poor capillary perfusion, oedema.
- Metabolic features of sepsis—hypo-/hyperglycaemia, acidosis, jaundice.
- Neurological signs—ventriculitis, meningitis (36% GBS, 31% *E. coli*, 5–10% *Listeria)*, cerebral vasculitis, cerebral oedema, cerebral infarction. Meningitis in early-onset sepsis occurs within 24–48h—signs of meningitis are present in only 30%, and CSF WCC may be normal. In late-onset disease, 80–90% have neurological features and CSF changes

may be markedly abnormal, especially with Gram-negative organisms. Neonates with meningitis are likely to be hypothermic.
- Haematological abnormalities—thrombocytopenia, DIC, high or low WCC (50% normal). The immature-to-total neutrophil ratio is a more useful marker of infection.
- GI—necrotizing enterocolitis has been associated with the presence of a number of species in the immature gut.

Investigations
- Blood tests—FBC, U&E, LFTs, CRP.
- Microbiological—blood, CSF, and urine cultures. Gram stain may provide early identification. Cultures may be negative if the mother received intrapartum antibiotics. If CSF is culture-positive, a follow-up LP is often performed at 24–36h after initiation of antibiotic therapy to document CSF sterility.
- Other tests—infection markers, such as IL-6, IL-8, and CD64, have been used in the evaluation of sepsis in neonates.
- Radiology—CXR may show lobar changes but more usually resembles respiratory distress syndrome, with a diffuse reticulogranular pattern. Cranial ultrasound may show evidence of ventriculitis and chronic changes. CT may be required in complex meningitis with obstruction and abscesses.

Management
- Medical emergency—IV antimicrobials should be commenced as soon as cultures are taken. Antibiotic choice should be guided by maternal history and local drug resistance patterns. A 2004 Cochrane review found no significant difference in outcome between various antibiotic regimes.[6] Generally, a glycopeptide is combined with an aminoglycoside. Treatment for 7–10 days may be appropriate, even in the absence of positive cultures.
- Cardiovascular, respiratory, and nutritional support may be required.
- Infants with bacterial meningitis require antibiotics capable of penetrating the blood–brain barrier to achieve therapeutic concentrations in the CSF, and longer courses of treatment (up to 3 weeks). If CSF is not sterile on a follow-up LP 24–36h after the initiation of therapy, consider modification of therapy.
- Surgical interventions—the development of hydrocephalus may require the placement of a VP shunt. Abscesses may require surgical drainage.
- With early diagnosis and treatment, prognosis is good, although residual neurological damage is seen in 15–30% of neonates with septic meningitis.
- Follow-up—hearing assessments before discharge and at 3 months if aminoglycosides have been given; follow-up for those at risk of developing neurological sequelae (with a paediatric neurologist).

Prevention
Some authorities recommend antibiotic prophylaxis should be given to certain groups of women at risk of carriage of GBS.

Reference

6 Mtitimila EI, Cooke RW (2004). Antibiotic regimes for suspected early neonatal sepsis. *Cochrane Database Syst Rev.* 4:CD004495.

Viral causes of childhood illness

(See Table 23.1.)

Table 23.1 Viral causes of childhood illness

Virus	Typical age	Features
HSV	Neonate: 90% of infections acquired perinatally, 5% congenitally, and the remainder post-natally (e.g. from an adult with herpes labialis)	Nearly all infected infants manifest disease. Incubation: 3–14 days. May be localized to the eye or CNS. 70% of untreated cases disseminate (hepatomegaly, jaundice, pneumonitis, encephalitis, vesicular rash). Neonates have the highest rates of visceral and/or CNS infection of any patient group
		70% of infected infants are born to mothers with no apparent disease. 70% of cases are due to HSV-2. 50% of babies delivered via an infected birth canal become infected. Most cases of HSV-1 follow maternal acquisition of genital HSV-1 late in pregnancy, with consequent neonatal contact with infectious secretions during delivery. Untreated, the death rate is 65%. Less than 20% of those with CNS infection develop normally. CNS morbidity is less severe with HSV-1 than HSV-2. For prevention, ➔ see Congenital infections, pp. 786–9. Systemic aciclovir is essential and has reduced the death rate of neonatal herpes to <25%
	Childhood (highest incidence of HSV-1 infection is seen in children aged 6 months to 3 years)	>80% of primary HSV infections are asymptomatic. Symptoms: fever, anorexia, sore mouth (ulcerative gingivostomatitis), local lymphadenopathy. Contamination of skin by infectious saliva may lead to secondary lesions on the perioral skin, eye, fingers, and vulva. Those with disseminated infection should be isolated. TOP aciclovir is of no benefit in acute primary infection of children. Systemic treatment can decrease healing time and is important in the immunocompromised

(*Continued*)

Table 23.1 (*Contd.*)

Virus	Typical age	Features
VZV	90% of cases occur in those under 13 years of age	Primary infection causes chickenpox, a maculopapular rash that forms pustulating vesicles. Complications: bacterial superinfection, cerebellar ataxia, and encephalitis. For the prevention and management of neonatal disease, ➔ see Preventing neonatal varicella, p. 795
Measles ('first disease')	Uncommon in those populations with vaccination	Acute, highly infectious disease characterized by cough, coryza, fever, and rash. Severe manifestations and complications include pneumonia, encephalitis, bacterial superinfection, and SSPE
Rubella ('third disease')	Prior to vaccination, incidence was highest in spring amongst children aged 5–9 years	Acute mild exanthematous viral infection of children and adults resembling mild measles, but with the potential to cause fetal infection and birth defects
Parvovirus B19 (slapped cheek disease, erythema infectiosum, 'fifth disease')	Infection common in childhood—50% are IgG-positive by 15 years	20% asymptomatic. Prodrome (5–7 days) of myalgia, arthralgia, malaise, rhinorrhoea, and fever, then a bright red rash on the cheeks, followed 1–2 days later by a maculopapular rash on the trunk, legs, arms, and buttocks. This clears after a few days, leaving a characteristic lacey pattern which fades/reappears over the following 3 weeks
HHV-6 (roseola, exanthem subitum, 'sixth disease')	Most children acquire infection between 4 months and 3 years of age	Abrupt onset of fever (± periorbital oedema) is followed 3–5 days later by a rash (rose-pink papules which are mildly elevated, non-pruritic, and blanch on pressure) on the back and neck and spreads to the chest and limbs, sparing the feet and face. Lasts ~2 days. Other features: malaise, vomiting, diarrhoea, cough, pharyngitis and lymphadenopathy, febrile convulsions (10% of primary infections). Meningitis and encephalitis are less commonly seen
Mumps	90% of cases occurred in those under 15 years prior to the introduction of vaccination. Many cases now occur in older children and those at university	Acute generalized viral infection of children and adolescents, causing swelling and tenderness of the salivary glands, and rarely epididymo-orchitis

Table 23.1 (*Contd.*)

Virus	Typical age	Features
Enteroviral infections	All age groups, but commoner in younger children	Accounts for the majority of childhood fever–rash syndromes, as well as meningitis, myocarditis, sepsis, hand, foot, and mouth disease, and herpangina
EBV (the cause of 90% of infectious mononucleosis)	~50% of UK children are infected by age 5 years, around 90% by age 25 years	Primary infection in childhood is asymptomatic. Infection in adolescence may present with an acute infectious mononucleosis syndrome
Other common viral infections of childhood	Adenovirus, molluscum, RSV, metapneumovirus, rhinovirus, rotavirus	

Enteroviral infections

The non-polio enteroviruses (including Coxsackie virus, enterovirus, echoviruses) cause a large number of different clinical syndromes, accounting for the majority of childhood fever–rash syndromes, as well as being important causes of meningitis, myocarditis, and even neonatal sepsis. Of the many clinical syndromes they cause, only hand, foot, and mouth (HFM) disease and herpangina have a clinical presentation distinct enough to allow identification.

Epidemiology

- Transmission is faeco-oral or via contact with discharging skin lesions. Respiratory and oral-to-oral routes occur in crowded conditions. Viruses can survive at room temperature for several days and tolerate the acidic pH of the GI tract.
- Found worldwide, affects all age groups, but highest infection rates are seen in children (secondary to exposure, hygiene, and immune status). Infection course is benign in older children, and more serious in neonates.
- Neonatal infections are probably acquired after birth.

Clinical features

- Incubation is 3–10 days, and the virus may be excreted in stool for weeks. Infection may be asymptomatic (90% of infections) or cause an undifferentiated flu-like illness or a more characteristic syndrome.
- Undifferentiated illness—low-grade fever of sudden onset, with or without upper respiratory and GI symptoms, e.g. flu-type syndrome of malaise, myalgias, sore throat, headache, conjunctivitis, nausea, vomiting, and diarrhoea. Orchitis and epididymitis can occur. Symptoms last 3–7 days.

- Herpangina (enteroviral vesicular pharyngitis)—typically seen during summer in children aged 3–10 years (may occur in young adults). Painful vesicles (usually 3–6) and ulcers of the posterior pharynx and tonsils with fever and a sore throat. There are no exudates present. Pain may make the child reluctant to eat. Symptoms last 3–7 days. Organism: Coxsackie virus group A and sometimes group B.
- HFM (enteroviral vesicular stomatitis with exanthema)—fever and vesicular eruption in the anterior pharynx, palms, and soles of toddlers/school-aged children. Oral vesicles not initially painful but later burst, leaving painful ulcers. Cutaneous vesicles heal by resorption of the fluid and do not crust. May develop characteristic rash. Organism: Coxsackie virus group A, serotype 16 (amongst others). Complications: HFM caused by enterovirus-71 has been associated with a higher incidence of neurological complications (polio-like syndrome, aseptic meningitis, encephalitis, encephalomyelitis, acute cerebellar ataxia, acute transverse myelitis, GBS, opsomyoclonus syndrome, and benign intracranial hypertension), rare cases of myocarditis, interstitial pneumonitis, and pulmonary oedema.
- Other—viral exanthems (pink, maculopapular, blanching rash, rarely urticarial, vesicular, or petechial—can mimic rubella and roseola, but with no significant adenopathy), aseptic meningitis, myocarditis/pericarditis, pleurodynia (lancinating chest pain attacks with fever and headache, also seen with Coxsackie B infection), and neonatal sepsis.

Diagnosis and management

- Diagnosis of herpangina and HFM is clinical (both are mild, self-limiting illnesses that do not warrant laboratory diagnosis), and management supportive (e.g. soft food for those with painful mouth ulcers, antipyretics, topical analgesics). See individual sections for the diagnosis and management of the more severe clinical presentations.
- The virus can be identified from respiratory secretions, cutaneous lesions, and stool. Paired serology will confirm recent infection. PCR tests are available.
- Hygiene—to prevent continued faeco-oral spread (handwashing, etc.).

Bacterial causes of childhood illness

Scarlet fever

A syndrome of exudative pharyngitis, fever, and scarlatiniform rash, caused by infection with an erythrogenic exotoxin-producing group A β-haemolytic *Streptococcus*. Once known as 'second disease'—the second exanthematous disease of childhood.

Clinical features

- Normal inhabitants of the nasopharynx, GAS may cause pharyngitis, skin infections, pneumonia, and bacteraemia. Scarlet fever usually occurs in association with pharyngeal infection.
- Usually seen in children aged 5–15 years.

- Rash appears 1–2 days after onset of sore throat, with a diffuse red blush with scattered points of deeper red. First noticed on the chest, it spreads to involve the trunk, neck, and extremities, sparing the palms, soles, and face. The face may, however, be flushed with circumoral pallor. Skinfolds in the neck, axillae, groin, elbows, and knees may appear as lines of deeper red. There may be petechiae and a sandpaper texture to the skin due to sweat gland occlusion. Examination of the oropharynx may reveal exudative pharyngitis, tonsillitis, and small red haemorrhagic spots on the palate. The tongue may be coated in early disease but then becomes beefy red ('strawberry tongue'). The skin rash fades over a week and is followed by desquamation which may last several weeks.
- Although common and fatal in the nineteenth and early twentieth century, it is rarely considered serious today. Severe scarlet fever may be due to haematogenous spread or systemic toxicity, with high fever which may be complicated by arthritis and jaundice.
- Complications—suppurative complications (e.g. abscess), rheumatic fever, post-streptococcal glomerulonephritis, erythema nodosum.

Diagnosis and management
- Throat swab for culture and ASOT.
- Treatment—phenoxymethylpenicillin PO or IV benzylpenicillin.
- Differential—consider measles, infectious mononucleosis, other viral infections with rash, Kawasaki's disease, staphylococcal infection.

Staphylococcal epidermal necrolysis

Also known as (staphylococcal) scalded skin syndrome (SSSS), this condition is caused by an exotoxin produced by *S. aureus* which leads to exfoliation of the upper layers of the epidermis; 98% of cases occur in children under 6 years of age, due to lack of immunity and immature renal clearance capability. Mortality is low in children (1–5%) but can be higher in adults who are usually immunocompromised or have renal failure.

Clinical features
- An infection commonly occurs at a site such as the oral or nasal cavities, throat, or umbilicus. Epidermolytic toxins are produced locally and act at a remote site, leading to the abrupt onset of generalized skin erythema.
- The epidermis beneath the granular cell layer separates due to binding of the toxins to desmoglein 1 in desmosomes. Bullae form, and diffuse sheet-like desquamation may occur 1–2 days later (Nikolsky sign positive). This leaves a raw and tender exposed surface.
- There may be associated conjunctivitis, stomatitis, and urethritis.
- Most patients do not appear very ill, but significant dehydration can develop. Healing occurs over 1–2 weeks.

Diagnosis and management
- *S. aureus* can usually be cultured from the site of remote infection; WCC is usually normal, but inflammatory markers may be elevated, a PCR test for the toxin is available. BCs are usually negative in children (but may be positive in adults).

- Differential diagnosis—toxic epidermal necrolysis (part of the disease spectrum that contains bullous erythema multiforme and Stevens–Johnson syndrome and associated with a deeper epidermal detachment than that of SSSS), erythema multiforme, burns.

Management

- Antibiotics—flucloxacillin, or erythromycin if penicillin-allergic.
- Fluids—patients can leak a lot of proteinaceous fluid through the skin and may require IV supplementation. Wound care is similar to that given for burns, and very severe cases may require specialist burns unit input. The skin damage can make patients vulnerable to secondary infection.

Pertussis

A highly contagious bacterial infection of the respiratory tract, spread by droplets and characterized by paroxysmal cough ('whooping cough'). Caused by *B. pertussis* (➔ see *Bordetella*, pp. 310–11), a Gram-negative pleomorphic bacillus of which humans are the sole reservoir, and less commonly *B. parapertussis*.

Epidemiology

- Infection is worldwide, but unusual in the UK and other countries with widespread vaccination. Neither infection nor vaccination provides complete or lifelong immunity. Protection against typical disease lasts 3–5 years, and immunity is not detectable after 12 years. The UK introduced a preschool pertussis booster in 2001 which has seen morbidity at the lowest levels yet in both vaccinated groups and infants too young to receive the vaccine.
- Most cases occur in infants/children (the majority infected by coughing adults and older children). Adults (10% of cases) experience milder disease. Children <1 year of age are most likely to require hospitalization.
- Worldwide, it remains a major cause of death. Around 50 million cases and 600 000 estimated deaths each year.
- Those at risk of severe disease (pneumonia, encephalopathy, death) include premature infants and those patients with underlying cardiac, pulmonary, and neuromuscular/neurological disease.

Clinical features

- Incubation—3–12 days. Patients are infectious from the onset of illness until towards the end of the paroxysmal phase.
- Pertussis is a 6-week illness of three stages, each lasting around 2–4 weeks. Older children and adults may not exhibit these distinct stages.
  - Stage 1 (catarrhal phase)—indistinguishable from the common cold: congestion, sneezing, mild fever, and rhinorrhoea. Patients are at their most infectious during this phase.
  - Stage 2 (paroxysmal phase)—paroxysms of intense coughing which can last several minutes may be followed by a loud whoop in older infants and toddlers. Infants <6 months may have apnoeic episodes but do not whoop. Vomiting is common after coughing. Subconjunctival haemorrhages and facial petechiae may occur. Most deaths occur in infants (coughing leading to choking and apnoea).

    - Stage 3 (convalescent phase)—chronic cough, which may last for weeks, triggered by intercurrent viral infections.
- Differential diagnosis—bronchiolitis, mycoplasmal pneumonia, chlamydial pneumonia, inhaled foreign body.
- Complications—pneumonia, secondary bacterial infection, pneumothorax, diaphragmatic rupture, surgical emphysema, neurological deficits secondary to hypoxia.

Diagnosis

- Laboratory confirmation is usually delayed. Diagnosis should be made clinically.
- General—leucocytosis (WCC >100 000 is associated with an increased risk of death); CXR may be normal or show peribronchial thickening, consolidation (secondary bacterial infection, rarely pertussis pneumonia), pneumothorax, pneumomediastinum, or air in the soft tissues.
- Microbiological culture—requires special media (e.g. Regan–Lowe or Bordet–Gengou agar). Culture specimens are best obtained by flexible swab or deep NPA during the catarrhal or early paroxysmal phase. Culture for 7 days. Usually negative in those previously immunized or given antibiotics.
- Serology is useful to confirm the diagnosis retrospectively. PCR-based tests are available.

Management

- General—supportive care is the mainstay. Consider admitting patients at risk of severe disease and complications plus those younger than 3 months or 3–6 months with severe paroxysms; 50% of infants require hospitalization. Infection control measures should be taken for those patients in the contagious phase of the disease.
- Antimicrobial therapy—erythromycin given early in the catarrhal phase shortens the duration of the paroxysmal stage. Once cough is established, antimicrobial agents do not alter the course of the illness but serve to limit the spread of disease. Treatment duration: 14 days. Patients should be isolated. Consider treating close contacts of pertussis cases (including children and staff at day centres) who are particularly vulnerable, unvaccinated, partially vaccinated, or under 5 years of age.
- Other agents—there is no evidence for any benefit from corticosteroids or β_2-adrenergic agents. Pertussis-specific immunoglobulin is an experimental therapy that may be effective in decreasing paroxysms of cough.

Prevention

- Vaccination is recommended for all babies at 2, 3, and 4 months, as part of the DTP vaccine. It may not prevent the illness entirely but lessens disease severity and duration.
- There is no transfer of protective maternal antibody, even from mothers with a documented history of infection or vaccination. Nearly all cases of fatal pertussis in developed countries occur in infants too

young to be immunized. In the UK and USA, children are given boosters at 3–4 or 11–12 years of age, respectively, with the aim of reducing transmission to pre-vaccination infants.

Other common causes of bacterial infection in childhood

- Bacterial meningitis, including *N. meningitidis* (➔ see Bacterial meningitis, pp. 718–22).
- Bacterial causes of pneumonia (➔ see Community-acquired pneumonia, pp. 611–5).
- Infectious diarrhoea (➔ see Infectious diarrhoea, pp. 647–9).
- UTIs (➔ see Urinary tract infections: introduction, pp. 678–9).
- URTIs (➔ see pp. 590–601).
- Superficial bacterial infections of the skin (e.g. erysipelas) (➔ see Skin and soft tissue infections: introduction, pp. 758–9).

Chapter 24

Immunodeficiency and HIV

Primary immunodeficiency 810
Antibody deficiency syndromes 810
Selective T-cell deficiency 811
Secondary immunodeficiency 812
Infections in asplenic patients 814
Neutropenic sepsis 815
Infections in transplant recipients 816
HIV epidemiology 819
HIV natural history 819
HIV classification 821
Initial evaluation of the HIV patient 824
HIV skin complications (1) 825
HIV skin complications (2) 827
HIV oral complications 828
HIV cardiovascular complications 829
HIV pulmonary complications 830
HIV gastrointestinal disease 833
HIV liver disease 835
HIV kidney disease 837
HIV neurological complications 838
HIV infection and malignancy 839
HIV prevention 840

Primary immunodeficiency

Most of these rare conditions are inherited as single-gene disorders and present in early infancy or childhood. They can be divided into three groups:

- antibody deficiency syndromes;
- selective T-cell deficiencies;
- mixed T- and B-cell defects.

Antibody deficiency syndromes

The lifetime prevalence of severe antibody deficiency syndromes is ~16 per million of the population in the West. Partial antibody deficiency occurs in about 1/700 Caucasians, most of whom are healthy.

X-linked agammaglobulinaemia

Presents with recurrent infections during the first 2 years of life. Affected children have very few B cells and low levels of circulating IgG. Prone to infections with the following pathogens: *H. influenzae, S. pneumoniae, Mycoplasma* spp., *Ureaplasma* spp., *C. jejuni, G. lamblia*, enteroviruses. Treatment is with IVIG. Prognosis is relatively good, with >90% survival at 30 years.

Common variable immunodeficiency

Peak incidence in early childhood and late adolescence. Serum Ig levels are variable, but IgA is virtually absent, IgG is <2g/L, and IgM is <0.2g/L (but may be normal or raised). There is often a family history of selective IgA deficiency and/or autoimmune disease. Associated with the MHC haplotype HLA A1, B8, C4A*QO, DR3 in 50% of patients. One-third of patients are severely lymphopenic, with CD4+ T-cell counts of $<0.4 \times 10^9$/L, low numbers of B cells, and a relative increase in CD8+ T cells; 70% of patients have features such as IBD, splenomegaly, lymphadenopathy, autoimmune diseases, and malignancies. Treatment is with IVIG. Prognosis is relatively good, with ~70% survival at 30 years.

Thymoma with hypogammaglobulinaemia

Thymoma occurs in patients >40 years and is associated with, or followed by, hypogammaglobulinaemia. Clinical features are similar to common variable immunodeficiency (CVID), but prognosis is poorer; patients usually die within 15 years of symptom onset.

Selective IgA deficiency

Complete absence of IgA occurs in ~1/700 Caucasians. Most people are healthy, and only ~5% suffer from recurrent respiratory tract infections. May be a mild variant of CVID and is also associated with the MHC haplotype HLA A1, B8, C4A*QO, DR3. There is a small increase of IgA deficiency in coeliac disease, Still's disease, rheumatoid arthritis, and epilepsy patients, but this may be drug-related, e.g. sulfasalazine, gold, penicillamine, or anti-epileptics.

IgG subclass deficiencies

IgG subclass deficiencies may be asymptomatic or associated with recurrent infections or a range of disorders.

- IgG1 subclass deficiency—usually results in hypogammaglobulinaemia (as IgG1 comprises two-thirds of total serum IgG). Often associated with other subclass deficiencies, e.g. IgG3. Symptomatic IgG1 subclass deficiency presents with pyogenic infections.
- IgG2 subclass deficiency—more prevalent in children than adults. Associated with increased risk of infections caused by encapsulated bacteria (e.g. *S. pneumoniae, H. influenzae, N. meningitidis*), autoimmune disorders (e.g. SLE, juvenile diabetes mellitus, defects in IFN-γ production, chronic mucocutaneous candidiasis), and secondary immune deficiency states (e.g. HIV, BMT).
- IgG3 subclass deficiency—commoner in adults than children. Often associated with IgG1 subclass deficiency and infections with *M. catarrhalis* and *S. pyogenes*. Other associations include asthma, chronic bronchitis, GI infections, and recurrent lymphocytic meningitis.
- IgG4 subclass deficiency—common and usually asymptomatic. May occur alone or in combination with IgG2 or IgA/IgG2 deficiencies. Has been associated with recurrent pulmonary infections, bronchiectasis, ataxia telangiectasia, chronic mucocutaneous candidiasis, growth hormone deficiency, allergic colitis, and Down's syndrome.

Selective IgM deficiency

- A rare immune disorder characterized by absence or deficiency of IgM and normal levels of other immunoglobulins.
- May be asymptomatic or present with recurrent bacterial and viral infections.
- Associated malignancies and haematological diseases include multiple myeloma and paraproteinaemias, clear cell sarcoma, Bloom's syndrome, lymphomatoid papulosis, ITP, and lymphocytic leukaemias.
- Associated rheumatological conditions include associated disorders, including SLE, Hashimoto's thyroiditis, ITP, autoimmune glomerulonephritis, and rheumatoid arthritis.
- Other associated conditions include Crohn's disease, GORD, interstitial lung disease, massive splenomegaly, inflammatory multifocal osteomyelitis, and inability to train in athletes.

Selective T-cell deficiency

These conditions are very rare. Infections associated with T-cell deficiency include HSV, VZV, CMV, adenovirus, papillomavirus, rotavirus, *Mycobacterium* spp, *C. neoformans, T. gondii, Candida* spp., *Aspergillus* spp., *P. jiroveci, Cryptosporidium* spp., and *Strongyloides* spp.

Thymic aplasia (di George syndrome)

Caused by fetal malformation of the third and fourth branchial arches during gestation. Most cases associated with chromosomal deletion at 22q11.2. The classic triad of features is cardiac abnormalities, hypoplastic thymus, and hypocalcaemia. Immunodeficiency can range from recurrent sinopulmonary infections to severe combined immunodeficiency (SCID). Severely affected infants usually die from associated cardiac abnormalities. Those that survive have a few circulating T cells (<10%) and remain healthy. Severely affected infants are prone to recurrent infections, especially life-threatening. An increased incidence of autoimmune and atopic disease is seen. CMV and VZV disease. Treatment is with a thymus graft.

Purine nucleoside phosphorylase deficiency

A rare autosomal recessive condition characterized by progressive immunodeficiency and neurological symptoms. Clinical presentation is with frequent bacterial, viral, and opportunistic infections, including sinopulmonary infections, disseminated VZV, progressive vaccinia, disseminated BCG, and PML. Neurological symptoms include developmental delay, spasticity, ataxia, and pyramidal signs. BMT is curative. Gene therapy is under investigation.

Severe combined immunodeficiency

This is due to rare mutations in genes that influence the maturation of B and T lymphocytes, e.g. adenosine deaminase deficiency, X-linked SCID, lymphocyte MHC class II deficiency, reticular dysgenesis, and multiple interleukin deficiency. Infections are usually much more severe than those seen in primary hypogammaglobulinaemia and selective T-cell deficiency, probably because macrophage function is affected. Infants present with failure to thrive, chronic diarrhoea, mucocutaneous candidiasis, and recurrent severe infections, e.g. adenovirus, CMV, EBV, rotavirus, norovirus, RSV, VZV, HSV, measles, influenza, parainfluenza, and *P. jiroveci*. Immunization with live vaccines, e.g. polio or BCG, may cause fatal infection. Patients may also suffer from GVHD. Most patients die within 2 years, unless they undergo BMT.

Secondary immunodeficiency

Secondary immunodeficiency is defined as a defect in the components or function of the immune system, occurring as a result of another disease or condition. It may affect humoral immunity, CMI, or both. HIV infection, drugs, and lymphoreticular malignancies are the most important causes (see Table 24.1).

Table 24.1 Causes of secondary immunodeficiency

Cause	Examples	Humoral immunity	CMI
Viruses	HIV	✓	✓
	Rubella	✓	
Drugs	Corticosteroids		✓
	Cyclophosphamide		✓
	Azathioprine		✓
	Ciclosporin		✓
	Mycophenolate		✓
	Anti-T-cell antibodies		✓
	Gold	✓	
	Penicillamine	✓	
	Sulfasalazine	✓	
	Phenytoin	✓	
	Methotrexate	✓	
	Bleomycin		✓
	Vincristine	✓	✓
	Cisplatin		✓
Malignancy	Chronic lymphocytic leukaemia	✓	
	Myeloma	✓	
Metabolic	Renal failure	✓	✓
	Liver failure	✓	✓
	Trauma	✓	✓
	Vitamin A deficiency		✓
	Vitamin B_{12} deficiency	✓	
	Zinc deficiency		✓
Ig loss	Nephrotic syndrome	✓	
	Protein-losing enteropathy	✓	
	Dystrophia myotonica	✓	

Infections in asplenic patients

The spleen is the largest lymphoid organ in the body and performs a wide range of immunological functions that protect it from severe infections. The relationship between an absent or hypofunctioning spleen and severe infection has long been recognized and is termed post-splenectomy sepsis (PSS) or overwhelming post-splenectomy infection (OPSI). Asplenia may be congenital but is usually acquired, e.g. traumatic or therapeutic. Other causes of hyposplenism include sickle-cell disease, haemoglobinopathies, collagen vascular disease, and allogeneic BMT.

Clinical features

- Patients are at risk of overwhelming sepsis caused by encapsulated organisms, e.g. *S. pneumoniae, H. influenzae, N. meningitidis*. Other organisms include *C. canimorsis, B. holmesii, Salmonella* spp., *P. falciparum, Babesia* spp., *Erlichia* spp., *B. bacilliformis*, and CMV.
- The highest risk of PSS is in the first few years after splenectomy, but it may occur up to 20 years post-splenectomy.
- PSS has a short prodrome with fever, chills, pharyngitis, muscle aches, vomiting, and diarrhoea. In adults, there is usually no obvious site of infection, whereas, in children, meningitis is common.
- Deterioration is usually rapid and occurs over hours with septic shock, DIC, seizures, and coma.

Diagnosis

- The diagnosis is clinical, and all asplenic patients with fever should be considered to have, and managed as, PSS.
- The presence of Howell–Jolly bodies (nuclear remnants) on the blood film confirms hyposplenism, but they may not always be present.[1]

Management

- Asplenic patients should be given a supply of prophylactic antibiotics for self-administration at the first sign of serious illness.
- If the patient presents acutely with PSS, they should receive immediate treatment with IV antibiotics, e.g. ceftriaxone plus vancomycin.[1]

Prevention

- Prophylactic antibiotics—lifelong PO penicillin V should be given to patients with an absent or dysfunctional spleen.
- Immunization against *S. pneumoniae, N. meningitidis, H. influenzae*, and influenza virus is recommended for all apslenic patients.[1]

Reference

1 Davies JM, Lewis MP, Wimperis J, *et al.*; British Committee for Standards in Haematology (2011). Review of guidelines for the prevention and treatment of infection in patients with an absent or dysfunctional spleen: prepared on behalf of the British Committee for Standards in Haematology by a working party of the Haemato-Oncology Task Force. *Br J Haematol*. **155**:308–17.

Neutropenic sepsis

Neutropenia is associated with an increased risk of bacteraemia and severe infection. Although neutropenia is defined as an absolute neutrophil count of $<0.5 \times 10^9$ cells/L, many experts believe that the risk of infection increases when the neutrophil count falls below 1×10^9 cells/L. In very immunocompromised patients, signs of infection may be absent, and the first and only sign of infection may be fever (>38°C). Febrile neutropenia is considered a medical emergency, and appropriate antimicrobial therapy should be started immediately, as the mortality of neutropenic patients with untreated Gram-negative sepsis approaches 40%.

Classification

Febrile neutropenia can be divided into four categories:
- microbiological documented infections (MDIs) with bacteraemia;
- MDIs with isolation of a significant pathogen from a well-defined site of infection, e.g. urine, respiratory, abscess;
- clinically documented infection without microbiological proof;
- unexplained fever without clinical or microbiological proof.

Aetiology

- Bacteraemia is documented in only 10–15% of neutropenic fever episodes.
- Although Gram-negative infections were commonest a few decades ago, Gram-positive pathogens now predominate.
- This is likely related to the use of long-term CVCs and antimicrobial prophylaxis against Gram-negatives.

Patient evaluation

The following factors should be considered:
- Underlying disease and any recent chemotherapy.
- Previous history of infections and risk of drug-resistant organisms.
- Co-morbidities.
- Non-infectious causes of fever, e.g. blood transfusion, disease progression.
- Symptoms—fever, organ-specific symptoms.
- Examination—skin and mucous membranes, IVC sites, lungs, abdomen, perianal region.
- Investigations—FBC, biochemistry, urinalysis, BCs (central and peripheral), other cultures (e.g. urine, stool, swabs, sputum, CSF, as clinically indicated), serum fungal markers (in high-risk patients).
- Imaging—CXR in low-risk patients and CT chest in high-risk patients.
- Risk stratification—high-risk patients are defined as those who are expected to be neutropenic for >7 days.

Management

- Febrile neutropenia is a medical emergency—broad-spectrum empiric antibiotic therapy should be commenced as soon as possible, ideally within 60min of presentation.

- Initial therapy—this should be guided by local antibiotic policies and take into account the patient's clinical presentation, recent antibiotic use and culture data, and antibiotic allergies. The IDSA guidelines recommend initiation of monotherapy with an antipseudomonal β-lactam agent, e.g. piperacillin-tazobactam or meropenem.[2] Vancomycin is not recommended as part of the initial regimen, unless there is suspected catheter-related infection, skin and soft tissue infection, pneumonia, or haemodynamic instability.
- Combination therapy—numerous combination regimens have been studied as initial empiric therapy, but none has been shown to be clearly superior to monotherapy or other combination regimens.
- Penicillin-allergic patients—for patients with immediate hypersensitivity, alternative regimens include vancomycin plus aztreonam or ciprofloxacin and clindamycin.
- Antifungal agents—empiric antifungal therapy should be added after 4–7 days in high-risk patients who have persistent fever. The IDSA guidelines recommend liposomal amphotericin, caspofungin, voriconazole, or itraconazole as suitable options.[2]
- Patients should be examined daily, and persistent/recurrent fever should prompt a search for occult infection.
- The duration of therapy is determined by the clinical syndrome and pathogen—in general, it is continued until the neutrophil count is $>0.5 \times 10^9$ cells/L.
- Colony-stimulating factors—these are generally not recommended for patients with febrile neutropenia, although there are some exceptions.

Outcomes

There has been a progressive decline in mortality rates since the introduction of empiric antibiotic therapy for neutropenic sepsis in the 1970s. Prior to this, mortality rates were >90%. In a US study of >40 000 patients with neutropenic sepsis, conducted between 1995 and 2000, the in-hospital mortality rate was 9.5%. Higher rates were seen in patients with co-morbidities.

Prevention

The IDSA guidelines recommend consideration of fluoroquinolone prophylaxis in patients at high risk for profound, prolonged neutropenia ($<0.1 \times 10^9$ cells/L for >7 days).[2]

Reference

2 Freifeld AG, Bow EJ, Sepkowitz KA, *et al.*; Infectious Diseases Society of America (2011). Clinical practice guideline for the use of antimicrobial agents in neutropenic patients with cancer: 2010 update by the Infectious Diseases Society of America. *Clin Infect Dis*. **52**:e56–93.

Infections in transplant recipients

The advent of immunosuppression has resulted in a marked growth in organ transplantation over the last 30 years. Apart from medical and surgical issues related to function and rejection of transplanted organs, infections are the most important problem. Most infections occur during the first 6 months after transplantation. The following risk factors have been identified:

- pre-transplant factors (underlying medical conditions, lack of immunity, prior latent infections, colonization with nosocomial organisms, prior medications, environmental exposures);
- transplantation factors (type of organ, trauma of surgery);
- immunosuppression (medication, chemotherapy, irradiation);
- allograft reactions (GVHD).

Clinical features

- The clinical manifestations are variable and depend on a number of factors, including prior immune status of the host, reason for transplant, type of transplant, preconditioning treatment, time after transplantation, degree of immunosuppression, likelihood of exposure, and infecting pathogen.
- BMT-associated infections:
  - pre-engraftment (<3 weeks)—the main risks are mucocutaneous damage, neutropenia with loss of phagocytosis, and organ dysfunction. Bacterial infections with aerobic Gram-positive and Gram-negative bacteria account for most infections. Fungal infections include *Candida* (especially azole-resistant), *Aspergillus, Fusarium*, and *Zygomycetes*. Viral infections include HSV and respiratory viruses;
  - immediate post-engraftment (3 weeks to 3 months)—B- and T-cell function starts to recover. Bacterial pathogens of note during this period are *L. pneumophila* and *L. monocytogenes. P. jiroveci* is rare but occurs at a median of 9 weeks post-transplantation. Invasive aspergillosis typically occurs 100 days post-engraftment and are commoner in allogeneic than autologous transplants. Other fungal infections include resistant *Candida, Fusarium*, and *Zygomycetes*. Viral infections include adenovirus, CMV, EBV, HHV-6, HHV-7, HHV-8, enteric viruses, and respiratory viruses. Parasitic infections include toxoplasmosis, strongyloidiasis, and cryptosporidiosis. Mycobacterial infections are rare;
  - late post-engraftment (100 days to 1 year)—B- and T-cell function continues to recover but may take 18–36 months to fully recover. Most infections seen in allogeneic transplants. Bacteraemia is usually *S. pneumoniae, H. influenzae, N. meningitidis*, and staphylococci Gram-negative bacteria. Reactivation of VZV, EBV, HBV, and HCV are common. Other viral infections include parvovirus B19 (anaemia) and BK/JC virus (haemorrhagic cystitis and PML).
- Solid organ transplant-associated infections:
  - 1 month post-transplantation—there are two major causes of infection: donor-derived infections and infectious complications of surgery/hospitalization:
    - —donor-derived infections include a wide range of viruses (e.g. CMV, EBV, HHV-6, HSV, VZV), bacteria (e.g. bacteraemia at time of transplantation, meningococcus, syphilis, mycobacteria), fungi (e.g. *Candida, Aspergillus, C. neoformans*, endemic mycoses), and parasites (e.g. *S. stercoralis, T. gondii, T. cruzi*, malaria, babesiosis);
    - —infections related to surgery include wound infection, pneumonia, UTI, and line-related infections. The causative organisms are often those that have colonized the donor or the recipient and

may include drug-resistant nosocomial pathogens, e.g. MRSA, VRE, MDR Gram-negatives, *C. difficile;*
- 1–6 months post-transplantation—patients are most at risk of opportunistic infections (e.g. *P. jiroveci*, toxoplasmosis, leishmaniasis, *T. cruzi*), fungal infections (e.g. histoplasmosis, coccidioidomycosis, cryptococcosis, blastomycosis), viral infections (respiratory viruses, HBV, HCV, BK virus, HHV-6, HHV-7, HHV-8), mycobacterial infections, and GI parasites (*Cryptosporidium* and *Microsporidium*);
- after 6 months—patients will have the same risk of bacterial infections as a minimally immunosuppressed patient in the community. In contrast, patients with rejection are at increased risk of opportunistic infections such as those seen prior to 6 months.

Pre-transplantation screening

Pre-transplantation screening of the donor, recipient, and/or blood products is performed, in order to try and prevent or predict transplant-related infections.

- Recipient screening:
  - ongoing or active infection;
  - serological testing for HBV, HCV, HIV, HSV, VZV, EBV, CMV, *T. pallidum*, and *T. gondii*;
  - in endemic areas, consider *T. cruzi, Histoplasma*, and *Strongyloides*.
- Donor screening:
  - serological testing for HBV, HCV, HIV, *T. pallidum*, and *T. gondii*;
  - culture of cadaveric organs, perfusates, and transport medium;
  - if living donor, take clinical and epidemiological history, and consider tuberculin testing and fungal serology;
  - in endemic areas, consider screening for malaria and *T. cruzi*.
- Blood products:
  - screening for HBV, HCV, HIV, and *T. pallidum*;
  - leucodepleted blood reduces the risk of CMV.

Post-transplantation surveillance

Post-transplantation surveillance is performed, in order to guide pre-emptive therapy and monitor response to treatment:

- CMV disease by PCR;
- *Candida* or *Aspergillus* infection by antigen tests;
- surveillance cultures for MDR pathogens.

Prevention of infection

- Routine immunizations for people with chronic diseases, e.g. pneumococcal and influenza immunization should be given prior to transplantation.
- Prophylatic antimicrobials are commonly given in the first few months following transplantation, e.g. co-trimoxazole, antivirals (aciclovir, valaciclovir, ganciclovir, or valganciclovir), and antifungals (nystatin, fluconazole, or itraconazole). Protocols differ between different transplant centres.

HIV epidemiology

There are an estimated 36.7 million people living with HIV/AIDS, with 2.1 million new infections and 1.1 million deaths in 2015. The majority of new infections occur in young adults (aged 15–24 years) in developing countries. Sub-Saharan Africa bears the brunt of the epidemic. Although the introduction of antiretroviral drug therapy has dramatically reduced morbidity and mortality in North America and Western Europe, there is still a treatment gap in developing countries.

HIV transmission

HIV may be transmitted via a number of routes:
- sexual transmission;
- perinatal transmission—intrapartum, peripartum, breastfeeding;
- blood transfusion;
- IDU/sharing needles;
- occupational transmission—needlestick injury or mucocutaneous exposure.

The risk of transmission differs with the route of infection (see Table 24.2).

Table 24.2 HIV transmission rates

Exposure	Risk per 10 000 exposures
Blood transfusion	9000
IDU	67
Receptive anal intercourse	50
Needlestick injury	30
Receptive vaginal intercourse	10
Insertive anal intercourse	6–7
Insertive vaginal intercourse	5

HIV natural history

The natural history of HIV infection is divided into the following stages (see Fig. 24.1):
- *primary infection*—diagnosis is based on a plasma HIV RNA level >10 000 copies/mL plus indeterminate or negative serology or recent seroconversion;
- *acute retroviral syndrome* (2–3 weeks)—clinical features include fever (96%), adenopathy (74%), pharyngitis (70%), rash (70%), myalgia (54%), diarrhoea (32%), headache (32%), nausea and vomiting (27%), hepatosplenomegaly (14%), weight loss (13%), thrush (12%), and neurological symptoms (12%). This is accompanied by rapid decline in CD4+ T-lymphocyte count and high concentrations of HIV RNA in the plasma;

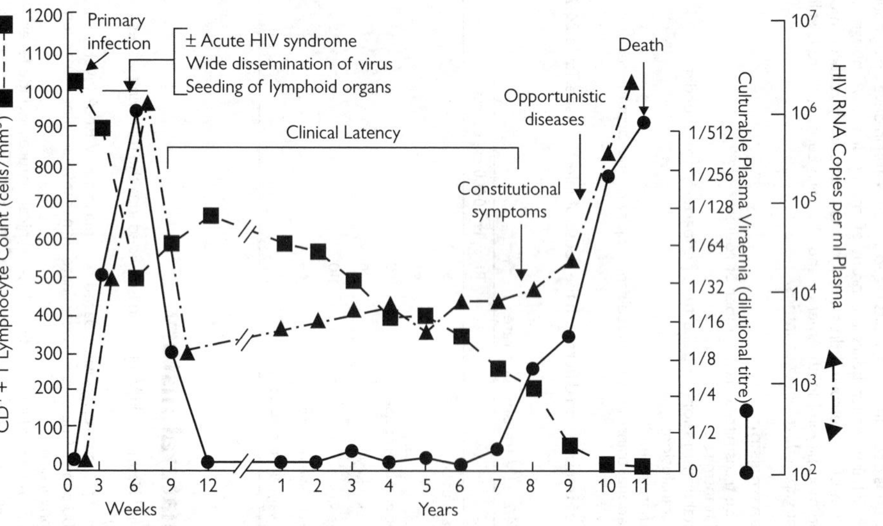

Fig. 24.1 Typical course of HIV infection.
Reproduced from Fauci AS, Patales G, Stanley S, Weuoman D. Immunopathogenic mechanisms of HIV infection. *Ann Intern Med* 1996;124(7):654–63.

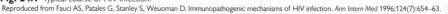

Table 24.3 CD4 count and HIV complications

CD4 count	Complications
>500/mm³	Acute retroviral syndrome, *Candida* vaginitis, persistent generalized lymphadenopathy (PGL), GBS, myopathy, aseptic meningitis
200–500/ mm³	Pneumococcal and other bacterial pneumonia, pulmonary TB, herpes zoster, oropharyngeal candidiasis, cryptosporidiosis, Kaposi's sarcoma, oral hairy leucoplakia, cervical intraepithelial neoplasia, cervical cancer, B-cell lymphoma, anaemia, mononeuritis multiplex, ITP, Hodgkin's lymphoma, lymphocytic interstitial pneumonitis (LIP)
<200/mm³	PCP, disseminated histoplasmosis, disseminated coccidioidomycosis, miliary/extrapulmonary TB, PML, wasting syndrome, peripheral neuropathy, HIV-associated dementia, cardiomyopathy, vacuolar myopathy, progressive radiculopathy, non-Hodgkin's lymphoma (NHL)
<100/mm³	Disseminated herpes simplex, toxoplasmosis, cryptococcosis, chronic cryptosporidiosis, microsporidiosis, oesophageal candidiasis
<50/mm³	Disseminated CMV, disseminated MAC, primary central nervous system lymphoma (PCNSL)

- *recovery and seroconversion* (2–4 weeks)—characterized by recovery of CD4 cell count and reduction in plasma HIV viral load to a set point;
- *asymptomatic chronic HIV infection* (average 8 years)—associated with gradual decline in CD4 cell count;
- *symptomatic HIV infection/AIDS* (average 1–3 years)—occurs when the CD4 count declines to <200/mm³ and the viral load begins to rise;
- death usually occurs 10–11 years after infection in untreated individuals.

Complications of HIV infection

As the CD4 count declines, the complications, shown in Table 24.3, may occur.

HIV classification

Centers for Disease Control and Prevention 1993 revised classification

This categorizes patients according to clinical categories A–C and CD4 count categories 1–3. Patients in categories A3, B3, and C1 to C3 are defined as having AIDS (see Table 24.4).[3]

- *Category B symptomatic conditions* include—bacillary angiomatosis, oropharyngeal candidiasis, persistent vulvovaginal candidiasis, PID, cervical dysplasia/carcinoma *in situ*, oral hairy leukoplakia, multidermatomal herpes zoster, ITP, constitutional symptoms >1 month, peripheral neuropathy.

- *Category C AIDS indicator conditions* include—recurrent bacterial pneumonia, candidiasis of the oesophagus, bronchi, trachea, or lungs, cervical carcinoma, coccidioidomycosis, extrapulmonary cryptococcosis, chronic intestinal cryptosporidiosis, CMV, HIV encephalopathy, chronic HSV, extrapulmonary histoplasmosis, chronic isosporiasis, Kaposi's sarcoma, Burkitt, immunoblastic, or primary CNS lymphoma, extrapulmonary MAC, extrapulmonary *M. kansasii*, MTB, *P. jiroveci*, PML, recurrent non-typhoidal *Salmonella* bacteraemia, CNS toxoplasmosis, and HIV wasting syndrome.

World Health Organization classification

This categorizes patients into four clinical stages with no CD4 count criteria. Patients with clinical stage 4 are defined as having AIDS (see Table 24.5).[4]

Table 24.4 CDC 1993 revised classification of HIV

	A (asymptomatic, acute HIV, PGL)	B (symptomatic)	C (AIDS indicator conditions)
CD4 ≥500/mm^3	A1	B1	C1
CD4 200–499/mm^3	A2	B2	C2
CD4 <200/mm^3	A3	B3	C3

Table 24.5 WHO classification of HIV

Stage	Symptoms
1	Asymptomatic
	PGL
2	Moderate unexplained weight loss, <10% of body weight
	Recurrent respiratory infections
	Herpes zoster
	Angular chelitis, recurrent oral ulceration
	Papular pruritic eruptions, seborrhoeic dermatitis, fungal nail infections
3	Unexplained severe weight loss, >10% of body weight
	Unexplained chronic diarrhoea, >1 month
	Unexplained persistent fever, >1 month
	Persistent oral candidiasis
	Oral hairy leukoplakia
	Pulmonary TB
	Severe presumed bacterial infections
	Acute necrotizing ulcerative stomatitis
	Unexplained anaemia (Hb <8g/dL)
	Neutropenia (neutrophils <500 cells/microlitre)
	Chronic thrombocytopenia (platelets <50 000 cells/microlitre)

(*Continued*)

Table 24.5 (*Contd.*)

Stage	Symptoms
4	HIV wasting syndrome, as defined by CDC[a]
	PCP
	Recurrent severe bacterial pneumonia
	Chronic HSV infection >1 month or visceral
	Candidiasis of the oesophagus, trachea, bronchi, or lungs
	Extrapulmonary TB
	Kaposi's sarcoma
	CMV retinitis or infection of other organs
	CNS toxoplasmosis
	HIV encephalopathy[b]
	Extrapulmonary cryptococcosis
	Disseminated NTM infection
	PML
	Chronic cryptosporidiosis
	Chronic isosporiasis
	Disseminated mycosis
	Recurrent non-typhoidal *Salmonella* bacteraemia
	Lymphoma, cerebral or B-cell non-Hodgkin's
	Cervical carcinoma
	Atypical disseminated leishmaniasis
	Symptomatic HIV-associated nephropathy
	Symptomatic HIV-associated cardiomyopathy
	Reactivation of American trypanosomiasis

[a]HIV wasting syndrome: weight loss of >10% of body weight, plus either unexplained chronic diarrhoea (>1 month) or chronic weakness and unexplained prolonged fever (>1 month).

[b]HIV encephalopathy: clinical finding of disabling cognitive and/or motor dysfunction interfering with activities of daily living, progressing over weeks to months, in the absence of a concurrent illness or condition other than HIV infection that could explain the findings.

References

3 Centers for Disease Control and Prevention (1992). 1993 revised classification system for HIV infection and expanded surveillance case definition for AIDS among adolescents and adults. *MMWR Recomm Rep*. **41**(RR-17):1–19.

4 World Health Organization (2007). *WHO case definitions of HIV for surveillance and revised clinical staging and immunological classification of HIV-related disease in adults and children*. Available at: http://www.who.int/hiv/pub/guidelines/HIVstaging150307.pdf.

Initial evaluation of the HIV patient

All newly diagnosed HIV patients should be carefully evaluated to determine the clinical stage of disease, coexistent infections, and laboratory abnormalities:

- FBC;
- biochemistry profile—renal and LFTs;
- fasting blood glucose and serum lipids;
- serology for HIV (if laboratory confirmation not available), hepatitis A, B, and C, CMV, syphilis, and *T. gondii*;
- urinalysis;
- cervical smear in women;
- testing for *C. trachomatis* and *N. gonorrhoeae* is optional but should be considered for those at high risk;
- TST (unless previous history of TB or positive test);
- CXR;
- *CD4+ T-cell count*—this is an indicator of immunocompetence and is a strong predictor of progression and survival. Once treatment starts, the CD4 count usually rises by 100–150 cells/mm^3 per year, with an accelerated response in the first 3 months. During treatment, it is monitored every 3–6 months, longer if established on ART and stable;
- *plasma HIV RNA*—numerous studies have shown an association between the decrease in plasma viraemia and improved survival. Baseline viral load may be a consideration in when to start treatment. It should be measured immediately before, and 2–8 weeks after, initiation of treatment. Its main role is in monitoring the response to therapy. HIV viral load should be checked every 3–4 months in patients on a stable antiretroviral regimen, or earlier if clinically indicated;
- *HIV drug resistance testing*—for patients with HIV RNA >100 000 copies/mL, genotypic drug resistance testing is recommended, regardless of whether the patient starts ART. If treatment is deferred, this should be repeated prior to commencing therapy. In antiretroviral-naïve patients, a genotypic assay is generally preferred. Drug resistance testing should also be performed in the setting of virological failure, to assist with choosing new drugs;
- *HLA-B*5701 screening*—the abacavir hypersensitivity reaction (ABC HSR) is a multiorgan clinical syndrome which occurs in 5–8% of patients within 6 weeks of starting abacavir therapy. Several studies have shown an association between the HLA allele HLA-B*5701 and ABC HSR. For this reason, all patients should be screened for this allele prior to commencing abacavir therapy, and those who are HLA-B*5701-positive should not be given the drug;
- *co-receptor tropism assays*—during acute/recent infection, most patients harbour a CCR5-tropic (R5) virus. In untreated patients, the virus shifts to using CXCR4 (R4-tropic) or both (dual/mixed-tropic). The CCR5 inhibitors (maraviroc and vicriviroc) prevent HIV entry into target cells by binding to CCR5. Co-receptor tropism assays should be performed prior to considering therapy with CCR5 receptor antagonists.

HIV skin complications (1)

Skin manifestations are common in HIV-infected patients and may be caused by bacteria, fungi, viruses, parasites, or drugs.

Bacillary angiomatosis

- Caused by *B. henselae* and *B. quintana* (➔ see *Bartonella* species, pp. 348–50).
- Lesions start as red or purple papules that expand into nodules or pedunculated masses. They appear vascular and may bleed with trauma.
- Skin biopsy shows vascular proliferation, inflammation, and typical organisms on Warthin–Starry silver stain. Serology (IFA or EIA) may be used to support the diagnosis.
- Treatment is with PO erythromycin or doxycycline for 3 months.

Cutaneous candidiasis

- Usually caused by *C. albicans*.
- Lesions are moist, red, and scaly, and may have satellite lesions. May also cause intertrigo, balanitis, glossitis, angular cheilitis, paronychia, and nail dystrophies.
- Diagnosis is usually clinical but may be confirmed by KOH preparation or wet mount.
- Treatment may be topical (e.g. ketoconazole, miconazole, clotrimazole, or nystatin) or systemic (e.g. ketoconazole or fluconazole).

Cryptococcosis

- Caused by *C. neoformans* (➔ see *Cryptococcus*, pp. 480–1) as part of disseminated disease.
- Lesions are nodular, papular, follicular, or ulcerated, and may resemble molluscum. Usually occurs on the face, neck, and scalp.
- Skin biopsy with Gomori methenamine silver stain shows typical budding yeasts and positive culture. Serum cryptococcal antigen is usually positive. LP should be performed in patients with positive cultures or cryptococcal antigen, to exclude cryptococcal meningitis.
- Treatment is with PO fluconazole 400mg/day for 8 weeks, followed by 200mg/day.

Dermatophyte infections

- Caused by a variety of fungi, e.g. *T. rubrum, T. mentagrophytes, T. tonsurans, Trychophyton soudanense, M. canis, E. floccosum*.
- May present with fungal nail infections (onychomycosis), athlete's foot (tinea pedis), or ringworm (tinea corporis, tinea cruris, tinea capitis).
- Diagnosis is confirmed by skin scrapings for KOH preparation and culture.
- Treatment is with PO terbinafine or itraconazole for nail infections, or topical agents (e.g. clotrimazole, ketoconazole, miconazole, terbinafine) for skin infections.

Drug eruptions

- Common causes include antibiotics (e.g. co-trimoxazole and β-lactams), anticonvulsants, and NNRTIs.
- Lesions occur within 2 weeks of a new drug and present as an itchy, morbilliform, exanthematous eruption ± fever. More severe forms include urticaria, toxic epidermal necrolysis, Stevens–Johnson syndrome, hypersensitivity reactions (especially abacavir and nevirapine), and anaphylaxis.
- Treatment of uncomplicated cases is with antihistamines and topical antipruritics and topical corticosteroids. For severe reactions, discontinue the drug, and administer supportive care.

Folliculitis

- Usually caused by *S. aureus*. Other causes include *Pityrosporum ovale* (intrafollicular yeast), *D. folliculorum* (intrafollicular mite), and eosinophilic folliculitis (unknown cause).
- Lesions are itchy, follicular papules and pustules on the face, trunk, and extremities. Occurs at CD4 count of 50–250 cells/mm^3. Often relapses and remits. May recur with immune reconstitution.
- Diagnosis is clinical and confirmed by skin biopsy.
- Treatment is of the underlying cause.

Herpes simplex

- Caused by HSV (➔ see Herpes simplex, pp. 396–9).
- Lesions begin as papules, which develop into vesicles and ulcerate and crust. They are usually found on the lip, in the mouth, or in the genital region. Recurrences are common.
- Diagnosis is usually clinical but may be confirmed by PCR, HSV antigen detection, viral culture, or Tzanck preparation.
- Treatment is with PO aciclovir, valaciclovir, or famciclovir for 7–10 days. Severe or disseminated disease may require IV aciclovir (➔ see Antivirals for herpes simplex virus and varicella-zoster virus, pp. 90–1).

Herpes zoster (shingles)

- Caused by reactivation of VZV (➔ see Varicella-zoster virus, pp. 399–402). This affects 5% of healthy adults but is 15–25 times commoner in HIV-infected adults.
- The rash is usually preceded by a painful prodrome in the region of a dermatome. This is followed by the development of a dermatomal vesicular rash.
- Diagnosis is usually clinical but may be confirmed by PCR, HSV antigen detection, viral culture, or Tzanck preparation.
- Treatment is with PO aciclovir, valaciclovir, or famciclovir for 7–10 days. Severe or disseminated disease may require IV aciclovir (➔ see Antivirals for herpes simplex virus and varicella-zoster virus, pp. 90–1).

HIV skin complications (2)

Kaposi's sarcoma

- Caused by HHV-8 (➔ see Human herpesvirus type 8, pp. 394–6). Can occur in the general population but is 20 000 times commoner in HIV-infected individuals.
- Lesions are purple to brown-black macules, papules, nodules, and patches, which occur on the legs, face, mouth, and genitalia. Complications include lymphoedema and visceral involvement.
- Diagnosis is clinical but may be confirmed by biopsy.
- Treatment—ART is associated with lesion regression, decreased incidence, and prolonged survival. Local therapies include intralesional vinblastine, radiation therapy, or topical alitret. Systemic therapy is used for advanced or rapidly progressive lesions, e.g. pegylated liposomal doxorubicin, liposomal daunorubicin, or paclitaxel (more toxic).

Molluscum contagiosum

- Caused by molluscum contagiosum virus.
- Spread by direct contact.
- Pearly, dome-shaped lesions with a central dimple.
- Treatment—salicylic acid or tretinoin cream for mild cases. Imiquimod showed no benefit in clinical trials. Cryosurgery, curette scraping, cantharidin, or pulsed laser dye therapy may be used for severe cases.

Prurigo nodularis

- Cause unknown.
- Lesions are hyperpigmented, hyperkeratotic papules and nodules which usually occur on the chest. They are usually intensely itchy, resulting in excoriation, ulceration, and scars.
- Diagnosis is usually clinical but may be confirmed by biopsy.
- Treatment is with topical steroids, intralesional corticosteroids, occlusive dressings, antihistamines, or phototherapy. Systemic therapies include thalidomide, ciclosporin, and methotrexate.

Scabies

- Caused by *S. scabiei*.
- Lesions are small, red papules that are intensely itchy; sometimes there are 'burrows'. Occur in the finger webs, wrists, periumbilical area, axillae, thighs, buttocks, genitalia, legs, and feet. A severe, crusted form (Norwegian scabies) may occur in immunocompromised patients.
- Diagnosis is clinical and confirmed by microscopic examination of the mite.
- Treatment—the patient and all close contacts should be treated simultaneously with TOP 5% permethrin cream, or PO ivermectin 200 micrograms/kg stat dose. Alternative agents: lindane, benzyl benzoate, crotamiton, malathion, and sulphur in petrolatum. Pruritus may respond to antihistamines. Bedding and clothing must be washed in hot water or dry-cleaned.

Seborrhoeic dermatitis

- Cause unknown, but *Malassezia* has been detected more frequently in affected skin.
- Lesions are erythematous plaques with greasy scales and indistinct margins. Usually occur on the scalp, face, sternum, and axillae, behind the ears, and sometimes in the pubic area.
- Diagnosis is clinical.
- Treatment is with a weak topical corticosteroid cream (e.g. hydrocortisone 2.5%), a topical antifungal agent (e.g. ketoconazole 2%), or a combination of the two. Scalp lesions may be treated with various shampoos, e.g. selenium sulfide 2.5%, ketoconazole 2%, or ciclopirox 1% shampoo.

HIV oral complications

A number of oral complications may occur in HIV-infected patients.

Aphthous ulcers

- Cause unknown. Differential diagnosis includes HSV, CMV, and drug-induced ulcers.
- Diagnosis is clinical. Biopsy recommended for non-healing ulcers.
- Treatment is with TOP lidocaine solution, carmellose dental paste, 5% amlexanox oral paste. Refractory cases may require PO prednisolone, colchicine, dapsone, pentoxifylline, or thalidomide.

Oral candidiasis (thrush)

- Caused by *Candida* spp., usually *C. albicans*.
- Lesions are white, painless plaques on the buccal and pharyngeal mucosa or the tongue. Risk factors include CD4 count <250 cells/mm^3, antibiotics, and corticosteroids.
- Diagnosis is clinical but may be confirmed by KOH preparation. Culture is only indicated for speciation and drug susceptibility testing, e.g. for refractory cases.
- Treatment is with PO clotrimazole, nystatin, or fluconazole. Most cases respond in 7–14 days, unless prior azole exposure and CD4 count <50 cells/mm^3. Refractory cases may require itraconazole suspension, amphotericin suspension, or IV amphotericin.

Oral hairy leukoplakia

- Caused by EBV and found almost exclusively in HIV-infected patients with low CD4 count.
- Presents as unilateral or bilateral adherent white frond-like patches on lateral margins of the tongue.
- Diagnosis is usually clinical; biopsy is rarely required.
- Treatment is not usually required, as is usually asymptomatic. Responds to ART. Occasionally treated for pain or cosmetic reasons, with TOP podophyllin, surgical excision, cryotherapy, or antivirals.

Salivary gland enlargement

- May be due to HIV-related lymphoid proliferation.
- Presents with unilateral or bilateral parotid enlargement. Usually asymptomatic but may present with pain or xerostomia.
- Diagnosis is by fine-needle aspiration (FNA) for microbiology, cytology, and decompression. Occasionally, a biopsy is required to exclude a tumour.
- Treatment is by FNA for decompression of fluid-filled cysts.

Other conditions

The oral cavity may be involved in a number of conditions, e.g.:

- HSV infections;
- Kaposi's sarcoma;
- leishmaniasis;
- syphilis.

HIV cardiovascular complications

Cardiac abnormalities, such as myocarditis and cardiomyopathy, have long been recognized as complications of HIV infection. In the ART era, patients are living longer, and hypertension, metabolic abnormalities (hyperlipidaemia, hyperglycaemia), accelerated atherosclerosis, and coronary artery disease are becoming increasingly important.

Dilated cardiomyopathy

- Cause unknown, but hypotheses include direct invasion of HIV into myocardial cells, drug toxicity (e.g. zidovudine, pentamidine), illicit drug use (e.g. cocaine, metamphetamine), *l*-carnitine deficiency, and selenium deficiency.
- Incidence declining—previously 30–40% of AIDS patients, now 3–15%.
- Clinical features include CCF, arrhythmias, cyanosis, syncope, and sudden death.
- Diagnosis is by echocardiogram which shows an ejection fraction ≤50% ± arrhythmias on ECG.
- Treatment is with ART and an ACE inhibitor. Diuretics, e.g. furosemide or spironolactone, are given for persistent symptoms. Digoxin may be given for refractory cases. Other options: treat hypertension and hyperlipidaemia; discontinue alcohol and cocaine; discontinue azathioprine; some recommend supplements of *l*-carnitine or selenium (if deficient).

Endocarditis

HIV has no effect on the incidence of endocarditis, apart from in IDUs, in whom it is commoner. Associated with increased mortality in AIDS patients (30%).

Myocarditis

The cause is unclear in most cases. HIV may have a direct effect; 20% associated with infections, e.g. cryptococcosis, CMV, EBV, HSV, TB, and *T. gondii*.

Pericardial disease

- Prior to ART, pericarditis was the commonest presentation of HIV-related cardiac disease.
- The commonest clinical presentation is a pericardial effusion, which may be asymptomatic or present with cardiac tamponade.
- Causes include mycobacteria, pyogenic bacteria (e.g. *S. aureus, S. pneumoniae*), lymphoma, Kaposi's sarcoma, viruses, and fungi.
- Aspiration and pericardial biopsy may yield a diagnosis.
- Treatment depends on the underlying cause.

Pulmonary hypertension

- Relatively uncommon complication that can occur at any stage of infection and carries a high mortality.
- Cause unknown, but HHV-8 has been implicated.
- Clinical features are similar to primary pulmonary hypertension with exertional dyspnoea, fatigue, cough, haemoptysis, chest pain, and syncope.
- Diagnosis—CXR shows enlarged pulmonary vessels, and right ventricular and right atrial hypertrophy. Echocardiography shows a dilated right atrium and ventricle ± tricuspid regurgitation. Cardiac catheterization shows increased pulmonary artery pressure, increased right atrial pressure, and normal pulmonary capillary pressure.
- Treatment is difficult, as the condition is usually progressive. Some studies report improvement with ART; others show no benefit. Other options include epoprostenol, diuretics, oral anticoagulant, sildenafil, and antiviral therapy (controversial).

HIV pulmonary complications

HIV infection may be associated with a number of pulmonary complications, some of which are considered AIDS-defining illnesses.

Pneumocystis jiroveci pneumonia

- Caused by *P. jiroveci* (formerly called *Pneumocystis carinii*), a ubiquitous environmental organism, transmitted by inhalation.
- Risk factors—associated with low CD4 count (<200 cells/mm^3). Other risk groups: bone marrow and solid organ transplant recipients, haematological malignancy, chemotherapy, glucocorticoid therapy, other immunosuppressive medications, severe malnutrition.
- Clinical features—fever, dry cough, progressive dyspnoea, chills, malaise, chest pain, weight loss. Examination reveals crepitations or wheeze but may be normal in 50%. Hypoxia is common. May desaturate on exercise.
- Imaging—CXR shows diffuse bilateral interstitial infiltrates; 25% are normal in early disease. CT scan shows ground-glass opacification.

- Diagnosis—induced sputum or BAL with specific stains (e.g. calcofluor white, Gomori methenamine silver, or toluidine blue). PCR of induced sputum or BAL increases sensitivity in HIV-uninfected, immunocompromised patients.
- Treatment[5,6]—high-dose co-trimoxazole for 21 days is the treatment of choice. Alternatives include: clindamycin and primaquine; dapsone, atovaquone, and IV pentamidine. Adjunctive corticosteroids should be given if PaO_2 <7kPa or alveolar–arterial (A–a) gradient >3.5 KPa. ART should be started within 2 weeks of PCP treatment.
- Secondary prophylaxis should be given to all patients who have had PCP, and continued until the CD4 count is >200 cells/mm^3 for ≥3 months.

Pulmonary tuberculosis

- Caused by MTB.
- A common presentation of HIV infection—may occur at any stage of disease, and present with pulmonary and extrapulmonary disease.
- Clinical features—presents in a similar way to HIV-negative patients, with fever, cough, night sweats, malaise, and weight loss. May have evidence of extrapulmonary or disseminated disease.
- Imaging—CXR may show apical cavitation or may be atypical or even normal, particularly in patients with advanced HIV disease. CT scan is helpful in patients with atypical or normal CXRs.
- Diagnosis—sputum smear microscopy for AFB. Sputum induction or bronchoscopy may be required to obtain specimens. Molecular tests, such as the automated Xpert® MTB/RIF assay, are increasingly being used. Urine antigen tests, e.g. urine lipoarabinomannan (LAM) test is useful in patients with low CD4 counts and disseminated TB.
- Treatment—similar to treatment of HIV-negative patients. Empiric therapy for drug-susceptible TB is rifampicin, isoniazid, pyrazinamide, and ethambutol for 2 months, followed by rifampicin and isoniazid for 4 months. For suspected drug-resistant TB, additional agents are required—seek expert help.
- ART—efavirenz-based regimens are preferred because of interactions between rifampicin and PIs. For patients with pulmonary TB and CD4 counts <50 cells/mm^3, ART should be started early, i.e. within 2 weeks of TB treatment. For patients with pulmonary TB and CD4 counts >50 cells/mm^3, in the absence of severe disease, ART may be started later, e.g. 8–12 weeks after starting TB treatment.
- Prevention—treatment of latent TB infection is effective in preventing active TB in HIV-infected patients. In resource-rich settings, most patients are treated with 9 months of isoniazid. In resource-limited settings, clinical trials have evaluated various regimens, ranging from 6 months to lifelong therapy.

Pneumonia

- Caused by a wide variety of pathogens, e.g. pyogenic bacteria (*S. pneumoniae, H. influenzae, P. aeruginosa, S. aureus*), *P. jiroveci*, MTB, *R. equi, Nocardia* spp., *C. neoformans, C. immitis, H. capsulatum, Aspergillus* spp., influenza, CMV.

- Clinical features—fever, cough, dyspnoea, pleuritic chest pain. Onset and duration of symptoms are short in bacterial pneumonia and longer in PCP, TB, and fungal infections.
- Examination—skin lesions may be helpful, e.g. in cryptococcosis. Retinal examination may show evidence of CMV, TB, or fungal disease. Lymphadenopathy may be seen with TB.
- CD4 count—a high CD4 count is usually seen with 'normal' pathogens, e.g. *S. pneumoniae*, TB, *S. aureus*, and influenza. A CD4 count <200 cells/mm^3 is associated with opportunistic pathogens.
- Imaging—CXR may appear to show typical or atypical appearances or may even be normal in patients, e.g. PCP and TB. Intrathoracic lymphadenopathy suggests TB, atypical mycobacteria, lymphoma, and Kaposi's sarcoma. CT chest is more sensitive for early interstitial lung disease, lymphadenopathy, and nodules.
- ABG analysis—useful to determine the degree of hypoxia, the A–a gradient, and exercise desaturation in PCP.
- Laboratory diagnosis—expectorated sputum is used for TB diagnosis. Induced sputum is better for PCP. Bronchoscopy has a yield of ~95% for PCP. PCR-based tests are available for TB and PCP. Tests to consider in patients who are not responding to treatment are *Legionella* urinary antigen, serum cryptococcal antigen, and *H. capsulatum* serum or urinary antigen. BCs for TB and *Histoplasma*.
- Treatment is of the underlying cause. Lung biopsy is rarely required.
- Primary prevention—co-trimoxazole reduces the incidence of PCP and bacterial pneumonia. Influenza vaccination appears to reduce the risk of influenza. The effects of pneumococcal vaccination are variable.
- Secondary prophylaxis—patients who present with AIDS-defining pulmonary infections, e.g. PCP, should be treated with co-trimoxazole until their CD4 count is >200 cells/mm^3 for 6 months.

Lymphoid interstitial pneumonitis

- A diffuse interstitial lung disease of unknown cause, characterized by a benign polyclonal lymphoid cell infiltrate in the alveolar septae. Most cases are idiopathic, but some may be associated with autoimmune diseases.
- It occurs in <1% of HIV-infected adults, but up to 40% of HIV-infected children.
- Clinical features—fever, weight loss, dyspnoea, pleuritic chest pain, fatigue, arthralgia. Adults may be asymptomatic. Chest examination shows bibasal crepitations. Children may have clubbing and adenopathy.
- Imaging—CXR shows bilateral reticulonodular shadowing. High-resolution CT scan shows ground-glass shadowing and pulmonary nodules.
- Diagnosis—BAL may show increased numbers of lymphocytes. Transbronchial lung biopsy is diagnostic in adults. In children, persistence of abnormalities for >2 months and exclusion of other infectious causes are considered diagnostic.
- Treatment—PO prednisolone is the treatment of choice. The optimal duration of treatment is unknown; 6–12 months is usually given. For patients who do not respond or who are intolerant of glucocorticoids,

additional immunosuppressive therapy (e.g. azathioprine or cyclophosphamide) may be required. The condition may improve with the institution of ART.

Pneumothorax

- The commonest cause in HIV-infected persons is *P. jiroveci* (PCP). Other causes include iatrogenic, Kaposi's sarcoma, IDU, toxoplasmosis, and bacterial, viral, fungal, and mycobacterial infections.
- Clinical features—presents with pleuritic chest pain, dyspnoea, and cough. On examination, there is hyper-resonance to percussion and reduced breath sounds.
- Imaging—CXR shows a rim of air around the lung.
- Treatment—aspiration or chest drain insertion. Persistent or recurrent pneumothoraces may require pleurodesis or surgery.

References

5 Nelson M, Dockrell D, Edwards S, *et al.*; BHIVA Guidelines Subcommittee (2011). British HIV Association and British Infection Association guidelines for the treatment of opportunistic infection in HIV-seropositive individuals 2011. *HIV Med.* **12** Suppl 2:1–140.

6 Panel on Opportunistic Infections in HIV-Infected Adults and Adolescents (2015). *Guidelines for prevention and treatment of opportunistic infections in HIV-infected adults and adolescents: recommendations from the Centers for Disease Control and Prevention, the National Institutes of Health, and the HIV Medicine Association of the Infectious Diseases Society of America.* Available at: http://aidsinfo.nih.gov/guidelines/html/4/adult-and-adolescent-oi-prevention-and-treatment-guidelines/0.

HIV gastrointestinal disease

Gingivitis/periodontitis

- Gum inflammation and bleeding, caused by oral anaerobic bacteria.
- Four phases—linear gingival erythema, necrotizing gingivitis, necrotizing periodontitis, necrotizing stomatitis.
- Diagnosis is clinical. Orthopantogram may show bony loss.
- Treatment—routine dental care plus antiseptic mouthwash. A dental opinion should be sought regarding curettage and debridement. Antibiotics, e.g. metronidazole, are given for necrotizing stomatitis.

Oropharyngeal candidiasis

Usually caused by *C. albicans*. Diagnosis is clinical. Treatment is with PO fluconazole.

Oesophageal candidiasis

- Caused by a number of *Candida* spp. Usually occurs in patients with CD4 count <100 cells/mm^3.
- Clinical features—dysphagia, odynophagia, and retrosternal pain.
- Diagnosis is clinical, but upper GI endoscopy may be performed if atypical presentation or poor response to treatment.
- Treatment—fluconazole or itraconazole for 14–21 days.
- Secondary prophylaxis may be considered in patients with >3 episodes in 1 year.

Nausea and vomiting

- Often due to medications (especially antiretrovirals, antibiotics, opiates). May also be due to abacavir hypersensitivity, nevirapine hepatotoxicity, and lactic acidosis. Other causes: adrenal insufficiency, uraemia, hypercalcaemia, CNS lesions, GI disease.
- Investigations—lactate level, ultrasound/CT abdomen, CT brain.
- Treat the underlying cause. If due to drugs, consider changing them. Otherwise symptomatic treatment.

Diarrhoea

- Often caused by medications, especially PIs.
- Acute diarrhoea may be due to a number of enteric pathogens, e.g. *Salmonella* spp., *Shigella* spp., *Campylobacter* spp., *E. coli, S. aureus*, viruses.
- Chronic diarrhoea may be due to *Cryptosporidium, Microsporidium*, MAC, *Cyclospora, Isospora, G. lamblia, E. histolytica*, or HIV enteropathy.
- Anorectal pain/tenderness may be due to infection with *Chlamydia*, gonorrhoea, or LGV.
- Clinical features—fever, abdominal cramps, diarrhoea, tenesmus, PR bleeding. Complications include electrolyte disturbance and malnutrition.
- Diagnosis—stool sample for microscopy, culture, ova, cysts, and parasites, and *C. difficile* toxin testing. An acid-fast stain is required for *Cryptosporidium, Isospora*, and *Cyclospora*. In patients with a CD4 count <100 cells/mm^3, a trichrome strain should be done for *Microsporidia*. BCs should be taken for MAI infection.
- Endoscopy—in patients with colitis and negative stool investigations, a colonoscopy and biopsy may be required to exclude CMV disease. In patients with advanced HIV disease and persistent diarrhoea, an endoscopy with small bowel biopsies may be required to look for MAI, cryptosporidiosis, microsporidiosis, histoplasmosis, lymphoma, or Kaposi's sarcoma.
- Imaging—CT abdomen may show evidence of colitis, hepatosplenomegaly, lymphadenopathy, or biliary tract disease.
- Treatment—treat the underlying cause. If due to drugs, consider changing them. Otherwise symptomatic treatment. Nutritional support may be required.

Peritonitis

- Infections that have been associated with peritonitis include TB, MAC, toxoplasmosis, cryptococcosis, and histoplasmosis.
- Amongst patients with ascites, abdominal paracentesis may help to establish the diagnosis, although laparoscopy/laparotomy may be required.
- NHL may also present with peritonitis.

HIV liver disease

Deranged liver function tests

These are common in HIV-infected patients and may be due to a variety of causes:

- drug toxicity, e.g. NNRTIs, PIs, co-trimoxazole, TB drugs, statins, paracetamol;
- alcohol toxicity or substance abuse;
- viral hepatitis (acute infection, flare of chronic disease, drug resistance);
- opportunistic infections, e.g. MAC, CMV, TB, histoplasmosis, *P. jiroveci*, *B. henselae*, and visceral leishmaniasis;
- tumours, e.g. Kaposi's sarcoma, NHL, metastases from primaries elsewhere.

Hepatic steatosis

HIV/HCV co-infected patients are at increased risk of hepatic steatosis, compared with HCV monoinfected patients.

Lactic acidosis

- Hyperlactataemia is defined as a venous lactate level of >2mmol/L.
- It can occur with any NRTI, but the main culprits are zalcitabine (withdrawn), didanosine (ddI), stavudine (d4T), and zidovudine (AZT).
- The mechanism is inhibition of DNA polymerase γ, leading to depletion of mitochondrial DNA.
- It can be asymptomatic or associated with a symptomatic, and sometimes fatal, acidosis.
- Asymptomatic elevations in lactate occur in 8–20% of patients on prolonged ART.
- Symptomatic hyperlactataemia occurs in 0.5–1/100 patient-years of NRTI exposure.
- Diagnosis—patients who have symptoms compatible with lactic acidosis (nausea, vomiting, abdominal pain) or abnormal LFTs/amylase should have their lactate levels measured. A lactate level >5mmol/L is considered diagnostic.
- Treatment—stop the NRTIs, and switch to another drug class. Substitution of abacavir (ABC), lamivudine (3TC), emtricitabine (FTC), or tenofovir (TDF) may be possible in patients who are not seriously ill.
- Prognosis is related to lactate level—7% if lactate 5–10mmol/L; >30% if lactate 10–15mmol/L, and >60% if lactate >15mmol/L.

Viral hepatitis

- All patients who develop deranged LFTs should be screened for the hepatitis viruses.
- Patients may acquire an acute hepatitis (e.g. HAV or HEV) transmitted by the faeco-oral route.
- HIV patients may be chronically infected with other blood-borne viruses such as HBV or HCV.
- All patients should be advised to avoid or limit their intake of alcohol. They should also be vaccinated against HAV and HBV, if non-immune when their CD4 count is >200 cells/mm^3.

- Treatment of HBV—in patients with normal renal function, tenofovir is recommended, as it is active against both HIV and HBV, including lamivudine-resistant HBV. Most patients receive combination therapy with tenofovir and emtricitabine (Truvada®). In patients with impaired renal function (CrCl <50mL/min), entecavir is recommended.
- Treatment of HCV—a recent development is the availability of IFN-free regimens. In ART-naïve HIV/HCV co-infected patients, ART is usually initiated 4–6 weeks before HCV therapy. For those with a CD4 count >500 cells/mm^3, it is reasonable to delay ART until HCV treatment is completed. For HIV/HCV genotype 1 infections, simepravir plus sofosbuvir for 12 weeks is recommended; interactions between simepravir and PIs, efavirenz, and nevirapine may limit its use. An alternative regimen is PEG-IFN, ribavirin, and sofosbuvir. For most HIV/HCV genotype 2 infections, sofosbuvir and weight-based ribavirin for 12 weeks is recommended. For most HIV/HCV genotype 3 and 4 infections, sofosbuvir and weight-based ribavirin for 24 weeks is recommended. There are no clinical data on HCV genotype 5 and 6 infections, although efficacy is expected to be comparable.

Cholangiopathy

- Syndrome of biliary obstruction caused by infection-associated strictures.
- Causes—*C. parvum* (commonest), *Microsporidium, C. cayetanensis, Isospora*, and *Giardia*; 20–40% idiopathic.
- CD4 count usually <100 cells/mm^3.
- Clinical features—right upper quadrant pain, fever, diarrhoea (if intestinal involvement).
- LFTs show raised ALP. Ultrasound shows dilated bile ducts. Diagnosis confirmed by ERCP.
- Treatment—sphincterotomy for papillary stenosis. Endoscopic stenting for isolated bile duct stricture. Ursodeoxycholic acid has been used experimentally in cholangiopathy without stenosis. Pathogen-specific therapy, if possible.
- Outcome—average survival is 9 months; worse if ALP >1000IU/L.

Atazanavir-associated cholelithiasis

- Atazanavir has been associated with cholelithiasis.
- Symptoms occurred after a median of 42 months.
- Complications included cholecystitis, cholangitis, and acute pancreatitis.

Pancreatitis

- Pancreatitis is a well-recognized complication in HIV-infected patients.
- In the pre-ART era, pancreatitis was due to opportunistic infections (e.g. CMV, MAC, TB, cryptosporidiosis, cryptococcosis, toxoplasmosis) or infiltrative diseases (e.g. lymphoma, Kaposi's sarcoma).
- Drug-induced pancreatitis has been reported with didanosine (commonest), stavudine, ritonavir, sulfonamides, and pentamidine.

- Diagnosis is based on amylase >3 times the upper limit of normal. A CT scan should be performed to stage the disease, detect complications, and exclude other diagnoses.
- Treatment is supportive—fluids, antibiotics, analgesia.
- Prognosis is related to the APACHE II score.

HIV kidney disease

Acute kidney injury

- The incidence of acute kidney injury (AKI) is higher in patients with HIV infection than those without, and has increased over time.
- Risk factors for AKI are similar to HIV-negative patients and include older age, diabetes mellitus, pre-existing chronic kidney disease (CKD), and acute or chronic liver disease.
- Causes of AKI are similar to HIV-negative patients and include pre-renal states (volume depletion, cardiac failure, cirrhosis), acute tubular necrosis (ischaemic, nephrotoxic), crystalluria with obstruction, and interstitial nephritis.
- Medication nephrotoxicity may occur with PIs (indinavir and atazanavir), tenofovir, aciclovir, foscarnet, cidofovir, co-trimoxazole, and pentamidine. Cobicistat and dolutegravir can interfere with tubular secretion of creatinine.
- HIV-associated thrombotic microangiopathy is a rare cause of AKI.

Chronic kidney disease

- The prevalence of CKD and end-stage renal disease (ESRD) is projected to rise, as HIV prevalence increases.
- Risk factors for CKD include HCV infection, low CD4 count, high HIV viral load, tenofovir, boosted PIs, diabetes mellitus, and hypertension.
- Causes of CKD include previous AKI, diabetes mellitus, hypertension, HIV-associated nephropathy (HIVAN), and HIV immune-mediated glomerulonephritis.

HIV-associated nephropathy

- First described in 1984.
- A collapsing form of focal segmental glomerulosclerosis with tubular microcysts and interstitial inflammation.
- Risk factors—black race, advanced HIV disease.
- Clinical features—heavy proteinuria, rapid decline in kidney function, haematuria, hypertension, oedema.
- Diagnosis—proteinuria (nephrotic range) is common. Renal ultrasound shows normal to large echogenic kidneys. Renal biopsy is diagnostic.
- Treatment—ART improves renal survival. Renin–angiotensin system inhibition with ACE inhibitors or angiotensin receptor blockers (ARBs). Treatment targets are a blood pressure of <130/80mmHg and proteinuria <1g/day. Glucocorticoids have been given in patients with rapidly progressive disease, despite ART and angiotensin inhibition.

HIV neurological complications

Peripheral neuropathy

Peripheral neuropathy is another relatively common complication of HIV therapy. There are a number of possible causes:

- distal sensory neuropathy (DSN)—pain and numbness in glove-and-stocking distribution. CD4 count usually <200 cells/mm^3;
- antiretroviral toxic neuropathy (ATN)—same as DSN, but associated with ddI, ddC, and d4T. Commoner in older patients with diabetes. Can occur at any CD4 count;
- tarsal tunnel syndrome—pain and numbness in the anterior part of the soles of feet;
- HIV-associated neuromuscular weakness syndrome—ascending paralysis with arreflexia ± cranial nerve or sensory involvement. Usually associated with d4T. Poor survival;
- HIV-associated myopathy (AZT myopathy)—pain, aching, and weakness of proximal muscles. Associated with AZT and raised CK. Can occur at any CD4 count;
- polyradiculitis—rapidly evolving weakness and numbness in legs, with bladder and bowel incontinence. May be caused by CMV or HSV. CD4 count <50 or >500 cells/mm^3;
- vacuolar myopathy—stiffness, weakness, and numbness in legs, followed by bowel and bladder incontinence. Need to exclude vitamin B_{12} deficiency and HTLV-1 infection. CD4 count <200 cells/mm^3. Physiotherapy, methionine, or ART may be helpful;
- inflammatory demyelinating polyneuropathies—weakness in arms and legs, with a minor sensory component. Can occur at any CD4 count. Treatment: plasmapheresis, IVIG, and/or ART;
- mononeuritis/mononeuritis multiplex—asymmetrical mix of motor and sensory defects occurring over weeks. CD4 count variable. Treat with steroids if CD4 count >200 cells/mm^3. Treat for CMV if CD4 count <50 cells/mm^3.

Central nervous system manifestations

CNS involvement may be due to HIV itself, opportunistic infections, or malignancies:

- *cryptococcal meningitis* (8–10% of all AIDS patients)—presents with fever, headache, visual changes, stiff neck, cranial nerve deficits, and seizures. Progresses over 2 weeks. CD4 count <100 cells/mm^3. CSF India ink-positive in 60–80%; CSF culture positive in 95–100%. Cryptococcal antigen >95% sensitive and specific;
- *HIV-associated dementia* (HAD, 7%)—presents with a triad of cognitive, motor, and behavioural dysfunction over weeks to months. Afebrile. CD4 count <200 cells/mm^3. Elevated β_2 microglobulin. Neuropsychological tests show subcortical dementia;
- *toxoplasmosis* (2–4%)—presents with fever, reduced conscious level, focal neurological deficits, and seizures. CD4 count <200 cells/mm^3. MRI scan shows ring-enhancing lesions. *Toxoplasma* IgG falsely negative

in 5%; 85% respond to empiric therapy in 7 days. Brain biopsy makes the definitive diagnosis;

- *primary CNS lymphoma* (2%)—clinical presentation afebrile, with altered mental status, focal neurological deficits, and seizures with progression over 2–8 weeks. CD4 count <200 cells/mm^3. Suspect if the patient has no response to anti-toxoplasma therapy. Thallium-201 SPECT scan 90% sensitive and specific;
- *PML* (1–2%)—presents with impaired speech, vision, and motor function. No fever or headache. CD4 count usually <100 cells/mm^3. MRI shows multifocal lesions in the subcortical white matter. CSF or brain biopsy positive for JC virus (➔ see Polyomaviruses, pp. 442–3);
- *CNS TB* (0.5–1%)—fever, headache, meningism, impaired conscious level, focal neurological deficits. CD4 count <100 cells/mm^3. CT/MRI scan shows meningeal enhancement, hydrocephalus, and tuberculomas. ZN smear positive in 20%. CXR shows active TB in 50%. Gold standard for diagnosis is positive CSF culture for MTB;
- *CMV encephalitis* (>0.5%)—presents with fever, lethargy, delirium, disorientation, headache, neck stiffness, photophobia, and cranial nerve deficits. CD4 count <100 cells/mm^3. May have CMV retinitis. CSF CMV PCR positive. Definitive diagnosis is made by brain biopsy;
- *neurosyphilis* (0.5%)—various clinical presentations: meningitis-like, tabes dorsalis, general paresis of the insane, meningovascular strokes/myelitis; ocular manifestations (iritis, uveitis, optic neuritis). Occurs at any CD4 count. Diagnosis positive CSF VDRL (60–70%);
- *HIV neurocognitive disorders*—here is a spectrum of cognitive deficits in HIV-infected patients, ranging from asymptomatic neurocognitive impairment (ANI) to mild neurocognitive disorder (MCD) to HAD. Risk factors include low CD4 count, older age at seroconversion, duration of HIV infection, and prior AIDS-defining illness. The use of ART has reduced the prevalence of HAD, but not of the milder forms.

HIV infection and malignancy

HIV-infected individuals have an increased risk of developing malignancies. An increase in the incidence of Kaposi's sarcoma was noted early in the AIDS epidemic, and it was classified as an AIDS-defining condition. NHL and invasive cervical carcinoma were subsequently added as AIDS-defining conditions. The use of ART has resulted in a relative increase in non-AIDS-defining cancers.

- *Kaposi's sarcoma*—caused by HHV-8. Commonest HIV-associated malignancy. Rate is 20 000-fold higher in HIV-positive than HIV-negative individuals, and 300-fold higher than in other immunosuppressed patients. It is commoner in MSM and women. Presents with purple/brown/black macules, nodules, and papules on the face, mouth, legs, and genitals. Visceral involvement affects the lungs and GI tract. ART associated with decreased incidence and regression of lesions. Treatment may be local, e.g. vinblastine injections, or systemic, e.g. liposomal anthracycline.

- *NHL*—50–80% are EBV-positive. CD4 count <100 cells/mm^3; 200–600 times commoner in HIV than in the general population. The majority are high-grade diffuse large-cell or Burkitt-like lymphomas. Usually present with advanced disease, sparse lymph nodes, and constitutional 'B' symptoms. Diagnosis is made by biopsy of the brain, lymph nodes, or bone marrow. CT better than endoscopy for assessing GI involvement. Treatment: ART plus chemotherapy. Initial response rates 60–80%, but median survival <1 year.
- *Primary CNS lymphoma* (➲ see HIV neurological complications, pp. 838–9).
- *Primary effusion lymphoma*—caused by HHV-8 and EBV. Very rare, accounting for <0.14% of NHL in AIDS. Presents with serous effusions (pleural, pericardial, peritoneal, and joint spaces). Diagnosis is made by examining the effusions. Treatment: ART plus chemotherapy.
- Invasive cervical cancer is associated with HPV types 16, 18, 31, 33, and 35. CIN and invasive cervical cancer are both commoner in HIV-positive than HIV-negative women. The frequency and severity of cervical dysplasia increases with progressive immune compromise. The US CDC recommends a gynaecological examination and Pap smear at baseline, at 6 months, and then yearly in HIV-infected women.

HIV prevention

There are an estimated 35.3 million people living with HIV/AIDS, with 2.3 million new infections and 1.6 million deaths in 2012. The majority of new infections occur in young adults (aged 15–24 years) in developing countries, and it is likely that a range of preventive strategies will be required to curb the epidemic.

Prevention of mother-to-child transmission (PMTCT)

Without preventative measures, the risk of perinatal HIV transmission is 15–45%. The three major factors associated with perinatal HIV transmission are: high maternal plasma HIV viral load, prolonged rupture of membranes, and breastfeeding. A number of studies have shown:

- ART of the mother during pregnancy and delivery reduces maternal viraemia and HIV transmission;
- ART of the child (*in utero* and after birth) reduces HIV transmission;
- delivery by Caesarean section has led to a decline in HIV transmission;
- continuation of ART in mothers who choose to exclusively breastfeed is beneficial.[7,8]

Prevention of sexual transmission

A number of factors have been identified to be important in sexual transmission: plasma HIV RNA level, genital HIV RNA level, acute infection versus advanced disease, degree of immunosuppression, genital ulcers, inflammatory STIs, cervical ectopy, uncircumcised status, host genetics, and levels of cytokines and chemokines. Interventions to reduce sexual transmission include:

- reduction of HIV RNA level—studies in Africa have shown that ART reduces the risk of HIV transmission between sero-discordant couples by >80%;
- HSV-2 suppression—treatment with valaciclovir was associated with reduction in plasma and genital HIV-1 levels and reduced incidence of HIV transmission. However, use of aciclovir was not associated with reduced HIV acquisition in two other studies;[7]
- male circumcision—several ecological studies and three RCTs have shown that male circumcision is associated with a 60–70% reduction in rates of HIV acquisition.[7] Circumcision also reduced the frequency of genital ulcer disease and HIV acquisition by female sexual partners. Modelling studies now suggest that male circumcision in sub-Saharan Africa could potentially prevent 5.7 million infections and 2 million deaths over the next 20 years, if the intervention could be delivered safely and cost-effectively;
- microbicides—whereas circumcision is a method that can protect men from HIV, there is an urgent need to develop female-controlled methods of protection. Numerous studies have investigated the effectiveness of female condoms, diaphragms, and microbicides but have failed to show benefit. In some studies, the use of microbicides has been associated with an increased risk of HIV acquisition;
- post-exposure prophylaxis following sexual exposure (PEPSE)—this is recommended where the individual presents within 72h after anal and/or vaginal intercourse with a known HIV-positive source or a source from a group or area of high HIV prevalence.[9,10]
- pre-exposure prophylaxis (PrEP)—a number of studies have shown that daily oral PrEP, with a fixed-dose combination of tenofovir and emtricitabine, is safe and effective in reducing the risk of sexual HIV acquisition in adults. The US CDC has therefore recommended the use of oral PrEP as a HIV prevention option in sexually active MSM, heterosexual men and women, and IDUs at substantial risk of HIV acquisition.[11]

HIV vaccines

Despite billions of pounds and over 20 years of research, an effective vaccine for the prevention of HIV remains elusive. Specific characteristics of the virus that hinder vaccine development include the extreme genetic variability in circulating viral isolates worldwide, the biological properties of HIV that impede an immune attack, and a high mutation rate that allows for rapid escape from adaptive immune responses.

References

7 Panel on Treatment of HIV-Infected Pregnant Women and Prevention of Perinatal Transmission (2015). *Recommendations for use of antiretroviral drugs in pregnant HIV-1 infected women for maternal health and interventions to reduce perinatal HIV transmission in the United States*. Available at: http://aidsinfo.nih.gov/contentfiles/lvguidelines/perinatalgl.pdf.

8 de Ruiter A, Taylor GP, Clayden P, *et al.*; British HIV Association (2014). British HIV Association guidelines for the managament of HIV infection in pregnant women 2012 (2014 interim review). *HIV Med.* **15** Suppl 4:1–77.

9 Smith DK, Grohskopf LA, Black RJ, *et al.*; *U.S. Department of Health and Human Services (2005). Antiretroviral postexposure prophylaxis after sexual, injection-drug use, or other nonoccupational exposure to HIV in the United States*. Available at: http://www.cdc.gov/mmwr/preview/mmwrhtml/rr5402a1.htm.

10 Benn P, Fisher M, Kulasegaram R; BASHH; PEPSE Guidelines Writing Group Clinical Effectiveness Group (2011). UK guideline for the use of post-exposure prophylaxis for HIV following sexual exposure. *Int J STD AIDS*. 22:695–708.

11 US Public Health Service (2014). *Preexposure prophylaxis for the prevention of HIV infection in the United States—2014: a clinical practice guideline*. Available at: http://www.cdc.gov/hiv/pdf/PrEPguidelines2014.pdf.

Chapter 25

Health protection

Immunizations *844*
Notifiable diseases *845*
Bioterrorism *846*
Migrant health *848*

Immunizations

Routine childhood immunizations

All children in the UK are entitled to free immunizations to protect them from childhood illnesses. The introduction of immunization has resulted in dramatic declines in certain diseases, e.g. meningitis caused by *H. influenzae* type B and *N. meningitidis* serogroup C. Routine childhood immunization schedules vary from country to country. The UK routine childhood immunization schedule is summarized in Table 25.1.

Non-routine immunizations

Some children who may be at increased risk of certain diseases (e.g. TB and hepatitis B) may be given additional vaccines, as may those in other risk groups. The indications shown in Table 25.2 are not exhaustive, and full guidelines can be found in the UK *Green Book*.

Table 25.1 Routine childhood immunization schedule

Child's age	Vaccine(s) given	Diseases protected against
2 months	DTaP/IPV/Hib, PCV, Rotavirus, MenB	Diphtheria, tetanus, pertussis, polio, *H. influenzae* type B, pneumococcal, and rotavirus infection. Meningococcal B from September 2015
3 months	DTaP/IPV/ Hib, MenC, Rotavirus	Diphtheria, tetanus, pertussis, polio, *H. influenzae* type B, meningococcal C, rotavirus
4 months	DTaP/IPV/Hib PCV, MenB	Diphtheria, tetanus, pertussis, polio, *H. influenzae* type B, pneumococcal infection, meningococcal B
12–13 months	Hib/MenC, MMR, PCV, MenB	*H. influenzae* type B, meningococcal C, measles, mumps, and rubella, pneumococcal infection, meningococcal B
2, 3, and 4 years	Flu (annually)	Influenza
3 years and 4 months	DTaP/IPV or MMR	Diphtheria, tetanus, pertussis, polio, measles, mumps, and rubella
Girls aged 12–13 years	HPV	Cervical cancer caused by HPV types 16 and 18
13–18 years old	Td/IPV Men ACWY	Diphtheria, tetanus, polio Meningococcal types A, C, W, Y
65 and over	Flu (annually), PPV	Influenza, pneumococcal infection
70 years	Shingles vaccine	Shingles

Table 25.2 Indications and vaccines for at-risk children

Recipient	Vaccine	Diseases protected against
At birth, for babies who are more likely to be exposed to TB	BCG	TB
At birth, for babies whose mothers are hepatitis B-positive	Hep B	Hepatitis B
IDUs, MSM, anyone receiving regular transfusions of blood products, sex workers, medical staff, etc.	Hep B	Hepatitis B
Those in close contact with the immunocompromised (e.g. children of someone undergoing chemotherapy)	Varicella	Chickenpox

Vaccinations in those infected with HIV

HIV-infected adults who are susceptible on serological screening should be considered for vaccination against hepatitis B, measles/mumps/rubella (if CD4 count >200), and varicella (if CD4 count >400).

Inactivated vaccines may be used safely in all HIV-infected adults, if required. These include cholera WC/rBS, hepatitis A and B, *Haemophilus* influenza, parenteral influenza, meningitis C and ACWY, pneumococcus PPV23, rabies, Td/IPV (tetanus, diphtheria, parenteral polio), and typhoid ViCPS. Certain live vaccines are contraindicated in all HIV patients, regardless of the CD4 count. These include cholera CVD103-HgR, intranasal influenza, oral polio (OPV), typhoid Ty21a, and BCG.

Further reading

British HIV Association (2008). Available at: ☞ http://www.bhiva.org/documents/Guidelines/Immunisation/Immunization2008.pdf.

The NHS Immunization information website http://www.immunisation.nhs.uk

Public Health England (2013). *Immunisation against infectious diseases (The Green Book)*. Available at: ☞ https://www.gov.uk/government/organisations/public-health-england/series/immunisation-against-infectious-disease-the-green-book.

Notifiable diseases

- The statutory requirement for the notification of certain infectious diseases (e.g. cholera, diphtheria, smallpox, and typhoid) started towards the end of the nineteenth century.
- Originally, the head of the family or landlord had the responsibility of reporting the disease to the local authority 'Proper Officer'; the attending medical practitioner now does this.
- The prime purpose of the notification system is to detect possible outbreaks or epidemics. Accuracy of diagnosis is secondary, and a clinical suspicion of a notifiable infection is all that is required. If a diagnosis later proves incorrect, it can always be changed or cancelled.

- Doctors in England and Wales have a duty to notify the Proper Officer of suspected cases of diseases shown in Table 25.3. They should not wait for laboratory confirmation. The notification certificate should be sent within 3 days or verbally within 24h for urgent cases. Requirements differ slightly for Scotland (excludes some of the diseases shown in Table 25.3, but specifically includes *E. coli* O157, meningococcal infection, *H. influenzae* type B, necrotizing fasciitis, and tularaemia).

Table 25.3 Notifiable diseases

Acute encephalitis (NS)	Malaria
Acute infectious hepatitis	Measles
Acute meningitis (NS)	Meningococcal sepsis
Acute polio	Mumps
Anthrax	Plague
Botulism	Rabies
Brucellosis	Rubella
Cholera	SARS
Diphtheria	Scarlet fever
Enteric fever (typhoid/paratyphoid)	Smallpox
Food poisoning	Tetanus
HUS	TB
Infectious bloody diarrhoea (NS)	Typhus
Invasive GAS (NS)	VHF
Legionnaires' disease	Whooping cough
Leprosy (NS)	Yellow fever

*NS, not Scotland.

Bioterrorism

Biological warfare has a long and unpleasant history. Around 400 BC, the Scythians were attempting to poison their arrows with blood and manure, and, in the fourteenth century, the Tartar catapulted the corpses of plague victims into the city of Kaffa, with the intention of initiating an outbreak. The years after the Second World War saw a race to develop more effective biological agents, before various treaties later led to the limitation, and even destruction, of biological weapon stockpiles by many nations (the UK 1957, the USA 1973). Today, around 17 countries are suspected of having biological weapons programmes. The threat of biological warfare is seen as issuing not primarily from states, but from independent organizations and terrorists. The term 'deliberate release' refers to any intentional spread of a biological or chemical agent. Such a release may be *overt* (e.g. a prior warning or the release may be apparent, either due to the use of an explosive device or because a suspicious substance is obviously visible) or *covert* (the release not becoming apparent until the first cases of disease arise). Only two proven deliberate releases have recently affected a large number of people: contamination of restaurant salads with *S. typhimurium* in Oregon in 1984 and dissemination of *B. anthracis* via the US mail in 2001.

Organisms with the potential to be used as weapons agents

The ideal biological weapon agent has low visibility and high potency, is accessible with a long shelf life, is relatively easy to deliver, and shows limited epidemic spread. A small amount of the agent may be capable of killing a large number of people (particularly in a metropolitan environment) and creating a disproportionate level of fear and disruption—a key part of their attractiveness to terrorist organizations.

- Category A agents—those organisms easily disseminated or transmitted from person to person, with high mortality rates and potential for major public health impact and requiring special action for public health readiness:
    - anthrax (➲ see *Bacillus anthracis*—ACDP 3, pp. 258–60)—pulmonary anthrax presents with a severe febrile illness or sepsis with respiratory failure (massive mediastinal lymphadenopathy). The organism may be identified in BCs or the sputum;
    - smallpox (➲ see Poxviruses, pp. 444–5)—the previously vaccinated lose protection after 10–20 years. Vaccination provides moderate protection if given within 2–4 days of exposure. Disease may develop 1–3 weeks after exposure;
    - botulism (➲ see *Clostridium botulinum*, pp. 267–8)—toxin may be inhaled or food-borne. Anti-toxin is available;
    - plague (➲ see *Yersinia pestis*—ACDP 3, pp. 314–5)—inhaled as aerosol, causing pneumonic plague;
    - tularaemia (➲ see *Francisella*—ACDP 3, pp. 317–8);
    - VHFs (➲ see Viral haemorrhagic fevers, pp. 459–61).
- Category B agents—moderately easy to disseminate, moderate morbidity rates and low mortality rates, require enhancement of both diagnostic capacity and disease surveillance. They include: glanders (➲ see Treatment, p. 303), melioidosis (➲ see *Burkholderia pseudomallei*—ACDP 3, pp. 302–3), brucellosis (➲ see *Brucella*—ACDP 3, pp. 311–3), psittacosis (➲ see *Chlamydophila psittaci*, pp. 354–5), and Q fever (➲ see *Coxiella burnetii* (Q fever), pp. 346–8).
- Category C agents—emerging pathogens that might be engineered for mass dissemination, e.g. SARS, H1N1 flu, hantavirus.

Recognizing an attack

In the absence of issued warnings or a very obvious release (e.g. explosive device), the first indicator of an outbreak may be a cluster of symptomatic cases. Such clusters may present acutely or over a period of days or weeks. Isolated fatalities due to undiagnosed febrile illness are not uncommon. Prompt epidemiological inquiry is essential. Features indicative of deliberate release include:

- an unusually large number of patients over a short time period;

- cases that are linked by epidemiological or geographical features;
- signs/symptoms that are unusual or very severe;
- unknown cause or an identified cause unresponsive to normal therapy or unusual in the UK or where acquired.

Remember that symptoms may also be due to radiological or chemical contamination.

Responding to an attack

Consider the risk of transmission to, or contamination of, staff and other patients—it may be appropriate to isolate affected patients and use PPE. Decontamination of potentially exposed individuals is vital for suspected releases of *B. anthracis*. Expert advice must be sought locally, and the HPU informed. Empirical antibacterial prophylaxis is indicated for possible exposure to certain bacterial agents such as anthrax, plague, and tularaemia (ciprofloxacin) or *Brucella, Burkholderia*, and Q fever (e.g. doxycycline). National agencies have stockpiles of suitable antibiotics for such emergencies. Early cases should be managed according to the best available advice, until more detailed epidemiological information and laboratory tests are available. In the UK, management of all incidents is led by the police, with involvement of other emergency and health services, as appropriate. All microbiological testing of suspect material must be done in *specialist* laboratories.

More information

The PHE website has extensive information on the management of deliberate release incidents, including clinical and diagnostic algorithms, antibiotic protocols, and guidelines for dealing with 'suspect packages'. See https://www.gov.uk/government/collections/deliberate-and-accidental-releases-investigation-and-management.

Migrant health

A mix of social, economic, and political factors mean more people are migrating across the world than ever before. The 2011 census of England and Wales demonstrated that 13% (7.5 million) of residents were born outside the UK (up from 4.6 million in 2001). Most are young healthy adults, but many will have a number of risk factors that put them at increased risk of ill health. These include:

- an early life in regions with a high prevalence of infectious disease. In the UK, <70% of new cases of HIV, TB, and malaria are diagnosed in those who were born overseas;
- frequent travel to the country of origin or contact with those who do;
- many may live in crowded or deprived regions of the UK, mixing with other at-risk groups;
- some people are at increased risk of diabetes and cardiovascular disease, particularly if moving to a 'Western' diet and lifestyle. In the UK, diabetes is three times more prevalent in those of Bangladeshi, Pakistani, or Indian origin, and the highest rates of heart disease are seen amongst the black Caribbean population;

- risk of preventable infections due to an incomplete vaccine history;
- mental health issues, perhaps related to the circumstances of the departure from their home country, social isolation, or exploitation in the UK.

New arrivals

New arrivals presenting to secondary care should be encouraged to find a GP. Those presenting to primary care should have the standard new patient check (e.g. medical history, allergies, social, smoking, alcohol, etc.). Attention should also be given to:

- the circumstances of their migration—are they likely to have specific economic or mental health needs? (e.g. refugee, persecution, human trafficking);
- their social situation in the UK;
- any specific infectious disease risk—those from high-prevalence countries should automatically be offered screening for HIV, TB, and hepatitis, as well as certain parasitic infections if symptoms suggest it;
- if immunizations are not in keeping with the UK schedule, then they should be brought up-to-date;
- any specific nutritional or metabolic concerns (e.g. vitamin D or A deficiency);
- education regarding lifestyle, diet, exercise, and sexual health;
- information about the structure and use of the NHS;
- visits back home—if they are planning to make trips home, they should be advised to seek travel advice, if relevant. For example, those from countries in which malaria is endemic may be unaware of their increased risk of acquiring malaria and the need for prophylaxis.

PHE have a comprehensive migrant health resource which includes country-specific health risks and advice for primary care. It is available at: ☞ https://www.gov.uk/government/collections/communicable-diseases-migrant-health-guide.

Index

The index entries appear in word-by-word alphabetical order.

1-3 beta-*D*
-glucan 472–3, 487–8
5-FC 473
5-fluorouracil/adrenaline gel 700–1

A

abacavir 104–6
abacavir hypersensitivity testing 824
abbreviations, infection control (UK) 131
abdominal angiostrongyliasis 568
Abelcet® 80–1
Abiotrophia 255
abscesses
amoebiasis 534–5
brain 534–5, 737–9
cutaneous 758
diverticular 666, 667
epidural 740–1
intra-abdominal 667–9
lateral pharyngeal 606
liver 670–1
lung 621–3
peritonsillar 594–5
prostatic 689
renal 685–6
retropharyngeal 593–4
absorption 15
Acanthamoeba species 536–7
accreditation, laboratory 231–3
aciclovir 90–1, 398–9, 401, 704, 736, 795
acid-fast bacilli (AFB) 222–4, 357–8
acid-fast cell walls 211
Acidominococcus species 280
acridine orange stain 222–4
acrodermatitis chronica atrophicans (ACA) 338
Actinobacter 297–9
Actinomadura 273
Actinomyces 271–2
actinomycetoma 273
actinomycosis 271–2
adamantanes 95–6
adefovir 98, 99, 416–17
adenocarcinoma, oesophageal 646
adenoidectomy 604–5
adenolymphangitis (ADL) 554
adenovirus 436–8
Adeoviridae 370
adhesins 216, 235
administration routes, antimicrobials 18–21
adrenaline, nebulized racemic 596–7
adult T-cell leukaemia/lymphoma (ATL) 449–50
adverse effects see toxicity/side effects
Advisory Committee on Dangerous Pathogens (ACDP) 160–3
Bacillus anthracis 207–362
Blastomyces dermatitidis 503–5
Brucella 311–13
Burkholderia pseudomallei 302–3
Coccidiodes immitis 505–8
Coxiella burnetii 346–8
Francisella 317–18
Histoplasma capsulatum 498–503
Mycobacterium leprae 359–61
Mycobacterium tuberculosis 355–9
Paracoccidioides brasiliensis 508–9
Penicillium marneffei 509–10
Rickettsia 344–8
Yersinia pestis 314–15
aerobic metabolism 215
Aerococcus 256
Aeromonas 325
aerosolized administration 20–1
aesculin hydrolysis test 226
African histoplasmosis 501–2
African tick bite fever 343, 345
agar, types of commercial chromogenic 219–20
Aggregatibacter
A. actinomycetemcomitans 307
A. aprophilus 306, 307
aggressins 216–17
agriculture, antibiotic use 7
Agrobacterium 294–5
air sampling 178
albendazole 119, 124
ascariasis 543, 586–7
clonorchiasis 565
cutaneous larva migrans 550
cysticercosis 561–2, 731–2
filariasis 555
Giardia lamblia 531
hookworm 545, 586–7
loiasis 556–7
pinworm 548
strongyloidiasis 547
toxocariasis 551
trichenellosis 553
trichuriasis 544
Alcaligenes 294–5
alcohols, disinfectants 173
alert organisms, surveillance of 140–1
allergic bronchopulmonary aspergillosis (ABPA) 485
allergic fungal sinusitis 600
alphaviruses 433–5
amantadine 95–6
Ambisome® 80–1
Ambler classification system 36
American Thoracic Society (ATS), atypical mycobacterial infection guidelines 363
amikacin 46–8, 74–5
aminoglycosides 24–5, 46–8, 74–5, 236
aminopencillins 33
amodiaquine 114–15
artesunate–amodiaquine 118–19
amoebae
amoebiasis 533–5
amoebic liver abscess 534–5, 670–1
amoebic lung abscesses 622
free-living 535–7
amoxicillin 712
AmpC β-lactamases 36
Amphocil 81
amphotericin 80–1, 481
amphotericin see amphotericin
amphotericin 80–1, 119
Candida 478
chromomycosis 497
Coccidioides immitis 507–8
cryptococcal meningitis 727–8
deoxycholate (AmB-d) 473, 727–9
Histoplasma meningitis 729–30
leishmaniaisis 529
lipozomal (LFAmB) 473, 504–5, 529

amphotericin (*Contd.*)
  Penicillium marneffei 509
  peritonitis 664, 665–6
ampicillin
  ampicillin–sulbactam 38
  enterococci 246–7
  meningitis 721
amplified fragment length polymorphism (AFLP) 230
Amsel criteria 696
anaemia 56, 545
anaerobic Gram-negative cocci 280
anaerobic Gram-positive cocci 255
anaerobic infections, synergy in 330
anaerobic metabolism 215
Analytical Profile Index (API) system 221–5
Ancylostoma duodenale 545–6
aneurysm, mycotic 634–5
Angiostrongylus cantonensis 568
anidulofungin 86
animals
  animal bites 320–1, 760
  animal scabies 573
  antibiotic use 7
  causes of encephalitis 733
anisakiasis 569
Anisakis 569
anogenital ulceration 695
anogenital warts 439, 440–1, 699–701
antagonism 17
anthrax 258–60, 770, 848
antibiotic resistance 6
  Acinetobacter 297–9
  aminoglycosides 46, 246–7
  anaerobic gram-negative rods 330
  antituberculous agents 71–4
  Burkholderia cepacia complex 301
  carbapenems 39, 40, 41
  cephalosporins 34
  chloramphenicol 55
  Citrobacter 287
  clonal expansion 12–13
  co-trimoxazole 61
  enteric fever 651
  Enterobacter species 286
  enterococci 246–7, 721
  Eschericihia coli 283
  fusidic acid 70
  glycopeptides 42–3, 239–40, 246–7, 254
  HACEK organisms 307–8
  Helicobacter pylori 329, 647
  ketolides 50
  Klebsiella species 284
  lipopeptides 53
  macrolide–lincosamide–streptogramin B (MLS_B) resistance 50
  macrolides 48–50, 244
  management of antibiotic-resistant organisms 164–6
  mechanisms of resistance 9–10
  metronidazole 65, 329, 647
  molecular genetics of 11–12
  mupirocin 70
  Mycobacterium tuberculosis 356
  Mycoplasma 352
  necrotizing fasciitis 764
  Neisseria gonorrhoeae 278, 709–10
  nitrofurans 66
  non-human use and 7
  overview of responses to 7
  oxazolidinones 54
  Pasteurella 317
  penicillins 4–5, 32–3, 244
  preventing development of 17–18
  Proteus species 285
  pyomyositis 765–6
  quinolones 63
  Salmonella enterica 651
  Serratia 288
  staphylococci 239–40, 241, 721; *see also* meticillin-resistant *Staphylococcus aureus* (MRSA)
  streptococci 243, 244, 249
  streptogramins 52
  sulfonamides 59
  tetracyclines 57
  trimethoprim 60–1
antibiotics
  aminoglycosides 24–5, 46–8, 74–5, 236
  with anaerobic cover 65
  antibiotic-associated diarrhoea/colitis 654–6
  antibiotic-coated/impregnated materials 27, 195–6
  antileprotics 75–7, 361
  antimicrobial stewardship 27–8
  antituberculous agents 71–5, 639
  bacterial vaginosis (BV) 696–7
  β-lactamase inhibitors 37–8
  β-lactamases 10, 35–7
  bite infections 760
  bone/joint infections 775–6, 777, 779–80
  brain abscess 738–9
  carbapenemases 39, 40, 41
  carbapenems 24–5, 39–41
  cephalosporins 24–5, 33–5
  chlamydia 712
  chloramphenicol 56, 651
  cholecystitis 657–8
  cholera 653
  chronic bronchitis 609
  clostridial gas gangrene 762
  community-acquired pneumonia (CAP) 614
  co-trimoxazole, see co-trimoxazole
  CSF shunt infection 742
  cystitis 680–1
  diverticulitis 667
  empyema 595
  enteric fever 651
  fidaxomicin 45–6, 200–1, 655–6
  fusidic acid 69–70
  global use 6–7
  glycopeptides, see glycopeptides
  gonorrhoea 711
  Helicobacter pylori 647
  heteroresistance 13
  history of 4–5
  HIV skin eruptions 826
  infective diarrhoea 649
  lipoglycopeptides 45
  lipopeptides 53–4
  liver abscess 671
  in liver impairment 23–4
  ketolides 50
  macrolides 24–5, 48–50
  mechanisms of action 8–9
  mediastinitis 641
  meningitis 720–2
  monobactams 41
  mupirocin 70–1
  neonatal sepsis 800–1
  neuroborreliosis 730–1
  neutropenic sepsis 815–16
  nitrofurans 66–7
  nitroimidazoles 64–6
  non-human use 7
  novobiocin 67
  ophthalmic infections 747–9, 750–1, 752, 756
  other cell wall agents 41–2
  otitis media 604–5
  outpatient parenteral antimicrobial therapy (OPAT) 28–9
  overview of human use problems 6

oxazolidinones 54–5
pancretitis 660
pelvic inflammatory disease (PID) 706
penicillins *see* penicillins
period of increased incidence (PII)prescribing review 144–5
peritonitis 662, 664, 665–6
pertussis 807
pharmacodynamics 16–18
pharmacokinetics 15–16
pharyngitis 592
polymyxins 68–9
in pregnancy 24–5
prophylaxis *see* antimicrobial prophylaxis
puerperal sepsis 798
pyelonephritis 682
quinolones 24–5, 62–4
in renal impairment 21–3
resistance to *see* antibiotic resistance
rifamycins 67–8
routes of administration 18–21
streptogramins 50, 52–3
subdural empyema 739–40
sulfonamides 4, 58–60
susceptibility testing 13–15
syphilis 716
tetracyclines 24–5, 56–8, 117, 124
trichomoniasis 713
trimethoprim 24–5, 59, 60–2
tropical genital ulceration 701–3
see also antimicrobials; *specific drugs*
antibody deficiency syndromes 810–11
antifolates 116
antifungals 79–87
Aspergillus 488, 521
Blastomyces dermatitidis 504–5
Candida 473, 478
chromomycosis 498
Coccidioides immitis 507–8
Cryptococcus 481
dermatophytes 494
echinocandins 85–6
eumycetoma 492
flucytosine 86, 481, 727–8
griseofulvin 86
Malassezia 478–9
mucormycosis 490
imidazoles 82
introduction to 80
neutropenic sepsis 815–16
Paracoccidioides brasiliensis 508–9
Penicillium marneffei 510
peritonitis 664, 665–6
Pneumocystis jiroveci 483–4
polyenes 80–1
in liver impairment 23–4
in renal impairment 21–3
resistance to 80, 82, 83–4, 86, 478, 492
Sporthrix schenckii 497
terbinafine 87
triazoles 83–4
see also antimicrobials; *specific drugs*
antigenic variation (shift/drift) 375–6
anti-HBc IgG 414–15
anti-HBc IgM 414–15
anti-HBe 414–15
anti-HBs 414–15
antihelminthic drugs 124–6
Ascaris lumbricoides 543
cestodes 559–62, 731–2
cutaneous larva migrans 550
Enterobius vermicularis 548
filariasis 555
Giardia lamblia 531
hookworm 545–6
loiasis 556–7
neurocysticercosis 731–2
onchocerciasis 558
Strongyloides stercoralis 547
toxocariasis 551
trematodes 563–8
trichenollosis 553
Trichuris trichiura 544
antileprotics 75–7, 361
antimalarials 112–13, 513–14
antifolates 116
artemisinin and its derivatives 117–19
in liver impairment 24
other agents and combination therapies 116–17
quinolines 113–15
in renal impairment 23
resistance to 112, 113–15, 116–17, 118
antimicrobial prophylaxis 25–7
anthrax 260
asplenic patients 814
bronchiectasis 626
Candida 475
chronic bronchitis 609
Cryptosporidium 522
in cystic fibrosis 624–5
cystitis 680–1
epiglottitis 597–8
group B *Streptococcus* 253
Haemophillus influenzae 305, 720–2
hepatitis A virus 412
Histoplasma capsulatum 502–3
HIV 154–6, 840–2
hookworm 546
influenza 379
intensive care unit (ICU) infections 183
leptospirosis 342
loiasis 557
lyme disease 340
malaria 112, 514
meningitis 276–7, 720–2
neutropenic sepsis 816
otitis media 604–5
peritonitis 662, 664, 666
plague 315
prosthetic joint infection 782–3
P. jiroveci 483–4
rabies 464–5
S. pneumoniae 245
toxoplasmosis 520
transplant recipients 818
urinary catheter-associated infection 190
whooping cough 311
antimicrobials
basics of *see* antimicrobials (basics of)
coated/impregnated catheters 195
definition of 4–5
prophylaxis *see* antimicrobial prophylaxis
resistance to *see* resistance (antimicrobial)
sepsis/severe sepsis management 581–2
see also antibiotics; antifungals; antiparasitic agents; antivirals
antimicrobials (basics of) 3–29
antimicrobial stewardship 27–8
clonal expansion 12–13
global antibiotic use 6–7
heteroresistance 13
history of antibiotics 4–5
in liver disease 23–4
mechanisms of action 8–9
mechanisms of resistance 9–10
molecular genetics of resistance 11–12
outpatient parenteral antimicrobial therapy (OPAT) 28–9

antimicrobials (basics of) (*Contd.*)
- pharmacodynamics 16–18
- pharmacokinetics 15–16
- in pregnancy 24–5
- prophylaxis see antimicrobial prophylaxis
- in renal impairment 21–3
- routes of administration 18–21
- susceptibility testing 13–15

antimony compounds 119

antiparasitic therapy 111–26
- antihelminthic drugs see antihelminthic drugs
- antimalarials see antimalarials
- antiprotozoal drugs see antiprotozoal drugs

antiprotozoal drugs 119–24
- anti-malarials see anti-malarials
- *Babesia* 516
- *Cryptosporidium* 521–2
- *Cystoisospora* 522–3
- *Entamoeba histolytica* 535
- free-living amoebae 535–7
- *Gardia lamblia* 531
- microsporidia 539
- *Trichomonas vaginalis* 533
- *Trypanosoma* 525, 527
- see also *specific drugs*

antipseudomonal penicillins 33

antiretroviral therapies (ARTs)
- *Cryptococcus* 481
- cytomegalovirus (CMV) 406–7, 408
- HIV protease inhibitors 102, 103, 108–9
- human herpesvirus type 8 396
- non-nucleoside reverse transcriptase inhibitors (NNRTIs) 102, 103, 106–8, 826
  - nucleoside/nucleotide analogue reverse transcriptase inhibitors (NRTIs) 102, 103, 104–6
- *Penicillium marneffei* 510
- *Pneumocystis jiroveci* 483
- prevention of HIV 840–2
- principles of HIV treatment 101–3
- pulmonary tuberculosis 831
- tuberculous meningitis 726–7

antiseptics, coated/impregnated catheters 195

antituberculous agents 39, 71–5, 639

antiviral resistance
- antiretroviral drug therapy (ART) 104, 106, 108, 824
- cytomegalovirus antivirals 92, 93–4, 408
- hepatitis B antivirals 97, 98–9, 416–17
- herpes simplex virus/varicella-zoster virus antivirals 91
- HIV resistance testing 429–30, 824
- influenza antivirals 94–6 378
- respiratory syncytial virus antivirals 96

antivirals 89–110
- aerosolized 21
- antiretroviral therapies see antiretroviral therapies (ARTs)
- cytomegalovirus (CMV) 92–4, 408
- dolutegravir (DTG) 110
- encephalitis 736
- enfuvirtide 110
- enterovirus 432
- Epstein–Barr virus (EBV) 405
- genital herpes 704
- hepatitis B 97–9, 416–17
- hepatitis 99–101, 420–1
- herpes simplex virus (HSV) 90–1, 704
- HIV protease inhibitors 102, 103, 108–9
- HIV treatment principles 101–3
- influenza 94–6, 378–9
- in liver impairment 23–4
- maraviroc (MVC) 110
- meningitis 724
- non-nucleoside reverse transcriptase inhibitors (NNRTIs) 102, 103, 106–8, 826
  - nucleoside/nucleotide analogue reverse transcriptase inhibitors (NRTIs) 102, 103, 104–6
- raltegravir (RAL) 110
- in renal impairment 21–3
- resistance to, see antiviral resistance
- respiratory syncytial virus (RSV) 96
- varicella-zoster virus (VZV) 90–1, 401
- see *also* antimicrobials; *specific drugs*

aphthous ulcers 828

aplastic anaemia 56

Arachnida 575–6

arboviruses 722–4

Arcanobacterium haemolyticum 267

Arenaviridae 370, 459

arenaviruses 462–3

Argentine haemorrhagic fever 459

Artekin 118–19

artemether–lumefantrine 118–19

artemisinins 112–13, 117–19

artemotil 118

artesunate 113, 118
- artesunate–amodiaquine 118–19
- artesunate–mefloquine 118–19
- artesunate–sulfadoxine–pyrimethamine 118–19

arthether 118

arthritis/arthralgia
- alphaviruses 433, 434
- reactive 776–8
- septic 774–5

arthrocentesis 781–2

arthroconidia 505

ascariasis 543, 586–7

Ascaris lumbricoides 543, 549

ascitic fluid 219, 661–2

Ascomycota 471

aseptic technique, CVC care 164

aspergilloma 484–7

aspergillosis 484–8

Aspergillus 85–6, 484–8, 766

aspiration pneumonia 617

asplenic patients 814

assembly, viral 368

Astroviridae 411

astroviruses 411

atazanavir 108–9
- associated cholelithiasis 836

atovaquone 116–17, 119, 516

auramine stain 222–4

autoclaves 175

azithromycin 49–50
- babesiosis 516
- chlamydia 712, 750–1
- cholera 653
- enteric fever 651

gonorrhoea 278
pelvic inflammatory disease (PID) 706
aztreonam 41

B

Babesia 515–16
babesiosis 515–16
bacillary angiomatosis (BA) 348–50, 771, 825
Bacillus species 257–8
B. anthracis 258–60, 770, 848
bacitracin 41–2
bacteraemia
Acinetobacter 298
Bacteroides 330–1
Bartonella 348–50
catheter-associated UTI 686–8
definition 580
endovascular infection and 634–6
enterococcal 246–7
Erysipelothrix rhusiopathiae 265–6
Escherichia coli 281
Gardnerella 309
group A *Streptococcus* (GAS) 250, 251
Listeria 263–5
primary/secondary 187
S. bovis 247–8
bacteria 207–362
automated diagnostics 228
basic bacteriology principles 209
biochemical tests 225–7
culture media 219–20
encephalitis diagnosis 736
genetics of 212–14
gram-negative cocci overview 274
gram-negative rods overview 293–4, 303
gram-positive cocci overview 233–4
gram-positive rods overview 256
growth and metabolism 214–16
hazard groups 160
identification of 221–5
microbiological specimens 218–19
molecular organism identification 229
molecular typing methods 229–31
quality assurance and accreditation (laboratory) 231–3
structure and function 210–12
virulence and pathogenicity 216–17
see also specific bacteria
bacterial folate synthesis 58–60
bacterial peliosis (BP) 348–50
bacterial vaginosis (BV) 309, 695–7
bactericidal antibiotics 13
bacteriophages 11–12, 213–14
bacteriostatic antibiotics 13
bacteriuria
asymptomatic 678, 686, 687–8
see also urinary tract infection (UTI)
Bacteroides 329–31
balanitis 695
Ballamuthia mandrillaris 537
Barrett's oesophagus 646
barrier nursing 163–4
Bartonella species 348–50, 770–1
bartonellosis 348–50
Basidomycota 471
Becton Dickinson 228
bedaquiline 74–5
beef tapeworm 559–60
Bell's palsy 340
benzathine benzyl pencillin 716
benzimidazoles 124–5
benznidazole 120, 525
benzylpenicillin 708–9, 716
β-galactosidase test 227
β-lactam ring 32
β-lactamase inhibitors 37–8
β-lactamases 10, 35–7
bioavailability 15
biochemical tests 225–7
biofilm formation 235
Biomerieux 228
biopsy samples 219
bone 779
liver 672–4
peptic ulcer disease 646
transbronchial 483
bioterrorism 258–60, 311–13, 317–18, 846–8
biothonol 566–8
bite infections 320–1, 760
BK virus 442–3
Blastomyces dermatitidis 503–5
bleach 173
blepharitis 746
blood agar 219–20
blood cultures 188–9, 218
blood fluke 563–4
blood transfusion *see* transfusion
bloodstream infection (BSI) 136, 187–9, 632–4
boceprevir 100
body fluids, infectivity of 151–3
Bolivian haemorrhagic fever 459
bone and joint infection 773–84
Blastomyces dermatitidis 503–5
Candida 477
Coccidioides immitis 506–8
diabetic foot infections 783–4
osteomyelitis 778–80
prosthetic joint infections 780–3
reactive arthritis 776–8
septic arthritis 774–5
septic bursitis 775–6
sporotrichosis 496–7
bone marrow suppression 56
bone marrow transplantation (BMT) 406–7, 437–8, 442–3, 817–18
borderline leprosy 360
Bordetella 310–11, 806–8
Borrelia 334, 337–40, 730–1
botulism 267–8, 848
bovine spongiform encephalopathy (BSE) 466–7
bowel surgery 187
brain abscess 534–5, 737–9
breakpoints 15, 17–18
breastfeeding, antimicrobials in 24–5
Brevundimonas 294
Brill–Zinsser disease 343, 345–6
British Society for Antimicrobial Chemotherapy (BSAC) 14–15
British Thoracic Society (BTS), atypical mycobacterial infection guidelines 363
bronchiectasis 625–6
bronchiolitis 21, 96, 381–2, 609–11
bronchitis
acute 606–7
chronic 607–9
Chlamydophila pneumoniae 355
tracheobronchitis 381–2, 486–8
bronchoalveolar lavage (BAL) 483, 487–8, 612–13

Brucella 311–13
brucellosis 311–13
Brugia species 554–5
bubonic plague 314–15
buccal space infection 605
buffered charcoal yeast extract (BCYE) agar 219–20
bulbar paralytic polio 446–7
Bunyaviridae 370, 435, 459
Burkholderia
B. cepacia complex 300–1, 623
B. gladioli 316
B. pseudomallei 302–3
Burkitt's lymphoma 404
bursitis, septic 775–6
Bush–Jacoby–Medeiros classification system 36

C

Calabar swelling 556–7
Calciviridae 410–11
Campylobacter 326–7
canaliculitis 746
Candida species 472–8
candidaemia/candidiasis, invasive 476
candiduria 477, 687–8
echinocandins 85–6
HIV complications 825, 828, 833
invasive infections (overview) 476–7
oesophagitis 475, 644–5
overview 472–3
skin infections 766–8, 825
superficial infections (overview) 475
treatment 473, 478
vulvovaginal candidiasis 475, 697–9
Capillaria philippinensis 569–70
capillariasis 569–70
Capnocytophaga 320–1
capsid 366
capsules, bacterial surface structure 211–12, 216–17
carbapenemase-producing Enterobacteriaceae (CPE) 167
carbapenemases 39, 40, 41
carbapenems 24–5, 39–41
carbon, bacterial growth 214
carbuncles 758–9
Cardiobacterium hominis 307–8
cardiovascular disease/ infections 629–41
candidiasis 476
cardiomyopathy 524–5, 829
congenital heart disease 738
Corynebacterium diphtheriae 260–1
endovascular infections 634–6
Entamoeba histolytica 534
HIV complications 829–30
infective endocarditis see infective endocarditis (IE)
intravascular catheter-related infections 632–4; see also central venous catheter (CVC)-related infections
mediastinitis 640–1
myocarditis 636–8
pericarditis 499–500, 502, 638–9, 830
syphilis 714–15
Trichenella species 552–3
valvular disease 347, 348, 476
care bundle approach see High Impact Interventions (Saving Lives)
caries, dental 603
carrier, definition 130
caspo 473
caspofungin 85–6, 488
Castleman's disease 394–6
cat-scratch disease 348–50, 770–1
catalase test 226
catheter-related infection
intravascular 193–6, 632–4; see also central venous catheter (CVC)-related infections; peripheral venous catheters (PVCs)
urinary 189–91, 686–8
CD4 T-lymphocyte count
Cryptococcus treatment 481
Cyclospora 523
HIV classification 821–2, 822
HIV complications and 821
HIV treatment principles 101–3
initial HIV patient evaluation 824
laboratory testing 429
microsporidia 538
natural history of HIV infection 819–21
Penicillium marneffei 510
Pneumocystis jiroveci prevention 483–4
Sporothrix schenkii 496
toxoplasmosis 517, 520
cefixime 651
cefotaxime 721, 730–1
ceftazidime 721, 738–9
ceftriaxone
bacterial meningitis 720–2
brain abscess 738–9
conjunctivitis 750–1
enteric fever 290, 651
gonorrhoea 278
neuroborreliosis 730–1
pelvic inflammatory disease (PID) 706
cell-mediated immunity (CMI) 470
cell walls
structure and function of bacterial 211
inhibition of synthesis 8
cellulitis 759, 783
Centers for Disease Control and Prevention , HIV classification 821–2
central European encephalitis (CEE) 453–4
central nervous system see neurological disease/ infection
central venous catheter (CVC)-related infection 632–4
bloodstream infection (BSI) 187–9, 632–4
catheter line tip specimens 219
high impact intervention no. 1 164, 188
sepsis 194–6, 581–2
cephalosporins 24–5, 33–5; see also specific types
cephamycins 34–5
cerebellar ataxia 735
cerebral aspergillosis 486–7, 487–8
cerebrospinal fluid (CSF)
bacterial meningitis (overview) 719–20
chronic meningitis 725–6
CJD protein markers 466–7
coccidioidal meningitis 728–9

cryptococcal
meningitis 727–8
CSF shunt infection 741–3
encephalitis 732–6
enterovirus diagnosis 432
Histoplasma
meningitis 729–30
microbiological
specimens 219
neuroborreliosis 730–1
neurocysticercosis 731–2
syphilis 715–16
tuberculous
meningitis 726–7
viral meningitis
(overview) 723–4
Cervarix® 441
cervical cancer,
invasive 839–40
cervical HPV 440–1, 839–40
cervical intraepithelial
neoplasia (CIN) 439,
440–1, 839–40
cervix, strawberry 713
cestodes 549, 559–62; *see also specific cestodes*
cetrimide agar 219–20
Chaga's disease 523–5
chagoma 524–5
chancroid 701
chemical sterilization 175–6
chemotherapy 450
chickenpox 399–402, 768–9,
791; *see also* varicella-zoster virus (VAV)
chikungunya 434, 459
children/infants 785–08
bacterial causes of illness
(overview) 804–8
botulism 267–8
cystitis 680, 681
encephalitis causes 733
enteroviral
infections 803–4
human herpesvirus
type 6 393
meningitis empirical
therapy 721
non-routine immunizations 844, 845
primary peritonitis 661
progressive disseminated histoplasmosis
(PDH) 500–1
renal scarring 683–4
routine immunizations 844
vesico-ureteric reflux
(VUR) 683–4
viral causes of illness
(overview) 801
see also congenital
infections; neonatal
infection; *specific infectious diseases*
Chinese liver fluke 565
Chlamydia 352–5
conjunctivitis 749–51
C. pneumoniae 355, 616
C. psittaci 354–5, 616
C. trachomatis 353–4,
701–2, 705–6, 711–12
keratitis 752
N. gonorrhoeae and 277–8
chloramphenicol 56, 651
chlorhexidine 173
chlorine bleach 175–6
chloroquine 113, 114
chloroxylenols 173
chlorproguanil
chlorproguanil–dapsone 117
chlortetracycline 56–8
chocolate agar 219–20
cholangiopathy
acute cholangitis 658
cholecystitis 656–8
HIV complications 836
cholera 321–2, 652–3
chorioamnionitis 796–7
chorioretinitis 518, 519–20
chromomycosis 497–8, 767
chronic mucocutaneous
candidiasis 766
Chryseobacterium 294–5
Chryseomonas 294–5
cidofovir 90, 93–4, 408, 438
Cierny–Mader system 778
ciprofloxacin 63–4, 120
anthrax 259
cholera 653
enteric fever 651
Neisseria
meningitidis 276, 720–2
circumcision, male 840–1
cirrhosis 416–17, 419–21,
661–2, 674
Citrobacter species 286–7
clarithromycin 49, 76, 120,
328–9, 647
classification
basic bacteriology
principles 209
β-lactamases 36
cephalosporins 34
corynebacteria 262
gram-positive cocci 233
gram-positive rods 256
HIV 821–3
non-tuberculous
mycobacteria 361–2
penicillins 32
streptococci 242, 248–9
sulfonamides 58–60
tetracyclines 56
viruses 366
clavulanate 37–8
ticarcillin–clavulanate 38
Clean Care is Safer
Care 146–50
cleaning, hospital *see* hospital
cleaning
Cleanyourhands
Campaign 150
CLED agar 219–20
clindamycin 51–2
antiprotozoal action 120
Babesia 516
bacterial vaginosis
(BV) 696–7
group A *Streptococci* 251
malaria 117
pelvic inflammatory disease
(PID) 706
in pregnancy 24–5
toxic shock
syndrome 708–9
clinical governance 142
Clinical Pathology
Accreditation (CPA) UK
Ltd 232
clinical specimens *see* microbiological specimens
clinical trials, infection
control 133
clinical waste 180–1
clofazimine 76
clonal expansion 12–13
clone 12–13
clonorchiasis 565, 567
Clonorchis sinensis 565, 567
Clostridium species 267–71
C. botulinum 267–8, 848
C. difficile infection
(CDI) 196–202, 654–6
C. sordellii 707–9
C. tetani 269
disease overview 268
gas gangrene 270–1, 762
clotrimazole 82
coagulase-negative staphylococci (CoNS) 240–1
coagulase test 226
co-amoxiclav 38
Coartem® 118–19
cocci
gram-negative 223
gram-positive 221, 233–4
see also specific groups/species
Coccidioides
immitis 505–8, 728–9
coccidioidomycosis 728–9
Cockroft and Gault
formula 22
cohorting (patient) 146
colistimethate
sodium 21, 68–9

colitis, antibiotic-associated 654–6
colonization
  colonial morphology 225
  definition 130
  MRSA nasal/extranasal 165
  small colony variants 235
common cold 590–1
common variable immunodeficiency 810
community infection
  community-acquired coronavirus 383
  community-acquired MRSA (CA-MRSA) 237–8
  community-acquired pneumonia (CAP) 611–617
  definition 130
  infection control in community 138, 202
comparative genomic hybridization 231
complement fixation tests 501–2
concentration-dependent killing 17
condylomata 439
congenital infections/disease 786–9
  congenital heart disease 738
  cytomegalovirus (CMV) 788
  enterovirus 787
  herpes simplex virus (HSV) 788–9
  parvovirus 787
  rubella 788
  syphilis 714–15
  toxoplasmosis 518, 519–20, 786
  varicella-zoster virus (VZV) 787
Congo–Crimean haemorrhagic fever (CCHF) 435–6, 459
conjugation 213–14
conjunctivitis 749–51
  inclusion 353–4
  kertatoconjunctivitis 353–4, 437–8
CONSORT (Consolidated Standards of Reporting Trials) 133
contact tracing 146, 694
containment levels (CL) 162–3
continuous ambulatory peritoneal dialysis (CAPD) 664–6
controls assurance 142
copreomycin 73–4
coronary artery bypass graft 187
Coronaviridae 370
coronaviruses 383–4
corticosteroids
  aspergillus 485
  bacterial meningitis 720
  bronchiolitis 610–11
  croup 596–7
  cysticercosis 561–2
  cytomegalovirus 405
  enteric fever 651
  neurocysticercosis 731–2
  septic arthritis 775
  TB pericarditis 639
  trichinellosis 553
corynebacteria
  C. diphtheriae 260–2
  non-diphtheria 262–3
co-trimoxazole 61–2, 120
  cholera 653
  Cystoisospora 522–3
  meningitis 721
  Penicillium marneffei 509–10
  Pneumocystis jiroveci 483–4
  in pregnancy 24–5
  toxoplasmosis prophylaxis 520
cough 596–7, 607–9
cowpox 444
Coxiella burnetii 346–8, 617
Coxsackie A/B viruses 430–2
crab louse 572–3
cranial nerve abnormalities 735
creatinine clearance (CrCl) 16, 22
creeping eruption 550
Creutzfeldt–Jakob disease (CJD) 169–72, 466–7, 467
crockery 152
croup 381–2, 596–7, 598
cryptococcosis 825
Cryptococcus 480–1
  C. neoformans 222–4, 480–1, 727–8, 825
  cryptococcal meningitis 480–1, 727–8, 838–9
cryptosporidiosis 520–2
Cryptosporidium 520–2
CSF *see* cerebrospinal fluid (CSF)
CSF shunt infection 741–3
CTX-M β-lactamases 36–7
Cullen sign 659
culture media, bacterial 219–20
CURB-65 score 590–1, 612–13
cutaneous infections *see* skin/soft tissue infections
cyclophosphilin inhibitors 101
cycloserine 42, 74
Cyclospora 523
CYP3A4 16
cystic fibrosis (CF) 20–1, 296, 300–1, 623–5
cysticercosis 561–2
cystitis 679–81
  candidal 473
  haemorrhagic 437–8
cysts 561–2, 731–2
cytoadherence 513
Cystoisospora 522–3
cytomegalovirus (CMV) 92–4, 405–8, 644–5, 788, 838–9
cytopathic effect, viruses 368
cytoplasm 210
cytoplasmic membrane 211
  disruption of 9

D

daclatasvir 101, 420–1
dacryoadenitis 747
dacryocystitis 747
dalbavancin 45
dalfopristin 52–3
  quinupristin–dalfopristin 52–3
danazol 450
dapsone 75–6, 120
  chlorproguanil–dapsone 117
daptomycin 53–4, 236, 238
dark-walled fungi 495
debridement and implant retention (DAIR) 782
decontamination 130
delamanid 74–5
delaviridine 106–8
Delftia acidovorans 294
demeclocycline 56–8
dementia
  encephalitis and 735
  HIV-associated 838–9
dengue fever (DF)/dengue haemorrhagic fever (DHF) 457–8
dengue virus 457–8
dental infection 605–6, 738, 833
deoxyribonuclease (Dnase) test 226
Department of Health guidance

blood cultures 188–9
Clostridium difficile infection (CDI) 199–200
infection prevention/ control in adult critical care 184
dermatolymphangioadenitis (DLA) 554
dermatophytes 492–4, 767, 825
developing world, antibiotic use problems 6
dexamethasone 720
diabetes patients
foot infections 783–4
mucormycosis 489–90
dialysis, infection control 158
diarrhoea (infective) 647–9
adenovirus 437–8
Aeromonas 325
antibiotic-associated diarrhoea 654–6
astroviruses 411
Bacillus 257, 258
Bacteroides 330–1
Campylobacter 326–7
cholera 322, 652–3
Clostridium difficile-associated (CDAD) 198–201, 654–6
Cryptosporidium 520–2
Cyclospora 523
Entamoeba histolytica 533–5
E scherichia coli 281, 282
Giardia lamblia 530–2
HIV complication 834
hospital epidemics 196–7
norovirus 410–11
Pleisomonas shigelloides 326
rotavirus 409–10
stool samples 219, 648–9
traveller's 281, 282, 647–8
tropical sprue/ enteropathy 675
Vibrios 322, 323, 324–5
viral gastroenteritis overview 408
virus overview 370
Yersinia enterocolitica 315
see also gastrointestinal (GI) infections/diseases; *specific causes/ diseases*
didanosine 104–6
Dienes phenomenon 284–5
diethylcarbamazine (DEC) 125, 555, 556–7, 558
di George syndrome 811–12
dihydroartemisinin 118
dihydroartemisinin–piperaquine 118–19
diloxanide furoate 120
dilution methods, susceptibility testing 14–15
diphtheria 260–2
Diphylobothrium latum 549, 560
Dipylidum caninum 549
Director of Infection Prevention and Control (DIPC) 138
disc diffusion, susceptibility testing 14–15
disinfection 172–4
Clostridium difficile 201
definition 130
distribution, pharmacokinetics 15
diverticulitis 666–7
DNA
bacterial structure and function 210
mechanisms of resistance 11–12
next generation sequencing (NGS) 228, 231
random amplification of polymorphic 230
DNA gyrase 62–3, 67
DNA viruses
genome 366–7
genome replication 367–8
overview of 370
see also specific viruses
dolutegravir 110
donovanosis 702–3
doxycycline 56–8, 117
anthrax 259
chlamydia 712, 750–1
cholera 653
filariasis 555
leptospirosis 342
lyme disease 340, 730–1
onchocerciasis 558
pelvic inflammatory disease (PID) 706
spotted fevers 344–5
dracunculiasis 553–4
Dracunculus medinensis 553–4
drainage
pyomyositis 765–6
septic arthritis 775
dressings, line infection minimization 195
drugs
drug eruptions in HIV 826
pharmacodynamics 16–18
pharmacokinetics 15–16
secondary immunodeficiency causes 813
see also specific drugs/ drug types
Duke criteria 631
duodenal ulceration 646
dwarf tapeworm 549, 561
dysentry 291–2

E

eagle effect 17
ear infection
mastoiditis 601–2, 738
otitis externa 602–3
otitis media 603–5, 738
East African trypanosomiasis 526–7
eastern equine encephalitis (EEE) 433–5
Ebola 459, 461–2
echino 473
echinocandins 85–6, 478
echinococcosis 562
Echinococcus 562
echoviruses 430–2
econazole 82
ecthyma 759
ectoparasites 571–6
education, infection control 153
Edwardsiella tarda 292–3
efavirenz 106–8
efflux pumps 10, 57
eflornithine 120–1, 527
EIA, toxin 198–9
Eikenella corrodens 294–5, 307, 308
elastography 419–20
Elizabethkingia meningoseptica 292–3
emphysematous pyelonephritis 684
empyema 619–21
subdural 739–40
emtricitabine 104–6
Encephalitazoon 537–9
encephalitis 732–7
adenovirus 437–8
alphaviruses 433–5
California encephalitis (CE) 435–6
chronic 725
clinical features and causes 735
enterovirus 431–2
epidemiological factors and causes 725, 733
flaviviruses 451–4
granulomatous amoebic (GAM) 536–7

encephalitis (*Contd.*)
herpes simplex virus (HSV) 397–9
HIV complication 838–9
human herpesvirus type 6 393–4
laboratory diagnosis 732–6
mumps 387–8
polioencephalitis 446–7
rabies virus 463–5
subacute sclerosing panencephalitis (SSPE) 385–6
virus overview 370
see also meningoencephalitis
endocarditis *see* infective endocarditis (IE)
endogenous infection 135
endophthalmitis 473, 485, 754–6
endoscopes, sterilization 175–6
endotoxins 217
enfuvirtide 110
Entamoeba histolytica 533–5
entecavir 98–9, 416–17
enteric fever 288–90, 649–51
Enterobacter species 285–6
Enterobacteriaceae
carbapenemase-producing (CPE) 167
see also specific species
Enterobius vermicularis 548, 549
enterococci 42–3, 245–7, 721
Enterocytozoon bieneusi 537–9
enteroviruses 430–2, 445–6, 722–4, 787, 801, 803–4
environmental disinfectants 172–4
environmental issues/factors
bacterial growth 215
infection control 137, 144–5, 162–3, 172–4, 176–8
ventilation systems 176–8
enzyme production
bacterial virulence factor 216–17
mechanism of resistance 10
eosinophilia 546–7, 568
pulmonary infiltrates with 619
epidemic influenza 376
epidemic typhus 343, 345–6
epidermodysplasia verruciformis 439, 440–1
Epidermophyton 492–4
epididymitis 689–90
epididymo-orchitis 387–8
epidural abscess 740–1
epiglottitis 596, 597–8
Epstein–Barr virus (EBV) 402–5, 801, 828
EQUATOR Network 133
equipment
containment level (CL) 162–3
Creutzfeldt–Jakob disease (CJD) 169–72
HIV/hepatitis B/hepatitis C patient care 152
period of increased incidence (PII) review 144–5
sterilization 174–6
transmissible spongiform encephalopathies (TSEs) 169–72
erlichiae 736
ertapenem 39–40
erysipelas 759
erysipeloid 265–6
Erysipelothrix rhusiopathiae 265–6, 770
erythema chronicum migrans (EM) 338–40
erythema infectiosum (EI) (parvovirus B19) 391–2, 787, 790–1, 792–4, 801
erythema nodosum leprosum 77, 360
erythromycin 49, 712, 750–1
Escherichia coli 280–3, 721
E-test 14–15
ethambutol 42, 72, 726–7
ethionamide 74
ethylene oxide (EO) sterilization 175–6
etravirine 106–8
eumycetoma 273, 491–2, 767
European Committee on Antimicrobial Susceptibility Testing (EUCAST) 14–15, 239
European Prevalence of Infection in Intensive Care (EPIC) study 182
exanthem subitum 393
excretion, pharmacokinetics 16
exit site infection 632
exogenous infection 135
exotoxins 217
extended-spectrum β-lactamases (ESBLs) 36–7
ESBL detection methods 37
extended-spectrum penicillins 33
eye infections *see* ophthalmological infections

F

famciclovir 90–1, 704
Fasciola hepatica 565–6, 567
fascioliasis 565–6, 567
fastidious gram-negative rods, overview 303
fatal familial insomnia (FFI) 468
fenticonazole 82
fetid foot 783
fever 579–87
eosinophilia in travellers 586–7
haemorrhagic *see* haemorrhagic fever
imported fever 584–6
introduction 580
puerperal pyrexia 797–8
pyrexia of unknown origin (PUO) 582–4
sepsis and severe sepsis *see* sepsis
fidaxomicin 45–6, 200–1, 655–6
filariasis 554–5
Filoviridae 370, 459
filoviruses 461–2
fimbriae 212, 280
financial/economic issues 130–5, 143, 181–2, 188, 189–91
fish tapeworm 549, 560
flagellae 212
Flagyl *see* metronidazole
Flavimonas oryzihabitans 294–5
Flaviviridae 370, 451–4, 459
flaviviruses 451–61
Flavobacterium 294–5
Fleming, Alexander 4–5
floppy child syndrome 267–8
flubendazole 125
flucloxacillin 236, 721, 747–8
flucon 473
fluconazole 83, 121
Candida 473, 475, 478, 698–9
coccidioidal meningitis 728–9
cryptococcal meningitis 727–8

flucytosine 86, 481, 727–8
fluids, microbiological specimens 219
flukes 563–8
fluoroquinolones 62–4, 74–5
folate synthesis, inhibition of 9
folliculitis 758, 826
  Malassezia 479
food poisoning 257–8, 267–8, 647–9
foot infection, diabetic 783–4
formaldehyde sterilization 175–6
fosamprenavir 108–9
foscarnet 93, 408
fosfomycin 42
Francisella 317–18, 848
free-living amoebae 535–7
fumagillin 121, 539
fungal antigen detection assays 472–3
fungi 469–510
  antifungals, *see* antifungals
  encephalitis 736
  hazard groups 160
  overview of 470
  skin infection overview 766–8
  see also specific fungi/ infections
furazolidone 66–7, 121, 531, 653
furuncles 758–9
furunculoid myiasis 574–5
fusariosis 495
Fusarium species 495, 767
fusidic acid 69–70
Fusobacterium 329–31, 332–3

G

gall bladder
  acute cholangitis 658
  cholecystectomy 657–8
  cholecystitis 656–8
gall stones 656–8
ganciclovir 92, 406–7, 408, 438
gangrene
  diabetic foot infections 783
  gas gangrene 270–1, 762
Gardasil® 441
Gardnerella 309
gas gangrene 270–1, 762
gastrointestinal (GI) infections/disease 643–76
  acute cholangitis 658
  anthrax 258–9
  botulism 267–8
  candidiasis 475, 644
  Chaga's disease 524–5
  cholecystitis 656–8
  cholera 322, 652–3
  Clostridium difficile 196–202, 654–6
  common organisms in hospital-acquired 136
  community-acquired coronavirus 383
  Cryptosporidium 520–2
  diverticulitis 666–7
  dysentery 291–2, 647–9
  enteric fever 288–90, 649–51
  Escherichia coli 281, 282
  food poisoning 257–8, 267–8, 647–9
  gastroenteritis 289–90, 315, 325–6, 327, 408, 647–9
  gastro-oesophageal reflux disease (GORD) 646
  haemorrhagic colitis 281, 282
  hepatitis, *see* hepatitis
  HIV complications 833–4
  hookworm 545–6
  hospital epidemics of diarrhoea/vomiting 196–7
  infective diarrhoea overview 647–9
  intestinal flukes 566
  intestinal nematode overview 542
  intra-abdominal abscess 667–71
  liver abscess 670–1
  malignancy 247–8, 646
  mesenteric adenitis 316, 674–5
  microsporidia 537–9
  mucormycosis 489–90
  oesophagitis 397–8, 473, 475, 644–5
  pancreatitis 659–60, 836–7
  peptic ulcer disease 327–9, 645–7
  peritoneal dialysis peritonitis 664–6
  pinworm 548
  primary peritonitis 661–2
  Salmonella 196–7, 288–90, 649–51
  schistosomiasis 563–4
  secondary peritonitis 662–4
  strongyloidiasis 546–7
  tropical sprue/ enteropathy 675
  typhlitis 675
  Whipple's disease 676
  Yersinia enterocolitica 315
  Yersinia pseudotuberculosis 316
  see also diarrhoea (infective); vomiting
gatifloxacin 64
genetics
  bacterial genetics overview 212–14
  gene transfer mechanisms 213–14
  genotypic susceptibility testing methods 14–15
  hepatitis B virus 413–17
  HIV genomic structure 426
  molecular genetics of resistance 11–12
  molecular organism identification 229
  molecular typing methods 229–31
  viral genome 366–7
  viral genome replication 367–8
  see also DNA
genital herpes 703–4
genital lumps 695
  genital warts 439, 440–1, 699–701
genital ulceration 695, 703–4
  tropical 701–3
genitourinary (GU) tract infection
  Blastomyces dermatitidis 503–4
  microsporidia 537–9
  see also urinary tract infection (UTI)
gentamicin 46–8, 706, 721, 742
Gerstmann–Sträussler–Scheinker syndrome 468
Ghon complex 356
Giardia lamblia 530–2
gingivitis 833
glanders 303
glass, disposal 180
global context, antibiotic use 6–7
Global Polio Eradication Initiative 446
glomerular filtration rate (GFR) 22
  estimated (eGFR) 22
Glucatell 472–3
glucocorticoids 777
glucose non-fermenters 294–5
glue ear 604–5

glutamate dehydrogenase (GDH) 198–9
glutaraldehyde sterilization 175–6
glycopeptides 42–4
  gram-positive organism resistance overview 254
  Leuconostoc resistance 254
  monitoring of 44–5
  MRSA treatment 238
  in pregnancy 24–5
  S. aureus resistance 42–3, 239–40
  see also specific drugs
gonorrhoea 277–8, 709–11
Gradenigo's syndrome 740
gram-negative cocci 223, 274; *see also specific groups/species*
gram-negative rods 224, 293–4, 303; *see also specific groups/species*
gram-positive cocci 221, 233–4; *see also specific groups/species*
gram-positive rods 222, 256; *see also specific groups/species*
Gram stain 210, 222–4
  positive/negative cell wall structure 211
granuloma
  conjunctival 749–50
  granuloma inguinale 702–3
  lymphogranuloma venereum (LGV) 353–4, 701–2
  mediastinal 499–500, 501–2
granulomatous amoebic encephalitis (GAM) 536–7
granulomatous prostatitis 689
grey baby syndrome 56
Grey Turner sign 659
griseofulvin 86
group A *Streptococcus* (GAS) 249–51, 591–2
group B *Streptococcus* (GBS)/*S. agalactiae* 252–3, 721
group C streptococci 254
group F streptococci 254
group G streptococci 254
growth, bacterial 214–16, 225
Guanarito virus 459
Guillain–Barré syndrome (GBS) 327
guinea worm infection 553–4
gummatous syphilis 714–15

H

H1N1 virus 375–6
HACEK organisms 306–8
haematuria 679
haemolysis 225, 242
haemophagocytic syndrome 391–2
Haemophilus 303–8
  H. ducreyi 306, 701
  H. haemolyticus 306
  H. influenzae 303–5, 306, 307, 720–2
  H. parahaemolyticus 306, 307
  H. parainfluenzae 306, 307
haemorrhagic colitis 281, 282
haemorrhagic fever
  Congo–Crimean haemorrhagic fever (CCHF) 435, 459
  dengue (DHF) 457–8, 459
  Omsk 454, 459
  overview of viral (VHF) 459–61
  with renal syndrome 435–6, 459
Hafnia alvei 292–3
Hamman's sign 640
hand, foot and mouth (HFM) 803–4
hand hygiene
  Clostridium difficile infection (CDI) 201
  handwashing 146–50
  high impact interventions (HII) 164
  period of increased incidence (PII) review 144–5
Hansen's disease, *see* leprosy
hantavirus 435–6, 459
Hartford nomogram 47–8
hazard groups 160
hazard versus risk 142
HBcAg 413–17
HBeAg 413–17
HBsAg 413–17
HBV DNA 413–17
HCV RNA 419–21
head infections 589–628
  dental infection 605–6, 738, 833
  mastoiditis 601–2, 738
  otitis externa 602–3
  otitis media 603–5, 738
  sinusitis 599–601, 738
  see also ophthalmological infections; respiratory infections; *specific infections*
head lice 572–3
head trauma 738
Health and Social Care Act 132
healthcare-associated/acquired infection (HCAI)
  meticillin-resistant *S. aureus* (HA-MRSA) 237–8
  prevention of *see* infection control
  see also hospital-acquired infection (HAI); nosocomial infection
healthcare workers (HCW)
  hospital-acquired infection risk factors 136
  hospital diarrhoea and vomiting epidemics 197
  management of risks from patients 151–3
  management of risks from virally infected 158–60
  tuberculosis transmission from 169
Healthcare-associated infections:prevention and control in primary and community care 202
health protection 843–9
  bioterrorism 258–60, 311–13, 317–18, 846–8
  immunization, *see* vaccination/immunization
  migrant health 848–9
  notifiable disease 845–6
Health Technical Memorandum (HTM) 03-01 177–8
Hektoen enteric (HE) agar 219–20
Helicobacter 327–9, 645–7
helminths 541–70
  antihelminthic drugs, *see* antihelminthic drugs
  encephalitis 736
  identification of ova 549
  see also specific helminths
HEPA filter 177
Hepadnaviridae 370
hepatic infection/disease see liver disease/infection; *specific diseases/infections*
hepatic steatosis 835
hepatitis
  acute 424, 671–3
  chronic 673–4
  encephalitis causes 735
  HIV and viral 835–6
  viruses overview 423–5
  see also specific viruses
hepatitis A virus (HAV) 411–12, 671–3, 835–6

hepatitis B immune globulin (HBIG) 154–6
hepatitis B virus (HBV) 413–17, 671–4
  antivirals for 97–9
  HIV complication 835–6
  infected health-care worker risk management 158–9
  management of risks to health-care workers 137, 151–2
  pregnancy 794, 795
hepatitis C virus (HCV) 418–21, 671–4
  antivirals for 99–101
  HIV complication 835–6
  infected health-care worker risk management 159
  management of risks to health-care workers 137, 152
  sharps injury from infected donor 137
hepatitis D virus (HDV) 417–18, 671–4
hepatitis E virus (HEV) 421–3, 671–4, 835–6
hepatitis G virus 424
herpangina 803–4
herpes gladiatorum 768
herpes labialis, recurrent 768
herpes simplex virus (HSV) 396–9
  antivirals for 90–1
  genital herpes 703–4
  HIV prevention and suppression of 840–1
  HIV skin complications 826
  keratitis 751, 752
  oesophagitis 644–5
  pregnancy and childhood 788–9, 801
  skin infections 768, 826
  tropical genital ulceration 701–3
herpes zoster (shingles) 399–402, 768–9, 791, 826; *see also* varicella-zoster virus (VZV)
Herpesviridae 370, 399
Herpesviruses 392
  cytomegalovirus (CMV) 92–4, 405–8, 644–5, 788, 838–9
  herpes simplex virus *see* herpes simplex virus (HSV)
  human herpesvirus type 6 393–4, 801
  human herpesvirus type 7 394
  human herpesvirus type 8 394–6, 827
  viral meningitis 722–4
herpetic whitlow 768
heterophile antibodies 404–5
Heterophyes heterophyes 566, 567
heterophyiasis 566, 567
heteroresistance 13, 239
Hexapoda 572–5
High Impact Interventions (Saving Lives) 132
  No. 1 central venous catheter care 164, 188–9
  No. 2 peripheral line care 194
  No. 4 preventing surgical site infection 186
  No. 5 ventilator care 193
  No. 6 urinary catheter care 190
  Nos. 7 and 8 *C. difficile* infection 199
hip joint replacement 187, 780–3
Histoplasma capsulatum 498–503, 729–30
  meningitis 729–30
histoplasmoma 499–500
histoplasmosis
  African 501
  progressive disseminated (PDH) 500–2
  pulmonary 499–500, 501–2
historical context, antibiotics 4–5
HIV/AIDS 809–42
  Candida infections 475, 825, 828, 833
  cardiovascular complications 829–30
  CD4 count see CD4T-lymphocytecount
  cerebral abscess 738
  classification 821–3
  Cryptococcus infections 480–1, 727–8, 825
  Cryptosporidium 521–2
  Cyclospora 523
  Cystoisospora 522–3
  cytomegalovirus (CMV) 406–8
  epidemiology 819
  Epstein–Barr virus (EBV) 404, 405
  gastrointestinal disease 833–4
  genital herpes 703, 704
  hepatitis 674, 835–6
  HIV protease inhibitors 102, 103, 108–9
  HIV-related pyrexia of unknown origin 583
  HIV RT 104–6
  human herpesvirus type 8 394–6, 827
  human papillomavirus (HPV) 439
  infected health-care worker risk management 159–60
  initial patient evaluation 824
  kidney disease 837
  laboratory tests 427–30
  liver disease (overview) 835–7
  management of risks to health-care workers 151–2, 666–7
  meningitis 722–4, 726–8
  microsporidia 538
  myocarditis 636
  natural history 819–21
  non-nucleoside reverse transcriptase inhibitors (NNRTIs) 102, 103, 106–8, 826
    nucleoside/nucleotide analogue reverse transcriptase inhibitors (NRTIs) 102, 103, 104–6
  oesophagitis 644, 645
  oral complications 828–9
  Penicillium marneffei 510
  Pneumocystis jiroveci 482–4
  pregnancy 794, 795
  prevention 840–2
  principles of HIV treatment 101–3
  progressive disseminated histoplasmosis (PDH) 500–1, 502–3
  pulmonary complications 830–3
  salmonellosis 289
  sharps injury from infected donor 154–7
  skin complications (overview) 825–8
  sporotrichosis 496–7
  syphilis 714–15, 716
  toxoplasmosis 517–20
  tuberculosis (TB) 356, 726–7
  typhlitis 675
  virology and immunology 425–7
HLA-B*5701 screening 824

hoarseness 596–7
hookworm 545–6, 549, 586–7
hospital-acquired infection (HAI)
bloodstream infection (BSI) 187–9
Clostridium difficile infection (CDI) 198–201
community infection and 202
control of see infection control
diarrhoea and vomiting epidemics 196–7
hospital-acquired pneumonia (HAP) 191, 192, 617–18
in intensive care 182–5
introduction to prevention of 181–2
line-related sepsis 193–6
organisms commonly involved in 136
pneumonia (HAP) 191, 617–18
surgical site infection (SSI) 185–7
surveillance 139–42
urinary catheter-associated infection 189–91
ventilator-associated pneumonia 191–3
see *also* healthcare associated/acquired infection (HCAI); nosocomial infection
hospital cleaning 137, 163–4
carbapenemase-producing *Enterobacteriaceae* 167
Clostridium difficilei infection (CDI) 199, 201
diarrhoea and vomiting epidemics 196–7
period of increased incidence 144–5
human African trypanosomiasis (HAT) 525–7
human bite infections 760
human coronavirus (HCoV) 383
human herpesvirus type 6 393–4, 801
human herpesvirus type 7 394
human herpesvirus type 8 394–6, 827
human hookworm infection 545–6, 549
human normal immuboglobulin (HNIG) 412
human papillomavirus (HPV) 439–41, 699–701
human scabies 573
human T-cell lymphotropic virus (HTLV-1/HTLV-2) 449–50
hydrocele 554
hydrogen peroxide 175–6, 201
hygienic hand disinfection 147
hygienic handwash 147
Hymenolepsis
H. diminuta 549
H. nana 549, 561
hyperinfection syndrome, strongyloidiasis 546–7
hyperparasitaemia 513
hyperplasia, pseudoepitheliomatous 503
hypochlorite 173
hypogammaglobulinaemia, thymoma with 810
hysterectomy 187

I

identification
bacteria 209, 221–5
see also specific techniques
imidazoles 82
imipenem 39–40
imiquimod 700–1
immunization, see vaccination/immunization
immunodeficiency 809–42
adenovirus 437–8
antibody deficiency syndromes 810–11
Aspergillus 486–7
asplenic patients 814
Blastomyces dermatitidis 503–5
cerebral abscess 738
Chaga's disease 524–5
Coccidioides immitis 506–8
Crypotococcus 480, 727–8
Cystoisospora 512–22
Epstein–Barr virus (EBV) 404
HIV/AIDS, see HIV/AIDS
human herpesvirus type 6 393
human papillomavirus (HPV) 439
immune-deficient pyrexia of unknown origin 583
infective diarrhoea 647–8
meningitis 727–8
microsporidia 538, 539
mucormycosis 489–90
myocarditis 636–8
neutropenic sepsis 815–16
Paracoccidioides brasiliensis 508
Penicillium marneffei 509–10
polyomaviruses 442–3
Pneumocystis jiroveci 482–4
primary immunodeficiency 810–12
progressive disseminated histoplasmosis (PDH) 500–1, 502–3
Pseudallescheria boydii 494–5
secondary immunodeficiency 812
selective T-cell deficiency 811–12
toxoplasmosis 517–20
transplant recipients see transplant recipients
varicella-zoster virus (VZV) 400–2
immunoglobulin (Ig) loss 813
immunoglobulin A (IgA) deficiency, selective 810
immunoglobulin G (IgG) deficiencies 811
immunoglobulin M (IgM) deficiency, selective 811
immunological reactions, *M. leprae* infections 77
immunotherapy 382, 406–7
impetigo 758
imported fever 584–6
inactivated polio vaccine (IPV) 448
India ink stain 222–4
indole test 227
inducible resistance 50
infants see children/infants
infection
basic epidemiology of 135–7
definition 130, 580
infection control 129–02
alert organisms' surveillance 140–1
antibiotic resistant organism management 164–6
basic epidemiology of infection 135–7
bloodstream infection–mandatory surveillance 187–9
carbapenemase-producing *Enterobacteriaceae* (CPE) control 167
Clostridium difficile infection (CDI) 198–201, 656

in community 202
containment levels (CL) 162–3
Corynebacterium diphtheriae 261
Creutzfeldt–Jakob disease (CJD) 169–72
definitions 130
diarrhoea epidemics 196–7
disinfection 172–4
environmental issues/ factors 137, 144–5, 162–3, 172–4
glycopeptide resistant *Staphylococcus aureus* 240
group A *Streptococcus* (GAS) 251
handwashing 146–50
hazard groups 160
infection control committee (ICC) 138
intensive care infections 182–5
introduction to 130–5
laundry 179
line-related sepsis 193–6
management of risks from virally infected health-care workers 158–60
management of risks to health-care workers from patients 151–3
nature of risk and its assessment 142–3
Neisseria meningitidis 276
outbreak management 144–6
overview of surveillance 139–40
patient isolation 150–1
prevention of hospital-acquired infection (introduction to) 181–2
renal dialysis units 158
respiratory syncytial virus 382
sharps risk management 153–7
sterilization 174–6
surgical site infection (SSI) 185–7
surveillance of hospital-acquired infection 141–2
transmissible spongiform encephalopathies (TSEs) 169–72
transplantation tissues (risk from) 157–8
tuberculosis (TB) 168–9
universal infection control precautions and barrier nursing 163–4
urinary catheter-associated infection 189–91
ventilation in health-care premises 176–8
ventilator-associated pneumonia (VAP) 191–3
viral haemorrhagic fevers (VHF) 460–1
vomiting epidemics 196–7
waste 180–1
infectious mononucleosis 402–5, 406–7
infective endocarditis (IE) 630–2
Abiotrophia 255
Bacteroides 330–1
Bartonella 348–50
Candida 473, 476
HACEK organisms 306–8
Histoplasma casulatum 502
HIV complication 829
prophylaxis 26–7
Q fever 347–8
Streptococcus bovis 247–8
inflammation
M. leprae infections 77
systemic inflammatory response syndrome (SIRS) 580
influenza 375–9
antivirals for 94–6
clinical features and diagnosis 377
introduction 375–6
parainfluenza 380
treatment/ prevention 378–9
inhalation, drug administration route 20–1
inhalational anthrax 258–9
insect bites, encephalitis causes 733
insect repellents 514, 527, 555
insecticide-treated bed nets 514, 555
insertion sequences (IS) 11–12
instruments see equipment
integrons 11–12
intensive care unit (ICU) infections in (overview) 182–5
neonatal (NICU) 184–5
ventilator-associated pneumonia (VAP) 191–3, 618–19
interferon (IFN) 416–17
interferon alfa 97, 99, 100, 450, 453, 700–1
PEG-IFN 420–1, 674
interferon gamma release assays (IGRA) 357–8
interstitial keratitis 752
intra-abdominal abscess 667–71
intra-abdominal infection 477
intracranial pressure (ICP), reduction of raised 720
intramuscular (IM) administration 19–20
intravascular catheter-related infections 632–4
intravenous (IV) administration 18–19
IV to oral switch 19
outpatient parenteral antimicrobial therapy (OPAT) 28–9
intravenous (IV) fluids, cholera 653
intravenous immunoglobulin (IVIG) 708–9
intussusception 437–8
iodine 173
iodoquinol 121
iron deficiency anaemia 545
isolate 12–13
isolation (patient) 150–1
antibiotic-resistant organism outbreak control 165
carbapenemase-producing *Enterobacteriaceae* (CPE) 167
Clostridium difficile infection 199
HIV/hepatitis B/hepatitis C patients 152
in intensive care unit (ICU) 183
outbreak management 146
routes of transmission and 137
tuberculosis (TB) 168–9
ventilation systems 176
isoniazid 42, 71–2, 358–9, 726–7
itraconazole 83–4
aspergillosis 485
Blastomyces dermatitidis 504–5
Candida 473
coccidioidal meningitis 728–9

itraconazole (*Contd.*)
Histoplasma meningitis 729–30
Paracoccidioides brasiliensis 508–9
Penicillium marneffei 510
Sporothrix schenckii 497
ivermectin 125
cutaneous larva migrans 550
filariasis 555
loiasis 556–7
onchocerciasis 558
pinworm 548
scabies 574
strongyloidiasis 547
trichuriasis 544

J

Japanese encephalitis (JE) 452
Jarisch–Herxheimer reactions 338
JC virus 442–3
joint infection *see* bone and joint infections
junin virus 459

K

K antigens 280–1, 283
Kanagawa phenomenon 323
kanamycin 46–8, 74–5
Kaposi's sarcoma (KS) 394–6, 827, 839–40
Katayama fever 563–4
keratitis 485, 751–2
amoebic 536–7
keratoconjunctivitis 353–214, 752
keratoconjunctivitis sicca 538
ketoconazole 82
ketolides 50
kidney infection/disease *see* renal infection/disease
kidney transplant *see* renal transplant
Kingella kingae 307, 308
Klebsiella 283–4
K. granulomatis 702–3
K. pneumoniae carbapenemase (KPC) 40, 41
Kluyvera 292–3
knee joint replacement 187, 780–3
koilocytosis 439
Koplik's spots 385–6
kuru 467
Kyasanur Forest disease 454, 459

L

laboratories
containment levels (CL) 162–3
pathology networks 233
quaity assurance and accreditation 231–3
lacrimal apparatus infection 746–7
lactic acidosis 835
laminar flow 177
lamivudine 97, 99, 104–6, 416–17
Lancefield groups 242
LapDap 117
larva migrans 550–1
laryngitis 598–9
lassa virus/lassa fever 459, 462–3
lateral pharyngeal abscess 606
laundry 152, 179
ledipasvir 101, 420–1
Lee and Waldvogel system 778
Legionella 318–20, 616
Legionnaires' disease 318–20
Leishmania 527–30
leishmaniasis 527–30
Lemierre's disease 333, 595
lepromatous leprosy 360
leprosy 359–61
antileprotics 75–7, 361
Leptospira 334, 340–2
leptospirosis 334, 340–2
Leuconostoc 254
leukaemia, adult T-cell (ATL) 449–50
levamisole 125
levofloxacin 63–4
lice 572–3
lincomycin 51–2
lincosamides 51–2
macrolide–lincosamide–streptogramin B (MLS_B) resistance 50
line-related sepsis 193–6, 581–2
linezolid 54–5, 246–7, 721
lipoglycopeptides 45
lipopeptides 53–4
lipozomal amphotericin B (LFAmB) 473, 504–5, 529
Listeria species 263–5, 721, 789
listeriosis 263–5, 789
liver disease/infection
antimicrobials in 23–4
cirrhosis 416–17, 419–21, 661–2, 674
deranged liver function tests 835
fibrosis 419–20
hepatic schistosomiasis 563–4
hepatic steatosis 835
hepatitis *see* hepatitis
HIV complications 835–7
liver abscess 534–5, 670–1
liver flukes 565–6
viruses overview 370
liver transplant
cytomegalovirus (CMV) 406–7
hepatitis 672–3, 674
Loa loa 556–7
local infiltration, antimicrobial prophylaxis 27
Löeffler's syndrome 545, 546–7
loiasis 555, 556–7
lopinavir 108–9
louse borne relapsing fever 334, 337–8
Ludwig's angina 605
lumbar puncture (LP) 737–8; *see also* cerbrospinal fluid (CSF)
lumefantrine 115
artemether–lumefantrine 118–19
lung abscess 621–3
lung fluke 566–8
lung transplant 301
lyme disease 334, 338–40
neuroborreliosis 730–1
lymecycline 56–8
lymphadenopathy
conjunctivitis 749–50
encephalopathy 735
onchocerciasis 557
lymphocytic choriomeningitis virus 432, 722–4
lymphocytoma 338–9
lymphoedema 554
lymphogranuloma venereum (LGV) 353–4, 701–2
lymphoid interstitial pneumonitis 832–3
lymphoma
adult T-cell lymphoma (ATL) 449–50
gastric 646
HIV complications 838–40

M

MacConkey agar 219–20
machupo virus 459

macrolides 24–5, 48–50
macrolide–lincosamide–streptogramin B (MLS_B) resistance 50
Madura foot, see mycetoma
mafenide acetate 58–60
malaria 112–19, 512–14
Malassezia
infections 478–9, 766
MALDI-TOF 228
malignancy
Candida
infections 475, 476
gastrointestinal (GI) 247–8
HIV complications 839–40
peptic ulcer disease and 646
progressive disseminated histoplasmosis (PDH) 500–1
secondary immunodeficiency causes 813
viruses and malignant change 369
mandibular infection 605
mannitol salt agar (MSA) 219–20
Mantoux test 357–8
maraviroc 110
Marburg virus 459, 461–2
masks
filtered 168–9
operating theatres 178
mastitis 798
mastoiditis 601–2, 738
MASTRING™ ID 331
maternal infection see pregnancy
mayaro 434
Mazotti test 558
measles 384–6, 790–1, 801
mebendazole 124, 531
ascariasis 543
hookworm 545
pinworm 548
trichenellosis 553
trichuriasis 544
mecA gene 237, 238
mechanisms/mode of action
aminoglycosides 46
antifungals 80, 82, 83, 85, 86–7
antihelminthic drugs 124
antileprotics 75–6
antimalarials 113–14, 118
antiretroviral drug therapy (ART) 108
antituberculous agents 71–3
basics of antimicrobials 8–9
carbapenems 39
cephalosporins 33–5
chloramphenicol 55
cytomegalovirus (CMV) antivirals 92, 93–4
fusidic acid 69
glycopeptides 42
herpes simplex virus antivirals 90
influenza antivirals 95–6
ketolides 50
lincosamides 51
lipopeptides 53
macrolides 48–50
metronidazole 65
mupirocin 70
nitrofurans 66
oxazolidinones 54
penicillins 32
polymyxins 69
respiratory syncytial virus (RSV) antivirals 96
streptogramins 52
sulfonamides 59
tetracyclines 57
trimethoprim 60
varicella-zoster virus antivirals 90
mediastinal fibrosis 499–500, 501–2
mediastinal granuloma 499–500, 501–2
mediastinitis 640–1
Mediterranean spotted fever 343, 345
mefloquine 114
artesunate–mefloquine 118–19
megacolon 524–5
megaoesophagus 524–5
Megosphora species 280
melarsoprol 121, 527
meliodosis 302–3
membrane (outer), alteration in permeability 10
meningitis
acute (overview) 718
Angiostrongylus cantonensis 568
aseptic meningitis syndrome 722–4
bacterial (overview) 718–22
Candida 473, 476
chronic 724–6
coccidioidal 506–8, 728–9
cryptococcal 480–1, 727–8, 838–9
enterovirus 431–2
herpes simplex virus (HSV) 397
Histoplasma 729–30
lymphocytic choriomeningitis virus 432
mumps 387–8
neonatal 286–7, 431
sporotrichosis 496–7
tuberculous 726–7
viral
(overview) 370, 722–4
meningoencephalitis
adenovirus 437–8
Listeria 263–5
primary amoebic 535–7
mepacrine 121–2
Merkel cell polyomavirus 442
meropenem 39–40, 721, 738–9, 742
mesenteric adenitis 316, 674–5
metabolism
alteration of metabolic pathways 10
bacterial 214–16
pharmocokinetics 16
secondary immunodeficiency causes 813
Metagonimus yokogawai 567
metacycline 56–8
metapneumovirus 384
meticillin-resistant *Staphylococcus aureus* (MRSA) 164–6, 237–9, 721
in the community 202
surgical site infection (SSI) 186
metrifonate 126
metronidazole 64–6, 122
bacterial vaginosis (BV) 696–7
brain abscess 738–9
Clostridium difficile 200–1, 655–6
Gardia lamblia 531
Helicobacter pylori 328–9, 329, 647
ophthalmic infections 747–9
pelvic inflammatory disease (PID) 706
in pregnancy 24–5
Trichomonas vaginalis 533, 713
micofungin 86
miconazole 82
micro-agglutination test (MAT) 341–2
microbicides 840–1
microbiological specimens 172, 218–19, 460–1

Micrococcus species 242
microscopy 222–4
microsporidia 537–9, 749–51
Microsporum 492–4
Middle East respiratory syndrome coronavirus 384
migrant health 848–9
mikamycin 52–3
milk, production standards 313
miltefosine 122
Milwaukee protocol 464–5
minimum bactericidal concentration (MBC) 14
minimum inhibitory concentration (MIC) 13
minocycline 56–8, 76–7
mites 575
mobile genetic elements (MGEs) 11–13
modification of diet in renal disease (MDRD) formula 22
molecular organism identification 229
molecular typing methods 229–31
molluscum contagiosum 445, 769–70, 827
monkeypox 445, 769
monobactams 41
mononeuritis/mononeuritis multiplex 838
Monospot test 404–5
Moraxella species 274, 279
Morganella 285
  M. morganii 292–3
moulds 484–95
moxifloxacin 63–4, 721
mucormycosis 489–90, 766–7
mucosal leishmaniaisis 527–30
mucous membrane infection, *Candida* 475
Mueller Hinton agar 219–20
multicentric Castleman's disease (MCD) 395–6
multidrug therapy (MDT), *M. leprae* infections 75
multilocus sequence typing (MLST) 231
multilocus variable-number tandem repeat analysis (MLVA) 230–1
multiple organ dysfunction syndrome (MODS) 580
multiresistant organisms, surveillance of 141
mumps 387–8, 691, 722–4, 801
mupirocin 70–1
murine typhus 343, 346
Murphy's sign 657
Murray Valley encephalitis 454
muscular diseases, overview of viruses 370
mutant prevention concentration 17–18
mutant selection window 17–18
mutation 213, 367–8
mycetoma 273, 491–2
  sinus 600
Mycobacterium
  encephalitis 736
  microscopy 222–4
  M. leprae 75–7, 359–61
  M. tuberculosis 63–4, 355–9, 627–8, 726–7, 831
  non-tuberculous (NTM) 361–2
Mycoplasma 350–2
  M. hominis 351–2
  M. pneumoniae 351–2, 615–16
mycosis, systemic progressive 508–9
mycotic aneurysm 634–5
myelopathy
  HTLV-1-associated 449–50
myiasis 574
myocarditis 636–8, 830
myonecrosis 270–1, 762
myopathy 838
myorhythmia 735
myositis 538–9
myringotomy 604–5

N

Naegleria fowleri 535–7
nail care 149
nail infections, dermatophytes 492–4
nalidixic acid 62–4
National Audit Office reports
  handwashing 146–50
  hospital-acquired infection 181–2, 188, 189–91
  infection control committees 138
  sharps' risk management 153
National Blood Service 158
National External Quality Assessment Service for Microbiology (NEQAS) 232
National Patient Safety Agency 150
nausea 834
Necataor americanus 545–6
neck infections 589–628
  bacterial tracheitis 598
  croup 596–7, 598
  laryngitis 598
  lateral pharyngeal abscess 606
  Lemierre's disease 333, 595
  pharyngitis 591–3
  quinsy (peritonsillar abscess) 594–5
  retropharyngeal abscess 593–4
  see also respiratory infections; *specific infections*
necrotizing fasciitis 763–4, 783
needlestick injuries 153–7
negative-pressure ventilation 177
Neisseria species 274–9
  N. gonorrhoeae 274, 277–8, 705–6, 709–11, 749–51
  N. meningitides 274–7, 720–2, 749–51
  non-pathogenic 274, 279
nematodes
  identification of ova 549
  overview 542
  see also specific nematodes
neomycin 46–8
neonatal infection
  Bacillus species 257
  Chlamydia trachomatis (pneumonia) 353–4
  chorioamnionitis and 796–7
  congenital, *see* congenital infections
  encephalitis 733
  Listeria species 264
  maternal infections associated with neonatal morbidity 789–90
  meningitis 287–8, 431
  pneumonia 353–4, 799–800
  prevention of perinatal infection 794–6
  rash contact in pregnancy 790–1
  rash illness in pregnancy 792–4
  sepsis 252–3, 281, 799–801
  viral causes of illness (overview) 801

neonatal intensive care unit (NICU) 184–5
nephropathy, HIV-associated 837
netilmicin 46–8
neuraminidase (NA) inhibitors 94–5, 378–9
neuroborreliosis 730–1
neurocysticercosis 731–2
neurological disease/infection
- *Blastomyces dermatitidis* 503–5
- brain abscess 737–9
- CNS candidiasis 476
- *Corynebacterium diphtheriae* 260–1
- CSF shunt infection 741–3
- cysticercosis 561–2
- encephalitis *see* encephalitis
- epidural abscess 740–1
- HIV complications 838–9
- meningitis *see* meningitis
- microsporidia 537–9
- mucormycosis 489–90
- neuroborreliosis 730–1
- neurocysticercosis 731–2
- neurosyphilis 714–16
- schistosomiasis 563–4
- subdural empyema 739–40
- toxoplasmosis 518, 519
- trichenellosis 552–3

neuropathy, peripheral 838
neurosurgery 738
neutropenia
- candidaemia in 473
- febrile 815–16
- neutropenic sepsis 815–16

nevirapine 106–8
New York City agar 219–20
next generation sequencing (NGS) 228, 231
NHS Blood and Transplant (NHSBT) Tissue Services 157
NICE guidance
- dyspepsia investigation and management 328–9
- *Healthcare-associated infections: prevention and control in primary and community care* 202

niclosamide 126, 559–61
Nidovirus 383–4
nifurtimox 122, 525
nigrosin stain 222–4
nitazoxanide 122, 521, 531, 539, 565–6
nitrofurans 66–7
nitrofurantoin 24–5, 66–7
nitrofurazone 66–7
nitrogen 214
nitroimidazoles 64–6
Nocardia species 272–3
nocardiosis 272–3
nomenclature 209–10
non-fermenters, gram-negative rods' overview 293–4
non-Hodgkin's lymphoma (NHL) 839–40
non-immune hydrops fetalis 391–2
non-nucleoside reverse transcriptase inhibitors (NNRTIs) 102, 103, 106–8, 826
non-steroidal anti-inflammatory drugs (NSAIDs) 777
norfloxacin 64
norovirus 410–11
Norwalk virus 410–11
Norwegian scabies 573
nosocomial infection
- *Acinetobacter* 297–9
- *Citrobacter* 286–7
- *Clostridium difficile* 196–201, 654–6
- control of *see* infection control
- definition 130
- enterococci 245
- *Escherichia coli* 281
- MRSA *see* meticillin-resistant *Staphylococcus aureus* (MRSA)
- *Proteus* 284–5
- pyrexia of unknown origin (PUO) 583
- respiratory syncytial virus (RSV) 381, 382
- *Stenotrophomonas maltophilia* 299–300
- *see also* healthcare-associated/acquired infection (HCAI); hospital-acquired infection (HAI)

Nosocomial Infection National Surveillance Scheme (NINSS) 141, 142
notifiable diseases 845–6
novobiocin 67
NS5A inhibitors 101
NS5B inhibitors 101
nucleic acid amplification test (NAAT)
- *Chlamydia trachomatis* 712
- *Clostridium difficile* 198–9
- *Neisseria gonorrhoeae* 277–8, 710–11

nucleic acid sequence-based amplification (NASBA) 428–9
nucleic acid synthesis, inhibition of 8–9
nucleocapsid 366
nucleoside/nucleotide analogue reverse transcriptase inhibitors (NRTIs) 102, 103, 104–6
nutritionally variant streptococci (NVS) 255
nystatin 80–1

O

O antigens 280–1, 283
Ochrobactrum 294–5
ocular onchocerciasis 557–8
ocular toxocariasis 550–1
ocular toxoplasmosis 518, 519–20
oesophageal infection/disease
- candidiasis 473, 475, 644, 833
- megaoesophagus 524–5
- oesophageal perforation 640–1
- oesophagitis 397–8, 473, 475, 644–5
- peptic ulcer disease and 646

ofloxacin 64, 76–7, 706, 712
Oligella 294–5
Omsk haemorrhagic fever 454, 459
Onchocerca volvulus 557–8
onchocerciasis 555, 557–8
onchercomata 557
ONPG test 227
onychomycosis 492–4
o'nyongnyong 434
oophoritis 387–8
operating theatres, ventilation systems 177–8
ophthalmological infections 745–56
- conjunctivitis *see* conjunctivitis
- endophthalmitis 473, 485, 754–6
- keratitis 485, 536–7, 751–2
- microsporidia 537–9
- onchocerciasis 557–8
- ophthalmomyiasis 574–5
- orbital 747–9
- periorbital 746–7
- retinitis *see* retinitis
- uveitis 753–4, 755

ophthalmomyiasis 574–5
opisthorciasis 565, 567
Opisthorcis 565, 567
optochin test 226
oral administration 18
IV to oral switch 19
oral candidiasis 475
oral complications, HIV 828–9
oral hairy leukoplakia 828
oral hydration salts (OHS) 649, 653
oral polio vaccine (OPV) 448
orbital infections 747–9
orbital (post-septal) cellulitis 748–9
orchitis 691
orf 445, 769
oriental liver fluke 565
ORION (Outbreak Reports and Intervention Studies of Nosocomial Infection) 133
oritavancin 45
ornidazole 122
oropharyngeal candidiasis 473, 833
oroya fever 348–50
Orthomyxoviridae 370, 375
ortho-phthalaldehyde sterilization 175–6
oseltamivir 94–5, 378–9
osteoarticular disease 496–7
osteomyelitis 778–80
otitis externa 602–3
otitis media 603–5, 738
outpatient parenteral antimicrobial therapy (OPAT) 28–9
overwhelming post-splenectomy infection (OPSI) 814
OXA β-lactamases 36–7
oxaminiquine 126
oxazolidinones 54–5
oxidase test 227
oxytetracycline 56–8
ozone sterilization 175–6

P

P450 16
PA824 74–5
PABA 58–60
pacemaker infections 635
palivizumab 382, 611
Paludrine 116
pancreatic abscess 668–9
pancreatitis 659–60, 836–7
pandemics, influenza 376, 378
Pantoea agglomerans 292–3
Panton–Valentine leucocidin (PVL) 235
Papovaviridae 370, 442
para-aminosalicylic acid (PAS) 73
paracentesis 661–2
Paracoccidioides brasiliensis 508–9
paragonimiasis 566–8
Paragonimus westermani 566–8
parainfluenza 380
paralysis
encephalitis and flaccid 735
enterovirus 431
poliovirus 446–7, 448
rabies 464
tick paralysis 576
Paramyxoviridae 370
measles 384–6
metapneumovirus 384
mumps 387
parainfluenza 380
respiratory syncytial virus (RSV) 21, 96, 381–2, 609–11
paraparesis, tropical spastic 449–50
parasites
antiparasitic therapy 111–26
hazard groups 160
helminths 541–70
see also specific parasites
parkinsonism 735
paromomycin 46–8, 122, 521, 531
parotitis 387–8, 735
partipoxviruses 445
Parvoviridae 370
parvovirus B19 390–2, 787, 790–1, 792–4, 801
Pasteurella 316–17
pathogenicity
bacterial 216
fungal 470
pathogenicity islands 235
pathology networks 233
viral 368–9
patient risk factors, hospital-acquired infection 136
Paul–Bunnell test 404–5
PCV7 (7-valent pneumococcal conjugate vaccine) 245
pediculosis 572–3
Pediculus 572–3
pelvic inflammatory disease (PID) 705–6, 711–12, 789
pelvic pain syndrome, chronic 689
penciclovir 90–1
penicillin-binding proteins (PBPs) 8, 10
penicillins 32–3
benzathine benzylpencillin 716
benzylpenicillin 708–9, 716
history of 4–5
neuroborreliosis 730–1
in pregnancy 24–5
benzylpenicillin 33, 721
phenoxymethylpenicillin 33
streptococci 244–5, 249, 251
Penicillium 4–5
P. marneffei 509–10
pentamidine 21, 122–3, 527
peptic ulcer disease 327–9, 645–7
peptidoglycan 235
peramivir 95, 378–9
perfusion, sepsis/severe sepsis management 581–2
pericardial disease 830
pericarditis 499–500, 502, 638–9, 830
perinephric abscess 685
period of increased incidence (PII) 144–5
periodontitis 833
periorbital infections 746–7
periorbital oedema 524, 746–7
peripheral neuropathy 838
peripheral venous catheters (PVCs)
bloodstream infection (BSI) 187–9
High Impact Intervention No. 2 194
line-related sepsis 193, 194, 195–6
peritoneal dialysis (PD) 477, 664–6
peritonitis 477
HIV complication 834
peritoneal dialysis peritonitis 664–6
primary 661–2
secondary 662–4
peritonsillar abscess 594–5
permethrin 573, 574
personal respiratory protection 168–9
pertussis 310–11, 806–8
phaeohyphomycosis 495
phages 11–12, 213–14
phagocytosis 216–17
pharmacodynamics 16–18

pharmacokinetics 15–16
pharyngeal abscess, lateral 606
pharyngitis 591–3, 803–4
pharyngoconjunctival fever 437–8
phenolics 173
phenotypic characteristics 209, 229–31
phlebitis 632
  visual infusion 193, 194
phlyctenules, conjunctival 749–50
Phocanema 569
Phoenix 228
Phthirus pubis 572
phylogenetic identification 209
physical sterilization 175
Picornaviridae 370, 445–6
pinworm 548
piperacillin–tazobactam 38, 708–9
piperaquine 115
  dihydroartemisinin–piperaquine 118–19
piperazine 125
pinta 334, 335–7
pityriasis versicolor 478–9, 766
plague 314–15, 848
plasmids 11–12, 210, 212–13, 216–17
  ColV 280
  F plasmid 213–14
Plasmodium species 512–14
Pleisomonas shigelloides 326
plenum ventilation 177
pleocytosis 723–4, 725, 726–8, 729–37
pleural fluid
  characteristics in empyema 620
  sampling 612–13
pneumococcal vaccination 604–5
Pneumocystis jiroveci 21, 482–4, 830–1
pneumonia
  aspiration 617
  atypical pneumonias 615–17
  Blastomyces dermatitidis 503–5
  Chlamydia 353–4, 355
  chronic fibrocavity 506
  Coccidioides immitis 506–8
  community-acquired (CAP) 611–17
  Friedlander's 283
  HIV complications 830–2
  hospital-acquired (HAP) 191, 617–18
  influenza 375–6, 377–9
  Legionnaires' disease 318–20
  necrotizing 266, 622
  neonatal 353–4, 799–800
  Pneumocystic jiroveci 21, 482–4, 830–1
  Q fever 347, 348
  respiratory syncytial virus (RSV) 96, 381–2
  ventilator-associated (VAP) 191–3, 618–19
pneumonic plague 314–15
pneumonitis 397–8, 400
  lymphoid interstitial 832–3
pneumothorax 833
pocket infection 632
podophyllin 700–1
podophyllotoxin 700–1
point mutations 11
poliovirus 445–8
polyclonal B-cell lymphoma 404
polyenes 80–1
polymerase chain reaction (PCR)
  16S rRNA 229
  18S rRNA 229
  Clostridium difficile diagnosis 198–9
  multiplex 229
  random amplification of polymorphic DNA (RAPD PCR) 230
  real-time/quantitative (qPCR) 229
  repetitive element (rep-PCR) 230
polymyxins 68–9; *see also specific drugs*
polyomaviruses 442–3
polyradiculopathy 406–7, 838
polysomes 210
pontiac fever 318–20
pork tapeworm 560, 561–2, 731–2
Porphyromonas 329–32
posaconazole 84
positive-pressure ventilation 176
post-antibiotic effect (PAE) 17
post-herpetic neuralgia 400, 401
post-kala-azar dermal leishmaniasis 527–30
post-lyme syndrome 340
post-poliomyelitis syndrome 446–7
post-splenectomy sepsis (PSS) 814
Powassan virus 453–4
Poxviridae 370
poxviruses 444–5, 769, 848
PPV23 (23-valent unconjugated polysaccharide vaccine) 245
praziquantel 125–6, 559–62, 563–5, 566–8, 731–2
pregnancy 785–08
  antimicrobials in 24–5
  bacterial vaginosis (BV) 696–7
  chickenpox 400
  chlamydia 712
  chorioamnionitis 796–7
  congenital infection overview 786–9
  cytomegalovirus (CMV) 788
  enterovirus 787
  hepatitis B 794, 795
  herpes simplex virus (HSV) 397–8, 788–9
  HIV 794, 795, 840
  Listeria infection 264, 789
  management of rash contact in 790–1
  maternal infections associated with neonatal morbidity 789–90
  measles 790–1
  neonatal sepsis 252–3, 281, 799–801
  parvovirus B19 391–2, 787, 790–1, 792–4
  polyomaviruses 442–3
  prevention of congenital/perinatal infection 794–6
  puerperal sepsis 797–8
  rubella 389–90, 788, 790–1, 792–4
  syphilis 786–7, 794
  toxoplasmosis 518, 519–20, 786
  varicella-zoster virus (VZV) 787, 791, 792–4, 795
  vulvovaginal candidiasis 698–9
  see also neonatal infections
premature rupture of membranes (PROM) 796–7
prescribing, antimicrobial stewardship 27–8
preseptal (periorbital) cellulitis 747–8
preterm labour 796–7
Prevotella 329–32
primaquine 113, 115, 123

primary effusion lymphoma (PEL) 394–6
primary immunodeficiency 810–12
prion diseases 465–8
prion proteins 169–72
pristinamycin 52–3
proctitis 701–2
progressive disseminated histoplasmosis (PDH) 500–2
progressive multifocal leukoencephalopathy (PML) 442–3, 838–9
proguanil 116
prophylaxis *see* antimicrobial prophylaxis; vaccination/immunization
prostatitis 688–9
prosthetic joint infections (PJI) 780–3
protease inhibitors (PI)
  hepatitis 100
  HIV 102, 103, 108–9
proteases 216–17
protective clothing/equipment 152, 163–4, 168–9
protective isolation 150–1; *see also* isolation (patient)
protein synthesis, inhibition of 8
proteinuria 679
Proteus species 284–5
prothionamide 74
proton pump inhibitors (PPI) 647
protozoa 511–39, 736
  antiprotozoals *see* antiprotozoal drugs
  see also specific protozoa
Providencia 285, 292–3
PrPc 465–8
PrPSc 465–8
prurigo nodularis 827
Pseudallescheria boydii 494–5, 767
pseudallescheriasis 494–5
pseudocowpox 445
pseudoepitheliomatous hyperplasia 503–5
pseudomembranous colitis 654–5
pseudomonads 293
Pseudomonas aeruginosa 184–5, 295–7, 623–5, 721
psittacosis 354–5
psoas abscess 669
pubic louse 572
Public Health England (PHE)
  bioterrorism 848
  blood donor infection surveillance 158
  infective diarrhoea 649
  migrant health 849
puerperal sepsis 252–3, 797–8
pulmonary cavities 506
pulmonary complications, of HIV 830–3
pulmonary cryptococcus 480–1
pulmonary histoplasmosis 499–500
pulmonary hypertension 830
pulmonary infiltrates with eosinophilia 619
pulmonary nocardiosis 272–3
pulmonary nodules 506
pulmonary sporotrichosis 496–7
pulmonary tuberculosis *see* tuberculosis (TB)
pulsed-field gel electrophoresis (PFGE) 229–30
pure red cell aplasia (PRCA) 391–2
purified protein derivative (PPD) 357–8
purine nucleoside phosphorylase deficiency 812
pyelonephritis 473
  acute 681–3
  chronic 683–5
pyogenic liver abscess 670–1
pyogranulomatous disease, systemic 503–5
pyomyositis 764–6
pyrantel 126, 548
pyrazinamide 72, 726–7
pyrexia
  puerperal 797–8
  pyrexia of unknown origin (PUO) 582–4
  see also fever
pyrimethamine 116, 123, 519–20
  artesunate–sulfadoxine–pyrimethamine 118–19
pyuria 679; *see also* urinary tract infection (UTI)

Q

Q fever 346–8
quality assurance, laboratories 231–3
quaternary ammonium compounds (QACs) 173
quinacrine 121–2, 531
quinine 112–4, 117, 516
quinolones 24–5, 62–4; *see also specific drugs*
quinsy 594–5
quinupristin 52–3
  quinupristin–dalfopristin 52–3

R

rabies virus 463–5
racemose cysticercosis 561–2
radiological imaging 519
  chest X-ray 627–8
raltegravir 110
Ramsay–Hunt syndrome 400
random amplification of polymorphic DNA 230
Raoultella 292–3
rapid plasma reagin (RPR) 715–16
rash
  alphaviruses 433, 434
  encephalitis 735
  herpesviruses 393–6
  hookworm 545
  measles 385–6, 790–1
  meningitis 719
  overview of viruses 370
  parvovirus B19 391–2, 790–1
  pregnancy and rash contact 790–1
  rubella 790–1
  scarlet fever 804–5
  strongyloidiasis 546–7
  syphilis 714–15
  varicella-zoster virus (VZV) 400
  see also specific infections
ravuconazole 84
recombination, of genetic material 367–8
recurrent respiratory papillomatosis 439, 440–1
refractory septic shock 580
rehydration
  cholera 653
  infectious diarrhoea overview 649
  pancreatitis 660
Reiter's syndrome 776–8
relapsing fever 334, 337–8
renal dialysis units, infection control 158
renal function, assessment of 22
renal infection/disease

acute kidney injury (AKI) 837
acute renal failure (ARF) 681, 683
antimicrobials in 21–3
Candida 477
chronic kidney disease (CKD) 837
filariasis 554
haemorrhagic fever with renal syndrome 435–6
HIV complications 837
pyelonephritis 681–3, 473
renal abscess 685–6
renal scarring 683
renal transplant
acute renal transplant pyelonephritis 683
asymptomatic bacteriuria 678
cytomegalovirus (CMV) 406–7
infection from transplant tissue 157–8
polyomaviruses 442–3
Reoviridae 370, 409
replication, viral 367–8
reproduction, fungal 470
resistance (antimicrobial)
antibiotics *see* antibiotic resistance
antifungals 80, 82, 83–4, 86, 478, 492
antimalarials 112, 113–15, 116–17, 118
antiprotozoal drugs 123, 513–14
antivirals *see* antiviral resistance
in the community 202
respiration management, sepsis/severe sepsis 581–2
respiratory/pulmonary infections 589–628
acute bronchitis 606–7
adenovirus 437–8
Aspergillus 484–8
aspiration pneumonia 617
bacterial tracheitis 598
Blastomyces dermatitidis 503–5
bronchiectasis 625–6
bronchiolitis 21, 96, 381–2, 609–11
Candida 477
cerebral abscess and 738
chronic bronchitis 607–9
Coccidioides immitis 505–8
common cold 590–1
common organisms in hospital-acquired 136
community-acquired coronavirus 383
community-acquired pneumonia (CAP) 611–17
Corynebacterium diphtheriae 260–2
croup 596–7
in cystic fibrosis *see* cystic fibrosis (CF)
empyema 619–21
encephalitis and 735
Entamoeba histolytica 533–5
epiglottitis 597–8
mucormycosis 489–90
pulmonary cryptococcus 480–1
hantavirus pulmonary syndrome 435–6
HIV complications 830–3
hookworm 545
hospital-acquired pneumonia (HAP) 191, 617–18
human herpesvirus type 6 393–4
influenza *see* influenza
inhalational anthrax 258–9
laryngitis 598–9
lung abscess 621–3
lung fluke 566–8
metapneumovirus 384
overview of viruses 370
Paracoccidioides brasiliensis 508–9
parainfluenza 380
pneumonia *see* pneumonia
pneumonic plague 314–15
pneumonitis 397–8, 400, 832–3
pulmonary cavities 506
pulmonary histoplasmosis 499–500, 501–2
pulmonary hypertension 830
pulmonary infiltrates with eosinophilia 619
pulmonary nocardiosis 272–3
pulmonary nodules 506
pulmonary sporotrichosis 496–7
recurrent respiratory papillomatosis 439, 440–1
respiratory syncytial virus (RSV) 21, 96, 381–2, 609–11
severe acute respiratory syndrome (SARS) 153, 383
sinusitis 486–8, 599–601, 738
strongyloidiasis 546–7
tracheitis (bacterial) 598
tracheobronchitis 381–2, 486–8
trichenellosis 552–3
tuberculosis *see* tuberculosis (TB)
ventilator-associated pneumonia (VAP) 191–3, 618–19
see also specific infections
respiratory samples 218
respiratory syncytial virus (RSV) 21, 96, 381–2, 609–11
Respirovirus 380
resuscitation, sepsis/severe sepsis 581–2
retinitis
chorioretinitis 518, 519–20
CMV 93–4, 406–7, 408
encephalitis and 735
retroperitoneal abscess 668
retropharyngeal abscess 593–4
Retroviridae 370
reversal reactions, *M. leprae* 77, 360
Reynold's pentad 658
Rhabdoviridae 370, 463
rhinocerebral disease 489–90
Rhodococcus equi 198–201
Rhodotorula species 479
rhomboencephalitis 735
Riamet® 118–19
ribavirin 21, 100
bronchiolitis 96, 382, 610–11
Bunyaviridae 436
derivative use in hepatitis C treatment 101
hepatitis C virus (HCV) 420–1, 674
respiratory syncytial virus (RSV) 96, 382, 610–11
ribosomes 210
rice water stool 652–3
Rickettsia 342–6, 736
rifabutin 68
rifamide 68
rifampicin 67
as antileprotic 76, 77
as antituberculous agent 72, 726–7
Clostridium difficile 655–6
epiglottitis 597–8
Haemophilus influenzae prophylaxis 305, 720–2
Neisseria meningitides prophylaxis 720–2

rifamycin SV 68
rifamycins 67–8; *see also specific drugs*
rifapentine 68
rifaximin 68
Rift Valley fever (RVF) 370, 435–6, 459
rilpivirine 106–8
rimantadine 95–6
ringworm 492–4
risk/risk assessment/risk management
  Creutzfeldt–Jakob disease (CJD) 170
  definitions 142
  line infection risk factors 195
  management of risks to health-care workers from patients 151–3
  nature of risk and risk assessment 142–3
  sharps-related 153–7
  viral haemorrhagic fever (VHF) 459
  virally infected health-care workers 158–60
ritonavir 108–9
river blindness 555, 557–8
RNA
  16S rRNA 229
  18S rRNA 229
  messenger (mRNA) 212–13
  transfer (tRNA) 212–13
RNA viruses
  genome 366–7
  genome replication 367–8
  overview of 370
  see also specific viruses
Rocky Mountain spotted fever 343, 344–5
rod bacteria, identification 222, 224
Romãna's sign 524–5
roseola exanthem 393–4, 801
Roseomonas 294–5
rosetting 513
Ross river syndrome 434
rotavirus 409–10
Rothia mucilaginosus 242
roundworms, *see* nematodes
rubella 389–90, 788, 790–1, 792–4, 801
Rubivirus 389
Rubulavirus 380
Russian spring–summer encephalitis (RSSE) 453–4

S

Sabouraud agar 219–20
salicylic acid 441
salivary gland enlargement 829
Salmonella 196–7, 288–90, 649–51
saquinavir 108–9
Saving Lives, *see High Impact Interventions* (Saving Lives)
scabies 573–4, 827
scalded skin syndrome 805–6
scarlet fever 804–5
Scedosporium prolificans 495, 767
Schistosoma species 563–4, 567
schistosomiasis 563–4
screening
  carbapenemase-producing *Enterobacteriaceae* (CPE) 167
  group B *Streptococcus* (GBS) 253
  hepatitis 421
  HIV 794
  human papillomavirus (HPV) 441
  meticillin-resistant *Staphylococcus aureus* 166, 186
  migrant health 849
  pre-transplantation 818
  viral haemorrhagic fever (VHF) 459
scrub typhus 343, 346
seborrhoeic dermatitis 479, 828
secondary immunodeficiency 812
seizures 561–2
selective decontamination of the digestive tract (SDD) 27, 183
selective IgA deficiency 810
selective IgM deficiency 811
selective T-cell deficiency 811–12
SENIC study (Study on Efficacy of Nosocomial Infection Control) 140
sepsis 580–2
  brain abscess and 738
  definitions 580
  group B *Streptococcus* (GBS) 252–3
  line-related 193–6, 478–9
  neonatal 252–3, 281, 799–801
  neutropenic 815–16
  post-splenectomy 814
  puerperal 252–3, 797–8
  septic shock 580
  severe 580–2
septicaemia 324, 580
  septicaemic plague 314–15
Serratia 287–8
serum blood samples 219
severe acute respiratory syndrome (SARS) 153, 383
severe combined immunodeficiency (SCID) 812
sexually transmitted infections (STIs) 693–716
  bacterial vaginosis (BV) 309, 695–7
  Chlamydia see *Chlamydia*
  epididymitis 690
  genital herpes 703–4
  genital warts 439, 440–1, 699–701
  gonorrhoea 277–8, 709–11
  HIV *see* HIV
  human papillomavirus (HPV) 439–41, 699–701
  human T-cell lymphotropic virus 449
  introduction 694–5
  Mycoplasma 351
  pelvic inflammatory disease (PID) 705–6, 711–12
  syphilis *see* syphilis
  toxic shock syndrome 707–9
  Trichomonas vaginalis 222–4, 532–3, 713
  tropical genital ulceration 701–3
  vulvovaginal candidiasis 697–9
sharps 152, 153–7, 163–4, 180, 421
Shewanella 294–5
shiga-like toxins 282
Shigella 196–7, 291–2
shingles (herpes zoster) 399–402, 768–9, 791, 826; *see also* varicella-zoster virus (VZV)
shock
  dengue shock syndrome 458
  septic 580
  toxic shock syndrome 707–9
  virus overview 370

SHOT (Serious Hazards of Transfusion) 158
SHV β-lactamases 36–7
side effects *see* toxicity/side effects
siderophore 216–17
SIGHT protocol 200
simepravir 100
sindbis syndrome 434
single locus sequence typing (SLST) 231
single nucleotide polymorphisms (SNPs) 11
sinusitis 486–8, 599–601, 738
skin disinfectants 172–4
skin flora 146–50
skin/soft tissue infections 757–71
  bacillary angiomatosis 348–50, 771, 825
  Bacteroides 330–1
  bite infections 320–1, 760
  Blastomyces dermatitidis 503–5
  cat-scratch disease 348–50, 770–1
  chromomycosis 497–8, 767
  clostridial gas gangrene 270–1, 762
  Coccinioides immitis 505–6
  Corynebacterium diphtheriae 260–1
  cutaneous anthrax 258–9, 770
  cutaneous candidiasis 766–8, 825
  cutaneous larva migrans 550
  cutaneous leishmaniaisis 527–30
  cutaneous myiasis 574–5
  cutaneous nocardiosis 272–3
  dermatophytes 492–4, 767, 825
  erysipeloid 265–6, 770
  fungal (overview) 766–8
  HIV skin complications 825–8
  introduction 758–9
  Malassezia 478–9
  mites 575
  mucormycosis 489–90, 766–7
  nectrotizing fasciitis 763–4
  onchocerciasis 557–8
  Paracoccidioides brasiliensis 509
  Pasteurella 316–17
  Prevotella and *Porphyromonas* 332
  pyomyositis 764–6
  scabies 573–4, 827
  schistosomiasis 563–4
  sporotrichosis 496–7
  surgical site infections (SSIs) 185–7, 760–1
  tissue nematode overview 542
  viral infections (overview) 768–70
slapped cheek (parvovirus B19) 391–2, 787, 790–1, 792–4, 801
sleeping sickness 525–7
slime substances, extracellular 216–17
smallpox 370, 444–5, 769, 848
social handwash 147
sodium stibogluconate 119
sofosbuvir 420–1, 674
source isolation 150–1
spectinomycin 46–8
Sphingobacterium 294–5
Sphingomonas paucimobilis 294–5
spills, infection control 152, 163–4
spinal paralytic polio 446–7
spiramycin 50, 123, 519–20
spirochaetes
  encephalitis 736
  overview 333
  see also specific spirochaetes
spleen
  asplenic patients 814
  splenic abscess 669
  splenic rupture 403–4, 405
Sporothrix schenckii 495–7, 767
sporotrichosis 495–7
spotted fevers 343, 344–5
St Louis encephalitis 453
staff, *see* health-care workers (HCWs)
stains, microscopy 222–4; *see also specific stains*
staphylococci 233–4
  coagulase-negative (CoNS) 240–1
  S. aureus see *Staphylococcus aureus*
  staphylococcal epidermal necrolysis 805–6
  staphylococcal toxic shock syndrome (TSS) 707–9
Staphylococcus aureus 234–6
  glycopeptide resistance 42–3, 239–40
  meningitis 721
  meticillin-resistant, *see* meticillin-resistant *Staphylococcus aureus* MRSA)
stavudine 104–6
Stenotrophomonas maltophilia 299–300
sterilization 130, 174–6
stool samples 219
strain, definition 12–13
streptococci 234, 242
  group A *Streptococcus* (GAS) 249–51, 591–2
  group B *Streptococcus* (GBS)/*S. agalactiae* 252–3, 721
  group C streptococci 254
  group F streptococci 254
  group G streptococci 254
  nutritionally variant streptococci (NVS) 255
  S. bovis 247–8
  S. pneumoniae 243–5
  streptococcal toxic shock syndrome (TSS) 707–9
  viridans streptococci 248–9
streptogramins 52–3
  macrolide–lincosamide–streptogramin B (MLS_B) resistance 50
Streptomyces species 273
streptomycin 46–8, 73
stridor 596–7
Strongyloides stercoralis 546–7, 586–7
strongyloidiasis 546–7
structure
  bacterial 210–12
  viral 366, 426, 451
Study on the Efficacy of Nosocomial Infection Control (SENIC) 182
subacute sclerosing panencephalitis (SSPE) 385–6
subdural empyema 739–40
sulbactam 37–8
  ampicillin–sulbactam 38
sulconazole 82
sulfacetamide sodium 58–60
sulfadiazine 58–60, 123
sulfadoxine 58–60
  artesunate–sulfadoxine–pyrimethamine 118–19
sulfamethoxazole 58–60, 61–2
sulfasalazine 58–60
sulfonamides 4, 58–60

suramin 123, 527
surgical scrub 147
surgical site infection (SSI) 185–7, 760–1
surveillance
  alert organisms 140–1
  blood donor infection 158
  bloodstream infection (BSI) 187–9
  hospital-acquired infection 141–2
  overview of 139–40
  surgical site infection 186
  tissue donor infection 157
Surviving Sepsis Campaign 581–2
susceptibility testing 13–15
sustained virological response (SVR) 420–1
swabs, microbiological specimens 219
swimmer's itch 563–4
swine flu virus 375–6
synergism 16, 330
syphilis 334, 335–7, 701–3, 714–16
  congenital 714–15, 786–7, 794
  HIV complication 838–9
  non-venereal endemic 334, 335–6
systemic inflammatory response syndrome (SIRS) 580

T

Taenia 549
  T. saginata 559–60
  T. solium 560, 561–2, 731–2
tafenoquine 115
tapeworms (cestodes) 559–62
target sites, alteration of antimicrobial 10
tarsal tunnel syndrome 838
taxonomy
  basic bacteriology principles 209
  see also classification
tazobactam 37–8
  piperacillin–tazobactam 38
Tazocin® 38, 708–9
T-cell deficiency, selective 811–12
tedizolid 54
teicoplanin 42–4, 44–5, 238, 241
telaprevir 100
telavancin 45
telbivudine 98, 416–17
telithromycin 50
TEM β-lactamases 36–7
tenofovir 98, 99, 104–6, 416–17, 674
teratogenesis 24–5; *see also* pregnancy
terbinafine 87
test of cure (TOC) 710–11
tetanus 269
tetracycline 653
tetracyclines 24–5, 56–8, 117, 124; *see also specific drugs*
Thayer–Martin agar 219–20
therapeutic window 16
thiazolidine ring 32
thioamides 74; *see also specific drugs*
thiocetazone 74
thrush 475, 828
thymic aplasia 811–12
thymoma with hypogammaglobulinaemia 810
tiabendazole 125
ticarcillin–clavulanate 38
ticks 576
  African tick bite disease 343, 345
  babesiosis 515
  Congo–Crimean haemorrhagic fever (CCHF) 435
  encephalitis causes' overview 733
  Kyasanur Forest disease 454
  lyme disease 334, 338–40, 730–1
  Omsk haemorrhagic fever 454
  tick-borne encephalitis 453–4
  tick-borne relapsing fever 334, 337–8
tigecycline 56–8
Timentin® 61
tinea capitis 492–4
tinea corporis 492–4
tinea cruris 492–4
tinea manuum 492–4
tinea pedis 492–4
tinea unguium 492–4
tinidazole 64, 124, 531, 533
Tinsdale agar 219–20
time-dependent killing 17
tioconazole 82
tipranavir 108–9
tobramycin 21, 46–8
Togaviridae 370, 433, 459
  rubella 389
Tokyo guidelines 658
tongue, strawberry 804–5
tonsils
  pharyngitis 591–3
  quinsy 594–5
topical (TOP) administration 20
TORCH infections 786–9
total quality management (TQM) 142, 231–3
toxic shock syndrome 707–9
toxicity/side effects
  aminoglycosides 48
  antifungals 80–2, 83–4, 85–6, 86–7
  antihelminthic drugs 124–5, 125–6, 126
  antileprotics 75–6
  antimalarials 113–15, 116–17
  antiprotozoal drugs 119–24
  antiretroviral drug therapy (ART) 105, 106, 107, 109
  antituberculous agents 71–4
  carbapenems 40
  cephalosporins 35
  chloramphenicol 56
  co-trimoxazole 62
  cytomegalovirus antivirals 92, 93–4
  fusidic acid 70
  glycopeptides 44
  hepatitis B antivirals 97, 98
  hepatitis C antivirals 100
  herpes simplex virus/varicella-zoster virus antivirals 91
  influenza antivirals 94–5, 95–6
  ketolides 50
  lincosamides 52
  lipopeptides 53–4
  mupirocin 71
  nitrofurans 67
  oxazolidinones 54–5
  penicillins 33
  polymyxins 69
  quinolones 64
  respiratory syncytial virus antivirals 96
  rifamycins 67
  streptogramins 53
  sulfonamides 60
  tetracyclines 58
  trimethoprim 61
toxins, bacterial 217
toxocariasis 550–1

Toxoplasma
gondii 517–20, 786
toxoplasmosis 517–20, 786, 838–9
tracheitis, bacterial 598
tracheobronchitis 381–2, 486–8
trachoma 353–4
transcription 367
transduction 213–14
transformation 213–14, 369
transfusion
blood donors' infection surveillance 158
Creutzfeldt–Jakob disease (CJD) transmission prevention 171–2
encephalitis 733
transient aplastic crisis (TAC) 391–2
transmissible spongiform encephalopathies (TSEs) 169–72
Creutzfeldt–Jakob disease (CJD) 169–72, 466–7
transmission routes, infection 137
transplant recipients 816–18
adenovirus 437–8
Aspergillus 486–7
bone marrow transplantation (BMT) 406–7, 437–8, 442–3, 817–18
Burkholderia cepacia complex colonization 301
Coccidioides immitis 506
cytomegalovirus (CMV) 406–7
encephalitis causes 733
infection in (overview) 816–18
liver see liver transplant
mucormycosis 489–90
polyomaviruses 442–3
pre-transplantation screening 818
renal see renal transplant
risk from tissues for 157–8
transposons 11–12
travellers
diarrhoea 281, 282, 647–8
encephalitis causes 733
esophilia in 586–7
imported fever 584–6
trematodes 563–8
Treponema 334, 335–7
T. carateum 335–6
T. pallidum 334, 335–7, 714–16, 786–7
triazoles 83–4
Trichenella species 552–3
trichenellosis 552–3
trichloroacetic acid 700–1
Trichomonas vaginalis 222–4, 532–3, 713
trichomoniasis 532–3, 713
Trichophyton 492–4
Trichosporon species 479
Trichostrongylus 549
trichuriasis 544
Trichuris trichiura 544
triclabendazole 125, 565–6
trimethoprim 24–5, 59, 60–2
Tropheryma whipplei 676
tropical genital ulceration 701–3
tropical spastic paraparesis 449–50
tropical sprue/ enteropathy 675
Trypanosoma 523
T. cruzi 523–5
T. brucei complex 525–7
tuberculosis (TB) 355–9, 627–8
antituberculous agents 39, 71–5, 639
HIV complications 831, 838–9
infection control 168–9
meningitis 726–7
microbiological specimens 218
non-pulmonary 168–9
open 168–9
pericarditis 638–9
peritonitis 665
tuberculoid leprosy 360
tularaemia 317–18, 848
tunnel infection 632
tympanostomy tube 604–5
type, definition 12–13
typhlitis 675
typhus 343, 345–6
typing techniques 199, 229–31

U

UK 5-year antimicrobial resistance strategy 2013–2018 28
UK Advisory Panel for Healthcare Workers Infected with Bloodborne Viruses (UKAP) 159
ulceration
diabetic foot infections 783–4
genital 695, 701–4
idiopathic oesophageal 644
peptic ulcer disease 327–9, 645–7
ultrasound
elastography 419–20
onchocerciasis 558
pelvic inflammatory disease (PID) 705–6
Unasyn 38
universal infection control precautions (UICP) 163–4
urea breath tests 328
Ureaplasma
urealyticum 351–2
urease test 227
urethral syndrome 681
urethritis 695, 713
urinary catheter
associated infection 189–91, 686–8
High Impact Intervention No. 6 190
urinary symptoms, encephalitis and 735
urinary tract infection (UTI) 677–91
acute pyelonephritis 681–3
brain abscess and 738
Candida 477
catheter-associated 189–91, 686–8
chronic pyelonephritis 683–5
common organisms in hospital-acquired 136
cystitis 437–8, 473, 679–81
epididymitis 689–90
Escherichia coli 281, 283
Gardnerella 309
introduction 678–9
orchitis 691
prostatitis 688–9
Proteus 284–5
renal abscess 685–6
schistosomiasis 563–4
urethritis 695, 713
urinary catheter-associated infection 189–91, 686–8
see also genitourinary (GU) tract infection
urine samples 191, 218, 679
uveitis 753–4, 755

V

vaccination/immunization 843–9
- adenovirus 438
- anthrax 260
- asplenic patients 814
- *Bordetella* 311, 806
- *Brucella* 313
- cholera 322, 653
- community-acquired pneumonia 615
- diphtheria 262, 844
- enteric fever 651
- *Francisella tularensis* 318
- group A *Streptococcus* (GAS) 251
- group B *Streptococcus* (GBS) 253
- *Haemophillus influenzae* (Hib) 303–4, 305, 844
- hepatitis A 412
- hepatitis B 156, 845
- hepatitis 101
- HIV 841–2, 845
- human papillomavirus (HPV) 441, 844
- influenza 379, 844
- Japanese encephalitis (JE) 452
- malaria 514
- measles (MMR) 386, 844
- meningitis 276–7, 303–4, 305, 720–2, 844
- migrant health 849
- mumps (MMR) 387, 388, 844
- *Neisseria meningitidis* 276–7
- non-routine immunizations (overview) 844, 845
- otitis media 604–5
- poliovirus 446, 448, 844
- rabies 463–5
- rotavirus 410, 844
- routine childhood immunizations (overview) 844
- rubella (MMR) 390, 844
- *Staphylococcus aureus* 236
- *Streptococcus pneumoniae* 245
- tetanus 269, 270, 844
- transplant recipients 818
- tuberculosis (BCG vaccine) 361, 845
- whooping cough (pertussis) 311, 806, 844
- varicella-zoster virus (VZV) 401–2, 844–5
- yellow fever 456

vaccinia 444

vaginal discharge 695
- bacterial vaginosis 695–7
- pelvic inflammatory disease 706
- trichomoniasis 713
- vulvovaginal candidiasis 698

valaciclovir 398–9, 401, 704

valganciclovir 93, 408

valvular disease
- cardiac candidiasis 476
- Q fever 347, 348

vancomycin 42–4
- brain abscess 738–9
- *Clostridium difficile* infection (CDI) 200–1, 655–6
- CSF shunt infection 742
- enterococci treatment/resistance 246–7, 254
- meningitis 721
- monitoring 44–5
- MRSA 238
- *Staphylococcus aureus* resistance 239
- streptococci 249
- toxic shock syndrome (TSS) 708–9
- vancomycin lock solutions 196

variable-number tandem repeats (VNTRs) 230–1

variably protease-sensitive prionopathy 169–72

varicella-zoster immune globulin (VZIG) 401–2, 795

varicella-zoster virus (VZV) 399–402, 768–9
- antivirals for 90–1
- HIV skin complications 826
- keratitis 752
- in pregnancy 787, 791, 792–4, 795, 801

variola 444–5

vascular access
- bloodstream infection – mandatory surveillance 187–9
- line-related sepsis 193–6
- *see also* central venous catheter (CVC)-related infection; peripheral venous catheters (PVCs)

vascular graft infection 635–6

vascular surgery 187, 635–6

Vasilchenko virus 453–4

Venereal Disease Research Laboratory (VDRL) test 715–16

Venezuelan equine encephalitis (VEE) 433–5

Venezuelan haemorrhagic fever 459

ventilation (health-care premises) 176–8

ventilator-associated pneumonia (VAP) 191–3, 618–19

ventilator care bundle 192–3

verotoxins 282

verrucous lesions 497–8, 503–4

veruga peruana 348–50

vesico-ureteric reflux (VUR) 681, 683–4

Vibrios 321–5
- *V. alginolyticus* 323, 324–5
- *V. cholerae* 321–2, 323, 652–3
- *V. parahaemolyticus* 323
- *V. vulnificus* 323, 324

Vincent's angina 605

viomycin 74–5

viral haemorrhagic fevers (VHF), overview 459–61

viridans streptococci 248–9

virulence
- bacterial 216–17
- *see also specific species*

viruria 442–3

viruses 365–468
- antivirals *see* antivirals
- basic virology principles 366–7
- childhood illness causes 801
- common cold aetiology/epidemiology 590
- hazard groups 160
- hospital diarrhoea and vomiting epidemics 196–7
- overview of 370
- pathogenicity 368–9
- resistance *see* antiviral resistance
- secondary immunodeficiency causes 813
- viral replication 367–8
- *see also specific infections/viruses*

visceral larva migrans (VLM) 550–1

visceral leishmaniasis 527–30

vitamin A 386

Vitek 2 228

vomiting
- *Bacillus* species 257
- HIV complication 834
- hospital epidemics 196–7
- norovirus 410–11
- *see also* gastrointestinal (GI) infections/diseases; *specific causes/infections*

voriconazole 84, 473, 488, 504–5, 507–8, 728–9
vulval irritation/pain 695
vulvovaginal candidiasis 697–9
vulvovaginitis 475

ward closure, infection control 145–6
warts
  genital 439, 440–1, 699–701
  human papillomavirus (HPV) 439–41, 699–701
waste 152, 180–1
water supply
  Legionella 318, 319–20
  Pseudomonas in taps in neonatal ICU 184–5
Weil–Felix test 344
Weil's disease 340–2
West African trypanosomiasis 526–7
Western equine encephalitis (WEE) 433–5
Whipple's disease 676
whole-genome sequencing (WGS) 228, 231
whooping cough 310–11, 806–8, 844
World Health Organization (WHO)
  hand hygiene 146–50
  HIV classification 822–3
  leprosy elimination programme 359
  trachoma grading 353
worms, helminths 541–70; *see also specific helminths*
wounds
  bite infections 320–1, 760
  botulism 267–8
  common organisms in hospital-acquired infection 136
  diabetic foot infections 783–4
  local infiltration for prophylaxis 27
  myiasis 574–5
  rabies post-exposure treatment 464–5
  surgical site infection (SSI) 185–7, 760–1
  tetanus 269
  Vibrios infection 323, 324–5
Wuchereria bancrofti 554–5

X

xanthogranulomatous pyelonephritis 684–5
x-linked agammaglobulinaemia 810
xylitol 604–5
xylose lysine deoxycholate (XLD) 219–20

yaws 334, 335–7
yeast infections 470–9; see *also specific infections*
yellow fever 455–6, 459
yellow fever vaccine-associated viscerotropic disease 456
Yersinia
  Y. enterocolitica 315
  Y. pestis 314–15, 848
  Y. pseudotuberculosis 316

Z

zanamivir 95, 378–9
zidovudine 104–6, 450
ZN stain 222–4
zygomycota 471

Date Due
